The JAAPA QRS Review for PAs

Study Plan and Guide for PANCE and PANRE

The JAAPA QRS Review for PAs

Study Plan and Guide for PANCE and PANRE

Editors

Reamer L. Bushardt, PharmD, PA-C, DFAAPA

Professor & Senior Associate Dean
School of Medicine & Health Sciences
The George Washington University
Washington, DC

Harrison L. Reed, MMSc, PA-C

Clinical Editor, JAAPA
Assistant Professor
Department of Physician Assistant Studies
School of Medicine & Health Sciences
The George Washington University
Washington, DC

Dawn Colomb-Lippa, PA-C, MHS

Departmental Editor, Quick Recertification Series, JAAPA
Senior Instructor of Biology
Quinnipiac University
Hamden, Connecticut

Amy M. Klingler, MS, PA-C, DFAAPA

Senior Clinical Editor, JAAPA
Physician Assistant
Salmon River Clinic
Stanley, Idaho

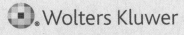 Wolters Kluwer

Philadelphia · Baltimore · New York · London
Buenos Aires · Hong Kong · Sydney · Tokyo

Acquisitions Editor: Matt Hauber
Development Editors: Kelly Horvath and Amy Millholen
Editorial Coordinator: Vinoth Ezhumalai
Marketing Manager: Phyllis Hitner
Production Project Manager: Kirstin Johnson
Design Coordinator: Steve Druding
Manufacturing Coordinator: Margie Orzech
Prepress Vendor: S4Carlisle Publishing Services
JAAPA Publisher: Marianne Kerr

9 8 7 6 5 4 3 2 1

Printed in Mexico

Library of Congress Cataloging-in-Publication Data

ISBN-13: 978-1-975143-81-7
ISBN-10: 1-975143-81-7

Library of Congress Control Number: 2021914094

shop.lww.com

Contributors

Alyssa Abebe, PA-C
Associate Program Director
Chatham University
Pittsburgh, Pennsylvania

Shekitta Acker, MS, PA-C
Academic Director
Physician Assistant Program
Mayo Clinic College of Medicine and Science
Rochester, Minnesota

Katelyn Adler, MSPAS, PA-C
Physician Assistant
Department of Surgery
Akron Children's Hospital
Alliance, Ohio

Amy Akerman, MPAS, PA-C
Assistant Professor
Department of Pediatrics
University of Colorado Denver—Anschutz Medical Campus
Aurora, Colorado

Corinne Isabelle Alois, MS, PA-C
Assistant Professor—Industry Professional
Physician Assistant Program
St. John's University
Jamaica, New York

Jeremy Amayo, MMSc, PA-C
Physician Assistant
Pulmonary/Critical Care Medicine
Department of Pulmonary, Critical Care, and Sleep Medicine
Piedmont Hospital: Piedmont Atlanta Hospital
Atlanta, Georgia

Alicia Andaloro, PA-C, MS
Physician Assistant
Department of Surgery
University of Pennsylvania
Philadelphia, Pennsylvania

Lauren Anderson, MMS, PA-C
Assistant Professor
PA School of Medical Sciences
Lincoln Memorial University
Harrogate, Tennessee

Renee Andreeff, EdD, PA-C, DFAAPA
Associate Professor, Program Research Director
Physician Assistant
D'Youville College
Buffalo, New York

Shane Ryan Apperley, MSc, PGCert, PA-R
Associate Professor
PA School of Medical Sciences
Lincoln Memorial University
Harrogate, Tennessee

Mary Beth Babos, PharmD, BCPS
Professor and Chair
Department of Pharmacology
Lincoln Memorial University—DeBusk College of Osteopathic Medicine
Harrogate, Tennessee

Jonathan Baker, PA-C
Physician Assistant
Laser Surgery Care
New York, New York

Sunny Torbett Baker, PA-MS
Physician Assistant
Department of Emergency Medicine
Texas Tech University Health Sciences Center El Paso
El Paso, Texas

Molly Band, PA-C
Physician Assistant
Department of Urology
Yale New Haven Hospital
New Haven, Connecticut

Adrian Banning, DHSc, MMS, PA-C
Associate Clinical Professor
Physician Assistant
Drexel University
Philadelphia, Pennsylvania

Nicole Bartoszewski, MPAS, PA-C
Physician Assistant
Department of Orthopaedics
Carthage Area Hospital
Carthage, New York

Katlin Bates, MSPAS
Advanced Practice Professional
Department of Surgery
Ruby Memorial Hospital
Morgantown, West Virginia

Nathan Bates, MMS, PA-C
Instructor
Department of PA Studies
Wake Forest School of Medicine
Winston-Salem, North Carolina

Teresa Bigler, DHEd, PA-C
Program Director, PA Program
Louisiana State University Health Sciences
    Center Shreveport
Shreveport, Louisiana

Maryellen Blevins, MPAS, PA-C
Physician Assistant
Samaritan Medical Center
Wound care
Watertown, New York

Janelle Bludorn, MS, PA-C
Clinical Assistant Professor
Duke University School of Medicine
Durham, North Carolina

Gayle Bodner, MMS, PA-C
Vice Chair and Assistant Professor
Department of PA Studies
Wake Forest School of Medicine
Winston-Salem, North Carolina

Ilana Borukhov, MSPAS, PA-C
Chief PA
Division of Pulmonary, Critical Care and Sleep Medicine
Mount Sinai Hospital
New York, New York

Brennan Bowker, MHS, PA-C
Senior Physician Assistant
Department of Surgery
Yale New Haven Hospital
New Haven, Connecticut

Alan Brokenicky, MPAS, PA-C
Academic Co-Director
Department of Education
Mayo Clinic College of Medicine and Science
Rochester, Minnesota

Gina Brown, MPAS
Associate Professor
Physician Assistant
Wichita State University
Wichita, Kansas

Michelle Brown, PhD
Associate Professor and Program Director
Department of Health Services Administration
University of Alabama at Birmingham
Birmingham, Alabama

Teri L. Capshaw, MBA
Principal Investigator, Adjunct Faculty Member
The George Washington University School of Medicine
    and Health Sciences
Washington, DC

Kara L. Caruthers, MSPAS, PA-C
M.S. Physician Assistant Studies, M.S. Molecular, Cellular and
    Systemic Physiology
Associate Professor and Associate Program Director
Department of Physician Assistant Sciences
Meharry Medical College
Nashville, Tennessee

Lindsey Caruthers, MS, PA-C
Assistant Professor
Physician Assistant Studies
Philadelphia College of Osteopathic Medicine
Suwanee, Georgia

Paige Cendroski, MPAS, PA-C
Assistant Professor
Physician Assistant Studies
Chatham University
Venetia, Pennsylvania

Sammy Cheuk
PA Student
Touro University California
Joint MSPAS/MPH Program
Vallejo, California

Pamela V. Chi, MMSc, PA-C
Physican Assistant
Mercer University—Atlanta Campus
Physician Assistant Studies
Atlanta, Georgia

Melissa Johnson Chung, MMS, PA-C
Director of Clinical Instruction and Assessment
Chicago College of Osteopathic Medicine
Midwestern University
Downers Grove, Illinois

Ryan Clancy, MSHS, MA, PA-C, DFAAPA
Assistant Clinical Professor
Physician Assistant
Drexel University College of Nursing and Health Professions
Philadelphia, Pennsylvania

Rebecca Clawson, PA-C
Master of Arts in Teaching, Bachelor of Science in Physician
    Assistant
Assistant Professor PA Program
School of Allied Health Professions
Louisiana State University Health Sciences Center
Shreveport, Louisiana

Kathy Clift, MSPAS, PA-C
Associate Professor
MSPAS-MPH Program
Touro University California
Vallejo, California

Leocadia Conlon, PhD, MPH, PA-C
Clinical Director
Hawai'i CARES
Hawai'i Department of Health & University of Hawai'i
   Thompson School of Social Work and Public Health
Honolulu, Hawaii

Johanna D'Addario, PA-C
Physician Assistant
Department of Gynecologic Oncology
Yale New Haven Hospital
New Haven, Connecticut

Stephanie Daniel, PhD
Professor
Family Medicine
Wake Forest School of Medicine: Wake Forest University
   School of Medicine
Winston-Salem, North Carolina

Jane Davis, DNP
Nurse Practitioner
Division of Nephrology
University of Alabama at Birmingham
Birmingham, Alabama

Melissa Day, DMS, MPAS
Associate Professor
Physician Assistant Studies
Lincoln Memorial University
Harrogate, Tennessee

Sondra M. DePalma, DHSc, PA-C
Director
Advocacy and Reimbursement
American Academy of Physician Assistants
Alexandria, Virginia

Nicole Dettmann, DSc, MPH, PA-C
Associate Program Director
PA Studies
Massachusetts College of Pharmacy and Health Sciences—
   Worcester Campus
Worcester, Massachusetts

Lisa Dickerson, MD
Medical Director and Clinical Associate Professor
Physician Assistant Studies
Mercer University
Atlanta, Georgia

Rebecca Dodd, DMSc, PA-C
Critical Care Medicine
Dignity Heart and Vascular Institute
Critical Care Medicine
Mercy General Hospital
Cardiac ICU
Sacramento, California

Bethany Dunn, PA-C, DC
Associate Professor
Physician Assistant
School of Health Professions
D'Youville College
Buffalo, New York

Jeanette Elfering, MHS, PA-C
Physician Assistant
Department of Neuro-Ophthalmology
Duke University Hospital
Durham, North Carolina

Kelsey Ellender-Barthel, MPAS
Physician Assistant
Department of Cardiothoracic and Thoracic Surgery
Christus Highland Medical Center
Shreveport, Louisiana

Bill Engle, DD, MS
Program Director
Medical Technology Program
Lincoln Memorial University
Harrogate, Tennessee

Rob Estridge, BA, BS, MPAS, PA-C
Advanced Practice Provider
Director, Cleveland Clinic Community Care, West
   Cleveland Clinic Community Care
Independence, Ohio

Jenny Fanuele, MMSc, PA-C
Faculty Instructor
Physician Assistant Studies
MGH Institute of Health Professions
Boston, Massachusetts

Tanya Fernandez, MS, PA-C, IBCLC
Assistant Professor
Pediatrics, Child Health Associate/Physician
   Assistant Program
University of Colorado Denver—Anschutz
   Medical Campus
Aurora, Colorado

Amie Fonder, MS, PA-C
Physician Assistant
Department of Hematology
Mayo Clinic Rochester
Rochester, Minnesota

Ashley Fort, MPAS
Assistant Professor
PA Program
Louisiana State University Health Sciences Center
Shreveport, Louisiana

Cassiopeia Frank, MMSc
Physician Assistant
Department of Medicine
University of North Carolina at Chapel Hill
Chapel Hill, North Carolina

Sarah Garvick, MS, MPAS, PA-C
Associate Program Director
Department of PA Studies
Wake Forest School of Medicine
Winston-Salem, North Carolina

David Gelbart, DO, MMS, MS, PA-C
Resident Physician
Department of Emergency Medicine
University of Kentucky Medical Center
Lexington, Kentucky

James A. Gerding, MS, PA-C
Physician Assistant
R Adams Cowley Shock Trauma Center
University of Maryland Medical Center
Baltimore, Maryland

Frank Giannelli, PhD, PA-C
Lecturer
Physician Assistant Studies and Practice
Rutgers, The State University of New Jersey
Piscataway, New Jersey

Chris Gillette, PhD
Associate Professor and Assistant Director of Scholarship and
    Research
Department of PA Studies
Wake Forest School of Medicine
Winston-Salem, North Carolina

Bart Gillum, DSc, MHS, PA-C
Assistant Professor
Department of PA Studies
The George Washington University School of Medicine and
    Health Sciences
Ashburn, Virginia

Thomas Gocke, DMSc, ATC, PA-C, DFAAPA
Physician Assistant
Department of Orthopaedic Surgery
West Virginia University Health Sciences Center
Morgantown, West Virginia

Paul Gonzales, MPAS
Assistant Professor
Physician Assistant Studies
Touro University California
Vallejo, California

Jill Gore, PA-C
Physician Assistant
RediClinic
San Antonio, Texas

Colleen Grassley, MSPAS
Physician Assistant
Department of Emergency Medicine
Mayo Clinic: Mayo Clinic Minnesota
Austin, Minnesota

Joel Hamm, MD, MPH
Assistant Professor Emergency Medicine
University of Kentucky
Lexington, Kentucky

Katie Hanlon, MMS, PA-C
Clinical Assistant Professor, Critical Care Physician Assistant
Department of Allied Health Sciences
University of North Carolina—Chapel Hill
Chapel Hill, North Carolina

Jennifer Harrington, PA-C, MHS
Associate Professor
Physician Assistant Studies
Lincoln Memorial University
Harrogate, Tennessee

Michelle Heinan, EdD, PA-C
Faculty
Physician Assistant Program
Lincoln Memorial University
Harrogate, Tennessee

Maureen Heneghan, PA-C, MSHS, MS
Physician Assistant
Hospital for Special Surgery LLC
New York, New York

Debra Herrmann, DHSc, MPH, PA-C
Assistant Professor
Physician Assistant Studies
George Washington University
Washington, DC

Patricia Higgins, DO
Associate Professor and Director of Clinical Education
Midwestern University
College of Health Sciences-PA Program
Downers Grove, Illinois

Timothy Hirsch, MS, PA-C
Physician Assistant
Littleton, Colorado

Eric Hochberg, MPAS, PA-C
Senior Physician Assistant I
R Adams Cowley Shock Trauma Center
University of Maryland Medical Center
Baltimore, Maryland

Chelsey Hoffmann, RD, PA-C
Physician Assistant
Department of Pain Medicine
Mayo Clinic
Rochester, Minnesota

Neil Howie, PGDip, MSc, SFHEA, PA-R
Senior Lecturer
Physician Associate Studies
Department of Paramedic Science and Physician Associate
    School of Allied Health and Community
University of Worcester
Worcester, UK

Sara Hoyle, MSPA
Physician Assistant
Student Health Services
Texas A&M University College Station
College Station, Texas

Stephanie Hull, EdS, MMS, PA-C
Associate Professor and Program Director, LMU-Knoxville PA
    Program
Physician Assistant Program
Lincoln Memorial University
Knoxville, Tennessee

Ryan Hunton, MSc, PA-C
Physician Assistant
Emergency Department
Frankfort Regional Medical Center
Frankfort, Kentucky

Joseph Janosky, MS, PT, ATC
Director of Sports Safety
Hospital for Special Surgery
Sports Medicine Institute
New York, New York

Jennifer Johnson, BS, MPAS, DMSc
Director of Simulation Education, Assistant Professor
Physician Assistant
Rocky Mountain University of Health Professions
Provo, Utah

Kelly Marie Joy, MS, MSPAS, PA-C
Assistant Professor
PA Program
Sullivan University
Louisville, Kentucky

Michelle Kavin, PA-C
Physician Assistant
Department of Orthopedics
Rothman Orthopaedic Institute
Philadelphia, Pennsylvania

Steven Kelham, DHSc, PA-C, DFAAPA
Clinical Assistant Professor
PA Studies
Mercer University—Atlanta Campus
Atlanta, Georgia

Julie Kinzel, MEd, PA-C, DFAAPA
Assistant Clinical Professor
Physician Assistant Department
Drexel University College of Medicine
Philadelphia, Pennsylvania

Amber Koehler, MPAS, PA-C
Physician Assistant
Department of Hematology
Mayo Clinic Minnesota
Rochester, Minnesota

Melodie Kolmetz, MPAS, PA-C
Assistant Professor
Physician Assistant Program
Ithaca College
Ithaca, New York

Paul "PJ" Koltnow, MS, MSPAS, PA-C
Assistant Professor
Department of Physician Assistant Studies
University of Tennessee Health Science Center
Memphis, Tennessee

Danielle Kruger, PA-C, MS Ed
Associate Professor and Academic Coordinator
Physician Assistant Education Program
College of Pharmacy and Health Sciences
Saint John's University
Queens, New York

Darcie Larimore-Arenas, MSPAS, MPH, PA-C
Assistant Professor
Touro University California
Joint MSPAS/MPH Program
Vallejo, California

Travis Layne, DMSc, MPAS, PA-C
PA Instructional Faculty
Rocky Mountain University of Health Professions
Provo, Utah

Viet T. Le, MPAS
Cardiovascular Research PA, Associate Professor of Research
Cardiovascular Research; Cardiology
Intermountain Heart Institute, Intermountain Healthcare
PA Faculty
Rocky Mountain University of Health Professions
Salt Lake City, Utah

Jon Levy, MD
Orthopaedic Surgeon
Greater Pittsburgh Orthopaedic Associates
Pittsburgh, Pennsylvania

Susan LeLacheur, DrPH, PA-C
Professor
Physician Assistant Studies
School of Medicine and Health Sciences
The George Washington University
Washington, DC

Madison Lewis, BS
Student, Master of Physician Assistant Studies
Chatham University
Pittsburgh, Pennsylvania

Kristin Lindaman, MMS, PA-C
Assistant Professor
Department of PA Studies
Wake Forest University School of Medicine
Winston-Salem, North Carolina

Sara Lolar, MS, PA-C, DFAAPA
Clinical Assistant Professor
Physician Assistant Studies
Wayne State University
Detroit, Michigan

Douglas D. Long, DMSc, PA-C
PA Clinical Liaison
Grace Hospital
Cleveland, Ohio

Victoria Louwagie, PA-C
Physician Assistant
Department of Gastroenterology and Hepatology
Mayo Clinic Health System in Mankato
Mankato, Minnesota

Kristy Luciano, PA-C
Assistant Professor and Director of Didactic Education
Physician Assistant
Midwestern University
Downers Grove, Illinois

Cheryl Ann Lugiano, MPAS, PA-C
Cardiac Surgery Physician Assistant
Department of Cardiac Surgery
St. Luke's University Hospital—Bethlehem Campus
Bethlehem, Pennsylvania

Shaun Lynch, MS, MMSc, PA-C
Academic Coordinator/Assistant Professor
Department of Physician Assistant Studies
Elon University
Elon, North Carolina

Stacey Lynema, PA-C
Physician Assistant
Department of Dermatology
Novartis Pharmaceuticals
Seattle, Washington

Stephanie Maclary, RN, MHS, PA-C
Director of Didactic Education
PA Studies
Massachusetts College of Pharmacy and Health Sciences—
   Worcester Campus
Worcester, Massachusetts

Kristopher Maday, MS, PA-C, DFAAPA
Program Director, Associate Professor
Physician Assistant Studies
University of Tennessee Health Science Center
Memphis, Tennessee

Ziemowit Mazur, EdM, MS, PA-C
Associate Program Director
Physician Assistant
Rosalind Franklin University of Medicine and Science College of
   Health Professions
North Chicago, Illinois

Ann McDonough-Madden, MHS, PA-C
Assistant Professor
Physician Assistant
Drexel University College of Nursing and Health Professions
Philadelphia, Pennsylvania

Natasha McKee, MMSc, PA-C
Physician Assistant
Western Montana Clinic
Missoula, Montana

Joshua Merson, MS-HPEd, PA-C
Assistant Professor
Department of PA Studies
MGH Institute of Health Professions
Boston, Massachusetts

Paula Miksa, DMS, PA-C
Assistant Dean and Program Director, DMS Program
Lincoln Memorial University
Harrogate, Tennessee

Christopher Miles, MD
Associate Professor
Department of Family and Community Medicine
Wake Forest University School of Medicine
Winston-Salem, North Carolina

Amanda Miller, MPH, MPAS, PA-C, AAHIVS
Physician Assistant
Department of Family Medicine
CentroMed
San Antonio, Texas

Lindsey Mitchell, MS, MPAS, PA-C
Student
PA Studies
Wake Forest School of Medicine: Wake Forest University
   School of Medicine
Winston-Salem, North Carolina

K. Alexis Moore, MPH, PA-C
Assistant Professor
Physician Assistant Studies
Elon University
Elon, North Carolina

Joy Moverley, DHSc, MPH, PA-C
Associate Program Director
Joint MSPAS/MPH Program
Touro University California
Vallejo, California

Melissa Murfin, PharmD, PA-C
Associate Professor
Physician Assistant Studies
Elon University
Elon, North Carolina

Dominique Murphy, MMSc, PA-C
Instructor
PA Studies
MGH Institute of Health Professions
Boston, Massachusetts

Sarah Neguse, PA-C
Assistant Professor
Physician Assistant Program
Rocky Vista University
Parker, Colorado

Bryan Nelson, DMSc
Instructor
Physician Assistant
Rocky Mountain University of Health Professions
Provo, Utah

Becky Ness, MPAS, PA-C
Physician Assistant
Department of Nephrology
Mayo Clinic Health System
Mankato, Minnesota

Erin Niles, PA-C
Physician Assistant
Department of Critical Care
R Adams Cowley Shock Trauma Center
Baltimore, Maryland

Stephen Noe, DMS, MPAS
Program Director
School of Medical Science
Lincoln Memorial University Carnegie Vincent Library
Harrogate, Tennessee

Carrie Smith Nold, MPA, PA-C
Assistant Professor and Coordinator of Didactic Studies
Department of Physician Assistant Studies
Philadelphia College of Osteopathic Medicine—Georgia
    Campus
Suwanee, Georgia

Jennifer Norris, MSPAS, PA-C
Assistant Professor
Physician Assistant Program
Towson University College of Health Professions
Phoenix, Maryland

Catherine Nowak, MS, PA-C, DFAAPA
Assistant Professor; Director of Clinical Education
Physician Assistant Program
Drexel University
Philadelphia, Pennsylvania

Robert O'Brien, MHS, PA-C
Physician Assistant
Department of Sports Traumatology
Hospital for Special Surgery LLC
New York, New York

Kevin Michael O'Hara, MMSc, MS, PA-C
Physician Assistant
Adult Bone Marrow Transplant
Memorial Sloan Kettering Cancer Center
North Merrick, New York

Danielle O'Laughlin, PA-C, MS
Physician Assistant, Clinical Skills Co-Director
Department of Internal Medicine
Mayo Clinic Minnesota
Rochester, Minnesota

Ryan Olivero, MMS, PA-C
Physician Assistant
Department of General Surgery
Saint John Providence Health System
Macomb, Michigan

Jonathan Parch, MPAP
Physician Assistant
Department of Surgery
Cedars-Sinai Medical Center
Los Angeles, California

Nata Parnes, MD
Director of Orthopedics
Department of Orthopaedics
Carthage Area Hospital
Carthage, New York

Marie Patterson, MSM, DHSc, PA-C
Program Director
Physician Assistant Program
Middle Tennessee State University
Murfreesboro, Tennessee

Brian Peacock, MMS
Program Director
Department of PA Studies
Wake Forest School of Medicine
Winston-Salem, North Carolina

Daniel Perez, MPAS
Physician Assistant
Carl R. Darnall Army Medical Center
Bennett Health Clinic
Fort Hood, Texas

Sonya Peters, PA-C
Physician Assistant
Department of Internal Medicine
Mayo Clinic
Rochester, Minnesota

Marie Pittman, DMSc, MPAS, PA-C, RDH
Principal Faculty
Physician Assistant
Rocky Mountain University of Health Professions
Provo, Utah

Daniel Podd, MPAS, PA-C
Associate Professor
Clinical Health Professions
St John's University
Fresh Meadows, New York

Antoinette Polito, MHS, PA-C
Associate Professor
Physician Assistant Studies
Elon University
Elon, North Carolina

Daniel Provencher, MS, PA-C
Assistant Professor
Physician Assistant
Midwestern University—Downers Grove Campus
Downers Grove, Illinois

Alicia Quella, PhD, PA-C
Program Director and Department Chair
Physician Assistant Studies
Augsburg University
Minneapolis, Minnesota

Andrea Rhodes, OTR, MPA, PA-C
Clinical Instructor
Physician Assistant
Louisiana State University Health Sciences
    Center Shreveport
Shreveport, Louisiana

Lendell Richardson, MD
Medical Director and Associate Professor
PA Program
Midwestern University
Downers Grove, Illinois

Melissa Ricker, PA-C
PA Fellowship Director
Center for Advanced Practice
Atrium Health
Charlotte, North Carolina

Brendan Riordan, MPAS, PA-C
Physician Assistant
Department of Cardiac Surgery
University of Washington Medical Center
Seattle, Washington

Tamara S. Ritsema, PhD, MPH, PA-C/R
Associate Professor
Department of PA Studies
The George Washington University
Washington, District of Columbia
Adjunct Senior Lecturer
Physician Associate Programme
St. George's, University of London
London, UK

Brian Robinson, MS, MPAS, M(ASCP)CM, PA-C
Assistant Professor
Department of PA Studies
Wake Forest School of Medicine
Winston-Salem, North Carolina

Sean Robinson, DHSc, PA-C
Assistant Professor
Physician Assistant Studies
The George Washington University
Washington, DC

Lorraine Sanassi, PA-C, DHSc
Physician Assistant
Urgent Care
One Medical
New York, New York

Teresa Sanders, MPAS, PA-C
Physician Assistant
Simmons Cancer Center
University of Texas Southwestern Medical Center at Dallas
Dallas, Texas

Jamie Saunders, MSc, FHEA, PA-R
Physician Associate
Haematology Department
Guy's and St Thomas' NHS Foundation Trust
London, UK

Rebecca Schettle, MSN, RN, APNP, FPN-BC
Nursing Instructor, Nurse Practitioner
Department of Nursing
University of Wisconsin Milwaukee
Milwaukee, Wisconsin

Sarah Schettle, PA-C, MBA, MS
MCSD Coordinator, Director of Development
Department of Cardiovascular Surgery
Mayo Clinic Minnesota
Rochester, Minnesota

Natalie Schirato, MPAS, PA-C
Assistant Professor
Physician Assistant Studies
Chatham University
Pittsburgh, Pennsylvania

Joel Schwartzkopf, MPAS, MBA
Associate Executive Director
CSU Health Network
Colorado State University
Fort Collins, Colorado

Chrystyna Senkel, MPAS, PA-C
Director of Clinical Education, Assistant Professor
PA Studies
Lincoln Memorial University
Harrogate, Tennessee

Mimoza Shehu, MPAS, PA-C
Physician Assistant
Lynn Community Health Center
Urgent Care
Lynn, Massachusetts

Joshua Shepherd, MMS, PA-C
Principal Faculty
PA Program
Lincoln Memorial University
Harrogate, Tennessee

Catherine Shull, PA-C, MPAS
Assistant Professor
PA Studies and Family and Community Medicine
Wake Forest School of Medicine
Winston-Salem, North Carolina

Caroline Sisson, MMS
Assistant Professor
Department of PA Studies
Wake Forest School of Medicine
Winston-Salem, North Carolina

Tonya Skidmore, DMS, PA-C
Associate Professor
PA SMS
Lincoln Memorial University
Harrogate, Tennessee

Jon Slaven, MMS, PA-C
Physician Assistant
Lincoln Memorial University Carnegie Vincent Library
PA School of Medical Sciences
Harrogate, Tennessee

Ian Smith, MMS, PA-C, APA-C
Assistant Professor
Department of PA Studies
Wake Forest School of Medicine
Winston-Salem, North Carolina

Taryn Smith, PA-C
Physician Assistant
Department of Urogynecology
Mercy Health
Edmond, Oklahoma

Russell Snyder, MD
Vice Chair
University of Texas Medical Branch
OB/GYN
Galveston, Texas

Tyler D. Sommer, MPAS, PA-C
Associate Program Director
Physician Assistant Program
Rocky Mountain University of Health Professions
Provo, Utah

Victoria Specian, MSCP, PA-C
Physician Assistant
Department of Psychiatry
Shreveport, Louisiana

Lauren Stanford, MPAS
Principal Faculty
Physician Assistant
Rocky Mountain University of Health Professions
Provo, Utah

Kristina Stanson, MMS, PA-C
Senior Physician Assistant
Hey Clinic for Scoliosis and Spine Care
Raleigh, North Carolina

Matthew Steidl, MPAS
Assistant Professor
Physician Assistant Studies
Lipscomb University
Nashville, Tennessee

Michael Stephens, DMS, PA-C
Assistant Professor
Physician Assistant Studies
School of Medical Sciences
Lincoln Memorial University
Harrogate, Tennessee

Joy Stevens, PA-C
Physician Assistant
Department of Internal Medicine
Mayo Clinic Minnesota
Rochester, Minnesota

Brittany Strelow, MS, PA-C
Clinical Co-Director of Development
Physician Assistant Program
Mayo School of Health Sciences
Rochester, Minnesota

Emily Thatcher, MPAS, PA-C
Physician Assistant
Children's National Emergency
Washington, DC

George Thompson, DMS, MMS
Assistant Professor
School of Medical Sciences
Lincoln Memorial University
Harrogate, Tennessee

Katherine Thompson, MCHS
Physician Assistant
Urgent Care
Kaiser Permanente Washington
Bellevue, Washington

Tracey Thurnes, EdD, MPAS, PA-C
Associate Professor and Director of Accelerated Pathways
   Program
Physician Assistant Studies
Elon University
Elon, North Carolina

Lauren Trillo, PA-C
Instructor
Physician Assistant Studies
Midwestern University—Downers Grove Campus
Downers Grove, Illinois

Judy Truscott, MPAS
Program Director; Associate Professor
PA Studies
Chatham University
Pittsburgh, Pennsylvania

Marianne Vail, DHSc, PA-C
Assistant Professor
Department of Physician Assistant Studies
School of Medicine and Health Sciences
The George Washington University
Washington, DC

Danielle Vlazny, PA-C, MS
Physician Assistant
Department of Vascular Medicine
Mayo Clinic Rochester
Rochester, Minnesota

Mark Volpe, MPH, MMSc, PA-C
Physician Assistant
Department of Internal Medicine
Suffield Medical Associates
Suffield, Connecticut

Jennifer Vonderau, MMS, PA-C
Physician Assistant
Department of Surgery
University of North Carolina at Chapel Hill
Chapel Hill, North Carolina

Lesley Evan Ward, DHSc, MHSc, PA-C
Assistant Professor
Department of Physician Assistant Studies
The University of Tennessee Health Science Center
Memphis, Tennessee

Elyse Watkins, DHSc, PA-C, DFAAPA
Associate Professor
School of PA Medicine
University of Lynchburg
Lynchburg, Virginia

Lauren Webb, DMSc, MSM, PA-C
Assistant Professor
Physician Assistant Studies
Lipscomb University
Nashville, Tennessee

Emily Weidman-Evans, PharmD, BC-ADM, CPE
Professor and Associate Program Director, LSU Health
Physician Assistant Program
Clinical Pharmacist, Department of Family Medicine and
    Comprehensive Care
School of Allied Health Professions

Holly Ann West, MPAS, DHEd, PA-C
Senior Medical Educator
Office of Educational Development
University of Texas Medical Branch
Galveston, Texas

Heather White, MPAS
Physician Assistant
Department of Nephrology
Delta Nephrology, LLC
Shreveport, Louisiana

Amber Whitmore, PA-C
Physician Assistant
Family Birth Center
Beaumont Health
Royal Oak, Michigan

Anne Wildermuth, MMS, PA-C, RD
Associate Program Director and Admissions Director
Division of PA Education
University of Nebraska Medical Center
Omaha, Nebraska

Lauren Wiley, PA-C
Lead Advanced Practice Provider
Department of Critical Care
Piedmont Healthcare Inc.
Atlanta, Georgia

Gladys Wilkins, MSPAS, PA-C
Physician Assistant
Waldorf Women's Care
Oxon Hill, Maryland

Kate Woodard, PA-C
Clinical Instructor
Department of Pediatrics
University of Colorado Denver—Anschutz Medical Campus
Aurora, Colorado

Kim Zuber, PA-C, MS
Executive Director
American Society of Nephrology PAs
St. Petersburg, Florida

Figure Credits

Figure 2.1A,B. Morton PG, Fontaine DK. *Essentials of Critical Care Nursing*. Wolters Kluwer; 2012: Fig. 8-21.

Figure 3.1. Kline-Tilford AM, Haut C. *Lippincott Certification Review: Pediatric Acute Care Nurse Practitioner*. Wolters Kluwer; 2015: Fig. 5-33.

Figure 3.2. Huff J. *ECG Workout*. 7th ed. Wolters Kluwer; 2016: Fig. 7-23.

Figure 4.1. Huff J. *ECG Workout*. 7th ed. Wolters Kluwer; 2016: Fig. 9-5.

Figure 5.1A-D. Wolfsthal S. *NMS Medicine*. 7th ed. Wolters Kluwer; 2011: Fig. 2-3.

Figure 6.1A,B. Perpetua EM, Keegan P. *Cardiac Nursing*. 7th ed. Wolters Kluwer; 2020: Fig. 12-70.

Figure 6.2. Kline-Tilford AM, Haut C. *Lippincott Certification Review: Pediatric Acute Care Nurse Practitioner*. Wolters Kluwer; 2015: Fig. 5-24.

Figure 7.1. American College of Sports Medicine. *ACSM's Clinical Exercise Physiology*. Wolters Kluwer; 2019: Fig. 6-43.

Figure 7.2. Honan L. *Focus on Adult Health*. 2nd ed. Wolters Kluwer; 2018: Fig. 17-16.

Figure 13.1A,B. Morton PG, Fontaine DK. *Essentials of Critical Care Nursing*. Wolters Kluwer; 2012: Fig. 14-2.

Figure 22.1. Daffner RH, Hartman MS. *Clinical Radiology*. 4th ed. Lippincott Williams & Wilkins; 2014: Fig. 2-48a.

Figure 48.1. Casanova R. *Beckmann and Ling's Obstetrics and Gynecology*. 8th ed. Wolters Kluwer; 2018: Fig. 29-4. From Wilkinson EJ, Stone IK. *Atlas of Vulvar Disease*. Williams & Wilkins; 2003:9.3.

Figure 48.2. Azar FM. *Orthopaedic Knowledge Update®: Sports Medicine 6 Print + Ebook with Multimedia*. 6th ed. Wolters Kluwer; 2021: Fig. 45-3. Reproduced from Centers for Disease Control and Prevention. Molluscum Contagiosum. http://www.cdc.gov/poxvirus/molluscum-contagiosum. Accessed September 28, 2020.

Figure 48.3A,B. Gonzales P. *The PA Rotation Exam Review*. Wolters Kluwer; 2018: Fig. 2-113. From Elder DE, Elenitsas R, Rubin AI, et al. *Atlas and Synopsis of Lever's Histopathology of the Skin*. 3rd ed. Wolters Kluwer; 2013: Fig. 2-118.

Figure 50.1A-C. Cohen BJ, Hull K. *Memmler's the Human Body in Health and Disease*. 13th ed. Wolters Kluwer; 2014: Fig. 6-10.

Figure 51.1. The Barankin Collection. Wolters Kluwer, 2005.

Figure 51.2. White AJ. *The Washington Manual of Paediatrics*. 2nd ed. Wolters Kluwer; 2016: Fig. 15-14a.

Figure 51.3. Edwards L, Lynch PJ. *Genital Dermatology Atlas*. 2nd ed. Wolters Kluwer; 2010: Fig. 11-21.

Figure 51.4A,B. A. Barankin Dermatology Collection. Image provided by Stedman's; Fig. Pityriasis rosea—anterior trunk. Nicol N. *Dermatology Nursing Essentials*. 3rd ed. Wolters Kluwer; 2016: Fig. 8-22. From Goodheart HP. *Goodheart's Photoguide of Common Skin Disorders*. 2nd ed. Lippincott Williams & Wilkins; 2003.

Figure 238.1. Yochum, TR and Rowe, LJ. *Yochum and Rowe's Essentials of Skeletal Radiology*, 3e. Philadelphia: Lippincott Williams & Wilkins, 2004; Fig. 9-108.

Figure 263.1A,B. Greenspan A, Beltran J. *Orthopaedic Imaging: A Practical Approach*. 7th ed. Wolters Kluwer; 2020: Fig. 7-11.

Figure 263.2A-C. Yochum TR, Rowe LJ. *Yochum and Rowe's Essentials of Skeletal Radiology*. 3rd ed. Lippincott Williams & Wilkins; 2004: Fig. 9-188.

Foreword

As the editor-in-chief of the *Journal of the American Academy of PAs*, I am so excited that my colleagues from the journal's editorial board have brought their vision for *The JAAPA QRS Review* for PAs to life for the benefit of readers like you and me. For more than a decade, the practical, timely content and self-assessments in the Quick Recertification Series (QRS) have made it one of the most popular departments in JAAPA.

While Amy Klinger and Dawn Colomb-Lippa initially developed the QRS to help new PAs navigate PANCE and experienced PAs excel on PANRE, what JAAPA readers have shared with me is that it has offered them so much more. QRS articles became a way for readers to reinforce general medical knowledge in medical and surgical specialties as well as a transition tool for those shifting from one specialty to another. When Harrison Reed led the journal, he also helped grow the QRS department and expand the breadth of topics it covered, encouraging the QRS editors to connect with talented clinicians from all over the United States (and beyond) to fill this book with exceptional content.

The editors of this book, each skilled in medical writing as well as experienced teachers, clinicians, and editors, also wanted to expand upon the original QRS series to develop a more comprehensive clinical resource and to introduce readers to a well-tested, efficient model for self-assessment, exam preparation, and success in certification and recertification testing. So, Reamer Bushardt tapped his former mentor and colleague Jennie Ariail to share a method she developed and perfected for health professionals and trainees preparing for high stakes exams.

This new book offers readers a blueprint and a broad array of clinical content that covers all material for the PANCE and PANRE. Students and clinicians now have everything needed for successful certification or recertification as well as an essential resource for maintaining your medical knowledge.

Richard Dehn, MPA, PA-C
Editor-in-Chief, *Journal of the American Academy of PAs*
Professor, Department of Physician Assistant Studies
Northern Arizona University
and
Professor of Practice, Department of Biomedical Informatics
University of Arizona College of Medicine

Contents

PART X: MUSCULOSKELETAL SYSTEM   401

Introduction

The Art (and Science) of Learning: What We Know About the Brain and What the Brain Must Have to Learn

Jennie C. Ariail, PhD Professor Emerita

As authors of this chapter, we have collectively taught health professional trainees—including PA, medical, nursing, pharmacy, dental medicine, physical therapy, and occupational therapy students plus more—for nearly 30 years. Additionally, we have worked closely with medical residents and health professionals, both new and seasoned ones, to prepare for high-stakes examinations required for entry to practice or maintenance of certification. The techniques and strategies we share with you here reflect what we have learned through these many years of experience, research, and the personal interactions with thousands of trainees, which includes hundreds and hundreds of PAs. Before you jump into the rich clinical content and assessments provided within this book, we encourage you to start with this chapter in order to equip you with the efficient, high-impact approach to learning and knowledge mastery that we have seen drive success for so many others facing a high-stakes examination or another impetus to strengthen their clinical knowledge and skills in patient care. This chapter is also designed to help you get the most value out of the rest of the content contained within this resource and individualize your approach for your success. An added benefit to this approach, and one that we have received much positive feedback about over the years, is that clinicians note it has helped them become more effective health educators with their patients when applied in conversations about their health, well-being, and living more healthful lifestyles. And in that we are counting on you!

Here is what we know about health professionals like you, whether you are new to practice or highly seasoned in your field:

- You have been studying and taking tests for many years.
- You have excelled in both these skills.
- You have a track record of success.
- You were accepted into a rigorous, competitive training program.
- You have limited time.
- You are focused on being an exceptional clinician and making a positive difference in the lives of the patients and families you serve.
- High-stakes exams are likely stressful for you.

The educational and clinical preparation of a PA, or any health professional for that matter, is to teach you to be excellent in gathering data, interpreting it, making decisions, and implementing those decisions in partnership with others (eg, patients, family members, other members of the healthcare team). And, that process requires most learners to incorporate different ways to learn to meet the cognitive and affective demands required for success.

We are going to introduce a little bit of theory here, so hold on tight because it is relevant to your goal in acquiring this book. And remember, a theory is just a system of ideas intended to explain something, and we use them every day. For many years, theories of learning were informed by the French philosopher and scientist Rene Descartes (1596-1650), who proposed a theory of a mind-body split. Until the latter part of the 20th century, his philosophy informed theories of cognition. Western scholars interpreted his philosophy as a split between cognition and affect, primarily privileging cognition and dismissing the role of affect in learning. As the neurosciences evolved more sophisticated techniques and approaches to help study and understand the functions of the human brain, Descartes's philosophy was questioned and replaced, notably through the work of Antonio DaMasio (*Descartes' Error*, 1994; *The Feeling of What Happens: Body and Emotion in the Making of Consciousness*, 1999). DaMasio's research resulted in a new understanding of the role of emotion in learning, the importance of affect in cognition, and how they can operate in tandem to ensure that what you are learning will be readily available to you as you care for patients.

Cognition refers to the higher order functions of the brain such as thinking, knowing, remembering, judging, and problem-solving. *Affect* is primarily concerned with intrinsic motivation and allows you to make connections to your life, to add emotional content such as pictures (from your life) and stories (from your patients) to both enable and enhance short-term and long-term memory. A line from an old song goes like this: "Love and marriage, love and marriage go together like a horse and carriage," but to learn, we need to change those words to "affect and cognition go together to make an outstanding clinician" (apologies for the corny joke). Significant evidence from the field of neuroscience affirms that engaging the amygdala, a structure with a primary role in emotional processing, can enhance memory. In fact, the engagement of the amygdala can enhance not only problem-solving but also working memory function (Gray et al 2006), solidifying an important connection between cognition and affect.

Equally important to mastering knowledge for a high-stakes examination or the demands and complexity of caring for patients is our ability to develop the critical thinking skill involved in metacognition (simply stated, the ability to think about our thinking). Let us ask ourselves: How do we process information? What are the best ways for us to learn and retain information vital to our health careers? As you become a lifelong learner, it is vital for you to analyze the way you take in knowledge and make it your own.

Over the past couple of decades, evidence points to the most effective and efficient method of study being retrieval practice (Roedinger and Karpicke 2006; Rohrer and Pashler 2011). Retrieval practice means just that, practicing the retrieval of information. Thus, a highly effective way to study is to practice answering questions about the material on which you will be tested or judged. By testing yourself on the information that you are trying to learn, you are better able to engage in metacognitive processing and reflection on your learning. Answering questions incorrectly allows you to reflect on the material you do not fully understand as well as identify specific target topics to learn, develop, or reinforce. Additionally, providing relevance for the information within incorrectly answered questions gives you a reason to know and motivation to master that information. When we know why or how something is relevant to a concept we are trying to learn, we can better hold onto that information. Evidence also suggests that repeated retrieval of information creates stronger memory traces, which physically manifests by enhanced synaptic connections at a cellular level (Bjork 1994, 1999).

We hope we have presented a compelling case for using this introduction and the techniques we will describe to develop an engaging, evidence-based, and personalized study plan that utilizes the most effective learning strategies available.

▶ THE ART OF TEST-TAKING: TABLE OF CONTENTS

Patient Encounter in the Clinic
Five Steps for Conquering Multiple-Choice Questions
Five Steps for Efficient and Effective Studying
Let's Consider the PANCE/PANRE

▶ PATIENT ENCOUNTER IN THE CLINIC

Scene: You are in your office, a busy clinical practice with walls freshly painted with a mural of your favorite things (eg, a breathtaking mountain view, a sandy beach)

Time: Late Friday afternoon
Characters: You, Harriette Blake, capable PA, but tired and patient, Rex Jones, middle-aged man in a white shirt and blue jeans.
Harriette knocks on the door.
Rex: "Come in."
Harriette: walks over and puts out her hand, "Hello, I am Harriette Blake, your PA. What brings you in today?"
Rex: "I am Rex Jones. Guess you see I didn't go to work (waving his hand at his jeans). I work at an airplane manufacturer. Woke up with a pain right here (points to right upper part of his body). It was bad. Thought I better see what you thought, and I need an excuse for missin' work. It eased off. I thought I might go play golf. I decided I was not having a heart attack (nervous laugh), but after lunch, it started again, and my wife insisted that ... shakes head."
Harriette: "I am sorry. Can you tell me more about that pain? When did it first start?"
Rex: "Well, I think I had a few twinges over the last few weeks, but last night it got really bad after dinner. We celebrated the birth of our first grandchild at a restaurant last night with a steak, onion rings, and a bottle of red wine."
Harriette: "How soon after you ate did the pain begin? On a scale from 1 to 10, how severe was the pain?" (Thinking to herself, pancreas? gallstones? Do I need to rule out a heart attack?)

What do you do next? Ask more questions? Fever? Nausea? Take a family history? Race? Order CBC? Recommend a scope? CT? MRI? ERCP?

What is your job? Diagnosis? Next step? Confirmatory test?

NOTE: Did Rex have:

A. Peptic ulcer
B. Duodenal ulcer
C. Biliary colic
D. Cholangitis

The process you go through to diagnose and treat this patient requires the same critical thinking and process you follow as you decipher and answer a test question. Think about that. Every question you worked in school is training you to be a clinician and training you to excel on that (often stressful) high-stakes exam. You have a test question, but the processes and approaches to it are the same approaches and processes that guide your interaction with your patients.

Therefore, we Begin at the End: Taking tests mimics patient encounters. One exception: Patients do not present with possible diagnoses written on their foreheads. If they did, you might need to shift to a psychiatric evaluation.

Five Steps for Conquering Multiple-Choice Questions:

1. *Always* cover up the answer choices! Use a rectangular sticky note or a note card or even a folded piece of paper. What you refer to as answers or possibilities are really your enemies. Professionals who study test construction (psychometrists) call these things *distractors*. And we need to knock anything like mosquitoes or flies out of our way because they distract us.

   The truth is that your education and the way you were assessed were built on your understanding enough specific details so that your faculty can be assured they had taught you and you had learned sufficiently to differentiate between similar diagnoses, confirmatory tests, treatment, etc. They assessed your mastery of material by choosing, for example, distractors that are closely related. They taught you and tested you to think critically by focusing on similarities and differences. Your study plan and test-taking strategies should follow those same techniques.

2. *Always* read the last sentence of the question first. Just as Harriette did, you began the session with your patient by asking what the patient needs from you; you must know why the patient is in your office. What does each patient want from their time with you? As you study with questions, keep a mental list of the types of questions being asked; sometimes those questions are course specific, sometimes, more general.

   For example, pharmacology questions might ask you to give the mechanism of action of a drug. What drug should you order? Route of administration? Condition for which the treatment is used or contraindicated? An adverse effect? One the other hand, other questions might ask: Diagnosis? Cause? Comorbidity? Risk? Effect? Prognosis? And, of course, basic science concept questions might focus on differences in location, function, nerve, blood supply, innervations, damage of such things as muscles, nerves, arteries.

   So, think and prepare and take tests as if you were the teacher (or a member of the question writing panel for a high-stakes exam). Think how they think as they write test questions.

3. Write the question in one or two of your own words. In the play, Harriette did not "repeat back" to the patient the cause for the visit, but one of the primary reasons test-takers miss questions is that they answer the wrong question. It is important for you to repeat what you are looking for as you read the case, the details of the question. You are excited to be a clinician, and a natural instinct is mentally trying to diagnose every question in the same way that you would try to diagnose every patient's problem. But if you do that, and the question is asking you for an enzyme, you will spend too much time looking for signs and symptoms instead of thinking *enzyme, enzyme, I am just looking for an enzyme.*
   Hint: Noun or the next noun after the word *following*; noun after the word *which*; noun after the word *what*. The noun is always the exact question.

4. Read the rest of the stem of the question the same way Harriette questioned Rex.

   Slowly and never more than once. As you are learning, we urge you to write down the three or four things in the stem that you need to answer the question. (Questions often have information that you may not need. For example, Rex told you he played golf with his buddies, and that information does not help you decide on a diagnosis for him.)

   To do your best, your scratch paper might look like this:

   > Dx?   pain, urq
   >   Fatty meal
   >   Few weeks

   In our experience, the amount of time the patient reports experiencing the problem is often ignored or not prioritized by test-takers, but it can be important.

5. Write a prediction, answer the question. Write down the first thing that comes into your mind. Usually, the first thing you think is correct, but if you don't write it down, you may forget what you first thought.

A Note on Writing

Our working memories are rather limited, and extensive research has suggested that we can hold about seven items (plus or minus two) for a brief period of time in order to engage in a task or solve a problem. With more complicated concepts (eg, not the digits of a phone number), that is reduced much further. The limited capacity of our working memory can create a bottleneck when we're trying to solve complex problems or apply our knowledge of concepts to a unique situation. In an effort to free up mental resources for problem-solving, one strategy is to offload some of what we're holding in our working memory to an external memory field, that is, a piece of scratch paper. Writing down the information you consider important as you answer questions can be referred to as cognitive offloading. Evidence suggests that engaging in cognitive offloading increases your accuracy when solving complex problems (Finley et al 2018). We encourage you to write as you answer test questions because this process both focuses your attention to the important parts of the question and allows you to free up mental processing power to retrieve knowledge of the relevant concepts.

Now your scratch paper may look something like this:

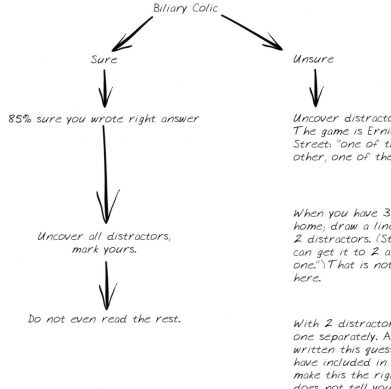

Biliary Colic

Sure

85% sure you wrote right answer

Uncover all distractors, mark yours.

Do not even read the rest.

Unsure

Uncover distractors, one at a time. The game is Ernie's game on Sesame Street: "one of these things is not like the other, one of these don't belong."

When you have 3 showing, one must go home; draw a line through it. Your goal is 2 distractors. (Students always state, "I can get it to 2 and choose the wrong one.") That is not true or you would not be here.

With 2 distractors left, work with each one separately. Ask yourself: "If I had written this question, what would I have included in the stem that would make this the right answer? If that does not tell you, then ask the same question of the remaining distractor. Choose the one closest to your prediction unless you have an epiphany."

Always choose one closest to your prediction.

Another way to visualize test questions as encounters with patients:

PA	Multiple Choice
• PA asks question: What's going on? How can I help you today?	• Student reads last sentence, actual question. What's going on here?

• PA probes:
  • When?
  • Where?
  • How long?
  • Complications?
	• Student reads rest of question once, noting concepts, pertinent facts that will aid in answering question.

• Takes notes as patient talks	• Selectively takes notes from question on scratch paper

PA	Multiple Choice

• Smart PA:
  • Refer to notes
  • Explores possibilities
  • Eliminates some based on findings
	• Smart student
	  • Refer to notes
	  • Explores possibilities
	  • Eliminates some based on findings

• Sure
  • Gives patient diagnosis, treatment, etc.
	• Sure
	  • Circles correct answer

PA	Multiple Choice
• Unsure?	• Unsure?

Smart PA:
  • Checks book in back room
  • Consults with another Physical Therapist
  • Sends patient to specialist
	Smart student:
	  • Eliminates distractors
	  • Explores two possibilities, one at a time
	  • Becomes specialist and writes, recalling buzz word

Whether learning to ride a bike, safely insert a chest tube, or share a compelling speech for your local professional society, the secret to success is practice, practice, and more practice. In this method, we are asking you to change the way you take tests. In fact, we are asking you to apply a type of practice that you probably took part in your medical education or other professional training (but may have never known it), called "deliberate practice" (a special type of practice that is purposeful and systematic requiring your focused attention). However, we know that much success on tests depends on having a strategy (and failure often involves the absence of a strategy or adoption of a faulty one). And having the structure of five steps and working them in order can also help mitigate potential test anxiety. You cannot be anxious and focus on working the steps, in order, for every question.

Because we know repetition is key; five steps: Cover, Read, Write, Read, Write (CRWRW)

▶ FIVE STEPS FOR EFFICIENT AND EFFECTIVE STUDYING

The other key to learning to become an efficient and effective physician assistant is to have a plan of study, daily and weekly, that incorporates practice questions, before and after every lecture.

We seem fixated on the number five, but here are five steps for effective study. Of course, these steps or activities are generic, so we suggest you think about how you learn (metacognition) and reshape or incorporate these suggestions into a study plan you can follow consistently.

One of us always wants a metaphor so you do not have to think about a plan. It is not rocket science. Think about eating an ice cream or snow cone—the shape of the cone gives you a memorable mental image as a structure for a plan.

Daily Plan of Study

1. Before class or a self-directed learning session: First licks of the ice cream—creating a structure for learning, 15–20 minutes
    A. Study the objectives and turn through the pages of the text or the lecture notes or PowerPoint to determine the amount of detail devoted to each objective.
    B. Organize the material in an outline or a concept map, listing main topics and subdivisions of each, leaving much white space to fill in class, the more you write during class (or your learning session), the more you will learn. We only remember about 10% of a lecture (or an online learning module) if we only sit and listen. Writing keeps us active in the process even if we are not able to write all the notes we will need.

Most lectures are linear, in other words, lectures cover one disease, syndrome, or muscle at a time, but your job is to learn differences. Find a way to take notes in class that will help you begin to learn those differences.

Insert blank concept map with specific topic in the middle of page, organizing discipline in the upper right-hand corner. Example: Muscles or Rashes or Drugs or ???? much blank space
    C. Quickly scan distractors on five to seven questions on the topic of the lecture to determine what a question writer perceives as important and what distractors are closely connected.

A Note on Scaffolding

Developing a scaffold for material prior to going to a lecture (or diving into a learning activity) allows for the experience to be significantly more memorable. By identifying the material that you are expected to learn, you will be better prepared to transfer that understanding and apply that information to a clinical scenario or test question.

You have spent 15–20 minutes that will save you much time after class.

2. In approximately 1-hour classes or study sessions, adjust the time for each additional hour: Level that wonderful ice cream at the top of the cone.
    A. Fill in the notes or concept maps or outline you made before class, write as much as you can because writing cements learning.
    B. Mark or star your notes for possible test questions, stressing the differences in concepts or details presented.
    C. Draw a silly picture from something in your life that reminds you or connects to the new information you must learn. The majority of us are more successful students when we connect things from the other parts of our lives, for example, some building on your college campus, a tree you climbed when you were a child, or a favorite movie character. Students often want to connect mental images of medical things they are learning to other medical things they are learning about. But first, try connecting something old to something new and drawing a quick silly picture. See how that works for you, noting our experience that it is generally very helpful. Both 1 and 2 are preliminary to studying, but *repetition* is vital to learning.
3. After class or study session: To ensure you learn, make careful study notes, 1.5–2 hours per 1 hour of lecture, eating that ice cream from the top of the cone through the widest part.

A. Our choice is to recreate or add to the concept maps you made: Maybe you prefer to rewrite or use tables or graphs or some method that will allow you to quickly see the similarities and differences in similarities, for example, drugs, or muscles, or childhood diseases, types of cancer including location of metastasis.

B. After you have completed the notes, review them by covering the information and seeing how much you remember. Please do not just read them over and think that it is an active review.

4. Note or ANKI cards: 15–20 minutes, almost to the end of that ice cream cone.

A. Do not overwhelm yourself with piles of cards that you will never find the time to review. The cards are only for specific details you could not recall as you review the notes you just made. Cards should be approximately 3 by 5 and have a title and the one thing you could not recall. Flip the card over and draw something silly in a color. Then put the card somewhere in your house, apartment, or room, picture-side up, that reminds you of the information you are trying to ensure you remember. The next morning pick up those five to seven cards while you are eating breakfast and getting ready to get to class and say, out loud if possible, what is on the other side of the card.

B. Aristotle taught the value of place in memory as he taught young males to memorize persuasive speeches concerning democracy in his peripatetic school. One of us suggests putting things in a memory palace.

5. Work questions, using the method you learned this chapter, 15–20 minutes, nearing the end of that ice cream cone.

A. Use that method to ensure you have learned. Work 10 questions (from the Pretests or the Comprehensive Exam[1]), most of those you skimmed before class, keep a record, do not get immediate answers, check answers by repeating the notes you made as you worked each question note and saying the word for the answer you choose. When you check using this method, you have had one more look at (another round of repetition) the information. When you answered correctly, give yourself three big checks, and move on; no need to read because you had enough information to figure it out. Good for you. However, every question you miss is a great *opportunity*. Say to yourself, "Oh, I am so glad I missed this question today instead of next week on the test." Every miss is an opportunity. Make notes on the differences of what you thought it was and what the correct answer was.

B. These steps are purposely generic, of course, but they provide a structure that follows a plan so you can adapt each of these steps to accommodate the way you learn best. Please remember that an important part of the learning process is to figure out what you do not know and learn that information. Our years of experience with thousands of students inform our belief that the best way to determine what you do not know is to work questions daily and weekly.

Weekly Plan

Review all of your notes for each class (or study session, every week, if possible). You have made excellent notes to review before each test. If you organized those notes according to similarities and differences, every concept map of notes arranged to highlight differences is a potential question.

And now you have a way to think about and visualize a plan for learning to be the best clinician you can be, a plan to enable you to focus on caring for and empathizing with your patients. It all fits together.

▶ LET'S CONSIDER THE PANCE/PANRE

You are ready. You have everything you need to excel on this test: a strategy for taking the test and a strategy for answering questions.

The only difference from daily and weekly study is that your entire study plan is built on questions and more questions, creating a review notebook, reviewing morning and night and one day a week for cumulative review of all your notes. We also suggest full-length practice tests.

You have been preparing for PANCE or PANRE with every note, every lecture, every question. Now it is time to put it all together.

During clinical rotations or clerkships, you might have tried to work every question for that body system or patient population you could find. The NCCPA Blueprints for PANCE and PANRE provide the best guide as you work questions in, for example, pediatrics, to evaluate questions based on tasks and organ systems. And, the review material and test questions in this book have been developed using the latest versions of those Blueprints.

The best way to approach this testing recommendation is to follow the advice we gave you earlier: Cover the distractors, read the last sentence, write the question in one or two of your own words, read the rest of the question slowly, taking a few notes on things in the question that will help you answer the question. Write a prediction. If you are sure of your answer, uncover all distractors,

---

[1]In this book, pretest questions have been developed by the authors and editors to help you focus in on the content that you determine needs your attention first. And the comprehensive examination developed by the authors and editors will support your preparation and enable practice for that upcoming high-stakes exam.

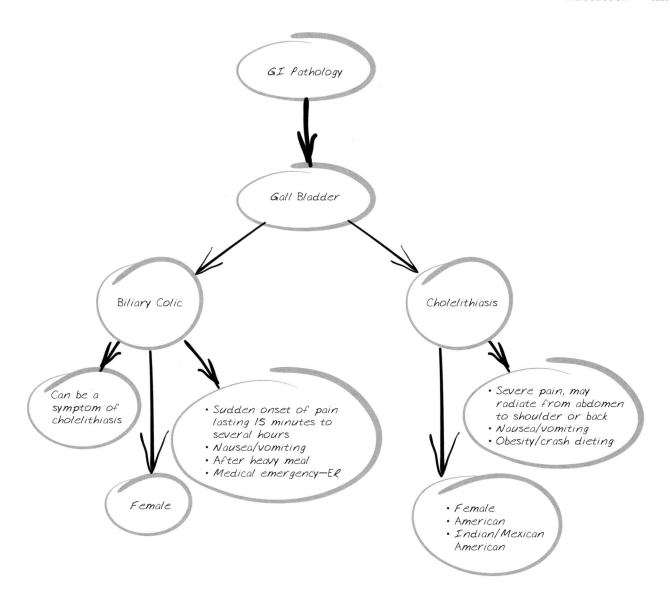

choose the one closest to your prediction, write the word(s) of that distractor, do not get the answer.

After working 5, 10, or 15 questions, use those question notes to review. Then repeat the word(s) of the distractor you chose. If correct, give yourself encouraging check marks. You are reviewing all that you know. If incorrect, "What an *opportunity*!" Make notes on what you thought the answer was and what it was, again, focusing on differences.

You can review them quicker if you only write on one side of the page and if they are organized according to tests, diseases, muscles, etc. Caution: Do not write down information that you know. That knowledge is not going anywhere. You are studying to make sure you have mastered what you were not sure of. No other way to figure it all out except to work questions and have a method for answering them.

Your goal is a well-organized review notebook for you to continue to do weekly cumulative reviews as you complete all of the questions. Review your notes before you stop studying and again a few minutes in the morning before your rotation. Try to do a cumulative review one day a week.

If you consistently follow this plan, you will be ready for that high-stakes exam with all the techniques, knowledge, and skills you need to be successful.

REFERENCE

Ericsson KA. Deliberate practice and the acquisition and maintenance of expert performance in medicine and related domains. *Acad Med.* 2004;79(10 Suppl):S70-S81. doi:10.1097/00001888-200410001-00022

Cardiovascular System Pretest

Section A Pretest: Conduction Disorders and Dysrhythmias

1. Which of the following would you most likely find on the history of a patient with premature ventricular contractions?

   A. Headache
   B. Shortness of breath on exertion
   C. The feeling of a "skipped" beat
   D. Loss of consciousness

2. A 54-year-old male complains of dyspnea and weight gain for 4 weeks. On physical examination, he has bilateral pitting edema and jugular venous distention (JVD). An ECG is performed and demonstrates sinus rhythm with an LBBB, which was not present on previous ECG. What is the most appropriate diagnostic test to evaluate a newly diagnosed LBBB?

   A. Cardiac rhythm monitor
   B. Transthoracic echocardiogram
   C. Coronary angiography
   D. Cardiac MRI

3. A 40-year-old man with a history of open aortic valve replacement 1 year ago presents with fatigue and dyspnea on exertion. He has a third-degree atrioventricular block. Which of the following is the most important treatment for him?

   A. Defibrillator implantation
   B. Hold all AV nodal-blocking agents
   C. Permanent pacemaker implantation
   D. Watchful waiting

4. A 78-year-old male is diagnosed with atrial fibrillation. He has a history of hypertension, hypothyroidism, and osteoarthritis. His renal and hepatic function are normal. An echocardiogram reveals mild LV hypertrophy and moderate aortic insufficiency. What is the most appropriate agent to reduce his risk of an embolic event associated with his arrhythmia?

   A. Aspirin 81 mg daily
   B. Clopidogrel 75 mg daily
   C. Rivaroxaban 20 mg daily
   D. Warfarin 5 mg daily

5. Which of the following is the appropriate management for ventricular fibrillation?

   A. Electrical defibrillation
   B. Beta-blockers
   C. Amiodarone
   D. IV magnesium

6. A 55-year-old male is diagnosed with asymptomatic atrial fibrillation with an average HR of 110 beats per minute. He is already taking warfarin because he has a mechanical mitral valve. He has no contraindications to any medications. Which of the following agents might you prescribe for rate-control therapy?

   A. Amlodipine 5 mg daily
   B. Metoprolol succinate 50 mg daily
   C. Flecainide 50 mg twice daily
   D. Propafenone 150 mg every 8 hours

7. Which of the following HR ranges is typically seen in a patient with a third-degree atrioventricular block?

   A. 20-40 beats per minute
   B. 40-60 beats per minute
   C. 60-80 beats per minute
   D. 80-100 beats per minute

8. Which of the following medications can cause an atrioventricular block?

   A. Dobutamine
   B. Lisinopril
   C. Metoprolol
   D. Warfarin

9. Regarding sick sinus syndrome (SSS), which of the following is true?

   A. Symptoms, when present, are specific for the disorder.
   B. Most symptomatic patients with confirmed SSS will need a pacemaker.
   C. Surface ECG allows direct assessment of sinus node activity.
   D. CAD is a common cause of SSS.

Section B Pretest: Congenital Heart Disease

1. A 4-week-old girl is diagnosed with coarctation of the aorta (CoA) after she became apneic during a feeding session and was rushed to the hospital. Which of the following murmurs would indicate a second condition, one which commonly occurs with CoA, in this patient?

   A. Blowing, systolic murmur heard best at the apex, radiating to the axilla
   B. Continuous, machine-like murmur heard best at the left upper sternal border
   C. Harsh, crescendo-decrescendo murmur heard best at the right upper sternal border
   D. Harsh, pansystolic murmur heard best at the left lower sternal border

2. Which of the following ECG findings may be seen in atrial septal defect?

   A. Inverted T waves
   B. J-point elevation
   C. Prolonged PR interval
   D. Right axis deviation

3. Which of the following is a common complication of ventricular septal defect repair?

   A. Aortic valve regurgitation
   B. Myocardial ischemia
   C. Right bundle branch block
   D. Ventricular wall rupture

4. Which of the following arrhythmias is associated with atrial septal defect?

   A. Atrial flutter
   B. Long QT syndrome
   C. SSS
   D. VT

5. A 2-week-old male presents to the ED after his mother reports that he has become irritable and breathless, especially during feeding. She reports a normal vaginal delivery with no complications. Physical examinations reveal 4+ carotid pulses bilaterally, 2+ brachial pulses bilaterally, and unpalpable femoral pulses. A loud, systolic ejection murmur is present. Based on the most likely diagnosis, which of the following interventions is considered the definitive treatment for this patient?

   A. Balloon angioplasty
   B. IV prostaglandin
   C. Stent implantation
   D. Surgical repair

6. Which of the following conditions is associated with ventricular septal defect?

   A. Congenital rubella
   B. Fetal alcohol syndrome
   C. Marfan syndrome
   D. Rheumatic heart disease

7. Which of the following etiologies is associated with ostium primum atrial septal defect?

   A. Maternal rubella infection
   B. Maternal varicella infection
   C. Trisomy 13
   D. Trisomy 21

8. Which physical examination finding correlates with the pulmonic stenosis seen in tetralogy of Fallot?

   A. Systolic ejection murmur heard best at the second intercostal space on the left sternal border
   B. Diastolic murmur heard best at the apex of the heart
   C. Muffled heart sounds
   D. Systolic murmur that radiates into the left axilla

9. Which infant is most likely to have respiratory compromise due to a PDA?

   A. A low-birthweight (LBW) female newborn who was delivered at 28 weeks' gestation diagnosed with respiratory distress syndrome
   B. A 3-week-old male born at 38 weeks gestation in the 65th percentile for weight with shortness of breath and tachypnea
   C. A 4-day-old female born at 30 weeks' gestation, normal weight, without signs or symptoms of respiratory distress
   D. A newborn male born at 40 weeks' gestation with normal height and weight with tachypnea, fever, and tachycardia.

10. Which of the following is NOT one of the four classic anomalies seen with tetralogy of Fallot?

    A. Right ventricular or pulmonic outflow obstruction
    B. Tricuspid atresia
    C. Right ventricular hypertrophy
    D. Ventricular septal defect

11. Which of the following is prevented by closing moderate-to-large ventricular septal defects before age 2 years?

    A. Anoxic brain injury
    B. Complete heart block
    C. Pulmonary hypertension
    D. Raynaud syndrome

Section C Pretest: Coronary Artery Disease

1. A 50-year-old man comes to your urgent care clinic for unrelenting chest discomfort over the past hour. He reports that over the past 6-8 months he has been experiencing chest discomfort along with increased shortness of breath with mowing his lawn as well as walking up two flights to his apartment. The symptoms resolve after 5 minutes of rest but occurs again with the same activity. The symptoms have become more easily provoked, last longer, and are more intense over the past day. An ECG demonstrates ST-elevation of 3 mm in leads V_3 and V_4. What do you suspect?

   A. Costochondritis
   B. STEMI
   C. NSTE-ACE
   D. Asthma

2. A patient presenting to the ED with exertional chest pain and high-risk features for CAD should promptly be evaluated for suspected myocardial infarction with which of the following?

   A. 12-lead ECG and troponin bloodwork
   B. Chest CT
   C. Invasive coronary angiogram
   D. Echocardiogram

3. Risk factor(s) generally associated with CAD include which of the following?

   A. Hypertension
   B. Diabetes
   C. Smoking
   D. All of the above

4. Which of the following history components increases the probability of Prinzmetal angina as the cause of a patient's chest pain?

   A. Hypercholesterolemia
   B. Metabolic syndrome
   C. Raynaud phenomenon
   D. Osteoarthritis

5. When ST-elevation of >2 mm is found in two contiguous leads on ECG, what is the treatment?

   A. Fibrinolytics within 30 minutes as a first-line treatment
   B. Beta-blockers, aspirin, and nitroglycerin and ICU admission

   C. Admission to a PCI-capable hospital for a goal of revascularization in 90 minutes or less (door-to-balloon)
   D. Further evaluation with stress testing to assess for coronary ischemia

6. A 65-year-old male with a known history of CAD is evaluated by his cardiologist for ongoing angina. He states the chest pain is provoked with physical activity and improves with sublingual nitroglycerin. He states he has been compliant with his metoprolol, atorvastatin, and aspirin, but he finds the anginal episodes to be lifestyle limiting. Coronary arteriography demonstrates 70% occlusion of his right coronary artery with a normal EF. The decision is made to place a stent in the patient's right coronary artery. Which of the following medication regimens should the patient go home on?

   A. Aspirin
   B. Aspirin and apixaban
   C. Apixaban
   D. Aspirin and ticagrelor

7. What physical examination finding is characteristic of Prinzmetal angina?

   A. Substernal chest pain
   B. Tachycardia with gallop
   C. Elevated serial troponins
   D. Transient ST-segment changes on ECG

8. Which of the following medications is NOT indicated in all patients with CAD (in the absence of contraindications)?

   A. Aspirin
   B. Beta-blocker
   C. ACEI
   D. Hydroxymethylglutaryl coenzyme A reductase inhibitor (statin)

9. In outpatient evaluation, if the ECG is normal, but the patient has ongoing chest pain, dyspnea, palpitations, or presyncope/syncope, which of the following is the best next step?

   A. The patient should be allowed to rest in the clinic room until symptoms abate.
   B. The patient can be sent home to recover.
   C. Send the patient via self-transport to the nearest ED for unresolving symptoms.
   D. Send the patient via EMS to the nearest ED for unresolving symptoms.

10. A 66-year-old female is being evaluated for intermittent chest pain and shortness of breath and is undergoing an exercise stress test. Presence of which of the following would be indicative of a positive stress test?

    A. Sinus arrhythmia
    B. ST depressions of 1 mm in precordial leads
    C. Reproduction of symptoms
    D. Sinus tachycardia

11. What is the most common description of angina-type chest pain?

    A. Pressure or tightness
    B. Sharp or stabbing
    C. Numbness and tingling
    D. Pleuritic

12. Which of the following patients would be most likely to present with atypical symptoms of CAD?

    A. An 86-year-old male with a history of tobacco use and type 2 diabetes mellitus
    B. A 45-year-old Caucasian male with a family history of CAD
    C. A 66-year-old African American male with a history of hypertension and hyperlipidemia
    D. A 55-year-old male with no prior medical history

13. Which of the following medications should be given for acute angina symptoms?

    A. Sublingual nitroglycerin
    B. Long-acting nitroglycerin
    C. Diltiazem
    D. Metoprolol

14. Which of the following is an indication for revascularization with CABG?

    A. History of prior coronary artery stent placement
    B. Single vessel disease involving the left circumflex coronary artery
    C. EF >45%
    D. Left main CAD

Section D Pretest: Heart Failure

1. Which of the following is the most common cause of cardiogenic shock?

    A. Pulmonary embolism
    B. Aortic dissection
    C. Acute MI
    D. Chest trauma

2. A 63-year-old female patient presents to the ED complaining of shortness of breath that has been progressive over the last several days. She states she was in the hospital last month for similar symptoms and last night woke up suddenly because she "could not breathe." She generally sleeps with two pillows but has recently needed three pillows. Physical examination: somnolent, exhibits exertional respirations, no use of accessory muscles, bibasilar crackles, grade II/VI systolic murmur best heard at left upper sternal border and 2+ bilateral lower extremity edema. Labs: Na 129, Cr 1.5, BNP >3500, otherwise normal. What is the most likely diagnosis?

    A. Pulmonary embolism
    B. Heart failure
    C. Acute MI
    D. Aortic dissection

3. A 47-year-old man presents to your office complaining of upper back pain that began last night. He has a medical history of hypertension and is a current smoker. He describes the pain as a "ripping" sensation that radiates to his neck. His family history is positive for sudden death. His vital signs are T: 97.8 °F, HR: 110 beats per minute, respiratory rate (RR): 20 breaths per minute, BP: 170/100 mm Hg, O_2 sat: 94%. What is the best plan for this patient?

    A. Start antihypertensive
    B. Pain control and observation
    C. Obtain stat CXR
    D. Urgent transfer to ED

4. Which of the following is NOT a sign of fluid retention?

    A. Ronchi
    B. Ascites
    C. JVD
    D. Pitting edema

5. A 65-year-old male patient presents to the clinic for an initial visit. His past medical history includes CAD, AMI status post PCI 3 years ago, obesity, hypertension, hyperlipidemia, diabetes mellitus type 2, and osteoarthritis. He has no other surgical history. He endorses four to five alcoholic beverages per week and recently quit smoking tobacco. He mostly works at his desk and computer as an office manager. He denies any chest pain, shortness of breath, orthopnea, paroxysmal nocturnal dyspnea, abdominal pain, fevers, or chills. Vitals: T: 98.8 °F, HR: 90 beats per minute, RR: 20 breaths per minute, BP: 138/92 mm Hg, O_2 sat 94%. Physical examination: appears comfortable, alert and oriented, obese, normal respiratory effort, normal heart rate with a regular rhythm, no murmurs, rubs or gallops, benign abdominal exam, no edema. His last echocardiogram 3 months ago showed an EF of 40% with no valvular abnormalities and normal right ventricular function. What initial medical strategies should you pursue?

A. Recommend repeat left heart catheterization to evaluate the severity of his CAD
B. Request cardiothoracic surgery consultation
C. Review and optimize his medications
D. Educate the patient about lifestyle modifications, including avoiding tobacco and minimizing alcohol use, exercising regularly, and following dietary guidelines.

6. A 68-year-old male patient presents for his follow-up visit. He has a history of mild-to-moderate mitral valve stenosis, heart failure with reduced EF, hypertension, esophageal dysmotility, and seborrheic keratosis. You have been managing his heart failure for over a year. His medications include aspirin 81 mg PO daily, carvedilol 6.25 mg PO twice daily, lisinopril 10 mg PO daily, atorvastatin 80 mg PO daily, furosemide 40 mg PO daily, potassium chloride 10 mEq PO twice daily, multivitamin daily, and vitamin C 500 mg PO twice daily. His last EF was 40% at his visit 3 months prior. Vitals: T: 99.0 °F, HR: 78 beats per minute, RR: 22 breaths per minute, BP: 130/88 mm Hg, O_2 sat 97%. What, if any, adjustments to the patient's medications are indicated?

A. Transition from lisinopril to the angiotensin receptor-neprilysin inhibitor (ARNI)
B. Decrease carvedilol to 3.125 mg PO daily
C. Increase furosemide to 40 mg PO twice daily
D. No changes indicated at this time

Section E Pretest: Hyperlipidemia

1. A 49-year-old male patient with a history of myocardial infarction comes in for follow-up on his lipids. Lipid panel reveals LDL 95 mg/dL and triglycerides (TGs) of 180 mg/dL. The patient currently is on high-intensity statin and takes it regularly. Which of the following would NOT be appropriate to consider adding to his medication regimen?

A. Ezetimibe
B. Icosapent ethyl
C. PCSK-9 inhibitor
D. Any of the following are reasonable additions to his care plan

2. What is the target LDL level for a patient with a history of a stroke?

A. ≤70 mg/dL
B. ≤100 mg/dL
C. ≤130 mg/dL
D. ≤190 mg/dL

3. Which of the following patients should be screened for lipid disorders?

A. A healthy 16-year-old female
B. A 40-year-old male seeking medical care for the first time
C. A 30-year-old female with low cardiovascular risk
D. A 47-year-old female who had normal lipid panel at age 45

4. Which of the following is NOT a risk factor for developing atherosclerotic cardiovascular disease (ASCVD)?

A. Age
B. Smoking
C. Hyperthyroidism
D. Diabetes

Section F Pretest: Hypertension And Hypotension

1. Which of the following patients would be most likely to develop orthostatic hypotension following a prolonged gastrointestinal illness?

    A. A 50-year-old male taking amlodipine for his BP and who recently started alfuzosin for his enlarged prostate symptoms
    B. A 25-year-old female with opiate use disorder who recently started naltrexone
    C. A 40-year-old depressed male on citalopram who added cetirizine for allergies
    D. A 22-year-old female with a DVT

2. Which of the following would be the most appropriate first step in the workup for orthostatic hypotension?

    A. MRI of the brain to check for Lewy bodies
    B. Basic metabolic panel to check for low sodium
    C. Stool guaiac for occult blood and hemoglobin/hematocrit to check for anemia
    D. Urinalysis and culture to check for occult urinary tract infection

3. Which direct vasodilator is associated with cyanide toxicity in patients with renal and liver disease?

    A. Nitroprusside
    B. Nicardipine
    C. Hydralazine
    D. Labetalol

4. A 42-year-old female has the following BPs recorded over the past month: 144/92 mm Hg, 138/92 mm Hg, and 140/90 mm Hg. Which of the following diagnoses and recommended treatments is the most appropriate?

    A. Prehypertension, start lifestyle modification only
    B. Prehypertension, start lifestyle modification and medication
    C. Hypertension, start lifestyle modification only
    D. Hypertension, start lifestyle modification and medication

5. Which of the following scenarios would be least likely associated with vasovagal hypotension?

    A. Syncope while having a bowel movement
    B. Syncope after a blood draw
    C. Syncope with associated nausea, diaphoresis, and feeling of impending syncope
    D. Syncope after exercise

6. A 55-year-old female has transferred to your clinic. She has a BP of 146/88 mm Hg and tells you this has improved over the past 3 months with lifestyle modification. Prior to nonpharmacologic intervention, she reports that her BPs were approximately 158/90 mm Hg. Which of the following is a recommended first-line agent for treating her hypertension?

    A. Chlorthalidone 12.5 mg once daily
    B. Metoprolol succinate 50 mg once daily
    C. Hydralazine 100 mg twice daily
    D. Prazosin 2 mg twice daily

7. A 60-year-old female has a sustained average BP of 144/88 mm Hg. She has stage III chronic kidney disease with albuminuria >300 mg/dL. Which of the following medications would be most appropriate to treat her hypertension with kidney disease?

    A. Amlodipine 5 mg once daily
    B. Bisoprolol 5 mg once daily
    C. Furosemide 40 mg once daily
    D. Lisinopril 10 mg once daily

8. A 65-year-old white male has an average BP on multiple readings over the past month of 160/92 mm Hg. He has no significant past medical history and has an otherwise normal physical examination and laboratory tests. Which of the following is a recommended first-line agent for treating his hypertension?

    A. Irbesartan 150 mg once daily
    B. Aliskiren 150 mg once daily
    C. Eplerenone 50 mg twice daily
    D. Atenolol 50 mg twice daily

9. Baroreceptor stretch causes which of the following to occur?

    A. Increased HR
    B. Increased vascular resistance
    C. Increased parasympathetic stimulation
    D. Increased stroke volume

10. Which of the following would decrease to maintain BP in a bleeding patient?

    A. HR
    B. Stroke volume
    C. Systemic vascular resistance
    D. Baroreceptor stretch

Section G Pretest: Infectious and Inflammatory Heart Disease

1. Which of the following findings is most likely to be present in a patient with cardiac tamponade?

   A. Sinus tachycardia
   B. Pericardial friction rub
   C. Flat neck veins
   D. Peripheral cyanosis

2. The diagnosis of cardiac tamponade is best confirmed by which of the following?

   A. Low voltage (diffuse) on ECG
   B. Chest radiograph showing cardiomegaly
   C. Presence of pericardial effusion on echocardiogram
   D. Hemodynamic and clinical response to pericardial fluid drainage

3. Which of the following cardiac valves is most commonly affected in IV drug users diagnosed with IE?

   A. Mitral
   B. Tricuspid
   C. Aortic
   D. Pulmonic

4. Which of the following echocardiography findings is consistent with the most common cause of restrictive cardiomyopathy?

   A. Obstruction of the LV outflow tract
   B. Pericardial thickening and calcifications
   C. Speckled myocardial pattern
   D. Ventricular interdependence

5. Which of the following is the definitive treatment for cardiac tamponade?

   A. Medical therapy with a positive inotropic agent
   B. NSAID plus colchicine
   C. Percutaneous or surgical drainage
   D. Avoidance of volume depletion

6. Which of the following IV medications should be used as empiric therapy in patients with suspected native valve endocarditis?

   A. Ampicillin
   B. Ciprofloxacin
   C. Vancomycin
   D. Rifampin

7. A 46-year-old male with no previous medical history is diagnosed with acute myocarditis. His symptoms include fatigue, dyspnea on exertion, and mild chest tightness. Physical examination reveals fine crackles at the base of both lungs, mild JVD, and lower extremity edema. ECG reveals sinus rhythm with a rate of 90 beats per minute. What treatment should he receive?

   A. Supportive treatment with acetaminophen and rest
   B. Supportive treatment, an ACE inhibitor, a beta-blocker, and a diuretic (as needed)
   C. Nonsteroidal anti-inflammatory and rest
   D. Antiarrhythmic and automatic implantable cardioverter-defibrillator (AICD) placement

8. A 20-year-old male presents for a preparticipation sports screening for college basketball. He reports that he is healthy and feels well today. His family history is notable for an older brother who experienced syncopal episodes due to a heart problem at age 22. He also reports a paternal uncle who died suddenly while running a marathon at age 30. The patient's ECG is notable for prominent inferior and lateral Q waves. Which physical examination finding would be consistent with the patient's most likely diagnosis?

   A. Resting severe hypertension
   B. Diastolic murmur with an opening snap
   C. Systolic murmur accentuated with squatting to standing
   D. Discrepant BPs in the upper and lower extremities

Section H Pretest: Valvular Disorders

1. Prompt recognition of giant cell arteritis and initiation of steroids is essential to prevent which complication of the disease?

   A. Severe vision loss or permanent blindness
   B. Persistent headaches
   C. Progression to polymyalgia rheumatica
   D. Stroke

2. Which of the following best describes the murmur of pulmonic stenosis?

   A. Systolic ejection murmur heard best at left sternal border
   B. Crescendo-decrescendo systolic murmur heard best at the right sternal border with radiation to carotid artery
   C. High-pitched holosystolic murmur heard best at the lower left sternal border
   D. Low, rumbling diastolic murmur and opening snap heard best at the left sternal border

3. Which of the following is NOT a risk factor for developing giant cell arteritis?

   A. Polymyalgia rheumatica
   B. Male
   C. Caucasian
   D. Age over 50 years

4. Which of the following situations is the most common cause of mitral stenosis in developed countries?

   A. Calcification of valve
   B. Drug toxicity
   C. Rheumatic fever
   D. Myocardial infarction

5. Which of the following most accurately describes the murmur heard with aortic valve regurgitation?

   A. Systolic ejection murmur heard best at the right second intercostal space
   B. Holodiastolic murmur heard best along the lower left sternal border
   C. Diastolic murmur heard best at the apex and radiating to the left axilla
   D. Machine-like continuous murmur heard best along the left sternal border

6. Which of the following maneuvers will accentuate the murmur of tricuspid stenosis?

   A. Standing
   B. Valsalva
   C. Inspiration
   D. Handgrip

7. Which of the following is considered a less common cause of aortic valve regurgitation?

   A. Marfan-related aortic root dilation
   B. Ventricular septal defect
   C. Inferior myocardial infarction
   D. Aortic valve sclerosis

8. Which of the following is a cause of functional tricuspid regurgitation?

   A. Ebstein anomaly
   B. Infective endocarditis
   C. Chronic hypoxemic lung disease
   D. Congenital CoA

9. What is the diagnostic test of choice for aortic valve regurgitation?

   A. Swan-Ganz catheterization
   B. Echocardiogram
   C. Electrocardiogram
   D. CXR

10. A 25-year-old man with known intravenous drug use presents to the ED with complaints of fatigue and ankle swelling. On examination, he is tachycardic but normotensive with an oral temperature of 38.4 °C. He has a visible pulsation in his neck veins, which appear distended, especially when you palpate over the right upper quadrant of his abdomen. Which diagnostic study will be most useful in confirming your suspected diagnosis?

    A. Peripheral blood cultures
    B. Transthoracic echocardiogram
    C. Electrocardiogram
    D. Chest CTA

11. Your elderly patient presents to the clinic with dyspnea, pulmonary edema, and murmur. Echocardiogram reveals aortic valve regurgitation. What is the definitive treatment of choice for this individual, assuming no contraindications?

    A. Beta-blocker and loop diuretics
    B. Heart transplant
    C. ACE inhibitor
    D. Aortic valve replacement

12. Which of the following is NOT a sign or symptom of severe aortic stenosis?
    A. Angina
    B. Dyspnea
    C. Syncope
    D. Claudication

13. An 80-year-old female has been diagnosed with aortic valve regurgitation and while sitting in the clinic, you notice that her head seems to bob up and down at a rate that matches her HR. What is the name of this clinical sign?
    A. Chadwick sign
    B. Musset sign
    C. Babinski sign
    D. Murphy sign

14. A 25-year-old man with known intravenous drug use presents to the ED with complaints of fatigue and ankle swelling. On examination, he is tachycardic but normotensive with an oral temperature of 38.4 °C. He has a visible pulsation in his neck veins, which appear distended, especially when you palpate over the right upper quadrant of his abdomen. Transthoracic echocardiography demonstrates a likely vegetation on the tricuspid valve with severe regurgitation and hepatic flow reversal. What is the most appropriate definitive treatment for this patient?
    A. Intravenous diuretics
    B. Broad-spectrum antibiotic therapy
    C. Balloon valvuloplasty
    D. Tricuspid valve replacement

15. Which of the following options is the definitive treatment for a patient with symptomatic mitral regurgitation (MR)?
    A. Mitral valve repair
    B. Mitral valve replacement
    C. Percutaneous valvuloplasty
    D. Symptomatic pharmacologic therapy

16. Which physical examination finding indicates severe aortic stenosis?
    A. Austin Flint murmur
    B. Pansystolic murmur with radiation to the left axilla
    C. Delayed carotid upstroke
    D. Opening snap following S2

17. What is the diagnostic tool of choice in diagnosing aortic stenosis?
    A. ECG
    B. CXR
    C. Echocardiogram
    D. Cardiac catheterization

18. Which of the following increases the likelihood of biopsy-positive giant cell arteritis?
    A. Elevated ESR and CRP, normochromic normocytic anemia, and elevated platelets
    B. Elevated ESR and CRP, low platelets, and normochromic normocytic anemia
    C. Vision loss, normal ESR and CRP, low platelets, and microcytic anemia
    D. Elevated CRP, ESR, platelets, and macrocytic anemia

19. Which of the following patients requires antibiotic prophylaxis before a dental procedure?
    A. Any patient with mitral valve disease
    B. A 35-year-old woman with severe symptomatic MR
    C. A 45-year-old man with MR and a history of IE
    D. A 50-year-old woman with MS and mitral valve repair 5 years ago

20. What is the gold standard for diagnosis of giant cell arteritis?
    A. Color Doppler ultrasound
    B. Elevated ESR and/or CRP
    C. Temporal artery biopsy
    D. Fundoscopic examination showing pale swollen optic disc

Section I Pretest: Vascular Disease

1. A 63-year-old male presents to the clinic for progressive lower extremity edema with pruritus and skin discoloration. He notes that his legs feel heavy by the end of the day after working and standing most of the day. He has not had any lesions on the legs and has not used compression. Which response below would NOT be part of conservative management for this patient?
    A. Daily moisturizing lotion
    B. Medical-grade compression
    C. Exercise
    D. Diuretic therapy

2. An ABI of less than which of the following values is consistent with occlusive arterial disease?

   A. 1.5
   B. 1.3
   C. 1.1
   D. 0.9

3. What is the most common location of an AAA?

   A. Infraceliac
   B. Infrailiac
   C. Inframesenteric
   D. Infrarenal

4. Which of the following is NOT a common symptom of polyarteritis nodosa?

   A. Systemic symptoms of fatigue, weight loss, weakness, fever, and arthralgia
   B. Skin lesions (livedo reticularis, purpura, ulcers)
   C. Abdominal pain
   D. Symmetric polyneuropathy

5. A 28-year-old female is admitted to the hospital for lower extremity swelling and was found to have DVT. The patient recently started on a form of birth control but does not recall the product's name. Which type of birth control may have caused her DVT?

   A. Mirena IUD
   B. Norethindrone
   C. Medroxyprogesterone
   D. Norgestimate/ethinyl estradiol

6. A 72-year-old male with familial hypercholesterolemia, medication-controlled diabetes and hypertension, chronic kidney disease, and GERD presents with a 3-hour history of right-sided facial droop and slurred speech. What is likely to be the source of his symptoms?

   A. Right temporal subdural bleeding
   B. Ruptured right cerebral aneurysm
   C. Bilateral carotid cholesterol plaque
   D. In situ thrombosis from a thrombotic disorder

7. A 70-year-old man presents with DVT 4 days after his total hip replacement. He was treated with enoxaparin prior to his surgery but still developed a DVT. You plan to increase his LMWH and initiate warfarin. Which tests should you order before starting therapy?

   A. Factor V Leiden
   B. Lupus anticoagulant
   C. Protein C and protein S
   D. None of the above

8. Which stage of polyarteritis nodosa is characterized by polymorphonuclear neutrophils infiltrating all layers of the vessel wall?

   A. Subacute stage
   B. Acute stage
   C. Chronic stage
   D. All stages

9. A 30-year-old female at 27 weeks' gestation presents with left lower extremity swelling. She recently returned from a trip to Asia. A Doppler of her left lower leg ultrasound confirms your diagnosis. Which of the following statements regarding anticoagulation in pregnancy is correct?

   A. Warfarin should be initiated and continued for at least 3 months during the pregnancy for the treatment of DVT.
   B. Dabigatran is recommended for anticoagulation therapy for the treatment of DVT.
   C. Inferior vena cava filters are the treatment of choice for preventing recurrent DVT during pregnancy.
   D. Anticoagulation with LMWH should be continued for at least 6 weeks postpartum (for a minimum of 3 months of treatment) for DVT diagnosed during pregnancy.

10. What is the main treatment for polyarteritis nodosa?

   A. Antivirals
   B. Corticosteroids
   C. Plasmapheresis
   D. Cyclophosphamide

11. Which of the following tests is considered the gold standard for diagnosing peripheral arterial disease?

   A. ABI
   B. Contrast angiography
   C. MRA of the lower extremities
   D. CTA of the lower extremities

12. What is polyarteritis nodosa (PAN)?

   A. Vasculitis of only the small arteries
   B. Vasculitis of only the medium arteries
   C. Vasculitis that affects small and medium muscular arteries
   D. Vasculitis that can affect any sized artery

13. Which of the following physical examination findings is associated with peripheral arterial disease?

   A. Bounding femoral pulses
   B. Lower extremity edema
   C. Dilated varicose veins
   D. Diminished dorsalis pedis pulses

14. A patient is diagnosed with a dissection that involves the aortic root and the ascending aorta. Which of the following interventions is the most appropriate?

   A. Endovascular stent repair
   B. IV diltiazem
   C. IV esmolol
   D. Surgical repair

15. Which of the following measurements is the cut-off value for referring a patient with an AAA to a surgeon?
    A. >4 cm
    B. >5 cm
    C. >6 cm
    D. >7 cm

16. An 80-year-old female presents with a pale, diffusely painful left foot. The pain developed rapidly over the last 2 hours with no history of trauma. Her medical history is significant for CAD status post CABG, previous tobacco use with a 75-pack-year history, osteoarthritis status post right knee replacement, and GERD. Her medications include daily aspirin 81 mg, Extra-strength Tylenol, omeprazole, and a multivitamin. What clinical evaluation will be most helpful to guide further evaluation?
    A. Nothing, go straight to CT imaging
    B. Bilateral lower extremity pulse examination and auscultation
    C. Lower extremity range-of-motion examination and palpation for point tenderness
    D. Cardiac auscultation and evaluation for carotid bruits

17. A 59-year-old woman with a history of diabetes presents with abdominal pain with nausea and vomiting that worsens after eating. This started approximately 48 hours ago and is getting worse. Her BP is 116/88, pulse 86, O_2 93% on room air. Pain is out of proportion to benign abdominal examination. She was a heavy smoker with a 60-pack-year history but quit 6 weeks ago. She does not drink alcohol and is postmenopausal. Her medications include lisinopril, insulin, atorvastatin, aspirin, and bupropion. CT scan demonstrates necrotic bowel, and she proceeds to surgical intervention. What additional finding was seen on the CT scan that contributed to her necrotic bowel?
    A. Left iliac artery aneurysm
    B. Inferior vena cava thrombus
    C. Renal artery aneurysm
    D. Thoracic aortic aneurysm

18. A 32-year-old woman is presenting to establish care in your clinic after recently moving. She tells you that she has been told she has a venous malformation. Which description below is likely to be the findings you encounter during your visit?
    A. A left lateral thigh area of purple discoloration that measures 10 cm × 15 cm, is not raised, and does not have calor
    B. Three small spots on the left forearm that are raised with a grayish discoloration, each measuring ~1 cm in diameter

    C. Bilateral areas just proximal to knees that have linear, dark red/blue lines and are scattered throughout an area ~5 cm in diameter
    D. A patch of skin on the left neck that is pale, the same temperature as the surrounding skin, and not raised, measuring 4 cm × 6 cm; several smaller areas are noted on the upper chest

▶ **ANSWERS AND EXPLANATIONS TO SECTION A PRETEST**

1. **C.** You most likely find the feeling of a "skipped" beat on the history of a patient with premature ventricular contractions.
2. **B.** Transthoracic echocardiogram is the most appropriate diagnostic test to evaluate a newly diagnosed LBBB.
3. **C.** Permanent pacemaker implantation is the most important treatment for this patient.
4. **C.** Rivaroxaban 20 mg daily is the most appropriate agent to reduce the risk of an embolic event associated with arrhythmia.
5. **A.** Electrical defibrillation is the appropriate management for ventricular fibrillation.
6. **B.** Metoprolol succinate 50 mg daily could be prescribed for rate-control therapy.
7. **A.** The HR range typically seen in a patient with a third-degree atrioventricular block is 20-40 beats per minute.
8. **C.** Metoprolol can cause an atrioventricular block.
9. **B.** Most symptomatic patients with confirmed SSS will need a pacemaker.

▶ **ANSWERS AND EXPLANATIONS TO SECTION B PRETEST**

1. **C.** Harsh, crescendo-decrescendo murmur heard best at the RUSB commonly occurs with CoA.
2. **D.** Right axis deviation may be seen on ECG in atrial septal defect.
3. **C.** Right bundle branch block is a common complication of ventricular septal defect repair.
4. **A.** Atrial flutter is an arrhythmia associated with atrial septal defect.
5. **D.** Surgical repair is considered the definitive treatment for this patient.
6. **B.** Fetal alcohol syndrome is associated with ventricular septal defect.
7. **D.** Trisomy 21 is associated with ostium primum atrial septal defect.
8. **A.** Murmurs associated with pulmonic outflow obstruction, such as pulmonic stenosis in tetralogy of Fallot, generally create turbulent blood flow through the pulmonic valve, which presents as a systolic murmur heard best at the pulmonic area (second intercostal space along the left sternal border).

9. **A.** Most cases of PDA are asymptomatic, involving no respiratory compromise or other systemic findings. However, PDA is very likely in a preterm and/or LBW newborn presenting with respiratory distress syndrome. Risk factors for the development of PDA include low or very low birthweight, preterm delivery (especially younger than 26 weeks' gestational age), female sex, and congenital rubella. Taken together, a LBW, preterm female newborn with respiratory distress syndrome is very likely to have a PDA as the cause of her presentation.

10. **B.** Tricuspid atresia is not part of the classic "tetrad," but rather a dilated, overriding aorta is characteristic.

11. **C.** Pulmonary hypertension is prevented by closing moderate-to-large ventricular septal defects before age 2 years.

▶ ANSWERS AND EXPLANATIONS TO SECTION C PRETEST

1. **B.** ST-segment elevation at the J-point of ≥2 mm in at least two contiguous leads is pathognomonic for myocardial infarction (STEMI).

2. **A.** As both STEMI and NSTEMI are acute events that may be fatal without early identification and treatment, in those presenting with chest pain or other anginal equivalent symptoms (eg, both exertional and nonexertional provoked heartburn-like feeling, unusual tiredness, nausea or vomiting, cold sweat, and sudden dizziness), a 12-lead ECG will quickly identify STEMI and prompt activation and delivery to the catheterization lab. In the absence of 12-lead ECG findings for STEMI, an elevated troponin should prompt admission and initiation of ACS treatment protocols for NSTEMI.

3. **D.** Identified primary risk factors for development of CAD include age >55 for men, >60 for women; hypertension, diabetes type 1 and 2, hypercholesterolemia, smoking, and a family history of premature coronary event in a primary relative (<55 for men, <60 for women).

4. **C.** Raynaud phenomenon increases the probability of Prinzmetal angina as the cause of a patient's chest pain.

5. **C.** ST-segment elevation of >2 mm most likely denotes ACS STEMI, acute full obstruction of a coronary artery(ies) in the region(s) identified on 12-lead ECG. The patient should be evaluated in a primary PCI center within 90 minutes of presentation as this is presumed STEMI until proven otherwise for revascularization, if indicated.

6. **D.** Given that a stent was placed, the patient requires dual antiplatelet therapy for at least 1 year with aspirin and a P2Y12 inhibitor, such as clopidogrel, ticagrelor, or prasugrel. Apixaban is a systemic anticoagulant that inhibits factor Xa and is not indicated for this patient.

7. **D.** Transient ST-segment changes on ECG are characteristic of Prinzmetal angina.

8. **C.** ACEIs are indicated in patients with a history of diabetes, LV dysfunction, or in the setting of uncontrolled hypertension in patients with CAD on beta-blockers. They are not routinely indicated in patients with stable CAD.

9. **D.** Symptoms are not resolved and should be further evaluated; given possibility of progression of symptoms, EMS transport is most appropriate. While the 12-lead ECG does not reflect obvious changes (ie, >2 mm ST-segment elevation in two contiguous leads) for STEMI, in the setting of ongoing symptoms and lack of troponin testing, NSTEMI or possible progression to STEMI has not been ruled out.

10. **C.** Reproduction of symptoms is considered a positive stress test. ST depression of >2 mm, hyper- or hypotension, and arrhythmias are also criteria for a positive stress test. Sinus arrhythmia is a normal variant and sinus tachycardia is an expected physiologic response to exercise.

11. **A.** Pressure or tightness is the most common description of angina-type chest pain.

12. **A.** Patients who are elderly, diabetic, or female are more likely to present with atypical symptoms of CAD or anginal equivalents. These patients are less likely to have the classic presentation of substernal chest pain and may present with fatigue, nausea, or shortness of breath only.

13. **A.** Sublingual nitroglycerin should be given for acute angina symptoms.

14. **D.** Indications for revascularization with CABG include left main CAD, symptomatic or critical stenosis triple-vessel disease, and reduced EF (<40%).

▶ ANSWERS AND EXPLANATIONS TO SECTION D PRETEST

1. **C.** AMI is the most common cause of LV dysfunction, resulting in cardiogenic shock and the heart's inability to pump a sufficient amount of oxygenated blood to the brain and vital organs.

2. **B.** The primary symptoms of HF are exertional dyspnea, orthopnea, paroxysmal nocturnal dyspnea, and fatigue, which are most commonly caused by volume overload. In patients with HF, reduced cardiac function results in reduced end-organ perfusion and function, causing volume retention and overload. Often, patients with HF have frequent hospitalizations for HF exacerbations. Most patients with HF require guideline-directed medical therapy, including diuretics, to reduce symptoms of volume overload.

3. **D.** This patient is presenting with signs of aortic dissection, which is a medical emergency. Urgent transfer to an ED is warranted for rapid workup and BP control. Should this patient not receive timely

medical therapy, his status may progress to a surgical emergency highlighted by aortic rupture, hypotension, and cardiogenic shock.

4. **A.** Ronchi is a physical examination finding caused by obstruction or secretions in larger airways. They are typically observed in patients with chronic obstructive pulmonary disease, bronchiectasis, pneumonia, chronic bronchitis, or cystic fibrosis. The other answers are all clinical signs of fluid retention.

5. **D.** Left heart catheterization is not indicated at this time because the patient is not exhibiting signs of acute coronary syndrome. Although reviewing and optimizing this patient's medications is appropriate, it is not the initial medical strategy indicated at this point. Educating the patient about the importance of lifestyle modifications is the first intervention clinicians should pursue.

6. **A.** The ARNI has demonstrated its superiority in the reduction of mortality and morbidity risk to ACEI. It is estimated that patients who are treated with the ARNI instead of an ACEI or ARB at adequate doses will gain an additional 1–2 years of life and have a significant reduction in hospitalizations. Patients with chronic HF, New York Heart Association (NYHA) class II-IV symptoms, an elevated plasma BNP or NT-proBNP level, and an LVEF of ≤40% should be considered for ARNI therapy rather than an ACEI or ARB.

▶ ANSWERS AND EXPLANATIONS TO SECTION E PRETEST

1. **D.** Ezetimibe, icosapent ethyl, and a PCSK-9 inhibitor are all appropriate to consider adding to this patient's medication regimen.

2. **A.** The target LDL level for a patient with a history of a stroke is ≤70 mg/dL.

3. **B.** A 40-year-old male seeking medical care for the first time should be screened for lipid disorders.

4. **C.** Hyperthyroidism is not a risk factor for developing ASCVD.

▶ ANSWERS AND EXPLANATIONS TO SECTION F PRETEST

1. **A.** A 50-year-old male taking amlodipine for his BP and who recently started alfuzosin for his enlarged prostate symptoms would be most likely to develop orthostatic hypotension following a prolonged gastrointestinal illness.

2. **C.** Stool guaiac for occult blood and hemoglobin/hematocrit to check for anemia would be the most appropriate first step in the workup for orthostatic hypotension.

3. **A.** Nitroprusside should not be used in patients with renal insufficiency and liver disease. It contains cyanide molecules that are released when the drug is administered.

4. **D.** Starting lifestyle modification and medication is the most appropriate treatment for this patient with hypertension.

5. **D.** Syncope after exercise would be least likely associated with vasovagal hypotension.

6. **A.** Chlorthalidone 12.5 mg once daily is a recommended first-line agent for treating her hypertension.

7. **D.** Lisinopril 10 mg once daily would be most appropriate to treat her hypertension with kidney disease.

8. **A.** Irbesartan 150 mg once daily is a recommended first-line agent for treating his hypertension.

9. **C.** Baroreceptor stretch causes increased parasympathetic stimulation.

10. **D.** Baroreceptor stretch would decrease to maintain BP in a bleeding patient.

▶ ANSWERS AND EXPLANATIONS TO SECTION G PRETEST

1. **A.** Of the findings listed, the most common in patients with cardiac tamponade is sinus tachycardia (note: elevated jugular venous pressure is also very common). Sinus tachycardia is seen in almost all patients with this disorder; however, its presence is not specific for tamponade. In addition, although electrical alternans is pathognomonic for cardiac tamponade (as it reflects the heart motion within a large effusion), it is actually only present occasionally.

2. **D.** While each of the abnormal test findings listed may be seen in patients with cardiac tamponade, they are only suggestive, or supportive, of the diagnosis. Recall that cardiac tamponade is a clinical diagnosis. Therefore, clinical and hemodynamic response to pericardial fluid drainage confirms the diagnosis.

3. **B.** In IE, right heart involvement (namely the tricuspid valve) is associated with IV drug use or indwelling vascular catheters. The aortic and mitral valves are most commonly associated with native valve endocarditis.

4. **C.** The most common cause of RCM is amyloidosis and the classic echo finding of this disease is a "speckled" myocardial pattern. LV outflow tract obstruction can occur in RCM, but this is much more likely in hypertrophic obstructive cardiomyopathy. Ventricular interdependence and pericardial thickening and calcifications are characteristic of constrictive pericarditis, a disease that otherwise mimics the presentation of RCM.

5. **C.** Percutaneous or surgical drainage is the definitive treatment for cardiac tamponade.

6. **C.** Optimal therapy is based on the pathogen, antimicrobial susceptibility testing, and the absence or presence of prosthetic material. However, empiric antibiotic treatment recommendations are based on the valve type. For native valve endocarditis,

vancomycin (IV) plus either ceftriaxone (IV) or gentamicin (IV or IM) is recommended.

7. **B.** This patient has symptoms of heart failure and should be started on a routine heart failure regimen. This includes an ACEI, a beta-blocker, and, when needed, a diuretic. Supportive treatment such as pain relief with acetaminophen and rest is also recommended. NSAIDs should be avoided in patients with myocarditis because of an associated worsening of the inflammation and subsequent increased risk of myocardial necrosis. Antiarrhythmics and an AICD would only be indicated if there was evidence of recurrent arrhythmias on ECG.

8. **C.** The patient's young age, family history of early, unexplained cardiogenic syncope and death, and prominent Q wave findings on ECG point to HCM as the most likely diagnosis. HCM often presents with a systolic murmur on physical examination that intensifies with provocative maneuvers that worsen LV outflow tract obstruction, such as standing up from a squatted position.

▶ ANSWERS AND EXPLANATIONS TO SECTION H PRETEST

1. **A.** Prompt recognition of GCA and initiation of steroids is essential to prevent severe vision loss or permanent blindness.

2. **A** Systolic ejection murmur heard best at the left sternal border describes the murmur of pulmonic stenosis.

3. **B.** Being male is not a risk factor for developing GCA.

4. **A.** The most common cause of mitral stenosis in the United States and other developed countries is calcification. In less developed countries, it is still rheumatic fever.

5. **B.** Regurgitant blood flows forcefully back into the left ventricle with aortic valve incompetence, causing a diastolic murmur heard best along the left sternal border.

6. **C.** Inspiration will accentuate the murmur of tricuspid stenosis.

7. **A.** Aortic valve sclerosis is generally the most common cause of aortic valve regurgitation, while Marfan-related aortic root dilation is one of the less common causes. The other two options are not specifically known or identified as causes of aortic incompetency.

8. **C.** Chronic hypoxemic lung disease is a cause of functional tricuspid regurgitation.

9. **B.** Echocardiogram is the diagnostic test of choice for valvular heart disease, including aortic valve regurgitation. It is cost-effective and harmless to the patient, while allowing significant visualization of the heart valves and chambers.

10. **B.** Transthoracic echocardiogram will be most useful in confirming your suspected diagnosis.

11. **D.** While treatment of symptomatic heart failure may be required for a time, including diuretics and other medications, the definitive treatment for symptomatic aortic valve regurgitation is aortic valve replacement surgery.

12. **D.** Claudication is not a sign or symptom of severe aortic stenosis.

13. **B.** Musset sign is a classic finding that may be present, although not always, in individuals with aortic valve regurgitation. It occurs secondary to a wide pulse pressure.

14. **D.** Tricuspid valve replacement is the most appropriate definitive treatment for this patient.

15. **A.** Symptomatic MR can be definitively treated through surgery; valve repair is preferred over replacement due to a decrease in recurrence.

16. **C.** Delayed carotid upstroke indicates severe aortic stenosis.

17. **C.** Echocardiogram is the diagnostic tool of choice in diagnosing aortic stenosis.

18. **A.** Elevated ESR and CRP, normochromic normocytic anemia, and elevated platelets increase the likelihood of biopsy-positive GCA.

19. **C.** Not all patients with MR or MS require prophylaxis prior to dental procedures—only those at highest risk of IE. This includes those with a prosthetic valve or prosthetic materials, history of IE, or history of valvuloplasty.

20. **C.** Temporal artery biopsy is the gold standard for diagnosis of GCA.

▶ ANSWERS AND EXPLANATIONS TO SECTION I PRETEST

1. **D.** Diuretic therapy generally does not help with venous insufficiency–related edema.

2. **D.** An ABI of <0.9 is consistent with occlusive arterial disease.

3. **D.** Most AAAs involve the renal arteries to some extent.

4. **D.** A common symptom at the onset of PAN is asymmetric (nonsymmetric) polyneuropathy.

5. **D.** Estrogen-containing forms of birth control are associated with DVT. The other answer choices are progesterone-only forms of birth control.

6. **C.** With familial hypercholesterolemia, the patient is likely to have cholesterol plaque deposition, and carotid plaques are a source of acute stroke.

7. **D.** If a patient has risk factors based on the Virchow triad, such as surgery or other periods of increase stasis, no further testing is required. If the DVT is unprovoked and no other risk factor is identified, further testing may be warranted.

8. **B.** The acute stage of PAN is characterized by polymorphonuclear neutrophils infiltrating all layers of the vessel wall.

9. **D.** All DOACs and warfarin are considered teratogenic. The best and safest option in a pregnant patient is LMWH such as Lovenox.
10. **B.** Corticosteroids are the main treatment for PAN.
11. **B.** Contrast angiography is the gold standard test for diagnosing peripheral arterial disease.
12. **C.** PAN is a systemic necrotizing vasculitis that affects small and medium muscular arteries.
13. **D.** Diminished dorsalis pedis pulses are associated with peripheral arterial disease.
14. **D.** The appropriate treatment for an aortic dissection of the aortic root and the ascending aorta is open, surgical repair. Endovascular stent repair would be appropriate if the dissection was more distal. Medical therapy is appropriate for a type B dissection, which involves only the descending aorta.

15. **B.** Patients with an aneurysm >5 cm should be referred to a vascular surgeon for surgical intervention.
16. **B.** A full pulse examination will help to determine if there is loss of large vessel perfusion and at what level that has occurred. This also may add clinical suspicion for popliteal aneurysm or the presence of bruits as a source of embolism to the foot.
17. **D.** Acute arterial occlusion of the mesenteric artery leads to acute bowel ischemia and necrosis and can come from a proximal embolus source such as a thoracic aortic aneurysm.
18. **A.** This is a venous malformation characterized by a large area of purple discoloration that is not raised, erythematous, or with calor.

Cardiovascular System

Conduction Disorders and Dysrhythmias

Bradycardia/Bradyarrhythmia and Sick Sinus Syndrome

Lendell Richardson, MD

▶ GENERAL FEATURES

- Sinus bradycardia
  - In sinus bradycardia, the rate of impulses being generated by the sinoatrial (SA) node is lower than expected (ie, <60 beats per minute).
  - This may be due to vagal effects on the normal SA node pacemaker or disease of the SA node itself.
  - Bradycardia can be a normal finding seen in healthy individuals who are well-conditioned or while sleeping, but sinus bradycardia seen in elderly patients or patients with underlying heart disease may represent true sinus node pathology.
  - Other potential causes of severe bradycardia include obstructive sleep apnea, exaggerated vagal activity, or acute myocardial infarction.
  - Most patients with sinus bradycardia are asymptomatic and generally do not require treatment. However, patients with severe bradycardia may develop low cardiac output, leading to symptoms or other complications.
  - Sinus bradycardia can be exacerbated by medications such as beta-blockers, calcium channel blockers, or antiarrhythmics.
- Sick sinus syndrome (SSS)
  - SSS is a condition of clinically significant bradycardia resulting from chronic dysfunction of the SA node (secondary to nodal aging and aging of the surrounding myocardial tissue in the atrium).
  - Patchy atrial fibrosis (scarring) affects the sinus node and impairs the cardiac conduction system.
  - Prevalence of SSS: 1 case per 600 adults over age 65 years
  - SSS manifests as one of several patterns:
    - Persistent or episodic sinus bradycardia
    - Inability to appropriately increase heart rate in response to increased exertion
    - Sinus pauses, sinus blocks, or sinus arrest
    - Atrial tachyarrhythmias
    - Or (commonly) some combination of these four patterns

- Patients with SSS frequently have abnormalities on electrocardiogram (ECG) such as bradycardia or sinus pauses in association with a variety of potential signs and symptoms such as chest pain, palpitations, or syncope.
- In addition to bradyarrhythmias and SA node dysfunction, SSS may also be accompanied by recurrent supraventricular tachyarrhythmias (SVTs) such as atrial fibrillation, atrial flutter, and atrial tachycardia.
- "Tachy-brady" syndrome can also be seen (eg, profound bradycardia associated with tachyarrhythmias such as atrial fibrillation with rapid ventricular response).
- Other potential etiologies of SSS include: sarcoidosis; amyloidosis; cardiomyopathy; Chagas disease; drug therapy with antiarrhythmic agents, calcium channel blockers, beta-blockers; digitalis, or sympatholytic agents; hypothyroidism; and coronary artery disease (rare).

▶ CLINICAL ASSESSMENT

- History
  - Patients with bradyarrhythmia or SSS may have nonspecific symptoms such as fatigue, dyspnea on exertion, palpitations, syncope, presyncope, light-headedness, or chest pain.
  - Symptoms are often intermittent with gradually progressive frequency.
  - Patients are usually elderly (seventh or eighth decade of life) and suffer from comorbid conditions.
- Physical examination
  - Clinical manifestations may include:
    - Periods of marked sinus bradycardia (<50 beats per minute)
    - Inadequate rise in heart rate with exercise
    - Sinus pauses (usually 3 seconds or longer) accompanied by symptoms of light-headedness, presyncope, or syncope.
    - Confusion due to poor perfusion
    - Clinical signs of heart failure

▶ DIAGNOSIS

- SSS is a clinical diagnosis made by establishing a "symptom-rhythm" correlation.
- A 12-lead ECG in SSS may show the P-wave rate abruptly fall by 50% or more followed by a rapid return to the baseline sinus rate.
- If the diagnosis of SSS is clinically suspected (but unconfirmed) following initial workup, consider exercise stress testing (EST) to identify abnormal sinus node function and rule out myocardial ischemia.
- Ambulatory ECG (continuous monitoring or event monitoring) may be useful to document symptom-rhythm correlation.

▶ TREATMENT

- Most symptomatic patients with confirmed SSS will require an implanted pacemaker.
- SSS accounts for approximately half of all pacemaker implantations.
  - Dual-chamber pacing (atria and ventricles) is preferred (associated with a lower incidence of subsequent atrial fibrillation or atrioventricular [AV] block than if the ventricles alone are paced).
  - Pacemaker insertion should precede pharmacologic therapy of tachyarrhythmias as medical treatment of these rapid rhythms can worsen bradycardia or SSS.
  - Unfortunately, symptomatic relief following pacemaker insertion is inconsistent.

CHAPTER 2

Bundle Branch Blocks

Sondra M. DePalma, DHSc, PA-C

▶ GENERAL FEATURES

- Bundle branch blocks are caused by intraventricular conduction abnormalities of the His-Purkinje system, resulting in the affected ventricle being activated slowly and erratically by propagation of electrical activity through the myocardium from the opposite ventricle.
  - In a left bundle branch block (LBBB), myocardial activation begins in the right ventricle, and left ventricular depolarization is delayed.
  - In a right bundle branch block (RBBB), myocardial activation begins in the left ventricle, and right ventricular depolarization is delayed.
- Blocks lead to changes in the duration, shape, and axis of the QRS complex on electrocardiogram (ECG).
- They may be persistent or intermittent.
- Incidence increases with age.
- They are associated with underlying heart disease and degenerative changes of the conduction system.
- Acute LBBB may be caused by anterior myocardial infarction (MI).
- Acute RBBB may be caused by pulmonary embolism.
- LBBB in older individuals is associated with an increased risk of cardiovascular mortality.

▶ CLINICAL ASSESSMENT

- Bundle branch blocks are usually asymptomatic.
- Patients with LBBB may present with syncope, exertional dyspnea, or signs of heart failure due to ventricular dyssynchrony, underlying cardiomyopathy, or complete atrioventricular (AV) block.
- RBBB may cause wide splitting of S2; LBBB may cause splitting of S2 during expiration.

▶ DIAGNOSIS

- ECG: delayed ventricular conduction is associated with widened, aberrant QRS complexes (Figure 2.1).

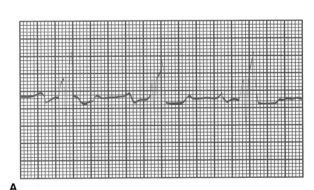

A

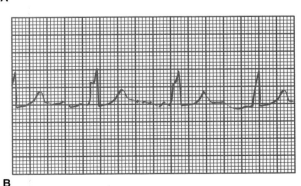

B

FIGURE 2.1 Bundle branch blocks. A, V1 tracing showing the wide QRS complex and double-peaked R wave characteristic of RBBB. B, A V6 tracing showing the wide QRS complex and double-peaked R wave characteristic of LBBB.

- LBBB: QRS duration of 120 milliseconds or more with broad, notched, or slurred R waves in leads I, aVL, V_5, and V_6 (left chest leads); small or absent initial R waves in V_1 and V_2 (right precordial leads) followed by deep S waves; and absent Q waves in leads I, V_5, and V_6.
  - RBBB: QRS duration of 120 milliseconds or more; prominent and notched R waves in leads V_1 and V_2 (right chest leads); and S waves in leads I and V_6 of 40 milliseconds or longer.
- LBBB may interfere with ECG evaluation of left ventricular hypertrophy, myocardial ischemia, and MI.
- Asymptomatic patients with RBBB generally do not require further diagnostic evaluation.
- A transthoracic echocardiogram should be performed in individuals with newly diagnosed LBBB to assess for structural cardiac abnormalities, including left ventricular systolic dysfunction.

- Ambulatory rhythm monitoring may be useful if there are other suspected conduction abnormalities such as symptomatic sinus node dysfunction or advanced heart block (eg, second-degree AV block type 2 or third-degree AV block).

▶ TREATMENT

- RBBB typically does not require treatment.
- Cardiac pacing may be indicated in certain patients with alternating bundle branch block or bifascicular block with accompanying AV block or syncope.
- Cardiac resynchronization therapy with a biventricular implantable cardiac device may be indicated in patients with LBBB and heart failure with reduced ejection fraction.

CHAPTER
3

Atrial Fibrillation, Atrial Flutter, and Multifocal Atrial Tachycardia

Sondra M. DePalma, DHSc, PA-C

▶ GENERAL FEATURES

- Supraventricular arrhythmias:
  - Atrial fibrillation (AF): uncoordinated atrial activation with ineffective atrial contraction and variable (irregularly irregular), often rapid, ventricular depolarization
  - Atrial flutter: coordinated, macroreentrant atrial tachycardia
  - Multifocal atrial tachycardia (MAT): irregular tachycardia from several atrial foci
- Common arrhythmias that are associated with increased morbidity (including embolic events, dementia, heart failure, hospitalizations, and decreased quality of life) and mortality.
- AF and atrial flutter are considered:
  - *Paroxysmal* if it terminates within 7 days (usually <48 hours) of onset (may recur with variable frequency)
  - *Persistent* if sustained for 7 days or more or requiring cardioversion
  - *Permanent* after attempts to restore and maintain sinus rhythm have ceased
- AF is often associated with structural heart disease and other chronic medical conditions, but the mechanisms sustaining the arrhythmia are often multifactorial.
- MAT is commonly associated with severe underlying conditions, especially pulmonary, valvular, and coronary diseases.

▶ CLINICAL ASSESSMENT

- Symptoms may be absent or include:
  - Palpitations
  - Dyspnea
  - Fatigue
  - Exercise intolerance
  - Light-headedness
- History may identify potentially reversible risk factors (eg, alcohol intake, uncontrolled hyperthyroidism).
- Cardiac examination may reveal an irregularly irregular and/or rapid heartbeat or pulse.
- Signs of concomitant cardiovascular conditions (such as heart failure, valvular heart disease, or ischemic heart disease) may include cardiac murmur or gallop, jugular venous distention, arterial bruits, crackles within lung fields, hepatomegaly, or peripheral edema.

▶ DIAGNOSIS

- Electrocardiogram findings include:
  - AF: rapid oscillatory/fibrillatory baseline with absent P waves and "irregularly irregular" ventricular response with variable R-R intervals and often a rapid ventricular rate (Figure 3.1)
  - Atrial flutter: regular and rapid atrial depolarizations at a rate of 250-350 beats per minute

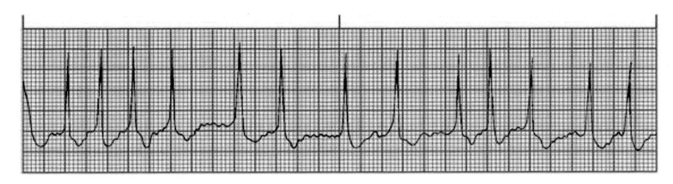

FIGURE 3.1   Atrial fibrillation.

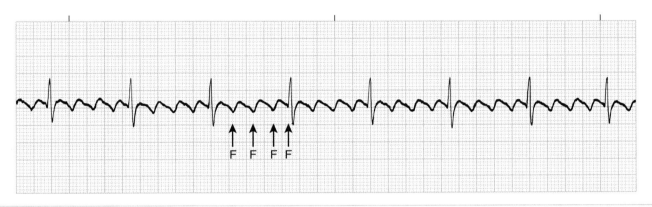

FIGURE 3.2   Atrial flutter.

(ventricular rate may be normal or rapid); classic "sawtooth" morphology of P waves may be present and regular or variable R-R intervals (Figure 3.2)
- MAT: irregular rhythm featuring P waves of several distinct morphologies and variable R-R intervals; may be accompanied by rapid ventricular depolarization
- Ambulatory rhythm monitoring is helpful for making the diagnosis of paroxysmal arrhythmia and for monitoring control of ventricular rate.
- Transthoracic echocardiogram is indicated to evaluate cardiac function and structure.

▶ TREATMENT

- AF and atrial flutter:
  - Medical management is often focused on either "rate control" or "rhythm control"; both strategies demonstrate similar outcomes regarding quality of life, morbidity, or mortality, but the rate-control approach is considered to have a more favorable safety profile with fewer adverse events and lower costs.
    - Rate control:
      - Reduces ventricular rate without changing the underlying cardiac rhythm

- Used for symptom management and to prevent tachycardia-mediated cardiomyopathy
- Goal average resting heart rate is <80 beats per minute and goal average ambulatory heart rate is <100 beats per minute
- Achieved by administering atrioventricular nodal blocking agents (eg, beta-blockers and nondihydropyridine calcium channel blockers)
  - Rhythm control:
    - Medication administered to maintain sinus rhythm; may be preferred in patients who have symptoms despite rate control, those with a rate that is difficult to control, or who develop tachycardia-mediated cardiomyopathy
    - Achieved with antiarrhythmic medications (eg, amiodarone, flecainide, propafenone, and sotalol), cardioversion, and/or transvenous catheter ablation
  - Embolism prevention:
    - Anticoagulation should be used in patients who are at high risk for embolic events and at low risk for bleeding complications.
    - Decision to use oral anticoagulants should be guided by risk of thromboembolism as determined by the CHA_2DS_2-VASc score (see Table 3.1).

TABLE 3.1   CHA$_2$DS$_2$-VASc Risk Stratification

For patients with AF or atrial flutter and an elevated CHA$_2$DS$_2$-VASc score of ≥2 in males or ≥3 in females, oral anticoagulants are recommended.		
	Definition	**Score**
C	(Congestive) heart failure or left ventricular dysfunction	1
H	Hypertension	1
A	Age 75 y or older	2
D	Diabetes	1
S	Stroke, transient ischemic attack, or thromboembolism	2
V	Vascular (eg, coronary artery disease, peripheral artery disease, arterial aneurysm)	1
A	Age 65-74 y	1
Sc	Sex category: Female	1

Adapted from January CT, Wann LS, Calkins H, et al. 2019 AHA/ACC/HRS focused update of the 2014 AHA/ACC/HRS guideline for the management of patients with atrial fibrillation. *J Am Coll Cardiol.* 2019;74(1):105-132.

- Anticoagulant options include coumadin/warfarin (INR target 2.0-3.0) and direct oral anticoagulants (eg, dabigatran, rivaroxaban, apixaban, and edoxaban).
- Left atrial appendage exclusion is an emerging strategy for embolic prevention and is indicated in patients at high risk of embolic events who are not candidates for anticoagulation.
- MAT
  - First-line treatment is optimized management of the underlying condition.
- Electrolytes, specifically potassium and magnesium, should be corrected. Magnesium infusion may be beneficial in suppressing ectopic atrial activity even in patients with normal serum magnesium levels.
- Beta-blockers or nondihydropyridine calcium channel blockers can be used to suppress ectopic foci in patients without contraindications.
- Patients with AF/atrial flutter and a rapid ventricular response causing hemodynamic compromise should be treated with immediate electric cardioversion.

CHAPTER

4

Premature Atrial and Ventricular Contractions

Tracey Thurnes, EdD, MPAS, PA-C

▶ GENERAL FEATURES

- Premature atrial contractions (PACs) are ectopic heartbeats resulting from early depolarization of atrial tissue heartbeat originating from somewhere other than the sinoatrial node.
- Premature ventricular contractions (PVCs) are ectopic heartbeats that occur when the underlying rhythm is interrupted by an early beat originating from the ventricles.
- PACs and PVCs may be caused by cardiac conditions including:
  - Coronary artery disease
  - Valvular heart disease
  - Cardiomyopathy
- PACs and PVCs may also be caused by noncardiac factors including:
  - Thyroid disease
  - Psychiatric disorders
  - Toxin or chemical exposures
  - Electrolyte disturbances
  - Pulmonary disease
  - Excessive alcohol or caffeine intake
- Although PACs or PVCs are often considered benign, patients with PACs or PVCs with or without symptoms should be evaluated for underlying cardiac disease.

▶ CLINICAL ASSESSMENT

- PACs and PVCs are often asymptomatic.
- Some patients present with a sensation of "skipping" or "flopping" in their chest or palpitations; rarely, patients will experience fatigue, dyspnea, chest pain, dizziness, or presyncopal episodes.
- The context of symptoms may hint at the underlying etiology; for example, palpitations that occur at rest or with exertion suggest cardiac etiologies, whereas palpitations occurring in stressful situations or in an individuals with a history of panic attacks may suggest a psychiatric etiology.
- History may also reveal contributing prescription medications, over-the-counter drugs and supplements, or illicit substance use.

▶ DIAGNOSIS

- The most common finding on physical examination is the presence of an irregular pulse: PACs may result in an early heart sound on auscultation, whereas PVCs may cause a compensatory pause after the premature beat.
- Electrocardiogram (ECG) manifestations include variations in the QRS complex depending on the origination site of the impulse.
  - PACs originate in the atria; therefore, the QRS complex may be narrow and similar in appearance to a normal QRS complex.
  - The impulse for a PVC originates in the ventricles, resulting in a widened QRS complex (Figure 4.1).
  - PACs/PVCs will often present in a patterned formation such as atrial or ventricular bigeminy or trigeminy.

- Normal physical examination or ECG in symptomatic patients does not exclude PACs, PVCs, or their underlying cardiac etiologies. Symptomatic patients benefit from ambulatory monitoring with a 24- to 48-hour Holter monitor.
- Echocardiogram is recommended to assess for cardiac structural abnormalities.
- Additional laboratory testing is warranted in patients with suspected noncardiac etiologies (eg, metabolic panel and electrolytes, thyroid-stimulating hormone, drug screen).

▶ TREATMENT

- Therapy varies based on the presence of symptoms and/or underlying structural heart disease.
- No therapy is needed in asymptomatic patients in the absence of heart disease or other contributing medical conditions.
- In symptomatic patients without contributing cardiac or noncardiac disease, reassurance and patient education such as avoiding or minimizing the use of caffeine, alcohol, and nicotine are important and often decrease symptoms.
- Medical therapy with a beta-blocker (first-line) or calcium channel blocker is suggested in patients with ongoing symptomatic PACs.
- PACs in the general population have been linked to a greater risk of atrial fibrillation, whereas PVCs have been associated with cardiomyopathy and sudden death, subsequently increasing cardiovascular mortality and morbidity.
- Prognosis varies based on the presence and extent of underlying disease.

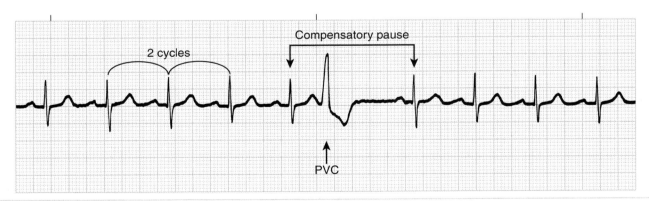

FIGURE 4.1 Normal sinus rhythm with one PVC.

Atrioventricular Blocks

Rebecca Clawson, PA-C

▶ GENERAL FEATURES

- Atrioventricular (AV) block is a collection of disorders in which conduction of impulses from the atria to the ventricles is delayed or completely blocked.
- Classified into four categories:
  - First-degree AV block (Figure 5.1A)
    - Prolonged PR interval only
    - Conduction from sinoatrial (SA) node to AV node impaired
  - Second-degree AV block, type 1 (Figure 5.1B)
    - Also known as Wenckebach or Mobitz type I
    - Progressively longer PR intervals followed by a dropped QRS
    - Conduction through the AV node and His bundle impaired
  - Second-degree AV block, type 2 (Figure 5.1C)
    - Also known as Mobitz or Mobitz type II
    - Consistent PR intervals followed by a dropped QRS
    - Conduction through the AV node and His bundle impaired
  - Third-degree AV block (Figure 5.1D)
    - Complete AV disassociation; no relay of electrical current through the AV node
    - P waves at a consistent rate, typically 60-100 beats per minute
    - QRS complexes also at a consistent, but different, rate, typically 20-40 beats per minute; complexes can be wide or narrow.

- First-degree and second-degree type I AV blocks are typically benign and reflect a functional problem.
- Second-degree type II and third-degree AV blocks are not benign and reflect an underlying structural problem.

▶ CLINICAL ASSESSMENT

- First-degree AV block
  - Typically asymptomatic
  - Incidentally discovered on telemetry/electrocardiogram (ECG)
- Second-degree AV block, type I
  - Typically asymptomatic; patient may experience palpitations as a result of the dropped QRS complex.
  - Incidentally discovered on telemetry/ECG
- Second-degree AV block, type II
  - Typically asymptomatic; patient may experience palpitations as a result of the dropped QRS complex.
  - Frequently dropped QRS complexes can cause the same symptoms as someone in third-degree block.
  - Discovered incidentally on telemetry/ECG
- Third-degree AV block
  - Symptoms include shortness of breath, chest pain, and/or light-headedness/near-syncope/syncope.
  - Symptoms may present/worsen with exertion.
  - May present with other symptoms from lack of perfusion and end-organ damage caused by bradycardia
  - Physical examination may reveal bradycardia, hypotension, or signs of hypoperfusion.

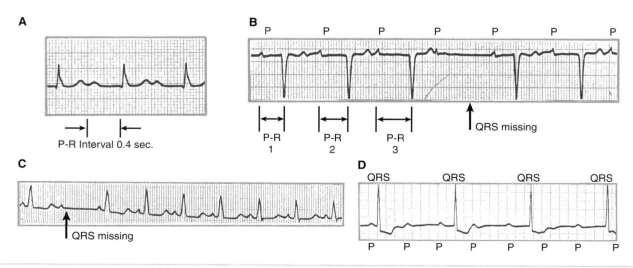

FIGURE 5.1 AV blocks. A, First-degree AV block. B, Type II AV block, Mobitz I. C, Type II AV block, Mobitz II. D, Third-degree/complete AV block.

▶ DIAGNOSIS

- Diagnosis is typically made with a 12-lead ECG alone.
- Additional diagnostics may be aimed at identifying underlying cardiac or systemic conditions.

▶ TREATMENT

- First-degree AV block
  - Monitor, progression unlikely
  - Stop AV nodal blocking drugs
    - Beta-blockers
    - Calcium channel blockers
    - Digoxin
- Second-degree AV block, type I
  - Monitor, progression unlikely
  - Atropine if symptomatic bradycardia (rare)
  - Stop AV nodal blocking drugs
- Second-degree AV block, type II
  - Can progress to third-degree block
  - Atropine if symptomatic bradycardia

- Permanent pacemaker (PPM)
- Until PPM implanted, stop AV nodal blocking drugs
- Third-degree AV block
  - Atropine if symptomatic bradycardia; consider beta-adrenergic agonists such as isoproterenol, dopamine, dobutamine, or epinephrine in symptomatic patients with low likelihood of coronary ischemia
  - Temporary pacing until a PPM is placed
  - Until PPM implanted, stop AV nodal blocking drugs
- Complications:
  - Almost exclusively seen in second-degree type II and third-degree AV blocks
  - Sudden cardiac death
  - Symptomatic bradycardia
    - Ischemia
    - Arrhythmias
    - Type II myocardial infarction
  - Falls due to syncope
  - PPM implantation can lead to site infection, endocarditis, or lead dislodgement.

CHAPTER 6

Supraventricular Tachycardia and Accessory Pathway Disorders

Rebecca Clawson, PA-C

▶ GENERAL FEATURES

- Supraventricular tachycardia (SVT) describes any tachyarrhythmia that originates from atrial or atrioventricular (AV) nodal tissue.
- SVT typically refers to either AV reentrant tachycardia (AVRT) or AV nodal reentrant tachycardia (AVNRT), with AVNRT being the most common.
  - AVNRT mechanism: two conduction pathways through the AV node, no accessory pathway
  - AVRT mechanism: two conduction pathways through the AV node, plus an accessory pathway; most common form of AVRT leads to a preexcitation syndrome called Wolff-Parkinson-White (WPW) syndrome
- Other forms of SVT include atrial tachycardia and multifocal atrial tachycardia.
- Risk factors include:
  - Atrial septal defects
  - Other congenital heart disease
  - Acute myocardial infarction
  - Intake of caffeine, alcohol, recreational drugs

▶ CLINICAL ASSESSMENT

- Symptoms typically include:
  - Palpitations
  - Angina
  - Dyspnea
  - Diaphoresis
  - Dizziness
  - Anxiety
- Symptoms may suddenly start or stop.
- On physical examination:
  - Patient may appear uncomfortable, diaphoretic, and dyspneic.
  - Tachycardia with heart rate 110 to >250 beats per minute
  - "Frog sign" or prominent jugular venous A waves
- WPW with a controlled rate is typically asymptomatic.
- If WPW is present with atrial fibrillation (AF), syncope and sudden cardiac death (SCD) may be the initial presentation; risk factors for this include:
  - Age <20

- History of an abnormal electrophysiology (EP) study
- History of other tachycardias

▶ DIAGNOSIS

- Diagnosis of SVT (Figure 6.1) and WPW is initially made on electrocardiogram (ECG).
- Holter monitor may be needed to capture arrythmia.
- SVT presents as a regular tachycardia with narrow QRS complexes and no P waves or P waves that are partially hidden in the QRS complexes.
- Three diagnostic criteria for WPW:
  - Presence of Delta waves (Figure 6.2)
  - Short PR interval
  - Wide QRS complex

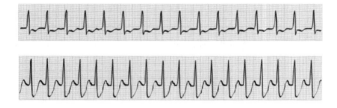

FIGURE 6.1   Two examples of SVT exhibiting narrow QRS tachycardia.

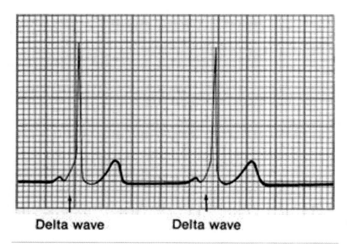

FIGURE 6.2   Delta waves seen in Wolff-Parkinson-White (WPW) syndrome.

- AF with WPW can be mistaken for ventricular tachycardia or AF with a left bundle branch block.
- Provocative EP studies may be useful in patients considering ablation or in patients with suspected WPW.
- Labs may reveal hypokalemia and/or hypomagnesemia; digoxin levels should also be checked, as toxicity can lead to SVT.

▶ TREATMENT

- Obtain "crash cart" and apply defibrillator/cardioverter pads to patients with SVT as a precaution.
- If patients with SVT are hemodynamically unstable (with hypotension or signs of organ hypoperfusion), direct current cardioversion (DCCV) is indicated.
- For hemodynamically stable patients with SVT:
  - Valsalva maneuvers may be attempted
  - Intravenous (IV) push of adenosine; 6 mg dose followed by 12 mg if unsuccessful
  - If unsuccessful: IV metoprolol or diltiazem to control rate
  - Cardioversion may be appropriate for refractory SVT or patients with contraindications to pharmacologic treatment.
- For WPW with a rapid rate, emergency consult to cardiology
  - Hemodynamically unstable: DCCV
  - Treatment involves IV ibutilide or procainamide
  - Avoid AV nodal-blocking agents, as this can lead to syncope and cardiac death.
- Patients with recurrent episodes of SVT:
  - Beta-blockers or non-dihydropyridine calcium channel blockers
  - If unsuccessful, cardiology consultation to manage with class IC or III antiarrhythmics
  - Catheter ablation of the slow pathway for AVNRT
  - Catheter ablation of accessory pathway for AVRT or WPW
- Complications of acute or recurrent SVT include:
  - Hemodynamic collapse
  - Thromboembolism
  - Heart failure
  - Catheter ablation carries a small risk for pericardial effusion and/or tamponade

Ventricular Arrhythmias

Tracey Thurnes, EdD, MPAS, PA-C

▶ GENERAL FEATURES

- Ventricular arrhythmias originate from cells capable of automaticity in the ventricles, therefore they appear as wide complex rhythms on an electrocardiogram (ECG) and include ventricular tachycardia (VT) and ventricular fibrillation.
- VT is defined as three or more successive ventricular complexes at a rate faster than 100 beats per minute (Figure 7.1).
  - Nonsustained VT terminates spontaneously within 30 seconds.
  - Sustained VT persists >30 seconds and/or requires intervention due to hemodynamic instability.
- Monomorphic VT features QRS complexes of the same morphology, indicating that each beat originates from the same source.

- Ventricular flutter is considered a monomorphic VT that occurs at a rapid rate around 300 beats per minute.
- Polymorphic VT has a continually changing QRS complex morphology.
  - Torsade de pointes is a polymorphic VT that occurs in the setting of QT prolongation, resulting in a "twisting of points" appearance of QRS complexes.
- Ventricular fibrillation involves no uniform activation of the QRS complex, resulting in electrical activity with no distinct QRS complexes or P waves (Figure 7.2).
  - It is a medical emergency and fatal if left untreated.

▶ CLINICAL ASSESSMENT

- Nonsustained VT may be asymptomatic, present as palpitations, or be incidentally found on ECG or cardiac telemetry.

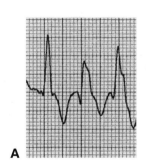
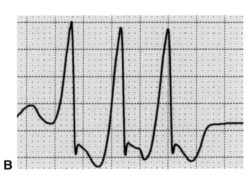
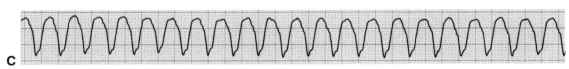

FIGURE 7.1 Ventricular tachycardia (VT). A, Nonsustained polymorphic VT (triplet). B, Nonsustained monomorphic VT (triplet). C, Sustained monomorphic VT.

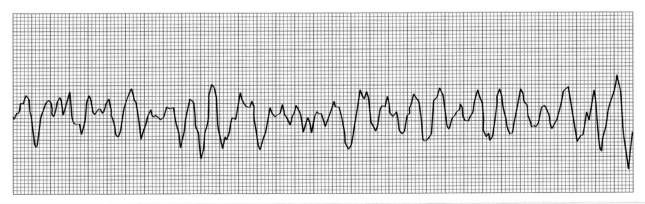

FIGURE 7.2 Coarse VF.

- Symptoms of ventricular arrhythmias commonly include palpitations, dyspnea, chest pain, light-headedness/presyncope, syncope, or sudden cardiac arrest.
- Syncope is often linked to an increased risk for cardiac arrest leading to sudden death, as it often indicates hemodynamic instability.
- Patients may have a known history of cardiac disease or cardiac risk factors.
- Review medications that may cause electrolyte imbalances or QT interval prolongation, as these can lead to polymorphic VT, especially torsades de pointes.
- Physical examination may be notable for tachycardia, hypotension, jugular venous distention (JVD) or prominent jugular venous pulsations ("frog sign"), peripheral edema, pallor, and diaphoresis.
- Other signs and symptoms present may be related to underlying structural cardiac disease.

▶ DIAGNOSIS

- Evaluation and management of ventricular arrhythmias is guided by the hemodynamic stability of the patient and presence of acute underlying cardiac disease.
- Obtain a 12-lead ECG and place patient on cardiac monitor.
- ECG will typically reveal a heart rate >100 beats per minute and wide QRS complexes.
  - The morphology of complexes will vary based on the specific type of arrhythmia.
  - Findings may additionally vary based on the presence of associated cardiac disease and metabolic disturbances.
- Transthoracic echocardiogram and additional workup for ischemic heart disease should be initiated based on clinical suspicion.
- Appropriate laboratory testing is warranted to rule out other contributing causes (eg, metabolic panel, electrolytes, thyroid-stimulating hormone, drug/toxicology screening).

▶ TREATMENT

- Underlying cardiac disease and metabolic derangements should be considered and corrected in all patients.
- Asymptomatic patients with nonsustained VT and no underlying cardiac comorbidities do not require additional therapy.
- Symptomatic patients with nonsustained VT without underlying cardiac disease may be treated with beta-blockers or calcium channel blockers to prevent recurrence.
- Sustained, monomorphic VT without hemodynamic compromise should be pharmacologically cardioverted with antiarrhythmic medications such as amiodarone or procainamide.
- Sustained, monomorphic VT with hemodynamic compromise or instability should be treated via advanced cardiac life support (ACLS) guidelines and may require cardioversion.
- Torsades de pointes is treated with intravenous (IV) magnesium, correction of electrolyte imbalances, and removal of any drugs that may have caused the arrhythmia; unstable patients require electrical cardioversion.
- Ventricular fibrillation is a medical emergency and requires immediate electrical defibrillation.
- Patients with recurrent sustained ventricular arrhythmias may benefit from radiofrequency ablation or an implantable cardioverter defibrillator (ICD).

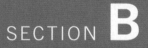

SECTION **B** *Congenital Heart Disease*

CHAPTER **8** **Tetralogy of Fallot**

Tyler D. Sommer, MPAS, PA-C

▶ GENERAL FEATURES

- Tetralogy of Fallot (TOF) is a complex congenital heart disorder and the most common of the cyanotic congenital heart anomalies.
- TOF represents ~10% of all congenital heart disorders with 3-6 cases per 10 000 births.
- It is a combination of four ("tetrad") different congenital anomalies:

- Ventricular septal defect (VSD)
- Right ventricular or pulmonic outflow obstruction
- Right ventricular hypertrophy
- Dilated aorta overriding the ventricular septum
- These defects allow deoxygenated blood from the hypertrophied right ventricle to be shunted into the left ventricle—bypassing the pulmonary circulation—resulting in systemic cyanosis

CLINICAL ASSESSMENT

- TOF is often diagnosed on routine fetal ultrasound.
- Infants born with TOF present with episodes of central cyanosis that are most obvious with crying or feeding, often accompanied with difficulty with feeding and failure to thrive.
- A systolic thrill may be palpated along the left sternal border, associated with the VSD.
- A harsh systolic ejection murmur may be heard over the pulmonic area, associated with the pulmonic outflow obstruction.
- Clubbing of the fingers generally appears at age 3-6 months
- Most adults in whom TOF has been repaired are relatively asymptomatic unless the right ventricle fails, or if arrhythmias arise.

DIAGNOSIS

- Doppler echocardiogram is the diagnostic test of choice.

- ECG typically shows right ventricular hypertrophy with signs of right axis deviation.
- Chest x-ray often reveals a classic "boot-shaped heart" due to prominence of the right ventricle, and an enlarged aorta is visible in about 25% of cases.

TREATMENT

- Patients with less severe pulmonic outflow obstruction may enter adulthood without obvious symptoms or ever having surgical correction of the anomalies.
- Most patients, however, will undergo surgical correction, often requiring serial surgical procedures, which involves closure of the VSD and alleviation of the pulmonic outflow obstruction, which sometimes includes infundibular muscle resection and insertion of an outflow tract transannular patch.
- In infants with significant cyanosis, an initial procedure may be performed to facilitate systemic arterial to pulmonary artery shunting.
- The surgical repair often results in pulmonic regurgitation, which can increase the likelihood of right ventricular failure over time; monitoring right ventricular size and function with serial echocardiograms is advised.
- Atrial fibrillation and ventricular ectopy are common.
- Patients should receive endocarditis prophylaxis throughout their lifetime.

CHAPTER

9

Coarctation of the Aorta

Rebecca Clawson, PA-C

GENERAL FEATURES

- Coarctation of the aorta (CoA) is a localized cardiovascular defect involving the media layer of the aorta and causing narrowing of the vessel lumen; it is typically severe.
- CoA is a common condition accounting for 5%-7% of all congenital heart defects.
- The most common site of stenosis is near the ductus arteriosus and pulmonary artery.
- Age at clinical presentation is inversely related to the severity of the defect.
- CoA is commonly associated with other congenital lesions; >50% of patients will also have a bicuspid aortic valve.

- A narrowed aorta increases cardiac afterload; this can occur acutely (such as with closure of ductus arteriosus) or gradually over years, leading to compensatory LVH.
- Heart failure develops when left ventricular contraction can no longer overcome vascular resistance.

CLINICAL ASSESSMENT

- Infants with severe stenosis present with heart failure, acidosis, and shock.
- Infants with more moderate stenosis present with sweating, dyspnea, tachypnea, irritability, pallor, and failure to thrive.

- Coarctation manifesting later in childhood or adulthood has less severe presentation due to formation of collateral blood vessels.
- Children often present with early-onset hypertension and/or a new murmur.
- Adults often present with hypertension, headaches, and/or claudication.
- Physical examination can reveal a brachiofemoral delay while palpating pulses, diminished femoral pulses, discrepancy in brachial and popliteal blood pressures, and a mid-to-late systolic murmur.
  - Murmur in infants/young children is heard best posteriorly between the scapulae.
  - Murmur in older children/adults is best heard in the lateral chest.

▶ DIAGNOSIS

- Diagnostic study of choice is transthoracic echocardiogram (TTE).
- Magnetic resonance imaging (MRI) and computed tomography (CT) can confirm diagnosis and aid in surgical planning.
- Chest x-ray may show aortic "3" sign and/or rib notching.
- Electrocardiogram (ECG) is usually nonspecific but may show LVH or signs of left ventricular strain.

▶ TREATMENT

- Definitive therapy:
  - Open surgical repair is the standard of care for infants in acute distress. Critically ill infants often require intravenous (IV) prostaglandin to keep the ductus arteriosus patent until they are stable for surgery.
  - Balloon angioplasty and stent implantation are options for patients not in acute distress.
  - Elective stent implantation is the preferred treatment for older adolescents and adults.
- Postsurgical follow-up:
  - ECG and transthoracic echocardiogram (TTE) every 2 years; a stress test every 3 years
  - Cardiac MRI (or CT angiogram, if contraindicated) every 2-5 years to screen for restenosis and aneurysm formation

▶ COMPLICATIONS

- Eisenmenger syndrome can develop if intervention fails or is delayed.
- Postsurgical complications include aneurysm, pseudoaneurysm, dissection, and restenosis.
- Intracranial and aortic aneurysms are common, with intracranial aneurysms mostly occurring in adults.

CHAPTER
10

Atrial and Ventricular Septal Defects

Stephanie Hull, EdS, MMS, PA-C

▶ GENERAL FEATURES

- Atrial septal defect (ASD):
  - ASD, the second most common congenital heart defect, is an opening between the right and left atria.
  - Ostium secundum, the most common type of ASD, is more common in females.
  - Ostium primum ASD, part of the spectrum of atrioventricular (AV) septal canal defects, is a common cardiac anomaly in trisomy 21 (Down syndrome).
  - Holt-Oram (heart-hand) syndrome is associated with ASD and abnormalities of the radius, carpal bones, and/or thumbs.
  - ASD is often asymptomatic until adulthood, with potential presenting complications of atrial arrhythmias and paradoxical embolization (typically resulting in stroke).
  - Late complications of larger defects may include right ventricular dilatation, tricuspid regurgitation, right heart failure, and pulmonary hypertension

that can become irreversible and lead to right-to-left shunting (Eisenmenger syndrome).
- Ventricular septal defect (VSD):
  - VSD are classified as a perimembranous (most common), muscular, or outlet openings between the ventricles.
  - Isolated VSD is the most common congenital heart defect (up to 50% of congenital heart disease).
  - VSD is associated with maternal exposure to phenytoin and fetal alcohol syndrome.
  - VSD is typically associated with a left-to-right shunt, the degree of which depends on the pressure gradient across the septum.
  - Smaller defects typically have a higher gradient and smaller degree of shunting; most close spontaneously by age 6 years.
  - Moderate and large defects with significant left-to-right shunting may cause increased pulmonary artery pressure; surgical correction in these patients

before age 2 years may prevent irreversible pulmonary hypertension.

- Eisenmenger syndrome is defined as cyanosis and pulmonary hypertension that occurs when the shunt reverses due to equalization of ventricular pressure in large, unrepaired shunts.
- Presentation of VSD in adulthood depends on the degree of shunting and protection of the lungs from systemic pressure and volume by pulmonic or subpulmonic stenosis.

CLINICAL ASSESSMENT

- ASD:
  - Most ASDs are small and do not cause symptoms in infancy or childhood.
  - Large ASDs occasionally present with symptoms of heart failure, recurrent respiratory infections, or failure to thrive in infancy or childhood.
  - Physical examination findings are dependent on the size of the defect, the degree of shunting, and the pulmonary arterial pressure.
  - Characteristic physical examination findings include a midsystolic pulmonary flow or ejection murmur accompanied by a fixed split S2.
  - The midsystolic ejection murmur is caused by increased flow across the pulmonic valve, not by flow across the ASD; a mid-diastolic murmur in the fourth intercostal space left sternal border (caused by increased flow across the tricuspid valve during diastole) suggests high flow with pulmonary-to-systemic blood flow ratio >2:1.
  - Atrial arrhythmias (atrial fibrillation and flutter) may be seen, especially in the third and fourth decades of life.
- VSD:
  - The high gradient associated with small defects results in a loud, harsh, holosystolic murmur best heard in the left third and fourth intercostal space along the sternum with radiation over the entire precordium.
  - In addition to a loud holosystolic murmur, a moderate degree of shunting results in slight prominence of the precordium with a left ventricular heave, systolic thrill, and, with larger defects, a mitral diastolic flow murmur.
  - Large defects associated with pulmonary hypertension result in precordial prominence, left and right ventricular heaves, systolic thrill, a palpable S2 in the pulmonic area, and accentuation of the pulmonary component; due to equalization of ventricular pressures, the holosystolic murmur may be difficult to hear in large defects.
  - Large defects usually present early in infancy as frequent respiratory infections, failure to thrive, and tachypnea and diaphoresis with feedings.

DIAGNOSIS

- ASD:
  - Dilatation of the right atrium, right ventricle, and main pulmonary artery and increased pulmonary vascular markings may be seen on chest radiography.
  - Right axis deviation and rSR' pattern of the right precordial leads (V_1-V_2) may be seen on electrocardiography.
  - Direct visualization of the anatomic location of the ASD by 2D echocardiography and demonstration of left-to-right shunting through the ASD by color-flow Doppler confirms the diagnosis.
- VSD:
  - 2D transthoracic echocardiography with Doppler is used to determine the size, anatomic location, and ventricular pressure difference of a VSD.
  - Cardiac catheterization is typically not needed but may be indicated in VSD associated with increased pulmonary vascular resistance.

TREATMENT

- ASD:
  - Secundum ASDs <8 mm in diameter typically close spontaneously by age 5 years.
  - Secundum ASDs ≥8 mm in diameter and other types of ASD are unlikely to close spontaneously, and the defect size tends to increase with age.
  - Left-to-right shunting increases with age due to relative increases in left versus right end-diastolic pressures; this increases the likelihood of developing symptoms and complications requiring surgical correction by age 40 years.
  - Treatment involves closure with percutaneous device or surgical repair depending on anatomic features of the defect and the patient's clinical context and preference.
- VSD:
  - All patients with VSD should be evaluated by a cardiologist with expertise in congenital heart disease.
  - Medical management may include the use of diuretics to relieve pulmonary congestion.
  - Surgical closure is indicated in moderate to large VSDs before age 2 years to prevent the development of pulmonary vascular disease/pulmonary hypertension.
  - Surgical closure is contraindicated if Eisenmenger syndrome is present.
  - Although the risk of infective endocarditis is low in patients with surgically repaired VSDs, education about appropriate skin and dental care is important.
  - Right bundle branch block is a common complication of surgical repair.

Patent Ductus Arteriosus

Sean Robinson, DHSc, PA-C

▌ GENERAL FEATURES

- Patent ductus arteriosus (PDA) is persistence (>2-3 days) of the ductus arteriosus, a communication between the pulmonary artery and the aorta that normally shunts blood away from pulmonary circulation during fetal development, maintained by the presence of prostaglandins.
- Allows blood from the descending aorta to pass into the pulmonary artery, thereby recirculating the blood from the pulmonary system.
- Effective cardiac output is lower due to partial redistribution of left ventricular (LV) output to the pulmonary system.
- Complications include intraventricular hemorrhage (due to ductal steal as blood moves more favorably through the shunt rather than through the arteries emanating off the aortic arch toward the brain), necrotizing enterocolitis, respiratory compromise due to pulmonary edema, and left heart failure.
- Chronically high pressures in the pulmonary circulation can result in bronchopulmonary dysplasia and pulmonary hemorrhage; eventually, pulmonary artery pressures surpass the pressures in the aorta resulting in a reversal of the shunt from left-to-right to right-to-left, commonly known as Eisenmenger syndrome.
- PDA is more common in premature births or low-birthweight infants.
- Spontaneous closure in the preterm infant (30-37 weeks) occurs in virtually all cases; rates decline significantly for very low–birthweight infants (<1500 g) or those born prior to 26 weeks gestational age.
- PDA is approximately twice as common in female infants.
- It is associated with congenital rubella.

▌ CLINICAL ASSESSMENT

- PDA is often asymptomatic and found incidentally on routine echocardiography.
- Symptoms include poor feeding, failure to thrive, and fatigue.
- Tachypnea and forceful respirations indicate pulmonary overcirculation with pulmonary edema.

- Physical examination may show characteristic wide pulse pressure, bounding pulse, and a continuous "machinery-type" murmur heard best in the left infraclavicular region; a hyperdynamic apical impulse and palpable thrill are common.
- In older children or adults with undiagnosed PDA with mild-to-moderate shunting, symptoms may not arise until shunt reversal due to gradually increasing pulmonary artery pressures; in that instance, differential cyanosis may occur resulting in cyanotic-appearing lower extremities (especially the toes) with warm and pink upper extremities.

▌ DIAGNOSIS

- Echocardiogram can confirm the presence of PDA and monitor treatment course.
- Chest x-ray may show diffuse pulmonary edema.
- B-type natriuretic peptide (BNP) may be elevated.
- Cerebral Doppler ultrasound can be performed to assess degree of ductal steal.
- Electrocardiogram (ECG) may show evidence of LV hypertrophy with persistent PDA (typically in older patients).

▌ TREATMENT

- Conservative treatment (watchful waiting with serial echocardiography, artificial ventilation until respiratory status improves) is the preferred approach for most patients.
- Pulmonary edema is treated with fluid restrictions and, if necessary, gentle diuresis with hydrochlorothiazide.
- Preterm, symptomatic, or hemodynamically compromised newborns with imaging evidence of PDA should receive a cyclooxygenase inhibitor to accelerate a decrease in prostaglandins; options include intravenous indomethacin or ibuprofen given as three doses over 36 hours.
- Failure to close with medical therapy warrants surgical ligation in the newborn or percutaneous closure for the older infant, child, or adult; complications to surgery include chylothorax, pneumothorax, and damage to the recurrent laryngeal nerve.

CHAPTER 12

Coronary Atherosclerosis

Katie Hanlon, MMS, PA-C

▶ GENERAL FEATURES

- Endothelial dysfunction typically from hemodynamic disturbance (hypertension), hypercholesterolemia, cigarette smoking, and increasing age
- Leads to lipid accumulation and leukocyte recruitment in coronary arterial tree
- Plaque progression results in restriction of vessel lumen, impeding blood flow and distal perfusion.
- Patients are symptomatic due to mismatch between available oxygen supply and metabolic demands of the cardiac tissue
- Location and extent of obstruction determine the severity of clinical presentation

▶ CLINICAL ASSESSMENT

- Evaluate patients for modifiable and nonmodifiable risk factors.
  - Modifiable: dyslipidemia, tobacco use, hypertension, diabetes, sedentary lifestyle, diet
  - Nonmodifiable: advanced age, heredity, gender (increased risk in males)
- Ensure optimization of modifiable risk factors as it pertains to current guidelines.
- Typical history
  - Crescendo-decrescendo substernal chest pain that is described as tightness or heaviness; onset often related to exercise, stress, or emotion.
  - Associated symptoms: nausea, shortness of breath, diaphoresis
  - Typically lasts 2-5 minutes and relieved with rest
- Atypical or anginal equivalent seen in women, elderly, and diabetic patients:
  - Typical chest pain may be absent and may report dyspnea, fatigue, nausea
- New-onset or changing features are more consistent with acute coronary syndrome (ACS).

▶ DIAGNOSIS

- Electrocardiogram (ECG)
  - Performed on patients with risk factors of coronary artery disease (CAD) for baseline and following acute coronary events or in patients with atypical or anginal equivalent symptoms
  - Typically normal in patients with stable ischemic heart disease; can have ST depressions or T-wave inversions if patient is symptomatic at the time of ECG
  - May demonstrate left ventricular (LV) hypertrophy due to chronic hypertension and remodeling of left heart
- Labs
  - Indicated as a baseline screening evaluation, annually in patients with a known history of CAD or following an acute coronary event
  - Complete blood count, basic metabolic panel (BMP), lipid panel, hemoglobin A1C
    - Lipid panel provides guidance in modifying the risk factor of dyslipidemia.
    - Hemoglobin A1C provides guidance in modifying the risk factor of hyperglycemia associated with diabetes mellitus.
  - Cardiac enzymes should be obtained if the patient is acutely symptomatic, either with "typical" or "atypical/anginal equivalent"; additionally, should be obtained on patients with new or changing features (such as lasting longer than 2-5 minutes, no longer relieved with rest). (*See Chapter 13: Acute Coronary Syndrome.*)
- Stress test: often the initial method to evaluate patients with known or suspected CAD for the extent and severity of coronary disease
  - Typically done on treadmill; positive stress test: ST depressions >2 mm, hypo- or hypertension, arrhythmias, development of symptoms
  - Pharmacologic stress test with coronary vasodilators: dobutamine, adenosine

- Radionuclide perfusion imaging: alternative in patients who are unable to exercise or have submaximal effort
- Coronary arteriography: indicated in patients with chronic stable angina with persistent angina or anginal equivalent that interferes with the patient's lifestyle, despite medical therapy; additionally, indicated in patients with findings suggestive of a high likelihood of severe ischemic disease (imaging, strongly positive stress test), depressed LV function (ejection fraction [EF] < 50%), and evidence of ischemia on noninvasive testing

▶ TREATMENT

- Anti-ischemic therapy
  - Beta-blockers: decrease myocardial oxygen demand and increase myocardial oxygen supply; first-line therapy to reduce anginal episodes and has been shown to improve exercise tolerance
  - Long-acting nitrates: decrease myocardial oxygen demand via systemic vasodilation; can be used as monotherapy or in conjunction with beta-blockers
    - Oral or dermal preparations improve exercise tolerance in patients with stable exertional angina
- Secondary prevention of disease progression
  - Antiplatelet therapy
    - Aspirin: interferes with platelet activation, which prevents progression from chronic stable angina to ACS; recommended for all patients with stable ischemic heart disease, in the absence of contraindications
    - Clopidogrel is an alternative to patients allergic to aspirin

- Lipid-lowering measures with high-intensity statin: goal low-density lipoprotein <70 mg/dL
  - Consider moderate-intensity statin in patients age >75 years who are unable to tolerate high-intensity therapy
- Angiotensin-converting enzyme (ACE) inhibitors or angiotensin-receptor blockers (ARBs) in select patients with diabetes, chronic kidney disease, LV dysfunction (EF < 40%), or uncontrolled blood pressure on beta-blockers and statins
- Risk factor reduction
  - Smoking cessation
  - Management of hypertension, goal blood pressure <130/80 mm Hg
  - Weight reduction through regular exercise and dietary changes with an emphasis of an increase in fresh fruits and vegetables
  - Glycemic control in diabetics
  - Cardiac rehabilitation referral
- Revascularization is indicated in patients with continued anginal symptoms, intolerant of medications or high-risk CAD (>50% left main, multivessel CAD with decrease in LVEF); two options:
  - Percutaneous coronary intervention: percutaneous opening of obstruction of coronary artery with stent placement to decrease rate of restenosis; can be done at time of coronary angiogram
    - Dual antiplatelet therapy with aspirin and a P2Y12 inhibitor (prasugrel, ticagrelor, clopidogrel) for at least 12 months following stent placement to prevent in-stent thrombosis
  - Coronary artery bypass grafting: indicated for patients with left main CAD, symptomatic or critical stenosis triple-vessel disease, and/or reduced EF (<40%)

CHAPTER 13

Acute Coronary Syndrome

Viet T. Le, MPAS

▶ GENERAL FEATURES

- Acute coronary syndrome (ACS) is a sudden decrease or cessation of blood flow to myocardial tissue generally caused by sudden plaque rupture or progressive atherosclerotic coronary plaque development leading to ischemia and/or infarction of myocardial tissue.
- Major risk factors for ACS include:
  - Hypertension
  - Smoking
  - Dyslipidemia
  - Diabetes
- Family history may show a premature coronary event.
- Cardiovascular disease is the leading cause of death in women and men.

▶ CLINICAL ASSESSMENT

- Common symptoms in both men and women include chest pain or discomfort (often described as burning, pressure, or tightness); tingling in the arms, back, neck, and jaw; and shortness of breath.
- Women are more likely to report a heartburn-like feeling, unusual fatigue, nausea or vomiting, cold sweat, and sudden dizziness.
- In the outpatient setting, high-risk features of continuing chest pain, severe dyspnea, syncope/presyncope, or palpitations should prompt immediate referral to the emergency department with transportation via emergency medical services.

- Coronary symptoms in those experiencing angina are often induced by activity or emotional stress in a consistent pattern; patients experiencing MI may experience unrelenting or worsening coronary symptoms at rest.
- When previously stable coronary symptoms (ie, stable angina) become more easily provocable, occur more frequently, and/or increase in intensity, angina has progressed to "unstable angina" (UA), which is now recognized as part of non-ST elevation acute coronary syndrome (NSTE-ACS).

▶ DIAGNOSIS

- Prompt ECG evaluation (within 5 minutes of presentation) with early troponin bloodwork should be completed. ST-segment elevation at the J point of ≥2 mm in at least two contiguous leads is pathognomonic for ST-elevation myocardial infarction (STEMI)); see Figure 13.1.

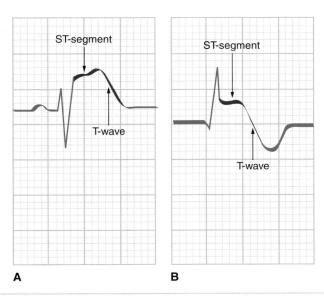

FIGURE 13.1 ST-segment elevation consistent with acute myocardial injury. A, Without T-wave inversion. B, With T-wave inversion.

- ACS symptoms in the absence of STEMI on ECG but in the presence of elevated troponin is suggestive of non-ST elevation myocardial infarction (NSTEMI) or NSTE-ACS; patients with NSTE-ACS should be admitted to the hospital under ACS treatment protocols for further evaluation and consideration for revascularization.
- Progressive ACS symptoms in the absence of ECG changes of STEMI or troponin elevation are suggestive of UA and should receive treatment similar to NSTE-ACS with consideration for functional testing (eg, stress test with or without imaging modality) to help further guide therapeutic decision-making.

▶ TREATMENT

- Patients with STEMI should be treated in a percutaneous coronary intervention (PCI)-capable hospital with a goal of reperfusion in ≤90 minutes.
- When a patient with STEMI presents to a non–PCI-capable hospital with known transfer-to-balloon time exceeding 120 minutes, fibrinolytics should be administered within 30 minutes of arrival to that non–PCI-capable hospital.
- Patients with NSTE-ACS should be treated with optimal medical management and be admitted for further evaluation for possible initial invasive reperfusion along with other ischemia-guided therapies; optimal medical management includes:
  - Aspirin 162-325 mg as soon as possible when ACS is suspected
  - Nitroglycerin (sublingual or titrated infusion) for ongoing ischemic discomfort
  - Beta-blocker within 24 hours unless contraindicated
  - Oral angiotension-converting enzyme inhibitor within 24 hours unless contraindicated
  - Statin therapy regardless of lipid levels
  - Oxygen in the setting of hypoxia
  - Continuous cardiac monitoring

CHAPTER 14

Stable Angina Pectoris and Prinzmetal Variant

Darcie Larimore-Arenas, MSPAS, MPH, PA-C
Joy Moverley, DHSc, MPH, PA-C

▶ GENERAL FEATURES

- Angina is chest pain/discomfort resulting from myocardial ischemia secondary to a myocardial oxygen demand/oxygen supply mismatch.

- Stable angina (also called exertional angina or stable ischemic heart disease) is angina that is predictable, typically provoked by exertion and relieved with rest (differentiated from "unstable angina," which is unprovoked or present at rest and should be urgently evaluated).

- Angina is most often caused by coronary artery disease (CAD); risk factors include tobacco use, older age, diabetes, hypertension, hyperlipidemia, sedentary lifestyle, obesity, and family history of heart disease.
- Stable angina is a risk factor for acute coronary syndrome (ACS) including myocardial infarction (MI).
- Prinzmetal angina, also known *as variant angina* or *vasospastic angina*, is an anginal syndrome that occurs as a result of focal or diffuse coronary artery spasm in the absence of advanced, permanent coronary stenosis.
  - Vasospasm restricts coronary blood flow and causes transient myocardial ischemia, producing angina; MI may develop if spasm persists; asymptomatic episodes can also occur.
  - It is associated with transient ST-segment elevation or depression that quickly resolves with sublingual nitrates.
  - Risk factors and triggers:
    - <50 years of age
    - Cigarette smoking
    - Multiple drugs can trigger vasospastic angina: ephedrine-based products, cocaine, marijuana, alcohol, butane, sumatriptan, and amphetamines.
    - Changes in autonomic activity and subsequent heart rate variability
    - Hyperventilation
    - Guidewire or balloon dilatation during percutaneous coronary intervention (PCI)
    - Food-borne botulism
    - Magnesium deficiency
    - Hypertension and hypercholesterolemia do not predict vasospastic angina.
  - The quality of pain in Prinzmetal angina is indistinguishable from other causes of angina, but the context differs.

▶ CLINICAL ASSESSMENT

- Stable angina history:
  - May be notable for conditions that provoke or exacerbate ischemia:
    - Cardiogenic: cardiomyopathy, aortic stenosis, tachycardia
    - Noncardiogenic: anemia, anxiety, hyperthermia, hyperthyroidism, hypoxemia (from pneumonia, asthma, chronic obstructive pulmonary disease, or obstructive sleep apnea), hyperviscosity (eg, hypergammaglobulinemia, leukemia, polycythemia), sickle cell disease, sympathomimetic use (eg, methamphetamine, cocaine)
  - Classic angina pectoris is a pressure or tightness beneath the sternum (but may be unilateral on either side or bilateral) that is triggered by physical exertion (or emotional stress) and relieved with rest.
    - The pain is typically not provoked or relieved by changes in body position or respiration.

- Episodes generally last 2-5 minutes.
- Radiation to jaw, shoulder, or arms is common.
- Accompanying symptoms may include dyspnea on exertion, decreased exercise tolerance, nausea, and diaphoresis.
  - Atypical angina symptoms include dyspnea alone, weakness, nausea and/or vomiting, epigastric pain or discomfort, palpitations, and syncope.
- Patients with a history of diabetes mellitus, women, and the elderly are at higher risk for silent ischemia and may present with atypical symptoms.
- Family history may include cardiac disease or risk factors.
- Important elements of the social history include sedentary lifestyle, substance use disorders including recreational drugs, alcohol, and tobacco use.
- Prinzmetal variant history:
  - Recurrent episodes of gradual-onset substernal chest pain are predominantly experienced at rest.
  - Episodes last 5-15 minutes but may persist longer and tend to occur more frequently during the night and early morning hours.
  - "Discomfort" reported more often than "pain" that does not change with respiration or position; may radiate to neck, throat, jaw, teeth, or left shoulder or arm.
  - Patients might also report nausea, sweating, dizziness, dyspnea, and palpitations.
  - Symptoms are reduced or relieved by short-acting nitrates.
  - It may accompany other vasospastic disorders, such as Raynaud phenomenon and migraine headache or its treatment.
- Physical examination in stable angina is typically normal but may be notable for new or changed heart sounds or murmurs, elevation in blood pressure or heart rate, or signs associated with risk factors.
- Physical examination in Prinzmetal variant is typically unremarkable, but:
  - Vital signs may be notable for hypertension.
  - Tachycardia and a gallop rhythm may be noted on cardiac auscultation.
  - Bradycardia and hypotension may occur if the sinoatrial or atrioventricular nodal and right ventricular arteries are involved in right coronary artery vasospasm.

▶ DIAGNOSIS

- Stable angina:
  - Acute chest pain should be worked up to rule out ACS (unstable angina, non-ST-elevation MI, or ST-elevation MI).
  - Electrocardiogram (ECG) should be obtained, but may be normal in the absence of symptoms or ACS.
  - Cardiac biomarkers (eg, troponin) will usually be in the normal range.
  - Chest radiograph is typically normal but may be useful in ruling out other causes of chest pain.

- Depending on risk factors and clinical presentation, additional workup for CAD should occur, including cardiac stress testing, echocardiogram, and referral to cardiologist for consideration for cardiac catheterization.
- Prinzmetal variant:
  - During an episode, ECG may demonstrate ST-segment elevation or depression in multiple leads that return to baseline after resolution of symptoms; baseline ECG when patient is symptom-free should be obtained for comparison.
  - Acute MI should be ruled out with serial troponin testing; troponin levels are typically in the normal range during an episode because of the brief duration of the vasospastic ischemia.
  - Patients without documented transient ST-segment changes are referred for stress ECG test to rule out fixed obstructive CAD; ambulatory ECG (7-14 days) with event recorder is recommended once coronary obstruction is ruled out.
  - Coronary arteriography with acetylcholine provocation can be performed to establish the diagnosis in complex cases.

▶ TREATMENT

- Stable angina:
  - Lifestyle modifications including moderate-intensity aerobic exercise, weight control, smoking cessation, healthy diet, and management of hypertension and diabetes.
  - Nitroglycerin (available as sublingual or spray) can be given as needed for acute symptoms.
  - For chronic stable angina, beta-blockers may reduce anginal episodes and improve exercise tolerance.
    - Calcium channel blockers can be given as an alternative if beta-blockers are poorly tolerated or contraindicated.
      - Nifedipine and other very short-acting dihydropyridines should be avoided.
    - Long-acting nitrates can be given if symptoms continue on a beta-blocker or calcium channel blocker.
    - Ranolazine can be considered as an alternative if symptomatic on long-acting nitrates and beta-blocker or calcium channel blocker.
  - Antiplatelet therapy with aspirin (or clopidogrel, if contraindicated) should be considered.
  - Statin therapy may reduce angina frequency.
  - Revascularization may be indicated in patients with significant CAD and unacceptable angina.
- Prinzmetal variant:
  - Sublingual nitroglycerin at onset of episode
  - Tobacco smoking cessation
  - Calcium channel blockers: diltiazem or amlodipine
  - Avoid beta-blockers (they can worsen vasospasm from unopposed alpha-receptor activity).

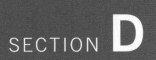

SECTION D

Heart Failure

CHAPTER 15

Heart Failure: Systolic Heart Failure, Diastolic Heart Failure, and Cardiogenic Shock

Jonathan Parch, MPAP

▶ GENERAL FEATURES

- Chronic heart failure (HF):
  - Systolic HF or HF with reduced ejection fraction (HFrEF) represents a decrease in the normal fraction of blood ejected from the left ventricle (LV).
  - It is commonly caused by ischemic heart disease and valvular disorders.
- Diastolic HF or HF with preserved ejection fraction (HFpEF) describes a decrease in the LV's capability to relax and fill with the normal volume of blood, although the fraction of blood ejected is preserved.

- It is commonly caused by chronic hypertension.
- Other causes include congenital heart defects, diabetes, anemia, and alcohol abuse.
- Acute HF and cardiogenic shock:
  - Cardiogenic shock is an acute decompensation in cardiac function, most commonly caused by acute myocardial infarction (AMI).
- Effective treatment of HF and cardiogenic shock requires identification and management of underlying causes.

▶ CLINICAL ASSESSMENT

- History
  - Chronic HF:
    - Primary symptoms are exertional dyspnea, orthopnea, paroxysmal nocturnal dyspnea, swelling of lower extremities, and fatigue.
    - Patients with HF exacerbation may report dyspnea with activity or at rest, decreased exercise tolerance, swelling of extremities, abdominal distension, or worsening of typical chronic symptoms.
  - Acute HF/cardiogenic shock:
    - Primary symptoms include dizziness, syncope, and signs/symptoms of decreased end-organ function (eg, anuria).
    - Symptoms of an acute underlying cause, such as chest pain from an AMI, may be present.
- Physical examination
  - Common clinical signs of HF include bibasilar crackles on auscultation of the lungs, diminished breath sounds or dullness to percussion indicating pleural effusions, tachycardia, S_3 gallop on cardiac auscultation, jugular venous distention, fluid wave or shifting dullness representing ascites, hepatomegaly, and pitting edema.

▶ DIAGNOSIS

- Initial labs and radiologic examinations:
  - Brain natriuretic peptide (BNP) will likely be elevated in HF exacerbation.
  - For patients <50, 50-75, and >75 years of age, the optimal plasma NT-proBNP cutoffs for diagnosing HF were 450, 900, and 1800 pg/mL, respectively.
- Cardiac troponins can be elevated in both cardiogenic shock and HF exacerbation.
  - Myocardial strain and myocyte death are the two primary mechanisms that lead to elevated troponin levels observed in HF exacerbation.
- Other labs may be useful in determining complications to other organs such as liver or kidneys.
- Electrocardiogram may show evidence of underlying cause such as ischemic changes or arrythmia

- Chest x-ray:
  - Cardiomegaly is often seen in patients with chronic HF.
  - Pleural effusions are commonly seen in patients with HF exacerbation.
- Transthoracic echocardiogram (TTE):
  - TTE should be obtained for patients with acute and chronic HF and cardiogenic shock.
  - It is useful to determine the function of left and right ventricles, the presence of valve disease, structural changes such as dilated cardiomyopathy, and the presence of diastolic dysfunction.
- Left heart catheterization may be useful to evaluate for the presence of coronary artery disease and may be therapeutic for appropriate coronary lesions contributing to acute HF or cardiogenic shock.
- Right heart catheterization is useful to evaluate cardiac output, volume status, and response to medical therapies for patients with cardiogenic shock.

▶ TREATMENT

- Chronic HF: goal is to control symptoms, optimize cardiac function, and prevent further cardiac remodeling
  - Lifestyle modifications and education: sodium intake restriction, exercise/cardiac rehab, and continuous positive airway pressure for patients with obstructive sleep apnea
  - Guideline-directed medical therapy:
    - First-line therapies:
      - Angiotensin receptor-neprilysin inhibitors, angiotensin-converting enzyme inhibitors, and angiotensin-receptor blockers
      - Beta-blockers (bisoprolol, carvedilol or metoprolol succinate) and ivabradine for sinoatrial modulation
    - Second-line therapies:
      - Diuretics, anticoagulants, and other antiarrhythmics and antihypertensives for subsets of HF patients
- Cardiogenic shock and acute/decompensated HF: goal is to remove cardiac insult and maintain or reestablish hemodynamic stability.
  - Intubation and mechanical ventilator support for patients with concomitant acute respiratory failure
  - Inotropic support until cardiac function improves
  - May require emergent use of mechanical support devices such as intra-aortic balloon pump, Impella device, or extracorporeal membrane oxygenation (ECMO)
  - Surgical intervention when refractory to medical therapy: left ventricular assist device, total artificial heart, orthotopic heart transplant

CHAPTER 16

Hypercholesterolemia and Hypertriglyceridemia

Mark Volpe, MPH, MMSc, PA-C

A 55-year-old male with type 2 diabetes and hypertension presents for his annual examination. He has no acute concerns, and his physical examination is unremarkable. Routine laboratory evaluation reveals an LDL of 140 mg/dL, HDL of 45 mg/dL, and triglycerides (TGs) of 200 mg/dL. What is the most appropriate treatment for his lipid levels?

▶ GENERAL FEATURES

- Hypercholesterolemia (elevated low-density lipoprotein [LDL]) and hypertriglyceridemia (elevated TGs) are independent risk factors for cardiovascular disease.
- Total cholesterol (TC):
  - <200 mg/dL is desirable
  - 200-239 mg/dL is borderline
  - ≥240 mg/dL is high
- LDL:
  - <100 mg/dL is optimal
  - 100-129 mg/dL is near/above optimal
  - 130-159 mg/dL is borderline high
  - 160-189 mg/dL is high
  - ≥190 mg/dL is very high
- TGs:
  - <150 mg/dL is normal
  - 150-199 mg/dL is borderline high
  - 200-499 mg/dL is high
  - ≥500 mg/dL is very high
- The estimated prevalence of dyslipidemia among U.S. adults is 30%-35%.
- Risk factors:
  - Hypercholesterolemia
    - Family history
    - Diabetes mellitus
    - Obesity
    - Diets high in fat, cholesterol, or sugar
    - Sedentary lifestyle
    - Increased age
    - Male gender
  - Hypertriglyceridemia
    - Family history
    - Diabetes mellitus
    - Excessive alcohol use
    - Hypothyroidism
    - Obesity
    - Diets high in fat or sugar
    - Nephrotic syndrome
    - Drugs (estrogen, tamoxifen, glucocorticoids, protease inhibitors, antipsychotics)

▶ CLINICAL ASSESSMENT

- Most patients with hypercholesterolemia or hypertriglyceridemia are asymptomatic and have no abnormal clinical features or examination findings.
  - Those with very high LDL may have xanthoma, xanthelasma, or arcus corneae.
  - Those with high TGs (usually >1000 mg/dL) may present with symptoms of pancreatitis such as epigastric abdominal pain/tenderness, nausea, and vomiting.

▶ DIAGNOSIS

- Diagnosis includes a fasting lipid panel of TC, LDL, high-density lipoprotein (HDL), and TGs.

▶ TREATMENT

- Goals:
  - Reduce morbidity and mortality from atherosclerotic cardiovascular disease (ASCVD), which includes coronary heart disease, cerebrovascular disease, peripheral artery disease, and aortic disease.
  - Reduce risk of pancreatitis in those with hypertriglyceridemia.

- Risk factor modification:
  - Low-fat and low refined-carbohydrate diet
  - Exercise
  - Weight loss
  - Smoking cessation
  - Diabetes control
- Medication management:
  - Elevated LDL:
    - The mainstay of therapy is statins (hydroxymethylglutaryl coenzyme A [HMG-CoA] reductase inhibitors), which reduce morbidity and mortality from ASCVD.
    - In patients with known ASCVD, high-intensity (or maximally tolerated) statin is recommended with a target LDL <70 mg/dL.
    - In patients with LDL ≥190 mg/dL, start high-intensity statin with goal LDL ≤100 mg/dL.
    - In patients age 40-75 with diabetes, start moderate intensity statin with goal LDL <70 mg/dL.
    - In patients age 40-75 who do not fall into the above categories and have a 10-year ASCVD risk of ≥7.5%, start moderate-intensity statin.
    - In all scenarios, if goal LDL is not met with statin alone, consider adding ezetimibe or PCSK-9 inhibitor.
    - Repeat lipid levels 1-3 months after initiation and, if at goal, every 3-12 months thereafter.
  - Elevated TGs
    - Treat underlying secondary causes.
    - If patient is a statin candidate based on their LDL and risk factors, initiate statin therapy first.
    - If still elevated >500 mg/dL, it is reasonable to add omega-3 fatty acids or fibrates (note increased risk of myopathy in statin/fibrate combination).
    - If patient has ASCVD or diabetes and two or more ASCVD risk factors and TGs >50 mg/dL on maximum tolerated statin, start icosapent ethyl to reduce cardiovascular morbidity and mortality.
- Screening lipid panel is recommended:
  - Once as a young adult
  - For patients with low cardiovascular risk in males at age 35 and females at age 45 and if normal, every 5 years after; if borderline normal, it can be repeated in 3 years.
  - For patients with high cardiovascular risk (hypertension, diabetes mellitus, smoking, or family history of premature coronary disease) screening should start by age 30 for men and age 35 for women, and if normal, every 5 years after; if borderline normal, it can be repeated in 3 years.
  - For patients with physical examination findings or clinical features of hypercholesterolemia or hypertriglyceridemia

---

Case Conclusion

The patient was initiated on moderate-intensity statin therapy. His lipid panel was checked 3 months later and revealed LDL, 68 mg/dL; HDL, 44 mg/dL; TGs, 145 mg/dL.

SECTION **F**

Hypertension and Hypotension

CHAPTER **17**

Primary (Essential) Hypertension and Secondary Hypertension

Sondra M. DePalma, DHSc, PA-C

▶ GENERAL FEATURES

- Hypertension (HTN) is a common cardiovascular condition characterized by elevated systemic blood pressure (BP) that affects nearly half (45%) of U.S. adults.
- HTN is associated with increased cardiovascular disease (CVD) risk and increased mortality when left untreated.
- Classifications and nomenclature vary, but the *2017 ACC/AHA/AAPA/ABC/ACPM/AGS/APhA/ASH/ASPC/NMA/PCNA Guideline for the Prevention, Detection, Evaluation, and Management of High Blood Pressure in Adult*s recommends the following BP categories and definitions (individuals meeting criteria for two categories should be classified in the higher category):
  - Normal: Systolic BP <120, diastolic BP <80 mm Hg

- Elevated: Systolic BP 120-129, diastolic BP <80 mm Hg
- Stage 1 HTN: Systolic BP 130-139, diastolic BP 80-89 mm Hg
- Stage 2 HTN: Systolic BP ≥140, diastolic BP ≥90 mm Hg
- Primary HTN is elevated BP that has no known secondary cause.
- Secondary HTN is elevated BP that has an identifiable cause.
  - Common causes of secondary HTN include obstructive sleep apnea, primary aldosteronism, renal vascular disease, renal parenchymal disease, and drug- or alcohol-induced.

CLINICAL ASSESSMENT

- HTN is most often asymptomatic.
- History may be notable for lifestyle factors that can increase BP, such as obesity, physical inactivity, excessive alcohol use or caffeine consumption, unhealthy diet, and high sodium intake.
- Patients may report taking substances that can elevate BP, such as nonsteroidal inflammatory drugs (NSAIDs), stimulants, oral contraceptives, decongestants, systemic corticosteroids, immunosuppressants (eg, cyclosporine), atypical antipsychotics (eg, clozapine, olanzapine), certain herbal substances (eg, ma huang, St. John's wort), or recreational drugs (eg, cocaine, methamphetamine).
- Features that suggest a secondary cause of HTN include:
  - Snoring, daytime sleepiness, fitful sleep, breathing pauses during sleep (obstructive sleep apnea)
  - Muscle cramps and weakness (primary aldosteronism)
  - Weight loss, heat intolerance, palpitations, diarrhea, and insomnia (hyperthyroidism)
  - Weight gain, cold intolerance, dry skin, and constipation (hypothyroidism)
  - Headache, sweating, and palpitations (pheochromocytoma)
- Other features that suggest secondary HTN include:
  - Abrupt onset of HTN or beginning in individuals <30 years
  - Exacerbation of previously controlled HTN
  - Drug-resistant HTN
  - Accelerated or malignant HTN
  - Disproportional target organ damage for degree of HTN
  - Onset of diastolic HTN in adults age ≥65 years
- Physical examination may be otherwise unremarkable or may show evidence of HTN-related target organ damage or physical features consistent with a secondary cause of HTN.

DIAGNOSIS

- Diagnosis is made using the average of two to three BP measurements obtained across multiple visits or occasions.
- Out-of-office BP measurements are recommended to confirm the diagnosis of HTN and for titration of BP-lowering medications.
- Basic laboratory and diagnostic tests should be obtained for all patients with a new diagnosis of HTN to rule out secondary causes and to assess for the presence of end-organ damage, including:
  - Fasting blood glucose
  - Complete blood count
  - Lipid profile
  - Serum creatinine
  - Serum electrolytes
  - Thyroid-stimulating hormone
  - Urinalysis
  - Electrocardiogram (ECG)
- Additional workup should be considered in patients with increased HTN severity, poor response to standard treatment approaches, a disproportionate severity of target organ damage for the level of BP, or historical or clinical features that support a secondary cause of HTN.

TREATMENT

- Nonpharmacologic intervention is recommended for all patients with elevated BP and HTN:
  - Nonpharmacologic therapy is the preferred therapy for adults diagnosed with elevated BP or stage 1 HTN who are not at elevated CVD risk (individuals without coronary heart disease, heart failure, stroke, or an estimated 10-year risk of CVD of 10% or greater calculated by the ACC/AHA Pooled Cohort Equation).
  - Nonpharmacologic therapy includes weight loss in adults who are overweight or obese, increased physical activity with a structured exercise program, a healthy diet (eg, Dietary Approaches to Stop Hypertension eating plan), reduced intake of dietary sodium, enhanced intake of dietary potassium, and moderation in alcohol intake (men ≤2 drinks daily and women ≤1 drink daily).
- Medications, along with nonpharmacologic intervention, should be used in individuals with stage 1 HTN and elevated CVD risk (individuals with coronary heart disease, heart failure, stroke, or an estimated 10-year risk of CVD of 10% or greater calculated by the ACC/AHA Pooled Cohort Equation) and in patients with stage 2 HTN.
  - Combination therapy with two or more drugs is recommended for patients with stage 2 HTN.
  - Antihypertensive agents:

- Primary first-line medications (in the absence of a specific indication for another agent) include thiazide or thiazide-type diuretics, ACE inhibitors, angiotensin-receptor blockers (ARBs), and calcium channel blockers (CCBs).
- In Black patients without heart failure or nephropathy, initial treatment with a thiazide diuretic and/or CCB is preferred over an ACE inhibitor or ARB.
- Agents for patients with HTN and specific co-morbid diseases:
  - Chronic kidney disease (stage 3 or higher, or stage 1 or 2 with albuminuria >300 mg per day): ACE inhibitors or ARBs
- Ischemic heart disease: beta-blockers and ACE inhibitors for patients with a history of myocardial infarction; beta-blockers with or without dihydropyridine CCBs for patients with angina
- Heart failure with reduced ejection fraction: ACE inhibitors, ARBs, angiotensin receptor neprilysin inhibitor-ARB combination, mineralocorticoid receptor antagonists, diuretics, and/or guideline-directed beta-blockers
- Atrial fibrillation: beta-blockers and non-dihydropyridine CCBs if needed for rate control, ARBs to reduce recurrence of atrial fibrillation
- Screen for and manage other modifiable CVD risk factors in adults with HTN.

CHAPTER 18

Hypertensive Emergencies

Corinne Isabelle Alois, MS, PA-C

▶ GENERAL FEATURES

- Hypertensive emergency is a medical emergency defined as elevated blood pressure (systolic >180 mm Hg or diastolic >120 mm Hg) with signs of end-organ injury.
  - Most commonly encephalopathy, cerebrovascular or cardiovascular events, pulmonary edema, renal injury, or aortic dissection
- In patients with a history of hypertension, the incidence of hypertensive emergency is 1%-3% and increases with age.
- Accompanied by significant morbidity and mortality:
  - Untreated hypertensive emergencies are associated with a 1-year mortality rate of >80%.
  - Hypertensive emergencies have a 1-year and 10-year survival of >90% and 70%, respectively.
- Risk factors
  - Hypertension: should identify baseline blood pressure, stage at diagnosis, and duration of known hypertension
  - Female gender
  - Obesity
  - Coronary artery disease
  - Renal disease
  - Preoperative or postoperative hypertension
  - Stroke
  - Head trauma
  - Eclampsia
  - Illicit drug use such as cocaine
  - Discontinuing or acute withdrawal from antihypertensive medications
  - Treatment with vascular endothelial growth factor
  - Pheochromocytoma

▶ CLINICAL ASSESSMENT

- Symptoms may include shortness of breath, chest pain, back pain, and acute mental status changes.
- Physical examination findings may include:
  - Bilateral blood pressure discrepancies
  - Fundoscopic examination notable for papilledema, acute hemorrhages, or exudates
  - Cardiac examination may have features of heart failure
  - Pulmonary examination may be notable for crackles in the setting of pulmonary edema
  - Neurologic deficits may be present in the setting of cerebrovascular accident

▶ DIAGNOSIS

- Diagnostic workup should be guided by the patient presentation and clinician judgment and should focus on potential areas of end-organ damage or dysfunction.
  - Radiology studies:
    - Head CT may reveal intracranial hemorrhage.
    - Chest imaging may reveal pulmonary edema.
    - Vascular studies may reveal aortic dissection.
  - Electrocardiogram (ECG) may reveal myocardial ischemia.
  - Laboratory studies:
    - Chemistry panel may reveal renal dysfunction.
    - Lactic acid level may be elevated in the setting of tissue hypoperfusion or ischemia.
    - Urinalysis may suggest glomerular injury.
    - Cardiac biomarkers may be elevated in the setting of cardiac ischemia.
    - Urine drug screen may identify contributing agents.

- Pregnancy test, in any woman of childbearing age, to evaluate for undiagnosed pregnancy and raise suspicion of preeclampsia
- Patients should be evaluated for possible secondary causes of hypertension, which may have precipitated the hypertensive emergency.

▶ **TREATMENT**

- Treatment requires the initiation of blood pressure reduction to prevent progression of target organ damage.
- Patients may require intensive care unit admission for continuous blood pressure monitoring and titration of intravenous agents.
- The American College of Cardiology and the American Heart Association 2017 guidelines recommend lowering the mean arterial pressure by no more than 25% within an hour of presentation and then, if the patient is stable, to titrate the blood pressure to the range of 160/110 mm Hg diastolic within the next 2-6 hours.
- After those goals have been met, blood pressure should be lowered to normal range over 24-48 hours.
  - Rapid or excessive blood pressure reduction may precipitate renal, coronary, or cerebral ischemia.
- Parenteral antihypertensive agents include:
  - Sodium nitroprusside
  - Nicardipine
  - Nitroglycerin
  - Hydralazine
  - Labetalol
- Once the target blood pressure is achieved, patient should be transitioned to oral antihypertension agents.
- Following hospital discharge, prompt outpatient follow-up is recommended to avoid recurrent episodes of hypertensive emergencies.

CHAPTER 19	**Orthostatic and Vasovagal Hypotension**

Bart Gillum, DSc, MHS, PA-C

▶ **GENERAL FEATURES**

- Orthostatic hypotension
  - Defined as a drop in measured systolic blood pressure of 20 mm Hg (or a 10 mm Hg drop in diastolic blood pressure) within 1-2 minutes of moving the patient from a supine to standing position.
  - Postural orthostatic tachycardia syndrome is defined as a rise in pulse rate by 30 beats per minute within 1-2 minutes of moving the patient from a supine to standing position or a persistent heart rate of >120 bpm.
  - Blood pressure is regulated by the autonomic nervous system and is a product of cardiac output—determined by stroke volume and heart rate—and systemic vascular resistance.
  - Baroreceptors are specialized nerve receptors in the carotid sinuses and the aortic arch that stimulate the sympathetic nervous system when these vessels are under low pressure and stimulate the parasympathetic nervous system when these vessels are under high pressure.
  - Etiology:
    - Transient or chronic volume depletion (eg, gastrointestinal bleed, dehydration, diuresis)
    - Vasodilation secondary to medications (eg, calcium channel blockers, beta-blockers, alpha blockers, nitrates, or anticholinergics)
    - Prolonged periods of inactivity (eg, paralysis)
    - Diseases affecting the autonomic nervous system (eg, Parkinson disease, dementia with Lewy bodies, primary autonomic failure, multiple system atrophy, diabetic or alcoholic neuropathies, Addison disease, paraneoplastic syndromes)
- Vasovagal hypotension
  - Precipitating event causes forceful myocardial contraction.
  - Results in an inappropriate decrease in sympathetic tone and increase in parasympathetic tone with a paradoxical decrease in heart rate, systemic vascular resistance, and contractility
  - Often results in syncope (represents 66% of syncope presentations)
  - Can be associated with:
    - Fear
    - Surprise
    - Strong emotional reaction
    - Prolonged standing
    - Micturition, cough, defecation

▶ **CLINICAL ASSESSMENT**

- Orthostatic hypotension
  - Common symptoms: light-headedness, dizziness, generalized weakness, fatigue, or syncope

- May involve an associated prodrome of diaphoresis, nausea, weakness, pale skin, feeling of impending syncope
- Often associated with comorbid conditions that produce volume loss (eg, hemorrhage, gastrointestinal illness, dehydration—especially in older patients)
- New neurologic symptoms such as sensory/motor dysfunction, neuropathic pain, or erectile dysfunction may point to primary autonomic failure or neurodegenerative disease
- Physical examination findings may include:
  - Pale skin
  - Diaphoresis
  - Abnormal tilt-table test
- Vasovagal hypotension
  - May be associated with a prodrome of progressive nausea, diaphoresis, and/or pallor

▶ DIAGNOSIS

- Orthostatic hypotension
  - Evaluated by manually measuring blood pressure with the patient lying flat and again within 2 minutes of standing
  - If the patient is unable to stand, or there is still strong suspicion of orthostatic hypotension despite nonsignificant changes in orthostatic vitals, a tilt-table test can be performed.
    - Specialized table with straps to secure patient as the table slowly rises from 180° to 60°-80°, measuring blood pressure and pulse every 3 minutes

- Electrocardiogram may be obtained to rule out an underlying arrhythmia, but should otherwise show sinus tachycardia.
- Vasovagal hypotension
  - Often made based on a suggestive history and lack of concerning features suggesting more serious disease
  - Tilt-table testing may be useful.

▶ TREATMENT

- Orthostatic hypotension
  - Correction of underlying etiology
  - Other steps can include:
    - Discontinue or change the dose/timing of contributing medications.
    - Avoid large, carbohydrate-rich meals if thought to be postprandial.
    - Limit or abstain from alcohol consumption.
    - Maintain adequate oral intake and hydration.
    - Keep symptom diary and avoid precipitating factors.
    - Sodium supplementation can be helpful in certain populations.
    - Lower extremity binders
  - Pharmacologic treatment includes:
    - Midodrine (peripheral selective alpha-1-agonist)
    - Pyridostigmine (cholinesterase inhibitor)
    - Fludrocortisone (mineralocorticoid effect)
- Vasovagal hypotension: management is often not needed or may resemble management of orthostatic hypotension.

SECTION **G**

Infectious and Inflammatory Heart Disease

CHAPTER
20

Hypertrophic Cardiomyopathy

Joshua Merson, MS-HPEd, PA-C
Dominique Murphy, MMSc, PA-C

▶ GENERAL FEATURES

- Hypertrophic cardiomyopathy is an autosomal-dominant genetic disorder characterized by left ventricular (LV) hypertrophy of various morphologies with impaired diastolic filling.
- Two types:
  - Obstructive: characterized by narrowing of the LV outflow tract due to a thickened interventricular septum

- Nonobstructive: characterized by a stiff LV, reducing the volume of blood the ventricle can hold without blocking blood flow
- Hypertrophic cardiomyopathy is the most common cause of sudden death in patients under age 35 years; prevalence of ~1:200 in the general population.

▶ CLINICAL ASSESSMENT

- Hypertrophic cardiomyopathy is commonly asymptomatic or with mild symptoms; correlation is not strong between the presence or magnitude of LV outflow tract obstruction, LV hypertrophy, and symptoms.
- Symptoms can include chest pain, fatigue, dyspnea on exertion, presyncope or syncope on exertion, or sudden cardiac death.
  - Syncope and/or sudden death may occur due to dysrhythmias secondary to abnormal cardiac myocytes.
- Examination may be normal or have nonspecific abnormalities.
  - Murmurs secondary to LV outflow tract obstruction are the most predominant examination abnormality.
    - Classically a crescendo-decrescendo systolic murmur that begins slightly after S1 is best heard at apex and left lower sternal border, and is exaggerated by standing up, inotropes, and vasodilators.
    - S3 or S4 is common in younger patients.
  - Other examination abnormalities may include a brisk arterial or carotid pulse, increased jugular venous distention (JVD) with a prominent "A" wave, and a diffuse and forceful LV apical impulse.

▶ DIAGNOSIS

- The following electrocardiogram (ECG) findings may be seen in hypertrophic cardiomyopathy but are nonspecific:
  - Prominent Q waves, P-wave abnormalities, left axis deviation, or deeply inverted T waves may be seen.
  - An LV hypertrophy pattern with or without abnormal Q waves is the most frequent ECG finding.
  - Atrial fibrillation (AF) is the most common dysrhythmia seen.
  - Ventricular tachycardia (VT) is the most common cause of death in patients with hypertrophic cardiomyopathy.
- Clinical diagnosis is confirmed by echocardiography when unexplained increased LV wall thickness is found in the absence of other cardiac or systemic disease.

- Additional risk stratification for dysrhythmias and myocardial ischemia may be assessed using ambulatory ECG monitoring, exercise stress testing, and cardiovascular magnetic resonance (CMR) imaging.

▶ TREATMENT

- First-degree relatives should be screened with history, physical examination, ECG, and echocardiogram.
- Pharmacologic therapy is not indicated for asymptomatic patients, as it does not change the disease course.
- For symptomatic patients, the goal of medical therapy is to manage LV outflow tract obstruction and systolic anterior motion.
  - Negative inotropic agents (beta-blockers, nondihydropyridine calcium channel blockers, or disopyramide).
  - Cautious use of diuretics and vasodilators due to the potential reduction in preload, which may exacerbate LV outflow tract obstruction, is recommended.
- Surgical myectomy or alcohol septal ablation is used for patients who do not respond to medical therapy.
- Heart transplantation may be considered in end-stage disease with patients showing advanced signs of heart failure.
- Prevent complications through use of antiarrhythmics, warfarin for patients with AF, or an implanted cardioverter-defibrillator (ICD) for patients with one or more of the following major risk factors for sudden cardiac death:
  - Prior aborted cardiac arrest or spontaneous sustained VT
  - Nonsustained VT
  - Unexplained syncope
  - LV thickness of ≥ 30 mm
  - Abnormal exercise blood pressure
  - Family history of premature sudden cardiac death
- Patients should avoid strenuous or intense competitive sports.

CHAPTER 21

Acute Pericarditis

Renee Andreeff, EdD, PA-C, DFAAPA

▶ GENERAL FEATURES

- Acute pericarditis is an inflammation of the pericardium, the fibroelastic sac that surrounds the heart.
- It may occur in isolation or as a component of systemic disease.
- It is most commonly caused by viral infections (such as coxsackievirus and echovirus) or is idiopathic.

- Other causes include acute myocardial infarction (MI); uremia; systemic diseases such as lupus, thyroid disease, and mixed connective tissue disease; fungal infections, especially in patients with HIV; medications such as dantrolene, hydralazine, isoniazid, phenytoin, and rifampin; bacterial infections and tuberculosis; malignancies such as breast and lung cancer, leukemia, and

lymphoma; radiation therapy of the lung or breast; invasive cardiac procedures; and chest trauma.
- Complications of acute pericarditis include pericardial effusion, cardiac tamponade, and myocardial involvement (myopericarditis and perimyocarditis).

▶ CLINICAL ASSESSMENT

- Often presents as sharp, sudden-onset pleuritic anterior chest pain
  - Exacerbated by coughing or inspiration
  - Relieved by sitting up and leaning forward
  - Pain may radiate to the back and trapezius ridge.
- If viral, may be preceded by flu-like respiratory or gastrointestinal symptoms
- Pericardial friction rub on cardiovascular auscultation over the left sternal border is common and highly specific, but not sensitive, for acute pericarditis.
- Ewart sign: dullness and bronchial breathing between the tip of the left scapula and the vertebral column
- Fever may be present.
- Patients may present with signs and symptoms of pericardial effusion and tamponade.

▶ DIAGNOSIS

- Electrocardiogram (ECG) typically shows widespread upward concave ST-segment elevation and PR-segment depression in the limb leads; T-wave depressions may be seen several days later, after ST-segments return to normal.
- Chest radiograph is typically normal but may have evidence of pericardial effusion.
- Laboratory signs of inflammation (elevated white blood cell count, elevated C-reactive protein, and erythrocyte sedimentation rate) may be present. Troponin I may be elevated due to epicardial cell damage.
- Chemistry panel may reveal uremia.
- Echocardiography may be normal but can rule out pericardial effusion.

- CT or MRI may reveal evidence of neoplastic causes:
  - Most sensitive method for the diagnosis of acute pericarditis is delayed enhancement of the pericardium on cardiac MRI.

▶ TREATMENT

- Most cases can be managed in an outpatient setting with medical therapy alone with the goal of reducing pain and resolving the inflammation.
- Medical therapy includes oral administration of nonsteroidal anti-inflammatory drugs (NSAIDs) such as ibuprofen (600–800 mg every 6–8 hours for 1–2 weeks, followed by gradual tapering of the dose by 800 mg per week for 3 additional weeks).
- Indomethacin (50 mg three times a day for 1–2 weeks followed by a slow tapering) also has shown efficacy in treating acute pericarditis (avoid in patients with coronary artery disease).
- Colchicine (0.5–0.6 mg twice daily for 3 months in addition to NSAIDs) should be considered in all patients with acute pericarditis, especially those who have not responded to NSAID therapy alone after 7 days.
- Refractory cases and patients with pericarditis due to connective tissue disease and failure of or contraindications for NSAID use can be treated with prednisone 0.25–0.5 mg/kg/day for 2 weeks (slow tapering) plus colchicine (0.5–0.6 mg twice daily for 6 months).
  - Corticosteroid use increases the risk for recurrent pericarditis.
  - NSAIDs (other than aspirin) and glucocorticoids should not be used in patients with post-MI pericarditis.
- Consider exercise restriction until resolution of symptoms.
- Hospitalization for patients with large pericardial effusion and/or signs of tamponade.
- Prognosis for acute pericarditis of idiopathic and viral origin is good, although following the initial episode of acute pericarditis, 24% of patients will experience a recurrence within the first few weeks.

CHAPTER 22

Pericardial Effusion and Cardiac Tamponade

Lendell Richardson, MD

▶ GENERAL FEATURES

- Pericardial effusion is an accumulation of fluid in the fibroelastic sac that surrounds the heart.
  - Effusions can develop secondary to acute pericarditis (viral, bacterial, tuberculous, uremic, or neoplastic), systemic disorders (eg, autoimmune disease, malignancy, myocardial infarction, myxedema, renal failure), or trauma.
- Cardiac tamponade is a compressive syndrome that occurs when significant fluid accumulation in the

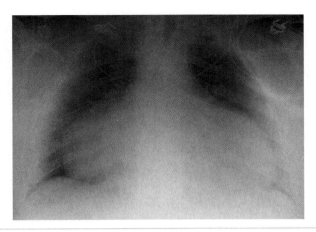

FIGURE 22.1 Enlarged cardiac silhouette with "water bottle" sign.

pericardial sac obstructs normal filling of the ventricles, leading to critical cardiovascular compromise.
- May be acute or subacute depending on the speed at which the pericardial fluid accumulates; the quantity of fluid required to cause tamponade varies:
  - With rapid development, as little as 200 mL of pericardial fluid can cause tamponade.
  - With slow development, more than 2000 mL may be needed to produce tamponade.
- Classic triad is used to describe acute tamponade:
  - Hypotension with or without pulsus paradoxus (systolic BP decreases >10 mm Hg during inspiration)
  - Muffled/distant heart sounds
  - Jugular venous distention (JVD)

▶ CLINICAL ASSESSMENT

- History
  - Acute tamponade: patients may present with chest pain, tachypnea, dyspnea, hypotension, cool extremities, peripheral cyanosis.
  - Subacute tamponade: patients may be asymptomatic early but later may develop dyspnea, edema, chest discomfort, and fatigue.
  - History may be notable for:
    - Pericarditis, cancer, renal disease, or infectious processes such as tuberculosis
    - Autoimmune disease or hypersensitivity
    - Trauma or recent invasive medical procedures
    - Bleeding disorders
    - Acute myocardial infarction (AMI)—as this can be associated with left ventricular free-wall rupture or hemorrhagic pericarditis
- Physical examination may be notable for:
  - Sinus tachycardia
  - Beck's triad: hypotension, JVD, and soft or absent heart sounds
  - Low/narrow pulse pressure (defined as the difference between systolic and diastolic pressures. The normal pulse pressure is between 30 and 40 mm Hg.)

- Signs of elevated jugular venous pressure
- Muted (distant) heart sounds
- Pulsus paradoxus (systolic BP decreases >10 mm Hg during inspiration)
- Pericardial friction rub (due to inflammation of the pericardium) on cardiac auscultation

▶ DIAGNOSIS

- Electrocardiogram (ECG)
  - Sinus tachycardia
  - May show low voltage (diffuse)
  - May show *electrical alternans* (amplitude of the P, QRS, or T waves varies from one beat to the next)
    - Fairly specific, but low sensitivity, finding for large pericardial effusion
- Chest radiograph
  - Cardiac silhouette may be enlarged, sometimes referred to as the "water bottle sign" (Figure 22.1); lung fields are typically clear.
  - Cardiomegaly may be absent acute tamponade due to the low volume of pericardial fluid required to cause obstruction.
- Echocardiogram (2D and Doppler) is the preferred imaging modality.
  - May show pericardial effusion; cardiac chamber collapse (particularly RV) during diastole; a dilated inferior vena cava; respiratory variations in cardiac blood volumes and flow rates
- Microscopic analysis and/or culture of pericardial fluid may aid in diagnosis when the etiology of the effusion is uncertain.

▶ TREATMENT

- Definitive treatment of cardiac tamponade is removal of the pericardial fluid via percutaneous drainage (pericardiocentesis) or surgical drainage.
  - Patients who exhibit clear hemodynamic compromise will need urgent/emergent pericardial fluid removal.
  - Pericardial fluid removal: three types
    - Percutaneous (catheter pericardiocentesis)
    - Open surgical drainage with or without pericardiectomy (pericardial "window")
    - Video-assisted thoracoscopic pericardiectomy
- Patients with suspected cardiac tamponade but minimal or absent hemodynamic compromise can be safely treated conservatively with serial echocardiograms, careful hemodynamic monitoring, avoidance of volume depletion, nonsteroidal anti-inflammatory drugs; colchicine; treatment of the underlying cause of the effusion.
  - Note: Pericardial fluid drainage may be required for refractory effusions, initially treated conservatively, or in patients with worsening symptoms.
- Follow-up echocardiogram is usually performed in these patients within 2 weeks of hospital discharge and again 6–12 months later.

Infective Endocarditis

Melissa Johnson Chung, MMS, PA-C

▶ GENERAL FEATURES

- Infective endocarditis (IE) occurs when bacteria or fungus infects a cardiac valve or tissue.
  - During bacteremia, microorganisms adhere to platelet-fibrin depositions on abnormal valves or at sites of endothelial injury or inflammation.
  - The mechanism of how bacteria or fungus infects intact endothelium is not well understood.
- Characteristic lesion is called a vegetation.
- Between 10,000 and 15,000 new cases per year in the United States
- Risk factors for developing IE:
  - Heart valve disease
  - Previous heart valve surgery
  - Congenital heart disease
  - Intravenous (IV) drug use
  - History of IE
  - Prolonged bacteremia
- Comorbid conditions include:
  - Previous history of IE
  - Prosthetic heart valve
  - Structural heart disease such as rheumatic heart disease, degenerative heart disease, and congenital heart disease
  - Chronic hemodialysis
  - Presence of an intravascular device
  - Cardiac implantable electronic devices such as pacemakers or implantable cardioverter-defibrillators
  - HIV
- In patients who use IV drugs, the tricuspid valve is the most commonly affected; in patients who do not use injection drugs, the mitral valve is most commonly affected.
- In patients who do not use IV drugs, in the United States, the 1-year mortality rate associated with IE is about 12%.
- *Staphylococci* and *Streptococci* account for most cases:
  - Staphylococcal IE is the most common cause of healthcare-associated IE.
  - Streptococcal IE is the most common cause of community-acquired IE.
  - *S. aureus* accounts for more than half of all cases of IE in patients who use IV drugs.

▶ CLINICAL ASSESSMENT

- The clinical presentation is variable and frequently nonspecific, with fever commonly present (90% of cases).
- Other symptoms may include chills, malaise, fatigue, anorexia, weight loss, cough, dyspnea, hemoptysis, chest pain, myalgias, arthralgias, headache, stroke symptoms, confusion, nausea/vomiting, abdominal pain, or back pain.
  - Symptoms may be the result of arterial, valvular, or cardiac damage. They also may be caused by embolization, metastatic infection, or immunologically mediated phenomena.
- Signs:
  - Fever, new heart murmur, neurologic abnormalities, splenomegaly, splenic infarct, clubbing, anemia, hematuria, evidence of embolic events
  - Classic signs associated with IE (minor criteria)
    - Petechiae: nonspecific, but the most common peripheral manifestation
    - Splinter hemorrhages: nonblanching, linear, reddish-brown lesions found under the nail bed
    - Osler nodes: painful, violaceous nodules found in the pulp of fingers and toes
    - Janeway lesions: macular, nonpainful, erythematous lesions on the palms and soles
    - Roth spots: exudative, edematous hemorrhagic lesions of the retina
  - Laboratory findings:
    - Anemia or leukocytosis is common
    - Elevated erythrocyte sedimentation rate in almost all patients
    - Elevated C-reactive protein
    - Rheumatoid factor is increased in about 50% of patients
    - Proteinuria and/or microscopic hematuria occurs in about 50% of patients

▶ DIAGNOSIS

- Obtain three sets of blood cultures from separate venipuncture sites, at least 1 hour apart and before antibiotics are started; bacteremia is the hallmark of the disease.
- Obtain the patient's score on the Modified Duke Criteria:
  - Definite endocarditis is defined by:
    - Pathology specimens from surgery or autopsy or
    - Two major criteria or
    - One major and three minor criteria or
    - Five minor criteria
  - Possible endocarditis diagnosis is defined by:
    - One major criterion and one to two minor criteria or
    - Three minor criteria
- Use transthoracic or transesophageal echocardiogram to visualize the vegetation.

▶ TREATMENT

- Empiric IV antibiotics pending culture if IE is highly suspected, and the patient is acutely ill:
  - Vancomycin for native-valve endocarditis (covers *Staphylococcus*, *Streptococcus*, and *Enterococcus*)
  - Vancomycin plus gentamicin and cefepime for prosthetic valve endocarditis
- Treat based on the organism found.
- Follow blood cultures until negative.
- IV antibiotics are the standard of care for all patients:
  - 4-6 weeks for native valve endocarditis
  - 6 weeks for prosthetic valve endocarditis
- Surgical consult:
  - All patients with prosthetic valve endocarditis
  - Patients with new valvular incompetence and heart failure
  - Patients with fungal infections
  - Patients with recurrent embolization
  - Patients with treatment failure or persistent vegetations
- American Heart Association guidelines for the prevention of IE:
  - Good oral hygiene
  - Antibiotic prophylaxis for patients at increased risk of experiencing adverse outcomes of IE prior to dental procedures that involve manipulation of the gingival tissue or the periapical region of teeth or perforation of the oral mucosa in patients with:
    - Prosthetic cardiac valves, including transcatheter-implanted protheses and homografts or
    - Prosthetic material used for cardiac valve repair, such as annuloplasty rings and chords or
    - Previous IE or
    - Unrepaired cyanotic congenital heart disease or repaired congenital heart disease, with residual shunts or valvular regurgitation at the site or adjacent to the site of a prosthetic patch or prosthetic device or
    - Cardiac transplant with valve regurgitation due to a structurally abnormal valve
- Prophylaxis may be considered in other scenarios and in consultation with the patient's cardiac specialist, for respiratory procedures with biopsy or incision of mucosa, procedures during active gastrointestinal or genitourinary infections, procedures on infected skin or musculoskeletal tissue, or placement of prosthetic valves or intravascular materials.
  - Antibiotic choice for dental procedures is oral amoxicillin 2 g, given 30–60 minutes prior to procedure; use clindamycin 600 mg if the patient is allergic to penicillin.

CHAPTER 24

Myocarditis

Sean Robinson, DHSc, PA-C

▶ GENERAL FEATURES

- Myocarditis is inflammation of the myocardium, usually in response to infection, resulting in infiltration, edema, and sometimes necrosis of myocytes and surrounding tissue.
- The most common etiology in the United States is viral infection; coxsackievirus, adenovirus, and parvovirus B19 are most common.
- Other infectious etiologies include bacteria (*Streptococcus*, *Staphylococcus*, *Borrelia burgdorferi*, and *Rickettsia rickettsii*, among others), fungi, and parasites (when involving *Trypanosoma cruzi*, the illness is known as Chagas disease).
- Noninfectious causes include autoimmune-mediated myocyte injury as seen in systemic lupus erythematosus (SLE) or sarcoidosis or after exposure to toxins such as certain medications or radiation.
- It is associated with increased risk of arrhythmias (current or remote history) and sudden cardiac death.
- Recurrent or chronic myocarditis is associated with increased risk of dilated cardiomyopathy.

▶ CLINICAL ASSESSMENT

- The presentation varies in degree and severity; it may be asymptomatic.
- Three major forms of myocarditis include:
  - Fulminant myocarditis:
    - More common in children
    - Rapid progression (days to weeks) of New York Heart Association (NYHA) Class IV heart failure symptoms (dyspnea at rest, unable to carry on any physical activity)
    - Refractory, sustained arrhythmias (such as ventricular fibrillation) are common.
    - Hypotension and cardiovascular shock may occur.
    - Increased risk of sudden cardiac death
  - Acute myocarditis:
    - Most common form
    - Generally occurs within 1-4 weeks after symptom onset of viral infection (usually upper respiratory infection [URI])

- May present with fatigue, palpitations, dyspnea, and chest pain
- Patients may not recall any recent URI symptoms, making the diagnosis by association a challenge.
  - Chronic myocarditis:
    - Characterized by heart failure symptoms (usually starting with an acute episode) lasting >3 months with no clearly identifiable cause
- Physical examination:
  - Tachycardia
  - Evidence of congestive heart failure (crackles, prominent S3, jugular vein distention, peripheral edema)
  - New systolic murmurs (mitral and tricuspid regurgitation)
  - Soft heart sounds and a pericardial friction rub indicate involvement of pericarditis

▶ DIAGNOSIS

- Generally a clinical diagnosis.
- Endomyocardial biopsy is considered the gold standard but is not commonly performed.
- Electrocardiogram (ECG) may show sinus tachycardia or nonspecific ST-segment changes (eg, ST-segment elevation in one or two noncontiguous leads)

- White blood cell count, inflammatory markers (erythrocyte sedimentation rate and C-reactive protein), and troponin levels may be elevated.
- Echocardiogram is useful to rule out other potential causes of heart failure.
- Cardiac MRI may show signs of acute myocardial inflammation but is only useful in select patients.

▶ TREATMENT

- Supportive care for acute cases with mild symptoms; nonsteroidal anti-inflammatory drugs should be avoided as they are associated with increased inflammation and myocardial necrosis.
- Heart failure symptoms should be treated with diuresis, afterload reduction (eg, angiotensin-converting enzyme inhibitor (ACEI)), and a beta-blocker as appropriate.
- For fulminant myocarditis, cardiovascular compromise may require inotropes and a vasopressor, mechanical circulatory support (eg, ventricular assist device), or extracorporeal membrane oxygenation (ECMO).
- For known viral myocarditis, IV immunoglobulins may be used but is generally restricted to children with fulminant myocarditis.

CHAPTER 25

Dilated and Restrictive Cardiomyopathy

Sean Robinson, DHSc, PA-C

▶ GENERAL FEATURES

- Dilated cardiomyopathy
  - Ventricular enlargement with an ejection fraction (EF) <40% in the absence of valve disease and ischemic, hypertensive, and congenital heart disease
  - Most common cardiomyopathy and cause of a third of all cases of heart failure
  - Multiple causes, idiopathic most common
  - Familial/genetic link, typically autosomal dominant
  - Nonfamilial causes include:
    - Toxic exposures such as chemotherapy, chronic alcohol consumption, and drugs (especially methamphetamine and cocaine)
    - Other medical conditions such as Duchenne muscular dystrophy, peripartum (onset in last trimester or as late as 6 months after delivery), chronic tachycardia, and nutritional deficiencies
  - Increased risk in patients with history of myocarditis or chronic restrictive cardiomyopathy

- Restrictive cardiomyopathy (RCM):
  - Impaired ventricular filling from thickened myocardium but no overall ventricular enlargement, resulting in diastolic dysfunction out of proportion to systolic dysfunction
  - Caused by abnormalities in the myocardium or endomyocardial surface
    - Infiltrative
      - Amyloidosis
      - Sarcoidosis
    - Noninfiltrative: from systemic diseases including hypertension, diabetes, scleroderma
    - Inflammatory: secondary to hypereosinophilia, a history of radiation therapy (especially for breast cancer or Hodgkin disease), or exposure to anthracyclines (eg, doxorubicin)
    - Storage diseases: Fabry, Gaucher, or hemochromatosis
    - Idiopathic disease

▶ CLINICAL ASSESSMENT

- Dilated cardiomyopathy:
  - Heart failure symptoms include dyspnea, dyspnea on exertion, orthopnea, paroxysmal nocturnal dyspnea (PND), cough, and lower extremity edema; may have history of syncopal episodes
  - Physical examination may show evidence of volume overload such as ascites, edema, jugular venous distention, pulmonary congestion.
  - Cardiac examination may have third heart sound and murmurs of mitral and/or tricuspid regurgitation that result from dilation of the annulus with increasing ventricular cavity size; may have pulsus alternans or narrow pulse pressure.
- RCM:
  - Symptoms: dyspnea on exertion (early), progressive worsening of breathing including PND and orthopnea, peripheral edema and ascites (late); fatigue and weakness are common.
  - Examination: signs of right heart failure (ascites, peripheral edema, jugular venous pressure [JVP]), Kussmaul sign (paradoxical increase in JVP with inspiration), absence of thrill or heaves that would normally be present in right-sided heart failure
  - Irregular pulse may be indicative of atrial fibrillation or heart block, both common due to amyloid and sarcoid deposition.

▶ DIAGNOSIS

- Dilated cardiomyopathy:
  - Electrocardiogram (ECG) will show left ventricular hypertrophy and left atrial enlargement and/or right atrial enlargement.
    - Sinus tachycardia and left bundle branch block are common.
    - Other tachyarrhythmias such as frequent premature ventricular contractions or atrial fibrillation with rapid ventricular response are common.
  - B-type natriuretic peptide (BNP) is typically elevated.
  - Chest x-ray will show enlargement of the cardiac silhouette; pulmonary edema and pleural effusions in advanced disease
  - Echocardiogram will show ventricular dilation with thinning of the ventricular walls; systolic dysfunction with EF <40% is required to make the diagnosis; evidence of pulmonary hypertension may be present.
- RCM:
  - Chest x-ray may show bilateral atrial enlargement with no or minimal ventricular enlargement.
  - ECG will often have nonspecific ECG changes but there are no findings specific for RCM.
  - Echocardiography shows biatrial enlargement; small, thickened LV walls; diastolic dysfunction; and, in the earlier stages, preserved systolic function; a "speckled" or "hyperrefractile" appearance to the myocardial pattern is nearly diagnostic for amyloidosis.
  - Cardiac MRI may be ordered to distinguish RCM from other infiltrative causes as well as constrictive pericarditis.
  - Biopsy is rarely needed.

▶ TREATMENT

- Dilated cardiomyopathy:
  - Begin usual medical management of heart failure including angiotensin-converting enzyme (ACE) inhibitor or angiotensin-receptor blocker (ARB) or ACE/neprilysin inhibitor combination; beta-blocker (mortality benefit with use of bisoprolol, carvedilol, or long-acting metoprolol succinate).
  - Salt-restricted diet (<2 g/day), cardiac rehabilitation, and exercise program
  - PRN loop diuretic for volume overload (limited due to kidney function)
  - Treat any concomitant coronary artery disease.
  - If heart failure symptoms persist despite initial therapy, consider addition of aldosterone receptor antagonist (eg, eplerenone or spironolactone).
  - Consider addition of digoxin (particularly if concomitant atrial fibrillation), vasodilators such as hydralazine, combination of long-acting nitrate (eg, isosorbide dinitrate) and hydralazine, or ivabradine if the maximum dose of beta-blocker has been achieved and heart rate >70 beats per minute.
  - If symptoms persist, EF <35%, and QRS duration is >150 milliseconds, consider cardiac resynchronization therapy with biventricular pacer.
  - Heart transplant if disease is severe and unresponsive to medical therapy; may need LV assist device as bridge to transplant or, if not a surgical candidate, as definitive therapy.
- RCM:
  - There is little evidence supporting any particular treatment of RCM, regardless of etiology.
  - Empiric therapy of heart failure symptoms may be beneficial:
    - Loop diuretics to decrease circulating volume
    - Non-dihydropyridine calcium channel blocker (eg, verapamil) or a beta-blocker useful to increase diastolic filling times
    - ACE inhibitors and ARBs are unproven in diastolic dysfunction but may be beneficial.
  - Avoid digoxin as there is an increased risk of arrhythmias.
  - Transplant is an option if patient fails medical therapy.

CHAPTER 26

Aortic Valve Regurgitation

Tyler D. Sommer, MPAS, PA-C

▶ GENERAL FEATURES

- Aortic valve regurgitation (AR) is characterized by the reflux of blood back through an incompetent aortic valve during ventricular diastole.
- Aortic valve incompetency generally occurs due to structural abnormalities of the aortic root or structural abnormalities of the valve itself, oftentimes a result of age-related degeneration.
- The most common causes include aortic sclerosis, congenital bicuspid valves, infective endocarditis, and chronic hypertension.
- Less common causes include Marfan-related aortic root dilation, aortic root dissection, widespread inflammatory conditions, and iatrogenic injury during cardiac surgery procedures.
- AR is most commonly seen in elderly individuals, and there is a correlation between degenerative calcific changes of the valve and atherosclerotic disease.

▶ CLINICAL ASSESSMENT

- Most cases are chronic rather than acute, and patients may be asymptomatic for long periods of time.
- Chronic symptomatic AR may present with signs and symptoms similar to heart failure, such as exercise intolerance or dyspnea on exertion
- Patients who develop severe acute AR generally present with signs of left ventricular (LV) failure, such as shortness of breath due to acute pulmonary edema, or signs of hypotension/poor perfusion such as syncope.
- Physical examination:
  - As pressurized blood from the aorta rushes through the incompetent aortic valve, the turbulent blood flow causes a holodiastolic murmur that is often loud and blowing.
  - The murmur of AR is generally heard best along the lower left sternal border and sometimes has a somewhat decrescendo characteristic.
  - An Austin Flint murmur is sometimes also heard (low-pitched, mid-diastolic murmur heard best at the apex).
- The heart gradually compensates for the increased LV pressure and volume due to regurgitant flow, resulting in a large stroke volume; this can manifest as a wide pulse pressure and a water hammer pulse.
- Patients' heads may nod or bob with each beat of the heart (Musset sign), a result of wide pulse pressure.

▶ DIAGNOSIS

- Echocardiogram (ECG) is the most important diagnostic tool for aortic valve disease and will reveal incompetent aortic valve with regurgitation; it may also reveal features of causative conditions or sequelae such as LV hypertrophy.
  - Transthoracic echocardiogram (TTE) is often sufficient to make the initial diagnosis.
  - Transesophageal echocardiogram (TEE) may be useful if TTE is suboptimal or for additional surgical planning.
- ECG may reveal evidence of ventricular hypertrophy and other nonspecific abnormalities.
- Chest x-ray may reveal evidence of cardiomegaly and can show signs of pulmonary edema in those who have developed LV failure.

▶ TREATMENT

- Patients without symptoms can be monitored with serial echocardiograms for progression of disease.
- Surgical aortic valve replacement is indicated in patients with symptoms, LV ejection fraction <50%, or if any other cardiac surgery is indicated; it may also be considered in patients with aortic root dilation.

CHAPTER 27

Aortic Valve Stenosis

Cheryl Ann Lugiano, MPAS, PA-C

▶ GENERAL FEATURES

- Aortic stenosis is the narrowing of the aortic valve caused by thickened, stiff leaflets that obstruct left ventricular (LV) outflow.
- Aortic stenosis is the most common valvular heart disease in adults that leads to sudden death.
- Untreated symptomatic aortic stenosis is associated with 25% annual mortality.
- The most common causes of aortic stenosis are congenital anomalies, rheumatic heart disease, and atherosclerosis/calcification (degenerative in older adults and early calcification in congenital bicuspid valves).

▶ CLINICAL ASSESSMENT

- Patients with mild-to-moderate aortic stenosis may be asymptomatic, and the disease may be incidentally detected by auscultation of a murmur.
- Severe aortic stenosis is described by the "classic triad" of SAD: *Syncope, Angina,* and *Dyspnea* (with or without exertion).
- Other symptoms may include exercise intolerance, dizziness, light-headedness, or orthopnea.
- Physical examination may feature the hallmark harsh, crescendo-decrescendo systolic ejection murmur heard best over the right upper sternal border with radiation to the carotid arteries.

- There may be a delayed carotid upstroke detected with simultaneous palpation of the apex and the carotid artery.

▶ DIAGNOSIS

- Diagnosis is made through transthoracic echocardiography, revealing an increased aortic jet velocity and increased mean transvalvular pressure gradient.
- Electrocardiogram (ECG) may demonstrate LV hypertrophy or a left bundle branch block.
- Chest radiograph may show calcification of the aortic valve and LV prominence.

▶ TREATMENT

- No medical treatment has been shown to prevent or delay disease progression.
- The "gold-standard" definitive treatment is surgical aortic valve replacement or transcatheter aortic valve replacement (TAVR).
  - Surgery is indicated in:
    - Symptomatic with severe aortic stenosis
    - Patients with moderate-to-severe aortic stenosis undergoing another form of heart surgery (eg, coronary artery bypass grafting or aortic reconstruction)
    - Patients with severe aortic stenosis and LV systolic dysfunction (ejection fraction <50%)

CHAPTER 28

Mitral Valve Disease

Rebecca Clawson, PA-C
Emily Weidman-Evans, PharmD, BC-ADM, CPE

A 68-year-old man with a history of hypertension presents with peripheral edema, dyspnea on exertion, and orthopnea. Physical examination is normal except for bibasilar crackles and a 3/6 blowing and holosystolic murmur with a decrescendo pattern heard best at the apex. What is the most likely diagnosis? Which test is the most appropriate next step to arrive at a definitive diagnosis?

▶ GENERAL FEATURES

- Mitral valve prolapse (MVP)
  - MVP is the malformation or degeneration of mitral valve characterized by superior displacement of one or both leaflets, resulting in excess leaflet motion.

- MVP is the most common cause of mitral regurgitation (MR).
- Often asymptomatic, MVP can present as atypical chest pain, dyspnea, palpitations, anxiety, and presyncope.
- Physical examination often reveals a murmur that begins in midsystole with a click and continues through systole.
- Diagnosis, treatment, and complications closely mirror those of MR, discussed later.
- The major predictor of outcomes in MVP is the degree of MR present and the complications that develop.
- MR
  - MR refers to the abnormal retrograde flow of blood from the left ventricle through the mitral valve to the left atrium.

- Varies in severity and may be acute or chronic
- Chronic MR is classified as primary or secondary:
  - Primary MR is degenerative in nature.
  - Secondary MR is due to functional or ischemic causes (atrial remodeling, cardiomyopathy, or myocardial infarction).
- MR occurs in ~2% of the U.S. population.
- More common in older populations, approaching 10% in those >70 years old
- Mitral stenosis (MS)
  - MS is narrowing of the mitral valve orifice, obstructing forward blood flow.
  - Rheumatic fever is the cause of approximately 85% of cases worldwide—predominantly in developing countries; symptoms usually do not present until 20-40 years after the infection.
  - Incidence of MS is low in the United States: ~1 in 100,000, most commonly caused by valve calcification.

▶ CLINICAL ASSESSMENT

- MR may present with:
  - Symptoms: exertional dyspnea, orthopnea, paroxysmal nocturnal dyspnea, peripheral edema, fatigue
  - Physical examination findings: holosystolic, decrescendo, blowing murmur heard best at the mitral area and can sometimes radiate to the axilla; laterally displaced point of maximal impulse; pitting edema; bibasilar rales
- MS presents with signs/symptoms of heart failure:
  - Symptoms: exertional dyspnea, orthopnea, paroxysmal nocturnal dyspnea, peripheral edema, and fatigue
  - Signs: mid-diastolic, crescendo, rumbling murmur heard best at the mitral area with the bell and the patient in left lateral decubitus—opening snap may be heard; diminished or irregular pulses, edema, jugular vein distention
  - Severe MS may also present with signs of poor perfusion and ischemia: chest pain, syncope, pallor, and dyspnea

▶ DIAGNOSIS

- Definitive diagnosis of MR is made by an echocardiogram.
  - Electrocardiogram (ECG) and chest x-ray may show signs of cardiomyopathy.
- Diagnosis of MS is made by echocardiogram.

▶ TREATMENT

- Asymptomatic mitral valve disease typically does not require treatment.
- MR
  - Secondary MR requires treatment of the underlying condition (eg, guideline-directed medical therapy [GDMT] for left ventricular dysfunction).
  - Surgery is first-line treatment for patients with symptomatic mitral valve disease. Patients with

decreased ejection fraction due to MVP or primary MR may require valve repair or replacement.
  - Mechanical valve replacement (MVR) requires lifetime anticoagulation with warfarin; international normalized ratio goal 2.5-3.5.
- Pharmacologic treatment for mitral valve disease is indicated based on symptoms and/or complications, consistent with current evidence and guidelines (eg, a loop diuretic for symptoms of volume overload, a beta-blocker and angiotensin-converting enzyme [ACE] inhibitor for decreased ejection fraction, or a vasodilator for pulmonary hypertension).
- All patients with a murmur should be referred to a cardiologist for workup; symptomatic valvular disease should be referred to a cardiologist immediately.
- Complications of both MVP and MR are related to increased atrial and ventricular pressures and the resulting decrease in function; common pathologies include atrial fibrillation and dilated cardiomyopathy.
  - Warfarin is indicated in some patients with MVP or MR, namely those with accompanying atrial fibrillation and a CHA_2DS_2-VASc score of 2 or greater. A direct oral anticoagulant (DOAC) can also be used.
  - Antibiotic prophylaxis against infective endocarditis during dental procedures is recommended for those at highest risk: prosthetic valve or prosthetic materials, history of infective endocarditis, or history of valvuloplasty.
- Prognosis
  - Patients with low- to moderate-grade, asymptomatic MR have an excellent prognosis; mortality increases significantly as the severity of valve dysfunction increases.
  - Outcomes are dependent on the change in ventricular and/or atrial dimensions, as well as the development of complications or severe symptoms.
- Patients with symptomatic MS typically undergo percutaneous valvuloplasty.
  - If this is contraindicated (due to severe regurgitation or the presence of a thrombus) or unsuccessful, MVR is indicated and requires lifetime anticoagulation with warfarin.
  - Complications of MS are related to increased atrial pressures and ischemia. They include atrial fibrillation (one-third of all patients), heart failure, and pulmonary hypertension.
  - The prognosis of MS is very good; overall 10-year survival rate is 80%. Survival is shortened if complications arise.

Case Conclusion

This patient is presenting with symptoms often associated with heart failure; that, paired with the quality of his murmur (holosystolic, decrescendo, blowing), should lead the clinician to suspect mitral regurgitation, which can be definitively diagnosed via an echocardiogram.

Giant Cell (Temporal) Arteritis

Colleen Grassley, MSPAS

A 74-year-old female presents to the emergency department for left-sided temporal headache, visual impairment, and jaw claudication. Her symptoms have been present for the last 2 weeks, but she is most concerned that her vision is worsening over the last several days. Her fundoscopic examination is reassuring, but you ordered labs that show an elevated ESR and CRP. What should you do next?

◗ GENERAL FEATURES

- Giant cell arteritis (GCA), also known as temporal arteritis, is a systemic vasculitis of the large- and medium-sized vessels with predilection for the vessels of the head and neck, particularly the extracranial branches of the carotid arteries.
- GCA is uncommon in young adults; risk increases every decade over the age of 50.
- GCA is more common in white patients, especially those of Scandinavian and northern European heritage.
- Polymyalgia rheumatica (PMR) occurs in 40%-50% of individuals with GCA, although only 10% of those with PMR will also have GCA.
- GCA is considered a medical emergency; the most feared complication is permanent and severe vision loss that can occur without prompt and early treatment.

◗ CLINICAL ASSESSMENT

- Consider GCA in patients older than 50 with new headache; abrupt visual disturbance; jaw claudication; or unexplained constitutional symptoms of fever, fatigue, or weight loss.
- The most common ocular presentations associated with GCA include transient monocular painless vision loss and anterior ischemic optic neuropathy in which ophthalmoscopic examination will show a pale swollen optic disc.
- Patients may have a palpable, tender temporal artery on the affected side.

◗ DIAGNOSIS

- Laboratory results suggesting temporal arteritis include elevated erythrocyte sedimentation rate (ESR) and C-reactive protein (CRP) level. The presence of normochromic normocytic anemia and elevated platelets increases the likelihood of biopsy-positive GCA; normal laboratory results do not rule out GCA.
- Diagnosis is confirmed by temporal artery biopsy.
- Color Doppler ultrasound of the head and neck can be used in conjunction with temporal artery biopsy to aid in diagnosis, but its utility is limited given variability in diagnostic criteria, equipment, and operator skill.

◗ TREATMENT

- GCA is treated with high-dose systemic steroids with a goal to preserve and prevent vision loss; treatment should be initiated immediately in the setting of high clinical suspicion rather than waiting for temporal artery biopsy results.
- Typically, individuals without vision loss will receive prednisone 1 mg/kg (maximum 60 mg) once daily, tapered over many weeks.
- For patients with vision loss or threated vision loss, methylprednisolone 500-1000 mg IV daily for 3 days is preferred.
- Patients with ocular symptoms should be referred to an ophthalmologist; otherwise, patients should be referred to rheumatology or neurology.

Case Conclusion

This patient has giant cell arteritis, which is considered a medical emergency. The most feared complication is permanent and severe vision loss that can occur without prompt and early treatment. Therefore, your next steps should be threefold: start steroid therapy immediately to prevent further vision loss, schedule her for the next available temporal artery biopsy, and refer her to ophthalmology.

Other Valve Disorders

Brendan Riordan, MPAS, PA-C

▶ GENERAL FEATURES

- Tricuspid regurgitation (TR)
  - TR is a malfunction of the tricuspid valve, allowing for retrograde flow of blood from the right ventricle (RV) to the right atrium (RA) during ventricular systole.
  - Further classified into primary (damage/dysfunction of the valve itself) or secondary/functional (RA/RV dilatation/pressure overload).
  - Secondary TR is far more common and is typically caused by underlying pulmonary hypertension; primary TR is often related to congenital disease (eg, Ebstein anomaly) or valvular destruction (infective endocarditis).
- Tricuspid stenosis (TS)
  - TS is a narrowing of the valve opening between the RA and RV, which impairs forward flow through the right side of the heart.
  - TS is a very uncommon condition and is rarely found in isolation (often concomitant with tricuspid/mitral regurgitation).
  - Most commonly seen with rheumatic heart disease
- Pulmonic stenosis (PS)
  - PS is a narrowing of the pulmonic valve or RV outflow tract (RVOT), which impairs blood flow from the RV into the pulmonary artery.
  - PS is a fairly common congenital condition that is often seen as an isolated anomaly.
  - Symptoms are tied to severity, and many cases go unrecognized until adulthood.

▶ DIAGNOSIS

- TR
  - TR is often asymptomatic unless acute and/or severe; may present with fatigue, exercise intolerance, abdominal fullness, or peripheral edema.
  - Specific physical examination findings for TR can include: a giant systolic jugular venous wave (Lancisi sign) and a high-pitched, holosystolic murmur auscultated over the left lower sternal border with radiation to the right sternal border; this murmur will increase during inspiration (Carvallo sign), which can help differentiate it from the murmur of mitral regurgitation.

- Other physical examination findings may be consistent with signs of RV dysfunction: increased jugular vein distention (JVD), hepatomegaly, lower extremity edema.
  - Echocardiography remains the gold standard for diagnosis; findings focus on the morphology of the valve leaflets and the presence of retrograde flow across the tricuspid valve; additionally, echocardiography can assess for the presence of RV dysfunction.
- TS
  - Severe, symptomatic TS will have similar features to TR with signs/symptoms of peripheral volume overload and RV dysfunction.
  - Physical examination findings may include prominence of JVD and a low rumbling diastolic murmur with an opening snap at the left sternal border; this murmur will be accentuated by maneuvers that increase venous return.
  - Definitive diagnosis is made by echocardiogram (increased pressure gradient across the tricuspid valve) and/or right heart/pulmonary artery catheterization.
- PS
  - Physical examination findings may be subtle and can include a systolic ejection murmur and a splitting of S2; this is heard best at the left sternal border in the second intercostal space.
  - Diagnosis is made by echocardiography, particularly pulse wave Doppler across and pressure gradient monitoring.

▶ TREATMENT

- TR
  - Treatment for secondary TR is management of underlying condition (eg, diuretic therapy for heart failure).
  - Patients with severe TR may be considered for procedural intervention (valve repair or replacement) if refractory to medical optimization or if undergoing concomitant surgery; severe primary TR will likely require surgical repair.
- TS: Treatment should be reserved for severe, symptomatic TS and requires interventional approach (valvotomy or valve repair/replacement).
- PS: Treatment is generally reserved for severe and/or symptomatic cases (balloon valvotomy or valve replacement/repair).

Deep Vein Thrombosis

Joy Moverley, DHSc, MPH, PA-C

▶ GENERAL FEATURES

- Deep vein thrombosis (DVT) is a blood clot that forms in the deep veins of the lower or upper extremities.
- Major mechanisms (Virchow triad):
  - <u>Stasis</u>: prolonged bedrest, immobility, long seated travel, congestive heart failure (CHF), obesity
  - <u>Hypercoagulability</u>: sepsis, inherited disorders of coagulation, presence of anticardiolipin antibodies and lupus anticoagulant, increased estrogens
  - <u>Endothelial injury</u>: trauma, surgery, IV catheters and procedures, other inflammatory processes, smoking
- Additional risk factors
  - Recent traveler
  - Bedridden patients
  - Patients with chronic indwelling IV lines
  - History of prior clot or vascular injury
  - Active malignancy
  - History of thrombophilias
- Clots can resolve spontaneously, remain in the originating vessel, propagate and grow, extend to the proximal veins, or break free and embolize to pulmonary circulation (pulmonary embolism [PE]).

▶ CLINICAL ASSESSMENT

- History:
  - The unilateral lower extremity may have:
    - Swelling/edema
    - Pain
    - Tenderness
    - Warmth
  - Assess for clinical symptoms of PE.
- Physical examination:
  - Lower extremity reveals warmth, erythema, tenderness, and/or dilated collateral veins.
  - Unilateral edema: measure calves at 10 cm below tibial tuberosity.
    - Asymmetry of >3 cm is considered significant.
  - Palpate all pulses.
  - Palpate for cord-like veins (especially in popliteal fossa).

▶ DIAGNOSIS

- Diagnosis is made based on clinical suspicion and diagnostic studies.
- Wells' criteria (for assessing pretest probability of DVT):
  - Active cancer (+1)
  - Bedridden >3 days or major surgery within 12 weeks (+1)
  - Calf swelling >3 cm compared to the contralateral leg (+1)
  - Superficial collateral veins present (+1)
  - Entire leg swollen (+1)
  - Localized tenderness along the deep venous system (+1)
  - Pitting edema, confined to symptomatic leg (+1)
  - Paralysis, paresis, or recent plaster immobilization of the lower extremity (+1)
  - Previously documented DVT (+1)
  - Alternative diagnosis as likely or more likely (−2)
    - Score of 0 = low probability (3%)
    - Score of 1-2 = moderate probability (17%)
    - Score of 3+ = high probability (75%)
- Laboratory evaluation: D-dimer is indicated for low-probability cases or cases with moderate to high probability and negative imaging findings.
- Imaging: Compression ultrasonography (CUS) is indicated for cases of moderate or high probability or low probability and a positive D-dimer.

▶ TREATMENT

- Treat outpatient if:
  - Hemodynamically stable
  - Low bleeding risk prior to anticoagulation therapy
  - Normal renal function
- Treat inpatient if:
  - High risk of bleeding while on anticoagulant therapy
  - Bleeding in the last 14 days
  - Active peptic ulcer disease (PUD)
  - Platelets <80k
  - Massive DVT (eg, DVT with the iliofemoral vein or inferior vena cava) causing acrocyanosis, edema of the entire limb, or phlegmasia cerulea dolens
  - High fall risk
  - Concurrent suspected or proven symptomatic PE
  - At risk for cardiopulmonary deterioration
- Outpatient management:
  - Selection of medication is based on comorbidities, cost, preference, convenience, and risk of bleeding.
    - Low-molecular-weight (LMW) heparin is the preferred agent if active malignancy or pregnancy.
    - Unfractionated heparin is the preferred agent in patients with severe renal failure (creatine clearance <30 mL/min).
  - For patients with no comorbidities, select one of the following regimens:
    - Initiate warfarin with parenteral LMW heparin until therapeutic international normalized ration (INR) of 2-3, then discontinue LMW heparin and continue warfarin therapy.
    - Initiate rivaroxaban or apixaban monotherapy; accompanying parenteral anticoagulation is not necessary.
    - LMW heparin for 5 days followed by either dabigatran or edoxaban
- Duration of treatment:
  - Most patients with a first episode of venous thromboembolism (VTE) should receive anticoagulation for a minimum of 3 months.
  - Anticoagulation >3 months is not recommended for patients who no longer have risk factors or for patients at high risk for bleeding complications.
  - Anticoagulation for 6-12 months is recommended in phlegmasia cerulea dolens.
  - Indefinite anticoagulation for patients with active malignancy, unprovoked recurrent VTE, antiphospholipid antibody syndrome, unprovoked proximal DVT, or symptomatic PE
- Additional therapies:
  - Ambulation: safe and encouraged
  - Compression stockings to prevent post-thrombotic syndrome
  - Thrombolytic therapy and thrombectomy rarely indicated unless phlegmasia cerulea dolens (massive iliofemoral DVT)
  - Inferior vena cava filter
    - Absolute contraindications to systemic anticoagulation in patients with acute proximal DVT or PE
    - New thromboembolic event while on adequate anticoagulation

---

CHAPTER 32

Peripheral Arterial Disease

Melissa Johnson Chung, MMS, PA-C

▶ GENERAL FEATURES

- Peripheral artery disease (PAD) is atherosclerotic stenosis or occlusion of the peripheral arteries causing luminal narrowing and decreased blood supply relative to demand.
- Lower extremity vessels are affected much more often than upper extremity vessels.
- Risk factors for lower extremity PAD include:
  - Coronary heart disease or atherosclerosis of other peripheral vessels
  - Increased age
  - Hypertension
  - Dyslipidemia
  - Cigarette smoking
  - Sex (more prevalent in men)
  - Diabetes
  - Metabolic syndrome
  - Erectile dysfunction (especially in younger men)
  - Family history of cardiovascular disease (CVD)

▶ CLINICAL ASSESSMENT

- History:
  - Frequently asymptomatic
  - Symptomatic patients may present with intermittent claudication (reproducible discomfort within a group of muscles induced by exercise and relieved by rest).
    - Symptoms may involve the buttocks, hips, thighs, calves, or feet.
    - Patients with critical limb ischemia may present with rest pain, nonhealing wounds/ulcers, or gangrene.
- Physical examination findings may include:
  - Cool skin temperature
  - Abnormal skin color
  - Hair loss
  - Dry, scaly, atrophic skin
  - Brittle and hypertrophic toenails

- Dependent rubor
- Nonhealing wounds or ulcers
- Gangrene
- Weak or absent lower extremity pulses
- Bruits (aortic, femoral, iliac)

▶ DIAGNOSIS

- Ankle-brachial index (ABI):
  - Ultrasound assessment comparing the ratio of systolic pressures in the lower versus upper extremities
  - 1.0-1.4 normal
  - 0.91-0.99 borderline
  - ≤0.9 indicates PAD (<0.5 indicates severe lower extremity PAD)
  - >1.4 indicates noncompressible vessels and warrants further testing (such as the toe-brachial index [TBI])
- Arterial ultrasound, CT angiogram, and magnetic resonance angiogram (MRA) may be used to confirm the diagnosis.
- Contrast angiography is the gold standard and should be performed in patients expected to undergo revascularization.

▶ TREATMENT

- Medical management:
  - Antiplatelet therapy (such as aspirin or clopidogrel) decreases the risk of myocardial infarction, stroke, and death.
  - High-intensity statin therapy is given in women and men age ≤75 years unless contraindicated (moderate intensity in patients age >75 years).
  - Risk factor modification includes smoking cessation, aggressive glycemic control, and aggressive blood pressure control.
  - Supervised exercise therapy
  - Cilostazol may improve symptoms and increase pain-free walking distances in patients with claudication.
- Revascularization:
  - Often reserved for patients with significant pain, disability, or those who do not adequately respond to exercise or pharmacologic therapy
  - Patients with critical limb ischemia require urgent revascularization.
  - Options include angioplasty with or without stenting, bypass surgery, or hybrid operations (combination endovascular and open surgery).

CHAPTER 33

Aortic Dissection and Thoracic and Abdominal Aneurysms

Kelsey Ellender-Barthel, MPAS
Rebecca Clawson, PA-C

A 65-year-old man with a past medical history of hypertension, hyperlipidemia, diabetes mellitus, and a 50 pack-year smoking history presents with new-onset 10/10 chest pain radiating to his back and described as "ripping" in nature. Vitals are heart rate (HR) 120s, blood pressure (BP) 81/50, respiration rate (RR) 18, O_2 sat 92%. ECG is unremarkable except for tachycardia. Physical examination reveals unequal BP in the upper extremities and a diastolic heart murmur auscultated at the right heart border. A chest x-ray reveals a widened mediastinum. What is the most likely diagnosis, and what is the nest step in treatment?

▶ GENERAL FEATURES

- Aortic dissection:
  - Characterized by a disruption of the aortic media layer causing separation of the aortic wall layers
  - Most common acute disease of the aorta

- Two types:
  - Stanford Type A (more common): dissection involving ascending aorta and/or arch
  - Stanford Type B: dissection involving only the descending aorta
- Causes:
  - Degenerative: uncontrolled hypertension, aneurysm, bicuspid aortic valve
  - Genetic: Turner syndrome, Marfan syndrome, aortic coarctation
  - Trauma
- Aortic aneurysm:
  - Thoracic aortic aneurysm (TAA) is permanent dilation of a segment of aorta, typically caused by degenerative disease of the media, >150% of the normal diameter.
  - Most TAAs are found in the ascending aorta; second-most in the distal aorta past the left subclavian.

- Abdominal aortic aneurysm (AAA) is an abnormal dilation of the abdominal aorta with a diameter >3 cm (or 50% more than normal vessel diameter).
- Most common location of an AAA is infrarenal.
- AAA is most common in men age >60 years who smoke or have a significant history of smoking.
- Risk factors are similar to aortic dissection with the addition of atherosclerosis.

▶ CLINICAL ASSESSMENT

- Aortic dissection:
  - Acute chest pain is often ripping or tearing in nature; can radiate to the back; may also present as back, flank, or abdominal pain.
  - Additional symptoms based on the involvement of specific vessels:
    - Neurologic symptoms: cerebrovascular accident, altered mental status, and/or weakness in ipsilateral arm (due to carotid involvement)
    - Pain, numbness, or weakness in extremities (due to subclavian or femoral artery involvement and limb ischemia)
    - Abdominal pain (due to abdominal aorta involvement or mesenteric ischemic)
  - Hemodynamic compromise, often due to myocardial infarction (MI) (due to coronary involvement), tamponade (from pericardial effusion), or aortic rupture:
    - Hypotension/syncope more likely with Type A
    - Hypertension more likely with Type B
  - Physical examination may be notable for:
    - Unequal pulses and BP in upper extremities (>20 mm Hg)
    - Possible murmur of aortic regurgitation
    - Focal neurologic deficits depending on vessels affected
- Aortic aneurysm:
  - Most TAAs are asymptomatic and found incidentally on imaging:
    - No routine screening recommended
    - No symptoms typically present
  - AAA:
    - Symptoms and signs may include abdominal pain, referred back pain, pulsatile abdominal mass; patient may also be asymptomatic.
  - Ruptured aortic aneurysm typically leads to hemorrhagic shock and rapid hemodynamic collapse.

▶ DIAGNOSIS

- Aortic dissection:
  - Laboratory studies may reveal evidence of organ ischemia, such as elevated lactic acid or elevated blood urea nitrogen/serum creatinine (BUN/SCr).
  - Chest x-ray may show a widened mediastinum.

- ECG will typically only reveal ischemic changes if coronary arteries are involved.
- Definitive diagnosis is made by a CT angiogram:
  - Notable finding is a dissection flap separating the false lumen from the true lumen.
- Aortic aneurysm:
  - TAA:
    - Definitive diagnosis on CT chest with contrast or CT angiogram, if available
    - Chest x-ray may show widened mediastinum.
  - AAA:
    - One-time screening with ultrasound is recommended for 65- to 75-year-olds with a history of tobacco use.
    - If aneurysm found:
      - <3 cm, no surveillance
      - 3-3.9 cm, ultrasound every 2-3 years
      - 4-5.4 cm, ultrasound every 6-12 months
    - Definitive diagnosis with ultrasound
    - CT abdomen needed for surgical planning
  - Referral:
    - TAA: If found, refer to CT surgery; surgical indications vary based on size, rate of growth, and location.
    - AAA: If aneurysm is >5.0 cm, refer to vascular surgery.

▶ TREATMENT

- Aortic dissection:
  - Type A dissection is a surgical emergency requiring emergent cardiothoracic surgical consultation and repair to prevent ischemic complications and high accompanying mortality. Additional emergent management includes HR and BP control to reduce shear force stress on the aorta and minimize continued dissection.
  - Type B:
    - Typically treated conservatively with observation and medical management
    - BP and HR should be controlled to reduce shear force stress on the aorta. Titrated infusions are preferred for immediate management with subsequent conversion to oral agents.
    - Surgical consultation is required, and surgery may be indicated for persistent symptoms or complications.
- Prognosis:
  - One in five patients die before reaching the hospital.
  - Type A: 5%-30% mortality rate during or after surgical intervention
  - Type B: 10% mortality rate after medical therapy
- Aortic aneurysm:
  - TAA:
    - Aortic root/ascending aorta with or without arch: surgical resection and root repair

- Arch/descending aorta: endovascular surgical repair, open versus closed
- Medical management: address risk factors, BP, smoking
- AAA:
  - Immediate intervention is warranted for AAA with symptoms or expanding >0.5 cm in 6 months.
  - Endovascular stent grafting by vascular surgery and/or interventional cardiology
  - If emergent, open surgery
  - Medical management: BP management and smoking cessation
- Complications:
  - Rupture
  - Acute arterial occlusion
  - Dissection
- Prognosis:
  - TAA annual risk of rupture/death:
    - 2% if <5 cm
    - 3% if 5-5.9 cm
    - 8%-10% if >6 cm
- AAA annual risk of rupture/death:
  - 0% if <4 cm
  - 1% if 4-4.9 cm
  - 5%-10% if 5-5.9 cm
  - 10%-20% if 6-6.9 cm
  - 20%-40% if 7-7.9 cm
  - 30%-50% if >8 cm

Case Conclusion

The patient presents with classic signs of a thoracic dissection: ripping chest pain, aortic regurgitation, and unequal pulses. Additionally, he has risk factors and an ECG that does not show any signs of ischemia. A widened mediastinum could be a thymic mass or a thoracic aneurysm, but with his other signs and symptoms, thoracic dissection is the most likely. Because the type is unknown, you should order a CT angiogram next to determine if this is a Type A or Type B dissection. This will guide your therapy toward surgical and medical management, respectively.

CHAPTER 34

Arterial Embolism and Thrombosis

Danielle Vlazny, PA-C, MS

A 67-year-old male with known tobacco use and hypertension presents with sudden onset of pain in his left leg 2 hours ago. His left leg is cool to touch and pale. Bedside Doppler was unable to identify a dorsalis pedis pulse signal. ECG demonstrates atrial fibrillation. What is the patient's most likely cause of left leg symptoms?

▶ GENERAL FEATURES

- Thrombosis is commonly caused by atrial fibrillation (AF) or another embolic source (eg, aneurysms, stents), including the showering of unstable cholesterol plaques (atheroemboli).
- Less commonly, thrombosis in situ can occur in the setting of hypercoagulable states and malignancy.
- Risk factors include AF, valvular heart disease, hyperlipidemia, smoking, aneurysms, and recent vascular procedures.

▶ CLINICAL ASSESSMENT

- Onset is typically sudden and intense with patients presenting within hours.
- Signs and symptoms of arterial thrombus causing limb ischemia are classically described as "the six Ps" in the affected extremity:

- Pain
- Paresthesia
- Paralysis
- Pallor
- Pulselessness
- Poikilothermia (coldness)
- Mesenteric embolus/thrombus may present as:
  - Abdominal pain out of proportion to the physical examination, worse after eating
  - Nausea, vomiting
  - Blood in stool
- Patients may report a history of claudication, recent vascular procedures such as stenting, or other symptoms suggestive of embolic source or low-flow states such as AF or myocardial infarction (MI).

▶ DIAGNOSIS

- Electrocardiogram (ECG) may reveal arrhythmia such as AF or signs of ischemia.
- Echocardiogram may reveal thrombotic source or underlying dysfunction leading to a low-flow state.
- Arterial thrombus in extremities:
  - Manual palpation and arterial Doppler of all pulses should be performed and documented.

- CT angiogram (CTA) is often obtained as it is fast and widely available. CTA of the chest, abdomen, and pelvis with lower extremity runoff may help differentiate arterial thrombus from aortic dissection.
- Angiography is often obtained prior to surgical intervention.
- Mesenteric embolus/thrombus
  - CTA of abdomen and pelvis, including mesenteric arteries, should be obtained.
  - If no source of thrombus is identified, a hypercoagulable workup and age-appropriate malignancy screening may be indicated.

▶ TREATMENT

- Immediate initiation of heparin unless contraindicated
- Emergent vascular surgery consultation
- Limb embolus/thrombus
  - Revascularization/reperfusion through:
    - Embolectomy
    - Endarterectomy
    - Surgical bypass
    - Catheter-directed thrombolysis
- Mesenteric
  - Bowel rest
  - Stenting of affected artery
  - Exploratory laparotomy with resection of affected bowel, if infarcted
- In all patients, continued anticoagulation (in the setting of AF or hypercoagulable state), antiplatelet therapy, and lipid management are typically indicated.
- Following treatment of limb ischemia, patients are at high risk of reperfusion injury, resulting in limb edema, compartment syndrome, metabolic acidosis, hyperkalemia, arrhythmia, pulmonary edema, myoglobinuria, renal failure, and potentially death.

Case Conclusion

This patient's most likely cause of left leg symptoms is a cardioembolic complication with the source being the left atrial thrombus.

CHAPTER
35

Phlebitis/Thrombophlebitis, Venous Insufficiency, Varicose Veins, and Venous Malformation

Danielle Vlazny, PA-C, MS

A 34-year-old female presents to her primary care provider with a 3-day history of a hot, red lump on the inner part of her right thigh that is about 4 cm long. Otherwise, she feels well. She is 1 week postpartum after delivering a healthy baby boy. She has no history of blood clots. What is your next step in management of this patient? What will be the first-line treatment if the patient presents with complications in 5 years without any further thrombotic events?

▶ GENERAL FEATURES

- Phlebitis/thrombophlebitis:
  - Often occurs due to the presence of one or more of the Virchow triad:
    - Stasis
    - Endovascular injury
    - Hypercoagulability
  - Common risk factors include:
    - Surgery
    - Hospitalization
    - Trauma
    - Exogenous estrogen
    - Inflammatory bowel disease
    - Malignancy
    - Sepsis
    - Inherited hypercoagulable states
- Venous insufficiency:
  - Venous hypertension/congestion, often a result of venous valve damage/dysfunction; may follow deep vein thrombosis (DVT) or surgery and can have a genetic component.
- Varicose veins:
  - Most common in women following pregnancy
  - Also associated with obesity, genetics, phlebitis, and prolonged sitting or standing
- Venous malformation:
  - Genetic mutations resulting in vein wall changes and low-flow states as a result of their dilation and tortuous appearance
  - Can be difficult to differentiate from other venous diseases when small

▶ CLINICAL ASSESSMENT

- Phlebitis/thrombophlebitis:
  - Pain, erythema, palpable cord, tenderness, and localized edema/induration in affected extremity, most commonly the lower extremities

- Phlebitis often occurs at sites of venipuncture, IV, or PICC lines.
- Concern for DVT is raised if unilateral extremity edema, erythema, or calor is present.
- Venous insufficiency:
  - History of DVT or surgery raises suspicion.
  - Symptoms include lower extremity edema (unilateral or bilateral), pruritus, pain (often relieved with elevation, walking, or compression), heaviness, aching, stasis dermatitis/skin changes, and ulceration.
  - Check for Villalta score or CEAP classification findings including telangiectasia, varicose veins, edema, pigmentation or eczema, and venous ulcers.
  - Physical examination may also reveal palpable cords, tenderness, induration, or bruits in the lower extremities; pedal pulses are typically intact and normal.
- Varicose veins:
  - Dilated, bulging veins visible at the skin surface are often associated with the great saphenous vein (GSV).
  - Dark colored reticular veins are smaller in caliber.
  - Telangiectasia and spider veins may also be present.
  - Sites may be asymptomatic or have tenderness or aching.
  - Veins may be flat when supine or with elevation and bulge with leg dependency.
- Venous malformation:
  - Most commonly seen on the extremities and face
  - Usually only located in one spot on the body
  - Blue/purple discoloration of the skin overlying soft tissue mass; discoloration deepens with dependent positioning, Valsalva, or exercise.
  - Discolored area is in the same temperature as surrounding skin.
  - Will grow with growth to adulthood and can become symptomatic, usually painful
  - Some areas may be thrombosed or calcified.

▶ DIAGNOSIS

- Phlebitis/thrombophlebitis:
  - No recognized scoring system
  - Diagnosis is often made by clinical examination.
  - Venous duplex ultrasound can confirm diagnosis and rule out DVT.
  - Strongly consider ultrasound evaluation of contralateral limb, even in the absence of symptoms.
- Venous insufficiency:
  - Diagnosis based on clinical suspicion and physical examination findings
  - Confirmed by duplex ultrasound
  - Venous plethysmography if ultrasound is inconclusive
- Varicose veins:
  - Ultrasound can determine if varicose veins are associated with underlying venous insufficiency that may need to be treated first.
  - CT venogram can evaluate for perforating veins or pelvic varicosities, although it is not routinely needed for diagnosis.

- Venous malformation:
  - Clinical appearance is usually all that is needed.
  - For extensive lesions, further imaging by ultrasound or MRI may be helpful for treatment planning and to determine involvement of adjacent structures.
  - D-dimer may be elevated and can indicate localized intravascular coagulopathy related to low-flow state.

▶ TREATMENT

- Phlebitis/thrombophlebitis:
  - Treatment aimed at symptom relief
    - NSAIDs (unless anticoagulation is prescribed)
    - heat
    - ice
    - compression
    - encourage mobility
  - Some professional societies recommend low-molecular-weight (LMW) heparin for large superficial venous thromboses to prevent propagation to deep veins, especially for high-risk patients.
  - Concurrent DVT will obligate use of anticoagulation.
- Venous insufficiency:
  - Compression therapy, leg elevation, exercise, and weight control
  - Treatment of ulcerative disease and dermatitis
    - Stasis dermatitis can be treated with topical steroids and moisturizing lotion; zinc oxide creams may be used for advanced cases.
  - Symptomatic disease treated with various ablative procedures (radiofrequency, thermal, nonthermal, and mechanical)
- Varicose veins:
  - Compression therapy, leg elevation, exercise, and weight control can be used for symptom management and in early or mild disease, though these do not address underlying reasons for venous reflux.
  - Sclerotherapy can be performed on varicose, reticular, and spider veins both for symptomatic relief and cosmetic purposes.
- Venous malformation:
  - Compression therapy for extremity lesions
  - Aspirin and/or nonsteroidal anti-inflammatory medications (NSAIDs) for pain and inflammation control
  - Sclerotherapy to reduce pain and extent of lesions
  - Surgical excision may be possible for larger lesions.

Case Conclusion

For the next step in treating this patient, recommend venous duplex ultrasound to see if there is DVT associated with the superficial phlebitis noted on examination. In 5 years, if she presents with complications, she will likely be suffering from varicose veins from the phlebitis, and the standard of care is compression therapy.

CHAPTER

36

Polyarteritis Nodosa

Maryellen Blevins, MPAS, PA-C
Nata Parnes, MD

▶ GENERAL FEATURES

- Polyarteritis nodosa (PAN) is a systemic necrotizing vasculitis that affects small- and medium-sized arteries.
- Although most cases are idiopathic, PAN is associated with hepatitis B, hepatitis C, and hairy cell leukemia.
- PAN is most commonly diagnosed in middle-aged to older adults.
- PAN is slightly more common in men.
- With treatment, the 5-year survival rate for idiopathic PAN is 80%; PAN caused by hepatitis B or C has a higher mortality rate.

▶ CLINICAL ASSESSMENT

- PAN commonly presents with systemic symptoms: fatigue, weight loss, weakness, fever, and arthralgia.
- Presentation may also include painful nodules and other skin lesions (livedo reticularis, purpura, ulcers), hypertension, renal insufficiency (elevated creatinine, hematuria, glomerulonephritis), and abdominal pain (due to inflammation of the mesenteric arteries leading to bowel infarction and perforation), especially after meals.
- Asymmetric polyneuropathy is common at onset and involves sensory and motor deficits; with time, it may affect additional nerve branches, progressing to distal symmetric polyneuropathy.

- The range of presenting complaints varies widely as any organ in the body can be affected: orchitis, ischemic retinopathy, splenic infarction, and inflammation of the bronchial arteries.

▶ DIAGNOSIS

- Diagnosis is typically clinical, based on history and examination; no lab tests or markers are specific for PAN.
- Biopsy confirms diagnosis.
- If there is no clear site for performing a biopsy, angiography is recommended to determine the presence of microaneurysms in the renal, hepatic, and/or mesenteric vessels.
- Alternative causes of vasculitis should be worked up and ruled out.

▶ TREATMENT

- Corticosteroids are the main treatment for PAN.
- If the disease is refractory to steroids or involves major organs, cyclophosphamide is added to treat idiopathic PAN.
- Treatment for hepatitis B– or hepatitis C–related PAN involves a combination of antivirals with steroids and plasmapheresis.
- Rheumatology consultation is recommended; other specialty consultations should be done according to the specific organ system that is affected.

Section A Pretest: Acneiform Disorders

1. Which of the following are noninflammatory acne lesions?
   A. Nodules
   B. Comedones
   C. Pustules
   D. All of the above

2. Exacerbating triggers for rosacea include which of the following?
   A. Alcohol
   B. Stress
   C. Sun exposure
   D. All of the above

3. Which of the following is associated with the pathogenesis of acne?
   A. Follicular hyperkeratinization
   B. Increased sebum
   C. C. acnes
   D. All of the above

4. Which medication is used to treat facial erythema associated with rosacea?
   A. Topical brimonidine
   B. Oral isotretinoin
   C. Oral doxycycline
   D. Topical adapalene

5. An 18-year-old male presents with mild comedonal acne on his forehead, chin, and jawline. There are no acne lesions on his upper back and chest. He is not using any over-the-counter acne products at home. Which of the following is the most appropriate initial acne treatment for this patient?
   A. Oral minocycline
   B. Oral isotretinoin
   C. Topical adapalene
   D. Oral spironolactone

6. Which physical examination feature differentiates acne from rosacea?
   A. Pustules
   B. Comedones
   C. Papules
   D. Erythema

7. Which of the following acne treatments is effective at treating the four main pathogenic features of acne including increased sebum production, follicular hyperkeratinization, inflammation, and C. acnes?
   A. Benzoyl peroxide
   B. Topical retinoids
   C. Oral isotretinoin
   D. Oral antibiotics

8. Which topical medication is most commonly used to treat papulopustular rosacea?
   A. Metronidazole
   B. Clindamycin
   C. Ketoconazole
   D. Sulfacetamide

9. Which class of oral antibiotics are used most often in the treatment of acne?
   A. Tetracyclines
   B. Fluoroquinolones
   C. Cephalosporins
   D. Macrolides

10. What is the most common facial location associated with phymatous changes in a patient with rosacea?
    A. Chin
    B. Glabella
    C. Nose
    D. Forehead

Section B Pretest: Desquamation Disorders

1. Which of the following is the most important component of treatment for patients with SJS or TEN?
   A. IV antibiotics
   B. Discontinue the causative drug
   C. IV corticosteroids
   D. Surgical debridement

2. How is the diagnosis of SJS, SJS-TEN overlap, and TEN differentiated?
   A. Percentage of BSA involved
   B. Progression to sepsis or shock
   C. Patient age
   D. Etiology of causative agent

3. A 5-year-old male with recent acute otitis media (AOM) presents with an extremely painful rash and oropharyngeal ulceration. His recent AOM, which demonstrated bullae on the tympanic membranes, was treated with amoxicillin and acetaminophen PRN. On examination, he has a positive Nikolsky sign. You suspect SJS. Which of the following is the most likely etiology of his SJS?
   A. Amoxicillin
   B. Acetaminophen
   C. *M. pneumoniae*
   D. Human herpes virus

4. In contrast to initial skin involvement seen in SJS and TEN, what is the primary location and description of skin lesions in erythema multiforme major?
   A. Face, thorax, and macular
   B. Face, thorax, and targetoid
   C. Face, extremities, and macular
   D. Face, extremities, and targetoid

Section C Pretest: Disorders of Skin Integrity

1. You are working in the ICU, taking care of a 49-year-old male patient, weighing 79 kg, who has second- and third-degree burns over ~15% of the body. When taking into consideration the fluid resuscitation for this patient using the Parkland formula, what is the approximate fluid volume to be given over the first 8 hours of care?
   A. 1.7 L
   B. 40 L
   C. None
   D. 3.5 L

2. Which of the following topical therapies is appropriate for short-term use in a flare of stasis dermatitis?
   A. Betamethasone dipropionate ointment 0.05%
   B. Clobetasol propionate cream 0.05%
   C. Fluocinonide gel 0.05%
   D. Triamcinolone acetonide ointment 0.1%

3. Which of the following is a preventative intervention that should be implemented for persons at risk for pressure ulcer development and those with existing pressure ulcers?
   A. While in a lateral decubitus position, patients should be placed at a 60° angle.
   B. Patients should be repositioned at a frequency of every 4 hours on a standard hospital bed.
   C. Use reactive mattress overlay support surfaces such as foam, gel, or alternating air pads.
   D. Perform routine inspection of the skin and pressure points every 2–3 days.

4. You are working in a postsurgical unit. You have a visit with a patient who is complaining of discharge from their abdominal surgical wound. This patient is 2 weeks postoperative from an exploratory laparotomy, denies fevers, and endorses a well-healing wound for the most part, until he noticed some yellow-brown discharge coming from a portion of the wound that also appeared to be opening slightly, per the patient description. When you expose the

area to examine it, the superior portion of the wound is slightly erythematous with brown discharge coming from an ~2 cm area of dehiscence. What is the next best step for the wound care of this patient?

A. Get a plastic surgery consult; this patient is going to need an immediate skin graft to cover the exposed tissue.

B. Gently free the involved area of the wound closure staples, clean the wound, take a culture of the fluid, place the patient on antibiotics, and use wet-to-dry dressings to begin healing this portion of the wound by secondary intention.

C. Call the general surgeon to take this patient back to the operation room to have the entire incision revised.

D. Do nothing; this is normal healing for large abdominal wounds.

5. The "inverted champagne bottle" appearance of the lower leg is associated with which of the following complications of venous stasis?

A. Acroangiodermatitis

B. Hemosiderin deposition

C. Kaposi sarcoma

D. Lipodermatosclerosis

6. Which of the following conditions is an established risk factor that contributes to the development of pressure wounds?

A. Urinary incontinence

B. Hypothyroidism

C. Lumbar spondylosis

D. Hyperalbuminemia

7. A 38-year-old female presents to your clinic complaining of discoloration of her lower leg. She experienced a deep venous thrombosis 6 months ago and was treated as an outpatient. What is the most important clinical intervention for this patient at this time?

A. Anticoagulation

B. Compression

C. Elevation

D. Topical corticosteroid application

8. What is the preferred treatment approach to a pressure ulcer that contains a thick, adherent, and large amount of nonviable tissue associated with cellulitis?

A. Application of topical silver sulfadiazine (Silvadene) cream

B. Hydrocolloid autolytic debridement

C. Mechanical debridement with wet-to-dry gauze dressings

D. Sharp debridement

9. Which of the following is the most common cause of stasis dermatitis?

A. Surgery

B. Thrombosis

C. Trauma

D. Venous insufficiency

10. An elderly male patient with a history of bed confinement is found to have a left posterior hip pressure sore. Further examination of the lesion reveals a full-thickness tissue loss with visible subcutaneous fat that extends to, but not through, the fascia. There is no visible slough, eschar, muscle, or bone. What is the correct ulcer stage according to NPUAP classification system?

A. Stage I

B. Stage II

C. Stage III

D. Stage IV

Section D Pretest: Disorders of the Hair and Nails

1. Onychomycosis is also known as which of the following?

A. Tinea manuum

B. Tinea pedis

C. Tinea unguium

D. Tinea cruris

2. Anagen effluvium is considered which type of hair loss?

A. Diffuse scarring

B. Diffuse nonscarring

C. Local scarring

D. Local nonscarring

3. You are seeing a patient with alopecia and suspect telogen effluvium as the cause. Which of the following is the best recommendation to give the patient about treatment?

A. Reassurance that the condition will resolve on its own is recommended.

B. Intralesional corticosteroid injections are needed.

C. Topical minoxidil will need to be used and continued indefinitely.

D. Oral antifungal medication is recommended.

4. You are seeing a patient who presents with redness and swelling of their second to fourth right nail folds for the past 8 months. The patient cleans houses for a living and uses a lot of cleaning products. You notice tender inflammation around the base of the nail fold. Which of the following is the best treatment for this condition?

A. An oral antibiotic with *S. aureus* coverage

B. Keep hands clean and dry and protected from irritants

C. Lance the nail folds

D. Topical antibiotic to affected areas

5. Oral antifungals are sometimes used to treat onychomycosis, but caution is warranted due to which of the following reasons?

A. They can cause acute kidney failure.

B. They increase the risk of heart attacks and strokes.

C. They are hepatotoxic.

D. They can cause blindness.

Section E Pretest: Envenomations and Arthropod Bite Reactions

1. A cluster rash noted on exposed skin upon waking is most likely due to which of the following?

A. Ant bites

B. Spider bite

C. Scorpion sting

D. Bedbugs

2. While gardening, a 22-year-old female was stung by a bee. She presents complaining of feeling dizzy, nausea, and shortness of breath. Physical examination reveals expiratory wheezing, a diffuse raised erythematous maculopapular rash, and a blood pressure of 82/50. Initial treatment of this patient would include which of the following?

A. Epinephrine 0.3 mg IM plus IV fluid bolus

B. Diphenhydramine PO plus famotidine PO

C. IV steroids plus IV fluid bolus

D. Six vials of CroFab IV

Section F Pretest: Infectious Diseases

1. Which of the following is an erythematous infection of the epidermis, upper dermis, and superficial lymphatics with distinct elevated borders?

A. Cellulitis

B. Folliculitis

C. Furuncle

D. Erysipelas

2. Incision and drainage is first-line treatment for all of the following, except:

A. Abscess

B. Furuncle

C. Folliculitis

D. Carbuncle

3. In cases of head lice in which the patient or the patient's parents are hesitant to expose their child to the chemicals of medical treatment, which of the following treatments would be most effective?

A. Nit comb for manual removal

B. Shaving the head

C. Mayonnaise to the hair shaft

D. Showering with very hot water

4. A 24-year-old sexually active female patient complains of vaginal pruritus and thick, cheese-like vaginal discharge. The most likely cause is which of the following?

A. Chlamydia

   B. Gonorrhea
   C. Bacterial vaginosis
   D. Vaginal candidiasis

5. An elderly woman has been living in a nursing home for the past 3 months. When visiting, her daughter notices a dry, flaking rash on her mother's forearms and learns that there is an outbreak of similar rash in the home. Which of the following is the recommended treatment of the most likely diagnosis?
   A. Permethrin 5% cream
   B. Lindane 1% lotion
   C. Ivermectin orally
   D. Ivermectin orally and permethrin 5% cream

6. Dermatophyte infections commonly affect all but which of the following areas?
   A. Groin
   B. Eye
   C. Scalp
   D. Nails

7. You are seeing a patient with a rash in the genital area for the past 3 weeks. On examination, you notice multiple discrete dome-shaped waxy lesions with umbilication. Which of the following is the most likely diagnosis?
   A. Condyloma acuminata
   B. Molluscum contagiosum
   C. Verruca vulgaris
   D. Verruca plantaris
   E. Verruca planus

8. Which of the following is first-line treatment for impetigo?
   A. Mupirocin
   B. Clindamycin
   C. Incision and drainage
   D. Penicillin

9. You suspect a patient of having a dermatophyte infection. Which is the best test to confirm your diagnosis?
   A. Wet mount
   B. Fungal culture
   C. KOH prep
   D. Anaerobic culture

10. Condyloma acuminata is caused by which of the following?
   A. Poxvirus
   B. Herpes simplex virus
   C. Herpes zoster virus
   D. Human papillomavirus

11. A child has a family heirloom teddy bear that was his great grandmother's, but the child was just diagnosed with scabies. What should you recommend the family do?
   A. Apply topical permethrin spray to the teddy bear.
   B. Wash the teddy bear on the highest temperature setting.
   C. Place the teddy bear outside in the sun for a couple of days.
   D. Seal the teddy bear in a plastic bag for at least 1 week.

12. A poxvirus causes which of the following?
   A. Verrucae plantaris
   B. Herpes simplex
   C. Molluscum contagiosum
   D. Verrucae vulgaris
   E. Condyloma acuminata

13. Esophageal candidiasis is most often associated with which disease process?
   A. AIDS
   B. Strep throat
   C. Endocarditis
   D. Gastroesophageal reflux disease

14. Which of the following areas is more likely affected in a child with scabies than in an adult?
   A. Webs of the fingers
   B. Axillae
   C. Genitalia
   D. Palms

15. Verruca plantaris is also known as which of the following?
   A. Plantar warts
   B. Common warts
   C. Flat warts
   D. Genital warts
   E. Molluscum

16. Skin infections are most often caused by which of the following pathogens?
   A. *Staphylococcus aureus*
   B. *Moraxella catarrhalis*
   C. *Salmonella*
   D. *Escherichia coli*

17. Which of the following is the single universally effective treatment of verrucae?
   A. Liquid nitrogen
   B. Ablation
   C. Excision
   D. Curettage
   E. There is no single universally effective treatment of verrucae

Section G Pretest: Keratotic Disorders

1. Actinic keratosis lesions may transform into which type of skin cancer?
   A. Basal cell carcinoma
   B. Squamous cell carcinoma
   C. Malignant melanoma
   D. All of the above

2. Treatment options for seborrheic keratosis may include which of the following?
   A. Topical imiquimod
   B. Liquid nitrogen cryotherapy
   C. Topical 5-FU
   D. All of the above

3. Risk factors for the development of actinic keratosis include which of the following?
   A. Increasing age
   B. Fitzpatrick skin types I, II, and III
   C. Chronic sun exposure
   D. All of the above

4. Common locations for seborrheic keratosis include which of the following?
   A. Face
   B. Back
   C. Extremities
   D. All of the above

5. A 65-year-old male presents with multiple AKs on his scalp. Which of the following treatment options would be appropriate to treat his current lesions as well as subclinical lesions?
   A. Liquid nitrogen cryotherapy
   B. Topical 5-FU
   C. Topical adapalene
   D. All of the above

6. Seborrheic dermatitis is associated with which skin microbe?
   A. *C. acnes*
   B. *M. furfur*
   C. *S. aureus*
   D. *Candida*

7. Treatment options for actinic keratosis may include which of the following?
   A. Liquid nitrogen cryotherapy
   B. Topical 5-FU
   C. Topical imiquimod
   D. All of the above

8. Which of the following statements regarding seborrheic keratosis is correct?
   A. Seborrheic keratosis is a precursor lesion of squamous cell carcinoma.
   B. Seborrheic keratosis lesions appear most frequently in young Caucasian women.
   C. Seborrheic keratosis is a benign epithelial tumor.
   D. All of the above

9. Common locations for seborrheic dermatitis include which of the following?
   A. Glabella
   B. Nasolabial folds
   C. Scalp
   D. All of the above

10. Common locations for the development of actinic keratosis include which of the following?
    A. Face
    B. Ears
    C. Scalp
    D. All of the above

11. A 22-year-old male complains of a mildly pruritic facial rash. On examination, there is erythema and maculopapular yellow-orange scaling lesions with a greasy texture of the nasolabial folds bilaterally. The remainder of the face is clear. A skin scraping demonstrates *M. furfur*. What is the most likely diagnosis?
    A. Seborrheic dermatitis
    B. Atopic dermatitis
    C. Perioral dermatitis
    D. Impetigo

12. A 22-year-old male complains of a mildly pruritic facial rash. On examination, there is erythema and maculopapular yellow-orange scaling lesions with a greasy texture of the nasolabial folds bilaterally. The remainder of the face is clear. A skin scraping demonstrates *M. furfur*. Appropriate treatment would include which of the following?
    A. Topical ketoconazole
    B. Oral metronidazole
    C. Oral doxycycline
    D. Topical adapalene

13. A 65-year-old male complains of a brown painless lesion on his back. On examination, there is a solitary discrete papular lesion with a stuck-on appearance. What is the most likely diagnosis?
    A. Seborrheic keratosis
    B. Actinic keratosis
    C. Seborrheic dermatitis
    D. Café-au-lait spot

14. Seborrheic dermatitis occurs more frequently in individuals with which underlying condition?
    A. Parkinson disease
    B. Diabetes mellitus
    C. Hypothyroidism
    D. Rheumatoid arthritis

15. Management options for seborrheic keratosis may include which of the following?
    A. Liquid nitrogen cryotherapy
    B. Curettage
    C. Observation
    D. All of the above

Section H Pretest: Malignancies

1. A 72-year-old man presents with a lesion on his shoulder that has doubled in size over the past several months. The lesion is nontender and does not bleed, but the patient's wife says it has been getting bigger and darker on one side. The macule is 7 mm in diameter. Which is the next best step?
   A. Liquid nitrogen cryotherapy
   B. Reassurance and observation
   C. Refer to dermatology for biopsy
   D. Topical imiquimod cream

2. Mohs micrographic surgery is the best treatment option in which of the following scenarios?
   A. A 6-mm superficial BCC located on the shoulder
   B. A 5-mm nodular BCC located on the infraorbital rim
   C. A 4-mm SCC located on the back
   D. A 5-mm SCC located on the abdomen

3. A 57-year-old woman presents with a nonhealing lesion on her back that has grown larger over the past few months. The 7-mm lesion is ulcerated and mildly bleeding with surrounding erythema. Squamous cell carcinoma is suspected. Which of the following interventions is part of the complete treatment plan?
   A. Topical imiquimod cream
   B. Excisional biopsy with a 6-mm margin
   C. Excisional biopsy with a 4-mm margin
   D. Cryosurgery only due to size of lesion

4. A 55-year-old female complains of a nonhealing lesion on her left cheek. Examination reveals a 6-mm pearly papule with surface telangiectasias and a central erosion. What is the most appropriate next step in management?
   A. Liquid nitrogen
   B. Curettage and electrodessication
   C. Observation and follow-up in 3 months
   D. Shave biopsy

Section I Pretest: Papulosquamous Disorders

1. What is the first line treatment of a patient with mild psoriasis?
   A. Broadband UVB
   B. Emollients
   C. Methotrexate
   D. Narrowband UVB

2. Which of the following is NOT a characteristic presentation of lichen planus?
   A. Pustular
   B. Planar
   C. Purple
   D. Pruritic

3. Which of the following is a common physical examination finding associated with psoriasis?
   A. Fatigue
   B. Nail pitting
   C. Pruritic lesions
   D. Xerophthalmia

4. Which of the following is the first-line treatment for adult atopic dermatitis?
   A. Topical emollients
   B. Systemic steroids
   C. Topical antifungal/steroid cream
   D. Extended bathing duration

5. How is psoriasis most commonly diagnosed?
   A. Biopsy
   B. Clinical impression
   C. Complete metabolic panel
   D. Diagnosis of exclusion

6. A 17-year-old male who is wearing jeans and a large belt buckle presents with a 4″ × 3″ red, papular lesion directly under his umbilicus. It has been present for 2 weeks. Which of the following is the most likely diagnosis?
   A. Contact dermatitis (from possible nickel in his belt buckle)
   B. Atopic dermatitis
   C. Lichen planus
   D. Pityriasis rosea

7. Which of the following is a risk factor for the development of psoriasis?
   A. Chronic skin irritation
   B. Dehydration
   C. Sun exposure
   D. Type 2 diabetes mellitus

Section J Pretest: Pigment Disorders

1. Vitiligo has a strong association with which type of disorders?
   A. Musculoskeletal
   B. Endocrine
   C. Pulmonary
   D. Cardiac

2. Which of the following is a first-line treatment for mild melasma?
   A. Hydroquinone 4% cream
   B. Chemical peel
   C. Oral tranexamic acid
   D. Laser or light therapy

3. Depigmentation therapy for vitiligo would include which of the following?
   A. Afamelanotide
   B. Phototherapy with wide-band UV light
   C. 20% monobenzylether of hydroquinone (MBEH, Benoquin)
   D. Topical steroids

4. Which patient would be the best candidate for laser treatment of melasma?
   A. Newly diagnosed with mild melasma
   B. Poor response to hydroquinone-only therapy
   C. Suboptimal melasma outcome after using topical treatment and chemical peels
   D. In the maintenance period after successful use of triple therapy and no melasma recurrence

5. Characteristics of vitiligo nonsegmental lesions include which of the following?
   A. Linear and unilateral distribution
   B. Lesions do not cross the midline
   C. Lacks association with autoimmune disorders such as thyroiditis
   D. Closely linked to autoimmune markers and thyroid disease

6. Triple therapy in treatment of melasma would include which of the following combinations?
   A. Skin-lightening compound, retinoid, steroid
   B. Skin-lightening compound, chemical peel, laser therapy
   C. Retinoid, chemical peel, laser therapy
   D. Skin-lightening compound, retinoid, laser therapy

7. Which of the following is a main component of maintenance therapy to prevent relapse of melasma?
   A. Use of hydroquinone 4% cream twice daily
   B. Aggressive use of broad-spectrum and visible-light sunscreens
   C. Monthly laser light therapy in darker individuals
   D. Use of oral tranexamic acid daily

8. A small localized areas of vitiligo would benefit best from first-line treatment with which of the following?
   A. Topical steroid and laser therapy
   B. Depigmentation therapy
   C. Afamelanotide
   D. MBEH

9. Vitiligo is best described as which of the following?
   A. Acute disorder associated with diffuse hyperpigmentation.
   B. Inherited disorder associated with melanocyte overproduction
   C. Acquired depigmentation disorder
   D. Acute depigmentation disorder affecting only males

Section K Pretest: Vascular Abnormalities

1. Which of the following is NOT a risk factor for cherry angioma and telangiectasia?
   A. Advanced age
   B. Use of anticoagulants
   C. Genetic predisposition
   D. Environmental exposure

2. The description the patient gives of skin appearance of a cherry angioma is?
   A. Painless red lacey skin pattern on the torso
   B. Painful large round skin lesion that is blanchable
   C. Round painless skin papule that is cherry red in color
   D. Painful red skin rash that presents in clusters in the lower extremities

3. What is true of cherry angiomas and telangiectasias?
   A. Biopsies are generally required to make the diagnosis.
   B. Laser treatment prevents progression of other associated medical conditions.
   C. Most cherry angiomas and telangiectasias are benign conditions.
   D. Younger men are at highest risk for developing these disorders.

4. What is the definitive treatment for telangiectasias?
   A. Sclerotherapy
   B. Skin grafting
   C. Topical steroids
   D. Vitamin E supplementation

Section L Pretest: Vesiculobullous Disease

1. Liz, a 12-year-old African American female who recently moved to the area, presents to the office with 3 × 2 patches of hard skin on her back. Mom says her previous pediatrician diagnosed Liz with scleroderma. What can be done with Liz's hard patches?
   A. Steroids to make the patches regress and disappear
   B. Moisturizer followed by stretching of the skin
   C. ACE inhibitor plus a PPI
   D. No treatment available

2. Diagnosis of pemphigoid or pemphigus requires which of the following testing?
   A. Blood work
   B. Skin biopsy
   C. Imaging
   D. No testing available

3. Who is most commonly diagnosed with scleroderma?
   A. Male Caucasian
   B. Female Caucasian
   C. Male African American
   D. Female African American

4. Robin, a 42-year-old Caucasian female, presents to the office with Raynaud phenomenon. She has also noticed that her hands feel stiff, but she attributes that to more computer time at work. What lab test would be appropriate to test for scleroderma?
   A. ANA
   B. SPEP/UPEP
   C. RA factor
   D. UACR

5. What does CREST stand for?
   A. **C**holesterol, **R**aynaud phenomenon, **E**mbolization, **S**clerodactyly, **T**elangiectasia
   B. **C**alcinosis, **R**aynaud phenomenon, **E**sophageal dysfunction, **S**clerodactyly, **T**elangiectasia
   C. **C**holesterol, **R**enal dysfunction, **E**mbolization, **S**clerodactyly, **T**elangiectasia
   D. **C**alcinosis, **R**aynaud Phenomenon, **E**mbolization, **S**clerodactyly, **T**elangiectasia

6. Alvin is a 58-year-old African American male with a history of shortness of breath. He presents to the office with worsening symptoms. His pulmonologist tells him that his pulmonary function tests are worse. Alvin tells you that he has noticed that he cannot make a fist as well with his left hand. On examination, you note the tough skin and decrease range of motion of the flexors. What is Alvin's most likely diagnosis?
   A. Scleroderma: localized disease
   B. Scleroderma: CREST syndrome
   C. Scleroderma: Diffuse systemic disease
   D. Tuberculosis

Section M Pretest: Other Dermatologic Disorders

1. What percentage of the population has a diagnosis of hidradenitis suppurativa?
   A. 50%-75%
   B. 25%-50%
   C. 10%-25%
   D. 1%-4%

2. A 44-year-old male patient reports a painful, rubbery 2-cm skin nodule that has been stable in size. He has a history of other similar but nonpainful lesions. You suspect he has which of the following?
   A. Lipoma
   B. Liposarcoma
   C. Angiolipoma
   D. Squamous cell carcinoma

3. Which of the following is NOT a trigger that could initiate a flare of hidradenitis suppurativa?
   A. Smoking
   B. Tight clothing
   C. Poor hygiene
   D. Stress

4. Photosensitivity reactions can be associated with which of the following systemic diseases?
   A. Diverticulitis
   B. Systemic lupus erythematosus (SLE)
   C. Hyperlipidemia
   D. Hodgkin lymphoma

5. While performing a routine physical for a healthy 17-year-old male patient, you note punctate pits at the midline of his gluteal cleft. There is no associated tenderness, fluctuance, or drainage, and he denies a history of pain in this area. What is the most likely diagnosis?
   A. Acute pilonidal disease
   B. Asymptomatic pilonidal disease
   C. Chronic pilonidal disease
   D. Pilonidal abscess

6. A 68-year-old male patient with a history of hypertension treated with lisinopril 40 mg daily is also being treated with doxycycline 100 mg BID for a methicillin-resistant *S. aureus* infection of the skin presents to the clinic with 1 day of vesicular lesions on both hands after fishing all day yesterday. He feels well otherwise and is afebrile. You suspect which of the following causes for the skin lesions?
   A. Herpes zoster
   B. Photosensitivity reaction
   C. Drug interaction between lisinopril and doxycycline
   D. Allergic reaction to doxycycline

7. Which of the following is a risk factor for acanthosis nigricans?
   A. Psoriasis
   B. Obesity
   C. Hypertension
   D. Chronic kidney disease

ANSWERS AND EXPLANATIONS TO SECTION A PRETEST

1. **B.** Comedones, including open and closed types, are noninflammatory lesions. Nodules and pustules are associated with inflammation.
2. **D.** Numerous triggers for rosacea have been identified, including sun exposure, spicy foods, alcohol, hot beverages, exercise, hot weather, wind, embarrassment, anger, stress, vasodilating medications, and topical skin irritants.
3. **D.** Follicular hyperkeratinizations, increased sebum, *C. acnes*, and inflammatory are the features associated with acne pathogenesis.
4. **A.** Two topical agents, brimonidine and oxymetazoline, have been approved to treat facial erythema associated with rosacea.
5. **C.** Topical retinoids (Tretinoin, Adapalene, Tazarotene) are the mainstay of treatment for mild comedonal acne.
6. **B.** Lack of comedones is the distinguishing feature between acne and rosacea. Acne has both open and closed comedones. Rosacea lacks comedones.
7. **B.** Topical retinoids (tretinoin, adapalene, tazarotene) are the mainstay of treatment for comedonal acne.
8. **A.** Topical metronidazole, ivermectin, and azelaic acid are used as treatment options for papulopustular rosacea.
9. **A.** The tetracyclines including doxycycline and minocycline are used most commonly for the treatment of acne.
10. **C.** The nose is the most common location for phymatous changes to occur.

ANSWERS AND EXPLANATIONS TO SECTION B PRETEST

1. **B.** Discontinuing the causative drug is the mainstay of treatment for SJS and TEN; early discontinuation reduces mortality. IV antibiotics, IV corticosteroids, and surgical debridement are not routinely indicated in these patients.
2. **A.** SJS, SJS-TEN overlap, and TEN all fall on the same disease continuum. The diagnosis is distinguished based on the percentage of BSA involved.
3. **C.** Although medications are the most common cause of SJS, this patient has not taken any high-risk causative medications. The second most common cause of SJS is *M. pneumoniae* infection, which is much more likely in this patient. *M. pneumoniae* is a common pathogen in AOM and may be associated with bullous myringitis.
4. **D.** Erythema multiforme major is a distinct disease process from SJS-TEN, with a different pathogenesis and different cutaneous appearance. Erythema multiforme major presents most commonly with targetoid, raised lesions that start on the extremities and face. SJS and TEN lesions are primarily erythematous macules, which typically affected the face and thorax first.

ANSWERS AND EXPLANATIONS TO SECTION C PRETEST

1. **A.** The Parkland formula is a common formula for the calculation of fluid volume repletion for burn patients. It is calculated as $3 - 4$ mL $\times$ %BSA burned $\times$ weight (kg). The first half should be given over the first 8 hours, and the second half over the subsequent 16 hours. Therefore, for this patient, 3 mL $\times$ 15 $\times$ 79 = 3555.0 mL; 3555.0/2 (first half) = 1775.5 mL/1000 = 1.775 L over the first 8 hours.
2. **D.** Medium-potency topical steroids can treat pruritus and inflammation associated with stasis dermatitis. High-potency steroids should be avoided due to increased risk of skin atrophy and ulceration.
3. **C.** The use of support surfaces instead of standard hospital mattresses results in a significant relative reduction in pressure ulcer incidence.
4. **B.** For a small portion of a surgical wound that has dehisced, the best choice for the patient is to allow that section to heal via secondary intention while monitoring the status of the wound and the rest of the patient's incision. Antibiotics are prudent, and keeping the area clean and covered is important to ensure healing and lack of infection.
5. **D.** Lipodermatosclerosis is deep, acute inflammation characterized by underlying fat necrosis that can resemble erythema nodosum. The appearance of the lower legs in lipodermatosclerosis has been described as an inverted champagne bottle.
6. **A.** The presence of moisture, from perspiration or incontinence, factors into the breakdown of tissue breakdown and maceration. These processes can initiate or worsen pressure ulcers. Furthermore, contaminants from urinary or fecal incontinence irritate skin and increase the risk of secondary wound infections.
7. **B.** Compression is first-line treatment for stasis dermatitis, but skin pigmentation may not resolve.
8. **D.** Sharp debridement is the treatment of choice for pressure wounds characterized by thick, adherent, and/or large amounts of nonviable tissue and when advancing cellulitis or signs of sepsis are present.
9. **D.** Venous insufficiency is the most common cause of stasis dermatitis. It may be caused by underlying vascular conditions such as congestive heart failure, medications such as amlodipine that cause lower extremity edema, and pregnancy.

10. **C.** According to NPUAP, the description identifies a stage III pressure wound. These wounds are characterized by a full-thickness skin loss involving damage or necrosis of subcutaneous tissue that may extend down to, but not through, the underlying fascia. There is no exposure of underlying muscle or bone. Clinically, this manifests as a deep crater with or without undermining of adjacent tissue.

▶ **ANSWERS AND EXPLANATIONS TO SECTION D PRETEST**

1. **C.** Tinea unguium is a fungal infection of the nail and is also known as onychomycosis.
2. **B.** Anagen effluvium does not scar and its distribution is diffuse.
3. **A.** Telogen effluvium is a temporary diffuse hair loss after a stressful event. It is self-limited and does not require any treatment. The hair will eventually regrow on its own.
4. **B.** This time frame and history of chemical exposure suggest chronic paronychia. While antibiotics, steroids, and antifungals are sometimes needed for this condition, the most important treatment is to keep the skin dry and protect it from chemical exposure. The skin will not heal if it continues to be macerated or exposed to chemicals.
5. **C.** Oral antifungals are known to cause hepatotoxicity, and it is recommended to monitor liver function when using them for treatment.

▶ **ANSWERS AND EXPLANATIONS TO SECTION E PRETEST**

1. **D.** Bedbugs feed at night while patients are sleeping and focus on exposed skin.
2. **A.** This patient is presenting in anaphylaxis and needs epinephrine 0.3 mg IM plus IV fluid bolus.

▶ **ANSWERS AND EXPLANATIONS TO SECTION F PRETEST**

1. **D.** Erysipelas is an infection of the epidermis, upper dermis, and superficial lymphatics and is erythematous with distinct elevated borders and generally associated with fever, lymphangitis, and regional lymphadenopathy.
2. **C.** Treatment of folliculitis is generally not indicated; however, if infection is moderate to severe, then treatment is based on the etiology.
3. **A.** A nit comb alone for manual removal of nits is effective, but tedious.
4. **D.** Vaginal candidiasis presents with vaginal pruritus and thick, white to yellow discharge.

5. **D.** The patient has symptoms of crusted scabies, which is difficult to treat. Both oral and topical therapies are indicated.
6. **B.** Tinea cruris (groin), tinea capitis (scalp), and tinea unguium (nail) are all common dermatophyte infections. Dermatophyte infections of the eye are not common.
7. **B.** Molluscum contagiosum presents as single or multiple flesh to pink-colored, dome-shaped, waxy umbilicated skin lesions.
8. **A.** Treatment of impetigo is to focus on reducing the spread of infection and improving the appearance of the lesion. Mupirocin or retapamulin for 5 days is the first-line therapy.
9. **C.** KOH prep of a skin scraping will reveal segmented hyphae.
10. **D.** The human papillomavirus causes condyloma acuminata.
11. **D.** Items that cannot be washed, or in this case is likely too delicate to wash, should be sealed in plastic for at least 1 week in the case of scabies.
12. **C.** Molluscum contagiosum is caused by the molluscum contagiosum virus, a poxvirus.
13. **A.** Esophageal candidiasis is an AIDS defining illness in patients who are HIV positive.
14. **D.** Children are affected on the neck, face, palms, and soles of the feet.
15. **A.** Plantar warts are also called verruca plantaris.
16. **A.** *S. aureus* is the most common pathogen found in skin infections.
17. **E.** There is no single universally effective treatment of verrucae.

▶ **ANSWERS AND EXPLANATIONS TO SECTION G PRETEST**

1. **B.** Actinic keratosis lesions can transform into squamous cell carcinoma.
2. **B.** Liquid nitrogen cryotherapy and curettage are the best treatment options for seborrheic keratosis.
3. **D.** Risk factors for the development of actinic keratosis include increasing age; Fitzpatrick skin types I, II, and III; and chronic sun exposure.
4. **D.** Seborrheic keratosis is commonly found on the face, back, and extremities.
5. **B.** Multiple current and subclinical actinic keratoses should be treated with topical 5-FU.
6. **B.** *M. furfur* is associated with seborrheic dermatitis.
7. **D.** Treatment options for actinic keratosis include liquid nitrogen cryotherapy, topical 5-FU, and topical imiquimod.
8. **C.** Seborrheic keratosis is a benign epithelial tumor that is more common in older men than women.
9. **D.** Seborrheic dermatitis may be found in the glabella, nasolabial folds, and scalp.

10. **D.** Actinic keratosis commonly develops on the sun-exposed areas of the face, ears, and scalp.
11. **A.** Seborrheic dermatitis presents as a mildly pruritic facial rash with erythema and maculopapular yellow-orange scaling lesions with a greasy texture. The nasolabial folds are a common site for seborrheic dermatitis.
12. **A.** Topical ketoconazole is the treatment of choice for seborrheic dermatitis.
13. **A.** Seborrheic keratosis commonly presents as a papular lesion that can range from light skin colored to black.
14. **A.** Patients with Parkinson disease are more likely to have seborrheic dermatitis.
15. **D.** Liquid nitrogen cryotherapy, curettage, and observation are all appropriate management options for seborrheic keratosis.

ANSWERS AND EXPLANATIONS TO SECTION H PRETEST

1. **C.** This lesion is suspicious for malignant melanoma, and the patient should be referred to dermatology for biopsy.
2. **B.** The preferred treatment for BCC on the head and face is Mohs surgery.
3. **C.** Treatment for squamous cell carcinoma is excision of the lesion with a 4-mm margin.
4. **D.** The lesion described has features of BCC. Biopsy is recommended to confirm the diagnosis.

ANSWERS AND EXPLANATIONS TO SECTION I PRETEST

1. **B.** Emollients should be prescribed before initiating other medical treatments for psoriasis.
2. **A.** Lichen planus lesions are characteristically planar, purple, pruritic, polygonal, papules, and plaques (the 6 Ps), but not pustular.
3. **B.** Nail pitting is a common physical examination finding seen in psoriasis.
4. **A.** Topical emollients are the first-line treatment for adult atopic dermatitis.
5. **B.** Psoriasis is most commonly diagnosed from the characteristic physical examination findings.
6. **A.** This patient presents with a classic presentation of a nickel allergy, causing contact dermatitis.
7. **A.** When skin is chronically irritated, it is more likely to develop psoriasis.

ANSWERS AND EXPLANATIONS TO SECTION J PRETEST

1. **B.** Vitiligo has been associated with endocrine system disorders, especially thyroid disorders.

2. **A.** Hydroquinone 4% is a recommended first-line treatment for melasma.
3. **C.** Depigmentation therapy is geared toward lightening normal skin to match the tone of the vitiligo lesion. 20% monobenzylether of hydroquinone (MBEH) is the only FDA approved depigmentation treatment.
4. **C.** Laser therapy may be used when first- and second-line treatments result in suboptimal outcomes.
5. **D.** Nonsegmental vitiligo is linked to thyroid disorders.
6. **A.** Triple therapy refers to a combination of topical agents consisting of skin-lightening compound (eg, hydroquinone), retinoid (eg, tretinoin), and steroid (eg, fluocinolone).
7. **B.** Sunscreens that block UV and visible light (such as from computers) are an important component of managing melasma, especially after active treatment.
8. **A.** Small, localized areas benefit from treatment with steroids and laser.
9. **C.** Vitiligo is an acquired depigmentation disorder that affects males and females equally and results in the destruction of epidermal melanocytes.

ANSWERS AND EXPLANATIONS TO SECTION K PRETEST

1. **B.** Use of anticoagulants is not generally associated with cherry angioma or telangiectasia.
2. **C.** Cherry angiomas are round, painless, papular lesions that are cherry red to purple color.
3. **C.** Most telangiectasias and cherry angiomas are benign. However, telangiectasias can be associated with other diseases such as scleroderma or SLE.
4. **A.** Sclerotherapy is used for definitive treatment of telangiectasias of the extremities.

ANSWERS AND EXPLANATIONS TO SECTION L PRETEST

1. **B.** In this age group, the most likely diagnosis is localized scleroderma, and the treatment that is most effective is moisturizer followed by stretching.
2. **B.** No blood test or imaging study can diagnose pemphigoid or pemphigus, and besides clinical suspicion, only a biopsy can make a definitive diagnosis.
3. **D.** There is a 4:1 female-to-male ratio in scleroderma. However, it is also more common in the African American population, so the patient who is most likely to present with scleroderma will be a female and more likely to be African American than Caucasian.
4. **A.** Although the ANA test is not 100% sensitive, it is an excellent screening test. If it is positive, Robin most likely has scleroderma. A negative test does not rule out the diagnosis.

5. **B.** The correct answer is: Calcinosis, Raynaud phenomenon, Esophageal dysfunction, Sclerodactyly, Telangiectasia. CREST syndrome is one of the two types of systemic scleroderma and makes up 50% of the systemic cases.

6. **C.** Alvin has systemic scleroderma as noted from his pulmonary symptoms plus his local hand symptoms. However, he does not have the other symptoms of CREST. Thus, while he has systemic disease, he is part of the 50% who have diffuse systemic disease.

▶ ANSWERS AND EXPLANATIONS TO SECTION M PRETEST

1. **D.** Only 1%–4% of the population has a diagnosis of hidradenitis suppurativa.

2. **C.** Angiolipomas have the classic features of a lipoma but are painful.

3. **C.** Smoking, tight clothing, and stress can all trigger a flare of hidradenitis suppurativa. Poor hygiene is not a cause of hidradenitis suppurativa flare.

4. **B.** Polymorphous light eruptions can be associated with SLE but are not routinely associated with diverticulitis, hyperlipidemia, or Hodgkin lymphoma.

5. **B.** Asymptomatic pilonidal disease typically presents with pits at the midline of the gluteal cleft but without tenderness, pain, fluctuance, or drainage.

6. **B.** Doxycycline commonly causes photosensitivity in patients. The patient in this question spent the prior day fishing likely with his hands exposed to the sun, resulting in the photoeruption.

7. **B.** Obesity is a risk factor for acanthosis nigricans.

CHAPTER
37

Acne Vulgaris

Marianne Vail, DHSc, PA-C

▶ GENERAL FEATURES

- Acne vulgaris is an inflammatory disorder of the pilosebaceous unit.
- Pathogenesis includes increased sebum production, increased colonization of *Cutibacterium acnes*, inflammation, and follicular hyperkeratinization.
- Acne is common in adolescent and young adults; it can persist or develop in adulthood, especially in females with flares associated with menses.
- Adolescent acne is more common in males, whereas postadolescent acne is more common in females.

▶ CLINICAL ASSESSMENT

- Acne is usually found on the face, neck, and trunk; it may also occur on the upper arms and buttocks.
- Clinical manifestations of acne vary widely and include:
  - Noninflammatory or comedonal acne, including open comedones (blackheads) and closed comedones (whiteheads)
  - Inflammatory acne or papulopustular acne consisting of papules and pustules
  - Nodular or nodulocystic acne consisting of inflamed cysts and/or tender nodules
  - Postinflammatory hyperpigmentation and scarring possible sequelae

▶ DIAGNOSIS

- Diagnosis is based on the history and physical examination; the presence of comedones strongly supports the diagnosis.

▶ TREATMENT

- Treatment usually requires 2–3 months of consistent use for clinical improvement.
- Treatment options vary based on factors including age, skin type, acne severity, and previous treatments.
- Multiple topical and/or oral agents can be used to target factors related to pathogenesis:

- Sebum production:
  - Hormonal therapy
  - Oral isotretinoin
- *C. acnes* colonization:
  - Benzoyl peroxide
  - Topical and oral antibiotics
  - Oral isotretinoin
- Inflammation:
  - Topical retinoids
  - Topical and oral antibiotics
  - Oral isotretinoin
- Follicular hyperkeratinization:
  - Topical retinoids
  - Oral isotretinoin
- Topical retinoids (tretinoin, adapalene, tazarotene) are the mainstay of treatment for comedonal acne.
  - Topical retinoids are used in combination with benzoyl peroxide or other topical antibiotics (clindamycin, etc.) for mild inflammatory acne.
  - Retinoids can also be used for maintenance after treatment with other therapies.
- Treatment for moderate-to-severe acne may include the addition of oral antibiotics to a topical regimen.
  - Tetracyclines (doxycycline and minocycline) are most common.
  - Topical and systemic antibiotics should not be used as monotherapy owing to the possibility of resistance.
  - Limit oral antibiotic use to 3–6 months.
  - Avoid concurrent use of topical and oral antibiotics.
  - Monotherapy with oral isotretinoin may also be used to treat moderate-to-severe or recalcitrant acne.
    - Oral isotretinoin is teratogenic and is administered through the iPLEDGE system.
    - Females are required to have two negative pregnancy tests before staring and monthly pregnancy tests thereafter while on treatment.
- Hormonal therapy with oral contraceptive pills or spironolactone is an alternative to oral antibiotics in adult women with moderate-to-severe acne, especially when acne is associated with menses.

Rosacea

Marianne Vail, DHSc, PA-C

▶ GENERAL FEATURES

- Rosacea is a chronic inflammatory condition of the pilosebaceous units, which may also have ocular manifestations.
- Rosacea is most common in adults over the age of 30 years, in fair-skinned persons with Fitzpatrick skin types I and II, and in women as compared to men, except for phymatous changes that occur more frequently in men.
- The pathogenesis is unclear but is associated with ultraviolet (UV) light exposure, innate immune system dysfunction resulting in vascular hyperreactivity (flushing, increased blood flow), chronic inflammation, and increased *Demodex folliculorum* infestation in sebaceous follicles.
- Exacerbating triggers include sun exposure, spicy foods, alcohol, hot beverages, exercise, hot weather, wind, embarrassment, anger, stress, vasodilating medications, and topical skin irritants.

▶ CLINICAL ASSESSMENT

- Rosacea predominantly occurs in a centrofacial distribution across the nose and cheeks.
- Skin manifestations include facial flushing to persistent erythema, inflammatory papules and pustules, telangiectasias, skin irritation (burning, stinging, dryness), and edema.
- A lack of comedones distinguishes rosacea from acne.
- Phymatous manifestations are caused by sebaceous gland hyperplasia with irregular contours, leading to disfigurement; these changes are most common on the nose (rhinophyma), but may also occur on the chin (gnathophyma), glabella (glabellophyma), forehead (metophyma), ears (otophyma), and eyelids (blepharophyma).
- Ocular manifestations may present independently or concurrently with skin lesions; findings may include lid margin telangiectasias, blepharitis, conjunctivitis, ocular irritation (burning, stinging), spade-shaped corneal infiltrates, scleritis, and keratitis.

▶ DIAGNOSIS

- Diagnosis is usually made by clinical assessment.
- Skin scrapings may show infestation of *D. folliculorum*.
- Biopsy is rarely used for diagnosis, and findings are nonspecific to rosacea.

▶ TREATMENT

- Prevention includes avoidance of triggers and daily use of a broad-spectrum sunscreen with an SPF of at least 30.
  - A gentle emollient-based moisturizer applied twice daily helps to maintain skin-barrier function.
  - In general, patients should avoid scrubbing of the face and use of facial irritants, including toners, astringents, and chemicals.
- Topical agents with antimicrobial, anti-inflammatory, and antioxidant properties are the mainstay of inflammatory papulopustular rosacea.
  - Improvement is usually seen over 1–2 months.
  - Common topical agents include metronidazole, ivermectin, and azelaic acid.
- Oral antibiotics may be added for a brief course (up to 3 months) for those who fail topical therapy or need quicker resolution of symptoms; doxycycline and minocycline are the most commonly used agents.
- Topical α-adrenergic receptor agonists (brimonidine and oxymetazoline) are used to treat facial erythema and flushing.
- Laser and intense pulsed light therapy can be used as supplemental therapy for vascular changes.
- Phymatous changes may be treated with oral isotretinoin, laser therapy, or surgical debulking.
- Patients with ocular manifestations should be referred to ophthalmology for evaluation and treatment.

CHAPTER

39

Stevens-Johnson Syndrome, Toxic Epidermal Necrolysis, and Erythema Multiforme

Anne Wildermuth, MMS, PA-C, RD

A 45-year-old man presents to the emergency department with a painful rash on his face and chest. He was prescribed trimethoprim-sulfamethoxazole 2 weeks ago. He has ulceration of his lips and widespread erythema on his face and chest. Skin sloughing occurs when traction is applied to uninvolved skin on his arm. What is the most likely diagnosis?

▶ GENERAL FEATURES

- Stevens-Johnson syndrome (SJS) and toxic epidermal necrolysis (TEN):
  - SJS and TEN are severe, sometimes fatal, mucocutaneous reactions, resulting in epidermal detachment and necrosis.
  - They are variants of same disease, with SJS defined as <10% body surface area (BSA) detachment, and TEN defined as >30% BSA detachment; SJS-TEN overlap refers to detachment of 10%–30% of BSA.
  - Nearly all patients have concurrent mucous membrane involvement.
  - Medications are the most common trigger, especially aromatic anticonvulsants (such as phenytoin, carbamazepine, and lamotrigine), allopurinol, sulfonamides, nevirapine, and meloxicam; symptoms can develop up to 8 weeks after medication exposure.
  - *Mycoplasma pneumoniae* infection is the second most common cause.
  - Mortality is most commonly due to septic shock; *Staphylococcus aureus* and *Pseudomonas aeruginosa* are common pathogens.

- SJS and TEN used to be considered part of a spectrum, including erythema multiforme (EM); however, now they are considered distinctly different than EM major.
- EM:
  - EM is a hypersensitivity reaction common in individuals aged 20–40 years.
  - Herpes simplex virus (HSV) is the most common cause; *M. pneumoniae* and fungal infections can also cause EM.
  - EM can be caused by drugs, including barbiturates, hydantoins, nonsteroidal anti-inflammatory drugs (NSAIDs), penicillin, phenothiazines, and sulfonamides.

▶ CLINICAL ASSESSMENT

- SJS and TEN:
  - Typically, an influenza-like prodrome occurs 1–3 days before skin changes; during this time, mucous membrane involvement may begin, manifesting as conjunctival burning or painful swallowing.
  - Classic cutaneous findings include painful, coalescing, erythematous macules, which are potentially targetoid, or diffuse erythema; the face and thorax are affected first, and widespread involvement can ensue.
  - Vesicles and bullae form, leading to epidermal sloughing.
  - Nikolsky sign, epidermal sloughing with traction to visibly uninvolved skin, is common.
  - The extent of BSA involvement, an important parameter, can be estimated using the rule of nines. The palm and fingers of the patient's hand represent about 1% BSA and are helpful to assess patchy areas.

- The oral mucosa and vermillion border are affected in nearly all patients, typically by erosion and ulceration.
- Ocular and urogenital involvement is common, manifesting as conjunctivitis and urethritis.
- As epidermal detachment occurs, dehydration develops, and infection risk increases; tachycardia and fever are suggestive of these processes.
- EM:
  - EM is usually self-limited and does not have a viral prodrome.
  - Itching and burning may be present.
  - Lesions appear first as sharply demarcated pink or red macules that progress to papules with vesicles or crusting in the center.
  - "Target" or "iris" lesions are characteristic and are round shape with concentric rings.
  - Lesions may be present on the oral mucosa.

▶ DIAGNOSIS

- SJS and TEN:
  - Diagnosis is clinical: ask patients about medications taken within 8 weeks of symptom onset.
  - Obtain a complete blood cell count and comprehensive metabolic panel.
    - Laboratory abnormalities generally are due to large transdermal fluid losses and a hypercatabolic state and may include anemia, lymphopenia, elevated liver transaminases, hypoalbuminemia, electrolyte disturbance, increased BUN, and hyperglycemia.
  - Skin biopsy is helpful for definitive diagnosis.
  - If infection is suspected, obtain a serum lactic acid and blood cultures.
- EM:
  - Diagnosis of EM is usually clinical.
  - Biopsy may be performed if diagnosis is uncertain or to rule out other causes.

▶ TREATMENT

- SJS and TEN:
  - The mainstay of treatment is discontinuing the causative drug; educate patients to avoid the causative

drug and related drugs for life because SJS and TEN can recur, especially with repeat drug exposure or reinfection with *M. pneumoniae*.
- Patients require aggressive crystalloid fluid resuscitation and electrolyte management; hypothermia is common and should be prevented.
- New research indicates that cyclosporine may reduce mortality significantly; although cyclosporine is not Food and Drug Administration (FDA) approved for these indications, consider giving 3–5 mg/kg per day as early as possible after diagnosis.
- Treat infection only if present; prophylactic antibiotics are not indicated.
- All patients require admission to the hospital, and nearly all require care in a burn unit or ICU.
  - The SCORTEN score is used in SJS and TEN to identify the most appropriate inpatient level of care and to predict mortality; this score should be calculated at the time of diagnosis.
- Provide ocular and wound care, pain management, and monitoring for development of infection; patients may need enteral nutrition support.
- Complications include acute respiratory failure, malnutrition, and abdominal compartment syndrome.
- EM:
  - Treat underlying cause.
  - Symptomatic relief can be achieved with antihistamines and/or topical steroids.
  - Oral steroid use for EM is controversial.
  - Recurrent EM can be treated with antiviral medications.
  - Refer to dermatology for severe or recurrent infections.

Case Conclusion

This patient most likely has SJS. Ulceration of the lips, recent exposure to a frequently implicated medication, and the presence of Nikolsky sign differentiate the most likely diagnosis of SJS from the cutaneous findings in EM minor, cellulitis, and erysipelas.

CHAPTER

40

Burns and Lacerations

Katherine Thompson, MCHS

A 28-year-old male presents after a kitchen accident. He states that he was attempting to empty a pot of boiling water when his hand slipped, causing the water to spill all over his feet. The patient complains of intense pain to both feet. In urgent care, you note multiple large vesicles with surrounding erythema. Some of the vesicles have sloughed open, revealing beefy red tissue underneath. What is a bedside procedure that you can do with local pain control that can help provide the best possible course of healing?

▶ GENERAL FEATURES

- Burns:
  - Burns are classified according to the percentage of body tissue involved, depth, whether the burn is circumferential, and what material created the injury.
  - The rule of nines is commonly used to estimate body surface area (BSA) percentage involved in a burn.
  - Burns are divided into three zones: zone of coagulation (most central area of the burn), zone of stasis (tissue likely to be lost secondary to inflammatory mechanisms), and zone of hyperemia.
  - Burns are caused by the following mechanisms: scalds, contact burns, fire, chemical, electrical, and radiation.
- Lacerations:
  - Lacerations are classified according to size, depth, shape, contamination status, foreign-body presence, and whether circulation, sensation, and motor control are present distal to the injury.
  - Important qualities to evaluate for lacerations include the amount of tissue involved, whether there is any tendon or bone involvement, and tetanus vaccination status.
- Three phases of wound healing are inflammation, proliferation (during which wound contraction and tissue fusing occurs), and maturation (formation of scar tissue, collagen production increases).

▶ CLINICAL ASSESSMENT

- Burns:
  - Differential diagnosis of burns is related to substance causing the burning, as this can radically change the treatment of the burn.
  - When examining a patient with burns, first assure the safety of the examiner: exposure to caustic substances or live wires must be mitigated before the examination can be continued.
  - Physical examination is centered on the area of burn, characteristics of depth, and area of the burn.
  - Lab studies depend on the overall condition of the patient; severely ill patient with large BSA percentages may require labs for electrolyte management, infection monitoring, and other advanced testing.
  - Rule of nines (adults): 9% of total body surface area (TBSA) each for the head, neck, and each upper extremity; 18% for the anterior and posterior trunk; 18% for each lower extremity; and 1% for the genital area
- Lacerations:
  - Physical examination of a laceration involves characteristics of the wound, contamination status, other injuries not initially noticed, and other factors depending on location (such as tendon or sensation examination).
  - Imaging may be performed to assess for radiopaque foreign bodies or bony involvement.

▶ DIAGNOSIS

- The diagnosis of the burn should include a description of the thickness of the burn (superficial, partial thickness, full thickness or a combination) and the percent of body surface area affected.
- Lacerations are diagnosed by physical exam and should be described by their shape, location, and the dimensions of the skin defect and affected skin layers.

▶ TREATMENT

- Burns:
  - Fluid resuscitation (Parkland formula): 3 − 4 mL × kg × %BSA; half should be given over the first 8 hours, half in the next 16 hours.
  - Low threshold for intubation: any sign of inhaled smoke (such as wheezing, coughing, singed nasal hairs, soot around nose or mouth, or even reasonable suspicion) should trigger informed discussion about intubation, given the likelihood of inhalation of toxic gases and/or superheated material in these cases.
  - Burn victims may require antibiotic prophylaxis.
- Lacerations:
  - Most lacerations should be closed to promote healing and reduce scar formation (with a few exceptions: puncture wounds, bite wounds without cosmetic concerns, exceptionally dirty wounds, and delayed presentation).
  - Suture technique should be chosen based on the structure and depth of wound, tension on the affected skin, patient condition, and psychosocial factors.
  - Nonabsorbable suture material is typically chosen for superficial closures, and absorbable material is often chosen for internal closures that are nonsurgical.
  - Skin staples and skin adhesives are alternatives to suture closure; there are exceptions to this general rule.
  - Vigilant cleaning of lacerations (plain water has been shown to be just as effective and less cytotoxic than substances such as iodine) is the best technique for avoiding infection and other complications; examination for foreign bodies should be completed on a bloodless field.
  - Antibiotics are not necessary for most lacerations unless the wound is grossly contaminated, it is a bite wound, or there are other clinical factors.
- Tetanus booster should be given for any vaccine status older than 10 years, although most clinicians routinely give a booster after ~6 years.
- If wound dehiscence occurs, monitor for infection and allow the wound to heal via secondary intention.

Case Conclusion

Simple debridement with adequate pain control is an effective technique for isolated burn areas that are not considered "complicated" burns (requiring transfer to a burn center). If debridement is not performed, the vesicles should remain fluid filled if possible to provide protection for the damaged skin underneath them. Burns should also be covered to prevent secondary infection.

CHAPTER 41

Stasis Dermatitis

Melodie Kolmetz, MPAS, PA-C

Mrs. White, a 73-year-old female, was recently admitted to the rehabilitation unit after a cerebrovascular accident (CVA). The staff has asked you to come assess her because they are concerned that she may have cellulitis of her lower legs. Her past medical history includes hypertension, type 2 diabetes, congestive heart failure, and this recent CVA. When you arrive at the bedside, you note that she has 2+ symmetrical edema to mid-calf with reddish skin discoloration to the anterolateral aspect of both lower legs and ankles. After you assess the patient, are you satisfied that the initial diagnosis is correct?

▶ GENERAL FEATURES

- Stasis dermatitis is a common skin disease of the lower extremities caused by chronic venous insufficiency and venous hypertension.
- It is usually seen in middle-aged or elderly patients, although it can occur after surgery, trauma, or thrombosis that leads to venous insufficiency; it can also occur during pregnancy.
- Incompetent venous valves, valve destruction, or venous obstruction can cause retrograde venous vascular flow, resulting in edema, dermatitis, hyperpigmentation, lipodermatosclerosis, and ulceration.
- Stasis dermatitis can frequently be misdiagnosed as cellulitis.

▶ CLINICAL ASSESSMENT

- Symptoms often begin at the medial ankle due to poor blood flow and can then progress to the foot and/or calf.
- Patients may complain of pruritus, affecting one or both extremities.
- Varicosities may be visible.
- Physical examination may reveal reddish brown discoloration due to hemosiderin deposition, dependent leg edema, erythema, scaling, and/or eczematous patches to the lower extremities.
- Severe cases can be characterized by exudative, weeping patches and plaques that can extend circumferentially around the extremity; skin ulcerations may also occur.

- Patients are at risk of secondary bacterial and fungal infections.
- Lipodermatosclerosis is a deep, acute inflammation characterized by underlying fat necrosis that can resemble erythema nodosum; the appearance of the lower legs in lipodermatosclerosis has been described as an inverted champagne bottle.
- Patients with congestive heart failure (CHF) are more prone to edema and, therefore, more likely to have associated venous stasis.
- Amlodipine can trigger or increase leg edema and contribute to stasis dermatitis.

▶ DIAGNOSIS

- Lab tests are generally not helpful, except in specific cases.
  - If cellulitis is a concern, then evaluating the white blood cell count can be helpful.
  - If venous thrombosis is a concern, then hypercoagulability workup may be indicated.
- In younger patients or patients with new-onset stasis dermatitis, venous Doppler studies can evaluate the deep venous circulation.
- Severe cases may have acroangiodermatitis that can resemble Kaposi sarcoma; biopsy is necessary to differentiate these two conditions.

▶ TREATMENT

- Pigmentation related to hemosiderin deposition does not resolve even when underlying stasis is well controlled.
- Compression therapy is a mainstay of treatment.
  - Other options include elastic wraps and compression boots, but these often require application by a health care professional.
  - Leg elevation is a beneficial adjunct to compression therapy.
  - Arterial circulation should be assessed clinically or with Doppler studies before initiation of compression therapy because compromising arterial circulation can risk ischemia.
- Topical therapy, specifically mid-potency corticosteroids such as triamcinolone 0.1% ointment, can help treat inflammation and itching in acute flares of stasis dermatitis; however, high-potency corticosteroids should be avoided owing to significant risk of steroid-induced skin atrophy that can contribute to ulceration.
- Underlying edema, inflammation, and pruritus can contribute to development of cellulitis, so clinicians should have a high index of suspicion for infection in patients with stasis dermatitis.

> **Case Conclusion**
>
> Your assessment tells you that this patient's clinical features and medical history suggest stasis dermatitis. Patients with stasis dermatitis are often misdiagnosed as having cellulitis.

CHAPTER
42

Pressure Injuries

Daniel Podd, MPAS, PA-C

An 84-year-old bedbound female with a past medical history of hypertension, hypoalbuminemia, anemia, cerebrovascular accident with left hemiplegia, congestive heart failure, urinary incontinence, dementia, and hypothyroidism is evaluated for a follow-up visit. Her skin examination is remarkable for a partial-thickness area of skin loss to the mid-sacral region measuring 4 cm × 3 cm × 0.5 cm. The ulcer has an erythematous wound base but is without any discharge, tenderness, odor, necrosis, or tunneling. Which diagnostic test would be most appropriate in the evaluation of this finding?

▶ GENERAL FEATURES

- The primary pathophysiology of decubitus ulcer formation is multifactorial and includes:
  - Local ischemia induced by occluded capillaries
  - Impaired lymphatic circulation in conjunction with increased metabolic waste production
  - Injury caused by reperfusion to previously devitalized tissue
  - Deformation of tissue cells
- Primary external factors are pressure (stress), shear, friction, and the presence of moisture.
- The most important risk factor that contributes to the development of ulcers is impaired mobility.
  - Concomitant conditions that increase the risk of development are diabetes, peripheral arterial disease, venous insufficiency, urinary or fecal incontinence, undernutrition, malnutrition, impaired mental status, altered pain or discomfort sensation, a negative nitrogen balance, dehydration, and weight loss.
- Pressure injuries may occur over any part of the body, but they most commonly develop on the hip and buttocks areas; more specifically, these involve the ischial tuberosities and trochanteric and sacral locations.
- An estimated 2.5 million cases are treated each year in acute care settings in the United States; although ulcers may occur across all health care settings, the patient populations at highest risk are those in critical care and orthopedics.

- Pressure injuries can lead to significant morbidity and mortality, due to the development of sinus tracts, septicemia, wound infection, cellulitis, and osteomyelitis.

▶ CLINICAL ASSESSMENT

- The National Pressure Ulcer Advisory Panel (NPUAP) has classified pressure injuries into a total of six stages according to the extent of soft-tissue damage:
  - Stage I pressure injury: nonblanchable erythema that usually exists over a bony prominence; skin remains intact
  - Stage II pressure injury: partial-thickness skin loss; the ulcer is superficial and may manifests as an abrasion, blister, or shallow crater
  - Stage III pressure injury: full-thickness skin loss involving damage or necrosis of subcutaneous tissue that may extend down to, but not through, underlying fascia
  - Stage IV pressure injury: full-thickness skin loss and the presence of exposed and/or directly palpable fascia, tendon, muscle, ligament, cartilage, or bone
  - Unstageable injury: obscured due to the presence of slough or eschar, the removal of which reveals a stage III or IV pressure injury
  - Suspected deep tissue injury: represents intact or nonintact skin with a localized area of persistent nonblanchable deep red, maroon, purple discoloration or epidermal separation that demonstrates a dark wound bed or blood-filled blister

▶ DIAGNOSIS

- The diagnosis is primarily made on clinical examination, with attention to physical characteristics, dimensions, and usual location over a bony prominence.
- Sequential photography and staging are crucial in the ulcer surveillance.
- Wounds are ordinarily heavily colonized by bacteria; routine wound culture is not recommended.
- A nutritional assessment is recommended in patients with pressure injury, especially those with stage III or IV pressure ulcers; recommended tests include hemoglobin, hematocrit, transferrin, prealbumin, albumin, and total and CD4+ lymphocyte counts.
- The presence of a fever and leukocytosis should raise suspicion of cellulitis, bacteremia, or underlying osteomyelitis.
  - Baseline studies recommended in the assessment of these complications include a complete blood count, blood cultures, and erythrocyte sedimentation rate or C-reactive protein.

▶ TREATMENT

- Medical management centers on reduction of pressure, debridement of necrotic and devitalized tissue, prevention and treatment of concomitant infection, and direct wound care.
- Pressure reduction is accomplished by incorporating frequent repositioning, protective padding and surfaces, and the use of support surfaces.

- Five methods of debridement:
  - Sharp debridement involves the use of a scalpel, scissors, or other sharp instruments to remove nonviable tissue.
  - Mechanical debridement involves the use of wet-to-dry dressings, whirlpool, lavage, or wound irrigation.
  - Autolytic debridement uses the body's own mechanisms to remove nonviable tissue.
    - Examples include transparent films, hydrogels, alginates, foams, hydrocolloids, and medical-grade honey.
  - Enzymatic debridement (eg, collagenase) involves applying a concentrated, commercially prepared enzyme to the surface of the necrotic tissue.
  - Biosurgery involves the application of maggots (disinfected fly larvae, *Phaenicia sericata*) to the wound typically at a density of 5–8/cm^2.
- For stage II injuries and beyond, adjunct wound cleansing with normal saline at an optimal force should accompany every dressing change.
  - Ulcer wounds should not be cleaned with skin cleansers or antiseptic agents such as povidone-iodine, hydrogen peroxide, or acetic acid, because these can destroy granulation tissue.
- Debridement is not recommended for heel ulcers that have stable, dry eschar without edema, erythema, fluctuance, or drainage.
- In addition to debridement, systemic antibiotics are indicated for patients with wound-related infections, such as sepsis, osteomyelitis, or cellulitis.
- Topical antibiotics such as silver sulfadiazine (Silvadene) cream should be used for up to 2 weeks for clean ulcers that are not healing properly after 2–4 weeks of optimal wound care.
- Pressure injury healing is supported by a high-calorie, high-protein nutritional supplement containing arginine; standard nutritional assessments should be performed in all malnourished patients (with or without ulcers) to identify deficits and nutritional treatment.
- Bedbound patients should be repositioned every 2 hours, and wounds checked each time position is changed.
- Use reactive overlay support surfaces such as foam, gel, or alternating air pads for all patients at risk of pressure injury.
- The use of vitamins to facilitate wound healing is regarded as controversial; no considerable evidence supports the use of vitamin C or zinc supplementation for the healing of pressure sores.

Case Conclusion

Nutritional screening should be part of the general evaluation of patients with pressure ulcers. As such, a comprehensive metabolic panel including a complete blood count and anemia and metabolic panels is useful in the initial assessment of a pressure wound without any findings concerning of associated infection.

Disorders of the Hair and Nails

Paronychia, Onychomycosis, and Alopecia

Marie Patterson, MSM, DHSc, PA-C

Mr. Alvarez is a 20-year-old male who presents with redness and swelling to his left third nail fold. He states it started 2 days ago and is very sore. He is a dishwasher at a local restaurant. He reports biting his nails when stressed. What should you consider?

▶ GENERAL FEATURES

- Paronychia:
  - Inflammation/infection around nail fold that is often painful
  - Can be acute with sudden onset or chronic with gradual onset and last for months
  - Acute form usually caused by *Staphylococcus aureus* and is common in people who bite their nails or pick their cuticles
  - Chronic form usually caused from an irritant or a fungus and often contains a mixture of yeasts and bacteria; it mainly occurs in people who have constantly wet hands
- Onychomycosis:
  - Also known as *tinea unguium*
  - Common fungal infection in the nails
  - Risk factors: older age, exposure to tinea pedis/onychomycosis, immunosuppression, nail dystrophy (psoriasis), and peripheral vascular disease or diabetes
- Alopecia:
  - Alopecia is also known as *hair loss*.
  - Hair loss is categorized as local or diffuse.
    - Local is then categorized as scarring or nonscarring.
      - Scarring is uncommon and is usually caused from inflammatory disorders such as systemic lupus erythematosus.
      - Nonscarring is usually from alopecia areata (autoimmune skin disease that causes hair

loss), tinea capitis (fungal infection of the scalp), traction alopecia (hair loss from constant pulling in same direction, such as tight braids or ponytails), or trichotillomania (obsessive-compulsive–type disorder with recurrent irresistible urges to pull hair).
- Diffuse hair loss can be from conditions causing excess shedding or thinning of the hair.
  - Diffuse alopecia areata (alopecia areata that extends beyond local patches), androgenic alopecia (male and female pattern baldness), telogen effluvium (temporary hair loss a few months after a stressful event), and anagen effluvium (pathologic hair loss in anagen/growth phase classically caused by chemotherapy or radiation to the scalp) are examples.

▶ CLINICAL ASSESSMENT

- Paronychia:
  - Nail fold can be painful, erythematous, swollen, and pus may form under cuticle.
  - Acute paronychia sometimes presents with fever and axillary lymphadenopathy.
  - Chronic paronychia often spreads to other nail folds and may distort the nails.
- Onychomycosis:
  - Nails are often thickened, deformed, and discolored yellow white.
- Alopecia:
  - Examine the scalp to look for areas of hair loss, scarring, erythema, or scaling.
  - Perform a full skin examination and thyroid examination.
  - Exclamation point hairs are indicative of alopecia areata and are found in areas of hair loss, are short, broken off, and narrower closer to the scalp, thus resembling exclamation points.

- Telogen effluvium is excessive shedding 3–4 months after a triggering/stressful event; may have a positive "pull test."

▶ DIAGNOSIS

- Paronychia:
  - Diagnosis is made from a detailed history about timing, behaviors, and risk factors.
- Onychomycosis:
  - Diagnosis is presumed by nail appearance and involvement.
  - Can be confirmed by KOH wet mount, culture, or polymerase chain reaction (PCR) of nail scrapings/clippings
- Alopecia:
  - A thorough history and physical examination is often diagnostic.
  - Consider basic lab work to rule out anemia and hypothyroidism.
  - Refer scarring alopecia to a specialist.

▶ TREATMENT

- Paronychia:
  - Often needs to be lanced to express pus
  - Mild cases of acute can be treated with antibiotic ointments, but most will need an oral antibiotic with *S. aureus* coverage.
  - Chronic cases are difficult to clear and often reoccur.
    - Hands must be kept clean and dry and protected from irritants.
    - Combination treatment with topical steroids, antifungals, and antibiotics is sometimes needed.
- Onychomycosis:
  - Treatment is not always needed because many cases are mild or asymptomatic.

- Treatment may be necessary in patients with previous cellulitis, diabetes, bothersome symptoms, or psychosocial concerns.
- Topical antifungals are less effective because there is poor penetration of the medication through the nail plate and into the nail bed.
- Treatment with oral antifungals may be curative but should be used selectively because they can be hepatotoxic; duration of treatment is 6 weeks for fingernails and 12 weeks for toenails.
- Nails can be removed if pharmacotherapy is unsuccessful; treat patients with antifungals after nail plate removal and warn about likelihood of recurrence.
- Prevent recurrence by keeping feet dry, nails short, and discarding old shoes.
- Alopecia:
  - Tinea capitis usually requires oral antifungal treatment.
  - Telogen effluvium, anagen effluvium, traction alopecia, and trichotillomania will resolve spontaneously when the offending agent is discontinued or the trigger has been resolved.
  - Intralesional corticosteroid injection is used for alopecia areata.
  - Topical minoxidil is used in androgenic alopecia but must be continued indefinitely to maintain hair regrowth.

Case Conclusion

Based on this patient's history, you suspect paronychia caused from an irritant or a fungus that mainly occurs in people who have constantly wet hands. You tell him to keep his hands clean, dry, and protected from irritants, such as by wearing gloves. If the condition does not resolve, you may prescribe a combination of topical ointments.

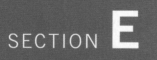

SECTION **E**

Envenomations and Arthropod Bite Reactions

CHAPTER
44

Envenomations and Arthropod Bite Reactions

Sunny Torbett Baker, PA-MS

A 23-year-old male presents to your rural facility following a snake bite to his left lower leg. The patient states he was hiking in the Arizona mountains about 40 miles from your location.

He was alone and noted acute pain in his leg. He then saw a snake moving away and found two small holes in his clothing. He hiked almost 5 miles back to his car and drove himself to the clinic. He had no contributing medical history, medications, or allergies. After removing his clothing, two small puncture wounds were noted to his right lower leg. He currently has some local swelling in the area, pain, redness, and is experiencing lower leg cramps/spams. What was the likely source of this patient's bite?

▶ GENERAL FEATURES

- Arthropods: includes insects and arachnids such as brown recluse spider, black widow spider, ticks, and bedbugs
- Hymenoptera: includes bees, hornets/wasps, and ants
- Scorpions: includes devil, bark, and Arizona hairy scorpions
- Snakes:
  - Crotalidae family: includes rattlesnakes, copperhead, and cottonmouths (aka, water moccasins)
  - Elapid family: includes coral snakes with three found in the United States (Eastern coral, Texas coral, and Arizona coral snakes)

▶ CLINICAL ASSESSMENT

- Arthropods:
  - Brown recluse:
    - Found in south-central United States, often seen indoors in dark space like closets or behind furniture
    - Has classic inverted violin-shaped marking on its back
    - Initial bites are often painless, followed by an erythematous lesion with central necrosis; occasionally fever, weakness, and rash
    - Not commonly fatal
  - Black widow:
    - Found nationwide, typically in yard debris, fields, gardens, and sheds
    - Has classic red hourglass mark on the abdomen
    - Initial bite from female that feels like a pinprick but progresses to intense pain, local muscle cramping that spreads to the chest or abdomen, weakness, headache, nausea and vomiting, diaphoresis, and edema
  - Ticks:
    - Many different species and habitats depending on location within the United States
    - Eight legs, small heads, large rounded bodies in various colors
    - Bites can result in multiple diseases such as Lyme disease, Rocky Mountain spotted fever, tick paralysis, and tularemia.

- Initial bite is typically painless but usually results in a characteristic rash.
  - Bedbugs:
    - Found nationwide in and around mattresses and headboards
    - Oval flat insects about 5 mm long
    - Bites are in groups or cluster over unclothed parts of the body and are noticed immediately after waking up
    - Self-limiting and not fatal
- Hymenoptera:
  - Bees:
    - Found throughout the United States
    - Number one cause of anaphylaxis due to insect bites
    - Usually not aggressive and only sting when threatened or provoked
    - Small subset of "Killer bees" and "Africanized bees" have migrated to Southwestern United States and can be aggressive and defensive, causing them to swarm their target; these account for many bee sting deaths.
    - Have barbed stingers that often remain attached in skin and can only sting once
  - Wasps/hornets:
    - Found nationwide
    - More aggressive than typical bees
    - Do not have barbed stinger and are able to sting multiple times
  - Ants:
    - Many species found nationwide.
    - Most ants bite with pincher-shaped mandibles, but some, such as fire ants, also have stingers that are used to administer doses of venom.
    - Bites may be single or multiple and cause pain.
    - Small sterile pustule can develop at bite site.
- Scorpions:
  - Crablike appearance with four legs and front pinchers; long segmented tail that curls up with stinger on end
  - Often in Southwestern states such as Arizona, Texas, California, and New Mexico; found in wood piles, trees, and moist indoor places such as blankets, clothing, and shoes
  - Stings are painful and cause local reactions similar to those of Hymenoptera.
  - Bark scorpion stings cause pain, then numbness, paralysis, muscle spasms, and respiratory problems; death may result in loss of airway and respiratory muscle control, acidosis, rhabdomyolysis, and hyperthermia (death more common in infants and elderly).
- Snakes:
  - Crotalidae family: account for >90% of all venomous bites; they have triangular heads, elliptical pupils,

hinged teeth, and often rattles; found throughout America

- Two puncture wounds noted with local swelling.
- Venom is hemotoxic/cytotoxic (attacking tissue and blood) and can cause pain, edema weakness ecchymosis, muscle spasms, thrombocytopenia, acute renal failure, disseminated intravascular coagulation, and shock.
- One in four bites is dry.
- Elapidae family: account for <10% of venomous bites; they are small, long, and thin with small fangs requiring them to chew when they bite.
  - Often but not always, striped with red, yellow, and black color
  - Those with red on black are not venomous in North America, but those with red and yellow colors are venomous.
  - Venom is neurotoxic (damaging nerves tissue), and symptoms often delayed up to 12 hours; symptoms can include minimal to no edema, local paresthesia, paralysis, respiratory depression, and, rarely, death.

▶ DIAGNOSIS

- Arthropods: based on clinical examination, history, location, or visualization of insect
- Hymenoptera: based on clinical examination, visual inspection of bite area, stinger, or insect
- Scorpions: based on clinical examination, history, or visualization of scorpion
- Snakes: based on clinical examination, history, or visualization of snake

▶ TREATMENT

- Arthropods:
  - Brown recluse: clean bite with soap and water, cold compress, elevation, loose immobilization.
    - If patient shows systemic reaction, admission may be needed.
    - For rapidly expanding or large lesions, extensive wound care, surgical debridement, or hyperbaric oxygen may be needed.
  - Black widow: aim of treatment is symptomatic relief with intravenous (IV) opioid analgesics and muscle relaxants such as benzodiazepines for spams; antivenom is available but reserved for severe reactions.
  - Ticks: remove tick using tweezers or commercially available tick remover without crushing or squeezing tick; clean area with soap and water.

- Doxycycline can be given in certain endemic regions.
- Watch for signs of transmitted diseases, such as Lyme disease.
- Bedbugs: topical hydrocortisone and oral antihistamines as needed and removal of bedbugs.
- Hymenoptera:
  - Uncomplicated minor reaction: if stinger remains, remove by scraping, wash area, ice packs, antihistamines, analgesics, and H1/H2 blockers.
  - Large local reactions: treat as minor reaction and add glucocorticoids over 3–5 days.
  - Systemic reactions: epinephrine 0.3–0.5 intramuscularly, corticosteroids, H1 and H2 antagonists, IV fluids, and admission.
- Scorpions:
  - Wash the area with soap and water, apply a cold compress, give analgesia and benzodiazepines, and monitor for decompensation.
  - Update tetanus status.
  - Antivenom (Anascorp) is available but only for severe cases.
- Snakes:
  - Not all snake bites result in envenomation.
  - Remove rings or constricting items and immobilize the extremity.
  - Wash and clean bite; determine tetanus status; and monitor and address ABC (airway, breathing, and circulation).
  - Give analgesics as needed.
  - Crotalidae: draw basic labs and monitor coagulation parameters, swelling, and systemic symptoms; start antivenom (CroFab or FabAV) for moderate or severe envenomations.
  - Elapidae: monitor for up to 12 hours for neurologic symptoms, such as generalized weakness, paralysis, salivation, and respiratory depression; if symptoms of neurotoxic envenomation are present, start antivenom.

Case Conclusion

The patient presents with classic symptoms of Crotalid envenomation. You clean the bite, give him an analgesic, determine his tetanus status, and monitor and address his ABCs. Because this patient was likely bitten by a Crotalid, labs including coagulation panels are needed to monitor his condition.

Bacterial Infections

Paula Miksa, DMS, PA-C

▶ GENERAL FEATURES

- Skin infections usually result from compromise of the epidermal layer that allows skin colonizers such as *Staphylococcus aureus* and *Streptococcus pyogenes* to infect the area.
- An abscess is a confined infection of purulent material in a cavity. A sterile abscess is an abscess without a causative pathogen.
- Abscesses, furuncles, and carbuncles are purulent skin infections and are generally caused by staphylococci, including methicillin-resistant *Staphylococcus aureus* (MRSA).
- Nonpurulent skin infections include erysipelas and cellulitis and are often caused by β-hemolytic streptococci.
- Impetigo can produce pus or exudate and is most often caused by *S. aureus* or β-hemolytic *Streptococcus*.
- Folliculitis is most often caused by *S. aureus* and Gram-negative bacteria.

▶ CLINICAL ASSESSMENT

- Abscesses are tender, erythematous, nodular, localized collections of pus within the dermis and subcutaneous fat; the collection of pus can often be felt as a fluctuant area under the skin.
- Furuncles are hair follicle–associated abscesses that extend into the dermis and subcutaneous tissue and are typically seen on the face, neck, and axilla.
- A carbuncle is an infection that extends subcutaneously to involve several furuncles.
- Erysipelas is an infection of the epidermis, upper dermis, and superficial lymphatics and is erythematous with distinct elevated borders and generally associated with fever, lymphangitis, and regional lymphadenopathy.
- Cellulitis involves the deeper dermis and subcutaneous fat tissue and is also erythematous, however, usually without distinct borders.

- Impetigo is a contagious superficial bacterial infection, commonly known for its honey-colored crust found on the face, and most often seen in children, but adults may also be affected.
- Folliculitis is an inflammation of the hair follicle with the classic clinical finding of follicular pustules and follicular erythematous papules on hair-bearing skin (superficial folliculitis); nodules are a hallmark of deep follicular inflammation.

▶ DIAGNOSIS

- Diagnosis generally established clinically by history and physical examination.
- Blood cultures rarely helpful in diagnosis of erysipelas and cellulitis.
- If an abscess, furuncle, or carbuncle is moderate to severe or if recurrent, a Gram stain and culture should be obtained from the purulent drainage to determine correct antibiotic coverage.

▶ TREATMENT

- Abscess should be treated with incision and drainage if drainable.
  - Smaller abscesses <2 cm may not need oral antibiotic therapy.
  - Antibiotics are indicated if the abscess is >2 cm; multiple lesions, extensive cellulitis, fever or signs of systemic infection, or significant comorbidities such as a prosthetic joint or pacemaker are present; or the patient is at high risk for endocarditis or spreading the infection to others.
- Primary treatment of furuncles and carbuncles is incision and drainage; moderate infections with systemic signs of infection require additional treatment with an antibiotic such as trimethoprim/sulfamethoxazole (TMP/SMX) or clindamycin.

- Treatment of uncomplicated erysipelas and cellulitis can be as short as 5 days but should last until the infection improves.
  - Consider risk of MRSA when choosing antibiotic therapy.
  - Treat mild cases with oral penicillin, cephalexin, TMP-SMX, or clindamycin.
  - Treat moderate cases with intravenous (IV) penicillin or cefazolin.
  - Treat severe cases with empiric IV vancomycin.
- Treatment of impetigo is to focus on reducing the spread of infection and improving the appearance of the lesion.
  - Topical therapy is for patients with limited skin involvement and oral therapy for patients with multiple lesions.
  - Mupirocin or retapamulin for 5 days is the first-line therapy.
- Treatment of folliculitis is generally not indicated; if infection is moderate to severe, then treatment is based on the etiology.
  - However, because *S. aureus* is most common, patients are often treated empirically.
  - Topical antibiotic therapy of mupirocin or clindamycin is the first-line agent.

CHAPTER 46

Parasitic Infections

Judy Truscott, MPAS

Lucy G. is a 10-year-old girl being evaluated for "constant scalp scratching." Her mother thinks that she might have dandruff. Her mother denies any new exposures to soaps, shampoos, or detergents, and no one at home has similar rash. She reports that the only new activity for Lucy is that she now plays on a softball team. Lucy says that she "loves softball and is always hugging her teammates when they score." What is the most likely cause of Lucy's infestation?

▶ GENERAL FEATURES

- Head lice (*Pediculus humanus capitis*):
  - The adult louse is small but visible, about 2 mm in length; it lays eggs on the hair shaft close to the scalp, and, until hatched, the egg is difficult to visualize.
  - An empty eggshell, or nit, appears opaque and white against dark hair and may be mistaken for dandruff or hair product.
  - Transmission occurs via direct contact when lice crawl and is unlikely without head-to-head contact; transmission is common in camps, schools, daycares, and households.
  - Indirect transmission may occur from shared items such as brushes, helmets, or hats but is less likely.
  - Girls are affected more than boys; typical age range is 3–11 years; African American individuals are affected less often because of increased hair shaft width and coarse texture.
  - Public perception of lice often carries a stigma of poor hygiene; however, neither hair cleanliness nor length plays a role in infestation.
  - A hypersensitivity reaction occurs as the louse injects saliva into the host's skin.
  - Psychological stress can occur due to the pruritus, stigma, or missed work or school.
- Scabies (*Sarcoptes scabiei*):
  - The scabies mite burrows into the skin where it propagates, laying eggs daily for up to 6 weeks, which hatch within a few days.
  - Transmission is due to direct skin-to-skin contact, such as with a sexual partner, household member, or between individuals in a crowded setting; common sites of outbreaks include nursing homes, daycare centers, and prisons.
  - Scabies has no predilection for age, race, or gender; a seasonal component exists in early winter because the mite survives longer in cooler temperatures.
  - In elderly or immunocompromised individuals, the infestation may evolve into crusted scabies (also known as *Norwegian scabies*) in which a thick and crusted rash develops; crusted scabies is more contagious because the crusted lesions can contain millions of mites.

▶ CLINICAL ASSESSMENT

- Head lice:
  - Rash is not necessarily noted, but excoriation may be apparent on the neck or behind the ears; nits or eggs are most easily seen in these areas.
  - Because the nit is adherent to the hair shaft, it can be distinguished from dandruff or hair product residue by trying to remove the substance.
  - Lice may be seen crawling through the hair, but rarely since they avoid light and move quickly.

- Scabies:
  - The patient's history may include a close contact with a similar papular rash.
  - The rash develops as a hypersensitivity reaction to the mite's feces, saliva, or eggs; short, wavy lines from the burrows may also be seen.
  - Distribution in adults occurs in the finger webs, axillae, wrists, elbows, and genitalia; in children, the rash may also occur on the neck, face, palms, and soles.
  - Signs of excoriation can be present due to the intense pruritus.
  - Crusted Norwegian scabies presents as a crusted plaque with skin flaking.

▶ DIAGNOSIS

- History and physical examination findings aid in a straightforward clinical diagnosis of lice and scabies.
- In cases where the diagnosis of scabies is unclear, perform a skin scraping; microscopic evaluation of the scraping may yield mites, ova, or feces from the mites.

▶ TREATMENT

- Head lice:
  - Permethrin 1% lotion (Nix) is an over-the-counter (OTC) treatment for lice that has been studied extensively and is effective with <1% resistance; a residue remaining after treatment is ovicidal.
  - Although not as effective as Permethrin, pyrethrins (Rid) is another topical treatment composed of plant extracts that are neurotoxic to lice, but safe for humans.
  - Malathion (Ovide) and others are prescription treatments that are costly and not first line.
  - Efficacy of occlusive products like mayonnaise or petroleum jelly is unknown.
  - After topical treatment, a louse comb should be used to remove the remaining nits and eggs; clinicians may recommend louse removal combs as the only treatment, which can be effective with careful combing.
  - Family members of those affected should be checked and treated, if indicated.
  - Although indirect transmission is unlikely, items in contact with the patient's head within 48 hours of treatment should be machine-washed above 130 °F; instruct patients to place items in a plastic bag for 2 weeks if they cannot be washed.
- Scabies:
  - Prescription Permethrin 5% topical cream is approved for use in those aged 2 months and older; it is ovicidal and kills live mites.
    - In cases of recurrent rash, a second treatment is necessary, although many clinicians recommend a second treatment regardless.
    - The cream should be applied on all skin surfaces for at least 8 hours before washing off.
  - Other medications include: Lindane lotion 1% and Crotamiton lotion and cream 10%; both are Food and Drug Administration (FDA) approved only for adults.
  - Crusted scabies requires both an oral and topical medication for resolution; Permethrin 5% cream and the antiparasitic, oral medication ivermectin are prescribed.
  - Clothing and bedding should be machine washed at high temperatures; if an item cannot be washed, it should be placed in a plastic bag for at least 1 week.
  - Sexual partners should be treated, and family members can be treated as indicated.
  - Instruct the patient that the pruritus may last for weeks after treatment.

Case Conclusion

Lucy reports hugging her teammates when they score at a softball game. The head-to-head contact that occurs during hugging is the most likely method of transmission for the lice she has picked up.

CHAPTER
47

Fungal Infections

Amy M. Klingler, MS, PA-C, DFAAPA

A 21-year-old college football player reports a 2-week history of pain, skin fissures, and pruritus between his toes. What is the proper treatment for this condition?

▶ GENERAL FEATURES

- Dermatophyte infection:
  - Also called *tinea*, most common cause of fungal infections of the hair, skin, and nails

- Most common subtypes are:
  - Tinea corporis: affecting body surfaces not otherwise specifically named
  - Tinea pedis: affecting the foot or feet
  - Tinea cruris: affecting the groin
  - Tinea capitis: affecting the scalp
  - Tinea unguium: affecting the nail (also called *dermatophyte onychomycosis*)
  - Other less common tinea infections include tinea faciei (face), tinea barbae (beard), and tinea manuum (hand(s)).
- If misdiagnosed and treated with corticosteroids, the appearance of these infections can change, making diagnosis based on clinical findings more difficult.
- Immunosuppression may contribute to development.
- Majocchi granuloma: rare infection of the subcutaneous tissue
  - Diagnosis requires biopsy and culture to identify the offending organism.
  - Treatment is aimed at the cause of the infection.
- Candidiasis:
  - Infection caused by *Candida* species that results in a spectrum of mild localized mucocutaneous infection to disseminated infection, causing multisystem organ failure.
  - Mild disease is common; more severe disease is usually only found in seriously ill or immunocompromised individuals.
  - Most common subtypes:
    - Oropharyngeal (also called *thrush*): affects the tongue and oral mucosa
    - Esophagitis: affecting the esophagus; this is an AIDS defining illness in patients who are HIV positive.
    - Vulvovaginitis: the most common candidal infection affecting the vulva and vagina; risk factors include the use of oral contraceptives, pregnancy, systemic antibiotics, and oral glucocorticoids.
    - Balanitis: affects the penis
    - Mastitis: affects the nipples of lactating women

▶ CLINICAL ASSESSMENT

- Dermatophyte infection:
  - Tinea corporis: pruritic, round, scaling patches or plaques that spread, often revealing central clearing and a raised border
  - Tinea pedis:
    - Interdigital: pruritic erosions and maceration of the skin between the toes
    - Hyperkeratotic: thickening of the skin of the foot in a moccasin distribution (plantar surfaces and sides of feet)
    - Vesiculobullous: erythematous bullous lesions that can be pruritic and/or painful, usually affecting the arch of the foot

- Tinea cruris: erythematous patches and satellite patches or pustules affecting the groin
- Tinea capitis: pruritic scaling and patchy hair loss of the scalp; most common in children
- Tinea unguium: thickening, discoloration, splitting, onycholysis, and/or splitting of the affected nail(s)
- Candidiasis:
  - Oropharyngeal: white patches and/or plaques on the tongue or buccal mucosa associated with cotton mouth sensation, decreased taste, and/or dysphagia
  - Esophagitis: odynophagia (lesions are not usually visualized without endoscopy)
  - Vulvovaginitis: vulvar erythema, edema, vulvar, and/or vaginal pruritus; thick or watery, white vaginal discharge
  - Balanitis: burning and/or pruritus associated with white patches on the penis. This infection can spread to the scrotum, groin, and thighs
  - Mastitis: breast pain and nipple skin changes; often found with concomitant vaginal candidiasis or oropharyngeal candidiasis of the breast-feeding infant

▶ DIAGNOSIS

- Dermatophyte infection: clinical findings in addition to finding segmented hyphae on skin scraping with potassium hydroxide (KOH) preparation
- Candidiasis: often made clinically; skin scrapings reveal budding yeast and/or pseudohyphae

▶ TREATMENT

- Dermatophyte infection:
  - Most can be treated with topical azoles 1–2 times per day for up to 4 weeks.
  - Systemic treatment can be used for individuals who fail topical therapy.
  - The gold standard treatment of tinea unguium is oral terbinafine for 12 weeks for toenails or 6 weeks for fingernails; however, topical therapies may be appropriate for certain patients. Consider referral to podiatry for evaluation and treatment.
  - Topical nystatin, which is effective in candida infections, is not effective.
- Candidiasis:
  - Oropharyngeal: topical antifungal therapy with nystatin, clotrimazole troches
  - Esophageal: systemic antifungal therapy for nonpregnant adults, amphotericin B for pregnant women; intravenous (IV) therapy for refractory disease
  - Vulvovaginal: topical vaginal antifungal suppositories and/or creams or oral fluconazole
  - Balanitis: improved hygiene and topical antifungals

- Mastitis: topical antifungal treatment or gentian violet; refractory cases may be treated with oral fluconazole. Infant is often treated for thrush at the same time as mother is treated.

Case Conclusion

This patient presents with tinea pedis. First-line treatments include topical azoles.

CHAPTER 48

Condyloma Acuminata, Molluscum Contagiosum, and Verrucae

Marie Patterson, MSM, DHSc, PA-C

Ms. Hopkins is a 20-year-old female who presents with new skin lesions to her pelvic area. She says she noticed one or two a few weeks ago and has since shaved the area multiple times. She says the skin lesions are now more numerous and seem to be spreading. What should be considered for a diagnosis?

▶ GENERAL FEATURES

- Condyloma acuminata (Figure 48.1):
  - Also known as *anogenital warts*, but they can also be found in the oral cavity, typically the tongue or lip.

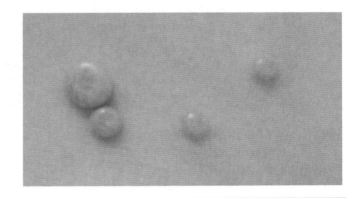

FIGURE 48.2 Molluscum contagiosum.

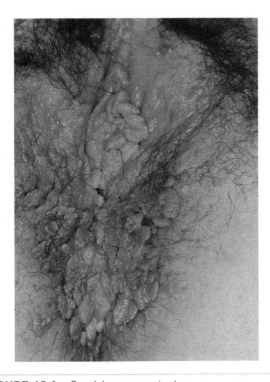

FIGURE 48.1 Condyloma acuminata.

  - These are caused by human papillomavirus (HPV) subtypes, typically HPV6 and HPV11.
  - Transmission occurs from skin-to-skin contact.
- Molluscum contagiosum: (Figure 48.2)
  - Caused by a poxvirus
  - Transmission occurs by direct skin-to-skin contact and by contamination with fomites.
  - In adults, most cases are transmitted through sexual contact.
  - Once a person is infected, lesions often spread by autoinoculation.
- Verrucae: (Figure 48.3)
  - Commonly known as warts
- Warts are caused by HPV, of which there are over 100 subtypes.
- Some of the most common types of verrucae are vulgaris (common warts), plana (flat warts), and plantaris (plantar warts).

▶ CLINICAL ASSESSMENT

- Condyloma acuminata:
  - Lesions are often asymptomatic and found incidentally.

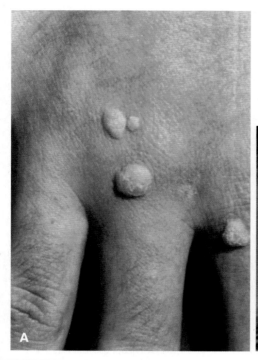
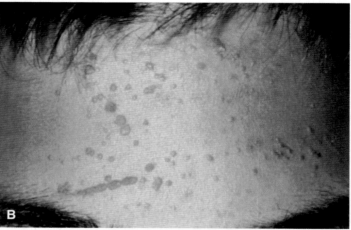

FIGURE 48.3   A, Verruca vulgaris. B, Verruca planae affecting the forehead.

- Lesions begin as soft pink or gray polyps that can enlarge, have rough surfaces, become pedunculated, and form in clusters.
- In women, mucosa of the vagina, urethra, and anus can be involved as well as the cervical epithelium.
- In men, the lesions often occur initially in the coronal sulcus but may be seen on the shaft of the penis, the scrotum, the perianal skin, the anus, or in the urethra.
- Molluscum contagiosum:
  - The lesions present as one or more dome-shaped, umbilicated, waxy papules.
  - The lesions are usually smooth and firm but can become soft; they appear whitish or pearly gray and may suppurate.
  - They are often seen on the face, extremities, abdomen, and genitals.
- Verrucae:
  - Verruca vulgaris is sessile, dome shaped, and usually about a centimeter in diameter; the surface is hyperkeratotic and consists of many small filamentous projections; it has a "cauliflower" appearance.
  - Verruca plana has a smooth, flat surface and are most common in children and young adults.
  - Verruca plantaris tends to grow inward and is covered by thick keratin.

▶ DIAGNOSIS

- Condyloma acuminata: diagnosis is usually made clinically but may require anoscopy or colposcopy to view internal areas.
- Molluscum contagiosum: diagnosis is made by clinical appearance.
- Verrucae: clinical appearance is diagnostic.

▶ TREATMENT

- Condyloma acuminata:
  - In immunocompetent patients, lesions may resolve on their own.
  - Sometimes, excision, cryotherapy, or topical treatments may be used to treat anogenital warts, but recurrence is common with all modalities.
  - Prevention with one of the HPV vaccines is recommended for children and young adults.
- Molluscum contagiosum:
  - The condition is viral and self-limited but may persist for 1–2 years before clearing.
  - Some patients may choose to have lesions removed by curettage or liquid nitrogen. Topical and oral therapies are also available.

- Immunocompromised individuals may have more widespread lesions and may not respond as well as immunocompetent patients to standard treatments.
- Verrucae:
  - Most warts in immunocompetent individuals resolve spontaneously in 1–2 years.
  - There are many modalities to treat verrucae, such as curettage, ablation, liquid nitrogen, topical acid, and excision.
  - Recurrence is common with all modalities, and no single treatment is universally effective.

Case Conclusion

Molluscum contagiosum and condyloma acuminata should both be considered in the differential diagnosis of a patient with skin lesions in the pubic area. Both can be spread by sexual contact and autoinoculation. Shaving can cause the lesions to initially resolve then return in greater numbers. Condyloma acuminata will appear as pink or gray polyps that may appear pedunculated and may have a rough texture while lesions of molluscum contagiosum will appear as white to pink, dome-shaped, waxy papules.

SECTION G *Keratotic Disorders*

CHAPTER 49

Actinic Keratosis, Seborrheic Dermatitis, and Seborrheic Keratosis

Marianne Vail, DHSc, PA-C

A 72-year-old male presents with multiple discrete to confluent erythematous maculopapular lesions with rough adherent scales scattered around his scalp and skin folds. What are the best treatment options for this condition?

▶ GENERAL FEATURES

- Actinic keratosis (AK):
  - AKs, also referred to as *solar keratosis*, are due to the proliferation of atypical keratinocytes.
  - AK is a precursor lesion to squamous cell carcinoma (SCC).
  - Lesions are more common in middle-aged to older adults, males more than females, and individuals with Fitzpatrick skin types I, II, and III.
  - Chronic sun exposure is the major risk factor for AK.
- Seborrheic dermatitis:
  - Seborrheic dermatitis is a chronic condition marked by flares and remissions with a predilection for body sites with increased number of sebaceous glands and may be associated with increased *Malassezia furfur* on skin.
  - Seborrheic dermatitis is seen in infants, adolescents, and adults. It is more common in males and in individuals with Parkinson disease and HIV.

- Seborrheic dermatitis is more common in winter months because of dry, indoor air.
- Seborrheic keratosis (SK):
  - SKs are benign epithelial tumors that usually develop gradually and increase with age.
  - SKs are more common in males than females.

▶ CLINICAL ASSESSMENT

- AKs:
  - Solitary to multiple lesions are most often identified on chronic sun-exposed skin areas, including the face and lips, balding scalp and ears, neck, and extremities.
  - Discrete, round-to-oval erythematous maculopapular lesions appear dry, with rough texture and adherent scales of varying degrees. Scales may appear skin colored, yellowish brown, dark brown, gray, or red tinged.
  - Some AKs may have cutaneous horns.
  - Lesions may be associated with pain.
- Seborrheic dermatitis:
  - Common distribution of seborrheic dermatitis includes the scalp and face, and trunk.
  - Facial lesions occur in nasolabial folds, glabella, forehead, ears, and in hair-bearing areas, including eyebrows, eyelashes, and beard.

- The presternal area is the most common trunk location.
- Intertriginous areas including the axillae, inframammary, genital, and gluteal areas may also be affected.
- Scalp lesions cause dandruff in adults and cradle cap in infants.
- Skin lesions are red-orange, well-demarcated patches and plaques associated with greasy scales. Scalp lesions vary from mild dandruff to marked scaling. Intertriginous lesions may be moist and erythematous.
- Pruritus is variable.
- SK:
  - SKs are commonly found on the face, trunk, and extremities.
  - Lesions may be single to multiple and vary in size from small papules to large plaques.
  - A Christmas-tree distribution may be found on the posterior trunk.
  - SKs may feel greasy or warty with a stuck-on appearance, with colors varying from skin colored, light tan to dark brown, and black.
  - Pruritus is variable, and SKs may be irritated from friction trauma, leading to pain and bleeding.

▶ DIAGNOSIS

- AKs:
  - Diagnosis can be made by clinical examination, but biopsy confirms AKs and rules out SCC.
  - Histopathologic features vary based on clinical presentation but may include pleomorphism, atypical keratinocytes, parakeratosis, orthokeratosis, and solar elastosis.
- Seborrheic dermatitis:
  - Seborrheic dermatitis is usually diagnosed by history and physical examination.
  - Biopsy may demonstrate nonspecific findings, including parakeratosis, neutrophils, acanthosis, and spongiosis.
- SK:
  - Diagnosis is usually made on clinical appearance and with dermatoscopy.

- Biopsy demonstrates proliferation of keratinocytes and melanocytes.

▶ TREATMENT

- AKs:
  - Lesions may spontaneously regress, persist as AKs, or transform to SCC.
  - Individual lesions may be treated with liquid nitrogen cryotherapy or curettage.
  - Areas with large surface involvement or subclinical lesions are often treated with 5-fluorouracil (5-FU), topical imiquimod, or photodynamic therapy (PDT).
  - Prevention includes the use of sunscreen.
- Seborrheic dermatitis:
  - Topical antifungals including creams, lotions, and shampoos are used for treatment; common agents include ketoconazole, selenium sulfide, and pyrithione zinc.
  - Low-potency corticosteroids help to reduce inflammation and erythema.
  - Keratolytics including salicylic acid and coal tar help to reduce dense scale.
  - Oral antifungals and isotretinoin may be used in severe, recalcitrant cases.
  - Cradle cap lesions may be treated with warm olive or mineral oil followed by baby shampoo.
- SK:
  - Lesions are benign, so they do not necessarily require treatment; patients may undergo treatment for cosmetic purposes or when lesions become irritated.
  - SKs are commonly treated with liquid nitrogen cryotherapy or curettage.

Case Conclusion

First-line treatment for seborrheic dermatitis includes topical antifungals, low potency corticosteroids, and keratolytics.

CHAPTER
50

Malignant Melanoma, Basal Cell Carcinoma, and Squamous Cell Carcinoma

Stacey Lynema, PA-C

A 55-year-old Fitzpatrick skin type II male presents with a new growth on his left temple that he noticed 3 months ago. Examination reveals a 1.0-cm light to dark brown patch with irregular border and marked asymmetry located on the left temporal area of the face and a background of photodamage. What would you expect to find in the patient's history?

▶ GENERAL FEATURES

- Skin cancer is the most common form of cancer diagnosed in the United States.
- The most common types of skin cancer in order of prevalence are as follows (Figure 50.1A–C):
  - Basal cell carcinoma (BCC)
  - Squamous cell carcinoma (SCC)
  - Malignant melanoma (MM)
- BCC arises de novo, with no known precursor lesion; it often presents on the head or neck but can arise on any sun-exposed site.
  - Males > females
  - Increasing incidence with age
  - Ultraviolet (UV) light exposure is the highest risk factor with intense episodes of burning being more important than chronic long-term exposure.

- Other risk factors include fair skin, previous skin cancer, previous cutaneous injury, immunosuppression, and exposure to radiation.
- SCC may arise de novo or from a precursor actinic keratosis.
  - Similar risk factors as BCC including male sex, increasing age, fair skin, UV exposure, immunosuppression, radiation exposure, previous cutaneous injury (particularly sites of human papillomavirus infection and scars).
- MM may arise de novo or within precursor melanocytic nevi.
  - It accounts for ~4% of skin cancers, but 80% of deaths resulting from skin cancer.
  - Males are 1.5 times more likely to develop MM than females.
  - MM is most common in Caucasian patients on sun-exposed sites: the back is most common site for men, and legs and arms for women.
  - Risk factors can be divided into three categories:
    - Genetic: family history of MM, lightly pigmented skin
    - Environmental: UV exposure including tanning bed use, immunosuppression
    - Phenotypic: >100 melanocytic nevi, atypical nevi, multiple solar lentigines, personal history of MM

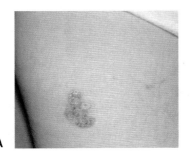

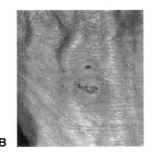

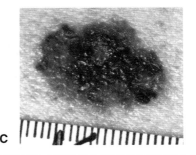

A   **B**   **C**

FIGURE 50.1 Skin cancer. A, Basal cell carcinoma. B, Squamous cell carcinoma. C, Malignant melanoma.

▶ CLINICAL ASSESSMENT

- Perform a full skin examination and take a thorough history of previous and current sun exposure as well as personal and family history of skin cancer.
- BCC classically presents as a pearly pink papule with telangiectasias that may ulcerate with time.
- SCC may present as a tender erythematous keratotic papule or nodule that arises within a background of sun-damaged skin, often with a history of rapid enlargement.
- MM is characterized by the ABCDE criteria: **A**symmetry, **B**order irregularity, **C**olor variegation, **D**iameter >6 mm, **E**volution; a history of a changing mole in an adult should prompt high suspicion.

▶ DIAGNOSIS

- Diagnosis is based on clinical suspicion followed by biopsy and subsequent histologic confirmation.
- The pathology report will list the diagnosis as well as the subtype, for example, superficial BCC or nodular BB.
- For a melanoma, additional features including Breslow thickness, Clark level of invasion, margins of excision, mitotic rate, and whether ulceration is present are also reported and are important indications of prognosis and treatment.

▶ TREATMENT

- Treatment of BCC/SCC is dependent on the histology (subtype, differentiation, depth of invasion, perineural spread) size, location, the number of lesions to be treated, primary versus recurrent, and patient factors such as immunosuppression and prior radiation therapy.
  - An elliptical excision with a 4-mm margin is appropriate for most BCC/SCC on the body.
  - Mohs micrographic surgery is a technique employed in high-risk areas of the head and neck and/or recurrent cancers because of its high cure rate.
  - Superficial BCC/SCC in situ may be treated with electrodessication and curettage, photodynamic therapy, radiotherapy, topical imiquimod, topical 5-fluorouracil, or cryotherapy.
  - Targeted therapy with oral hedgehog pathway inhibitors is used for locally advanced primary, metastatic, or recurrent BCC.
- Treatment of MM involves wide local excision with 0.5 cm (for in situ) to 1.0 cm margins; the need for sentinel lymph node biopsy, adjuvant chemotherapy, and/or radiation are dictated by Breslow thickness.

Case Conclusion

You would expect to find dysplastic nevi in the patient's history. Dysplastic nevi are a risk factor for MM, which this patient presents with.

SECTION **I**   *Papulosquamous Disorders*

CHAPTER **51**

Contact Dermatitis, Eczema/Atopic Dermatitis, Lichen Planus, and Pityriasis Rosea

Adrian Banning, DHSc, MMS, PA-C

A 34-year-old woman presents to her primary care physician assistant complaining of a new-onset, slightly pruritic rash on her torso that appeared 2 days ago and appears to be "spreading" to her arms and neck. She noticed the first lesion on her upper chest her while trying on clothes in a clothing store fitting room. The patient has been under a considerable amount of stress. The lesions are scattered across her anterior and posterior torso in no apparent pattern and spread outward distally with less density onto her neck and beyond her elbows and knees. The lesions are oval and vary in size from 0.5 to 7 mm. They are red and surrounded by a scaling, lacy collarette. How do you diagnose and treat her?

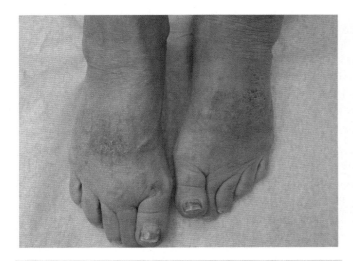

FIGURE 51.1 Shoe allergic contact dermatitis.

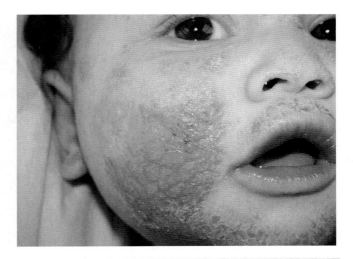

FIGURE 51.2 Atopic dermatitis. Infantile eczema with oozing plaques on the cheeks.

▶ GENERAL FEATURES

- Contact dermatitis:
  - Allergic contact dermatitis (ACD) is a type IV, cell-mediated, hypersensitivity reaction due to contact with an allergen or irritant in the patient's environment (Figure 51.1).
  - Irritant dermatitis is due to repeated insult to the skin without sufficient time to heal between insults and is common in occupations with repeated exposure to chemicals, radiation, water, detergents, and mechanical friction.
  - Complete occupational, social, and environmental histories are important to determine the irritant(s) in question.
    - Inquire about new personal hygiene products, new household or laundry cleaners, recent travel, outdoor activities, and wardrobe irritants such as nickel present in accessories like jewelry and belt buckles.
- Eczema/atopic dermatitis:
  - Usually presents in children <2 years old but can present in adulthood; may resolve with age (Figure 51.2)
  - Presents on cheeks, knees, and elbows of younger children
  - Presents on hands, wrists, ankles, backs of knees, and neck in older children and adults
  - Often associated with atopic triad: eczema, asthma, history of allergies
- Lichen planus (Figure 51.3):
  - Rare, <1% of US population
  - Etiology unknown; may have a genetic component
  - Autoimmune, T-cell–mediated response that causes skin change
- Pityriasis rosea (Figure 51.4A,B):
  - Characterized by a large, raised scaly patch called the "herald patch" that precedes the generalized skin eruption

- Most common in ages 10–35 years
- Often described as following a Christmas-tree pattern along skin Langer lines, but this pattern can easily be indistinguishable clinically depending on the number of lesions
- Etiology unknown, but possibly related to human herpes virus (HHV) 6 or HHV7
- Relationship to stress reported, but no definitive relationship has been demonstrated

▶ CLINICAL ASSESSMENT

- Contact dermatitis:
  - ACD may present as erythematous lesions corresponding in size or greater than the area that contacted the allergen; vesicles or bullae in more severe cases may be present along the erythematous base.

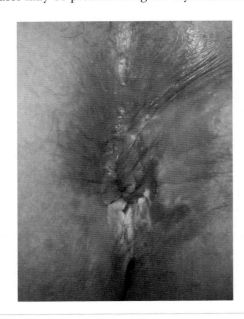

FIGURE 51.3 Anogenital lichen planus.

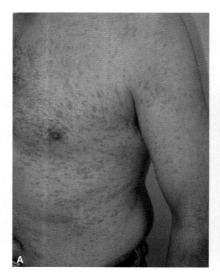
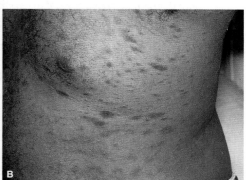

FIGURE 51.4 Pityriasis rosea.
A, Adult white male. B, Eruption is
typically distributed on the chest and/or
back in a Christmas-tree pattern.

- Lesions can be spread by moving the allergen along the skin during regular activity after exposure or via excoriation secondary to pruritis.
- Irritant contact dermatitis presentation depends on the type of irritant, duration and concentration of exposure, and can vary from mild erythema or scaling to full-thickness ulceration.
- Eczema/atopic dermatitis:
  - Patches of dry skin, pruritic, sometimes painful areas of skin; sometimes exacerbated by allergen exposure, cold temperatures, hay-fever, excessive hot water exposure
  - Red, scaling, pinpoint macules; can become ulcerated or crack
- Lichen planus:
  - Follows the "6 Ps": **P**urple, **P**ruritis, **P**lanar (flat), **P**olygonal, **P**apules, and **P**laques
  - Can be extremely pruritic and can leave hypopigmented scarring, both complications can severely affect the patient's quality of life
  - Prone to Koebner phenomenon, meaning lesions appear over areas of trauma
  - Can involve the tissue of multiple body systems, including the eyes, mouth, scalp, hands, feet, and genitalia
  - Can become sclerosing or ulcerative, leading to considerable disability and discomfort
  - Ability to progress to a malignant process is controversial; if possible, risk is considered low.
- Pityriasis rosea:
  - Annular, papular rash of lesions that are pink in color and vary in size from roughly <1–10 mm; lesions are generally confined to the trunk and may have classic, lacy collarette
  - May be pruritic
  - Viral prodrome may precede appearance of herald patch.

▶ DIAGNOSIS

- All are clinical diagnoses.
- No testing is necessary to diagnose these dermatologic conditions.
- Skin scrape or biopsy might be done in any of the above conditions if the diagnosis is unclear, possibly overlapping with another dermatologic condition, or to pursue differential diagnoses.

▶ TREATMENT

- Contact dermatitis:
  - Identification and removal of the causative agent is necessary in allergen and irritant contact dermatitis.
  - ACD can be treated with oral and/or topic antihistamines or steroids, appropriate to the severity of the dermatitis.
  - Irritant contact dermatitis must be treated according to the presentation and severity of symptoms.
  - Secondary infections due to skin disruption should be treated with appropriate antimicrobials that cover common skin pathogens like *Staphylococcus aureus*.
- Eczema/atopic dermatitis:
  - Avoid prolonged exposure to hot water; bathing should be done in warm water, for as short a duration as possible, using gentle soap on areas that require cleaning.
  - After bathing, pat skin dry and copiously apply a thick emollient cream or ointment.
  - Reapply emollient cream throughout the day as needed.
  - Topical steroids do not need to be avoided and should be used appropriately, avoiding high-potency topical steroids to the face.
  - Parental education may be needed to encourage appropriate use of topical steroids.

- Identification and avoidance of allergens is encouraged; oral antihistamines may be useful during allergy season.
- Scratching or rubbing can lead to skin lichenification; encourage patients to avoid scratching.
- Lichen planus:
  - Self-limited, but owing to the possibility of extensive dermal involvement, multitude of areas that can be affected, and severity of disability that might result, comprehensive, coordinated multidisciplinary care is encouraged, focusing on symptoms and immunosuppression.
- Pityriasis rosea:
  - Pityriasis rosea is self-limited, usually resolving in 5–8 weeks.

- No treatment is necessary.
- Acyclovir and ultraviolet (UV) light may hasten resolution.
- UV light exposure should be medically supervised if utilized.

Case Conclusion

This patient likely has pityriasis rosea based on her presentation. These lesions are generally annular, papular, pink in color, and vary in size from roughly <1–10 mm. They may have a classic lacy collarette, and the general distribution may be preceded by a herald patch. You should reassure her that pityriasis is generally self-limited and no treatment is necessary at this time. The lesions will resolve on their own over the next several weeks.

CHAPTER 52

Psoriasis

Lauren Anderson, MMS, PA-C
Tonya Skidmore, DMS, PA-C

Mrs. Owens, a 24-year-old woman, comes to you for evaluation of a rash on her elbows and knees. It does not itch, but the patient is embarrassed by the rash. She has tried over-the-counter (OTC) lotions without success. What should you consider?

GENERAL FEATURES

- Psoriasis is a common, benign skin disease due to chronic inflammation.
- Injury and/or irritation at the skin site tend to induce lesions.
- There are several variants, with the plaque type being the most common.

CLINICAL ASSESSMENT

- Psoriasis is usually asymptomatic, but lesions may be pruritic; scratching causes more lesions.
- Major sites include the scalp, elbows, knees, palms, soles of the feet, and nails.
- Lesions are pink to red, sharply defined plaques with a silvery scale.
- Pitting of the nails is highly suggestive for psoriasis; nail plates may separate from the nail bed, and oil spots may be present.
- Psoriasis variants:
  - Chronic plaque psoriasis: lesions are typically well-demarcated, raised, red plaque with a white scaly surface.
  - Guttate psoriasis: lesions manifest as small papules over the upper trunk and proximal extremities, found frequently in young adults.
  - Erythrodermic psoriasis: lesions can present on all body sites; erythema with superficial scaling is the most prominent feature of the lesions.
  - Pustular psoriasis: lesions are preceded by fever that lasts several days, then, a sudden generalized eruption of small pustules develops on the trunk and extremities; the pustular lesions become confluent as the disease progresses.

DIAGNOSIS

- Diagnosis is typically based on clinical impression.
- Biopsy should be performed only when the clinical history and physical examination are not diagnostic.
- Biopsy is rarely necessary to confirm the diagnosis.
- Laboratory abnormalities are nonspecific and of little value.
- Chronic psoriasis is divided into three severities based on the amount of body surface area (BSA) involved:
  - Mild: <10% BSA
  - Moderate: >10% to <30% BSA
  - Severe: >30% BSA

TREATMENT

- Treatment is driven by severity.
  - Mild:
    - First line: emollients, glucocorticoids, vitamin D3 analogs
    - Second line: salicylic acid, dithranol, tazarotene, tar

- Moderate:
  - First line: narrow-band ultraviolet (UV)B light, broadband UVB
  - Second line: psoralen and UVA light, excimer, climatotherapy
- Severe:
  - First line (in addition to treatments for mild and moderate): methotrexate, acitretin, apremilast, biologics, and biosimilar drugs (etanercept, adalimumab, infliximab, ustekinumab, secukinumab, ixekizumab)

- Second line: fumaric acid ester, cyclosporine A, and other agents such as hydroxyurea, 6-thioguanine, mycophenolate mofetil, sulfasalazine

Case Conclusion

You diagnose Mrs. Owens with psoriasis based on your clinical impression of her characteristic physical examination findings. You prescribe her emollients to use that are more effective than her OTC lotions.

SECTION **J**   *Pigment Disorders*

CHAPTER
53

Melasma and Vitiligo

K. Alexis Moore, MPH, PA-C

Ms. Harrison is a 48-year-old Afro-Latino woman who presents to a family practice office with concerns about darkening of her face over a 2-year period. Moderate hyperpigmented patches are noted on the left cheek and under the chin. What is the likely diagnosis?

▶ GENERAL FEATURES

- Melasma:
  - Melasma is a symmetric hyperpigmentation disorder that is marked by darkened macules and patches commonly encountered on the face in the areas of the cheek, bridge of the nose, and chin.
  - Increased melanocyte production of melanin is the primary dysfunction leading to hyperpigmentation.
  - It is most prominent in women and darker skin individuals with skin tones IV–VI based on Fitzpatrick skin typing classification.
  - The exact cause of melasma is unknown, but sun exposure (ultraviolet [UV] light), hormones, genetic predisposition, and drugs such as oral contraceptive pills play a role.
  - Conditions that share a similar appearance to melasma include freckles, postinflammatory hyperpigmentation, solar lentigo, pigmented contact dermatitis, drug-induced hypersensitivity, and cutaneous erythematous lupus.

- Melasma is a chronic condition that can be managed, but not cured; aggressive sun protection is required to avoid relapse.
- Vitiligo:
  - Vitiligo is an acquired chronic depigmentation disorder that occurs due to destruction of epidermal melanocytes.
  - The exact cause is unknown; several theories have been promoted, including autoimmune activation and oxidative stress.
  - There is a clinical association with autoimmune conditions in children: thyroid disease (commonly Hashimoto thyroiditis and Graves disease), rheumatoid arthritis, and diabetes mellitus type 1.
  - Vitiligo tends to cluster in families.
  - It has equal distribution among males and females; incidence can be higher in children.

▶ CLINICAL ASSESSMENT

- Melasma:
  - Hyperpigmented areas can assume three distribution patterns: malar (limited to the cheek or nose), centrofacial (forehead, cheek, upper nose, or lip), and mandibular (along the jawline).
  - Macules range from brown to tan or black depending on the level of dermal (epidermis or dermis) involvement and base skin tone.

- Vitiligo:
  - Patients typically present with well-demarcated, depigmented macules or patches often described as "milk or chalk white" in color.
  - Lesions may be round, oval, or linear in shape and exhibit a discrete or confluent distribution.
    - Depending on the extent of spread, lesions may be surrounded by normal-appearing skin.
    - Vitiligo lesions may be classified as segmental or nonsegmental.
      - Segmental lesions have a unilateral dermatomal distribution on one side of the body and do not cross the midline. Segmental lesions are not associated with autoimmune or thyroid disorders.
      - Nonsegmental vitiligo is more closely linked to autoimmune markers and thyroid disease and constitutes all other vitiligo patterns that are not segmental; lesions can appear and spread anywhere on the body but are most commonly found on the face (with a propensity for perioral and periocular presentations), neck, dorsum of hands, genitals, and orifices.
  - Inspection during physical examination is usually sufficient to begin workup.

▶ DIAGNOSIS

- Melasma:
  - Inspection and a history of insidious development are usually sufficient for diagnosis; if indicated, other conditions should be ruled out.
  - Wood's light may be used to determine the depth of melasma penetration.
  - Dermoscopy can aid in evaluating severity.
- Vitiligo:
  - Wood's light may assist with detecting vitiligo on lighter skinned patients.
  - Biopsy is rarely required but may be indicated to distinguish vitiligo from other hypopigmenting disorders.
  - Histology may be used to confirm the absence of melanocytes and inflammatory cell-mediated changes.
  - Order a thyroid panel (thyroid-stimulating hormone [TSH], triiodothyronine [T3], free thyroxine [T4]); also consider antinuclear antibody screening.

▶ TREATMENT

- Melasma:
  - Treatment is difficult: symptoms frequently rebound with the cessation of topical agents and other modalities.
    - Melasma may be worsened by the same agents used to treat it.
    - Sun exposure worsens the disease.

- Treatment is targeted at skin depigmentation, early skin cell turnover, and inflammatory responses.
- For mild melasma, topical skin lightening agents such as hydroquinone 4% are recommended first-line treatment.
- Second-line therapy for moderate cases or those with poor response to a single agent includes "triple therapy": a combination of a skin-lightening compound (hydroquinone), retinoid (tretinoin), and low-dose topical steroid (fluocinolone) or tranexamic acid, an antifibrinolytic that inhibits the plasminogen pathway, resulting in slowing of melanin synthesis.
- Third-line treatment with laser and light therapy is indicated when suboptimal outcomes have occurred from topical treatment and chemical peels. Laser and light therapy may cause hyperpigmentation, especially with overuse in darker skinned individuals.
- Active treatment periods of 4–6 months alternate with maintenance periods when topical agents are used less frequently.
- Maintenance treatment can include non–hydroquinone-based skin-lightening agents, such as azelaic and kojic acid or niacinamide.
- Continuous sunscreen use is emphasized in all individuals with melasma.
- Vitiligo:
  - Treatment of vitiligo is geared toward managing cosmetic effects by targeting pigmentation and stopping inflammatory or immune-mediated responses.
  - Phototherapy (narrow-band UVB): repigments skin, rendering a more even tone and appearance:
    - Phototherapy is indicated for vitiligo that is generalized and covering a wide area.
    - Localized vitiligo benefits from treatment with laser therapy.
    - Phototherapy can induce tanning of normal surrounding skin, especially in lighter individuals, which can lead to more distressing cosmetic outcomes.
  - Depigmentation therapy reverses phototherapy by depigmenting normal skin to match vitiligo lesions; 20% monobenzylether of hydroquinone (MBEH, Benoquin) is the most common agent and can be applied BID for up to 12 months.
  - Afamelanotide is a melanocyte-stimulating hormone analog that is delivered by subcutaneous implant and is intended to produce rapid return of pigment, particularly to vitiligo facial lesions.
  - Topical steroids are first line to treat lesions covering smaller areas and negate inflammatory activity.
  - Calcineurin inhibitors inhibit cytokine and T-cell activity; tacrolimus ointment (0.03% or 0.1%) and pimecrolimus cream are used on vitiligo lesions, specifically those on the head and neck.

- Other treatments interrupt immune activities such Janus kinases (JAK), which compromise cytokinase signaling, thereby reducing outcome of immune cell–mediated activity.
- Vitiligo management almost always combines more than one treatment modality for optimal effect.

Case Conclusion

Ms. Harrison most likely has melasma, given her darker skin tone and the location of her hyperpigmented patches on the left cheek and under the chin. Women develop melasma more often than men, and women with darker skin tones are most likely to develop melasma.

SECTION K

Vascular Abnormalities

CHAPTER 54

Cherry Angioma and Telangiectasia

Sarah Schettle, PA-C, MBA, MS
Rebecca Schettle, MSN, RN, APNP, FPN-BC

▶ GENERAL FEATURES

- Cherry angiomas (CAs):
  - Benign, painless, macular or papular skin lesions
  - Composed of dilated capillaries and may be flat or slightly raised on the skin.
  - Environmental factors may influence development, including some chemical or gas exposures.
  - Genetic predisposition also plays a role.
  - CAs are most noticeable on individuals with fair skin.
  - CAs tend to occur later in life and may increase in frequency with age.
- Telangiectasias (TGs):
  - Small blood vessels below the skin surface that are red, blue, or purple and may appear in a lacy pattern
  - Typically painless, but there may be an associated sensation of burning
  - Visible on the skin or mucosal surfaces but may also be located in the intestines or brain
  - More common in women than men and tend to be more prevalent after age 40 years
  - Causes include aging, sun exposure, radiation, trauma, genetic predisposition, topical steroid applications, oral contraceptives, rosacea, pregnancy, and varicose veins
  - May also be associated with features of other medical conditions, including hereditary hemorrhagic TG, ataxia-telangiectasia, lupus, and scleroderma
  - Attributed to insufficient blood flow to the area where they present and may be a harbinger of vessel injury

- Can be exacerbated with alcohol, smoking tobacco, hot or spicy foods and drinks, and temperature extremes

▶ CLINICAL ASSESSMENT

- CAs are small, round, or oval shaped painless skin papules or macules that are typically bright cherry red in color but may also appear blue to purple that can be found anywhere on the body and are often located on the trunk.
- TGs present as fine pink or red lines on the skin that blanch when touched.

▶ DIAGNOSIS

- CA:
  - Primarily clinical, based on general features of the lesion(s)
  - Confirmation, although rarely indicated or required, can be elicited through a biopsy
- TG:
  - Diagnosis is usually made clinically based on the presence of characteristic features.
  - Additional testing including biopsy, blood tests, genetic testing, and imaging studies may aid in diagnosis of other diseases that may have TG as a feature.

▶ TREATMENT

- CA:
  - Intervention is rarely indicated, but some patients may elect to undergo treatment if a CA is injured and bleeds or for cosmetic reasons.

- Treatment options consist of cryotherapy, laser treatment, cautery, electrodessication, or excision.
- Often, treatment of CAs will result in minimal to no scarring.
- TG:
  - Intervention is typically not indicated, but patients who are bothered by TG for cosmetic reasons may also elect to have them removed.

- Treatment options consist of sclerotherapy when TGs are located on the legs and laser treatment or intense pulse light treatment when TGs are on the face.

SECTION **L**

Vesiculobullous Disease

CHAPTER
55

Pemphigus and Pemphigoid

Sunny Torbett Baker, PA-MS

A 60-year-old male comes in for evaluation of tender blisters on his body. He noted them getting worse over the past few months. He denies injury or burns and states they do not itch but are painful. He has only a history of arthritis and hypertension and no new medications or allergies. Physical examination notes blister-likes sacs filled with clear fluid. During examination of a number of these blisters, they rupture, and underlying skin is noted to be red and denuded. What is the likely diagnosis, and what medication must be initiated for the patient?

▶ GENERAL FEATURES

- Pemphigus and pemphigoid are both rare autoimmune diseases that cause blistering of the skin and mucous membranes that can be life-threatening.
- PemphiguS (Superficial) affects the epidermis and is caused by autoantibodies that affect cell–cell adhesion signaling.
  - Desmoglein 1 and 3 are the most common auto-antibodies in pemphigus vulgaris and pemphigus foliaceus
  - There are multiple subtypes of pemphigus:
    - Pemphigus vulgaris
    - Pemphigus foliaceus
    - Immunoglobulin A (IgA) pemphigus
    - Pemphigus vegetans
    - Paraneoplastic pemphigus
    - Epidermolysis bullosa acquisita

- PemphigoiD (Deep) affects the subepidermis and is caused by anti–bullous-pemphigoid antigen (anti-BPA)-2 and anti–BPA-1 antibodies that affect the basement membrane of the epidermis.
  - There are multiple subtypes of pemphigoid:
    - Bullous pemphigoid
    - Cicatricial pemphigoid
    - Gestational pemphigoid
    - Mucous membrane pemphigoid
- Men and women are equally affected, but higher rates can be seen in certain ethnic groups: Ashkenazi Jews and people of Mediterranean, North Indian, and Persian decent.
- Symptoms often present between the ages of 40 and 60 years in pemphigus and >60 years of age in pemphigoid, but children have reportedly been affected.

▶ CLINICAL ASSESSMENT

- Pemphigus:
  - Almost all patients have oral lesions that can affect the buccal mucosa, pharynx, and larynx; pharyngeal lesions cause painful swallowing, and laryngeal lesions cause hoarseness.
  - Examination demonstrates flaccid bullae filled with clear fluid in the oropharynx.
  - The initial oral eruption may be followed by a cutaneous bullous eruption over weeks to months.
  - Cutaneous bullae rupture easily, resulting in painful erosions and raw-exposed skin that may crust over.

- The lesions are usually painful, but not pruritic, and may become infected.
- When large areas are affected, electrolyte loss can occur.
- Nikolsky sign: upper layers of epidermis move laterally and slip away with slight pressure or rubbing of the skin.
- Hansen sign: gentle pressure on intact bullae causes fluid to spread away from the site of pressure and beneath the adjacent skin.
- Pemphigoid:
  - Pemphigoid often starts as a nonspecific urticarial or papular red rash for weeks that then develop to deep blisters.
  - Pemphigoid mostly affects skin around skinfolds of axilla, groin, and abdomen; lesions are rarely found in the mouth.
  - Blisters are large (>10 mm) and filled with serous or hemorrhagic fluid, but do not rupture easily.
  - Blisters are painful and pruritic.
  - Nikolsky sign is negative.

▶ DIAGNOSIS

- Skin biopsy of margin of bulla will demonstrate suprabasilar blister with acantholysis.
- Direct and indirect immunofluorescence of skin sample will detect desmoglein autoantibodies, which are indicative of pemphigus.

▶ TREATMENT

- Remission is possible, but no cure exists.
- Referral to dermatologist with experience in treating this disorder is recommended.
- Open skin lesions are treated in same manner as partial-thickness burns with antibiotics as needed.
- Treat skin infections with antibiotics as needed.
- Corticosteroids are the primary initial treatment.
- Start high-dose prednisone (1 mg/kg/day) with or without immunosuppressive medications until the Nikolsky sign is no longer present and no new bullae form, then taper to maintenance dose.
- Topical steroids may be used for local recurrence or mild cases.
- Immunomodulatory agents such as azathioprine, rituximab, methotrexate, or cyclosporine can be added for adjuvant therapy.
- Plasma exchange or intravenous immunoglobulin (IVIG) can be done.

Case Conclusion

This patient has painful blisters that do not itch but are fragile to the touch and contain clear fluid. This is the classic presentation of pemphigus. Had this same patient described blisters that were itchy and not easily ruptured, pemphigoid would be the most likely diagnosis. Biopsy would be needed to confirm the diagnosis. He also needs to be started on systemic steroids to mediate the reaction of pemphigus.

CHAPTER 56

Scleroderma

Kim Zuber, PA-C, MS
Jane Davis, DNP

Mary, a 55-year-old African American woman, presents to your office for her annual checkup. She complains of fatigue and difficulty holding a pen or pencil. She also mentions that in the winter, her toes and fingers often feel numb and turn blue. She also notes that her face is feeling dry and tight but denies chemical or facial surgery. On further questioning, she admits she has some difficulty swallowing dry foods such as crackers. Physical examination: looks younger than stated age, all other examination within normal limits.

▶ GENERAL FEATURES

- Scleroderma is an autoimmune disease that can cause small vessel changes, leading to skin and soft-tissue changes.
- The name comes from the Greek meaning "hard skin," the most common manifestation.
- Two types are localized or systemic.
  - Localized disease is more common in children.
  - Of the 300,000 Americans (all age groups) with the disease, two-thirds have the localized disease.
- Women are more often affected than men at a 4:1 ratio; African Americans are more commonly affected than Caucasians.
- Systemic disease, also referred to as CREST (Calcinosis, Raynaud phenomenon, Esophageal dysfunction, Sclerodactyly, Telangiectasia) syndrome, can be limited or diffuse; CREST syndrome can lead to pulmonary hypertension and shortness of breath.

▶ CLINICAL ASSESSMENT

- The most common presentation is Raynaud syndrome (70% of presentations); the most common age at presentation is 25–55 years.
- Distinct patches of hard, tight skin may be present on the body.
- Hardening of the internal vessels leading to pulmonary artery hypertension (PAH) or kidney failure are the more serious outcomes of the diffuse version of the disease.
- Digestive symptoms may include heartburn, dysphagia, cramps, bloating, diarrhea, and/or constipation.
- Many patients look young for stated age as the lines or wrinkles in the face are diminished.
- The disease is often a diagnosis of exclusion.

▶ DIAGNOSIS

- Antinuclear antibody (ANA) test is almost always positive.
- The diagnosis is often made clinically, as no specific test can rule scleroderma in or out.

▶ TREATMENT

- There is no cure.
- In the case of systemic disease, treatment is often directed to the affected organ:
  - Raynaud syndrome: calcium channel blockers
  - Kidney disease: angiotensin-converting enzyme inhibitors
  - Gastrointestinal disease: proton-pump inhibitors
  - Lung disease: steroids
- Depending on the subtype, patients with scleroderma have a shortened lifespan.
- Stretching exercises to increase and maintain range of motion are vitally important.

Case Conclusion

Mary has scleroderma, as evidenced by her Raynaud phenomenon, age, and appearance of being younger than she really is. You give her calcium channel blockers to address the Raynaud phenomenon, and educate her about stretching exercise to maintain her range of motion.

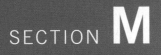

SECTION **M**   *Other Dermatologic Disorders*

CHAPTER **57**

Hidradenitis Suppurativa

Sunny Torbett Baker, PA-MS

A 22-year-old female presents to the clinic for the evaluation of multiple skin abscesses in her right axilla described as starting small but becoming large, red, swollen, and draining over a period of 2 weeks. The patient states she has been seen and treated for similar abscesses to both axillae in the past by multiple providers, but they always return. She presented today due to the pain and smell of the discharge. On assessment, a draining abscess is noted with scarring seen in the area. She is obese and has a past medical history of prediabetes and polycystic ovary syndrome. She smokes 1/2 pack per day and takes oral birth control pills daily. What is her diagnosis, and at what stage should she be classified?

▶ GENERAL FEATURES

- Hidradenitis suppurativa is also known as *acne inverse*; less commonly, hidradenitis axillaris, acne conglobata, apocrine acne, and apocrinitis.
- It is characterized by chronic, recurrent, and debilitating skin infections with abscesses in skinfolds such as axillae, groin, and the anal areas.
- Once believed to be a disorder of the apocrine sweat glands, new research demonstrates chronic follicular occlusion due to hyperkeratosis that progresses to inflammation, abscess, and, ultimately, follicular rupture, resulting in scarring and sinus track development.

- Its prevalence is between 1% and 4%; it begins after puberty, peaks between 20 and 30 years, and women are affected more often than men.
- Predisposing factors include obesity, metabolic syndrome, irritable bowel syndrome (IBS), and genetics.
- Triggers include smoking, tight or irritating clothing, deodorants, shaving, stress, sweating, heat and humidity, and oral contraceptives.
- Complications include secondary infection, fistula, and severe or keloid scaring.

▶ CLINICAL ASSESSMENT

- Differential considerations include simple cutaneous abscesses of the anal and perirectal regions, carbuncle, pilonidal cysts, furuncle, follicularis, and epidermoid or dermoid cysts.
- Patients describe single or multiple red painful nodules, often with burning or itching that lasts weeks to months, and may describe previous similar episodes with similar nodules.
- Individual lesions may be indistinguishable from cysts, simple abscesses, or other more common lesions; however, patients with hidradenitis suppurativa often have multiple lesions, double-ended comedones, draining sinus tracts, fistula, and previous scarring or lesions in more than one site.
- Some patients may note spontaneous drainage of malodorous discharge.
- Patients may have a family history of hidradenitis suppurativa or similar conditions.

▶ DIAGNOSIS

- Diagnosis is largely clinical and based on history and assessment looking for typical lesions in typical locations and chronicity.
- Typically affected areas demonstrate multiple lesions or recurrence of previously treated nodules or abscesses, sinus tracts, fistula, and scarring.
- No laboratory tests are needed for diagnosis.
- Biopsy is not required but may assist in further diagnosis.
- Hurley staging system may be used for further classification and treatment guidance:
  - Stage I (mild): solitary or multiple abscess formation without scarring or sinus tracts
  - Stage II (moderate): recurrent abscesses, single or multiple widely separated lesions with or without sinus tracts

- Stages III (severe): broad insolvent across a large area with multiple abscesses or sinus tracts
- The Hidradenitis Suppurativa Score (HHS) is a more detailed classification system often used to measure the efficacy of the treatments.

▶ TREATMENT

- Treatments vary widely depending on source referencing, but none are curative.
- Incision and drainage may be used for acute situation or lesions that are fluctuate or for those already draining.
- Lifestyle modifications and minimizing triggers are a focus.
- Give anti-inflammatory medications for pain.
- Early surgical and/or dermatological referral as needed.
- Stage I treatment:
  - Warm compresses
  - Topical clindamycin (1% solution or gel twice daily) and oral tetracycline (500 mg twice daily)
  - Intralesional steroid injection with triamcinolone (10 mL/mL varied volumes)
  - Topical resorcinol (15% cream once or twice daily)
- Stage II treatment:
  - Antibiotics such as doxycycline (100 mg twice daily) or minocycline (100 mg twice daily) or clindamycin (300 mg twice daily) and rifampicin (300 mg twice a day)
  - Intralesional steroid injections
  - Hormonal therapy in women with cyproterone acetate (100 mg daily) or ethinyl estradiol
  - Retinoids such as acitretin with caution
- Stage III treatment:
  - TNF-α inhibitor adalimumab (Humira) in those refractory to other treatments
  - Surgical treatments

Case Conclusion

Based on this patient's presentation, past medical history, and lifestyle factors that are triggers, she has hidradenitis suppurativa. She is obese and has a past medical history of prediabetes and polycystic ovary syndrome. She presents with recurrent abscesses, single or multiple widely separated lesions with or without sinus tracts, indicating Hurley stage II.

CHAPTER 59

Lipoma, Epidermal Inclusion Cysts, and Photosensitivity Reactions

Amy M. Klingler, MS, PA-C, DFAAPA

A 34-year-old female presents to the clinic with concerns about a soft, rubbery skin nodule on her left arm for several years. It is nontender and has not changed significantly in size. She is concerned that it may be cancerous. What is your advice to her?

GENERAL FEATURES

- Lipoma:
  - Benign tumor composed of mature adipose tissue that grows in the subcutaneous layer of skin
  - Can be single or multiple
  - Generally develop in adulthood but may appear in children
  - Transformation to the malignant liposarcoma is rare
- Epidermal inclusion cyst (EIC):
  - Benign encapsulated skin nodule filled with keratin material originating from the upper area of a hair follicle; a central punctum is often visible without magnification
  - Also known as *epidermoid cyst* or *epidermal cyst*
  - Can occur anywhere on the body but are most often found on the face, neck, or trunk
  - Range in size from a few millimeters to a few centimeters
  - Usually asymptomatic but can become infected with skin flora
  - Commonly misidentified as sebaceous cysts, but they do not contain sebum and do not originate from sebaceous glands
  - In rare cases can be malignant, with squamous cell carcinoma being the most common malignancy developed from EIC
- Photosensitivity reaction:
  - Abnormal skin response caused by exposure to ultraviolet (UV) or visible light
  - Types:
    - Solar urticaria: urticarial wheals that develop after sun exposure
    - Chemical photosensitization: drug-induced photosensitivity from oral or topical medications
    - Polymorphous light eruption (PMLE): an idiopathic photodermatitis that often recurs in susceptible individuals and resolves
  - Often a positive family history of similar reactions

- Obtain complete history to narrow the differential diagnosis, including age at onset, duration and location of symptoms, description of cutaneous findings, seasonal variation, oral medications and any products applied topically to the skin, similar past episodes, and family history of similar episodes.
- Some photosensitivity reactions can be associated with systemic lupus erythematosus (SLE) or porphyria.

CLINICAL ASSESSMENT

- Lipoma:
  - Smooth, soft, mobile nodule found under the skin
  - Usually asymptomatic; if painful, consider the diagnosis of angiolipoma, which is a similar benign nodule of adipose tissue and capillaries
- EIC:
  - 0.5 cm to several centimeters firm, subcutaneous nodule with visible central punctum
  - If infected, may appear erythematous, tender, and fluctuant
- Photosensitivity reaction: pruritic, erythematous skin lesions (wheals, papules, vesicles) on sun-exposed skin, often with sparing of areas of the skin that are shaded from the sun such as upper lip, nasolabial folds, posterior auricular area, and parts of the neck

DIAGNOSIS

- Lipoma:
  - Diagnosis is usually made by clinical findings, but biopsy or ultrasound can confirm the diagnosis.
  - Biopsy should be performed if the lesions are increasing in size or if the nodule is firm rather than soft.
- EIC:
  - Diagnosis is usually made clinically based on the appearance of a discrete, freely moveable cyst, often with a visible central punctum; cysts can occur anywhere on the body and typically present as nodules directly underneath the patient's skin.
  - If infected, culture is recommended before initiating antibiotics.
- Photosensitivity reaction: requires evaluation of history and physical examination findings and may include evaluation for with ANA, anti-dsDNS, anti-Ro (SSA), anti-LA (SSB) titers, and porphyrin studies if SLE or porphyria is suspected.

◗ TREATMENT

- Lipoma:
  - Surgical excision can be performed for cosmesis or bothersome lesions, but it is also appropriate to monitor.
  - Once excised, lipomas do not usually recur.
- EIC:
  - For clinically stable EIC, can monitor or excise
  - Ideal time to excise the nodule is before it becomes infected.
  - It is important to remove the cyst with cell wall intact to prevent recurrence.
- Photosensitivity reaction:
  - Prevention of sun exposure by avoiding direct exposure to sunlight, use of protective clothing and broad-spectrum sunscreens, window films to block UV light
  - Solar urticaria may respond to H1 blockers.
  - PMLE may respond to oral or topical corticosteroids or hydroxychloroquine.

Case Conclusion

The patient's examination demonstrates a 3-cm rubbery, smooth skin nodule that is mobile. It is not tender and not compressible. There is no fluctuance or central punctum. You reassure her that her skin nodule is likely a benign lipoma. It can be excised for cosmetic purposes, or she can monitor it and return for further evaluation if it changes size or becomes painful.

CHAPTER
59

Acanthosis Nigricans

Sarah Schettle, PA-C, MBA, MS

Mr. Menken is a 32-year-old male who presented for a primary care visit at the insistence of his girlfriend owing to the presence of a chronic dark, velvety patch on the fatty folds of his neck. What might be causing this skin issue in this patient?

◗ GENERAL FEATURES

- Acanthosis nigricans (AN) is a diffuse, dark brown or black, velvety appearance of skin that tends to appear most commonly in body folds.
- The neck and axilla are the most commonly affected areas.
- AN has a strong association with obesity.
- Risk factors for AN include: familial AN, Native American ethnicity, endocrine syndromes, obesity and insulin resistance, malignancy related to paraneoplastic syndromes, certain medications (oral contraceptives [OCPs], vitamin B3, steroids), and greater skin pigmentation.

◗ CLINICAL ASSESSMENT

- AN initially presents as darkening of the skin that progresses to thick, velvety skin with obvious skin lines.

◗ DIAGNOSIS

- AN is diagnosed on clinical examination.
- Although rarely indicated, skin biopsy can confirm the diagnosis.
- There are no specific lab tests or imaging studies used to diagnose AN.

◗ TREATMENT

- Address underlying conditions.
- Recommend weight loss for obese patients.
- Laser therapy and topical prescription lightening creams can provide aesthetic relief.
- Avoid scrubbing the affected skin areas or using abrasive agents to treat AN.
- In patients who take certain medications (OCPs, vitamin B3, steroids), consider whether medications can be discontinued or transitioned to different agents.
- When AN is related to underlying malignancy, surgical tumor removal may result in skin change resolution.

Case Conclusion

Mr. Menken's skin findings of a diffuse, dark, velvety appearance at a body fold (his neck) suggest acanthosis nigricans (AN). You suggest that he try to lose weight, which will help Mr. Menken's AN resolve.

chapter 60

Acute Urticarial Eruptions and Drug Eruptions

Anne Wildermuth, MMS, PA-C, RD

A 27-year-old female with a past medical history of bipolar disorder treated with lamotrigine presents to the emergency department with a rash. She has experienced an intermittent fever around 101 °F the past several days and feels fatigued. In the past day, she has noticed that her face is "puffy." On examination, you note a morbilliform rash with follicular accentuation on examination and desquamation of her palms. What is the most likely diagnosis?

▶ GENERAL FEATURES

- Urticaria:
  - Commonly referred to as *hives*, the intensely pruritic skin lesions are typically self-limited and resolve spontaneously.
  - Individual urticarial lesions disappear within 24 hours; however, the presence of urticaria can persist.
  - Acute urticaria is defined by lesions present for l to <6 weeks.
  - Urticaria may have an identifiable trigger, such as drugs, foods, infection, insect bites, or stress.
  - Exercise, exposure to the sun, cold temperatures, or water may also cause urticaria.
  - A clear etiology is frequently not found.
- Dermatologic drug eruptions:
  - These common adverse reactions to medications can be considered simple or complex depending on the degree of morbidity and mortality.
  - Simple reactions include a maculopapular or morbilliform rash without associated systemic signs or symptoms.
  - Antibiotics, especially penicillins, β-lactams, and sulfa and sulfonamide medications are common causes of urticarial and maculopapular reactions.
  - Complex drug eruptions are systemic and include Stevens-Johnson syndrome and DRESS (drug reaction with eosinophilia and systemic symptoms).
    - The most commonly implicated drug in DRESS is lamotrigine; carbamazepine, allopurinol, and phenytoin are also common causes.
    - DRESS is a systemic, drug-induced hypersensitivity reaction, frequently associated with reactivation of latent human herpesvirus, and is potentially life-threatening; acute liver failure is the most common cause of death in DRESS.
    - Involvement of internal organs occurs in nearly all patients with DRESS, and the majority of

patients have two or more organs involved; the liver is most commonly affected, followed by the kidneys and lungs.
    - DRESS typically resolves after drug withdrawal; however, some cases can persist for months with relapses and remissions even when the causative agent is avoided.

▶ CLINICAL ASSESSMENT

- Urticaria:
  - Raised, clearly demarcated erythematous plaques may exhibit central pallor.
  - Lesions come in a variety of shapes, including round and serpiginous, and vary in size.
  - Urticaria may be confluent and can affect any area of the body.
- Maculopapular or morbilliform drug reactions:
  - These are the most common skin reaction to medications; typically, rashes start on the thorax and spread to extremities.
  - Drug reactions usually occur 1–2 weeks after starting a medication but may occur up to a week after stopping a medication; the eruption typically clears within 3–5 days after discontinuing the offending medication.
  - DRESS frequently begins with a prodrome of fever, malaise, lymphadenopathy, and mucous membrane pain without ulceration for several days before cutaneous changes.
    - The rash in DRESS is morbilliform in nature with follicular accentuation; it starts on the face, upper trunk, and extremities first and typically spreads to cover at least 50% of body surface area (BSA).
    - Exfoliative dermatitis and desquamation of the palms and soles are possible.
    - DRESS organ involvement can present from asymptomatic to severe symptoms.
    - An asymptomatic increase in serum liver function tests (LFTs) is the most common manifestation. Hepatitis, acute liver failure, acute interstitial nephritis, respiratory symptoms, interstitial pneumonitis, and myocarditis are possible.

▶ DIAGNOSIS

- Acute urticaria is a clinical diagnosis:
  - A careful history should be taken to search for a trigger and evaluate for any signs of anaphylaxis.

- Referral to an allergy specialist for testing is warranted in cases of anaphylaxis, unresolving urticaria, and/or a suspected food or drug allergy.
- Simple drug eruptions are a clinical diagnosis:
  - Diagnosing DRESS requires a high degree of clinical suspicion and is suggested when the eruption is ≥50% BSA and/or includes two or more of facial edema, infiltrated lesions, scaling, and purpura.
  - Laboratory evaluation in DRESS confirms the diagnosis and allows for evaluation of visceral involvement:
    - Diagnostic studies should include a complete blood count (CBC) with differential, peripheral smear, comprehensive metabolic panel (CMP), urinalysis, and ECG.
      - The white blood count (WBC) differential and the peripheral smear will reveal eosinophilia.
      - CMP may show increased LFTs or abnormal renal function.
      - Urinalysis may be consistent with nephritic syndrome and show abnormal urinary sediment with eosinophils.
      - ECG and troponin may be abnormal in the case of myocarditis.
  - A skin biopsy can be completed if the diagnosis remains uncertain.

▶ TREATMENT

- Acute urticaria:
  - Treatment is focused on relief of pruritus, typically with H1 antihistamines:
    - First-generation H1 antihistamines include diphenhydramine and hydroxyzine, and second-generation agents include cetirizine and loratadine.
    - Second-generation H1 antihistamines are preferred, as first-generation drugs often cause significant drowsiness and anticholinergic side effects.
  - A short course of corticosteroids may be beneficial if the urticaria persists for several days.
  - If a clear trigger of urticaria is identified, educate patients on avoiding the causative agent.
  - Simple drug exanthems are managed by stopping the causative agent; oral antihistamines can be used for any associated pruritus.
- DRESS:
  - The mainstay and most important treatment in DRESS is withdrawal of the causative drug; patients must be counseled to avoid the causative agent for life.
  - DRESS warrants admission, preferably to an intensive care unit or burn unit.
  - Systemic corticosteroids, such as methylprednisolone intravenous (IV) or prednisone PO, are indicated for 3–6 months and are slowly tapered to prevent relapse.
  - Cutaneous lesions should be treated with high-potency steroids, such as betamethasone or clobetasol, for 1 week.
  - Organ involvement in DRESS should be managed as indicated depending on the location and severity of involvement.

Case Conclusion

This patient is most likely having DRESS (drug reaction with eosinophilia and systemic symptoms). The most common drug to cause DRESS is lamotrigine, which the patient takes. She also has three of the classic symptoms, facial edema, desquamation of the palms, and a morbilliform rash with follicular accentuation. You immediately discontinue her lamotrigine and admit her to the hospital for additional care.

CHAPTER 61

Pilonidal Disease

Janelle Bludorn, MS, PA-C

A 20-year-old overweight man seeks evaluation at the student health clinic for 2 days of pain and swelling near his tailbone. He reports moderate discomfort worsened by sitting for long periods of time while driving for a ride-sharing service. He cannot recall preceding trauma to the area, nor has he noted any drainage. Today, he experienced a low-grade fever and began feeling generally ill, prompting him to seek care. His examination is remarkable for tenderness and fluctuance in the gluteal cleft without surrounding erythema or induration. What is the likely diagnosis, and how should he be treated?

▶ GENERAL FEATURES

- Pilonidal disease is a skin and soft-tissue condition of the sacrococcygeal region between the upper buttocks; this area is sometimes referred to as the *gluteal cleft* or *natal cleft*.
- Derived from Latin *pilus* (hair) and *nidus* (nest), pilonidal disease is characterized by midline pits or sinus tracts that amass hair or other debris and may become acutely or chronically infected.
- Acute pilonidal disease occurs when an abscess forms in a gluteal cleft pit or sinus. Chronic pilonidal disease is an iterative or persistent manifestation of such infection.
- Pathogens in pilonidal abscesses are typically anaerobes. Aerobic organisms are the most common cause of chronic pilonidal disease.
- Pilonidal disease is 3–4 times more likely to affect males than females and usually occurs in the late teens or early twenties, with an incidence of 26 cases per 100,000 people.
- Individuals who are sedentary, overweight/obese, have increased body hair, or who have a family history of pilonidal disease may be at higher risk.

▶ CLINICAL ASSESSMENT

- History and physical examination findings for pilonidal disease depend on whether an individual is experiencing asymptomatic, acute, or chronic manifestation of the condition:
  - Asymptomatic:
    - No symptoms reported, but incidental findings of midline pits or sinus tracts in the gluteal cleft.
  - Acute:
    - Pain in the sacrococcygeal region is acute, especially when sitting, bending at the waist, or performing other activities that stretch the skin of the gluteal cleft.
    - Pain is moderate to severe and may be accompanied by swelling, purulence, blood-tinged drainage, malaise, or fever.
    - Physical examination reveals a tender area of fluctuance at the gluteal cleft consistent with abscess; a midline sinus tract with purulent or bloody material or protruding hair may be present.
  - Chronic:
    - History shows repeated or prolonged episodes of acute pilonidal disease.
    - Physical examination demonstrates one or multiple gluteal cleft sinus tracts with or without purulent or bloody drainage, accompanying abscess(es), or protruding hair.

▶ DIAGNOSIS

- Diagnosis is clinical and can be made based on a characteristic history and physical examination findings.

- History ranges from asymptomatic to acute, chronic, or recurrent episodes of gluteal cleft pain, swelling, or drainage; may be associated with malaise or fever.
- Physical examination of the gluteal cleft reveals a combination of midline pits, tenderness, fluctuance, and one or more sinus openings with or without the presence of purulent or bloody drainage.
- Laboratory and imaging studies are not essential for diagnosis.

▶ TREATMENT

- Asymptomatic pilonidal disease does not require treatment.
- If abscess is present, management of acute and chronic pilonidal disease is incision and drainage (I&D) with the following considerations:
  - Incision should be made lateral to midline to decrease risk of midline pits interfering with wound healing.
  - Thorough debridement of hair and debris is necessary.
  - Allow healing via secondary intention; the clinician may elect to pack the wound with packing material.
- Counsel patients that treatment with I&D may not be definitive, as the recurrence rate is 10%–55%, but risk of recurrence may be decreased with gluteal cleft hair removal and hygiene measures.
- The definitive management for chronic pilonidal disease is surgical excision of the sinus tracts; multiple surgical techniques exist, without clear evidence for an optimal approach, yet these trends have emerged:
  - Primary-closure procedures promote more rapid healing, whereas delayed-closure procedures decrease risk of recurrence.
  - Off-midline suture placement is superior to midline considering healing time and likelihood of recurrence.
- Antibiotics are reserved for individuals with:
  - Associated cellulitis
  - Immune compromise
  - Underlying medical conditions that increase their risk of systemic infection

Case Conclusion

This patient has acute pilonidal disease with abscess, most likely caused by an anaerobic organism. Imaging studies are not necessary for this diagnosis. These abscesses occur more often in men than women. You plan to treat the abscess with incision and drainage (I&D) and debridement to prevent recurrence. Optimal wound healing and infection treatment are achieved by making an off-midline incision and allowing healing by secondary intention.

Section A Pretest: Ear Disorders

1. Which of the following is NOT a clinical finding in acute otitis externa?
   A. Pain with tragus or auricle movement
   B. Discharge from affected ear
   C. Fever
   D. Decreased hearing

2. Which of the following is a known risk factor for the development of acoustic neuroma?
   A. Leisure noise exposure
   B. Frequent ear infections
   C. Chronic cerumen impaction
   D. Swimming in cold water

3. Which of the following is NOT an indication to perform a culture of the external auditory canal?
   A. Patient who is HIV positive
   B. Recurrent otitis externa infections
   C. When selecting an empiric antibiotic treatment
   D. Otitis externa diagnosed 1 week after ear surgery

4. What is considered the imaging test of choice for diagnosis of cholesteatoma?
   A. CT
   B. MRI
   C. US
   D. Otoscopy

5. A 27-month-old female presents with unilateral otalgia, fever, and irritability that has worsened over the past 7 days. Symptoms started with sudden onset of fever, malaise, and nasal drainage 1 week ago. Which of the following organisms is most likely causing this patient's symptoms?
   A. *Streptococcus pneumoniae*
   B. *Staphylococcus aureus*
   C. *Clostridioides difficile*
   D. *Streptococcus pyogenes*

6. What is the treatment of choice for a cholesteatoma?
   A. Surgical excision
   B. Oral amoxicillin
   C. Topical ciprofloxacin
   D. Vestibular therapy

7. Which of the following is considered first-line treatment for acute otitis media (AOM)?
   A. Azithromycin
   B. Penicillin
   C. Amoxicillin
   D. Cephalexin

8. Which topical otic medication can be used in a patient with otitis externa and tympanic membrane (TM) perforation?
   A. Chloroxylenol, pramoxine, and hydrocortisone
   B. Ciprofloxacin and dexamethasone
   C. Ciprofloxacin and hydrocortisone
   D. Polymyxin B, neomycin, and hydrocortisone

9. Tyler is a 3-year-old male with otitis media with effusion (OME) that has been persistent for >6 months. He is now experiencing language delay from the chronic presence of middle ear fluid. What should Tyler's PA recommend as next steps to his parents?
   A. Intranasal corticosteroids
   B. 10-Day course of antibiotics
   C. Tonsillectomy
   D. Tympanostomy tubes

10. Which of the following is a risk factor for AOM?
    A. Breastfeeding
    B. Attending day care
    C. Female gender
    D. Sensorineural hearing loss

11. Which of the following is most likely to lead to the development of an acquired cholesteatoma?
    A. Allergic rhinitis
    B. Otitis media
    C. Otitis externa
    D. Acoustic neuroma

12. Which of the following studies is NOT included in the workup of a patient who is suspected to have mastoiditis?
    A. Audiogram
    B. Complete blood count
    C. CT scan of the mastoid
    D. Culture of middle ear aspirate
    E. MRI

13. Which of the following findings would most closely correlate with a potential diagnosis of cholesteatoma?
    A. Painless, recurrent otorrhea
    B. Ear pain, otorrhea, and tinnitus
    C. Presence of aural polyp on the TM
    D. Purulent otorrhea with granulation tissue

14. Which of the following is a risk factor for obstructive-type eustachian tube dysfunction (ETD)?

    A. Weight loss
    B. Allergies
    C. GERD
    D. Anxiety

15. Which of the following statements is true regarding cholesteatomas?

    A. Hearing loss is typically reversible.
    B. Recurrence rate after surgical removal is ~5%.
    C. They are made of keratin.
    D. They are localized to the external auditory canal.

16. A 66-year-old man presents with asymmetric bilateral sensorineural hearing loss. MRI shows bilateral acoustic neuromas. Which of the following systemic conditions does this patient most likely have?

    A. Neurofibromatosis type 2
    B. Ménière disease
    C. Marfan syndrome
    D. Sjögren syndrome

17. An acoustic neuroma arises from what anatomic structure?

    A. Myelin covering of the vestibular portion of cranial nerve VIII
    B. Myelin covering of the cochlear portion of cranial nerve VIII
    C. Neuronal cells in the cerebellopontine angle (CPA)
    D. Bone cells of the ossicles

18. Which of the following is the best long-term management for obstructive-type chronic eustachian tube dysfunction in a patient with chronic otitis media with effusion?

    A. Corticosteroids
    B. Tympanocentesis
    C. Systemic decongestants
    D. Tympanostomy tubes

19. What is the differentiating factor between labyrinthitis and vestibular neuritis?

    A. Presence or absence of headache and ataxia
    B. Presence or absence of hearing loss and tinnitus
    C. Presence or absence of nausea and vomiting
    D. Presence or absence of vertigo and nystagmus

20. Which of the following descriptions of an adult patient's symptoms would lead you to consider patulous eustachian tube dysfunction at the top of your differential diagnosis?

    A. Tinnitus, vertigo, and unilateral hearing loss
    B. Otorrhea and external canal pain
    C. Unusually loud hearing of a person's own voice
    D. Clicking noise in ear, ear pressure, and pain with opening jaw wide

21. A 67-year-old patient with lifelong allergic rhinitis presents with complaints of unilateral ear pressure, pain, and muffled hearing that has not improved with 12 weeks of intranasal corticosteroids and systemic antihistamines. Which of the following imaging studies should be considered in this patient?

    A. Ultrasound of the neck
    B. MRI of the brain without contrast
    C. CT with contrast of the head and neck
    D. Sinus plain film x-rays

22. Which of the following is part of the classic triad of Ménière disease?

    A. Headache
    B. Tinnitus
    C. Otorrhea
    D. Otalgia

23. Which of the following statements regarding the prognosis of labyrinthitis is true?

    A. Severe vertigo typically last for 3–4 months.
    B. BPPV or panic disorder may subsequently develop.
    C. Future recurrences are common.
    D. Hearing loss always resolves.

24. Which of the following is an appropriate daily maintenance therapy for Ménière disease?

    A. Hydrochlorothiazide and triamterene
    B. Atenolol
    C. Intratympanic gentamycin
    D. Ofloxacin otic

25. Which of the following treatment regimens is most appropriate for labyrinthitis?

    A. Intratympanic gentamycin
    B. Hydrochlorothiazide and triamterene
    C. Oral prednisone
    D. Azithromycin

26. Which of the following lifestyle modifications is recommended for Ménière disease?

    A. Potassium restrictions
    B. Calorie restrictions
    C. Cessation of lactose-containing products
    D. Cessation of nicotine-containing products

27. What is the diagnostic test of choice for hearing impairment?

    A. Weber and Rinne
    B. MRI
    C. Tympanometry
    D. Audiometry

28. Which of the following is NOT used for cerumen impaction removal?

    A. Ultrasound
    B. Ear curette
    C. Water irrigation
    D. Suction

Section B Pretest: Eye Disorders

1. A 40-year-old female patient presents to the office after fasting glucose returns >126 mg/dL for the second time. She has no visual or medical complaints. Her visual acuity is 20/20 OU. When should this patient be referred to an ophthalmologist for ocular screening and evaluation?

   A. Immediately at the time of this visit
   B. When she develops visual symptoms
   C. Within 2 years of this visit
   D. Within 3 years of this visit

2. Posterior blepharitis is an inflammatory process that involves which of the following structures?

   A. Anterior eyelashes
   B. Glands of Zeis
   C. Glands of Moll
   D. Inner lid at the level of the meibomian glands

3. A 70-year-old female with a 35-pack-year history of smoking reports 2 months of progressively worsening bilateral painless central vision loss. She also describes frequent partially distorted images. Which of the following findings are you most likely to find on funduscopic examination?

   A. Copper wiring, arteriovenous (AV) nicking, hemorrhages, and cotton-wool patches
   B. Crescents or rings of light along the temporal borders of the optic discs
   C. Hyperemic and swollen optic discs with hazy edges with green-gray macula
   D. Scattered hard drusen with clearly defined edges and areas of depigmentation

4. Dacryocystitis can occur in infants due to which of the following?

   A. Persistent membrane covering the valve of Hasner
   B. Persistent membrane covering the posterior lacrimal crest
   C. Persistent membrane covering the canaliculi
   D. Persistent membrane covering over the puncta

5. Fundoscopy will identify which of the following in the early stages of hypertensive retinopathy?

   A. Arteriolar constriction
   B. Arteriolar wall thickening
   C. Copper wiring
   D. Vascular wall hyperplasia

6. In what population does nasolacrimal duct obstruction commonly occur?

   A. Premenopausal women
   B. Older men
   C. Young men
   D. Postmenopausal women

7. What part of the lacrimal drainage system is generally affected in dacryocystitis?

   A. Puncta
   B. Canaliculi
   C. Lacrimal gland
   D. Nasolacrimal duct

8. A patient diagnosed with a hordeolum returns in 3 days after attempting conservative management at home with warm compresses and lid massage. The patient is afebrile, but there is swelling, tenderness, erythema of the entire eyelid and periorbital area. There is no proptosis or pain with eye movements. Which of the following is the next step in treatment?

   A. Continue warm compresses
   B. Massage the eyelid
   C. Start oral antibiotics
   D. Start topical antibiotics

9. Which of the following is NOT a common characteristic of dacryocystitis?

   A. Tearing
   B. Pain
   C. Swelling
   D. Double vision

10. Which of the following terms describes inward curling of an eyelash?

    A. Blepharitis
    B. Chalazion
    C. Entropion
    D. Ectropion

11. Which of the following is the definitive treatment for ectropion?

    A. Lubricating eye drops
    B. Surgery
    C. Taping the eyelid in place
    D. Warm compresses for exposed lid margins

12. Your patient presents with a sudden onset of right eye pain and discharge. The discharge is copious and constant. She is sexually active with a new partner and does not use barrier protection. She complains of burning with urination and vaginal discharge. What is the most likely diagnosis?

    A. Allergic conjunctivitis
    B. Gonococcal conjunctivitis
    C. Nongonococcal bacterial conjunctivitis
    D. Viral conjunctivitis

13. Mild cases of dacryocystitis can typically be treated with which of the following?

    A. Clindamycin
    B. Amoxicillin
    C. Sulfamethoxazole/trimethoprim
    D. Azithromycin

14. What is the appropriate treatment for a patient with gonococcal conjunctivitis who denies any allergies to medications?

    A. Artificial tears 4–5 times per day
    B. Ceftriaxone 1 g IM
    C. Prednisolone acetate 1% drops for 5–7 days
    D. Trimethoprim/polymyxin B drops for 5–7 days

15. Your patient presents with complaints of red, irritated eyes daily for 2 weeks. Her eyes are very itchy, and she rubs her eyes frequently. Her eyelids are red and irritated, and there is a watery discharge. She does not have any eye pain or photophobia, and there is no preauricular lymphadenopathy. She just adopted a cat. She is not sexually active. What is the most appropriate treatment?

    A. Await results from culture and Gram stain
    B. Ceftriaxone 1 g IM and azithromycin 1 g by mouth
    C. Oral antihistamine such as loratadine
    D. Topical antibiotic such as trimethoprim/polymyxin B

16. A 27-year-old male patient with suspected corneal abrasion should be treated with which of the following medications?

    A. Topical NSAIDs
    B. Topical antibiotics
    C. Oral antibiotics
    D. Topical anesthetic drops

17. Your 72-year-old Caucasian male patient with a history of diabetes and a 40-pack-year history of smoking complains of decreased visual acuity, blurred vision, and difficulty driving at night. On physical examination with an ophthalmoscope, you note a yellowish opacity of the lens of both eyes and a distorted red reflex. What is the best treatment for his condition?

    A. Surgical removal and replacement with an intraocular lens
    B. Antibiotic eye drops
    C. Steroid eye drops
    D. Vision correction with glasses

Section C Pretest: Nose and Sinus Disorders

1. Children who develop nasal polyps should be tested for which of the following conditions?

    A. Cystic fibrosis
    B. MS
    C. Cerebral palsy
    D. Inverted papilloma

2. Which medication has been known to induce rhinitis?

    A. Antihistamines
    B. Antipsychotics
    C. Opioids
    D. Oral contraceptive pills

3. Which of the following is recommended to minimize polyp recurrence after surgical management?

    A. Oral antibiotic maintenance therapy
    B. Long-term oral glucocorticoids
    C. Intranasal corticosteroid spray
    D. Monthly nasal endoscopy evaluation

4. Allergic rhinitis is which type of hypersensitivity reaction?

    A. Type I
    B. Type II
    C. Type III
    D. Type IV

5. Which of the following symptoms is common in patients with nasal polyps?

   A. Nasal obstruction
   B. Decreased congestion
   C. Hyperosmia
   D. Decreased postnasal drainage

6. What is the first-line medication indicated in patients with allergic rhinitis?

   A. Nasal anticholinergic
   B. Nasal antihistamine
   C. Nasal steroid
   D. Oral antihistamine

7. What is the imaging study of choice for nasal polyps?

   A. Coronal MRI
   B. Indirect nasopharyngoscopy
   C. Sweat chloride test
   D. Nonenhanced coronal CT scan

8. Viral rhinitis typically resolves within what time frame?

   A. 3 days
   B. 7 days
   C. 10 days
   D. 21 days

9. Which of these symptoms is most concerning for head and neck cancer?

   A. Nausea
   B. Decreased sense of smell
   C. Unexplained otalgia
   D. Dental caries

10. Which of the following is a risk factor for the development of nasal polyps?

    A. Acute upper respiratory infection
    B. Chronic seasonal allergies
    C. Acute bronchitis
    D. Chronic adenitis

11. Which test is indicated if you suspect rhinitis containing CSF?

    A. β-2-Transferrin
    B. Complete blood count
    C. Complete metabolic panel
    D. Erythrocyte sedimentation rate

12. A 36-year-old female presents with 12 days of sinus pressure, nasal congestion, purulent nasal drainage, and halitosis. She has not had a sinus infection in several years and has tried treating her symptoms with acetaminophen, topical intranasal corticosteroid, and pseudoephedrine. Which of the following organisms would most likely cause this patient's symptoms?

    A. *Pseudomonas aeruginosa*
    B. *Haemophilus influenzae*
    C. *S. aureus*
    D. *S. pyogenes*

13. What is the diagnostic study of choice for a patient with extensive nasal and facial trauma?

    A. Plain films
    B. MRI
    C. CT scan
    D. Ultrasound

14. Which of the following is considered the first-line treatment for acute bacterial rhinosinusitis?

    A. Clarithromycin
    B. Trimethoprim/sulfamethoxazole
    C. Azithromycin
    D. Amoxicillin-clavulanate

15. Seasonal predominance of epistaxis in the winter months is contributed to which of the following?

    A. Stress
    B. Changes in humidity levels
    C. Increased use of nasal corticosteroids
    D. Hypertension

16. Which of the following is an indication for imaging following nasal trauma?

    A. Absence of septal hematoma
    B. Trauma limited to the bridge of the nose
    C. Visible nasal displacement
    D. No change in ability to breathe

17. Which of the following should be NOT done as first-line treatment for minor epistaxis?

    A. Pinch the tip of the nose for 10–15 minutes.
    B. Use an ice pack.
    C. Tilt the head back.
    D. Use a topical vasoconstrictor.

18. What is the most common anatomic location for a patient presenting with foreign-body insertion?

    A. Ear
    B. GI tract
    C. Lower respiratory tract
    D. Nasal passage

19. Which of the following is responsible for head and neck cancers increasingly occurring in nonsmoking, nondrinking young adults?

    A. Gonorrhea
    B. Chlamydia
    C. HPV
    D. Herpes simplex virus

20. What demographic has the highest incidence demographic for nasal foreign-body insertion?

    A. Infant
    B. Toddlers and preschoolers
    C. Teenager
    D. Adult

21. If an anterior bleeding source is visualized, first-line treatment includes which of the following?

    A. Packing with petroleum gauze
    B. Insert nasal tampon
    C. Cautery using silver nitrate sticks
    D. Application of topical thrombin gel

22. What type of visualization or imaging should be used to confirm the presence of an inorganic nasal foreign body?

    A. CT of the head and neck
    B. Direct otoscopic visualization
    C. Fiberoptic rhinoscopy
    D. Plain radiograph of the head and facial bones

23. What is the preferred treatment approach for a 2-year-old patient with an occlusive bead in the right nare?

    A. Balloon or Katz extractor
    B. Cyanoacrylate glue
    C. Plastic umbrella suction
    D. Positive pressure "parent's kiss"

24. Which of the following statements regarding nasal trauma is true?

    A. The central location of the nose on the face predisposes it to fracture.
    B. Nasal fractures occur more commonly in females.
    C. Young children experience nasal fractures more commonly than adults.
    D. The bones of the nasal bridge are thick and difficult to fracture.

25. Which of the following descriptions of a patient's symptoms should lead you to put acute bacterial rhinosinusitis on the top of your differential diagnosis?

    A. Clear nasal drainage, nasal congestion, headache, and cough present <7 days
    B. Frontal sinus pain, clear nasal drainage, and fatigue for 8 days
    C. Purulent nasal drainage, maxillary sinus pain, and persistent headache for 12 days
    D. Headache, bad breath, and cough for 10 days

26. Which of the following examination findings is commonly associated with nasal fracture?

    A. Supraorbital ecchymosis
    B. Trismus
    C. Nasal crepitus and tenderness
    D. "Hot-potato" voice

27. What is the appropriate management of a septal hematoma?

    A. Refer to otolaryngology for evaluation 3–7 days after the injury
    B. Nasal septal reconstruction
    C. Immediate incision and drainage with packing
    D. Observation with follow-up in 5 days

28. What is the most common patient presentation of an inorganic nasal foreign body?

    A. Black nasal discharge
    B. Difficulty breathing
    C. Facial pain and/or swelling
    D. History concerning for foreign-body insertion

29. Which of the following is a risk factor for the development of squamous cell carcinoma (SCC) of the head and neck?

    A. Iced beverages
    B. Mandibular tori
    C. Smokeless tobacco
    D. Caffeine

30. Which of the following is considered the best treatment for chronic rhinosinusitis?

    A. Daily saline irrigation
    B. Amphotericin B
    C. Levaquin
    D. Watchful waiting

31. What is the imaging study of choice for head and neck cancers?

    A. Ultrasonography
    B. Contrast CT scan
    C. MRI
    D. Plain films

32. Which of the following is a risk factor for acute bacterial rhinosinusitis?

    A. Younger age
    B. Allergies
    C. Excessive alcohol use
    D. Chronic use of intranasal decongestants

33. Why is it necessary to visualize all aspects of the tongue and the mucosa under the tongue?

    A. Mandibular tori frequently transform into SCC.
    B. Herpes simplex virus lesions are common in these locations.
    C. The tongue is a common site of malignancy for lung cancer.
    D. Smokeless tobacco users hold the product in these locations.

Section D Pretest: Oropharyngeal Disorders

1. What is the most common causative organism of epiglottitis?
   A. *Moraxella catarrhalis*
   B. *Haemophilus influenzae* type B (Hib)
   C. *P. aeruginosa*
   D. *Corynebacterium diphtheriae*

2. What is the most common bacteria that causes cavities?
   A. *P. aeruginosa*
   B. *Actinomycosis viscosus*
   C. *Porphyromonas gingivalis*
   D. *Streptococcus mutans*

3. More serious signs of airway compromise in epiglottitis may include which of the following?
   A. Sore throat
   B. Pleurisy
   C. Stridor
   D. Nasal congestion

4. A patient experiences a sore throat and a fever. Two days later, a rash appears. On examination, you note Pastia lines and circumoral pallor. The patient develops a positive antistreptolysin O (ASO) titer. The patient takes no medications. What is the most likely diagnosis of this patient's symptoms?
   A. Rubella
   B. Infectious mononucleosis
   C. Scarlet fever
   D. Erythema infectiosum

5. Which of the following is the classic acute epiglottitis radiographic finding on lateral neck x-ray?
   A. McConnell sign
   B. "Steeple" sign
   C. "Thumb-print" sign
   D. "Spine" sign

6. Which of the following is NOT a recommended antibiotic treatment for GAS pharyngitis?
   A. Penicillin V
   B. Cefdinir
   C. Clindamycin
   D. Sulfamethoxazole/trimethoprim

7. What is the most appropriate next step in the management of a 39-year-old male patient with a confirmed painless, large dental abscess that is not putting pressure on the airway?
   A. Penicillin VK 500 mg TID for 7 days
   B. Referral to a dentist
   C. Penicillin VK 500 mg TID for 7 days and referral to a dentist
   D. Incision and drainage with PenVK Rx

8. Which of the following is NOT included in the Centor criteria?
   A. Fever >38 °C (100.4 °F)
   B. Pharyngeal erythema
   C. Pharyngotonsillar exudate
   D. Tender anterior cervical lymphadenopathy

9. Which of the following is an example of abnormal dental findings that typically are associated with systemic disease?
   A. Palpation of the left lower molar that moves inferiorly and laterally on palpation in a 45-year-old female
   B. Generalized erythematous gingival margins that bleed on light palpation
   C. Knife-edged interdental papilla that does not bleed on palpation
   D. Teeth with generalized slightly yellow color where all enamel appears to be intact

10. Which of the following is a characteristic finding in a patient with a peritonsillar abscess?
    A. Gray pseudomembrane on the pharynx
    B. "Strawberry tongue"
    C. Uvular deviation
    D. Kissing tonsils

11. What is the most common sign of gingivitis?
    A. Gingival bleeding
    B. Tooth mobility
    C. Dental decay
    D. Fissures and halitosis

12. Which of the following is a typical presentation of minor aphthous ulcers?
    A. 5 lesions, 4 mm in diameter each
    B. 20 lesions, 10 mm in diameter each
    C. 6 lesions, 12 mm in diameter each
    D. 12 clustered lesions, 2 mm in diameter each

13. What is the most appropriate management for leukoplakia?
    A. It is benign, no further follow-up is needed
    B. Radical neck dissection
    C. Oral nystatin suspension
    D. Surgical removal with serial monitoring

14. Which of the following is potential complication of deep neck infections?
    A. Inverted papilloma
    B. Mediastinitis
    C. Chronic tonsillitis
    D. Rheumatoid arthritis

15. What should be suspected as the most likely cause in an unvaccinated pediatric patient with bilateral parotitis and flulike symptoms?
    A. Measles
    B. Mumps
    C. HIV
    D. Rhinovirus

16. In a patient who presents with recurrent unilateral salivary gland swelling and pain that acutely worsens when eating, what would be the best option for definitive resolution of symptoms?
    A. Antibiotics
    B. Sialendoscopy
    C. Surgical removal of the gland
    D. Supportive care

17. What is the imaging study of choice for deep neck infections?
    A. Intraoral ultrasound
    B. MRA
    C. MRI
    D. Contrast CT

18. In a patient with acute-onset unilateral salivary gland swelling, tenderness, induration, and erythema, what is the most likely infectious etiology?
    A. *S. aureus*
    B. *Streptococcus*
    C. *Klebsiella*
    D. *H. influenzae*

19. Which of the following examination findings is associated with oral candidiasis?
    A. Lesions do not rub off
    B. Erythematous rim around lesion with yellow-gray center
    C. Lesions rub off with tongue depressor
    D. Midline pharyngeal bulge

20. What should be suspected in a patient with acute sialadenitis with pus expressed from the duct?
    A. Acute suppurative sialadenitis
    B. Viral sialadenitis
    C. Sialolithiasis
    D. Salivary gland neoplasm

21. A 14-year-old male presents with sore throat and fever but denies cough. Examination reveals elevated temperature, tender anterior cervical lymphadenopathy, and pharyngeal exudates. What is the most likely diagnosis?
    A. Epiglottitis
    B. Infectious mononucleosis
    C. Peritonsillar abscess
    D. Streptococcal pharyngitis

22. Which salivary gland disorder should be suspected in a patient with a painless, slowly enlarging gland?
    A. Acute suppurative sialadenitis
    B. Viral sialadenitis
    C. Sialolithiasis
    D. Salivary gland neoplasm

▶ ANSWERS AND EXPLANATIONS TO SECTION A PRETEST

1. **C.** Fever is not a clinical finding in acute otitis externa but may be present with a complication, such as periauricular otitis externa or malignant otitis externa. Tenderness with tragal or auricle movement is the hallmark of the condition; other signs and symptoms include ear pain, discharge, and hearing loss.

2. **A.** Leisure noise exposure such as listening to loud music on headphones has been linked to the development of an acoustic neuroma.

3. **C.** Cultures are reserved for patients with severe cases of otitis externa, recurrent otitis externa, chronic otitis externa, immunosuppressed patients, otitis externa in a patient after ear surgery, and in patients who do not respond to initial therapy.

4. **A.** High-resolution CT is the diagnostic imaging test of choice because of its ability to identify the soft tissue and bony involvement in a cholesteatoma.

5. **A.** Like many infections of the upper respiratory tract, *S. pneumoniae*, *H. influenzae*, and *M. catarrhalis* remain the three leading bacterial pathogens in AOM.

6. **A.** Surgical excision is the treatment of choice for cholesteatoma.

7. **C.** Although there is a growing consensus for watchful waiting of uncomplicated AOM, amoxicillin continues to be the first-line antibiotic treatment for AOM.

8. **B.** Ciprofloxacin/dexamethasone or ofloxacin alone is recommended for patients with TM perforation or if the membrane is not visible due to canal swelling or debris.

9. **D.** Placement of tympanostomy tubes in the affected ear is recommended for those patients without improvement at 3-month follow-up, or if they develop speech, hearing, or language impairments.

10. **B.** Daycare attendance, cigarette smoke exposure, bottle-feeding, and male gender are risk factors for children to have recurrent AOM.

11. **B.** Acquired cholesteatomas are thought to arise due to ETD following middle ear disease.

12. **E.** Audiogram, complete blood count, CT scan of the mastoid, and culture of middle ear aspirate are all included in the workup of a patient suspected of having mastoiditis.

13. **C.** The pathognomonic examination finding of cholesteatoma includes the presence of a white, round, compressible lesion (aural polyp) on the posterior superior quadrant of the TM.

14. **B.** There are numerous risk factors for obstructive-type ETD, but all of these listed are related to patulous ETD, except for allergies, which affects both obstructive and patulous ETD.

15. **C.** Cholesteatomas are composed of keratin. Hearing loss caused by cholesteatomas is typically not reversible. Recurrence rate is close to 50% following surgical removal. They are found on the middle ear and mastoid not the external auditory canal.

16. **A.** Only 5% of patients with an acoustic neuroma present with bilateral lesions. Almost all also have neurofibromatosis type 2.

17. **A.** Acoustic neuromas arise from the Schwann cells that function as part of the myelin covering the vestibular portion of the eighth cranial nerve. Acoustic neuromas are also known as vestibular schwannomas. They grow to occupy the space in the CPA.

18. **D.** Patients with obstructive ETD with associated chronic OME of >3 months duration, especially those with hearing loss, will benefit from tympanostomy tubes. For adults with chronic OME, additional workup should be completed to rule out any underlying obstruction, such as nasopharyngeal neoplasms.

19. **B.** Vestibular neuritis is a spontaneous postinfectious inflammation affecting only the vestibular nerve, so the primary symptoms will be vertigo. Labyrinthitis has the same cause but inflammation is located throughout the entire vestibular canal (including the cochlea), so the patient will have vertigo in addition to hearing loss and tinnitus.

20. **C.** Patulous ETD is present when the valve fails to close properly. Patients may hear themselves talk loudly, through the open ET, which is called autophony.

21. **C.** CT or MRI scan with contrast is indicated in patients with >3 months of unilateral symptoms or a middle ear effusion. These raise suspicion for a neoplasm that may be obstructing the eustachian tube and should be evaluated with diagnostic imaging.

22. **B.** The classic triad of Ménière disease is tinnitus, hearing loss, and episodic vertigo.

23. **B.** Most patients experience severe symptoms for 1–2 weeks, and hearing loss may be permanent. Most patients do not experience a recurrence of symptoms. However, labyrinthitis patients are at an increased risk for developing panic disorder and BPPV.

24. **A.** Daily maintenance therapy with diuretics may reduce the frequency of attacks.

25. **C.** Initial treatment consists of a 10-day prednisone taper. Antiemetics and vestibular suppressants may be prescribed for symptom relief.

26. **D.** Lifestyle modifications should include salt restrictions, caffeine restrictions, alcohol restrictions, and cessation of nicotine products.

27. **D.** Audiometry is the diagnostic test of choice for hearing impairment in children and adults.

28. **A.** An ultrasound is not needed for cerumen impaction removal. Ear curette, water irrigation, and suction are all methods or equipment used for cerumen removal.

▶ ANSWERS AND EXPLANATIONS TO SECTION B PRETEST

1. **A.** Many patients with diabetic retinopathy are not symptomatic until late stages of disease. In 20% of patients with type 2 diabetes mellitus (T2DM), retinopathy is presents at the time of diagnosis. It is important for patients to be evaluated promptly after the initial diagnosis of T2DM is made.

2. **D.** Posterior blepharitis involves the inner lid.

3. **C.** Wet macular degeneration characterized by hyperemic and swollen optic discs with hazy edges with green-gray macula is a cause of central vision loss. Many patients also complain of metamorphopsia or abnormal size of images and scotomas. There are many risk factors for developing AMD, including age >50, smoking, heavy alcohol use, and long-term aspirin use.

4. **A.** In infants, dacryocystitis is usually caused by a persistent membrane covering the valve of Hasner, which does not allow the tears to drain into the nasal cavity.

5. **A.** In the early stages, fundoscopy identifies arteriolar constriction, with a decrease in the ratio of the width of the retinal arterioles and the retinal venules. Arteriole wall thickening typically requires years of uncontrolled hypertension.

6. **D.** Postmenopausal women are most commonly affected by nasolacrimal duct obstruction.

7. **D.** In dacryocystitis, the lacrimal duct is affected.

8. **C.** Start oral antibiotics. This patient is presenting with preseptal cellulitis, a possible complication of a hordeolum.

9. **D.** Blurred vision, tearing, pain, and swelling are common characteristics of dacryocystitis. Double vision does not occur with dacryocystitis.

10. **C.** Entropion is the inward curling of an eyelash.

11. **B.** Surgery is the definitive treatment for ectropion and entropion. Other treatment modalities are temporizing and for patient comfort.

12. **B.** Gonococcal conjunctivitis is vision-threatening and should be considered in this patient. The patient may be presenting with other less dangerous forms of conjunctivitis, but you should rule out a vision-threatening diagnosis first.

13. **A.** Clindamycin is a first-line treatment for mild dacryocystitis.

14. **B.** This patient should be treated for gonorrhea conjunctivitis STI following CDC guidelines, currently 1 g ceftriaxone IM in a single dose.

15. **C.** The patient is presenting with allergic conjunctivitis. The treatment includes artificial tears, topical antihistamines or mast cell stabilizer drops, and oral antihistamines.

16. **B.** Topical antibiotics are prescribed for patients with corneal abrasion to prevent infection in the affected eye. Topical NSAIDs and topical anesthetic drops can delay healing. Oral antibiotics are not indicated.

17. **A.** The definitive treatment for cataracts is removal of the affected lens and replacement with an intraocular lens.

▶ ANSWERS AND EXPLANATIONS TO SECTION C PRETEST

1. **A.** Children who develop nasal polyps should be tested for cystic fibrosis (sweat chloride test or genetic testing) and asthma.

2. **D.** Oral contraceptive pills can cause rhinitis.

3. **C.** Intranasal corticosteroid sprays are recommended to minimize polyp recurrence following surgical treatment.

4. **A.** Allergic rhinitis is a type I hypersensitivity reaction caused by exposure to an allergen.

5. **A.** Patients with nasal polyps report worsening nasal congestion, nasal obstruction, decreased sense of smell, and postnasal drainage.

6. **C.** Nasal steroids are first-line medications for allergic rhinitis. The other treatments listed are second-line therapies.

7. **D.** Nonenhanced coronal CT scan is the imaging study of choice for nasal polyps.

8. **C.** Most case of viral rhinitis will resolve in 10 days.

9. **C.** Concerning symptoms include a nonhealing ulcer or an ulcer that recurs in the same spot, loosening teeth, dysphonia that persists for >3 weeks, chronic cough, hemoptysis, unexplained otalgia, and unexplained weight loss.

10. **B.** Risk factors for nasal polyp growth include chronic sinusitis, chronic allergic rhinitis, aspirin hypersensitivity, asthma, and cystic fibrosis.

11. **A.** The presence of β-2-transferrin in nasal discharge indicates CSF leak.

12. **B.** The most common causes of ABRS are *S. pneumoniae, H. influenzae,* and *M. catarrhalis.*

13. **C.** If extensive nasal and facial trauma is present, CT scan is the imaging study of choice.

14. **D.** The first-line treatment for the diagnosis of uncomplicated ABRS in children and adults is amoxicillin-clavulanate.

15. **B.** Low humidity causes mucous membranes to dry out, which will increase the chances of epistaxis.

16. **C.** Imaging is not required if the patient can breathe through each nostril, septal hematoma is absent, trauma is limited to the bridge of the nose; however, it is required if displacement is visible.

17. **C.** Do not allow the patient to tilt the head back during examination, which will obscure the nasal cavity from view.

18. **D.** The nasal passage is the most common anatomic location for a patient presenting with foreign-body insertion.

19. **C.** The increasing prevalence of the HPV over the past several decades has resulted in an increased prevalence of head and neck cancers in nonsmoking, nondrinking young adults.

20. **B.** Toddlers and preschoolers have the highest incidence demographic for nasal foreign-body insertion.

21. **C.** Cautery is the first-line treatment of anterior bleeding.

22. **B.** Direct otoscopic visualization should be used to confirm the presence of an inorganic nasal foreign body.

23. **D.** The positive pressure "parent's kiss" is the preferred treatment approach for a 2-year-old patient with an occlusive bead in the right nare.

24. **A.** Factors that predispose the nose to fractures include central location on the face, prominent protrusion, and a lack of structural support.

25. **C.** The conventional criteria for the diagnosis of ABRS is based on the presence of at least two major symptoms, including nasal congestion or obstruction, purulent nasal drainage, fever, anosmia, facial fullness, pressure, or pain. The diagnosis may also be met if the patient has one major symptom and at least two minor symptoms, including headache, ear pain/pressure, halitosis, dental pain, cough, or fatigue. Symptoms of ABRS will persist for a minimum of 10 days and may worsen 10 days after initial improvement.

26. **C.** Examination of a nasal fracture reveals laceration, swelling, infraorbital swelling, epistaxis, or gross nasal deformity.

27. **C.** A septal hematoma should be incised and drained immediately to express the clot, followed by anterior packing and referral to otolaryngology.

28. **D.** The most common patient presentation of an inorganic nasal foreign body is a history concerning for foreign-body insertion.

29. **C.** Risk factors for the development of head and neck cancers include tobacco products, alcohol, HPV, radiation exposure, environmental exposures, wood dust exposure, periodontal disease, and genetic factors.

30. **A.** Patients with chronic rhinosinusitis should use daily saline irrigation with optional topical intranasal corticosteroids and should not receive topical or systemic antifungal treatment.

31. **B.** CT scan of the head and neck with contrast is the imaging study of choice.

32. **B.** People with allergic rhinitis are at higher risk for developing rhinosinusitis.

33. **D.** These recesses are common sites for SCC development because smokeless tobacco users hold the product in these locations.

▶ ANSWERS AND EXPLANATIONS TO SECTION D PRETEST

1. **B.** Hib is the most common causative organism of epiglottitis, although much less in the modern medical era of vaccines.

2. **D.** *S. mutans* is the main cavity-causing bacteria.

3. **C.** Stridor, which is high-pitched turbulent airflow on inspiration through a narrow airway.

4. **C.** Sore throat, fever, and a positive ASO titer are all suggestive of a recent streptococcal infection. Pastia lines and circumoral pallor are commonly seen in scarlet fever rash caused by group A β-hemolytic streptococcal (GABHS) infection.

5. **C.** The "thumb-print" sign is the soft-tissue swelling on the epiglottis posterior to the hyoid bone.

6. **D.** Appropriate antibiotic treatment for GAS pharyngitis includes penicillins, cephalosporins, macrolides, and clindamycin.

7. **C.** Penicillin or clindamycin has been the antibiotics of choice for dental abscesses. Antibiotics should be started, and referral given to a dentist at the initial assessment of an abscess.

8. **B.** Centor criteria includes fever >38 °C (100.4 °F), pharyngotonsillar exudate, tender cervical lymphadenopathy, and the absence of cough.

9. **B.** The oral cavity has many clues to the overall health of a patient. Gingivitis and periodontitis, which present commonly with erythema and bleeding on gingival manipulation, will note that the oral cavity is not healthy and can imply systemic disease.

10. **C.** Deviation of the uvula should alert the provider that a peritonsillar abscess is likely present. A gray pseudomembrane on the pharynx is seen with diphtheria, and a "strawberry tongue" is seen with scarlet fever caused by GAS.

11. **A.** Gingivitis is the diagnosis associated with inflammation of the gingiva, resulting in bleeding due to the increased irritation at the gingival margin.

12. **A.** The morphology of the lesions is classified as minor (<1 cm in diameter), major (>1 cm in diameter), or herpetiform (2 mm, numerous lesions occurring in clusters).

13. **D.** Leukoplakia lesions should be surgically removed, and the patient monitored for recurrence or progression of the mucosa to SCC.

14. **B.** As a result of contiguous anatomic routes, deep neck infections can quickly spread to the mediastinum and chest. If mediastinitis occurs, mortality approaches 50%, irrespective of antibiotic therapy.

15. **B.** Mumps often presents as bilateral parotitis with other viral symptoms. Individuals who have not received the measles, mumps and rubella vaccine are susceptible.

16. **B.** Sialendoscopy can be diagnostic and therapeutic for sialadenitis caused by a salivary stone.

17. **D.** CT scan of the neck with contrast is the imaging study of choice.

18. **A.** *S. aureus* is the most common pathogen that causes bacterial parotitis.

19. **C.** The white lesions of oral candidiasis can be removed with a tongue depressor, revealing erythematous, painful, and friable mucosa.

20. **A.** Acute suppurative sialadenitis presents with acute infection and purulent discharge from the duct.

21. **D.** Fever, pharyngotonsillar exudates, tender anterior cervical lymphadenopathy, and lack of cough are most suggestive of GABHS infection.

22. **D.** Neoplasm of the salivary gland typically presents as a firm, painless, slowly enlarging salivary gland.

CHAPTER
62

Otitis Externa

Jill Gore, PA-C

A 9-year-old male accompanied by his mother presents to his primary care provider's office complaining of right ear pain for 3 days. Since summer vacation started 2 weeks ago, he has been swimming in his local pool nearly every day. His mother adds that when he is not in the pool, he is playing on a personal electronic device and wearing his ear buds. On examination of the affected ear, he has pain with both auricle and tragus movement, and the external auditory canal is erythematous, macerated, and 25% swollen. The tympanic membrane is visible, intact, and pearly. What is the recommended treatment for this patient?

▶ GENERAL FEATURES

- Otitis externa (OE), commonly called swimmer's ear, is an inflammation of the external auditory canal (EAC) most commonly caused by an acute bacterial infection; other causes include fungus (otomycosis), virus, allergy, or a dermatologic disease.
- Affects 10% of the population, most commonly children
- Highest incidence is during the summer.
- Risk factors:
  - Swimming or other water exposure
  - High temperature or humidity
  - Absence of cerumen
  - Trauma from excessive cleaning or scratching of the EAC
  - Objects that occlude the EAC, including hearing aids, earphones, or diving caps
  - Dermatologic conditions such as psoriasis and eczema
  - Allergic contact dermatitis from earrings or chemicals in cosmetics or shampoos can extend to the EAC
  - Previous radiation therapy
- *Pseudomonas aeruginosa, Staphylococcus epidermidis,* and *Staphylococcus aureus* are the most common causes of OE; anaerobes also can be present.

- Up to 10% of OE is due to fungus, most commonly *Aspergillus*; candidal infections typically affect patients who wear hearing aids.
- Possible complications include:
  - Periauricular cellulitis
    - Severe form of OE is characterized by intense pain and EAC swelling plus periauricular erythema, lymphadenopathy, and fever.
    - Addition of oral antibiotics is necessary for treatment.
  - Necrotizing (malignant) OE:
    - Life-threatening condition in which bacteria invade the deeper underlying structures and cause osteomyelitis; overall mortality is 50%.
    - More common in patients who have diabetes, are immunocompromised, have had radiotherapy to this region, or whose OE is not treated
    - Should be suspected if the patient's pain is out of proportion to the clinical appearance or if granulation tissue is seen in the ear canal

▶ CLINICAL ASSESSMENT

- Symptom onset is usually rapid, generally within 48 hours.
- Ear pain, discharge, and hearing loss are the most common symptoms; in patients with otomycosis, pruritus is more common than pain.
- On examination, the patient may have a conductive hearing loss due to swelling and narrowing of the EAC.
- Tenderness with tragal or auricle movement is the hallmark of OE.
- On otoscopic examination, the EAC may be edematous and erythematous.
  - Debris, discharge, or maceration may be present.
  - The tympanic membrane, if visible, may be erythematous.
- In otomycosis caused by *Aspergillus*, the EAC will have a fine, white mat topped with dark spheres. In *Candida* otomycosis, a white, sebaceous-like material will be present.

▶ DIAGNOSIS

- Clinical, based on history and physical examination
- Cultures are reserved for patients with severe cases of OE, recurrent OE, chronic OE, immunosuppressed patients, OE in a patient after ear surgery, and in patients who do not respond to initial therapy.

▶ TREATMENT

- Ear canal cleaning
  - Removal of cerumen, desquamated skin, and purulent material from EAC facilitates healing and enhances penetration of ear drops into inflamed skin.
  - If tympanic membrane is intact, irrigate EAC with 1:1 solution of hydrogen peroxide and warm water.
  - If tympanic membrane is not intact (ruptured), refer to otolaryngologist.
- Antimicrobials:
  - Because the infection is limited to the EAC, a topical antibiotic, with or without a corticosteroid, is the mainstay of treatment.
  - Minimal clinical difference between various topical agents.
    - Frequency of dosing depends on the agent used.
    - Treatment duration is for 7 days and may continue for up to 14 days for unresolved symptoms.
  - Fluoroquinolones (ofloxacin and ciprofloxacin) and aminoglycosides (tobramycin, gentamicin, and neomycin/polymyxin B) are effective against the two most common causes of OE; ototoxicity is a concern with aminoglycosides.
  - Topical corticosteroids (hydrocortisone, dexamethasone, prednisolone) decrease inflammation, resulting in less pruritus and pain; these can be prescribed either separately or in combination with antibiotics.

- If the tympanic membrane is perforated or is not visible due to canal swelling or debris, ofloxacin or ciprofloxacin/dexamethasone is recommended.
  - For otomycosis, topical clotrimazole 1% solution, applied twice daily for 10–14 days, is recommended.
- Most patients begin to improve within 48–72 hours, with full resolution of symptoms within 7–10 days.
- Wick placement:
  - Patients with severe EAC swelling should have a wick placed in the canal to allow topical medication to reach the site of infection; replace the wick every 2–3 days until the swelling has improved.
- Pain control: nonsteroidal anti-inflammatory drugs (NSAIDs) are the mainstay of therapy to treat associated pain.
- Activities:
  - The EAC should be kept dry during treatment and for 1–2 weeks after treatment; an earplug or a cotton ball coated with petroleum jelly can be placed in the EAC during bathing or showering.
  - Recreational water activities may be resumed in 7–10 days; patients involved in aquatic activities may return 2–3 days after starting treatment so long as they keep their heads above water or wear earplugs.
  - Hearing aids and earphones may be worn once pain and discharge have resolved.

Case Conclusion

The patient most likely has moderate otitis externa (OE). Treatment includes a topical fluoroquinolone or aminoglycoside antibiotic with or without a corticosteroid for 7–14 days. To relieve his ear discomfort, NSAIDs can be administered as needed. Patient education regarding risk factors for OE and avoidance of water activities during the treatment period should be discussed.

CHAPTER 63

Acute and Chronic Otitis Media

Amy Akerman, MPAS, PA-C

Leo Thompson is an 18-month-old male who is brought to his primary care physician assistant by his parents with concerns of his recent onset of frequent ear pulling that started after 7 days of a viral upper respiratory infection. Why is it so important to consider acute otitis media?

▶ GENERAL FEATURES

- Acute otitis media (AOM):
  - AOM is the most commonly diagnosed ear, nose, and throat (ENT) childhood disease.
  - The incidence for AOM is highest in male children aged <2 years.

- Risk factors for recurrent AOM include daycare attendance, cigarette smoke exposure, bottle-feeding, and male gender.
- Eustachian tube dysfunction is the most important factor in the pathogenesis of middle ear infections in all ages.
  - Anatomic changes throughout childhood improve eustachian tube patency and contribute to the decline in incidence of AOM with age.
  - However, poor tubal function can persist into adulthood, and AOM can still occur at any age due to eustachian tube dysfunction.
- Recurrent and chronic AOM infections are often implicated in those with hearing deficits and language delays.
- Chronic otitis media with effusion (OME):
  - OME is the presence of mucoid or serous effusion in the middle ear without the presence of infection occurring over 3 months and is often attributed to eustachian tube dysfunction.

▶ CLINICAL ASSESSMENT

- AOM:
  - The stereotypical presenting complaint of AOM is ear pain or pulling on the affected ear, usually preceded by viral upper respiratory infection symptoms.
  - AOM should be on the differential diagnosis in all patients aged <2 years with hearing loss.
  - Common associated symptoms include fever, purulent nasal drainage, nasal congestion, nonproductive cough, irritability, poor feeding, and malaise.
  - The leading bacterial pathogens in AOM are *Streptococcus pneumoniae*, *Haemophilus influenzae*, and *Moraxella catarrhalis*.
- Chronic OME may be asymptomatic, may provide a painless sensation of pressure in the affected ear, or may cause a conductive hearing loss.

▶ DIAGNOSIS

- AOM:
  - All patients in whom AOM is suspected should undergo pneumatic otoscopy with proper visualization of the tympanic membrane (TM).
  - In most cases, AOM can be diagnosed correctly when an erythematous, bulging, nonmobile TM is present along with local or systemic signs or symptoms.
  - Other forms of otitis media may cause the presence of middle ear fluid, erythema, or otalgia, but reduced mobility of the TM is a common feature of a bacterial cause of AOM.

- Recent evidence suggests that the color of the TM is not the defining feature in AOM because the TM may appear red or yellow.
- Opaque middle ear fluid may suggest the presence of AOM.
- Lab tests or diagnostic imaging is not necessary for accurate diagnosis of AOM in most cases.
- OME:
  - The best initial test for patients with chronic OME is pneumatic otoscopy to assess the mobility of the TM.
  - Patients with chronic OME will usually have an intact TM with air-fluid level behind the TM and impaired mobility of the TM.
    - Patients who have recurrent AOM or chronic OME may have hearing loss or delayed speech and language development.

▶ TREATMENT

- AOM:
  - Correct diagnosis and differentiation from other causes of otalgia is crucial to providing correct treatment in patients with AOM.
  - There is a growing consensus for watchful waiting of uncomplicated AOM, as it may be appropriate in most cases; patients should be re-examined at regular intervals to monitor for any persistent effusion.
  - Antibiotic treatment is generally aimed at *S. pneumoniae*, which accounts for 25%–50% of AOM cases.
  - Amoxicillin continues to be first-line antibiotic treatment choice for AOM, and several studies have shown that shorter courses are acceptable in low-risk children.
  - With increasing resistance to first-line antibiotics, second-line antibiotic choices include amoxicillin-clavulanate, cefprozil, ceftriaxone, and cefdinir.
- OME:
  - Management of chronic OME includes watchful waiting for 3 months for those without speech or language deficits.
  - Placement of tympanostomy tubes in the affected ear and/or adenoidectomy is recommended for patients without improvement at follow-up, or if they develop speech, hearing, or language impairments.

Case Conclusion

It is important to consider AOM in Leo's case because patients who have recurrent AOM may suffer hearing loss or delayed speech and language development.

Cholesteatoma

Lauren Webb, DMSc, MSM, PA-C

Mr. Robertson is a 62-year-old patient presenting with left ear drainage for 10 days. He reports that he has had similar symptoms many times over the past 2–3 years and has been diagnosed with "swimmer's ear." Upon further questioning, he states he has had tinnitus and muffled hearing in that same ear for years. Close examination of the tympanic membrane is necessary to rule out what possible lesion?

▶ GENERAL FEATURES

- Cholesteatomas are non-neoplastic, destructive cysts that arise within the temporal bone and may invade the middle ear, mastoid, and external auditory canal.
- They are made up of desquamated keratin and squamous debris, can be either congenital or acquired, and are typically unilateral.
- Acquired cholesteatomas are thought to arise due to eustachian tube dysfunction following middle ear disease and also may be secondary to prior surgery or traumatic injuries.
- Over time, these lesions cause destruction of the middle ear bones responsible for normal hearing and can spread to adjacent structures in the face, neck, and brain with the potential for serious complications.

▶ CLINICAL ASSESSMENT

- The most common presenting symptom is painless otorrhea that is often persistent or recurrent and may be purulent; this diagnosis should be considered in anyone with persistent or recurrent ear drainage.
- Ear pain before the onset of otorrhea is common, and other common associated symptoms include hearing loss, dizziness, and tinnitus that may have been present for years.

- Examination often reveals granulation tissue with drainage in the external auditory canal.
- The pathognomonic examination finding includes the presence of a white, round, compressible lesion (aural polyp) on the posterosuperior quadrant of the tympanic membrane.

▶ DIAGNOSIS

- High-resolution computed tomography (CT) is considered the imaging test of choice and is important in surgical candidates because of its ability to provide bony detail.
- Magnetic resonance imaging (MRI) may be performed to provide additional soft-tissue detail and when intracranial complications are suspected.

▶ TREATMENT

- Surgical excision is the mainstay of treatment, although up to 50% of cholesteatomas recur after surgical removal.
- Surgical removal often does not improve hearing, and hearing loss secondary to cholesteatoma is often permanent.

Case Conclusion

Thorough examination of Mr. Robertson's tympanic membrane is important to rule out cholesteatoma. Over time, these lesions cause destruction of the middle ear bones responsible for normal hearing and can spread to adjacent structures in the face, neck, and brain with the potential for serious complications.

Acoustic Neuroma

Antoinette Polito, MHS, PA-C

A 52-year-old man presents to clinic because of his complaints "my hearing is getting worse." Over the past year, he finds it more difficult to hear what others are saying in conversation, particularly if the ambient environment is noisy. His wife confirms that she more often has to repeat herself. Physical examination is consistent with unilateral sensorineural hearing loss on the left and normal hearing on the right. These findings are subsequently confirmed by audiometry. What is the most likely diagnosis and preferred treatment for this patient?

▶ GENERAL FEATURES

- Acoustic neuromas, also known as *vestibular schwannomas*, affect the vestibular portion of the eighth cranial nerve and are one of the most common types of intracranial tumors.
- These are benign lesions that arise from the Schwann cells covering the nerve and primarily affect the cerebellopontine angle.
- Incidence in the United States is approximately 1 per 100,000 person-years.
- Median age at diagnosis is 50 years old.
- Over 90% acoustic neuromas are unilateral.
- About 5% of acoustic neuromas present bilaterally; these are most often associated with hereditary syndromes, including neurofibromatosis type 2.
- Most studies show some correlation with noise exposure, with higher risk associated with leisure noise (eg, loud headphones) than occupational noise exposure.

▶ CLINICAL ASSESSMENT

- Acoustic neuromas typically present with unilateral hearing loss accompanied by deterioration of speech discrimination out of proportion to the degree of tone loss.
- Hearing loss is greater in higher frequency ranges and does not necessarily correlate with tumor size.
- Tinnitus is present in >60% of patients with an acoustic neuroma.
- Approximately 60% of patients also have involvement of the vestibular portion of the nerve with symptoms including unsteady gait; spinning vertigo is uncommon.
- Atypical presentations are not uncommon; they may include sudden unilateral hearing loss or asymmetric sensorineural hearing loss.

▶ DIAGNOSIS

- Anyone presenting with a unilateral or asymmetric sensorineural hearing loss should be evaluated for an intracranial mass lesion.
- The differential diagnosis includes presbycusis, meningioma, facial nerve schwannomas, gliomas, cholesterol cysts, cholesteatomas, hemangiomas, aneurysms, arachnoid cysts, lipomas, and metastatic tumor.
- Diagnosis is made by contrast-enhanced MRI.

▶ TREATMENT

- Treatment may consist of observation, surgical excision, or stereotactic radiosurgery depending on the size of the tumor and patient age and comorbidities.
- Complete tumor removal is possible in most patients, and tumors rarely if ever regrow if removed completely.
- Typically, these tumors are very slow growing, and observation may be an appropriate course for patients who are elderly or poor surgical candidates.
- In addition to their impact on hearing, acoustic neuromas can cause hydrocephalus if left to grow.
- Patients presenting with subjective hearing loss, regardless of age, should have a screening hearing examination and referral for audiometry. Those with confirmed unilateral or asymmetric sensorineural hearing loss should be further evaluated with an MRI to rule out acoustic neuroma.

Case Conclusion

The patient is found to have a left-sided acoustic neuroma on MRI. Most patients who are younger and motivated to preserve their hearing will benefit from surgical excision of the acoustic neuroma. If complete excision is possible, the lesion is very unlikely to grow back.

CHAPTER 66

Eustachian Tube Dysfunction

Amy Akerman, MPAS, PA-C

Mrs. Thompson is a 56-year-old female who presents with bilateral intermittent ear pressure, as if her ears are plugged. She recently had resolution of mild upper respiratory infection symptoms including malaise, nasal drainage, and unproductive cough. She denies any recent flying or scuba diving and has not experienced fever, ear drainage, or sinus pain. Why is it so important to consider eustachian tube dysfunction?

▶ GENERAL FEATURES

- Eustachian tube dysfunction (ETD) occurs when the functional valve of the tube fails to open (obstructive) or close properly (patulous), causing a wide variety of symptoms.
- People with ETD may have obstructive causes, leading to inadequate ventilation of the middle ear and improper clearance of middle ear secretions.

- Many of the common causes of ETD are obstructive, leading to negative pressure within the middle ear causing symptoms of fullness, aural pressure, popping, pain, hearing loss, vertigo, or tinnitus.
- Obstructive ETD is commonly preceded by an upper respiratory infection or allergic rhinitis, and there may be an associated otitis media.
- Etiologic factors for obstructive types of ETD include inflammation due to allergies, environmental irritants, laryngopharyngeal and gastroesophageal reflux (GERD), infections, hormonal changes, and nasopharyngeal masses.
- Patulous dysfunction occurs when the valve fails to properly close.
  - Patulous dysfunction is found to be caused by allergies, weight loss, gastroesophageal reflux, and stress/anxiety.

CLINICAL ASSESSMENT

- The stereotypical presenting complaint of ETD in adults is unilateral or bilateral ear pressure.
- ETD should be on the differential diagnosis in all adult patients with ear pain, intermittent ear pressure, and reduced hearing acuity; other diagnoses may include Ménière disease and temporomandibular disorders.
- ETD is an important factor in the development of acute otitis media (AOM) and otitis media with effusion (OME), especially in children.
  - AOM will usually present with ear pain and fever, but OME can be subtle and may cause long-term delays in speech and language development.
- Providers may fail to consider ETD in their differential diagnosis when the chief complaint is the patient's own voice is quite loud (autophony), and they can hear themselves breathe.
- Patulous dysfunction often fluctuates and can be difficult to diagnose: Patients will often attempt to close their eustachian tubes by constantly sniffing, generating negative pressure to temporarily close the valve.
  - This can lead to a vicious cycle in which the absence of opening makes it increasingly difficult to dilate the tube, and the failure to open increases the negative pressure.
- On examination of the ear, abnormal signs of inflammation may include dullness of the tympanic membrane (TM); mild erythema; the presence of clear, yellow, or amber fluid behind the TM; reduced light reflex; or retraction of the TM.
- Other components of the primary care physical examination should include pneumatic otoscopy, inspecting the nasal cavity for masses or polyps and the neck for masses or enlarged lymph nodes, and evaluating hearing with tuning forks.

DIAGNOSIS

- In most cases, adult and pediatric patients with persistent symptoms should have audiometric assessment to measure middle ear pressure (tympanogram) and to measure hearing (pure tone audiometry).
- Chronic ETD should be assessed by an otolaryngologist using fiberoptic nasal endoscopy to inspect the nasal cavity, nasopharynx, oropharynx, hypopharynx, and larynx and then finally examining the eustachian tube; the patient will be asked to swallow and yawn to observe the valve opening and closing.
- CT or MRI with contrast is indicated in patients with chronic unilateral symptoms or persistent middle ear effusion as these may indicate the presence of a neoplasm.

TREATMENT

- Appropriate treatment for ETD requires determining the underlying etiology.
- Trials of oral and topical decongestants, intranasal corticosteroids, antihistamines, antibiotics, and surgery have been studied, but none have been consistently effective.
- Treatment is generally aimed at managing the underlying etiology:
  - Use of topical and systemic medications is only recommended if the patient's ETD symptoms are found to be caused by a specific etiology (nasal congestion, GERD, chronic sinus inflammation, allergic rhinitis, OME).
  - Surgery may be indicated when medical management fails.
    - Tympanostomy tubes are first-line treatment to reduce the negative pressure within the middle ear and may improve the obstructive and patulous symptoms.
    - The addition of balloon dilation eustachian tuboplasty (BDET) has been shown to improve long-term outcomes in those patients with ETD with chronic suppurative OME (CSOME).
    - For adults with chronic OME, additional workup should be completed to rule out any underlying obstruction, such as nasopharyngeal neoplasms.

> **Case Conclusion**
>
> It is important to consider ETD in Mrs. Thompson's case to rule out any underlying obstruction, such as nasopharyngeal neoplasms.

Labyrinthitis and Ménière Disease

Jennifer Johnson, BS, MPAS, DMSc

> Mr. Eaton is a 32-year-old male who presents to the clinic for evaluation of dizziness. He reports sudden-onset, severe dizziness that began yesterday. His left-sided hearing is diminished. He cannot walk due to severe vertigo and has been vomiting consistently since his symptoms began. He had an upper respiratory infection the previous week that resolved before the onset of dizziness. What are the potential causes of this patient's symptoms?

▶ GENERAL FEATURES

- Labyrinthitis:
  - Labyrinthitis is a viral inflammatory disorder of the vestibular portion of the eighth cranial nerve.
  - Characteristic symptoms include rapid onset of debilitating vertigo, unilateral hearing loss, and severe nausea with vomiting.
  - Patients often report symptoms of an upper respiratory infection before the onset of vertigo.
  - Labyrinthitis rarely occurs in children.
- Ménière disease:
  - Ménière disease is a diagnosis of exclusion caused by endolymphatic hydrops of the labyrinthine of the inner ear, which results in distention of the membranous portions of the labyrinthine.
  - The classic triad is tinnitus, hearing loss, and episodic vertigo.
  - Hearing loss in Ménière disease is usually unilateral, fluctuating, and sensorineural, often progressing to permanent hearing loss within 10 years of disease onset.
  - It typically occurs in adults aged 20–40 years.
  - Presentation can be variable; some patients experience frequent, debilitating attacks, and others experience sporadic, mild attacks.
  - Attacks often occur in clusters with prolonged periods of remission between clusters.

▶ CLINICAL ASSESSMENT

- Labyrinthitis:
  - Physical examination reveals significant imbalance with patients swaying toward the affected side.
  - Horizontal nystagmus is often visible, with the fast phase beating away from the affected side.
  - Weber and Rinne tests with a 512-Hz tuning fork reveal a unilateral sensorineural hearing.
  - The head thrust test (patient attempts to maintain visual focus on a fixed, central point, while the examiner quickly turns the patient's head 15° to one side) will be positive toward the affected side.

- Ménière disease:
  - Clinical presentation will vary depending on whether the patient is experiencing an acute attack or is in remission.
  - Acute symptoms include significant vertigo, imbalance, nausea, vomiting, and signs of mild distress; spontaneous nystagmus may be noticeable with observation.
  - Perform a complete neurological examination: the Fukuda step test and Romberg test may reveal balance abnormalities.
  - During remission, the physical examination is often normal.

▶ DIAGNOSIS

- Labyrinthitis:
  - The diagnosis is usually made clinically without additional diagnostic studies; if the diagnosis is not consistent with the classic presentation of labyrinthitis, magnetic resonance angiography (MRA) and magnetic resonance imaging (MRI) are indicated to rule out other potential causes.
  - Audiometry will confirm the presence of a unilateral sensorineural hearing loss.
- Ménière disease:
  - There is no single diagnostic test.
  - Diagnostic criteria include:
    - Episodic vertigo lasting 20 minutes to 12 hours
    - Fluctuating sensorineural hearing loss, tinnitus, and/or sensation of aural fullness
  - Rule out autoimmune conditions, HIV, and syphilis; if indicated by patient history, test for West Nile virus and cat-scratch disease.
  - Serial audiometry will reveal a fluctuating, low-frequency sensorineural hearing loss in the affected ear.
  - Videonystagmography (VNG) will reveal decreasing vestibular function. Abnormal electrocochleography (ECoG) and vestibular evoked myogenic potential (VEMP) results will further increase the likelihood of the diagnosis.
  - A contrast MRI of the internal auditory canals is indicated to rule out retrocochlear pathology, such as an acoustic neuroma or other disorders.

▶ TREATMENT

- Labyrinthitis:
  - Initial treatment consists of a 10-day prednisone taper.

- Consider adding an oral antiviral medication if a viral cause is identified.
- Antiemetics and vestibular suppressants may be prescribed for symptom relief; commonly prescribed medications include ondansetron and diazepam.
- Vestibular rehabilitation exercises are recommended.
- Provide education about the natural disease progression of labyrinthitis; often, patients experience severe symptoms for 1–2 weeks, although imbalance may persist for several months, and hearing loss may be permanent.
- Most patients do not experience a recurrence of symptoms; however, labyrinthitis patients are at an increased risk for developing panic disorder and benign paroxysmal positional vertigo (BPPV).
- Ménière disease:
  - There is no cure for Ménière disease.
  - Treatment is aimed at symptom relief and reducing the number and frequency of attacks and patient expectations and providing support resources.
- Lifestyle modifications include cessation of nicotine products and salt, caffeine, and alcohol restrictions.
- Vestibular rehabilitation is also recommended to strengthen the vestibular system.
- Daily maintenance therapy with diuretics may reduce the frequency of attacks.
- During an acute attack, treatment is aimed at suppressing the vestibular system and minimizing nausea; beneficial medications include clonazepam, diazepam, and ondansetron.
- Refractory patients should be referred to otolaryngology.

> **Case Conclusion**
>
> This patient has labyrinthitis, a viral inflammatory disorder of the vestibular portion of the eighth cranial nerve. His history is notable for a recent upper respiratory infection.

CHAPTER 68

Hearing Impairment

Jennifer Johnson, BS, MPAS, DMSc

> Mr. Duncan is a 56-year-old man who presents to the clinic for evaluation of his hearing. He states that his spouse is frustrated with his difficulty hearing, which has worsened over several years. The patient reports that he turns the television volume louder than usual, has a hard time with conversations, and does not hear well in crowded restaurants. He works as a machinist in a manufacturing plant, and he notes that he enjoyed rock concerts as a young adult. What should you recommend for this patient?

▶ GENERAL FEATURES

- Hearing impairment affects both children and adults.
- Hearing loss may present as distorted sound, ear fullness, ear numbness, or ear pressure.
- Thee three types of hearing loss are as follows:
  - Sensorineural hearing loss: involves the inner ear structures, cochlea, or auditory nerve; ototoxic medications, brain injury, aging, and illness are common causes of this inner ear damage.
  - Conductive hearing loss: caused by an irregularity originating in either the external or middle ear that prevents external sound stimuli from reaching the inner ear, such as cerumen or ossicular chain discontinuity.
  - Mixed hearing loss: is a combination of sensorineural and conductive hearing loss.

- Hearing loss in children may be hereditary or nonhereditary. It can be caused by congenital malformation or congenital infection, such as rubella.
- Many children, and some adults, experience transient hearing loss at some point from eustachian tube dysfunction or otitis media.
- Common causes of hearing impairment in adults include cholesteatoma, otosclerosis, trauma, noise exposure, illness (such as Ménière disease), and presbycusis.
- As the popularity of cell phones and ear buds increases, the incidence of noise exposure hearing loss in adolescents and young adults is increasing.
- One cohort study found the prevalence of hearing impairment is 25% between the ages of 55 and 64 years and 43% between the ages of 65 and 84 years.
- Many patients with hearing impairment experience depression and social isolation from impaired ability to communicate.
  - Safety concerns also arise, such as difficulty hearing fire alarms or car horns.
  - For children, difficulty hearing in a school environment can negatively impact academic performance and socialization.
- A sudden change in hearing is considered an otologic emergency until proven otherwise and warrants prompt evaluation.

CLINICAL ASSESSMENT

- Obtain a thorough history, including over-the-counter (OTC) and prescription medications.
  - Many common medications are ototoxic, including aminoglycoside antibiotics, antimalarials, loop diuretics, nonsteroidal anti-inflammatory drugs (NSAIDs), and some chemotherapy agents.
- Perform a thorough head and neck examination.
- Evaluate the external auditory canals for cerumen or exostosis.
- Inspect the tympanic membranes and assess tympanic membrane mobility using pneumatic otoscopy or tympanometry.
- Hearing should be screened using the whisper test and a tuning fork.
  - Using a 512-Hz tuning fork, perform the Weber and Rinne tests to determine whether hearing loss is sensorineural or conductive; abnormal findings warrant a thorough auditory evaluation.
  - Weber test:
    - Normal hearing: midline; no lateralization
    - Sensorineural: lateralizes to unaffected ear
    - Conductive: lateralizes to affected ear
  - Rinne test (affected ear):
    - Normal or sensorineural hearing loss: air conduction > bone conduction
    - Conductive hearing loss: bone conduction > air conduction

DIAGNOSIS

- Audiometry is the diagnostic test of choice for hearing impairment in children and adults.
- Infants, toddlers, and patients unable to provide necessary feedback during audiometry may be tested by otoacoustic emissions (OAEs) or auditory brainstem response (ABR).

- These methods of testing are also useful if deception for secondary gain is suspected, as no verbal responses are required by a patient during testing.
- Conductive hearing loss with notching present at 4000 Hz is usually indicative of otosclerosis.
- Abnormal, sudden, or asymmetric sensorineural hearing loss warrants further evaluation with a contrast magnetic resonance imaging (MRI) of the internal auditory canals to rule out retrocochlear pathology.

TREATMENT

- Treatment is dependent on the type and cause of hearing impairment.
- Many forms of hereditary and sensorineural hearing loss are irreversible.
  - Management options for these patients include occupational therapy, sign language, lip reading, hearing aids, or cochlear implants.
- Some forms of hearing impairment may be corrected:
  - Chronic eustachian tube dysfunction can be managed by ear, nose, and throat (ENT) referral for myringotomy tube placement.
  - Cholesteatoma and otosclerosis should be referred to otology for surgical procedures, such as tympanomastoidectomy or ossicular chain reconstruction.
- School-aged children with hearing impairment should be provided accommodations to sit at the front of the classroom and to use hearing amplification devices.
- Re-evaluate every 6–12 months with audiometry to monitor hearing for further decline.

Case Conclusion

Mr. Duncan is experiencing sensorineural hearing loss from noise exposure. You assess his hearing with the Weber and Rinne tests and confirm the diagnosis. You educate him on the management options available to him, such as hearing aids.

CHAPTER
69

Ear Trauma: External Structures, Tympanic Membrane Perforation, and Barotrauma

Jennifer Johnson, BS, MPAS, DMSc

Mr. Hall is a 16-year-old male who presents to the clinic for evaluation of left ear trauma. He is a member of the high school wrestling team, and he injured his ear during practice today. He was not wearing protective headgear. The external ear is painful, with the anterior aspect of the pinna swollen and fluctuant. What is the most appropriate treatment for this patient?

▶ GENERAL FEATURES

- External ear trauma:
  - This is a common athletic injury; auricular hematoma is especially common in wrestling, boxing, and martial arts.
  - Auricular hematoma results from the shearing forces of a direct hit to the ear.
  - The cartilaginous structures of the external ear are particularly susceptible to hematoma formation from trauma.
  - Direct trauma to the ear separates the cartilage from the perichondrium, severing the perichondrial blood vessels and allowing blood to pool in the subperichondrial space.
  - An improperly treated auricular hematoma results in new, asymmetrical cartilage formation and cosmetic deformity known as "cauliflower ear" or "wrestler's ear."
- Tympanic membrane (TM) perforation:
  - Perforation of the TM can result from infection, trauma, or iatrogenic causes.
  - Residual perforation can persist following extrusion of myringotomy tubes.
  - Irrigation of the external auditory canals by primary care providers for cerumen removal can lead to perforation.
  - Risk factors for tympanic perforation include eustachian tube dysfunction, recurrent otitis media, recurrent otomycosis, cotton swab use, and instrumentation of the external auditory canal.
  - Patient presentation will vary depending on the size, location, and cause of the perforation.
  - Small residual perforations may be asymptomatic, with little effect on hearing.
  - Patients with tympanic perforation often report ear fullness, decreased hearing, audible whistling when sneezing, and sanguineous discharge from the ear followed by decreased pain.
  - Improperly treated tympanic perforations can progress to cholesteatoma formation.
- Barotrauma:
  - Barotrauma of the TM occurs when the air pressure lateral to the TM differs from the air pressure in the middle ear space; pressure is normally equal, and minor inequalities are corrected by opening the eustachian tube through yawning or swallowing.
  - The pressure difference between environment and middle ear space can cause TM distortion, TM bruising, or accumulation of serosanguineous exudate in the middle ear space.
  - Activities that often result in barotrauma include scuba diving, flying, blast injuries, and waterskiing.
  - Hyperbaric wound care is a common iatrogenic cause of TM barotrauma; eustachian tube dysfunction and chronic allergies are also risk factors.
  - Severe barotrauma can result in damage to the oval window, round, window, and ossicles; damage to these structures results in vertigo and potentially irreversible hearing loss.
  - Barotrauma can also lead to TM rupture.

▶ CLINICAL ASSESSMENT

- External ear trauma:
  - Patients usually present immediately following the injury.
  - Palpation of the pinna confirms a focal area of fluctuance and tenderness.
- TM perforation:
  - Physical examination reveals a visible defect in the TM.
  - Tympanic perforations are described by quadrant, margin involvement, and the percentage of the TM surface involved.
  - Otorrhea may be actively draining through the perforation if infection is present.
- Barotrauma:
  - Otoscopy reveals a dull TM with decreased light reflex.
  - Anatomic landmarks may be distorted.
  - Bloody middle ear effusion gives the TM a dark blue-purple appearance.
  - Pneumatic otoscopy confirms decreased or absent movement of the TM.

▶ DIAGNOSIS

- External ear trauma: Diagnosis is made clinically based on a history of ear trauma and characteristic appearance of the hematoma.
- TM perforation:
  - Labs and imaging are not indicated for uncomplicated tympanic perforations.
  - Audiometry may reveal conductive hearing loss.
  - If infection is refractory to treatment, obtain cultures and consider a noncontrast computed tomography (CT) scan of the temporal bone.
- Barotrauma:
  - Diagnosis is generally based on history and physical examination findings.
  - Audiometry confirms conductive hearing loss.
  - Further labs and imaging studies are not indicated in uncomplicated barotrauma.

▶ TREATMENT

- External ear trauma:
  - Initial treatment consists of cold compresses and moderate compression.
  - The hematoma should be incised and drained in either the emergency department or outpatient clinic setting.

- Following evacuation of the hematoma, apply a compression dressing to the medial and lateral aspects of the auricle and leave dressing in place for 3–5 days.
- Oral antibiotics should be prescribed for 7–10 days.
- Re-examine the patient every 24 hours until resolution.
- TM perforation:
  - Most tympanic perforations heal spontaneously within 3 months.
  - Dry ear precautions and periodic follow-up until resolution are recommended.
  - Large marginal perforations are less likely to heal spontaneously.
  - Occasionally, only one layer of the TM heals, resulting in a monomeric membrane.
  - Refer persistent perforations to otolaryngology for TM patching, myringoplasty, or tympanoplasty.
- Barotrauma:
  - Initial treatment consists of observation, Valsalva maneuvers, decongestants, and antihistamines.

- Most cases of barotrauma will resolve spontaneously within 1–3 months.
- Educate the patient about prevention and equalizing ear pressure.
- Patients with persistent middle ear effusion, underlying ear pathology, or chronic eustachian tube dysfunction should be referred to otolaryngology for further evaluation and treatment.
- Patients undergoing hyperbaric therapy who develop barotrauma should be referred to otolaryngology for myringotomy tube placement.

Case Conclusion

Mr. Hall has sustained an auricular hematoma. The hematoma should be incised and drained in either the emergency department or outpatient clinic setting. Following evacuation of the hematoma, a compression dressing to the medial and lateral aspects of the auricle should be applied.

CHAPTER 70

Cerumen Impaction and Foreign Body

Joy Stevens, PA-C

A 75-year-old female presents to clinic with a 2-week course of progressive fullness sensation, discomfort, tinnitus, and decreased hearing of the right ear. The patient admits to using cotton swabs daily after her shower. Her family has noted that she requests having the TV volume turned up louder than normal.

▶ GENERAL FEATURES

- Cerumen is normal in the ear to aid in lubrication and protection of the ear canal.
- A foreign body in the ear can occur in all ages.
- Patients with hearing aids may be more prone to cerumen impaction.
- Patients should be counseled to avoid use of cotton swabs, because repeated use can lead to more cerumen impactions.

▶ CLINICAL ASSESSMENT

- On examination, cerumen may be either crusty and dry or a soft wax–like material.

- Visualization of the cerumen or foreign body is needed to diagnose.
  - Visualize the ear canal with your otoscope by gently retracting the helix of the ear.
  - In children, you may need assistance of an adult to make sure the head is secure to see inside the ear canal.
  - Cerumen impaction or removal of a foreign body can be performed in the primary care physician office in most cases.
- Refer to ear, nose, and throat (ENT) for cerumen removal if the patient has had prior ear surgeries, a tympanostomy tube in the affected ear, cholesteatoma, possible tympanic membrane (TM) perforation, or provider cannot adequately visualize anatomic landmarks of the ear.
- Refer to ENT for foreign body removal from the ear; the foreign body has a risk of expanding in the ear canal, such as beans or seeds, because these objects may expand if water from ear irrigation is attempted, the ear canal is swollen, and the foreign body is deep and too close to the TM.

DIAGNOSIS

- Clinical diagnosis can be made from an examination showing cerumen impacted or foreign body in the ear canal.
- No additional testing is typically needed.

TREATMENT

- Cerumen or ear foreign body can be removed with ear curette, water irrigation, or suction.
- It is important to have direct visualization of the canal during the procedure.
- When performing ear irrigation, use of body temperature water is advised to avoid stimulating the vestibular reflex, which may cause symptoms of nystagmus and nausea.
- If cerumen is too impacted or dry, consider using hydrogen peroxide or docusate sodium drops in the ear and attempting ear irrigation again in 15–30 minutes.

- If cerumen is still not able to be removed, consider having patient use ear wax softener drops or mineral oil drops and returning in 3–5 days to repeat office procedure.
- For foreign body removal in the ear, use an alligator forceps if able to visualize the foreign body; gently pull back on the helix of ear or possibly have someone assist for better view of the canal to remove foreign body.

> **Case Conclusion**
>
> This patient on examination had a right ear cerumen impaction. The office procedure for ear irrigation was done, and the patient's hearing improved and her tinnitus decreased by the end of the clinic appointment.

CHAPTER 71

Vertigo

Chrystyna Senkel, MPAS, PA-C

GENERAL FEATURES

- *Vertigo*, the most common cause of dizziness, is defined as an illusion of movement, usually rotational.
- Etiologic causes are divided into physiologic vs. pathologic vertigo, based on intersensory mismatch between the visual, somatosensory, and vestibular systems vs. lesions or pathology in one or more of these spatial systems, respectively.
- Vestibular vertigoes are the most common and are divided into central vs. peripheral sources of vertigo, based on symptoms resulting from focal or diffuse lesions in the brainstem or cerebellum vs. symptoms resulting from a lesion or irritation in the peripheral vestibular nerves or organs, respectively.
  - Central (life-threatening) and peripheral (primarily benign) vertigoes present similarly, they must be differentiated.
    - The differential diagnosis and pathophysiology of peripheral vestibular vertigoes include:
      - Benign paroxysmal positional vertigo (BPPV): calcium carbonate crystals moving in the semicircular canals causes repeated episodic unwanted action potentials triggered by changes in head position.

  - Ménière disease: spontaneous increased endolymph causes episodic increased pressure throughout the entire inner ear.
  - Perilymphatic fistula: a tear in the oval window following an inciting traumatic event (sneeze, trauma, barotrauma pressure changes, or infection)
  - Vestibular neuritis: a spontaneous postinfectious inflammation to the vestibular nerve; labyrinthitis is the same cause but located in the entire vestibular canal (including the cochlea). Infectious causes can be viral or bacterial acute otitis media, meningitis, or upper respiratory infection.

CLINICAL ASSESSMENT

- Once the patient confirms a sensation of spinning, it should be noted if the vertigo occurs in episodes or is continuous; also note if the vertigo triggered (head position change, noise/pressure change, trauma, Hx prior episodes) or if it occurs spontaneously.
- Associated symptoms point toward a peripheral etiology of vertigo; absence does not rule out a peripheral etiology.

- Considering the pathophysiology of the underlying disorder and the middle/inner ear anatomy helps to predict associated symptoms.
  - BPPV is an episodic, triggered vertigo with associated nausea > vomiting and a sense of imbalance during head position changes; prior episodes are common.
  - Ménière disease includes episodic attacks of severe, spontaneous vertigo associated with nausea and vomiting, sense of imbalance and/or drop attacks, fluctuating hearing loss, "roaring" tinnitus, and aural fullness or otalgia; prior episodes are common.
  - Perilymphatic fistula presents as episodic, recurrent, provoked attacks of severe, spontaneous vertigo with associated hearing loss and tinnitus upon application of inner ear pressure or sound.
  - Vestibular neuritis and labyrinthitis present as moderate-severe continuous, spontaneous vertigo and associated symptoms of nausea > vomiting, sense of imbalance, with or without hearing loss, and tinnitus as applicable to condition.
- Any cranial nerve deficit, numbness, weakness, ataxia, pronounced gait impairment, diplopia, dysarthria, or headache and emesis point toward a central etiology of vertigo; absence does not rule out a central etiology.
- Nystagmus is present with vestibular and central vertigoes as it represents the physical manifestation of the patient's vertigo; peripheral nystagmus varies greatly from central:
  - Peripheral vertigo: nystagmus is episodic and triggered or only occurs when vertigo occurs; there will be a 5- to 20-second latency before the nystagmus begins.
    - The fast component is almost always unidirectional.
    - Peripheral-sourced nystagmus is rarely vertical, improves with fixed gaze, fatigues with attempts to reproduce, and has no visual acuity change.
  - Central vertigo: nystagmus is continuous and spontaneous without provocation; there is no latency.
    - The fast component is almost always bidirectional.
    - Central-sourced nystagmus is commonly vertical, does not improve with fixed gaze, will not fatigue, and may be accompanied by defects, such as diplopia and extraocular muscle (EOM) palsies.
- Physical examination components include HEENT (head, ears, nose, and throat) examination with possible hearing tests and neurologic examination to include cranial nerves II–XII, full assessment of cerebellar function, and special tests: Dix-Hallpike, assessment of Hennebert/Tulio, and HINTS (Head Impulse-Nystagmus-Test of Skew).

▶ DIAGNOSIS

- BPPV is a clinical diagnosis confirmed by the reproduction of vertigo and nystagmus with Dix-Hallpike maneuver.
- Ménière disease is a clinical diagnosis confirmed by audiometry and electronystagmography if needed.
- Perilymphatic fistula is a clinical diagnosis established by reproduction of vertigo with pressure over the tragus (Hennebert) or sound (Tulio) outside the affected ear or with noncontrast temporal bone computed tomography (CT) in cases of trauma; definitive diagnosis is made intraoperatively.
- Vestibular neuritis and labyrinthitis are a clinical diagnosis confirmed by results of all three components of a HINTS examination: abnormal HIT, unidirectional nystagmus, and no vertical skew.
- Central source of vertigo is a clinical diagnosis of neurologic symptoms and/or deficit with continuous, spontaneous vertigo and nystagmus confirmed by any component of a HINTS examination: normal HIT, bidirectional nystagmus, and vertical skew; it will need further imaging with CT or magnetic resonance imaging (MRI).

▶ TREATMENT

- Vestibular suppressants (antihistamines, anticholinergics, or benzodiazepines) along with antiemetics may be tried if symptoms are severe, but use will delay central compensatory mechanisms; ideally, should be in conjunction with proven treatment and only for short term.
- BPPV is best treated by particle repositioning therapy (Epley and associated maneuvers) to fatigue the vertiginous response.
- In Ménière disease, the goal is to reduce episodes by reduction of endolymph: restrict salt, alcohol, and caffeine, and prescribe hydrochlorothiazide/triamterene daily.
- Perilymphatic fistula will need surgical patch of the fistula.
- Vestibular neuritis and labyrinthitis: underlying infection should be treated with antimicrobials as applicable; prednisone taper may help.
- Central sources of vertigo need immediate neurologic evaluation and treatment for underlying pathology.

Acute Mastoiditis

Jennifer Harrington, PA-C, MHS

▶ GENERAL FEATURES

- Acute mastoiditis is a rare, potentially life-threatening complication of otitis media caused by a spread of infection beyond the mucosa of the middle ear cleft to the mastoid process.
- Acute mastoiditis is more common in children than in adults; children aged <5 years are at highest risk.
- Occurs in five stages:
  a. Mastoid mucosal cell hyperemia
  b. Pus formation within mastoid cells
  c. Necrosis of mastoid bone
  d. Loss of cell wall and abscess coalescence
  e. Extension of infection to adjacent areas
- Early diagnosis with aggressive intravenous (IV) antimicrobial treatment is required to treat infection, prevent progression, and reduce complications.
- The most common causative organism is *Streptococcus pneumoniae*, accounting for 25% of cases.

▶ CLINICAL ASSESSMENT

- Common feature: persistence of ear pain despite antibiotic treatment of otitis media and hearing loss
- Clinical findings: fever, ear pain, erythema over the mastoid bone, otorrhea, edema of the pinna, and a displaced auricle
- Perform audiometry before and after treatment owing to the high risk for conductive hearing loss.

▶ DIAGNOSIS

- Diagnosis can be made clinically.
- Perform computed tomography (CT) if mastoiditis is suspected, but characteristic findings are not present or for staging of disease or assess complications; positive findings include coalescence of mastoid air cells due to destruction of bony septa.
- Perform myringotomy or tympanocentesis to obtain specimens for culture and sensitivity testing.
- Perform complete blood count and audiometry.
- Perform lumbar puncture if intracranial extension of infection is suspected.

▶ TREATMENT

- Hospital admission and empiric treatment with IV antibiotics including coverage for *Staphylococcus aureus*, *Pseudomonas*, enteric Gram-negative rods, *S. pneumoniae*, and *Haemophilus influenzae*.
- In most cases, tympanostomy tube should be placed to allow for drainage of entrapped pus and aeration of the middle ear.
- If a tympanostomy tube is placed, topical antibiotics with steroids may be administered to decrease swelling and deliver antimicrobial therapy directly to the middle ear.
- High-dose IV steroids can decrease mucosal swelling and promote drainage.
- Give analgesics and antipyretics for pain and fever control.
- Patients should be treated with IV antibiotics initially; a patient who responds well to IV antibiotics, as demonstrated by a return to afebrile status and decreased swelling for 48 hours, and who has culture confirmed susceptibility may be switched to oral antibiotics; duration of treatment is usually 2–4 weeks.
- A patient who is nonresponsive to initial treatment should be referred for debridement and drainage of the infection via mastoidectomy.

CHAPTER
73

Retinal Disorders

Nicole Dettmann, DSc, MPH, PA-C

▶ GENERAL FEATURES

- Age-related macular degeneration (AMD):
  - AMD is a leading cause of blindness in industrialized countries.
  - AMD is the degenerative disease of the macula, the central portion of the retina; degeneration of this area results in painless acute or chronic central vision loss with unaffected peripheral visual fields.
  - Patients complain of metamorphopsia or abnormal size of images and scotomas.
  - Risk factors for developing AMD: age >50, smoking, heavy alcohol use, and long-term aspirin use.
  - AMD is more prevalent in Caucasians and females and has a predominance in patients with lighter irises and red or blond hair.
  - A genetic defect in the complement factor H gene explains ~50% of cases of AMD.
- Retinopathies:
  - Retinopathies occur when blood vessels in the retina become damaged by swelling of the retina or abnormal growth of new blood vessels, resulting in blurred vision, vision loss, or blindness.
  - The main causes of retinopathy are diabetes and hypertension.
    - Blood dyscrasias including severe thrombocytopenia, severe anemia, sickle cell anemia, and HIV infection/AIDS may also be precursors to retinopathies.
    - High doses of the antipsychotic drugs chlorpromazine and thioridazine have also been linked to retinopathies.
  - There are two forms of diabetic retinopathy (DR): nonproliferative diabetic retinopathy (NPDR) and proliferative diabetic retinopathy (PDR) named for the absence or presence of abnormal new blood vessels in the retina; each patient with DR has a unique combination of symptoms and findings on physical examination and rate of progression.

- Most patients who develop DR and hypertensive retinopathy (HR) have no symptoms until the late stages of the disease.
- Screen patients with diabetes mellitus and hypertension annually for ocular complications and the development of retinal disease.
- Refer pregnant patients with hypertension to ophthalmologist in the first trimester, then every 3 months until delivery.

▶ CLINICAL ASSESSMENT

- AMD:
  - Patients are often asymptomatic in early disease.
  - For clinical purposes, AMD is classified as dry (atrophic) or wet (exudative or neovascular); in some patients, dry AMD progresses to wet.
  - Patients with dry AMD usually complain of gradual loss of vision in one or both eyes due to atrophy and degeneration of the outer retina and retinal epithelium.
  - Patients with wet AMD may present with acute vision changes or loss of central vision.
    - These patients have neovascular degeneration.
    - New vessels grow between the Brunch membrane and the retinal epithelium, which leads to the accumulation of fluid, fibrosis, and hemorrhage.
    - Acute changes in vision, often in one eye, are more common with wet AMD.
- Retinopathies:
  - Patients with DR may have variable symptoms and physical examination findings.
  - Patients who have symptoms may complain of decreased visual acuity and color vision over time or symptoms associated with vitreous bleeds (floaters, curtain falling over the eye, sudden vision loss).
    - NPDR:
      - Microaneurysms are the earliest sign of DR and appear as small red dots in the superficial retinal layers.

- Macular edema is the leading cause of visual impairment in patients with diabetes due to damage and necrosis of retinal capillaries.
- Flame-shaped hemorrhages may be present.
- Retinal edema and hard exudates are caused by the breakdown of the blood-retina barrier, allowing seepage of serum proteins, lipids, and protein from vessels.
- Cotton-wool spots result from occlusions in the precapillary arterioles.
- PDR:
  - In addition to the previous findings, patients with PDR also have evidence of neovascularization, usually near the optic disc; preretinal hemorrhages often appear boat shaped; hemorrhage into the vitreous may appear as a diffuse haze or as clumps of blood clots.
  - Fibrovascular tissue proliferation is usually seen associated with the neovascular complex that can cause traction on the retina and places these patients at higher risk for retinal detachments.
- HR:
  - Patients may have gradual onset of reduced vision, subconjunctival hemorrhages, or double vision.
  - Physical examination findings include irregular narrowing of the retinal arterioles, arteriolar wall thickening, arteriovenous nicking, hemorrhages, exudates and cotton-wool patches, copper and silver wiring, and microaneurysms; papilledema will be present in patients with malignant hypertension.

▶ DIAGNOSIS

- AMD:
  - Acute vision loss requires urgent ophthalmic evaluation with an ophthalmologist.
  - A thorough ocular history should include the type of vision change, the rate of vision loss, and if one or both eyes are affected.
  - Dry AMD patients exhibit drusen.
    - Hard drusen appear on ophthalmoscopic examination as discrete yellow deposits, whereas soft drusen are larger, paler, and less distinct.
    - On dilated examination, areas of depigmentation may be visible, which is a sign of retinal atrophy.
  - In wet AMD, a dilated examination likely will reveal subretinal hemorrhage or fluid and neovascular changes, which look like greenish gray discoloration of the macula.

- Further testing with fluorescein retinal angiography and/or optical coherence tomography (OCT) can better characterize changes.
- Retinopathies:
  - The mainstay of diagnosis is a complete ophthalmic examination and dilated retinal examination by an ophthalmologist.
  - Fluorescein angiography is often performed to examine patterns of retinal blood flow.

▶ TREATMENT

- AMD:
  - Modifications in diet have not been shown to prevent the development of AMD; however, antioxidant vitamins (C, E), carotenoids (lutein, zeaxanthin), copper, and zinc have been shown to reduce the progression of disease in patients with moderate-to-severe disease.
  - Encourage smoking cessation.
  - Patients with AMD often benefit from referrals to low-vision specialists who are familiar with visual aids that may benefit patients.
  - There are currently no specific treatments for dry AMD.
  - Intravitreous injection of a vascular endothelial growth factor (VEGF) inhibitor and photodynamic therapy are two effective treatments for wet AMD.
- Retinopathies:
  - Treatment should include good glycemic control for patients with DR and blood pressure control for patients with HR; the presence of papilledema in patients with hypertension necessitates the rapid lowering of blood pressure.
    - In addition to glycemic control, local laser photocoagulation is the mainstay treatment for NPDR and is aimed at targeting the breaks in the retina blood vessels to prevent additional seepage or hemorrhage and causes regression of new blood vessels.
    - Panretinal photocoagulation is the preferred form of treatment for PDR. This involves applying laser burns over the entire retina, sparing the central macular area.
    - Vitrectomy may be recommended in cases of long-standing vitreous hemorrhage or tractional retinal detachment from fibrovascular tissue proliferation.

Lacrimal Disorders and Dacryocystitis

Shekitta Acker, MS, PA-C

GENERAL FEATURES

- The drainage system of the eye is composed of the puncta, canaliculi, lacrimal sac, and nasolacrimal duct.
- *Dacryostenosis* refers to a blocked tear duct.
- Dacryocystitis is an infection of the lacrimal sac secondary to the obstruction of the nasolacrimal duct; it typically occurs unilaterally.
- Chronic cases of dacryocystitis are more common than acute infection.
- Congenital dacryostenosis can occur in infants due to the persistent membrane covering the valve of Hasner, which is located at the opening of the inferior nasal meatus that empties into the nasal cavity.
- Microorganisms involved in chronic and acute infantile dacryocystitis include *Streptococcus pneumoniae*, *Staphylococcus* species, *Haemophilus influenzae*, and *Enterobacteriaceae* species.
- Causes of dacryostenosis include narrowing of the puncta (which often occurs with age), infection or inflammation, injury, surgery or trauma, tumor, chemotherapy, and chronic use of eye drops for the treatment of glaucoma.
- In adults, nasolacrimal duct obstruction typically occurs in postmenopausal women.
- Acute and chronic dacryocystitis in adults are usually caused by *Staphylococcus aureus*, *Staphylococcus epidermidis*, *Pseudomonas aeruginosa*, or anaerobic organisms such as *Peptostreptococcus* and *Propionibacterium* species.
- Complications that require emergent referral may include conjunctivitis, cellulitis, and orbital cellulitis.

CLINICAL ASSESSMENT

- Patients typically presents with unilateral eye tearing and discharge.
- They may also experience redness/inflammation, pain, swelling, tenderness in the area of the lacrimal sac, and blurred vision.

- In the chronic form, tearing and matting of lashes may be the only presenting symptom.

DIAGNOSIS

- In most cases, dacryocystitis is a clinical diagnosis.
- On physical examination, erythema and tenderness will be seen over the lacrimal sac.
- Purulent material can be expressed through the lacrimal puncta by direct pressure on the sac.
- Cultures of the ocular surface, nose, and lacrimal sac discharge may be useful in determining the appropriate antibiotic therapy.
- X-rays may be useful in viewing facial skeletal anomalies or foreign bodies as the cause of the lacrimal disorder.
- Computed tomography (CT) scans are useful in patients when there is a suspicion of malignancy or mass as a cause of dacryocystitis.
- Dacryocystography (DCG) and dacryoscintigraphy are useful adjunctive diagnostic modalities when anatomic abnormalities of the nasolacrimal drainage system are suspected.

TREATMENT

- Dacryocystitis responds well to appropriate systemic antibiotics.
  - Mild cases can typically be treated with clindamycin.
  - Severe cases can be treated with vancomycin or third-generation cephalosporin.
- Treatment with warm compresses may help in the resolution of the disease.
- Incision and drainage of the lacrimal sac may be necessary.
- Surgical correction of nasolacrimal duct obstruction is usually achieved by dacryocystorhinostomy, in which a permanent fistula is formed between the lacrimal sac and the nose.

Lid Disorders

Sara Lolar, MS, PA-C, DFAAPA

A patient presents with a painful swelling on the upper eyelid that began suddenly 2 days ago. There is no fever and no changes in vision or photophobia. On visual inspection, you see a localized, erythematous swelling on the upper eyelid that has a pointing pustule. What is the likely diagnosis?

▶ GENERAL FEATURES

- Hordeolum, also known as "stye":
  - Inflammatory or infectious process that results in abscess of the lid
    - Often *Staphylococcus* species; may be sterile
    - May be complicated by underlying skin conditions (eg, blepharitis, seborrheic dermatitis) or contaminated eye makeup
  - External hordeola involve the sebaceous gland of Zeis or the apocrine gland of Moll, which are associated with eyelash follicles.
  - Internal hordeola involve the meibomian gland, which is associated with the tarsal plate on the conjunctival aspect of the lid.
- Chalazion:
  - May be chronic; may progress to a severe chalazion
  - Granulomatous inflammation of the meibomian gland
  - Noninfectious
- Entropion/ectropion:
  - Usually involves the lower lid
  - Ectropion: outward turning of the lid and lashes
  - Entropion: inward turning of the lid and lashes
  - Prevalence increases with age.
  - Secondary causes: trauma, rubbing (usually from allergies), cranial nerve VII palsy, chronic blepharospasm, and skin conditions, such as blepharitis or contact dermatitis
- Blepharitis:
  - Inflammation of the eyelid margins; two types:
    - Posterior blepharitis: inflammation of the inner lid at the level of the meibomian gland; most common type
    - Anterior blepharitis: inflammation at the base of the eyelashes; usually, *Staphylococcal* type or seborrheic type
  - More common in older adults
  - Allergies, cigarette smoking, and contact lens wearing may exacerbate.

▶ CLINICAL ASSESSMENT

- Hordeolum:
  - Painful; remember "h"ordeolum "h"urts
  - Typical appearance of localized, erythematous, painful swelling on the upper or lower eyelid
  - May evolve into a preseptal cellulitis
- Chalazion:
  - Nonpainful; like a hordeolum, but less erythematous and angry appearing
  - Typical appearance of localized, painless rubbery nodule under the lid; best seen with lid eversion
- Entropion:
  - Inward turning of eyelid pushes eyelashes onto globe
  - Causes foreign-body sensation, conjunctival injection, and tearing
  - Dry eye symptoms are common.
- Ectropion:
  - May be asymptomatic
  - Symptoms secondary to exposure because of inadequate lid closure and lubrication
  - If symptomatic, usually minor tearing and irritation
- Blepharitis:
  - Significant overlap of symptoms in all types
  - Symptoms usually worse in the morning
  - Eyelid examination:
    - Red, swollen lids with crusting/matting of eyelashes; may be greasy if seborrheic
    - Flaking or scaling of the eyelid skin
    - Plugging of meibomian glands with thickened waxy secretions
  - Possible conjunctival injection, especially on the palpebral conjunctiva
  - Chronic inflammation may lead to changes of the eyelashes, including loss or misdirection of the eyelashes or ectropion/entropion.
  - Dry eye disease is frequent complication.

▶ DIAGNOSIS

- All are primarily a clinical diagnosis based on typical appearance.
- Hordeolum: assess for symptoms of preseptal cellulitis.
- Chalazion: persistent or recurring chalazion should be assessed for carcinoma.
- Entropion/ectropion: slit-lamp examination to evaluate for corneal and conjunctival involvement from exposure or mechanical damage from eyelashes.
- Blepharitis: culture of eyelid margins may be considered for recurrent blepharitis or if not responding to therapy.

▶ TREATMENT

- Hordeolum:
  - Often will resolve spontaneously in a few days with conservative management
  - Warm compresses for 10 minutes 3–5 times a day
  - Light massage over lesion may aid in drainage.
  - Consider a short course of topical antibiotics if draining; treat secondary causes such as complicating skin diseases.
  - Refer to specialist if worsening for definitive treatment, including incision and drainage.
- Chalazion:
  - Inflammatory/granulomatous condition; no role for topical or oral antibiotics
  - Warm compresses for 10 minutes 3–5 times a day
  - Light massage over the lesion may aid in opening the gland.
  - Refer to specialist if not resolved in 3–4 weeks for definitive treatment, including incision and curettage or intralesional steroid injection.
- Entropion/ectropion:
  - Medical management is temporizing:
    - Aggressive eye lubrication
    - Antibiotic ointment and warm compresses for exposed lid margins
    - Taping eyelid into proper position

- Definitive treatment is referral to specialist for surgery.
- Blepharitis:
  - Chronic condition; daily treatment may be needed indefinitely to manage symptoms.
  - Lid hygiene, including lid washing/scrubbing with mild shampoo and lid massage
  - Warm compresses for 5–10 minutes 3–4 times a day
  - Artificial tears 4–8 times per day if associated with dry eyes
  - If not improving with symptomatic treatment, may add topical antibiotic ointment (eg, bacitracin, erythromycin) at bedtime
    - Consider oral antibiotics (eg, doxycycline or tetracycline) for severe blepharitis not responsive to topical antibiotics.
  - If severe or refractory, refer to specialist for topical steroids or cyclosporine.

Case Conclusion

This patient has a hordeolum, which is usually an acute, painful presentation of a stye. You advise the patient to apply warm compresses for 10 minutes 3–5 times a day. A hordeolum often will resolve spontaneously in a few days with conservative management.

CHAPTER 76

Conjunctivitis

Sara Lolar, MS, PA-C, DFAAPA

A patient presents with complaints of red, irritated eyes for 4 days. It started in the left eye and then spread to the right eye yesterday. She also complains of a runny nose and scratchy throat. She is not sexually active. On examination, the eyes are injected, and there is a watery discharge. There are no epithelial defects or ulcers on the cornea. There is tender, bilateral preauricular lymphadenopathy. What is the most appropriate treatment?

▶ GENERAL FEATURES

- Commonly referred to as "pink eye"
- Highly contagious; spreads by direct contact with secretions or by contaminated fomites

- Three types:
  - Viral: most common; caused by an adenovirus of multiple serotypes
  - Bacterial
    - Nongonococcal:
      - Usually *Staphylococcus* or *Streptococcus* in adults; *Haemophilus* in children
    - Gonococcal:
      - Vision threatening
      - Seen in sexually active individuals and in neonates
      - Neonatal: gonococcal usually presents within 1–7 days after birth; chlamydial presents within the first 5–19 days after birth.
  - Allergic: often have a history of seasonal allergy, atopy, or specific allergy (eg, to cats)

CLINICAL ASSESSMENT

- Viral:
  - May report a prodrome of upper respiratory infection (URI)–type symptoms or exposure to someone with conjunctivitis
  - Itching, burning, tearing, or gritty sensation
  - Watery discharge
  - Often bilateral; starts in one eye and spreads to other
  - Presence of inferior palpebral conjunctival follicles
  - Ipsilateral, tender preauricular lymphadenopathy may be present.
- Bacterial:
  - Nongonococcal:
    - Often unilateral
    - Scant mucopurulent discharge, thick and globular
    - Discharge is continuous throughout the day and reaccumulates quickly after wiping, itching less prominent
  - Gonococcal:
    - Hyperacute onset (within 12-24 hours).
    - Severe purulent discharge
    - Presence of risk factors for sexually transmitted infections (STIs); concomitant urethritis usually present
- Allergic:
  - Itching is cardinal symptom.
  - Red, swollen eyelids; usually bilateral
  - May have stringy discharge or conjunctival chemosis/edema
  - No preauricular lymphadenopathy

DIAGNOSIS

- Rule out other causes of a red eye, including glaucoma, uveitis, corneal abrasion or foreign body, keratitis, scleritis, trauma, subconjunctival hemorrhage, etc.
  - "Red-flag" symptoms that warrant further evaluation include reduced visual acuity, photophobia, fixed pupil, corneal defects, or severe headache.
- Recommend slit-lamp/corneal staining to ensure no corneal involvement and/or herpetic signs (dendrites, skin vesicles).
- Viral:
  - Not necessary to perform culture or Gram stain
  - Presence of preauricular lymphadenopathy along with conjunctivitis symptoms is pathognomonic for viral conjunctivitis
- Bacterial:
  - Routine culture and gram stain not recommended unless concern for STI
    - Gonococcal conjunctivitis: Gram-negative intracellular diplococci
  - If severe, recurrent, or not improving despite adequate treatment, refer to specialist for further evaluation.
- Allergic: usually a clinical diagnosis with pruritus, stringy discharge, swollen eyelids, and/or allergic shiners

TREATMENT

- Viral:
  - Course is self-limited (much like a common cold).
  - Contagious while eyes are red or have active watering/tearing; consider work/school restrictions.
  - Stress importance of not touching face or rubbing eyes; stress frequent handwashing and disinfecting of household.
  - Artificial tears or antihistamine drops for comfort.
  - Routine use of topical antibiotics or steroids not recommended.
- Bacterial:
  - Nongonococcal:
    - Often self-limited, but early use of topical antibiotic may shorten the clinical course.
      - Empiric, topical broad-spectrum antibiotic therapy for 5–7 days
      - Antibiotic therapy can be adjusted based on culture results.
    - Should be followed closely initially, every 2–3 days until resolved
  - Gonococcal:
    - Administer the treatment for STIs as stated by the Centers for Disease Control and Prevention:
      - Current recommendation is ceftriaxone 1 g IM plus azithromycin 1 g by mouth.
      - Treat sexual partners.
    - If corneal involvement, patient should be hospitalized for parental antibiotics.
    - Consider topical fluroquinolone drops.
    - Saline irrigation may help with comfort and inflammation.
- Allergic:
  - Eliminate the underlying inciting agent.
  - Cool compresses for comfort
  - Mild symptoms: artificial tears 4–8 times a day for comfort
  - Moderate symptoms: consider antihistamine and/or mast cell stabilizer eye drops.
  - Severe symptoms: consider mild topical steroid for a short period of time in addition to the preceding regimens.
  - Oral antihistamines (including newer second-generation preparations like loratadine) can be helpful in moderate-to-severe infection.

Case Conclusion

The patient presents with a viral conjunctivitis. The treatment is mainly symptomatic, as the course is self-limited, so you advise her to use artificial tears for comfort. Antibiotics are not indicated for a viral conjunctivitis, and cultures are not necessary.

Corneal Disorders

Neil Howie, PGDip, MSc, SFHEA, PA-R

A 27-year-old male patient who does not wear glasses for vision reports foreign-body sensation to the left eye ~4 hours before arrival when he was working in construction without wearing eye protection and may have gotten sawdust in his eye. The affected eye has been tearing, red, and sensitive to light. What is the most likely cause of his symptoms?

▶ GENERAL FEATURES

- Cataracts:
  - Caused by the breakdown of proteins in the lens of the eye
  - Leading cause of blindness worldwide
  - Most common cause is aging; some cataracts can be congenital.
  - Risk factors include increased age, tobacco use or history of use, eye injury, chronic UV/sun exposure, long-term use of corticosteroids or statins, and diabetes.
  - Symptoms: blurred or double vision, photosensitivity, difficulty with night vision, vision change where bright colors appear faded
- Corneal abrasion:
  - Usually the result of minor eye trauma
  - Often associated with foreign body or contact lens use
- Keratitis:
  - Caused by inflammation and edema of the cornea
  - Infectious causes include bacteria, viruses, fungi, or parasites.
  - Noninfectious causes include foreign body, trauma, or inappropriate contact lens wear.
  - Risk factors include dry eyes, overexposure to UV light, immunocompromise, and contact lens wear.
  - For contact lens users, prevention involves keeping to a schedule for wearing and cleaning contact lenses and not swimming while wearing contact lenses.

▶ CLINICAL FINDINGS

- Cataracts:
  - Patients often complain of gradual decrease in vision.
  - Appear as opacities in the lens of the eye that can be gray, white, or yellow brown in color
  - Can cause distortion in the red reflex
- Corneal abrasion:

- Patients complain of foreign-body sensation, tearing of the affected eye, photophobia, injection and blepharospasm, or difficulty keeping eye open.
- Blurred vision is common; record visual acuity before and after treatment.
- Keratitis:
  - Painful red eye with tearing and photosensitivity; patients may complain of blurred vision.
  - Constricted pupil, corneal opacity, and/or ciliary flush may be present.
  - Fluorescein stain may reveal a white spot indicating bacterial keratitis or the classic dendritic lesion characteristic of ocular herpes simplex virus.

▶ DIAGNOSIS

- Cataracts: characteristic findings on slit-lamp examination, retinal examination with dilated pupils, and refractory and visual acuity tests
- Corneal abrasion:
- Application of topical anesthesia almost always resolves the pain.
- Slit-lamp examination will demonstrate a clear cornea; fluorescein stain will reveal an epithelial defect of the cornea.
- Keratitis:
  - Slit-lamp examination and fluorescein stain demonstrate corneal opacity or infiltrate along with the classic findings of a foreign-body sensation and photophobia.
  - Corneal culture or biopsy may be necessary to determine the cause of infectious keratitis.

▶ TREATMENT

- Cataracts:
  - Definitive treatment with surgical removal of the natural lens and replacement with intraocular lens; indications for surgery include worsening visual acuity or decrease in ability to perform activities of daily living owing to limitations in vision.
  - Protecting eyes from sunlight, vision correction with glasses/contacts, and treatment of underlying conditions such as diabetes and tobacco dependence can slow the development of cataracts.
- Corneal abrasion:
  - Topical anesthesia provides temporary relief of pain but should not be used for treatment because it can delay healing.
  - Saline irrigation can help remove foreign body.

- Prescribe topical antibiotics to prevent infection; avoid topical corticosteroids and topical nonsteroidal anti-inflammatory drugs (NSAIDs) because they can delay healing.
- Treat pain with oral medications if needed.
- Patching is usually not necessary.
- Expect improvement each day and refer to ophthalmology for evaluation if it fails to heal.
  - Keratitis:
    - For noninfectious keratitis, treatment usually involves lubricating eye drops; for more severe cases, a bandage contact lens or anti-inflammatory eye drops may be prescribed.

- For infectious causes, treat the underlying infection with topical; in more severe cases, treat with oral antibiotics.
- Emergent referral is recommended when hyphema or hypopyon is present because these findings can indicate a sight-threatening infection.

Case Conclusion

The patient presents with symptoms of a corneal abrasion likely caused by sawdust and working without eye protection. He should be evaluated with a visual acuity test, slit lamp, and fluorescein stain of the affected eye to confirm the diagnosis.

CHAPTER 78

Orbital Cellulitis

Jeanette Elfering, MHS, PA-C

A 6-year-old boy presents to his primary care provider with an erythematous, edematous right eye that has progressively worsened over the past 3 days. His mother reports that he recently had an upper respiratory infection (URI), and he was improving until yesterday when he became febrile and started complaining of eye pain and a headache. His examination was notable for significant right lid edema and erythema, with decreased visual acuity and pain with extraocular muscle examination. What is the most likely diagnosis of this patient's symptoms?

▌ GENERAL FEATURES

- Infection of soft tissue surrounding the eye socket behind the orbital septum
- Isolated infection anterior to the orbital septum is considered preseptal cellulitis.
- Etiologic factors include:
  - Periorbital structures: 90% caused by infection of the adjacent sinuses; other causes include skin, dental, and intracranial infections.
  - Exogenous sources (trauma or postsurgical)
  - Intraorbital infection (endophthalmitis or dacryoadenitis)
  - Bacteremia: most common pathogens are Grampositive *Staphylococcus aureus* and *Streptococcus* species.
    - Anaerobes are much less common and are associated with dental abscesses.
    - Consider fungal infections in immunocompromised or diabetic patients.

- Complications include subperiosteal or orbital abscess (10%), exposure keratopathy, secondary glaucoma, retinal disease, optic neuropathy, cranial nerve palsies, blindness, meningitis, subdural or brain assess, and death.

▌ CLINICAL ASSESSMENT

- History:
  - Risk factors: history of recent upper respiratory infection (URI), acute or chronic bacterial sinusitis, ocular trauma, ocular/periocular infection, recent facial or eye surgery, and systemic infection
  - Symptoms: pain with eye movement, lid edema, painful erythematous eye, decreased vision, fever, nausea, vomiting, diplopia, headache, sinus pain, upper respiratory symptoms, or lethargy
- Physical examination:
  - Decreased visual acuity could indicate optic nerve involvement or secondary exposure keratopathy.
  - Dilated fundus examination to evaluate for optic nerve or retinal pathology
  - Ocular motility (rule out cavernous sinus involvement), pupillary function, and assessment of proptosis via Hertel exophthalmometry should also be assessed.
  - Thorough orbital examination to include the direction of displacement of the globe, resistance to retropulsion (gently palpate globe through the lid, a positive result is resistance), and unilateral vs. bilateral involvement

- Oral and nasal examination in immunocompromised patients to assess for black eschar, suggesting fungal infection

▶ DIAGNOSIS

- Substitute: Orbital cellulitis is a clinical diagnosis based on exam findings of edema and erythema in the periorbital region, but computed tomography (CT) (preferred) or magnetic resonance imaging (MRI) of the orbits should be obtained to help differentiate between orbital cellulitis and preseptal cellulitis, identify the presence of an abscess, and determine whether surgical intervention is necessary.
  - Indications to perform imaging: proptosis, ophthalmoplegia, bilateral edema, unable to successfully assess vision or worsening vision, no improvement of symptoms after 24 hours of initiation of intravenous (IV) antibiotics, or clinical indications of central nervous system (CNS) involvement

- Laboratory tests: complete blood count (CBC) will show leukocytosis. Blood cultures and nasal/throat swabs can help identify source and causative organism.

▶ TREATMENT

- Hospital admission with broad-spectrum IV antibiotics for empiric treatment with modification of antibiotic regimen based on culture results
- Improvement monitored by temperature, white blood cell count, patient's symptoms, visual acuity, optic nerve function, degree of proptosis, and extraocular motility

Case Conclusion

Given his history and the examination, our patient has orbital cellulitis. He has erythema and edema surrounding his eye, but what differentiates this from preseptal cellulitis is the pain with eye movement, decreased vision, and fever. You admit him to the hospital for intravenous antibiotics.

CHAPTER
79

Retinal Detachment and Retinal Vascular Occlusion

Sara Lolar, MS, PA-C, DFAAPA

A 56-year-old male presents with a 1-hour history of sudden, painless vision loss in the right eye. The patient has a history of diabetes and hypertension and smokes tobacco. He reports seeing flashes of light and had a brief loss of vision in the right eye yesterday. You note a cherry-red spot on fundoscopic examination. What diagnosis is most likely?

▶ GENERAL FEATURES

- Retinal detachment:
  - Separation of the retina from the underlying retinal pigment epithelium (RPE) and choroid, which is the vascular supply to the retina
  - Causes:
    - Tear or hole in the retina that allows fluid from the vitreous chamber to collect in the subretinal space and pulls the retina away from the underlying RPE and choroid

  - Most common, usually atraumatic but also caused by trauma
  - Risks: myopic eye ("near-sighted"), increasing age, personal/family history of detachment
  - Accumulation of fluid between the retina and the RPE without a hole or tear
    - Usually caused by infectious or inflammatory conditions such as sarcoidosis, syphilis, or ocular cancers
  - Traction pulling the retina away from the RPE
    - Usually associated with diabetic retinopathy or previous trauma that causes adhesions/scarring
- Retinal vascular occlusion:
  - Central retinal artery and vein are the sole blood supply and return of the retina; occlusion results in a central retinal artery occlusion (CRAO) or central retinal vein occlusion (CRVO).
    - CRAO is a form of stroke and considered an ophthalmologic emergency.

- Risk factors are similar to other vascular disorders, including increasing age, male sex, history of hypertension, diabetes, obesity, and tobacco use.
  - Atherosclerotic disease and cardiogenic embolism are the most common causes of CRAO.
  - Hypercoagulable states are associated with both CRAO and CRVO.
  - Giant cell arteritis is associated with CRAO.
  - Glaucoma is associated with CRVO; the increased intraocular pressure prevents retinal vein outflow.

CLINICAL ASSESSMENT

- Retinal detachment:
  - Hallmark is painless loss of vision in the affected eye, either peripheral or central or both.
    - Depending on the site of the detachment, may present as a visual field deficit
  - May initially see floaters ("cobwebs" or "spots") or flashes of light
  - As the tear progresses, may see a shadow or curtain drawn over the field of vision
- Retinal vascular occlusion:
  - Presents with unilateral, painless acute vision loss or blurred vision
    - Vision loss is usually severe, patients may only be able to sense light or finger movement.
    - If a branch artery or vein, visual loss may be restricted to a visual field.
  - May have a history of amaurosis fugax
  - Often will have a relative afferent pupillary defect
  - Funduscopic examination:
    - CRAO: ischemic retinal whitening with a "cherry-red" fovea; may see retinal emboli
    - CRVO: diffuse retinal hemorrhages resulting in a "blood-and-thunder" fundus; possible optic disc edema and cotton-wool spots

DIAGNOSIS

- Retinal detachment:
  - Urgent ophthalmology referral should be considered in any patient presenting with flashers, floaters, or painless visual loss and/or with the following high-risk features such as decreased visual acuity or visual field deficits.
  - Fundoscopic examination may demonstrate the retinal detachment, seen as a flap in the vitreous humor.
    - Bedside ultrasound may assist in the diagnosis of a retinal detachment.
- Retinal vascular occlusion:
  - Workup to determine the underlying etiology of occlusion may include:
    - Screening for cardiovascular risk factors, including hemoglobin A1C and lipid panel
    - Carotid artery imaging
    - Cardiac evaluation: may include electrocardiogram (ECG) for atrial fibrillation, echocardiography, and Holter monitoring
    - Exclusion of giant cell arteritis with erythrocyte sedimentation rate (ESR)
    - Hypercoagulable testing

TREATMENT

- Retinal detachment: emergent referral to ophthalmology for definitive treatment, ranging from surgery to vitrectomy
- Retinal vascular occlusion:
  - Spontaneous recovery from CRAO or CRVO is rare.
    - Branch retinal or venous occlusion has better prognosis.
  - CRAO should be treated like an acute stroke:
    - Urgent neurology consult
    - Consideration of intra-arterial thrombolytic therapy
  - Treatment is directed to risk modification to prevent long-term management and to prevent recurrent vascular events.
  - May consider treatment with antiplatelet therapy

Case Conclusion

This patient most likely has central retinal arterial occlusion (CRAO). CRAO and central retinal vein occlusion (CRVO) are both associated with risk factors of vascular disease, including diabetes, hypertension, tobacco use, and heart disease. Both may present with painless of vision. However, in CRAO, a cherry-red spot is seen on fundoscopy because of ischemia of the retina. CRVO will usually present with retinal hemorrhage.

Optic Neuritis

Jeanette Elfering, MHS, PA-C

A 26-year-old healthy female presents to the emergency department complaining of visual changes that she describes as a "black spot" in the central vision of her left eye that started yesterday and has progressively worsened. On examination, you note decreased vision in her left eye, 20/60, when compared to her right eye, 20/20, and pain when she fully abducts and adducts her eye. Her pupil examination is remarkable for a relative afferent pupillary defect (RAPD) in the left eye. Fundus examination and neurologic examination were normal. What do you suspect is the diagnosis?

▶ GENERAL FEATURES

- Optic neuritis (ON) is an immune-mediated inflammatory demyelinating process that affects the optic nerves.
- The myelin that surrounds the optic nerves becomes damaged, causing axons to poorly conduct impulses.
- There is a female-to-male ratio of 3:2; it most commonly affects patients between the ages of 20 and 40 years.
- The most common cause is multiple sclerosis (MS); other causes include:
  - Neuromyelitis optica (NMO)
  - Myelin oligodendrocyte glycoprotein (MOG)
  - Varicella-zoster virus (VZV)
  - Herpes simplex virus (HSV)
- Differential diagnosis: ischemic optic neuropathies, syphilis, sarcoidosis, cat-scratch disease, Lyme disease, and systemic lupus erythematosus
- Certain medications: ethambutol and chloramphenicol

▶ CLINICAL ASSESSMENT

- History:
  - >90% of patients present with abrupt loss of central vision that occurs over several hours to days, and pain in and around the affected eye.
  - Other symptoms: photopsias, dyschromatopsia, and Uhthoff phenomenon

- Physical examination:
  - Decreased visual acuity, color vision, and contrast sensitivity in the affected eye (typically, monocular but can present binocularly)
  - Visual field deficits (central or peripheral)
  - Notable relative afferent pupillary defect (RAPD) (only present with unilateral ON) on pupil examination
  - Fundus examination can appear unremarkable (suggestive of retrobulbar ON, 67% of cases) or show optic nerve edema (33% of cases)

▶ DIAGNOSIS

- Diagnosis is usually clinical with central vision loss, decreased visual acuity, visual field defects, and RAPD. However, further workup is required to rule out potential demyelinating, infiltrative, or infectious processes.
- Magnetic resonance imaging (MRI) of the brain and orbits with and without contrast will demonstrate optic nerve enhancement/enlargement of the affected optic nerve; MRI of the brain may reveal ovoid periventricular white matter lesions suggestive of MS.
- Based on history, it may be necessary to rule out other potential causes.
- The role of cerebrospinal fluid (CSF) analysis is unclear; however, the presence of oligoclonal banding in CSF is associated with MS, and CSF studies are most useful to rule out other inflammatory or infectious etiologies.

▶ TREATMENT

- Acute ON is treated with high-dose (1 g) intravenous (IV) Solu-Medrol (methylprednisolone) for 3 days, followed by an oral prednisone taper.

Case Conclusion

This patient has signs and symptoms consistent with optic neuritis. The best imaging modality to confirm this diagnosis is a magnetic resonance imaging of the brain with and without contrast to visualize the optic nerve.

CHAPTER 81

Traumatic Eye Disorders

Shekitta Acker, MS, PA-C

A 26-year-old male presents to the emergency department complaining of a "bloody eye." He was in an altercation this morning and was hit in the right eye. You examine him, and his visual acuity in the affected eye is blurry and he only can slightly see your waving hand. He has moderate edema of the lids and ecchymosis but can open his eyes. You can see blood in the anterior chamber (but it is not completely occluded), the pupil appears unequal, and there is no diplopia. What should you consider?

▶ GENERAL FEATURES

- Hyphema: ocular injury that damages the blood vessels of the iris, causing hemorrhage in the anterior chamber of the eye
- Globe rupture: ocular injury that results in a full-thickness defect in the cornea and/or sclera, exposing the intraocular compartments to the external environment
- Orbital blowout fracture: direct impact with the transmission of force through the bones or indirectly by injury to the thin bone of the orbital walls from the elevation of intraorbital pressure
  - Commonly affects the orbital floor
  - May result in entrapment of orbital tissue
  - Signs and symptoms may include enophthalmos or exophthalmos, paresthesias, numbness in the first and second divisions of the trigeminal nerve, diplopia, and orbital crepitus.
- Foreign body/corneal abrasion: presents with pain, foreign-body sensation, and light sensitivity

▶ CLINICAL ASSESSMENT

- Hyphema: decreased vision, unequal pupils, injected conjunctiva/sclera, blood in the anterior chamber, and increased intraocular pressure (IOP)
- Globe rupture: teardrop pupil and/or subconjunctival hemorrhage
- Orbital blowout fracture: limited upward gaze due to inferior rectus muscle entrapment
- Foreign body/corneal abrasion: tearing, photophobia, and injected conjunctiva

▶ DIAGNOSIS

- Hyphema:
  - Can be evaluated with gross examination of the eye with good lighting
  - Classified according to the amount of blood in the anterior chamber:
    - Grade 1: <1/3 of the anterior chamber, most common
    - Grade 2: 1/3 to 1/2 of the anterior chamber
    - Grade 3: 1/2 to almost full
    - Grade 4: Full

- Can be a sign of an open globe injury; thorough examination needs to be completed, and computed tomography (CT) scan recommended
- Globe rupture:
  - On the slit-lamp examination, aqueous humor flow may be visible on fluorescein testing (Seidel sign).
  - CT scan is recommended.
  - Do not check IOP with tonometry if globe rupture is suspected.
- Orbital blowout fracture: CT scan will show a teardrop sign that indicates the muscle is herniated.
- Foreign body/corneal abrasion: area of fluorescein dye uptake or a vertical or zigzag pattern may present on slit-lamp examination; foreign body may still be present.

▶ TREATMENT

- Hyphema:
  - Most resolve in 5–7 days
  - Eye protection and rest with the head of the bed at 30° at all times
  - Acetaminophen for pain, but avoid aminosalicylates and nonsteroidal anti-inflammatory drugs (NSAIDs)
  - Refer patients if they have elevated IOP or for suspicion of globe rupture.
  - Surgical intervention recommended for persistent grade 4 hyphema or prolonged elevated IOP.
- Globe rupture:
  - Emergent referral for surgical repair; eye protection, elevate the head of the bed.
  - Provide medications for pain, nausea, and antibiotics of potential infections.
- Orbital blowout fracture: emergent referral; surgical intervention
- Foreign body/corneal abrasion:
  - Removal of the foreign body
  - Cornea can be anesthetized with a topical anesthetic drop with a 27-guage needle or greater.
  - Broad-spectrum antibiotic eye drops
  - Eye protection such as patching
  - Limit use of topical anesthetics and avoid topical steroids because they can lead to corneal ulcers.
  - Consider referral if you are unable to remove foreign body or for follow-up.

Case Conclusion

The patient presents with grade 3 traumatic hyphema because blood is present in more than half of the anterior chamber. Hyphema can cause vision changes and it increases a patient's risk of glaucoma and corneal damage.

Amaurosis Fugax

Jeanette Elfering, MHS, PA-C

A 56-year-old male current smoker with a past medical history of hypertension and hyperlipidemia presents to an urgent care clinic complaining of monocular vision loss in his right eye that lasted for about 60 seconds and then his vision returned. Your examination was overall unremarkable; ophthalmologic and neurologic examination was completely normal. What is the likely diagnosis of his symptoms?

▶ GENERAL FEATURES

- Amaurosis fugax is monocular (more common) or binocular transient vision loss (TVL) caused by vascular insufficiency that leads to hypoperfusion of the optic nerve or retina lasting seconds to minutes followed by complete visual recovery; often precipitated by a postural change or cardiac arrhythmia.
- Monocular TVL indicates a disorder anterior to the optic chiasm; binocular TVL is indicative of a posterior process involving either the visual cortex, optic chiasm, or the optic radiations.
- Causes of monocular TVL:
  - Vascular: cardioembolic or carotid pathology (most common)
  - Inflammatory: giant cell arteritis
  - Hypercoagulable/hyperviscosity state
  - Neurologic: migraine or occipital seizure
  - Ophthalmic: angle-closure glaucoma, central retinal vein occlusion, orbital mass, papilledema
- Binocular TVL differential: migraine (more common), seizure, and vertebrobasilar ischemia
- Precipitating factors: severe carotid occlusive disease, ocular movement to a specific gaze, exercise, hot shower, and postural changes

▶ CLINICAL ASSESSMENT

- History:
  - Important to differentiate between monocular vs. binocular TVL
  - Risk factors: age, cardiovascular disease risk factors (hypertension, hyperlipidemia, previous vascular surgery), diabetes, smoking, clotting disorders, use of cocaine, or oral contraceptive use
  - Associated symptoms: headache, periocular pain, extremity weakness, contralateral hemiplegia, vertigo, and diplopia
- Physical examination:
  - Dilated fundus examination to visualize the retina, optic nerve, and blood vessels

- Depending on the cause will be normal or could show optic nerve edema, torturous/dilated vessels, hemorrhages, cotton-wool spots, or macula edema
- Confrontation and formal visual field testing to rule out a homonymous defect (patients tend to report a homonymous visual field defect as monocular deficit)
- Full neurologic examination to assess for a neurologic deficit

▶ DIAGNOSIS

- Ophthalmic examination needed to rule out ocular pathology
- Laboratory workup may include:
  - Inflammatory markers: erythrocyte sedimentation rate (ESR) and C-reactive protein (CRP)
  - Complete blood count (CBC)
  - Lipid profile
  - Hemoglobin A1C
  - Hypercoagulability testing
- Imaging to rule out cardioembolic process or vascular abnormality may include:
  - Electrocardiogram (ECG)
  - Magnetic resonance imaging (MRI) of the brain with and without contrast
  - Carotid ultrasound (US)
  - Echocardiogram (transesophageal or transthoracic)
  - Magnetic resonance angiogram (MRA) or computed tomography angiogram (CTA) of the head and neck
  - Consider electroencephalogram (EEG) if bilateral TVL or if seizure activity is suspected

▶ TREATMENT

- Depends on the cause of the visual disturbance:
  - Control arteriosclerotic risk factors (hypertension, diabetes, dyslipidemia)
  - Consider 81–325 mg of aspirin
  - Vascular surgery/cardiology consult
  - Lifestyle modifications
  - Consider antiplatelet or anticoagulation therapy

Case Conclusion

The patient presents with multiple risk factors for amaurosis fugax, such as hypertension and hyperlipidemia. You discuss lifestyle modifications to control his arteriosclerotic risk factors and arrange a cardiology consult.

CHAPTER 83

Glaucoma, Amblyopia, and Strabismus

Shekitta Acker, MS, PA-C

> A 67-year-old female presents to the ophthalmologist with severe nausea, vomiting, right eye pain, and blurred vision. She reports the symptoms began about 2 hours ago. She has no significant past medical history. On gross examination, her visual acuity is OD 20/200, her right eye is injected, and her right pupil is larger than her left. What are the next steps?

▶ GENERAL FEATURES

- Glaucoma:
  - Acquired chronic optic neuropathy characterized by optic disc cupping and visual field loss
  - Loss of retinal ganglion cells characterized by either normal or increased intraocular pressure (IOP)
  - Two types:
    - Open-angle (most common): increased IOP due to resistance of trabecular meshwork that impedes outflow and is treated by reducing IOP with eye drops
    - Closed-angle: acute increased IOP from a mechanical obstruction that needs to be treated immediately
  - Risk factors:
    - >50 years old
    - First-degree relative
    - African descent
    - Chronic use of systemic or topical steroids
- Strabismus:
  - Misalignment in which only one eye fixates with the fovea on the object of interest
  - May occur in any direction—inward (eso-; cross-eyed), outward (exo-; wall-eyed), up (hyper-), down (hypo-), or torsional
    - Tropia (manifest strabismus) is strabismus present under binocular viewing conditions.
    - Phoria (latent strabismus) is a deviation present only after binocular vision has been interrupted by occlusion of one eye.
  - Seen in ~4% children:
    - Horizontal ocular deviations are common during the first few months of life, especially transient exotropia.
    - Gradually improving visual acuity and maturating of the ocular motor system typically produces normal ocular alignment by age 2–3 months; ophthalmologist should investigate ocular misalignment after this age.
    - Associated with abnormal sensory phenomena such as diplopia, visual confusion, amblyopia, and eccentric fixation
- Amblyopia:
  - Referred to as "lazy eye"
  - Reduced visual acuity in excess of that explicable by organic disease
  - In children, generally caused by other disorders of vision or the eye
  - Four main causes: strabismus, refractive errors, congenital cataract, ptosis
  - In esotropia, amblyopia is common and severe, whereas exotropia is uncommon and mild.

▶ CLINICAL ASSESSMENT

- Glaucoma: assess visual acuity; perform slit-lamp examination, tonometry, and examination of visual fields.
- Strabismus and amblyopia:
  - Evaluate visual acuity in all patients.
  - Refractive error is measured by retinoscopy.
  - Perform all four components of cover/uncover testing:
    - Cover test
    - Uncover test
    - Alternate cover test
    - Prism and alternate cover test
  - Assess patient's ability to fixate on a target, which may be in any direction of gaze at distance or near.
  - On examination, the patient's eyes are not gazing in the same direction at the same time.

▶ DIAGNOSIS

- Glaucoma:
  - Acute open-angle glaucoma can be asymptomatic but may present with injection of the conjunctiva, cloudy cornea; large cup-to-disc ratio may be seen when evaluating the optic disc by direct ophthalmoscopy.
  - Acute closed-angle glaucoma presents with a painful red eye, vision loss, headache, nausea, vomiting, and halos around the light; typically unilateral.
  - Tonometry is used to measure IOP (normal range = 11-21 mm Hg).

- Visual field loss involves mainly the central 30° of field during visual field examination.
- The anterior chamber angle width is best determined by gonioscopy but can be estimated by oblique illumination with a penlight or by slit-lamp observation of the depth of the peripheral anterior chamber.
- Strabismus and amblyopia: based on history and confirmed when there is abnormality of alignment, visual acuity, refraction, and/or cover tests

▶ TREATMENT

- Glaucoma:
  - Commonly treated with a combination of eye drops
  - Nonspecific β-blockers to decrease development of aqueous humor (eg, timolol 0.5%, once or twice a day)
  - Prostaglandin analogs for facilitation of aqueous humor outflow (eg, latanoprost 0.005%, once a day)
  - Carbonic anhydrase inhibitors for chronic glaucoma used to suppress aqueous production (eg, dorzolamide 2%, 2-3 times a day); acetazolamide is the more commonly used systemic oral medication and is more effective than topical treatment

- α-Agonists used to inhibit aqueous production and increases aqueous outflow (eg, brimonidine 1.0%, 2-3 times a day)
  - Surgical and laser treatment may be recommended when other therapies fail: peripheral iridotomy, iridectomy, and iridoplasty
- Strabismus: nonsurgical; includes treatment of amblyopia, the use of optical devices (prisms and glasses), pharmacologic agents, and orthoptics
- Amblyopia:
  - Two stages:
    - Occlusion is the "gold standard"; the better eye is covered with a patch for 2–14 h/day to stimulate the amblyopic eye.
    - Atropine, as ophthalmic drops or ointment, is instilled in the better eye 2–7 days/week to inhibit its accommodation and promote use of the amblyopic eye during near viewing.

Case Conclusion

Given the patient's typical presentation of acute angle-closure glaucoma with headache and vomiting, you perform a slit-lamp examination and confirm the diagnosis. You discuss treatment options.

SECTION C   *Nose and Sinus Disorders*

CHAPTER 84   Nasal Polyps

Jennifer Johnson, BS, MPAS, DMSc

Ms. Anderson is a 32-year-old woman who presents to the clinic for evaluation of nasal congestion. Breathing through her nose has become more difficult over the past month. She also notes anosmia and postnasal drainage as well as a long history of seasonal allergies. What are the most likely causes of this patient's symptoms?

▶ GENERAL FEATURES

- Nasal polyposis is an inflammatory condition that results in hyperplasia of the paranasal mucosa, leading to benign nasal growths.
- The exact cause of nasal polyps is unclear.

- Nasal polyps usually develop near the middle meatus in the nasal cavity.
- Risk factors for nasal polyposis include chronic sinusitis, chronic allergic rhinitis, aspirin hypersensitivity, asthma, and cystic fibrosis.
- If left untreated, progression of aggressive nasal polyps may lead to erosion of the bones of the sinus cavities, a rare but serious complication.

▶ CLINICAL ASSESSMENT

- Patients with nasal polyps report worsening nasal congestion, nasal obstruction, decreased sense of smell, and postnasal drainage.

- Associated symptoms may include headache or facial pain and pressure.
- Decreased or absent sense of smell in patient with nasal polyps is a direct result of nasal obstruction.
- Physical examination reveals single or multiple pale, gray, polypoid masses with the appearance of a peeled grape in the nasal cavity.
- Polyps may occur unilaterally or bilaterally.

▶ DIAGNOSIS

- Polyps are visible via direct nasal endoscopy in an outpatient clinic.
- Nonenhanced coronal computed tomography (CT) scan is the imaging study of choice for nasal polyps.
- Children who develop nasal polyps should be tested for cystic fibrosis (sweat chloride test or genetic testing) and asthma.

▶ TREATMENT

- Nonsurgical treatment of nasal polyps includes intranasal corticosteroid sprays and brief courses of oral glucocorticoids; antibiotics are indicated only if there is a concomitant infection.
- Treat chronic allergic rhinitis and sinusitis aggressively.
- Many patients with nasal polyps are symptomatic despite appropriate medical treatment; these patients require otolaryngology referral for surgical polypectomy or treatment with biologics.
- Intranasal corticosteroid sprays are recommended to minimize polyp recurrence following surgical treatment.
- Despite adequate medical and surgical treatment, nasal polyps tend to recur.

Case Conclusion

As indicated by her presentation, such as nasal obstruction as evidenced by her difficulty breathing through her nose, loss of smell, postnasal drainage, and seasonal allergies, you suspect this patient has nasal polyps. After confirming with nonenhanced coronal computed tomography scan, you prescribe seasonal allergy medication and an intranasal corticoid spray.

CHAPTER 85

Rhinitis

Brian Robinson, MS, MPAS, M(ASCP)CM, PA-C

Mr. Jones, a 32-year-old Asian man, presents to his primary care physician assistant for "runny nose." He states that it has been worse since the start of spring. He also states that it is worse when he is at work. He describes a clear drainage associated with nasal congestion. He denies fever or chills. What is the first-line treatment for this condition?

▶ GENERAL FEATURES

- Rhinitis (inflammation of the nose) is one of the most common chronic conditions in the United States.
- Symptoms of rhinitis include edema of mucous membranes of the nose, rhinorrhea, and nasal congestion.
- Rhinitis may be grouped according to etiology:
  - Infectious rhinitis is caused by a viral infection and involves inflammation and infection of the nasal and sinus mucosa causing acute rhinitis.
    - Sneezing and malaise are often associated, but patients generally present without fever.
    - Symptoms typically resolve within 10 days.
    - Acute rhinitis can progress beyond 10–14 days to secondary bacterial infection, causing purulent nasal drainage, fever, and facial pain; this may also be seen with a worsening of symptoms following an initial improvement (double worsening).
  - Allergic rhinitis is an immunoglobulin E (IgE)–mediated mast cell degranulation, type I hypersensitivity reaction, following acute or chronic exposure to an allergen causing rhinitis.
    - Fatigue is a common symptom associated with nasal congestion, nasal and ocular pruritis, and sneezing.
    - Symptoms can be seasonal (associated with exposure to various pollens) or perennial (associated with exposure to dust mites, molds, and animal dander) and typically do not resolve until the allergen is removed.
  - Noninfectious/nonallergic rhinitis can have a variety of causes, but common etiologic factors include

gustatory rhinitis (associated with taste or consumption of certain foods), rhinitis medicamentosa (overuse of certain nasal medications such as oxymetazoline), pregnancy, medications (such as birth control pills), hypothyroidism, nasal mucosa atrophy, and vasomotor rhinitis (diagnosis of exclusion but associated with nasal congestion and triggers such as certain smells or cold air).

▶ CLINICAL ASSESSMENT

- History and physical examination are key to categorizing the patient's complaints and grouping them into the appropriate category.
- Social history including home and work environment and the timing of symptoms are critical to distinguish diagnoses.
- Allergic rhinitis may have additional physical examination findings, including pale to bluish nasal turbinates, transverse nasal creasing, mouth breathing, crease-like wrinkles under the lower eyelids, and dark circles under the eyes.
- Severity of symptoms and impact on activities of daily living (ADLs) may help guide diagnosis and treatment.
- A reliable and validated tool, such as Sino-Nasal Outcome Test (SNOT), may be completed by the patient to help distinguish allergic vs. nonallergic symptoms and impact of symptoms on the patient.
- Patients should be concurrently assessed for chronic comorbid conditions, including asthma, atopic dermatitis, otitis media, sleep-disordered breathing, conjunctivitis, and rhinosinusitis.
- Acute rhinitis following a head and neck procedure or trauma may be indicative of a cerebrospinal fluid (CSF) leak and is an emergency.

▶ DIAGNOSIS

- Diagnosis of infectious, allergic, or nonallergic rhinitis is frequently a clinical diagnosis thorough history and physical examination.
- Imaging (plain film or computed tomography [CT]) is not recommended for patients with suspected allergic etiology; this should be reserved with suspected

anatomic pathology as the source (eg, rhinitis with suspected basilar skull fracture or chronic sinusitis).
- Allergy testing, including specific IgE skin or blood testing, should be performed on a patient who fails to improve with empiric treatment or when the diagnosis/etiology is uncertain.
- Suspected CSF leak may be diagnosed with head and neck imaging (CT/MRI [magnetic resonance imaging]) and by collecting a sample of the rhinitis with analysis for β-2 transferrin.

▶ TREATMENT

- Nasal saline rinses can be initiated twice daily for congestion and drainage.
- Intranasal steroids, such as fluticasone, budesonide, triamcinolone, or mometasone, are first-line treatment for patients with allergic rhinitis and symptoms affecting ADLs.
- Nasal antihistamines, such as azelastine, are an additional treatment for patients diagnosed with allergic rhinitis.
- Oral antihistamines should be added for patients with primary complaints of sneezing and/or itching.
- Intranasal anticholinergics, such as ipratropium bromide, may be used in patients with infectious, allergic, or nonallergic rhinitis for symptom management.
- A combination of treatment options may be needed to control symptoms.
- Avoidance of allergens is recommended when specific allergens are either identified in the history or confirmed on skin or blood testing.
- Immunotherapy, either subcutaneous or sublingual, should be recommended for patients without improvement on pharmacologic therapy or avoidance of allergen(s).

Case Conclusion

Mr. Jones presents with allergic rhinitis. Intranasal steroids, such as fluticasone, budesonide, triamcinolone, or mometasone, are first-line treatment for patients with allergic rhinitis and symptoms affecting activities of daily living.

Acute and Chronic Sinusitis

Amy Akerman, MPAS, PA-C

> Mr. Thompson is a 43-year-old male who presents to urgent care with complaints of maxillary and frontal sinus pain, purulent nasal drainage alternating with nasal congestion, and a persistent headache for 10 days. He acknowledges a history of allergic rhinitis due to environmental triggers throughout his adult life. What diagnosis should you consider?

▶ GENERAL FEATURES

- Acute rhinosinusitis is most commonly caused by viral (90%-98%) and bacterial infections (2%-10%).
- Risk factors: older age, allergies, smoking, air travel, exposure to changes in atmospheric pressure (eg, deep sea diving), asthma, and immunodeficiency
- The most common cause for acute bacterial rhinosinusitis (ABRS) is a preexisting upper respiratory viral infection, especially causing a "double-sickening" presentation with a return of fever, headache, or rhinorrhea after 6 days of initially improving.
- The most common bacterial agents that cause ABRS: *Streptococcus pneumoniae*, *Haemophilus influenzae*, and *Moraxella catarrhalis*.
- Rhinosinusitis is considered chronic when symptoms and objective findings are present consecutively for at least 12 weeks.
- The most common causes of chronic rhinosinusitis: *Staphylococcal aureus*, *Pseudomonas aeruginosa*, and fungal species.

▶ CLINICAL ASSESSMENT

- Criteria for the diagnosis of ABRS are based on the presence of at least two major symptoms: nasal congestion or obstruction, purulent nasal drainage, fever, anosmia, facial fullness, pressure, or pain.
- The diagnosis may also be met if the patient has one major symptom and at least two minor symptoms: headache, ear pain/pressure, halitosis, dental pain, cough, or fatigue.
- ABRS should be on the differential diagnosis in all patients with purulent nasal drainage, nasal congestion or obstruction, and maxillary or frontal sinus pain.
- Symptoms of ABRS will persist for a minimum of 10 days and may worsen 10 days after initial improvement.

- Overdiagnosis of ABRS is common as many providers treat with antibiotics when a viral cause is more likely.
- Sinus computed tomography (CT) is the preferred method for workup of chronic rhinosinusitis symptoms; it may also be used as a physical examination tool and help the provider with surgical planning in patients with chronic symptoms.

▶ DIAGNOSIS

- All patients suspected of having ABRS should have a full HEENT (head, eyes, ears, nose, and throat) physical examination, including the tympanic membranes and the nasal mucosa.
- In most cases, the timing and description of all symptoms will help guide the diagnosis.
- Lab tests or diagnostic imaging are rarely necessary for the diagnosis of primary, uncomplicated rhinosinusitis.
  - Nasopharyngeal cultures are unreliable and not recommended for the diagnosis of ABRS.
  - Radiography is not recommended in the evaluation of uncomplicated acute rhinosinusitis.
- An otolaryngologist should be consulted for patients with chronic rhinosinusitis as they may require endoscopy cultures or sinus surgery to improve sinus drainage and relieve sinonasal inflammation.

▶ TREATMENT

- The first-line treatment for the diagnosis of uncomplicated ABRS in children and adults is amoxicillin-clavulanate.
- Doxycycline or a respiratory fluoroquinolone, such as levofloxacin or moxifloxacin, may be used as an alternative therapy for those who cannot tolerate or have an allergy to amoxicillin-clavulanate.
- Treatment is aimed at eradicating infection and preventing complications and chronic disease.
- Treatment for uncomplicated ABRS in adults is 5–7 days and 10–14 days in children.
- Important adjunct treatments include saline irrigation and intranasal corticosteroids.
- Consider alternative treatment for patients who fail to improve after 3–5 days or worsen after 48–72 hours of initial antimicrobial therapy.

- Patients with chronic rhinosinusitis should use daily saline irrigation with optional topical intranasal corticosteroids and should not receive topical or systemic antifungal treatment.
- If medical management fails, sinus cultures should be obtained endoscopically while assessing the patient for allergies, immune dysfunction, or additional chronic conditions that would require changes to management.

Case Conclusion

Mr. Thompson should be evaluated for acute bacterial rhinosinusitis based on his presentation of purulent nasal drainage, nasal congestion and obstruction, and maxillary or frontal sinus pain. He also has the minor associated symptom of headache. You should perform a full HEENT physical examination and conform the diagnosis. You start him on amoxicillin-clavulanate for a 7-day course.

CHAPTER

87

Epistaxis

Renee Andreeff, EdD, PA-C, DFAAPA

▶ GENERAL FEATURES

- Epistaxis is an acute hemorrhage from the nostril, nasal cavity, or nasopharynx and can be classified as anterior or posterior based on the location of the bleeding.
- Epistaxis occurs in about 60% of the general population.
- Epistaxis can occur at any age, but has a bimodal distribution, occurring most often in children up to age 10 years and adults over age 50 years.
- Seasonal variation; predominance in the winter months is due to the incidence of upper respiratory infections, allergic rhinitis, and changes in temperature and humidity levels.
- Causes can be divided into categories:
  - Trauma: nose picking, facial trauma, foreign body
  - Neoplastic: squamous cell, adenoid cystic carcinoma, melanoma, inverted papilloma
  - Hematologic: leukemia, AIDS, liver disease, hemophilia, von Willebrand disease, thrombocytopenia
  - Vascular malformation: Osler-Weber-Rendu syndrome, angioma, aneurysm of the carotid artery
  - Environmental: dry air, barotrauma
  - Drug induced: nonsteroidal anti-inflammatory drugs, aspirin, warfarin, clopidogrel, nasal sprays, chronic intranasal drug use
  - Inflammatory: sinusitis, allergy, irritants such as cigarette smoke
- Anterior epistaxis is the most common type and occurs in 90% of cases.
  - Most of these cases occur in Little's area (the anterior inferior quadrant of the nasal septum) where the Kiesselbach plexus is located.
  - Most cases are self-limiting.
- Posterior epistaxis generally arises from the posterior nasal cavity via branches of the sphenopalatine arteries at an area known as Woodruff plexus.

- Most cases occur behind the posterior portion of the middle turbinate or at the posterior-superior roof of the nasal cavity.
- Posterior epistaxis can result in significant hemorrhage.

▶ CLINICAL ASSESSMENT

- Initial assessment should focus on the patient's general appearance, mental status, vital signs, and cardiopulmonary stability; if these are normal, then a more thorough history can be obtained.
- Ask about timing, frequency, and severity of epistaxis; bleeding lasting >15 minutes requires medical intervention.
- Obtain a complete past medical history:
  - Conditions that predispose the patient to bleeding, recent trauma or surgery, medications, and systemic diseases such as HIV, cirrhosis, coagulation disorders, and hypertension
  - Nausea, hematemesis, anemia, melena, or hemoptysis, which are more indicative of posterior epistaxis
  - Dyspnea, sweating, chest pain or pressure, pain that radiates, and syncope
  - Blood loss from epistaxis may complicate existing cardiopulmonary disease.
- Examine the patient's skin for signs of coagulopathy (ecchymoses, petechiae, and telangiectasias).
- Use anesthesia (2% lidocaine) and proper lighting when examining the patient's nose; the patient should be examined in a dental chair if possible.
- To identify the location of the bleeding, use a nasal speculum and have the patient look straight ahead; do not let the patient to tip the head back, which will obscure the nasal cavity from view.
- Inspect Little's area for bleeding, ulceration, and/or erosion.
- Posterior bleeding is harder to visualize owing to its location.

TREATMENT

- The patient should don a gown and have an emesis basin readily available.
- Compression is recommended for all stable patients and can be done as the history is being taken:
  - The patient should pinch the tip of the nose between the thumb and the forefinger for 10–15 minutes.
  - A locally applied topical vasoconstrictor (oxymetazoline) and anesthetic can be placed in the anterior cavity before compression.
  - An ice pack can also be applied.
- Clots can be cleared using gentle suction or by having the patient gently blow the nose.
- If a vasoconstrictor was not used for compression, apply one locally (such as oxymetazoline) and anesthetize the nasal cavity (eg, using 2% lidocaine) using cotton pledgets.
- Anterior bleeding that does not respond to compression and topical vasoconstrictors can be treated using one or more of the following in succession:
  - Cautery (silver nitrate sticks for 10 seconds or less or electrocauterization); avoid bilateral cautery
  - Nasal packing (nasal tampon, petroleum-gauze, balloon catheters, or thrombogenic agents such as fibrin glue or topical thrombin gel):
    - After packing, perform a thorough examination to ensure that bleeding has stopped.
    - Packing should remain in place for 3–5 days; prophylactic antibiotics can be considered to cover possible staphylococcal infection.
- Unilateral anterior packing can be performed in an outpatient manner unless the patient has serious comorbidities.
  - Patients requiring bilateral packing should be admitted for monitoring.
  - An ear-nose-throat (ENT) evaluation is recommended for all patients requiring packing.
- Posterior epistaxis requires the following treatment:
  - Immediate ENT consultation
  - Local application of a vasoconstrictor such as oxymetazoline and anesthetization of the nasal cavity using 2% lidocaine and cotton pledgets
  - Anteroposterior packing with petroleum-impregnated gauze or a posterior balloon catheter as first-line treatment for posterior bleeding
  - Patients with posterior bleeding require hospitalization with cardiac monitoring.
  - Posterior packing should be removed in 24–48 hours for re-evaluation and possible repacking or surgical intervention.
- Complications:
  - Minor: anosmia, breathing difficulties, nasal septum hematomas, septal perforations, sleep apnea symptoms
  - Moderate: abscesses, sinusitis, syncope, necrosis, intranasal adhesions
  - Severe: toxic shock syndrome, uncontrollable bleeding, hypotension, bradycardia, aspiration, angina, hypovolemia

CHAPTER
88

Nasal Foreign Body

Janelle Bludorn, MS, PA-C
Joshua Merson, MS-HPEd, PA-C

Dalton, a 22-month-old male, is brought into the clinic with his mother with malodorous nasal discharge from the right nare. The mother reports they were cleaning the house 2 days ago and is concerned about possible dust allergy. What is important to consider in a toddler presenting with unilateral nasal discharge?

GENERAL FEATURES

- The most common anatomic location for foreign bodies is the nasal passage, surpassing all other respiratory and digestive tract sites.
- Most intranasal foreign bodies are located anteriorly or inferiorly to the inferior turbinate or anteriorly to the middle turbinate.
- The right nare is more commonly affected due to the prevalence of right handedness in the general population.
- Inorganic foreign bodies (beads, small toys, stones) are more common than organic foreign bodies (seeds, food items, gum).
- Two items that are prone to cause significant damage are button batteries, which can cause tissue necrosis, and disc magnets, which may lead to perforation if located on either side of the septum.
- The key demographic for nasal foreign-body incidence is toddler- and preschool-aged children but can also be seen in older children and adults, especially those who have developmental delays.

▶ CLINICAL ASSESSMENT

- Most inorganic nasal foreign bodies have few or no symptoms; most present with the patient or caregiver providing a history or concern of nasal foreign-body insertion.
- If symptoms are present, they may include discharge or odor from the nare, epistaxis, nare obstruction, sneezing, or facial pain and swelling.
- Organic foreign bodies often produce malodorous unilateral nasal discharge.
- Black nasal discharge in the setting of nasal foreign body should raise the suspicion for necrosis caused by a button battery.
- Physical examination should include inspection of the nare with otoscope, headlamp, or other external light source.
- Other physical examination components should include:
  - Facial palpation to assess for sinusitis
  - Inspection of the ear canals and contralateral nare to assess for foreign bodies at these sites

▶ DIAGNOSIS

- This is a clinical diagnosis based on history and visualization of the intranasal foreign body using an otoscope or other external light source.
- Fiberoptic rhinoscopy may be required, rarely.
- Radiographs are not generally required to confirm the diagnosis but may be helpful in the setting of button batteries, magnets, or other radiopaque foreign bodies not easily visualized on examination.

▶ TREATMENT

- Most foreign bodies can be removed at the bedside. Two common techniques include:
  - Positive pressure techniques:
    - Preferred with soft or smooth nasal foreign bodies that completely occlude the nasal cavity
      - Children under age 3 years, consider oral positive pressure by having the parent blow in the patient's mouth while occluding the unaffected nostril ("parent's kiss").

- Children over age 3 years, have the patient blow his/her nose while occluding the unaffected nostril.
  - Instrumentation:
    - Preferred on nonocclusive foreign bodies in the anterior nasal cavity:
      - Light, restraint, and proper equipment are needed to ensure successful removal.
      - Use topical anesthesia as instrumentation may be painful (avoid on button batteries).
      - Extract compressible objects using alligator or similar forceps, avoid with noncompressible objects as forceps may push object deeper into the nasal cavity.
      - Remove smooth objects or objects that cannot be grasped using a blunt right-angled hook or catheter such as balloon or Katz extractor.
      - Other considerations may include the use of a metal suction catheter with a plastic umbrella or cyanoacrylate glue.
- Otolaryngology consultation is indicated in the setting of:
  - Failed attempt(s) of bedside retrieval
  - Inability to visualize foreign body on inspection, suggestive of posterior location
  - Presence of significant inflammation
  - Penetration of the septum or ala(e)
- Button batteries and paired disc magnets should be removed urgently to avoid damage to nasal structures; other foreign bodies can be removed electively.
- Aspiration is an uncommon risk of removal.

Case Conclusion

The mother attempted the "parent's kiss" technique by forcibly blowing into the patient's mouth while occluding the unaffected nostril. The technique did not work, requiring the patient to be restrained using a sheet wrap. The nose was anesthetized using a lidocaine, epinephrine, oxymetazoline mixture. After anesthesia was achieved and with appropriate lighting, a small bead was successfully removed from the right nare using a balloon catheter, which was well tolerated by the patient.

CHAPTER 89

Nasal Trauma

Jennifer Johnson, BS, MPAS, DMSc

▶ GENERAL FEATURES

- Nasal fractures typically result from athletic activities, motor vehicle accidents, falls, or physical altercations.
- The bones of the nasal bridge are thin and fracture easily.
- Factors that predispose the nose to fractures include central location on the face, prominent protrusion, and a lack of structural support.
- Nasal fractures occur more frequently in males.
- Young children experience displaced nasal fractures less frequently than adults as a result of more elastic bones and more nasal cartilage present.
- Displaced nasal fractures may result in cosmetic deformity and deviated septum.

▶ CLINICAL ASSESSMENT

- Patients may present with a history of trauma, bruising, epistaxis, nasal airway obstruction, or a perceived change in nasal appearance.
- Physical examination reveals laceration, swelling, infraorbital swelling, epistaxis, or gross nasal deformity.
- Palpation of the nose may illicit abnormal movement, crepitus, and tenderness.
- Thoroughly evaluate the nasal septum for signs of septal hematoma, specifically widening of the septum or a dark blue or purple mass on the septum.
- Assess the patient for a potential cerebrospinal fluid (CSF) leak if rhinorrhea is present.

▶ DIAGNOSIS

- Imaging is not required if the patient can breathe through each nostril, septal hematoma is absent, trauma is limited to the bridge of the nose, and no displacement is visible.
- Plain films are the preferred imaging study if trauma is isolated to the nasal bridge and the above criteria are not met.
- If facial trauma is more extensive, computed tomography (CT) is the imaging study of choice.

▶ TREATMENT

- Elevation of the head and ice compresses are recommended.
- Patients should be evaluated within 12 hours of injury to determine whether a septal hematoma is present.
  - If present, it should be incised and drained immediately to express the clot, followed by anterior packing and referral to otolaryngology.
  - If no septal hematoma is present, the patient should be seen by otolaryngology within 3–7 days following the injury.
- If the appearance of the nose is acceptable to the patient and breathing is unchanged, no additional intervention is required.
- If the appearance of the nose is unacceptable to the patient or if breathing through one or both nares is more difficult than before the injury, closed nasal reduction is recommended.
- Fractures older than 10 days that resulted in cosmetic changes deemed unacceptable by the patient, referral to a surgeon specializing in rhinoplasty is recommended.

CHAPTER 90

Head and Neck Cancer

Jennifer Johnson, BS, MPAS, DMSc

Mr. Gordon is a 62-year-old male who presents to the clinic for evaluation of hoarseness that is progressively worsening. It has been constant for 10 weeks. Associated symptoms include right ear pain, a frequent cough, and weight loss of 10 pounds. He smokes tobacco, 1–2 pack-day for 43 years, and drinks alcohol 3 or 4 times per week. What is the most appropriate next step in evaluating this patient?

▶ GENERAL FEATURES

- Squamous cell carcinoma (SCC) accounts for >90% of head and neck cancers.
- In addition, >70 lymph nodes are present on each side of the neck, making the neck a common site for metastasis.

- The incidence of head and neck cancer is highest in older men; however, owing to the increasing prevalence of human papilloma virus (HPV) over the past several decades, head and neck cancers are increasingly occurring in young adults without other risk factors.
- Risk factors for the development of head and neck cancers: use of tobacco products, alcohol use, HPV, radiation exposure, environmental exposures, wood dust exposure, periodontal disease, and genetic factors
  - Alcohol and tobacco have a synergistic effect on risk of SCC development; patients who use both tobacco products and consume alcohol have a significantly higher risk of developing SCC than patients who use one or the other.
- Concerning symptoms include a nonhealing ulcer or an ulcer that recurs in the same spot, loosening teeth, dysphonia that persists for >3 weeks, chronic cough, hemoptysis, unexplained otalgia, persistent pharyngitis, and unexplained weight loss.
- The most common site for laryngeal cancer is the glottic region.
- Common sites of oropharyngeal SCC include the lower lip, lateral margins of the tongue, and the floor of the mouth.
- SCC of the head and neck frequently metastasize to cervical lymph nodes.

▶ CLINICAL ASSESSMENT

- Perform a thorough head and neck examination:
  - Assess all lymph nodes and visualize all of the oral mucosa.
  - Visualize all aspects of the tongue as well as the mucosa beneath the tongue; these recesses are common sites for SCC development as smokeless tobacco users hold the product in these locations.
  - Perform a thorough bimanual examination of the oral cavity using your gloved, nondominant hand to assess for any thickened, indurated, or fixated areas.
  - Palpate the floor of the mouth, the base of the tongue, and assess for loosening teeth.
- SCC often appears as red or red and white lesions with an ulcerated appearance that persist for >3 weeks.
- Urgent referral to otolaryngology for in-office endoscopy if unable to perform complete examinations of these areas.

▶ DIAGNOSIS

- Biopsy visible, concerning lesions promptly; a common error is to delay biopsy of concerning lesions in high-risk patients in favor of observation.
- Computed tomography (CT) scan of the head and neck with contrast is the imaging study of choice; magnetic resonance imaging (MRI), positron emission tomography (PET), or PET/CT may also be performed.

▶ TREATMENT

- Refer patients to otolaryngology and radiation and medical oncology.
- Management and prognosis vary depending on the location and stage of the tumor.
  - Early carcinomas with no metastasis may require removal with clean margins or definitive radiation only.
  - Advanced carcinomas will require radical neck dissection, radiation, and/or chemotherapy.
- Advanced cancer of the oropharynx, hypopharynx, or larynx will be managed using an organ-sparing, function-sparing approach in an effort to preserve speech and swallowing; however, laryngectomy may be required in severe cases.
- Many patients will require rehabilitative therapies following treatment of head and neck cancers to improve function and speech.
- A significant number of patients continue to consume alcohol and use tobacco products following a diagnosis of head or neck cancer; it is paramount that supportive resources and patient education on cessation are provided.
- The HPV vaccine may be indicated for some patients and may prevent the acquisition of additional harmful strains, and there is some evidence that routine administration of the HPV to older children and adolescents may reduce the overall incidence of SCC of the head and neck.

Case Conclusion

You suspect Mr. Gordon has squamous cell carcinoma and order a computed tomography scan of the head and neck with contrast. If the test comes back positive, you will refer him to otolaryngology and radiation and medical oncology.

CHAPTER
91

Epiglottitis

Eric Hochberg, MPAS, PA-C

▶ GENERAL FEATURES

- Epiglottitis is swelling or edema of the epiglottis, the structure at the base of the tongue that protects the lower airway during swallowing.
- Acute epiglottitis usually has an infectious cause with *Haemophilus influenzae* type b (Hib) as the most common organism.
- Bacterial causes of other upper and lower airway disease can also cause epiglottitis, such as *Moraxella*, *Streptococcus pneumoniae*, and group A streptococci.
- Other and rare etiologic factors include viruses, exposures, and inhalation injuries and connective tissue diseases.
- Since the introduction of the Hib vaccine to the childhood schedule of vaccinations in the late 1980s, the incidence of acute epiglottitis has declined significantly; the incidence of acute epiglottitis in adults has remained stable-low over the past 30 years.

▶ CLINICAL ASSESSMENT

- Symptoms of epiglottitis are common to other upper airway disease such as fever, sore throat or hoarseness, and odynophagia.
  - In children, symptoms may be rapidly progressive (<12-24 hours).
  - Serious signs of upper airway obstruction can include drooling, stridor (high-pitched airflow on inspiration), intercostal retractions, or cyanosis.
  - Children may appear "toxic" and sitting in the "tripod" position often restless or irritable; they may have a hoarse, muffled, or "hot potato" voice.
- Physical examination may reveal lymphadenopathy, a relatively near-normal oropharyngeal examination, or anterior neck pain, specifically over the hyoid bone.
- Acute epiglottitis should be suspected in any patient with sore throat, an unimpressive oropharyngeal examination and anterior neck pain.

- Laboratory studies may reveal leukocytosis, which is nonspecific.
  - Rapid screen for group A *Streptococcus* should be performed.
  - Blood cultures should be obtained.

▶ DIAGNOSIS

- The method of diagnosis must be weighed against the risks and benefits in the setting of the patient's clinical status; an adult with mild symptoms does not pose the same risks as a "toxic" appearing child who is drooling with intercostal retractions.
- The gold standard for diagnosis of epiglottitis is direct visualization best performed in a controlled environment such as emergency department, intensive care unit, or the operating room by a skilled practitioner while securing the patient's airway.
- Direct or indirect laryngoscopy or tongue depressor examination may be attempted with extreme caution because this may cause spasm of the edematous airway necessitating a surgical airway (cricothyrotomy).
- Lateral neck radiograph may reveal enlargement of the epiglottis or the classic "thumb-print" sign; other findings may include enlargement of the aryepiglottic folds, distension of the hypopharynx, decreased vallecular air space, or straightening of the cervical spine lordosis.
- Computed tomography (CT) scanning may be useful to evaluate for other pathologies, such as peritonsillar or retropharyngeal abscess or foreign body.

▶ TREATMENT

- If epiglottitis is suspected, treatment should not be delayed while awaiting confirmatory testing or diagnostic imaging.

- Treatment should focus on maintaining patency of the patient's airway via noninvasive or invasive means (not discussed here).
- Causative infectious organisms should be targeted with antibiotics such as third- or fourth-generation cephalosporin or ampicillin/sulbactam plus extended coverage if methicillin-resistant *Staphylococcus aureus* (MRSA) is suspected with an anti-staphylococcal agent such as vancomycin.
- Although controversial, corticosteroid therapy is also sometimes used as adjunct.

- Infectious disease consultation should be obtained for the immunocompromised patient with suspected acute epiglottitis.
- Patients with acute epiglottitis are best served with admission to an observed unit such as an intensive care unit with skilled personnel and appropriate equipment readily available.
- Epiglottic edema typically starts to resolve in 48 hours; treatment failure should raise the suspicion of incorrect antibiotic choice, alternative diagnosis, or abscess formation.

CHAPTER 92

Acute Pharyngitis

Jill Gore, PA-C

An 8-year-old male, accompanied by his mother, presents to his primary care provider's office complaining of a sore throat for 3 days. Yesterday, he developed nasal congestion, occasional sneezing, ear pressure, malaise, and mild myalgias. He has had a fever (T_{max} 99.8 °F orally). His mother states that a few of his classmates have been diagnosed with strep throat. What is his most likely diagnosis?

▶ GENERAL FEATURES

- Pharyngitis is inflammation of the pharynx and surrounding lymph tissue and accounts for 1%–2% of ambulatory care visits annually; 50% of cases occur in children.
- Viral causes are most common: rhinovirus, adenovirus, and coronavirus account for 25%–45% of all infections; parainfluenza, respiratory syncytial virus (RSV), coxsackie, and Epstein-Barr virus (EBV), influenza A and B, HIV, and enterovirus are less common.
- Group A β-hemolytic streptococcal (GABHS or GAS) infection is the most common bacterial cause of pharyngitis and accounts for <15% of adult pharyngitis and <30% of pediatric pharyngitis; GABHS infection is a focus of diagnosis because of its potential to lead to rheumatic sequelae if not treated appropriately.
- Other bacterial etiologies include *Neisseria gonorrhoeae*, *Corynebacterium diphtheriae*, *Haemophilus influenzae*, and groups C and G *Streptococcus*.
- Fungal organisms, including *Candida albicans*, can also cause pharyngitis.
- Noninfectious causes, including allergic rhinitis; mouth breathing; acid reflux; exposure to dry air; trauma; vocal strain, foreign body; irritation from smoking, alcohol, and marijuana; neoplasms; and subacute thyroiditis, may contribute to pharyngitis.

- Adequate antibiotic treatment of GABHS infection usually avoids complications, including scarlet fever, glomerulonephritis, poststreptococcal reactive arthritis, streptococcal toxic shock syndrome, rheumatic fever (carditis, valve disease, arthritis), and local abscess formation.

▶ CLINICAL ASSESSMENT

- Sore throat is the primary complaint; fever, anorexia, malaise, pain with swallowing (odynophagia), and headache may be present.
- Patients with pharyngitis caused by a virus typically have other symptoms of an upper respiratory tract infection, such as fatigue, nasal congestion, conjunctivitis, cough, sneezing, coryza, hoarseness, ear pain, and sinus pressure.
- Clinical features most suggestive of GABHS, known as the Centor criteria, include:
  - Fever >38 °C (100.4 °F)
  - Pharyngotonsillar exudate
  - Tender anterior cervical adenopathy
  - Lack of cough
  - When these four features are present, GABHS is highly likely.
- Other signs of GABHS include erythematous pharynx and enlarged, erythematous tonsils; soft palate petechiae may be present.
- GAS infection may be accompanied by scarlet fever rash, a "sandpaper" rash that presents as a fine, pinhead-sized exanthem that is more pronounced in a linear pattern along the major skin folds in the axillae and antecubital fossae (Pastia sign). It typically starts in the groin and axillae, expands to cover the trunk and extremities, and then desquamates.
  - The palms and soles are usually spared.
  - Circumoral pallor may be present.
  - "Strawberry tongue," a thick white-coated tongue with hypertrophied red papillae, may be noted.

- Although uncommon in the United States, pharyngitis due to diphtheria presents with a gray pseudomembranous exudate that bleeds when removed.
- Pharyngitis due to EBV, the major cause of infectious mononucleosis, manifests with a classic triad of fever, exudative pharyngitis, and adenopathy, particularly posterior cervical adenopathy; fatigue, headache, palatal petechial rash, and splenic enlargement may be present as well.
- Now rare in the United States, epiglottitis is a life-threatening upper airway obstruction caused by *H. influenzae*; other symptoms include high fever, stridor, drooling, and a toxic appearance.
- Pharyngeal abscess and peritonsillar abscess are potentially life-threatening infections and present with difficulty swallowing (dysphagia), fever, and trismus; a deviated uvula is highly suspicious for peritonsillar abscess.
- *C. albicans* pharyngitis may occur after antibiotic use or in an immunocompromised patient; thin, diffuse, or patchy exudate on mucous membranes is present.

DIAGNOSIS

- A positive throat culture or rapid antigen detection test provides confirmation of GABHS infection; throat culture may be considered for some patients, particularly pediatrics, when there is clinical suspicion and a negative rapid test.
- If gonococcal pharyngitis is suspected, culture needs to be performed on Thayer-Martin medium, or nucleic acid amplification test of an oropharyngeal swab may be ordered.
- If EBV mononucleosis is suspected, consider performing heterophile agglutination, also known as a Monospot test; specific EBV antibody tests can also be performed.
- To diagnose diphtheria, a culture of the pseudomembrane is needed in Loeffler or tellurite selective medium, followed by testing for toxin production.

- A complete blood count may be performed to aid in the diagnosis; typically, leukocytosis occurs with bacterial infection, and leukopenia occurs with viral infection.
- Following an active streptococcal infection, an antistreptolysin O (ASO) titer will be positive.

TREATMENT

- Viral causes, including infectious mononucleosis, are treated symptomatically with oral and topical analgesics, anesthetic lozenges, saltwater gargles, and a cool-mist humidifier.
- For patients with GABHS infection, antibiotic treatment is prescribed to prevent rheumatic sequelae:
  - First-line treatment is penicillin V or amoxicillin.
  - Second-line treatment includes cephalosporins, macrolides, or clindamycin for penicillin-allergic patients.
- Patients diagnosed with GABHS infection are contagious for 24 hours after the start of antibiotic therapy; toothbrushes should be changed 48–72 hours after beginning antibiotics.
- Topical treatment is usually sufficient for candidal pharyngitis: nystatin oral suspension, or for adolescents and adults, clotrimazole 10-mg buccal troches.
- Pharyngeal gonorrhea is treated with ceftriaxone, and chlamydia is treated with azithromycin or doxycycline.
- Treatment for diphtheria involves antibiotics and diphtheria antitoxin; seek specialist consultation and report cases to the state health department and Centers for Disease Control and Prevention.

Case Conclusion

The patient likely has viral pharyngitis as a symptom of his viral upper respiratory tract infection as evidenced by the additional symptoms of nasal congestion, sneezing, ear pressure, malaise, myalgias, and low-grade fever.

CHAPTER
93

Diseases of Teeth and Gums

Marie Pittman, DMSc, MPAS, PA-C, RDH
Jennifer Johnson, BS, MPAS, DMSc

GENERAL FEATURES

- Tooth and gum health depend on preventative measures, such as brushing, flossing, dental imaging, orthodontics, and denture prevention.

- Professional teeth cleaning and checkups are recommended every 6 months.
- Risk factors for cavity development include high acidity food, hard or sticky candy, sugar, the presence of *Streptococcus mutans*, baby bottle when sleeping, and lack of saliva protection.

- Protective measures include adequate saliva, fluoride, consistent oral hygiene, and antibacterial treatments to decrease the bacterial load on the teeth.
  - Salivary flow helps with remineralization of the enamel and cleansing the teeth and digesting food.
- Gum disease can result in local and systemic infections.
  - Gum disease ranges from gingivitis to periodontitis, superficial gum disease to gum disease affecting the supporting structures of the teeth, respectively.
  - Local infections can erode the periodontium, the connection of the tooth and bone, leading to tooth and bone loss.
- Be familiar with what a normal oral anatomy is so variations are recognized.
  - Healthy teeth:
    - The visible portion of a tooth is the crown and is typically smooth and made of enamel.
    - The neck of the tooth should not be visible on examination.
    - Tooth structure with any variable coloration (eg, extra white, yellow, brown, black, or red) should be evaluated closer.
    - Deciduous teeth are typically whiter in color than adult teeth and shorter in crown height.
  - Healthy gingiva:
    - Typical healthy gingival features include pink, tight, stippled, nonbleeding, and sharp/knife-edged interdental papilla.
    - Some generalized pigmentation is normal depending on ethnicity.
    - Gingiva can be connected or free-floating.
    - Connected gingiva is sensitive to the examination if bumped with the tongue depressor, for example.
- Unilateral lesions are concerning and often indicate disease.
- Other abnormal oral findings include:
  - Rampant caries in an adult (should raise suspicion for illicit drug use, typically methamphetamines)
  - Baby bottle tooth decay
  - Gastroesophageal reflux disease (GERD) or bulimia and erosions on the palatal maxillary teeth
  - Vigorous brushing and wearing away gum and tooth structure
  - Natal teeth
  - Gingival overgrowth from medications
  - Malocclusion
- Oral bacteria can cause endocarditis during dental procedures in at-risk patients; prophylactic antibiotics are recommended before dental treatment in certain groups at increased risk.

CLINICAL ASSESSMENT

- An extensive assessment of the oral cavity is critical at each visit.
- Ensure the physical examination is completed by looking at the lips, teeth, gums, hard and soft palate, lingual surface of teeth and gums, tongue, buccal mucosa, and saliva presence.
- Any lesion that is noted as changed from healthy, whether painful or painless, should be examined further.

DIAGNOSIS

- Tooth disease is assessed by physical examination and with radiographs.
- Gingival assessment is noted with a physical examination by a dental or medical professional, noting color, contour, and connection of the gums to the teeth; dental professionals can better assess the periodontal ligament.
- Assess for diseases associated with the development of dental abnormalities.

TREATMENT

- Preservation of teeth and gingiva is important, so patient education and prevention are crucial; brushing and flossing are the basis of prevention.
- Tooth disease:
  - Cavities: tooth structure repair is necessary to preserve the tooth; options include, but are not limited to, a small repair such as a filling, or extensive repair involving replacement of the whole crown.
  - Abscesses are managed with endodontic treatment; PenVK is the antibiotic of choice unless the patient is allergic.
  - Assessment and treatment of malalignment and malocclusion are foundational in oral and mental health; refer to orthodontics for management.
  - Any breakdown of teeth warrants education on brushing, flossing, and fluoride treatments; fluoride recommendations vary by location and are usually available online or at the local health department.
- Gingival disease:
  - Ranges from gingivitis to periodontitis. Close dental follow-up is recommended to preserve the teeth and their supporting bone structures.
- Many medications cause xerostomia, which is harmful for enamel. Select an alternative medication if possible and recommend over-the-counter (OTC) sialogogues.

Aphthous Ulcers, Oral Leukoplakia, Oral Candidiasis, and Deep Neck Infection

Jennifer Johnson, BS, MPAS, DMSc

▶ GENERAL FEATURES

- Aphthous ulcers:
  - Recurrent aphthous stomatitis, or "canker sores," is an inflammatory condition characterized by multiple, discrete oral lesions that are typically <10 mm in diameter; the lesions are round and painful with a well-defined erythematous rim surrounding a yellow-gray center, and many patients note a prodromal burning sensation.
  - Aphthous ulcers often begin during childhood or adolescence and recur through adulthood, with many patients experiencing gradual improvement in symptoms over time.
  - The etiology and pathophysiology are not well understood.
- Oral leukoplakia:
  - Leukoplakia (not to be confused with hairy leukoplakia) is an oral potentially malignant disorder; in some patients, these lesions progress over time and transform into oral squamous cell carcinoma (SCC).
  - Leukoplakia is a diagnosis of exclusion after the lesion has persisted for at least 6 weeks; other potential causes of white oral lesions must be ruled out in order to make the diagnosis.
  - Leukoplakia plaques are bright white, clearly demarcated, and slightly raised; they are not painful or bothersome.
  - Risk factors include tobacco, alcohol, denture use, and human papillomavirus (HPV).
- Oral candidiasis:
  - Also known as "thrush," oral candidiasis is a fungal infection of the oral cavity caused by *Candida albicans*.
  - It is common in infants, immunocompromised patients, and after antibiotic or oral steroid use; it is also associated with the use of inhaled corticosteroids and the use of upper dentures.
  - Patients with oral candidiasis may present with a burning sensation in the oropharynx, altered sense of taste, or for evaluation of a white coating in the mouth.
- Deep neck infection:
  - Occur in the submandibular, parapharyngeal, and retropharyngeal spaces:
    - The submandibular space is located inferior to the mucosa of the floor of the mouth and superior to the deep cervical fascia.
    - The parapharyngeal space extends from the hyoid bone to the base of the skull.
    - The retropharyngeal space is located posterior to the pharynx and esophagus and extends from the base of the skull to the mediastinum.
  - Patients are ill appearing and may be toxic.
  - Submandibular infections result in swelling of the tongue, airway obstruction, and spread to the retropharyngeal space; Ludwig angina is an example of a submandibular infection.
  - Parapharyngeal infections result from dental infections, tonsillitis, parotitis, and mastoiditis; patients report trismus and swelling below the angle of the mandible.
  - Retropharyngeal infections can result from local or distant infections' patients often note trismus and unilateral neck stiffness.
  - Deep neck infections are particularly dangerous owing to an anatomic route leading to the mediastinum: submandibular space → parapharyngeal space → retropharyngeal space → mediastinum.
  - In addition, the "danger space" lies posterior to the retropharyngeal space and extends from the base of the skull to the mediastinum.
    - As a result of these contiguous routes, deep neck infections can quickly spread to the mediastinum and chest.
    - If mediastinitis occurs, mortality approaches 50%, irrespective of antibiotic therapy.

▶ CLINICAL ASSESSMENT

- Aphthous ulcers:
  - Multiple lesions are usually visible on examination.
  - The morphology of the lesions is classified as minor (<1 cm in diameter), major (>1 cm in diameter), or herpetiform (2 mm, numerous lesions occurring in clusters).
  - Residual scarring is common after major and herpetiform lesions heal.
- Oral leukoplakia:
  - On physical examination, a bright white, well-defined plaque is observed that cannot be rubbed off with a tongue depressor.
  - It can be associated with erythroplakia (erythema), which carries a higher risk of dysplasia or carcinoma.
- Oral candidiasis: typically begins as small, focal lesions that progress to large, white plaques on the tongue and oral mucosa.
- Deep neck infection:

- With any deep space infection, patients may present with sore throat, trismus, dysphagia, and/or odynophagia.
- Physical examination of submandibular infections reveals sublingual swelling and lymphadenopathy.
- With parapharyngeal infections, bulging of the pharyngeal wall is noted medially; edema and induration below the angle of the mandible is present.
- Clinical findings associated with retropharyngeal abscess include bulging of the posterior pharyngeal wall, often unilateral or midline; torticollis may be present.

▶ **DIAGNOSIS**

- Aphthous ulcers:
  - Diagnosis is made based on history and clinical findings.
  - Biopsy, serologic testing, or diagnostic studies may be utilized to rule out the causes of similar-appearing lesions (herpes simplex virus, HIV, Behçet syndrome, Crohn disease, ulcerative colitis).
- Oral leukoplakia:
  - Diagnosis is suspected based on history and clinical findings and confirmed by histopathology after biopsy.
  - Serologic testing and diagnostic studies may be utilized to rule out the causes of similar-appearing lesions or candidiasis.
- Oral candidiasis:
  - The diagnosis is usually made based on clinical findings without biopsy or culture.
  - Wet prep with potassium hydroxide can confirm clinical findings.
  - Suspicion is confirmed by scraping the plaque with a tongue depressor; the white lesions are not difficult to remove and reveal erythematous, painful, and friable mucosa.

- Deep neck infection:
  - Complete blood count with differential is indicated, and blood cultures should be obtained before the administration of intravenous (IV) antibiotics.
  - Computed tomography (CT) scan of the neck with contrast is the imaging study of choice.
  - Anteroposterior (AP) and lateral films can confirm the diagnosis of mediastinitis.

▶ **TREATMENT**

- Aphthous ulcers: treatment consists of avoidance of trauma to the oral mucosa, topical numbing agents, topical corticosteroids, topical antiseptics, and topical antimicrobials.
- Provide education on expected course and likely recurrence.
- Oral leukoplakia:
  - Surgical removal of lesions and close follow-up for recurrence or progression to SCC
  - If a lesion cannot be removed, it should be closely monitored by frequent clinical observation with photographic documentation.
  - Counsel patients on tobacco and alcohol cessation.
- Oral candidiasis:
  - Treatment consists of topical oral antifungal therapy for 7–14 days.
  - Common medications include clotrimazole troches and nystatin oral suspension (swish-and-spit or swish-and-swallow).
  - Systemic oral antifungal treatment may be used for resistant cases.
- Deep neck infection:
  - Admit patients for treatment with broad-spectrum IV antibiotics.
  - Assess the airway and secure if needed.
  - Consult with otolaryngology for surgical treatment.

CHAPTER
95

Salivary Disorders

Lauren Webb, DMSc, MSM, PA-C

A 45-year-old male presents with 2 days of "jaw swelling." On examination, you note the patient is febrile with moderate right parotid gland swelling, tenderness, and induration. What should you consider?

▶ **GENERAL FEATURES**

- Salivary gland disorders include viral, bacterial, inflammatory, and neoplastic conditions.
  - Sialadenitis is an inflammation of the salivary glands and can be secondary to viral, bacterial, autoimmune conditions, or salivary stones (sialolithiasis).

- The most common bacterial causative organism is *Staphylococcus aureus*.
- Common viral causes include mumps and HIV.
- Parotitis is one form of sialadenitis, defined as inflammation of the parotid gland, and can be unilateral or bilateral.
  - Mumps should always be considered in a patient with bilateral parotitis, but mumps can involve any of the salivary glands.

CLINICAL ASSESSMENT

- Sialadenitis presents in differently depending on the underlying causes; it is more common in individuals who have dry mouth due to age, poor fluid intake, medications, or underlying disease, such as Sjögren syndrome.
- Acute suppurative sialadenitis is due to a bacterial infection and presents with sudden onset of pain and swelling of the affected salivary gland; on examination, the gland is often swollen with overlying erythema, induration, and tenderness, and purulence may be visible from the duct.
- Chronic or recurrent sialadenitis is often due to obstruction, either from a stone or from stricture of the duct.
  - This typical patient presentation involves repeated episodes of pain and swelling, often acutely worsening with meals.
  - On examination, the gland often appears swollen and firm.
- Parotitis is sialadenitis localized to the parotid glands.
- Salivary gland neoplasms may be benign or malignant and typically present as a painless, firm, slow-growing mass.

DIAGNOSIS

- Based on clinical presentation
- Viral serologies may be used if a viral cause is suspected; cultures should be performed with any purulent drainage to direct antibiotic therapy.
- Computed tomography (CT) or ultrasound may be helpful with visualizing a calculus or dilated duct with sialolithiasis.
- CT or magnetic resonance imaging (MRI) is used if a neoplasm is suspected.

TREATMENT

- Treatment is based on the suspected underlying cause.
- Gland massage, sialagogues, and warm compresses can help return the normal flow of saliva and often relieve symptoms.
- Further supportive care is used for viral infections as needed, and the addition of antibiotics with suspected bacterial infections.
- If a stone is suspected, sialendoscopy or open surgery may be required for removal.
- A salivary gland neoplasm requires surgical removal of the gland.

Case Conclusion

The patient presents with an acute case of bacterial parotitis. The most likely cause is infection with *Staphylococcus aureus*, and antibiotic therapy should be directed appropriately.

Section A Pretest: Diabetes Mellitus and Metabolic Syndrome

1. Which laboratory values is most consistent with a diagnosis of DKA?
   A. Glucose <250 mg/dL, bicarbonate <15 mEq/L, and pH <7.3
   B. Glucose >250 mg/dL, bicarbonate >15 mEq/L, and pH <7.3
   C. Glucose >250 mg/dL, bicarbonate <15 mEq/L, and pH <7.3
   D. Glucose <250 mg/dL, bicarbonate >15 mEq/L, and pH >7.3

2. Which of the following traits is least likely to be seen in metabolic syndrome?
   A. Impaired glucose
   B. Elevated triglycerides
   C. Elevated waist circumference
   D. Low blood pressure

3. Which of the following is NOT a main goal when treating a patient with DKA?
   A. Correcting hypovolemia and electrolyte abnormalities
   B. Correcting ketonemia
   C. Correcting acidosis
   D. Treating the glucose level

4. In metabolic syndrome, what parts of the lipid screen are essential for classification?
   A. LDL
   B. Triglycerides
   C. HDL
   D. Both B and C

5. Which of the following statements is NOT true regarding cerebral edema as a complication of DKA treatment?
   A. It typically develops 12–24 hours after treatment.
   B. Deterioration in neurologic function is the main manifestation.
   C. Diagnosis is clinical without imaging required.
   D. It typically occurs in older adults.

6. Which intervention is most effective at treating metabolic syndrome?
   A. Physical activity
   B. Diet
   C. Pharmacotherapy
   D. Both A and B

7. Hypoglycemia and a hyperosmolar hyperglycemic state are distinguished from DKA by which of the following?
   A. Absence of significant ketosis
   B. Normal glucose levels
   C. Moderate ketonemia
   D. Serum bicarbonate <15 mEq/L

8. What A1c level is considered diagnostic for T2DM?
   A. ≥5.6%
   B. ≥6.0%
   C. ≥6.5%
   D. ≥7%
   E. ≥8%

9. What is the choice class of medication after metformin for a patient with TWD at risk for chronic kidney disease?
   A. SGLT2 inhibitors
   B. DPP-4 inhibitors
   C. Sulfonylureas
   D. Thiazolidinediones
   E. α-Glucosidase inhibitors

10. When should patients with T2DM be referred to ophthalmology?
    A. At initial diagnosis
    B. Within 6 months of diagnosis
    C. 1 year after diagnosis
    D. 5 years after diagnosis

11. Which BMI is classified as obesity (class 1)?
    A. 25-29.9 kg/m^2
    B. 30-32.9 kg/m^2
    C. 35-39.9 kg/m^2
    D. >40 kg/m^2

12. Which of the following is NOT considered a risk factor for screening for diabetes?
    A. First-degree relative with T2DM
    B. Pacific Islander ethnicity
    C. Polycystic ovarian syndrome
    D. Pregnant in last 6 months
    E. Hypertension

13. Which of the following is NOT a weight-related comorbidity?

    A. Hypertension
    B. COPD
    C. Sleep apnea
    D. Gastroesophageal reflux

14. When can the diagnosis of T2DM be made?

    A. A1C ≥6.5% and fasting glucose ≥126 mg/dL
    B. A1C ≥5.7% and fasting glucose ≥126 mg/dL
    C. A1C ≥7.0% and fasting glucose ≥101 mg/dL
    D. A1C ≥6.4% and fasting glucose ≥124 mg/dL

15. Which of the following is NOT a common cause of DKA?

    A. Insulin-pump catheter dislodgement or occlusion
    B. Infection
    C. Pregnancy
    D. Medications including ACE inhibitors and β-blockers

Section B Pretest: Hypogonadism

1. Primary hypogonadism is best characterized by which of the following?

    A. Abnormal function of one or both testes
    B. Abnormal function of the hypothalamus or pituitary gland
    C. Abnormal levels of prolactin hormone
    D. Abnormal level of thyroid hormone

2. A normal level of luteinizing hormone (LH) in conjunction with a low level of serum testosterone can indicate what condition?

    A. Primary hypogonadism
    B. Secondary hypogonadism
    C. Tertiary hypogonadism
    D. Low-T syndrome

3. What medication is used to treat hypogonadism?

    A. Cortisol derivative
    B. Thyroxine
    C. Testosterone
    D. Bioidentical hormones

4. Which of the following should be the main consideration(s) when selecting testosterone formulation?

    A. Avoidance of preparations requiring injections
    B. Patient body habitus
    C. Cost is most important
    D. There are multiple factors

Section C Pretest: Pituitary Disorders

1. Which of the following hormones causes an increase in cortisol hormone production?

    A. PRL
    B. ACTH
    C. GH
    D. TSH

2. Which sign or symptom of acromegaly is more commonly seen in women versus men?

    A. Enlarged hand and feet size
    B. Elevated glucose levels
    C. Protrusion of the jawline (prognathism)
    D. Galactorrhea

3. Which of following symptoms are present in 50% of patients with endocrine-active pituitary adenomas?

   A. Recurrent infections
   B. Hirsutism
   C. Weight gain
   D. Fatigue

4. Which hormone is the most reliable biochemical indicator of gigantism and can be used to monitor treatment?

   A. Glucose
   B. IGF-1
   C. Calcium
   D. GH

5. Other than blood and urine testing, as well as imaging, what other diagnostic test should be performed if the patient with an endocrine-active pituitary adenoma also complains of associated headaches?

   A. Visual testing for impairment or loss of central or peripheral vision
   B. Ultrasound of the carotids for potential thrombus
   C. PET scanning for potential metastasis
   D. Dexamethasone suppression test

6. Which of following is a risk factor for the development of gigantism?

   A. Delayed-onset puberty
   B. Female gender
   C. Family history of pituitary adenomas
   D. Premature gestation

7. A 41-year-old female is evaluated for polyuria 1 day after transsphenoidal pituitary surgery for a craniopharyngioma. The patient reports increased thirst over the past 12 hours, and urine output is currently 300 mL/hr. She takes no medications. On physical examination, vital signs are normal, except for dry mucous membranes. Lab results show a sodium level of 147 mEq/L (147 mmol/L). Which of the following is the most appropriate diagnostic test to perform next?

   A. Desmopressin challenge
   B. Urine and serum osmolality
   C. Urine electrolytes
   D. Water deprivation test

8. Which of the following should be considered when using radiation therapy for pituitary adenoma management?

   A. The adenoma is growing slowly.
   B. The tumor shrinks with medication.
   C. The surgery has minimal risk.
   D. The adenoma is not completely surgically removed.

9. What hormone plays an important role in diabetes insipidus?

   A. TSH
   B. PRL
   C. ACTH
   D. ADH

10. Headaches and visual changes are the most common signs and symptoms caused by which of the following?

    A. The mass effect of the pituitary tumor
    B. The secondary development of diabetes mellitus from the elevated IGF-1 secretion
    C. The bony remodeling of the head, resulting in prominent supraorbital ridges
    D. Uncontrolled hypertension that developed from the excess GH secretion

11. Which type of medication is used to lower the hormone levels of both GH and IGF-1?

    A. GH antagonist drugs
    B. Oral hypoglycemic drugs
    C. Somatostatin
    D. Dopamine agonists

Section D Pretest: Polyendocrine and Neoplastic Disorders

1. What is the curative treatment of choice for most pituitary adenomas?

   A. Thyroidectomy
   B. Transsphenoidal surgery
   C. β-Blockers or calcium channel blockers
   D. Hormonal therapy

2. A 32-year-old female presents to the clinic with palpitations, diaphoresis, and headache. In addition to TSH, what other testing would you recommend for evaluation of her symptoms?

   A. Hgb A1C
   B. Serum Prolactin
   C. 24-hour urine collection for fractionated metanephrines and catecholamines
   D. Psychiatric evaluation

3. MEN syndromes are caused by what type of inheritance pattern?

   A. Autosomal dominant
   B. Autosomal recessive
   C. X-linked dominant
   D. X-linked recessive

4. A 20-year-old male recently diagnosed with MEN2A reports a history of renal calculus. You review his labs and see that his serum calcium is elevated. What is the most likely reason for this?

   A. Hyperparathyroidism
   B. Adrenal insufficiency
   C. Increased dietary intake of calcium
   D. Pituitary adenoma

5. What findings best describe the presence of SIADH?

   A. Isovolemic hypotonic hypernatremia
   B. Isovolemic hypotonic hyponatremia
   C. Isovolemic hypertonic hypernatremia
   D. Isovolemic hypertonic hyponatremia

6. Which medication is commonly associated with the development of SIADH?

   A. Amitriptyline
   B. Furosemide
   C. Sertraline
   D. Spironolactone

7. Large nonfunctional pituitary adenomas typically cause what symptom?

   A. Central vision loss
   B. Balance disturbance
   C. Sensorineural hearing loss
   D. Bilateral loss of peripheral vision (hemianopsia)

8. What is the initial treatment of choice if inadequate water restriction?

   A. Demeclocycline
   B. Furosemide
   C. Tolvaptan
   D. Urea

9. Rapid correction of serum sodium can result in which complication?

   A. Liver disease
   B. Orthostatic hypotension
   C. Osmotic demyelination
   D. Prerenal disease

Section E Pretest: Primary Adrenal Insufficiency

1. What is the most common cause of primary adrenal insufficiency?

   A. Infections
   B. Autoimmune conditions
   C. Inherited disorders
   D. Medications

2. What is a feature consistent with Cushing syndrome?

   A. Hypercortisolism
   B. Hypocortisolism
   C. Hypoaldosteronism
   D. Hypoglycemia

3. What finding is consistent with primary adrenal insufficiency?

   A. Weight gain
   B. Weight loss
   C. Hypertension
   D. Glucose intolerance

4. What is the most common cause of Cushing syndrome?

   A. Adrenal tumor
   B. Pituitary tumor
   C. Ectopic secretion
   D. Idiopathic

5. Which laboratory result is most consistent with primary adrenal insufficiency diagnosis?

   A. Hyperkalemia
   B. Hypokalemia
   C. Hypernatremia
   D. Hyperglycemia

Section F Pretest: Thyroid Disorders

1. A 19-year-old female student presents to the university student health center complaining of anxiousness. She denies acute stressors and is overall experiences pleasure with outdoor activities and spending times with her friends and family. In the review of systems, she endorses excessive sweating, unintentional weight loss, palpitations, and heat intolerance. Physical examination reveals resting tachycardia, lid lag, and exophthalmos. Her thyroid is nontender, smooth, but mildly enlarged. What is the first-line treatment to address the most likely cause of her symptoms?

   A. Methimazole
   B. Levothyroxine
   C. Radioactive iodine ablation treatment
   D. Propranolol

2. Which is the first-line treatment for a patient with subacute thyroiditis?

   A. Methimazole
   B. Levothyroxine
   C. Radioactive iodine ablation treatment
   D. Propranolol

3. A patient has undergone a thyroidectomy to treat her refractory hyperthyroidism. In addition to being on levothyroxine and synthetic parathyroid hormone, what supplement is required?

   A. Iron
   B. Vitamin B12
   C. Vitamin B6
   D. Calcium

4. What will clinicians most likely see on the thyroid scan of a patient with Graves disease?

   A. Diffusely increased uptake
   B. Uniformly decreased uptake
   C. Patchy uptake with areas of concentrated uptake
   D. Even uptake with concentrated area of no uptake

5. A 36-year-old male with severe persistent asthma atopic dermatitis comes in for a yearly follow-up. He says he was recently at the pulmonologist who prescribed him albuterol, budesonide, and prednisone. All routine lab work resulted within normal limits, except that his TSH was high at 8 mIU/L (range 0.28-5.00). Which of the following medications do you suspect could be contributing to his high TSH?

   A. Albuterol
   B. Budesonide
   C. Prednisone
   D. Triamcinolone ointment

6. Which type of thyroid cancer is associated with the lowest survival rate?

   A. Papillary
   B. Follicular
   C. Medullary
   D. Anaplastic

7. You are counseling a 22-year-old female patient about her new diagnosis of hypothyroidism. You explain that she will be tested after starting hormone replacement therapy but could also have some future fluctuations in her TSH level during what circumstances?

   A. Dehydration
   B. Pregnancy
   C. Eating foods with high fat content
   D. Exercise

8. Which of the following labs should be ordered to evaluate a thyroid nodule?

   A. Thyroglobulin
   B. Total T4
   C. Free T4
   D. TSH

9. A 42-year-old woman presents complaining of recent weight gain, heavy periods, fatigue, and constipation. The patient has a hoarse voice, brittle hair, and a slow heart rate. Lab tests show an elevated TSH and a low serum free T_4. She is not pregnant. What is the most appropriate initial treatment?

   A. Propylthiouracil
   B. Levothyroxine
   C. Surgical resection
   D. Radio-iodide ablation

10. A 43-year-old female presents to the office for a TSH level check. You find her TSH level is out of range and prescribe an increased dose of levothyroxine. When should the patient's TSH level be rechecked?

    A. 6 weeks
    B. 12 weeks
    C. 6 months
    D. 12 months

11. Thyroid nodules are most commonly present in which of the following patients?
    A. 45-year-old male smoker
    B. 12-year-old female with type 1 diabetes
    C. 56-year-old female with family history of goiter
    D. 22-year-old male with hyperthyroidism

▶ ANSWERS AND EXPLANATIONS TO SECTION A PRETEST

1. **C.** Laboratory values of glucose >250 mg/dL, bicarbonate <15 mEq/L, and pH <7.3 confirm a diagnosis of DKA.
2. **D.** Low blood pressure is not a likely trait of metabolic syndrome. The presence of at least 3 out of 5 metabolic risk factors supports diagnosis of metabolic syndrome (eg., large waistline, high triglycerides, low HDL cholesterol, high fasting blood sugar, and high blood pressure).
3. **D.** Treating the glucose level is not a main goal when treating a patient with DKA.
4. **D.** Classification of metabolic syndrome looks at serum triglycerides ≥150 mg/dL (1.7 mmol/L) and serum HDL cholesterol <40 mg/dL (1 mmol/L) in men and <50 mg/dL (1.3 mmol/L) in women.
5. **C.** Cerebral edema is a serious, major complication that may occur during treatment of DKA, primarily affecting children. Deterioration of the level of consciousness despite improved metabolic state is indicative. MRI is typically used to confirm the diagnosis. In most cases, symptoms are apparent between 3 to 12 hours after initiation of treatment of DKA, and rarely occur later than 24 hours.
6. **D.** Although pharmacotherapy can be utilized to help with metabolic syndrome, the most effective treatment is diet and increased physical activity.
7. **A.** Absence of significant ketosis distinguishes hypoglycemia and a hyperosmolar hyperglycemic state from DKA.
8. **C.** An A1c level ≥6.5% is considered diagnostic for T2DM.
9. **A.** SGLT2 inhibitors are the choice class of medication after metformin for a patient at risk for chronic kidney disease.
10. **A.** Patients with T2DM should be referred to ophthalmology at initial diagnosis.
11. **B.** A value of 25–29.9 kg/m^2 is considered overweight, 30–32.9 kg/m^2 is obesity class 1, 35–39.9 kg/m^2 is obesity class 2, and >40 kg/m^2 is obesity class 3.
12. **D.** Being pregnant in the last 6 months is not considered a risk factor for screening for diabetes.
13. **B.** Weight-related comorbidities include hypertension, T2DM, elevated fasting blood glucose, dyslipidemia, sleep apnea, degenerative joint disease of weight-bearing joints, gastroesophageal reflux, nonalcoholic fatty liver disease, and polycystic ovary syndrome.
14. **A.** The diagnosis of T2DM can be made when A1C is ≥6.5% and fasting glucose ≥126 mg/dL.
15. **D.** Medications including ACE inhibitors and β-blockers are not a common cause of DKA.

▶ ANSWERS AND EXPLANATIONS TO SECTION B PRETEST

1. **A.** Primary hypogonadism is best characterized by abnormal function of one or both testes.
2. **B.** Normal LH in conjunction with a low level of serum testosterone can indicate secondary hypogonadism.
3. **C.** Testosterone is used to treat hypogonadism.
4. **D.** When selecting a testosterone formulation, consider multiple factors.

▶ ANSWERS AND EXPLANATIONS TO SECTION C PRETEST

1. **B.** ACTH causes an increase in cortisol hormone production.
2. **D.** Galactorrhea is more commonly seen in women with acromegaly.
3. **C.** Weight gain is present in 50% of patients with endocrine-active pituitary adenomas.
4. **B.** Elevated insulin-like growth factor 1 (IGF-1) is used to diagnose gigantism along with tracking growth (eg., growth chart shift from normal growth curve). IGF-1 is also the most reliable biochemical indicator of acromegaly, and it is also useful in monitoring the efficacy of treatment.
5. **A.** Visual testing for impairment or loss of central or peripheral vision should be performed if the patient with an endocrine-active pituitary adenoma also complains of associated headaches.
6. **C.** Family history of pituitary adenomas is a risk factor for the development of gigantism.
7. **B.** Urine and serum osmolality are the most appropriate diagnostic tests to perform next.
8. **D.** When using radiation therapy for pituitary adenoma management, consider that the adenoma is not completely surgically removed.
9. **D.** ADH plays an important role in diabetes insipidus.
10. **A.** Headaches and visual changes are the most common signs and symptoms caused by the mass effect of the pituitary tumor.
11. **D.** Dopamine agonists are used to lower the hormone levels of both GH and IGF-1 in acromegaly.

ANSWERS AND EXPLANATIONS TO SECTION D PRETEST

1. **B.** Transsphenoidal surgery is the treatment of choice for pituitary adenomas.
2. **C.** Pheochromocytomas can be imaged with CT or MRI and/or diagnosed with 24-hour urine, fractionated metanephrines, and catecholamines, or plasma-fractionated metanephrines.
3. **A.** Syndromes of MEN are inherited autosomal dominant traits that cause predisposition to the development of tumors of two or more different endocrine glands.
4. **A.** Primary hyperparathyroidism is present in 10%–25% of MEN2A patients.
5. **B.** The hallmark of SIADH is isovolemic hypotonic hyponatremia. An increase in ADH increases water retention and impairs water excretion, leading to hyponatremia, causing inadequate urinary dilution by the kidneys and concentrated urine.
6. **C.** Medications are the most common cause of SIADH, most commonly including SSRIs and thiazide diuretics. Loop diuretics are used for treatment, and potassium-sparing diuretics and TCAs are not associated with SIADH.
7. **D.** Nonfunctional pituitary adenomas cause symptoms due to mass effect such as headache, bitemporal hemianopsia, and hypopituitarism.
8. **A.** Demeclocycline inhibits ADH action. Tolvaptan is well tolerated but cost prohibitive and associated with liver toxicity. Loop diuretics decrease volume expansion, preventing concentrated urine and limiting hyponatremia, but can be used as adjunct therapy. Oral urea increases water excretion but is limited by unpalatable taste.
9. **C.** Overly aggressive treatment and too-rapid of correction in serum sodium can result in neuronal damage and osmotic demyelination. Liver disease, prerenal disease, and orthostatic hypotension can be adverse effects of some of the treatment regimens for SIADH, but not a complication from rapid correction.

ANSWERS AND EXPLANATIONS TO SECTION E PRETEST

1. **B.** The most common cause of primary adrenal insufficiency is autoimmune.
2. **A.** Hypercortisolism is consistent with Cushing syndrome.
3. **B.** Weight loss is the finding most consistent with primary adrenal insufficiency.
4. **D.** Cushing syndrome is most commonly idiopathic.
5. **A.** Hyperkalemia is the lab result most consistent with primary adrenal insufficiency diagnosis.

ANSWERS AND EXPLANATIONS TO SECTION F PRETEST

1. **A.** Methimazole or propylthiouracil are anti–thyroid-modulating drugs used to reduce hormone production.
2. **D.** The first-line treatment is propranolol. NSAIDs also may be used. Methimazole and radioactive iodine ablation are used to treat Grave disease. Levothyroxine is used to treat hypothyroidism.
3. **D.** In addition to being on levothyroxine and synthetic parathyroid hormone, this patient requires calcium supplementation.
4. **A.** Graves disease is characterized by diffusely increased uptake on thyroid scan. Uniformly decreased uptake is seen in subacute thyroiditis, and patchy uptake with areas of concentrated uptake is seen in toxic multimodal goiter. Even uptake with concentrated areas of no uptake requires further workup.
5. **C.** High-dose glucocorticoids suppress serum TSH in hypothyroid patients and euthyroid patients.
6. **D.** Anaplastic thyroid cancer is the least common but most deadly form of thyroid cancer. It accounts for about 2% of all thyroid cancers but up to 50% of thyroid cancer deaths in the United States.
7. **B.** TSH levels can fluctuate with pregnancy because Human Chorionic Gonadotropin (HCG) stimulates the production of T4 and T3. In counseling a patient who was hypothyroid before pregnancy, one would describe how HCG can increase the T4 and T3, resulting in lower than usual TSH levels during the pregnancy. Adjusted TSH ranges for use during pregnancy are available to help guide clinicians.
8. **D.** TSH should be ordered to evaluate a thyroid nodule.
9. **B.** Levothyroxine is the first-line treatment for patients whose signs and symptoms are consistent with primary hypothyroidism, defined as an elevated TSH and a low serum free T4. Propylthiouracil, surgical resection or thyroidectomy, and radio-iodide ablation are treatments for hyperthyroidism.
10. **A.** Any change in levothyroxine dose requires a recheck in 6 weeks.
11. **C.** A thyroid nodule would be most likely in the 56-year-old female with family history of goiter.

CHAPTER 96

Diabetic Ketoacidosis

Timothy Hirsch, MS, PA-C

▶ GENERAL FEATURES

- Diabetic ketoacidosis (DKA) is a metabolic emergency, primarily occurring in individuals with uncontrolled type 1 diabetes mellitus, that is associated with hyperglycemia, metabolic acidosis, and ketonemia.
- DKA may occur in patients with other forms of diabetes.
- DKA results from insulin deficiency (absolute or relative) and elevated levels of counterregulatory hormones.
- Hyperglycemia, in the absence of insulin, causes cellular starvation, ketogenesis, and metabolic gap acidosis.
- Important causes of DKA:
  - Gastrointestinal (GI) hemorrhage
  - Heat illness
  - Hyperthyroidism
  - Infection
  - Insulin pump catheter dislodgement or occlusion
  - Medications including thiazides, corticosteroids, sympathomimetics, and antipsychotics
  - Myocardial infarction
  - Pancreatitis
  - Pregnancy
  - Pulmonary embolism
  - Reduced use or omission of daily insulin
  - Stroke
  - Substance abuse
  - Trauma or surgery
  - Complications include cerebral edema, hypokalemia or hyperkalemia, hypoglycemia, shock, and death.
  - Mortality is generally low overall (<1%), but higher rates occur in frail, elderly, or patients with significant comorbidities.

▶ CLINICAL ASSESSMENT

- Commonly presents with recent onset of polydipsia, polyuria, nocturia, fatigue, unintended weight loss, nausea, vomiting, abdominal pain, and abdominal tenderness.
- Patients may have altered mental status and decreased level of consciousness.
- Fruity breath odor and Kussmaul respirations are characteristic and occur from acetone excretion via the lungs.
- Osmotic diuresis causes dehydration with subsequent tachycardia, orthostatic hypotension, and poor skin turgor.
- Patients may be normothermic despite infection.

▶ DIAGNOSIS

- Initial rapid assessment of the patient using the CAB framework allows clinicians to identify any immediate and life-threatening concerns, which is essential when treating DKA patients.
- Initial testing of patients suspected to have DKA includes:
  - Laboratory testing:
    - Arterial blood gas analysis including serum pH and bicarbonate looking for acidosis
    - Glucose
    - Electrolytes (sodium, potassium, magnesium, and phosphorus)
    - Anion gap
    - Urine and serum ketones
    - BUN and creatinine
    - Complete blood count
    - Urinalysis: evaluate for ketones, glucose, and screening for urinary tract infection (UTI)
    - Pregnancy testing
- ECG to assess for abnormalities linked to electrolyte abnormalities like hypokalemia or hyperkalemia
- Chest radiograph: looking for fluid overload or infection

- Cultures: consider urine, blood, and throat cultures as indicated
- Diagnosis is based on clinical presentation and laboratory values:
  - Serum glucose of >250 mg/dL
  - Serum bicarbonate <15 mEq/L
  - pH <7.30
  - Moderate ketonemia (β-hydroxybutyrate)
  - Anion gap >12
- Ketonemia causing a high anion gap metabolic acidosis is characteristic.
- Sodium, chloride, calcium, phosphorus, and magnesium levels may be low due to diuresis.
- Pseudohyponatremia is common:
  - For each 100 mg/dL increase in glucose level, there is a 1.6 mEq/L decrease in sodium.
- Serum potassium may be low, normal, or high.
- Despite normal or low potassium level, significant depletion of total body potassium.
- Differential diagnosis includes all other causes of an anion gap metabolic acidosis.
  - Ingestions (methanol, ethylene glycol, salicylates)
  - Alcoholic or starvation ketoacidosis
  - Renal failure
  - Lactic acidosis
- Consider hypoglycemia and a hyperosmolar hyperglycemia state; these are distinguished from DKA by the absence of significant ketosis.

▶ TREATMENT

- Goals:
  - Treat metabolic acidosis.
  - Close the anion gap.
  - Monitor glucose and electrolytes.
  - Patients generally require hospital admission.
- First priority is replacing fluids:
  - 1–2 L bolus of 0.9% NS in first hour followed by 500 mL/hr

- Goal 3–4 L of fluid over initial 4 hours
- Avoid fluid overload in patients with cardiac disease.
- Monitor:
  - Cardiac monitor and pulse oximetry if patient is unstable
  - Venous blood gas, pH, anion gap, potassium, and bicarbonate hourly until recovery
- Correct hypovolemia, ketonemia, acidosis, and electrolyte abnormalities.
- Initial potassium level determines further therapy:
  - Potassium administration is essential, and insulin should be delayed until K^+ >3.5 mEq/L.
  - Typical total body K^+ deficit of 3–5 mEq/kg
  - Closely monitor potassium every 1–2 hours during the first 4–6 hours of treatment.
  - Adequate urine output is essential before starting potassium.
- Insulin:
  - Reverses ketogenic state
  - Regular insulin should be initiated as continuous intravenous (IV) infusion at 0.1 U/kg/h.
  - Adjust insulin infusion in response to anion gap and glucose changes.
  - Continue insulin drip until pH >7.3 and anion gap closes.
  - Serum glucose will normalize more rapidly than resolution of acidosis.
    - Keep glucose >250 mg/dL using glucose-containing fluids like D5 45% NS.
- Complications:
  - Cerebral edema is an important complication of treatment of DKA that mostly occurs in children.
    - Associated with rapid correction of glucose, sodium, and hypovolemia
    - Develops 4–12 hours into treatment
    - Deterioration in neurologic function is main manifestation.
    - Treatment with mannitol is needed.
    - Diagnosis is confirmed by computed tomography (CT).

CHAPTER
97

Type 2 Diabetes Mellitus

Joy Moverley, DHSc, MPH, PA-C
Sammy Cheuk
Joy Stevens, PA-C

▶ GENERAL FEATURES

- Type 2 diabetes mellitus (T2DM) is the most common type of diabetes worldwide.
- According to the Centers for Disease Control and Prevention (CDC), 34.2 million people in the United States have diabetes, more than 90% of which is T2DM.

- T2DM leads to hyperglycemia as a result of a progressive loss of β-cell insulin secretion with insulin resistance.
- Although many people are asymptomatic at the time of diagnosis, hyperglycemia symptoms of T2DM include polydipsia, polyphagia, and polyuria.
- Risk factors:

- First-degree relative with diabetes
- High-risk race/ethnicity (eg, African American, Latino, Native American, Asian American, Pacific Islander)
- History of cardiovascular disease (CVD)
- Hypertension
- Low high-density lipoprotein (HDL) level (<35 mg/dL) and/or elevated triglyceride level (>250 mg/dL)
- Polycystic ovary syndrome (PCOS)
- Physical inactivity
- Insulin resistance signs (eg, severe obesity, acanthosis nigricans)
- T2DM can lead to complications such as CVD, vision loss, and kidney disease.

▶ CLINICAL ASSESSMENT

- Multiple guidelines exist for screening and managing T2DM.
- American Diabetes Association Screening Recommendation:
  - Without any previous risk factors, begin screening at age 45 years.
  - Screen for prediabetes and/or T2DM in all patients aged ≥10 years who are overweight or obese (body mass index [BMI] ≥25 or ≥23 kg/m² in Asian Americans) and one or more additional risk factors (see earlier).
  - For women with a history of gestational diabetes, repeat testing every 3 years, regardless of age.
  - U.S. Preventive Services Task Force recommends screening for abnormal blood glucose in adults aged 40–70 years who are overweight or obese.
- Targets for clinical assessment and treatment include:
  - Managing glycemia control
  - Supporting weight loss (if obese or overweight) and increased activity
  - Preventing microvascular (eg, retinopathy, nephropathy, neuropathy) and macrovascular (eg, CVD, cerebrovascular, and peripheral artery disease) complications

▶ DIAGNOSIS

- Criteria for T2DM:
  - A1C ≥6.5%
  - Fasting plasma glucose ≥126 mg/dL
  - Random plasma glucose ≥200 mg/dL in a patient with classic hyperglycemic symptoms or crisis
  - Oral glucose tolerance test ≥200 mg/dL
- Differential diagnosis:
  - Type 1 diabetes (autoimmune β-cell destruction causing insulinopenia)
  - Gestational diabetes (diabetes diagnosed in the second or third trimester of pregnancy)
  - Monogenic diabetes
  - Latent autoimmune diabetes of adulthood
  - Cushing syndrome
- Upon diagnosis of T2DM:
  - Develop a patient-centered plan for continuity of care to address psychosocial, self-management, and routine health maintenance needs.
  - Glycemic targets:
    - Perform the A1C test at least 2 times a year if patient is meeting treatment goals.
    - Quarterly A1C test with therapy changes or if not meeting glycemic goals
    - Supplemental self-monitoring of blood glucose (SMBG) and continuous glucose monitoring (CGM) can be helpful in assessing treatment effectiveness.
  - Individualized A1C target based on age, comorbidities, hypoglycemia risk, and patient factors:
    - A1C goal of <7% (American Diabetes Association or ADA) or <6.5% (American Association of Clinical Endocrinologists or AACE) appropriate for most nonpregnant adults, adolescents, and children with T2DM if achieved without hypoglycemia
    - A less stringent A1C recommended (ADA <8%) for patients with history of severe hypoglycemia, limited life expectancy, advanced vascular complications, extensive comorbidities, or long-standing uncontrolled diabetes despite extensive treatment
  - Identify and treat atherosclerotic cardiovascular disease (ASCVD) risk factors through:
    - Blood pressure control
    - Lipid management
    - Antiplatelet treatment

▶ TREATMENT

- Individualized patient-centered care managed by multidisciplinary team to achieve glycemic control and reduce microvascular complications:
  - Behavioral changes:
    - Diabetes self-management education and support
    - Medical nutrition therapy
    - Smoking cessation
    - Routine physical activity of 150 minutes or more of moderate- to vigorous-intensity aerobic activity per week
    - Psychosocial care including assessment of diabetes distress and disordered eating using validated tools
  - Pharmacologic interventions:
    - In addition to diet and exercise therapies, consider antidiabetic medication to control blood sugar:
      - Target A1C of <7% in most patients

- Consider target A1C <8.0% in elderly patient's or those with other chronic medical conditions who may be at risk for hypoglycemia
- Fasting/preprandial glucose goal 80–130 mg/dL
- Metformin, a biguanide, is the initial medication of choice for hyperglycemia in T2DM:
  - Contraindicated in severe renal impairment (estimated glomerular filtration rate [eGFR] <30 mL/min) and acute or chronic metabolic acidosis, to minimize risk of lactic acidosis
  - Discontinue for iodinated contrast imaging procedures for 72 hours
- In patients with or at high risk for ASCVD, heart failure, or diabetic kidney disease, consider addition of either:
  - Glucagon-like peptide 2 (GLP-2) receptor agonist
  - Sodium-glucose cotransporter-2 (SGLT2) inhibitor
- Without these risks, consider metformin in combination with other drugs if needed to achieve glycemic control:
  - Sulfonylurea
  - Thiazolidinedione
  - Dipeptidyl peptidase IV (DPP-4) inhibitor
  - SGLT2 inhibitor
  - GLP-1 receptor agonist
- Patient-centered approach to guide choice in pharmacologic agents including cost, weight, hypoglycemia risk, and comorbidities (heart failure, ASCVD, or kidney disease)
- Older adults have increased risk of hypoglycemia.
- Insulin should be considered if evidence of catabolism (weight loss), hyperglycemia symptoms, elevated A1C (>10%):
  - Consider beginning 0.1–0.2 units per kg of basal insulin such as glargine or detemir in the evening with appropriate titration schedule every 3–7 days.
- T2DM patients with ASCVD or risk of kidney disease have benefitted from an SGLT2 or GLP-1.
- Weight loss:
  - Strive for weight loss of 5%–10% body weight, if indicated.
  - Consider bariatric surgery referral in patients with T2DM and a BMI ≥35 kg/m².
- Preventing and managing complications of diabetes:
  - Vaccinations according to the CDC including influenza, Tdap, pneumococcal, and hepatitis B
  - Hypoglycemia:
    - Glucose (15-20 g) is the preferred treatment for conscious individuals with blood glucose <70 mg/dL; repeat treatment if still hypoglycemic after 15 minutes.

- Glucagon to treat level 2 hypoglycemia, a blood glucose <54 mg/dL
- ASCVD:
  - Blood pressure:
    - Regularly measure blood pressure and target blood pressure at <130/80 mm Hg for high-risk patients; <140/90 mm Hg for lower risk patients.
    - Treat hypertension with lifestyle intervention consisting of weight loss, DASH style eating, alcohol intake moderation, and increased physical activity.
    - Pharmacologic treatment should include medication classes proven to decrease CVD risk in patients with diabetes: angiotensin-converting enzyme (ACE) inhibitors, angiotensin receptor blockers (ARBs), thiazides, and calcium channel blockers.
  - Lipids:
    - American Cardiology Association/American Heart Association Guidelines: consider a moderate statin therapy in all patients over aged 40 years with diabetes; calculate 10-year ASCVD risk and select a high-intensity statin if indicated.
    - Use lifestyle modification and statin therapy in patients with elevated triglyceride levels (≥150 mg/dL) and/or low HDL cholesterol (<40 mg/dL for men, <50 mg/dL for women).
  - Antiplatelet agents: use aspirin therapy (75-162 mg/day) as secondary prevention strategy in those with diabetes and history of ASCVD.
- Microvascular complications:
  - Chronic kidney disease (CKD):
    - Screen urinary albumin and eGFR annually.
    - Optimize glucose control and blood pressure control to reduce the risk or slow CKD progression.
    - For nonpregnant patients with diabetes and hypertension, ACE-inhibitor or ARB use is recommended.
  - Diabetic retinopathy:
    - Refer patients at the time of diabetes diagnosis.
      - Refer patients at the time of diabetes diagnosis.
      - Screen every 1–2 years if no evidence of retinopathy.
      - Repeat screening more often if signs of retinopathy.
    - Optimize glycemic control, blood pressure, and serum lipid control to slow or reduce risk of the progression of diabetic retinopathy.
  - Neuropathy:
    - Screen patients for peripheral neuropathy at diagnosis of T2DM.

- Optimize glucose control to prevent or delay the development of neuropathy.
  - Neuropathic pain can be treated with pregabalin and duloxetine per the U.S. Food and Drug Administration.
- Foot care:
  - Perform a comprehensive foot evaluation at least annually to identify risk factors for ulcers and amputations.
  - If risk factors are present, foot inspections should occur at every visit.
  - Examination should include skin inspection, deformity assessment, neurologic, and vascular assessment in feet and legs.
- Treat foot neuropathy and plantar pressure signs with well-fitting shoes that cushion the feet and redistribute pressure.

CHAPTER 98

Metabolic Syndrome and Obesity

Brittany Strelow, MS, PA-C

▶ GENERAL FEATURES

- The Centers for Disease Control and Prevention (CDC) defines body mass index (BMI) as (body weight [in kg] divided by height [in meters] squared):
  - <18.5 kg/m^2 underweight
  - 18.5-24.9 kg/m^2 normal weight
  - 25-29.9 kg/m^2 overweight
  - 30-32.9 kg/m^2 obesity (class 1)
  - 35-39.9 kg/m^2 obesity (class 2)
  - >40 kg/m^2 obesity (class 3)
- Metabolic syndrome is a group of concurrent metabolic risk factors:
  - Atherogenic dyslipidemia
  - Central obesity
  - Elevated blood pressure
  - Insulin resistance
- Complications:
  - Cardiovascular disease
  - Chronic kidney disease
  - Diabetes
- Associated with increased morbidity and mortality, including cardiovascular events and certain cancers
- Risk factors:
  - Mexican American ethnicity
  - Higher incidence in women than men for:
    - African Americans
    - Mexican Americans
  - Increased body weight
  - Large waist circumference
  - Increased soft-drink and sugar-sweetened beverage consumption
  - Medications:
    - Antipsychotic medications
    - Corticosteroids
    - Antidepressants
  - Poor cardiorespiratory fitness status

▶ CLINICAL ASSESSMENT

- Identification of patients at high metabolic risk:
  - Blood pressure
  - Waist circumference
  - Fasting lipid profile
  - Fasting glucose:
    - Re-check at 3-year intervals those with one or more risk factors
- Overnight oximetry
- Aspartate aminotransferase and alanine transaminase level
- Thyroid-stimulating hormone

▶ DIAGNOSIS

- Two widely accepted definitions of metabolic syndrome:
  - The National Cholesterol Education Program (NCEP) Adult Treatment Panel III (ATP III) criteria define metabolic syndrome as the presence of any three of the following five traits:
    - Abdominal obesity, defined as a waist circumference ≥102 cm (40 in) in men and ≥88 cm (35 in) in women
    - Serum triglycerides ≥150 mg/dL (1.7 mmol/L) or drug treatment for elevated triglycerides
    - Serum high-density lipoprotein (HDL) cholesterol <40 mg/dL (1 mmol/L) in men and <50 mg/dL (1.3 mmol/L) in women or drug treatment for low HDL cholesterol
    - Blood pressure $\geq130/85$ mm Hg or drug treatment for elevated blood pressure
    - Fasting plasma glucose (FPG) ≥100 mg/dL (5.6 mmol/L) or drug treatment for elevated blood glucose

- International Diabetes Federation defines metabolic syndrome as the presence of any three of the following five criteria:
  - Increased waist circumference, with ethnic-specific waist circumference cut-points
  - Triglycerides ≥150 mg/dL (1.7 mmol/L) or treatment for elevated triglycerides
  - HDL cholesterol <40 mg/dL (1.03 mmol/L) in men and <50 mg/dL (1.29 mmol/L) in women, or treatment for low HDL
  - Systolic blood pressure ≥130, diastolic blood pressure ≥85, or treatment for hypertension
  - FPG ≥100 mg/dL (5.6 mmol/L) or previously diagnosed type 2 diabetes

▶ TREATMENT

- Overall management of metabolic syndrome includes targeting the individual components of the syndrome with the goal of preventing cardiovascular-, kidney-, and diabetes-related complications.

- Aggressive lifestyle interventions:
  - Weight reduction:
    - Diet:
      - Mediterranean diet
      - Dietary Approaches to Stop Hypertension (DASH) diet
      - Foods with a low glycemic index
      - High-fiber diet
    - Physical activity: 30 minutes moderate-intensity daily
    - Pharmacologic therapy
- Weight-related comorbidities:
  - Hypertension
  - Type 2 diabetes mellitus
  - Elevated fasting blood glucose
  - Dyslipidemia
  - Sleep apnea
  - Degenerative joint disease of weight-bearing joints
  - Gastroesophageal reflux
  - Nonalcoholic fatty liver disease
  - Polycystic ovary syndrome

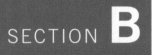

SECTION **B**

CHAPTER **99**

Hypogonadism

Hypogonadism

Ziemowit Mazur, EdM, MS, PA-C

▶ GENERAL FEATURES

- Hypogonadism results from disrupted activity of ≥1 hormone levels of the hypothalamic-pituitary-testicular axis, resulting in low serum testosterone and/or sperm levels.
  - If the testes are affected, this is termed *primary hypogonadism*; if the hypothalamus or pituitary is affected, this is termed *secondary hypogonadism*.
  - Each type of hypogonadism can be congenital or acquired.
- To distinguish between primary and secondary hypogonadism, measurement of luteinizing hormone (LH) and follicle-stimulating hormone (FSH) is necessary.

▶ CLINICAL ASSESSMENT

- Symptoms of hypogonadism in children can include appearance younger than chronological age and

additional signs of delayed puberty, including low muscle weight and lack of expected voice changes.
- In adults, the clinical findings are consistent with decreased mood and libido.
- Gynecomastia and infertility are most commonly found in secondary hypogonadism.

▶ DIAGNOSIS

- If history and physical examination are suspicious for hypogonadism, laboratory tests including total serum testosterone concentration and LH and FSH levels should be ordered.
  - Levels of FSH and LH are key to help differentiate primary and secondary causes of hypogonadism.
  - If infertility is a concern, then semen analysis should be performed.

- Primary hypogonadism is characterized by below-normal serum testosterone and/or the sperm count and serum level of LH and/or FSH above normal.
- Secondary hypogonadism is characterized by below-normal serum testosterone and/or the sperm count, but serum level of LH and/or FSH can be normal or low.
- Pituitary function testing for suspected secondary hypogonadism should include serum concentrations of cortisol, thyroxine, and prolactin.
  - If pituitary functions are abnormal or if there are any significant neurologic deficiencies noted on physical examination, brain magnetic resonance imaging (MRI) should be the imaging of choice.

▶ TREATMENT

- Adult males who are hypogonadal should be treated with testosterone, which is available in multiple preparations, including topical/transdermal and parenteral formulations.
- Choice of testosterone preparation should take into consideration factors including patient preference, convenience, and insurance coverage.

SECTION C   *Pituitary Disorders*

CHAPTER 100   Pituitary Adenomas

Kara L. Caruthers, MSPAS, PA-C

▶ GENERAL FEATURES

- The pituitary is an essential organ in the body's endocrine function and plays a critical role in the feedback axis between the hypothalamus and other endocrine organs.
- It is divided into an anterior and posterior lobe and produces and secretes several hormones: antidiuretic hormone (ADH), oxytocin, prolactin (PRL), growth hormone (GH), thyroid-stimulating hormone (TSH), follicular-stimulating hormone (FSH), luteinizing hormone (LH), and adrenocorticotropic hormone (ACTH).
- Pituitary adenomas are generally benign tumors that occur spontaneously; most develop in the anterior lobe, and ~1 in 10 people will develop an adenoma during their lifetime.
- Pituitary adenomas are classified as endocrine-active (functioning) or endocrine-inactive (nonfunctioning), with >50% of adenomas producing excess amounts of one or more hormones.
- Endocrine-active pituitary adenomas can cause excessive secretion of ACTH, resulting in elevated cortisol secretion, as well as excessive secretion of GH, TSH, and PRL.

▶ CLINICAL ASSESSMENT

- Patients with pituitary adenomas often present with symptoms of headache, visual changes, unintended weight gain, easy bruising and/or bleeding of the skin, changes in bone structure, menstrual irregularities, decreased sex drive, and lactation in the absence of pregnancy.
- Pituitary adenomas are typically <5 mm in size; however, 5%–10% of adenomas are large enough to cause a mass effect in which the patient will present with headaches and visual loss.
- 50% of patients will present with weight gain, but may also present with fatigue, hypertension, easy bruising, striae, poor wound healing, decreased sex drive, amenorrhea and hirsutism in women, and frequent infections.
- A detailed history and thorough physical examination is necessary because many symptoms of endocrine-active adenomas share the same presentation as other diseases and disorders.

DIAGNOSIS

- Diagnostic blood, urine, and imaging may be performed; as the pituitary produces multiple hormones, more than one hormone may be impacted by the development of an adenoma.
- Prolactin, GH, insulin-like growth factor 1 (IGF-1), free thyroxine, cortisol, and testosterone levels may be elevated and should be evaluated based on history and clinical presentation.
- If there are symptoms secondary to mass effect, visual testing should be performed to determine the specific visual deficit.

TREATMENT

- For optimal patient care and management, a multidisciplinary team of neurosurgery, otolaryngology, endocrinology, and radiation oncology should be considered.

- Some pituitary adenomas do not require treatment; treatment depends on adenoma size, specific pituitary area, the presence of mass effect, and the specific elevated hormone(s) secreted.
- Surgery is often done from a nasal approach, which can be performed through minimally invasive techniques.
- Radiation therapy may be considered if the surgery is deemed too risky or if the adenoma is growing rapidly, does not shrink with medication, or cannot be completely removed surgically.
- Medication is used to suppress excessive production of specific hormones, shrink the adenoma, or replace specific pituitary hormones after tumor resection, radiation treatment, or if the body is no longer able to produce a specific hormone.

CHAPTER

101

Central Diabetes Insipidus

George Thompson, DMS, MMS

GENERAL FEATURES

- Central diabetes insipidus (CDI) is a relatively uncommon disease caused by a deficiency in arginine vasopressin (AVP), also called *antidiuretic hormone* (ADH), that causes free water loss from the kidneys.
- Multiple causes:
  - Idiopathic
  - Pituitary injury (eg, surgery, trauma, autoimmune disease)
  - Genetic
- Primary CDI (without an identifiable lesion noted on the magnetic resonance imaging [MRI] of the pituitary and hypothalamus) accounts for about one-third of all cases.
- Secondary CDI is due to damage to the hypothalamus or pituitary.
- Absent ADH, complete diabetes insipidus, and reduced ADH, partial diabetes insipidus, prevent the reabsorption of water in the kidneys, resulting in polyuria and polydipsia.
- Reversible CDI can occur during chemotherapy with temozolomide and in myelodysplastic preleukemic phase of acute myelogenous leukemia.

CLINICAL ASSESSMENT

- Signs and symptoms:
  - Polyuria

- Nocturia
- Polydipsia (consecutive)
- Intense thirst
- Hypernatremia (rare)
- Urine is typically normal, except for large volumes and low specific gravity.
- The serum sodium concentration in untreated CDI is often in the high-normal range.
- High-dose corticosteroids increase renal free water clearance and may aggravate diabetes insipidus.
- A number of familial and congenital diseases have been associated with CDI, including familial CDI, Wolfram syndrome, and congenital diseases, such as congenital hypopituitarism and septo-optic dysplasia.

DIAGNOSIS

- Suspect CDI in a patient producing a large volume of dilute (hypotonic) urine.
  - Obtain a 24-hour urine sample: urine volume <2 L/24 hours (in the absence of hypernatremia) rules out diabetes insipidus.
- Inappropriately low urine osmolality in the setting of an elevated serum osmolality and hypernatremia in a patient with polyuria (>50 mL/kg/24 hours in the absence of glucosuria) is diagnostic.

- With CDI and primary polydipsia, the plasma AVP level is usually low (<1 pg/mL), whereas the urine osmolarity is also low (<300 mOsm/L).
- In nephrogenic diabetes insipidus, the plasma AVP level is normal or elevated (>2.5 pg/mL), whereas the urine osmolarity is low (<300 mOsm/L).
- Patients with CDI will respond to a "vasopressin challenge test" with a reduction of thirst and polyuria; serum sodium usually remains normal.
- A hypertonic 3% saline-stimulated measurement of copeptin test may help distinguish CDI from primary polydipsia; a copeptin level of <4.9 pmol/L helps confirm the diagnosis.

▶ TREATMENT

- Treatment of choice is desmopressin (DDAVP), a synthetic analog of AVP, administered intranasally, orally, or subcutaneously; caution should be taken to avoid over replacement as this can result in hyponatremia, water intoxication, and volume overload.
- Mild cases of diabetes insipidus require no further treatment than adequate fluid intake.
- Polyuria can be improved with the reduction of aggravating factors (eg, corticosteroids).
- Start with low doses at bedtime: in adults, 5 µg DDAVP intranasally and titrate up by 5 or 50 µg DDAVP orally and titrate up by 50 µg; adjust to control polyuria and polydipsia.
- Typical maintenance oral doses are 100–800 µg/day in divided doses in adults or children aged ≥4 years; typical maintenance intranasal doses are 5–20 µg once or twice daily in adults and 5–30 µg/day in children aged ≥4 years.
- Monitor serum sodium levels frequently in the first 48 hours to adjust dose in all patients.
- MRI of the pituitary and hypothalamus is useful in distinguishing primary CDI from primary polydipsia.
- Once a stable dose of DDAVP is achieved, annual or biannual monitoring of the serum sodium may be performed.

CHAPTER 102

Acromegaly and Gigantism

Kara L. Caruthers, MSPAS, PA-C

▶ GENERAL FEATURES

- Growth hormone (GH)–secreting adenomas are one of the most common types of functioning pituitary adenoma; this specific adenoma occurs in both children and adults, causing gigantism and acromegaly, respectively.
- The primary risk factor for acromegaly is a history of a pituitary tumor; ~50% of patients with gigantism have an underlying inherited genetic disorder.
- Clinical manifestations of excess GH secretion are often subtle, taking years before a patient will present with complaints.
- In cases of gigantism, there are a few soft-tissue symptoms, but often a long delay in diagnosis in male children, resulting in lower disease control, although they are more likely affected.
- Although clinical manifestations (taller height in children/adolescence, glove/shoe size changes, and prominent facial features in adults) are more noticeable, increased secretion of insulin-like growth factor 1 (IGF-1) must also be monitored.
- IGF-1 increases protein synthesis in chondrocytes (linear growth in puberty), muscle (increase in lean body mass), and in most organs (increasing organ size).

▶ CLINICAL ASSESSMENT

- A common sign of acromegaly is an increase in the size of the hands and/or feet.
  - Patients may have difficulty wearing rings or a pair of shoes that they previously worn.
  - Patients may also present after noticing a drastic change in appearance from old photos.
- Headaches and visual changes are the most common symptoms due to mass effect.
- Facial structural changes (prognathism, macroglossia, prominent supraorbital ridges), hyperhidrosis, glucose intolerance or diabetes mellitus development, and the presence of cardiovascular disease develop as a result of GH concentration and increase in IGF-1.
- Women with acromegaly may also present with galactorrhea and menstrual disorders in the absence of pregnancy and/or breastfeeding.

▶ DIAGNOSIS

- Measurement of serum GH 1 hour after oral administration of 75–100 g of glucose, with levels elevated >10 mg/mL, is considered the gold standard.

- IGF-1 is considered the most reliable biochemical indicator for acromegaly and is useful for both diagnosis and treatment monitoring.
- Magnetic resonance imaging (MRI) of the head should be obtained *after* a laboratory data demonstrates the diagnosis of acromegaly; however, if no pituitary tumor is uncovered, consider computed tomography (CT) to look for GH-secreting tumors in other parts of the body.

▶ TREATMENT

- The overall goal is to decrease GH levels and remove as much of the GH-secreting tumor as possible; thus, for optimal management, a multidisciplinary team approach should be implemented, with inclusion of neurosurgery and endocrinology.

- Surgical removal of the pituitary tumor may be sufficient to resolve the excess GH secretion and the symptoms from the mass effect of the tumor.
- If all the tumor cannot be removed or GH levels remain elevated, additional surgery, medication, and/or radiation treatments may be necessary for disease management.
- The common medications used to manage acromegaly include drugs that reduce GH production (somatostatin analogs), lower hormone levels of GH, and IGF-1 (dopamine agonists) and block the action of GH (GH antagonist).
- Management of glucose tolerance, cardiovascular disease, and other systemic alterations must occur until GH and/or IGF-1 return to nonpathologic levels.

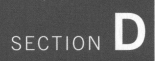

SECTION D *Polyendocrine and Neoplastic Disorders*

CHAPTER 103 Primary Endocrine Malignancies

Jenny Fanuele, MMSc, PA-C
Joshua Merson, MS-HPEd, PA-C

▶ GENERAL FEATURES

- Primary adrenal malignancies include adrenocortical adenomas, adrenocortical carcinomas (ACC), and pheochromocytomas.
- Primary thyroid malignancies include papillary carcinoma, follicular carcinoma, and medullary carcinoma.
- Primary pituitary malignancies include pituitary adenomas.
- Syndromes of multiple endocrine neoplasia (MEN) are inherited autosomal-dominant traits that cause predisposition to the development of tumors of two or more different endocrine glands.

▶ CLINICAL ASSESSMENT

- Adrenocortical adenomas are either functional (hormone secreting) or nonfunctional and can be benign or malignant.
  - Majority are benign, nonfunctional.

- Functional adrenocortical adenomas secrete steroids independently from the influence of adrenocorticotropic hormone (ACTH), causing Cushing syndrome.
- Nonfunctional adrenocortical adenomas can cause abdominal symptoms secondary to mass effect.
- ACC are rare, more aggressive tumors that may be functional or nonfunctional.
  - Functional adrenocortical adenomas secrete steroids independently from the influence of ACTH, causing Cushing syndrome.
  - Nonfunctional adrenocortical adenomas can cause abdominal symptoms secondary to mass effect.
- Pheochromocytomas are catecholamine-secreting tumors that can cause the classic triad of episodic headache, diaphoresis, and tachycardia, with or without paroxysmal hypertension; severe heart failure, cardiovascular collapse, and sudden death can occur due to paroxysms and cardiac arrhythmias.

- Thyroid papillary and follicular carcinomas usually initially present as a thyroid nodule.
- Pituitary adenomas can be functional or nonfunctional:
  - Functional pituitary adenomas present with pituitary hormone hypersecretion.
  - Nonfunctional pituitary adenomas cause symptoms due to mass effect such as headache, bitemporal hemianopsia, and hypopituitarism.
- MEN syndromes are categorized into types 1–4; the presentation of MEN syndromes is variable, and affected patients are prone to many different tumors, including parathyroid, endocrine pancreas and duodenum, pituitary, thyroid, and adrenal:
  - MEN1 presentation is variable; most commonly presents with tumors of the parathyroid glands, endocrine pancreas and duodenum, and anterior pituitary.
  - MEN2A is characterized by medullary thyroid cancer (MTC), bilateral pheochromocytomas, and primary parathyroid hyperplasia.
  - MEN2B/3 is characterized by mucosal and gastrointestinal ganglioneuromas, MTC, and pheochromocytomas, but not by hyperparathyroidism.
  - MEN4 is associated with pituitary adenomas, parathyroid adenomas, pancreatic neuroendocrine tumors (NET), adrenocortical adenomas, neuroendocrine cervical carcinoma, and testicular cancer.

▶ DIAGNOSIS

- Nonfunctional adrenocortical adenomas and ACCs are most often discovered as an abdominal mass on physical examination and/or with imaging with CT of the adrenal glands.
- Functional secreting adrenocortical adenomas and carcinomas secrete cortisol and cause signs and symptoms of Cushing syndrome; laboratory evaluation includes serum dehydroepiandrosterone sulfate (DHEAS) and dexamethasone suppression test (DST).
- Pheochromocytomas can be imaged with CT or MRI, also diagnosed with 24-hour urine fractionated metanephrines and catecholamines, or plasma-fractionated metanephrines.
- Thyroid nodules can be assessed by ultrasound to confirm the presence of nodules and lymphadenopathy; thyroid function tests are often normal.
- Pituitary adenomas are evaluated with brain MRI, labs to measure pituitary hormones, and clinical assessment to screen for symptoms of hypersecretion/hyposecretion.
- MEN syndromes are diagnosed based on clinical signs and symptoms of tumor types, family history, DNA testing of patient and first-degree relatives, and labs to screen for hormonal and chemical abnormalities.

▶ TREATMENT

- Complete surgical resection is the only potentially curative treatment for adrenocortical adenomas or ACC.
- Medical treatment for hypertension and tachyarrhythmias associated with pheochromocytomas includes use of α-blockers and calcium channel blockers with or without β-blockers; surgical removal of pheochromocytomas is the definitive treatment of choice.
- Transsphenoidal surgery is the treatment of choice for most pituitary adenomas.
  - Medical management can include hormone replacement for hypopituitarism.
  - Prolactin-secreting adenomas are treated with bromocriptine or cabergoline.
- MEN syndromes:
  - MEN1:
    - Parathyroidectomy is recommended for symptomatic hypercalcemia, nephrolithiasis, and diminished bone density.
    - Pituitary adenomas are treated the same as sporadic pituitary adenomas.
    - Active Zollinger-Ellison syndrome is treated with proton-pump inhibitors.
    - Surgical excision is indicated for insulinomas located in the pancreas.
  - MEN2A:
    - Total thyroidectomy is the only way to cure MEN2-related MTC.
    - Adrenalectomy is necessary for pheochromocytomas.
    - Indications for surgical intervention for hyperparathyroidism are like those in patients with sporadic primary hyperparathyroidism (symptomatic hypercalcemia, nephrolithiasis, hypercalciuria, and diminished bone density).
  - MEN2B/3:
    - Treat hormone dysfunction.
    - Treat symptoms.
    - Genetic counseling.
    - Surgical resection is often challenging as most tumors are small, difficult to detect, multiple, and/or ectopic.
  - MEN4:
    - Treat hormone dysfunction.
    - Treat symptoms.
    - Genetic counseling.
    - Surgical resection is often challenging as most tumors are small, difficult to detect, multiple, and/or ectopic.

Syndrome of Inappropriate Antidiuretic Hormone Secretion

Melissa Day, DMS, MPAS

A 65-year-old female with progressive macular hypomelanosis of tobacco abuse and chronic back pain was admitted 4 days ago for treatment of pneumonia. Broad-spectrum antibacterial agents were started. Initial labs revealed hyponatremia with a sodium of 128 mEq/L, plasma osmolality 245 mOsm/kg, urine osmolality 600 mOsm/kg H_2O, and urine sodium of 95 mEq/L. BUN was 8, creatinine 1.0, cortisol 26, and thyroid-stimulating hormone of 2.7. Despite fluid restriction, repeat sodium was 120 mEq/L. Chest computed tomography showed a large central mass. She denies headache, nausea, and vomiting. Physical examination is consistent with euvolemia. What is your differential diagnosis based on her symptoms and laboratory findings?

▶ GENERAL FEATURES

- Normally, hypovolemia or hyperosmolarity increases antidiuretic hormone (ADH) secretion; syndrome of inappropriate antidiuretic hormone secretion (SIADH) causes an inappropriate increase in ADH secretion.
  - This change in ADH increases water retention and impairs water excretion, leading to hyponatremia, causing inadequate urinary dilution by the kidneys and concentrated urine; hyponatremia occurs from excess water, not a deficiency of sodium.
- The hallmark of SIADH is isovolemic hypotonic hyponatremia.
- Cause is often medication related:
  - Antidepressants (eg, selective serotonin reuptake inhibitor), antipsychotic agents, anticonvulsants (eg, carbamazepine), diuretics (eg, thiazides), pain medications (eg, narcotic analgesics, nonsteroidal anti-inflammatory agents), and cytotoxic agents (eg, intravenous [IV] cyclophosphamide)
- Other causes to consider: central nervous system (CNS) diseases (eg, stroke, infection, malignancy, post-op), pulmonary disease (eg, small cell lung cancer secretes ectopic ADH), endocrine disease (hypothyroidism, glucocorticoid deficiency or excess), and in addition, it may be idiopathic or seen in endurance exercise.

▶ CLINICAL ASSESSMENT

- Symptoms vary with underlying cause.
- Neurologic symptoms stem from the severity and presence of cerebral edema, cerebral tumor, or head injury.
  - Symptoms can include confusion, disorientation, delirium, generalized muscle weakness, myoclonus,

tremor, asterixis, hyporeflexia, ataxia, dysarthria, Cheyne-Stokes respirations, pathologic reflexes, generalized seizures, and coma.
- May present with pulmonary symptoms, signs of infection, malignancy, or various endocrine symptoms
- There may be no signs of edema; the patient may or may not have weight gain because natriuresis prevents edema despite volume expansion.

▶ DIAGNOSIS

- Diagnostic studies should include a computed tomography (CT) of the head to rule out a CNS disease and to detect complications such as cerebral edema and radiography of the chest to rule out lung pathology.
- Laboratory diagnostics should include a complete blood count and complete metabolic panel looking for infection, renal function abnormalities, and electrolyte abnormalities; also look at serum cortisol, thyroid-stimulating hormone, uric acid, osmolality, and urine for sodium.
- The patient should have normal cardiac, hepatic, thyroid, adrenal, and renal functions.
- Diagnostic criteria include:
  - Hyponatremia: serum sodium <135 mEq/L
  - Serum osmolality: hypotonic; <275 mOsm/kg H_2O
  - Urine osmolality: >100 mOsm/kg H_2O
  - Volume status: isovolemic
  - Elevated urine sodium (>20 mEq/L) under conditions of normal salt and water intake
  - Absence of adrenal, pituitary, thyroid, renal insufficiency, or diuretic use

▶ TREATMENT

- Treatment is determined by severity of symptoms and rapidity of decline.
  - Asymptomatic or mild-to-moderate symptoms (eg, headache, lethargy)
  - Symptomatic with an acute duration (<48 hours) and an acute decrease in serum sodium
  - Significant neurologic symptoms (eg, seizures, coma) with a chronic duration (>48 hours) and decline in serum sodium.
- Treatment options:
  - Fluid restriction is mainstay.
    - <800 mL to1 L/day is recommended, but usually not tolerable.
  - Pharmacologic therapy if there is inadequate water restriction.

- Demeclocycline: inhibits ADH action; associated with photosensitivity and gastrointestinal symptoms
- Tolvaptan: ADH antagonist; well tolerated but cost is prohibitive, and it is associated with liver toxicity; can be used in acute and chronic settings
- Loop diuretics: decrease volume expansion, preventing concentrated urine and limiting hyponatremia
- Salt tablets: associated with volume depletion
- Oral urea: increases water excretion; limited by unpalatable taste
  - Fluids:
    - 3% hypertonic saline, 100 mL bolus, with a loop diuretic to increase serum sodium by 2–4 mEq/L.
    - For persistent symptoms, repeat the bolus once or twice at 10-minute intervals.

- Overly aggressive treatment and too-rapid correction in serum sodium can result in neuronal damage and osmotic demyelination (ie, central pontine myelinolysis).
  - Sodium should not be increased >8–10 mEq/L in 24 hours.
  - Sodium should not be increased >0.5 mEq/L per hour.

Case Conclusion

Although pneumonia potentially could have contributed to the patient's symptoms, the central lung mass, which is likely lung cancer, is the main cause of her syndrome of inappropriate antidiuretic hormone secretion.

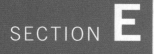

SECTION E   *Primary Adrenal Insufficiency*

CHAPTER 105   Primary Adrenal Insufficiency and Cushing Syndrome

Ziemowit Mazur, EdM, MS, PA-C

▶ GENERAL FEATURES

- Adrenal insufficiency is a life-threatening clinical syndrome that most commonly results from an autoimmune process, leading to the destruction of the adrenal cortex.
- Primary adrenal insufficiency usually presents with signs and symptoms consistent with mineralocorticoid and glucocorticoid deficiency.
- Cushing syndrome is synonymous with hypercortisolism and has several causes: iatrogenic (most common), pituitary tumor (Cushing disease), adrenal masse, and ectopic adrenocorticotropic hormone (ACTH)–secreting tumor.
- Presentation of Cushing syndrome is consistent with that of excess cortisol.

▶ CLINICAL ASSESSMENT

- Primary adrenal insufficiency is most commonly caused by an autoimmune destruction of the adrenal cortex (Addison disease), followed by infectious causes.

- Presenting signs and symptoms are due to chronic or acute deficiency of adrenal cortex hormones and range from fatigue, weight loss, abdominal pain, nausea and vomiting, skin hyperpigmentation, postural hypotension, fever, confusion, and coma.
- Adrenal insufficiency may reveal hyponatremia and hyperkalemia.
- Most common signs and symptoms due to hypercortisolism are central obesity, round face, abnormal glucose intolerance, ecchymoses, hirsutism, hypertension, and a dorsal fat pad.
- If acute adrenal insufficiency is suspected, begin treatment immediately (before diagnostic test results are available).

▶ DIAGNOSIS

- Measurement of serum cortisol, ACTH, sodium, and potassium are key to investigate primary adrenal insufficiency.

- Laboratory findings consistent with primary adrenal insufficiency demonstrate low total serum cortisol, very high level of ACTH, hyponatremia, and hyperkalemia.
- An ACTH stimulation test with synthetic ACTH (cosyntropin) helps to further identify the source of adrenal insufficiency.
- Suspect Cushing syndrome in a patient presenting with common features including weight gain, depression, muscle weakness, headache, osteoporosis, diabetes, easy bruising, facial plethora, and menstrual irregularity and in patients with unusual features for their age, such as hypertension or osteoporosis in younger patients, as well as in children exhibiting weight gain and decreased linear growth.
- An initial diagnosis of Cushing syndrome, after excluding exogenous glucocorticoid intake, can be established with the following laboratory tests: late-night salivary cortisol, 24-hour urinary free cortisol excretion, or overnight 1 mg dexamethasone suppression test.

▶ TREATMENT

- For acute adrenal crisis, immediately give 100 mg intravenous (IV) by appropriate fluid resuscitation and hydrocortisone 200 mg/day as continuous IV infusion or 50 mg IV every 6 hours for 24 hours.
- For chronic adrenal insufficiency, in addition to patient education, glucocorticoid therapy is recommended in all patients with confirmed diagnosis of primary adrenal insufficiency.
- Treatment of Cushing syndrome is directed at the primary cause:
  - Idiopathic: stop glucocorticoids
  - Pituitary tumor: transsphenoidal surgery
  - Adrenal mass: adrenalectomy
  - Ectopic ACTH-secreting tumors: surgical excision of tumor

---

SECTION **F**   *Thyroid Disorders*

CHAPTER
106

Hyperthyroidism and Graves Disease

Frank Giannelli, PhD, PA-C

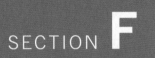

A 19-year-old female student presents to the university student health center complaining of anxiousness. She denies acute stressors and overall experiences pleasure with outdoor activities and spending times with her friends and family. In the review of systems, she endorses excessive sweating, unintentional weight loss, palpitations, and heat intolerance. Physical examination reveals resting tachycardia, lid lag, and exophthalmos. Her thyroid is nontender, smooth, but mildly enlarged. What common clinical concerns should you consider?

▶ GENERAL FEATURES

- Hyperthyroidism, the condition of overproduction of thyroid hormone, has a prevalence of about 1.2% and is far less common than hypothyroidism; it can occur at any age, with peak incidence at age 30–60 years.

- The most common cause of hyperthyroidism (60%-80% of patients) is Graves disease, followed by toxic multinodular goiters and toxic adenomas.
  - Graves disease is an autoimmune disorder caused by anti–thyrotropin receptor antibodies.
  - Graves disease is 5 times more common in females than men and results in thyroid gland growth and excessive thyroid hormone production.
  - Toxic multinodular goiters are the most common cause of hyperthyroidism in patients aged >40 years; they are caused by hyperfunctioning thyroid nodules.
- Thyroiditis is inflammation of the thyroid gland and may be acute, subacute, or chronic.
  - Subacute thyroiditis, thought to be caused by a viral infection, causes transient hyperthyroidism and, in some patients, may be followed by transient hypothyroidism before resolution.

- Secondary causes of thyrotoxicosis include increased iodine levels, excessive levothyroxine, drugs such as amiodarone, and increased production of thyroid-stimulating hormone (TSH).

▶ CLINICAL ASSESSMENT

- Clinical presentation varies depending on the age of onset, severity, and duration of hyperthyroidism, sex, and comorbidities.
- Symptoms may include sudden onset of tachycardia, anxiety, fine tremor, wide pulse pressure hypertension, and unintentional weight loss; delirium is more common in older adults.
- Physical examination findings can include an enlarged or nodular thyroid.
  - Exophthalmos may occur in patients with Graves disease.
  - Pain on palpation of the thyroid suggests subacute thyroiditis. Some patients present with no physical examination findings.
- Ask about previous intake or current use of iodine, immune-modulating medications, and amiodarone.

▶ DIAGNOSIS

- Diagnosis is based on characteristic clinical features and biochemical abnormalities.
  - Initial screening laboratory tests for hyperthyroidism are TSH and T4 levels.
  - A low TSH and a high T4 are diagnostic for hyperthyroidism.
- Additional initial laboratory work includes T3, complete blood cell count, and ECG.
- The presence of anti–thyrotropin receptor antibodies helps to differentiate Graves disease from other causes and is the most sensitive diagnostic test.
- A positive thyroid-stimulating immunoglobulin (TSI) also helps diagnose Graves disease.
- Thyroid imaging is helpful in distinguishing the various causes of hyperthyroidism:
  - A thyroid scan measures radioiodine uptake of nodules in the thyroid.
  - A thyroid ultrasound is used to evaluate the anatomic features of the thyroid and does not give information about thyroid function.
- Diffuse active uptake is typical in Graves disease patients.
- Patients with toxic multimodal goiter will show patchy uptake with pockets of concentration (hot nodules) near the goiter.

- Patients with subacute thyroiditis will show a diffuse decreased iodine uptake.
- The differential diagnosis for thyrotoxicosis includes anxiety disorders, cardiac tachyarrhythmias, and neurologic disorders with tremor.

▶ TREATMENT

- Graves disease: initial treatment of choice in young adults and teens is an anti–thyroid-modulating drug such as methimazole or propylthiouracil; radioactive iodine ablation or thyroidectomy may be required if remission is not achieved.
- Toxic multimodal goiter and toxic adenomas: permanent tissue destruction with radioactive iodine ablation or thyroidectomy
- Subacute thyroiditis: short-term symptomatic relief with nonsteroidal anti-inflammatory drugs and β-blockers such as propranolol
  - β-Blockers play a role with symptomatic relief of anxiety and tachycardia but have no effect on the underlying cause.
- Radioactive iodine ablation is contraindicated during pregnancy and breastfeeding.
- Patients undergoing radioactive iodine ablation or thyroidectomy may require lifelong thyroid hormone replacement and monitoring for parathyroid hormone levels and calcium deficiency.

▶ COMPLICATIONS

- Thyroid storm, a life-threatening condition, may occur in patients with untreated hyperthyroidism who are under stress, such as from an infection or surgery; the condition is treated emergently with propylthiouracil, β-blockers, IV fluids, iodine, glucocorticoid treatment, and rapid cooling.
- Optic complications and blindness are consequences of untreated exophthalmos in patients with Graves disease.

Case Conclusion

Graves disease is the most common cause of hyperthyroidism in young females. Thyroid-stimulating hormone (TSH) and T4 are used to diagnosis Graves disease. We would expect a low TSH and high T4.

Hypothyroidism

Joshua Merson, MS-HPEd, PA-C
Emily Thatcher, MPAS, PA-C

A 57-year-old white transgender male presents to the primary care clinic with complaints of generalized fatigue and inability to lose weight. He is attempting to exercise and diet but is not losing weight at the same rate as his partner. He endorses periodic constipation and dry mouth. He states that he has been feeling this way for some time, but it has worsened over the past year. His examination reveals several pertinent findings: body mass index is 31, heart rate is 52 bpm, and there is slight thinning of the eyebrows. No thyromegaly or nodules are noted. What potential endocrine conditions should you consider?

▶ GENERAL FEATURES

- Hypothyroidism, or a deficiency of thyroid hormone, occurs in 0.1%–2% of patients in the United States; prevalence increases with age.
- In the United States, the prevalence of clinical hypothyroid disease is ~0.3%, and the prevalence of subclinical hypothyroid prevalence is ~4%.
- Hypothyroidism is 5–8 times more common in women than men.
- Primary thyroid disease accounts for >95% of cases of hypothyroidism:
  - Hashimoto thyroiditis (autoimmune thyroiditis) is the most common cause of hypothyroidism in iodine-sufficient populations.
  - Other common causes of primary hypothyroidism include surgical thyroid excision, thyroid radioablation secondary to treatment for Graves disease, radiation therapy to the neck, or an adverse reaction to certain medications known to affect thyroid function.
- Suspect secondary or tertiary (central) hypothyroidism in patients with:
  - Known hypothalamic or pituitary disease
  - Mass lesion present in the pituitary gland
  - Signs and symptoms of hypothyroidism associated with other hormonal deficiencies

▶ CLINICAL ASSESSMENT

- Clinical manifestations are highly variable depending on the onset, duration, and severity of hypothyroidism.
- Patients may be asymptomatic, especially subclinical hyperthyroidism.
- Symptoms are nonspecific, especially in older adults who present with fewer and less classic signs; most common symptoms are fatigue, cold intolerance, weight gain, constipation, dry skin, myalgia, hoarse voice, and irregular menstruation.
- The most common physical findings include goiter, bradycardia, hypertension, pretibial edema, and delayed relaxation phase of deep tendon reflexes.
- Thyroid nodules are common in patients with Hashimoto thyroiditis.
- The thyroid gland may be enlarged, atrophic, or of normal size.
- Signs and symptoms of severe hypothyroidism may include carpal tunnel syndrome, obstructive sleep apnea, and hyponatremia.
- Ask about the use of medications associated with thyroid dysfunction, including iodine, amiodarone, lithium, tyrosine kinase inhibitors, interferon-alfa, and thalidomide.

▶ DIAGNOSIS

- Thyroid-stimulating hormone (TSH) level remains the most valuable initial test for hypothyroidism.
  - The reading may be inaccurate in patients after acute or chronic illness or those taking medications, such as glucocorticoids, dobutamine, or octreotide.
  - TSH level also may vary depending on factors, such as age, sex, iodine intake, or pregnancy.
  - TSH level generally is considered elevated if it is above 4–5 mU/L; however, the accepted upper limit of normal is controversial.
- Measuring free thyroxine (FT4) may help distinguish between primary and secondary or tertiary hypothyroidism.
- Primary hypothyroidism is defined as a high TSH level and a low serum FT4 level (normal range, 0.7-1.9 ng/dL).
- Subclinical (asymptomatic) hypothyroidism is defined as a normal free T4 level in a patient with an elevated TSH level.
- Secondary and tertiary (central) hypothyroidism are defined as inappropriately low TSH in a patient with a low or low-normal serum FT.
- Patients with hypothyroidism also may have hyperlipidemia and hyponatremia.
- Testing for thyroid peroxidase antibody is positive in 95% of patients with Hashimoto thyroiditis.
- All pregnant women should be asked about any history of thyroid dysfunction or the use of thyroid hormones.
- Women planning to become pregnant or who are newly pregnant should be tested for TSH level if they have any of the following risk factors: personal or family

history or symptoms of thyroid disease; history of head or neck radiation or thyroid surgery; age over 30 years; type 1 diabetes or other autoimmune disorder; history of preterm delivery, miscarriage, or two or more previous pregnancies; morbid obesity; use of amiodarone, lithium, or recent use of iodinated contrast; or if they live in an area of known iodine insufficiency.

▶ TREATMENT

- Thyroid hormone (T4) replacement therapy is the recommended treatment.
  - Healthy adults will require about 1.6 µg/kg per day (about 1 µg/kg per day in adults age >50 years, depending on comorbidities).
  - Younger, healthy patients may be started at the full anticipated dose, but patients aged >50 years or those with a history of coronary artery disease should be started at 25–50 µg/day.
  - Recheck the patient's TSH level 6 weeks after initiation and 6 weeks after any change in levothyroxine dose. Make gradual changes in levothyroxine dosing to achieve a normal TSH level.
  - When the TSH level is within normal limits and the patient is asymptomatic, recheck the TSH level in 6 months.

- Patients with subclinical hypothyroidism should be treated if their TSH levels are 10 mU/L or greater; treating patients with subclinical hypothyroidism and TSH levels between 5 and 10 mU/mL remains controversial.
- All pregnant women with newly diagnosed hypothyroidism should be treated with thyroid hormone (T4) to restore euthyroidism as soon as possible.
  - Women typically have an increased requirement for T4 during pregnancy.
- Women with preexisting hypothyroidism who plan to become pregnant should achieve euthyroidism before conceiving.

Case Conclusion

The patient's sign and symptoms are consistent with Hashimoto thyroiditis, the most common cause of hypothyroidism in the United States. Patients with thyroid carcinoma present with a lump, swelling, or pain in the front of the neck, voice changes, or trouble swallowing. Most patients with a thyroid (follicular) adenoma or goiter are euthyroid and are asymptomatic.

CHAPTER 108

Benign Thyroid Nodules

Melissa Murfin, PharmD, PA-C

▶ GENERAL FEATURES

- Palpable thyroid nodules are found in up to 50%–65% of healthy individuals; 5% of women and 1% of men in countries replete with iodine; ultrasound may detect thyroid nodules in as many as 19%–68% of people.
- Most thyroid nodules are benign and asymptomatic; only 7%–15% are found to be cancerous.
- Thyroid nodules are 4 times more common in women than men and occur more frequently with increasing age; family history is also a risk factor.

▶ CLINICAL ASSESSMENT

- Diagnosis is made through a detailed history, including patient age, personal and family history of thyroid disease and thyroid cancer, prior irradiation to the head or neck, anterior neck pain, dysphonia, dysphagia,

dyspnea, any symptoms of thyroid dysfunction, and the use of any drugs or supplements that contain iodine.
- The differential diagnosis includes thyroid cancer, goiter due to autoimmune thyroid disease, subacute thyroiditis, lymphoma, and neck infection.
- Physical examination should include thyroid and cervical lymph node palpation. Assessment of thyroid size and consistency; the location, size, and number of thyroid nodules; the presence of neck tenderness or neck pain; and any cervical lymphadenopathy should be documented.
- Thyroid-stimulating hormone (TSH) should be measured to determine if the nodule is functional.
  - If the TSH is low, a radionuclide scan should be performed.
  - Thyroid nodules identified as "hot" on radionuclide scanning are considered hyperactive and are rarely malignant.

▶ DIAGNOSIS

- Thyroid ultrasound should be performed; cervical lymph nodes should also be assessed during ultrasound.
- Nodules are assessed on ultrasound based on size and echogenic pattern.
- Perform fine-needle aspiration (FNA) to determine malignancy:
  - Nodules that do not appear suspicious on ultrasound should be biopsied when size is ≥1.5–2 cm.
  - Nodules that appear suspicious for thyroid cancer should undergo FNA if size is ≥1 cm. Suspicious echogenic features include:
    - Hypoechoic to surrounding thyroid tissue
    - Irregular margins
    - Microcalcifications, rim calcifications
    - Taller than wider shape
    - Evidence of extrathyroidal extension
- Nodules that appear fully cystic do not require FNA.
- Hyperactive thyroid nodules generally do not require FNA unless suspicious features are present.

▶ TREATMENT

- Benign, nonfunctional thyroid nodules do not require treatment; annual ultrasound, symptom assessment, and TSH are sufficient for monitoring.
- Ultrasound may be repeated in 2 years if no change in size, symptoms, or functionality is present after the first year.
- FNA is repeated if suspicious features are noted on follow-up, nodule volume increases by >50%, or becomes symptomatic.
- Surgery may be needed when symptoms of dysphagia, dysphonia, or dyspnea are present or develop over time.
- Hyperactive nodules may require treatment with radioactive iodine ablation or thyroid-suppressive medication therapy.

CHAPTER 109

Thyroid Cancer

Melissa Murfin, PharmD, PA-C

▶ GENERAL FEATURES

- Thyroid nodules are very common, but only 7%–15% are cancerous; most nodules are asymptomatic.
- More than 50,000 patients are diagnosed with thyroid cancer annually in the United States; it is the most common cancer in patients aged 15–29 years and is the fifth most common cancer in women.
- Four types:
  - Papillary thyroid cancer (PTC)
  - Follicular thyroid cancer
  - Medullary thyroid cancer
  - Anaplastic thyroid cancer
- Differentiated cancers such as PTC and follicular thyroid cancer comprise 85% of cases and are associated with the best overall disease-specific survival rates.
- The overall 5-year survival rate for differentiated thyroid cancer is 98%.
- Medullary thyroid carcinoma, present in 1%–2% of thyroid cancers, is associated with elevated calcitonin levels; the 10-year survival rate is dependent on staging at diagnosis and ranges from 21% to 100%.
- Anaplastic thyroid cancer is diagnosed in ~1.7% of thyroid cancer cases and is the most concerning thyroid malignancy, with a median survival of only 5 months; the 1-year survival rate is 20%.

- Risk factors for thyroid cancer include female gender, family history of thyroid cancer, history of radiation to the head or neck, and increased age.

▶ CLINICAL ASSESSMENT

- A detailed thyroid history should include patient age, personal and family history of thyroid disease and thyroid cancer, prior irradiation to the head or neck, anterior neck pain, dysphonia, dysphagia, dyspnea, any symptoms of thyroid dysfunction, and the use of any drugs or supplements that contain iodine.
- Differential diagnosis includes benign thyroid nodule, goiter due to hypothyroidism or hyperthyroidism, subacute thyroiditis, neck infection, lymphoma, and metastatic disease.
- Physical examination involves assessing thyroid and cervical lymph nodes via palpation; thyroid size and consistency; the location, size, and number of thyroid nodules; the presence of neck tenderness or neck pain; and any cervical lymphadenopathy should be documented.
- Thyroid-stimulating hormone (TSH) should be measured to determine whether the nodule is functional.
  - If TSH is low, a radionuclide scan should be performed.

- Thyroid nodules identified as "hot" on radionuclide scanning are considered hyperactive and are rarely malignant.

▶ DIAGNOSIS

- Thyroid ultrasound should be performed to further characterize the location, size, number of nodules, nodule shape, texture, and echogenicity; cervical lymph nodes should also be assessed during ultrasound.
- Ultrasound-guided, fine-needle aspiration (FNA) is performed based on sonographic characteristics to determine whether the nodule is benign or malignant:
  - Nodules with no suspicious features on ultrasound should be biopsied when the size is ≥1.5–2 cm.
  - Nodules that are ≥1 cm and appear suspicious for thyroid cancer should be assessed via FNA.
  - Suspicious echogenic features include:
    - Hypoechoic echogenicity compared to surrounding thyroid tissue
    - Irregular margins
    - Microcalcifications or rim calcifications
    - Taller than wider shape
    - Evidence of extrathyroidal extension
- Fully cystic and hyperactive thyroid nodules generally do not require FNA unless suspicious features are present.

▶ TREATMENT

- Thyroidectomy is generally indicated for malignant nodules.
- Active surveillance may be employed for patients with very low-risk tumors (no evidence of metastases or aggressive disease) or shortened lifespan.
- Dissection of lateral cervical lymph nodes is needed for patients with metastatic lymphadenopathy.
- Radioactive iodine ablation may be considered postoperatively to reduce the risk of recurrence in patients with metastatic disease or extrathyroidal extension.
- Patients require treatment with levothyroxine after total thyroidectomy for iatrogenic hypothyroidism; the TSH goal is initially 0.1–0.5 mU/L.
- Monitor patients after surgery by testing thyroglobulin and performing neck ultrasound to detect metastases or recurrence; if no recurrence is noted, the TSH goal may be relaxed to 0.5–2 mU/L.

▶ COMPLICATIONS

- Vocal cord paralysis and laryngeal nerve dysfunction may occur after thyroidectomy. Preoperative voice evaluation is recommended to establish a baseline, then postoperatively to determine any impairment.
- Thyroid surgery can result in iatrogenic hypoparathyroidism and hypocalcemia; calcium levels are monitored postoperatively to determine the need for calcitriol treatment.

CHAPTER 110

Hyperparathyroidism and Hypoparathyroidism

Kristopher Maday, MS, PA-C, DFAAPA

▶ GENERAL FEATURES

- Parathyroid hormone (PTH) is created and stored in the parathyroid gland and secreted in response to low serum calcium.
- Three main actions:
  - Skeletal: increases osteoclastic activity to mobilize calcium stores from the bone
  - Renal:
    - Increases reabsorption of calcium
    - Inhibits reabsorption of phosphate
    - Synthesizes calcitriol
  - Intestinal: increases calcium absorption by calcitriol
- Hyperparathyroidism:
  - Primary hyperparathyroidism is a common endocrine disorder caused by overproduction of the PTH by abnormal parathyroid glands and characterized by hypercalcemia without appropriate suppression of plasma PTH levels.
  - Secondary hyperparathyroidism is caused by a failure of calcium, phosphate, and vitamin D homeostatic mechanisms, resulting in elevated PTH levels. It is common in patients with chronic kidney disease (CKD), calcium malabsorption, or vitamin D deficiency.

- Hypoparathyroidism:
  - Rare condition characterized by absent or inappropriately low PTH resulting in hypocalcemia and serum phosphate levels in the upper normal or elevated range
  - Most common cause is surgery-associated removal of, damage to, or devascularization of parathyroid tissue.
  - Iatrogenic (most common):
    - Postsurgical
    - Postradiation
  - Autoimmune:
    - Autoimmune polyglandular syndrome
    - Calcium-sensor receptor antibodies
  - Genetic:
    - Abnormal development
    - Mutations in the calcium-sensing receptor

▶ CLINICAL ASSESSMENT

- Hyperparathyroidism: ~80% of patients are asymptomatic, and the disease is detected by an incidental finding of hypercalcemia on a laboratory test. Symptomatic patients present with findings related to chronic hypercalcemia, including renal, skeletal, neuromuscular and cardiovascular findings in addition to neuropsychiatric symptoms:
  - "Stones": nephrolithiasis
  - "Bones": decreased bone mineral density and nonspecific bone pain
  - "Abdominal groans": nausea, vomiting, anorexia, and pancreatitis
  - "Porcelain thrones": polyuria and constipation
  - "Psychiatric moans": depression, psychosis, and delirium
  - "Fatigue overtones": lethargy and fatigue
- Hypoparathyroidism: varies from an asymptomatic laboratory finding to a severe, life-threatening condition, with symptoms of hypocalcemia due to both serum level and rate of change of serum calcium levels
  - Acute:
    - Due to postsurgical hypocalcemia
    - Perioral numbness, paresthesias, muscle cramps, tetany
    - Dysrhythmias (torsades de point)
    - Chovstek sign: facial spasms with percussion of facial nerve
    - Trousseau sign: carpopedal spasm with insufflation of blood pressure cuff
  - Chronic:
    - Dental abnormalities: dental hypoplasia, defective enamel
    - Cataracts
    - Basal ganglia calcifications
    - Dry, puffy skin
    - Coarse, brittle hair and nails

▶ DIAGNOSIS

- Laboratory tests are the first step to diagnose a parathyroid disorder and differentiate between hyperparathyroidism and hypoparathyroidism:
  - Serum PTH
  - Serum calcium
  - Urinary calcium
  - Primary hyperparathyroidism: increased PTH, increased serum calcium, increased urinary calcium
  - Secondary hyperparathyroidism: increased PTH, normal serum calcium, decreased urinary calcium
  - Hypoparathyroidism: decreased PTH, decreased serum calcium, decreased urinary calcium
- Radiographic:
  - If an adenoma or malignancy is suspected, ultrasound is the initial test of choice.
  - Sestamibi nuclear medicine scan is used if ultrasound inconclusive.

▶ TREATMENT

- Patients presenting with hypercalcemic crisis (rapid-onset albumin-corrected serum calcium >14 mg/dL and signs or symptoms of multiorgan dysfunction) require immediate management.
  - Primary hyperparathyroidism:
    - Surgical indications:
      - Age <50 years
      - Serum calcium >1 mg/dL above upper limit of normal
      - DXA T-score ≤−2.5
      - Vertebral fracture
      - 24-hour urine calcium ≥400 mg/day
      - Creatinine clearance <60 mL/min
      - Presence of nephrolithiasis
    - Nonoperative:
      - Bisphosphonates
      - Calcimimetics
      - Vitamin D supplementation
  - Secondary:
    - Phosphate binders
    - Vitamin D supplementation
- Hypoparathyroidism: acute management may be required.
  - Intravenous (IV) calcium indications for acute cases include:
    - 10 mL ampule of 10% calcium gluconate in 50 mL of D5W over 10–20 minutes
    - Oral calcitriol and calcium carbonate
  - Chronic cases:
    - Goal is to treat until asymptomatic
    - Oral calcium carbonate or citrate
    - Oral calcitriol

Section A Pretest: Disorders of the Penis

1. Which of the following penile abnormalities should be treated urgently to prevent serious complication?

   A. Epispadias
   B. Phimosis
   C. Hypospadias
   D. Paraphimosis

2. Of the following, which best describes erectile dysfunction?

   A. Pain with erection
   B. Prolonged erection
   C. Inability to maintain an erection
   D. Abnormal curvature of erection

3. Which of the following conditions occurs in 75% of patients with epispadias?

   A. Vesicoureteral reflux
   B. Urinary incontinence
   C. UTI
   D. Balanitis

4. Erectile dysfunction may also indicate the presence of which underlying disease state?

   A. Thyroid disease
   B. Prostatic disease
   C. Cardiovascular disease
   D. Pulmonary disease

5. Which of the following aspects of a patient's history is important to address in patient education following the diagnosis of phimosis?

   A. Family history of phimosis
   B. History of urinary catheter placement
   C. Poor personal hygiene
   D. History of recurrent UTI

6. Which of the following is a risk factor for the development of penile cancer?

   A. Chlamydia
   B. Circumcision
   C. HPV
   D. Tinea cruris

7. Which of the following treatments is recommended for hypospadias?

   A. Surgical correction
   B. Urinary catheter placement
   C. Antibiotic treatment
   D. Improvement of hygiene

8. Of the following, which represents an organic etiology of erectile dysfunction?

   A. Anxiety
   B. Peyronie disease
   C. Stress
   D. Depression

9. What is the 5-year survival rate for stage II penile cancer?

   A. 99%
   B. 90%
   C. 85%
   D. 75%

10. Of the following, which medication is a reversible cause of erectile dysfunction?

    A. Atorvastatin
    B. Levothyroxine
    C. Metoprolol
    D. Metformin

11. Which is the name of the fascial layer surrounding both the penis and the testicles?

    A. Vas deferens
    B. Tunica albuginea
    C. Epidermis
    D. Seminal vesicle

12. Of the following, which is the best initial management for Peyronie disease?

    A. PDE5 inhibitor
    B. Urology referral
    C. Penile prosthesis
    D. Vitamin E

13. If urethral injury is suspected in a male patient with genital trauma, what is the best next step?

    A. Place a Foley catheter at the bedside.
    B. Consult urology to perform a cystoscopy.
    C. Monitor conservatively for signs of bleeding.
    D. Place a condom catheter.

14. A 45-year-old male presents for evaluation of a lesion on the penis that has been present for 6 months. The lesion occasionally bleeds but is not painful. The patient reports a history of genital warts but has not seen any lesions in the past year or so. The patient is sexually active with 1 partner and sometimes uses condoms. On examination, you note an uncircumcised penis, and upon retraction of the foreskin, there is a friable ulcerated lesion on the glans. What is the next best step in the management of this patient?

    A. Biopsy of the lesion
    B. Cryotherapy
    C. Culture for HSV
    D. Prescribe a topical steroid

15. Which of the following is true of penile cancer?

    A. Basal cell carcinoma is the most common subtype
    B. Lesions grow rapidly
    C. Most common in the third decade of life
    D. Association with HPV-16

16. Which of the following is NOT a sign or symptom of penile fracture?

    A. Snap-pop sensation
    B. Eggplant deformity
    C. Urinary retention
    D. Phimosis

17. Which of the following is the most appropriate treatment for penile cancer presenting as a bulky T3 tumor?

    A. Amputation
    B. Cryotherapy
    C. Laser ablation
    D. Topical therapy with imiquimod

18. Which of the following is NOT an initial sign/symptom of traumatic urethral injury?

    A. Hematuria
    B. Urinary retention
    C. Pyuria
    D. Bloody meatus

19. Which of the following is most likely to reduce long-term complications of genital injury?

    A. Prompt operative intervention in <8 hours
    B. Broad-spectrum antibiotic coverage
    C. Conservative management
    D. Placement of a Foley catheter at the bedside

Section B Pretest: Disorders of the Prostate

1. Which of the following diagnostic tests helps to rule out causes of lower urinary tract symptoms that are NOT related to BPH?

    A. Postvoid residual volume measurement
    B. Cystoscopy
    C. Transrectal ultrasound of the prostate
    D. Urinalysis

2. Which factor increases a patient's risk of developing prostate cancer?

    A. Age
    B. Family history of prostate cancer in a first-degree relative
    C. Ethnicity
    D. All of the above

3. Which of the following characteristics of nonspecific α-blockers makes them more difficult for patients to tolerate?

    A. Takes 6 months for maximum effect
    B. Often causes orthostatic hypotension
    C. Can cause changes to visual perception of color
    D. Increases risk of UTI

4. Which of the following DRE findings would be indicative of acute bacterial prostatitis?

    A. Tender, boggy prostate
    B. Firm, nodular prostate
    C. Normal prostate
    D. Enlarged prostate

5. A patient is diagnosed with both lower urinary tract symptoms likely secondary to BPH and erectile dysfunction. Which of the following medications is indicated to address both of these problems?

   A. α-1a-blockers such as tamsulosin
   B. 5-α-reductase inhibitors such as finasteride
   C. PDE5 inhibitor tadalafil
   D. Gonadotropin-releasing hormone agonist such as leuprolide

6. A 58-year-old Caucasian man with no significant past medical or family history comes to you to establish care after recently moving to the area. He asks about getting a PSA test. He has no symptoms to report and no significant findings on digital rectal examination. What is the next most appropriate step?

   A. Order the lab without further discussion.
   B. Reassure him that his risk is very low and advise against routine PSA screening.
   C. Discuss the risks vs. benefits of screening and weigh the patient's preference in the decision to screen.
   D. Refer to urology.

7. Which of the following interventions should be completed for a patient in urinary retention secondary to prostatic obstruction?

   A. Foley catheter placement
   B. Prostate biopsy
   C. Transurethral resection of the prostate
   D. Supportive therapy with analgesics

8. A repeat PSA test 1 month after a level of 5.1 ng/mL is now 5.3 ng/mL. What is the next most appropriate step in the management of this patient?

   A. MRI of the prostate
   B. Referral to urology to discuss TRUS-guided biopsy
   C. Repeat PSA testing in 6 weeks
   D. CT imaging of the pelvis

9. Which of the following is a risk of prostate cancer screening?

   A. Overdiagnosis of prostate cancer in men who would have never been affected by the cancer
   B. Reduced risk of death from prostate cancer
   C. Early detection of aggressive disease
   D. None of the above

10. Which of the following types of prostatitis should a prostate massage NOT be performed as part of the physical examination?

    A. Chronic bacterial prostatitis
    B. Asymptomatic prostatitis
    C. Chronic nonbacterial prostatitis
    D. Acute bacterial prostatitis

11. A patient's PSA result is 5.1 ng/mL. You call him to discuss his results. What is your recommendation?

    A. MRI of the prostate
    B. Referral to urology
    C. Repeat PSA testing in 4 weeks
    D. CT imaging of the pelvis

12. Which of the following treatments is considered first-line therapy for chronic bacterial prostatitis?

    A. Sitz bath
    B. Amoxicillin
    C. Fluoroquinolone
    D. α-Blocker

13. A 74-year-old man with a history of BPH currently managed with tamsulosin 0.8 mg daily comes to your clinic complaining daily episodes of urinary incontinence. On physical examination, the patient's lower abdomen is mildly distended and firm. Which of the following is the most appropriate next step in the management of this patient?

    A. Check PSA level
    B. Add a 5-α-reductase inhibitor such as finasteride
    C. Check a postvoid residual volume
    D. Order a CT scan of the pelvis

Section C Pretest: Disorders of the Testes and Related Structures

1. A 15-month-old boy was brought to a clinic by his father. He complains that while bathing his child, he noticed that his child's testes were not present in the scrotal sac. During the physical examination, you are able to palpate the testes in the inguinal canal. Which of the following age ranges is the most appropriate time to perform an orchiopexy in a child affected with cryptorchidism?

   A. 12-24 months
   B. 36-48 months
   C. 3-5 years
   D. >7 years

2. Overcoming the cremasteric reflex by holding tension on the testis in the scrotum for ~1 minute is the treatment of choice for which of the following disorders of the testis?

   A. True undescended
   B. Ectopic
   C. Retractile
   D. Atrophic

3. Which of the following laboratory studies should be performed on all patients suspected of acute epididymitis?

   A. Urinalysis with culture
   B. Complete blood count
   C. Ultrasound of the scrotum
   D. Gram stain of urethral discharge

4. Males are most at risk for testicular torsion in which age group?

   A. 10-20 years
   B. 20-30 years
   C. 30-40 years
   D. 40-50 years

5. A diagnosis of bilateral cryptorchidism cannot be made until which of the following is ruled out?

   A. Micropenis
   B. Female congenital hyperplasia
   C. Tunica vaginalis disorder
   D. Hypospadias

6. A 14-year-old male presents with acute-onset testicular pain and swelling that woke him up from sleep. Initially embarrassed to tell his parents, he now presents to the emergency department after 14 hours of pain and vomiting. You suspect testicular torsion. What is the most appropriate treatment at this point?

   A. Pain management
   B. Scrotal support
   C. Surgical exploration
   D. Urgent color Doppler ultrasound

7. A mother has brought her 7-month-old child to his follow-up appoint for an orchiopexy secondary to an empty scrotal sac. She is hesitant to consent the clinician advised orchiopexy and concerned about the procedure. Which of the following conditions is most frequently associated with an untreated bilateral undescended testis?

   A. Congenital inguinal hernia
   B. Chronic hydrocele
   C. Sterility
   D. Erectile dysfunction

8. Best practices for manual detorsion advise that the testis should be rotated laterally to how many degrees?

   A. 180
   B. 360
   C. 720
   D. 900

9. Why should all adolescent boys who present for abdominal pain and vomiting have their testicles examined?

   A. Testicular torsion has been diagnosed in boys who do not initially complain of abdominal pain.
   B. Undiagnosed testicular torsion can result in infertility.
   C. They might be embarrassed to tell their parents or a stranger that their testicles hurt.
   D. All of the above.

10. What is the most common cause of male infertility that can be corrected surgically?

    A. Varicocele
    B. Hydrocele
    C. Testicular cancer
    D. Spermatocele

11. A 25-year-old presents with a painless nodule of the right testicle. He reports he had a surgical repair as a child for an undescended testicle. What condition would be most consistent with these findings?

    A. Varicocele
    B. Epididymitis
    C. Testicular cancer
    D. Spermatocele

12. Acute-onset unilateral testicular pain and swelling that comes and goes is most concerning for which of the following?

    A. Epididymitis
    B. Torsion of the appendix testis
    C. Orchitis
    D. Intermittent testicular torsion

13. You obtain tumor markers in a patient whom you suspect has testicular cancer based on your physical examination and ultrasound results. If all the tumor markers were negative, what would be the most likely type of cancer found after orchiectomy and subsequent histology was performed?

    A. Nonseminoma
    B. Seminoma
    C. Nongerminal
    D. Lymphoma

14. You are examining a 70-year-old patient with an acute onset of right-sided scrotal swelling. Your examination reveals a "bag-of-worms" consistency to the mass that does not reduce when in the recumbent position. What is the most appropriate next step at this point?

    A. Observation only as this is a classic presentation of a varicocele.
    B. Recommend surgery as this is more than likely a noncommunicating hydrocele.
    C. Obtain an immediate scrotal ultrasound and CT of the abdomen and pelvis.
    D. Antibiotics and re-evaluate in 2 weeks as this is likely a reactive hydrocele.

15. You are evaluating a 6-month-old with unilateral scrotal swelling. Upon ultrasound, it is found to be the noncommunicating type of hydrocele. What would be the most appropriate next step?

    A. Immediate surgery to repair the hydrocele
    B. Antibiotics as this is likely reactive in nature
    C. Observation as most resolve by age 12 months
    D. No concern, normal variant in infants

16. Which of the following emergent medical conditions should be considered in any patient presenting with an acute onset of scrotal pain?

    A. Mumps
    B. Acute epididymitis
    C. Hydrocele
    D. Testicular torsion

17. A 33-year-old well-appearing male presents to your clinic with a gradual onset of left testicular pain and swelling over past 2 days. Symptoms are worse with standing and alleviated by lying down. The patient denies dysuria, fever or chills, nausea, or vomiting. However, recently, he was engaged in unprotected intercourse. On examination, he is noted to have tenderness at the posterior left testis with scrotal swelling and scrotal erythema without masses or nodules. What is the most likely diagnosis?

    A. Testicular torsion
    B. Testicular cancer
    C. Acute epididymitis
    D. Fournier gangrene

18. What is the preferred treatment regimen in a patient with acute epididymitis caused by sexually transmitted chlamydia or gonorrhea?

    A. Ceftriaxone 250 mg IM in a single dose plus doxycycline 100 mg orally twice a day for 10 days
    B. Levofloxacin 500 mg orally daily for 10 days
    C. Ceftriaxone 250 mg IM in a single dose plus metronidazole 500 mg orally twice a day for 7 days
    D. Doxycycline 100 mg orally twice a day for 10 days plus levofloxacin 500 mg orally daily for 10 days

19. Which of the following pathogen is the most common cause of acute epididymitis in a 22-year-old sexually active male?

    A. *Escherichia coli*
    B. *Chlamydia trachomatis*
    C. Cytomegalovirus
    D. *Pseudomonas aeruginosa*

Section D Pretest: Disorders of the Urinary Tract

1. A woman reports leakage of urine when she jumps, sneezes, or coughs. What type of urinary incontinence do her symptoms suggest?

   A. Stress incontinence
   B. Urge incontinence
   C. Mixed incontinence
   D. Overflow incontinence

2. Which of the following types of bladder cancer is the most common?

   A. Squamous cell carcinoma
   B. Urachal carcinoma
   C. Adenocarcinoma
   D. Transitional cell carcinoma

3. Which of the following is NOT a risk factor for incontinence in women?
   A. Cystocele
   B. Obesity
   C. Dysmenorrhea
   D. Vaginal atrophy

4. Which of the following stones form in the presence of an upper UTI with a urease-producing organism?
   A. Calcium oxalate
   B. Struvite
   C. Cystine
   D. Uric acid

5. Mixed incontinence is a combination of which of the following types of incontinence?
   A. Neurogenic and overflow incontinence
   B. Stress and urge incontinence
   C. Urge and overflow incontinence
   D. Neurogenic and stress incontinence

6. Which of the following positive physical examination findings is associated with urolithiasis?
   A. Murphy sign
   B. Obturator sign
   C. Rovsing sign
   D. CVA tenderness

7. The first-line treatment for stress incontinence is which of the following?
   A. Botulinum toxin injection
   B. Oxybutynin
   C. Pelvic floor exercises
   D. Mirabegron

8. Which of the following dietary recommendations should be made for patients with recurrent calcium oxalate stones?
   A. Increase animal protein intake
   B. Increase fluid intake
   C. Decrease calcium intake
   D. Decrease potassium intake

9. Which risk factor is most common for female patients complaining of bladder prolapse?
   A. Multiparity
   B. Bladder cancer
   C. History of sexually transmitted infections
   D. Frequent UTIs

10. Congenital abnormalities are frequently responsible for which urinary-related condition, common in children?
    A. Vesicoureteral reflux
    B. Bladder prolapse
    C. BPH
    D. Interstitial cystitis

11. Initial treatment considerations for a 6-year-old girl with a circular mass noted at her urethral meatus and spotting on her underwear but is otherwise asymptomatic include which one of the following?
    A. Estrogen cream and sitz baths
    B. Surgical excision
    C. Stent placement
    D. Oral antibiotics

12. Which of the following aspects of a patient's social history is most strongly associated with a risk of bladder cancer?
    A. Illegal drug use
    B. Alcohol use
    C. Smoking history
    D. Occupation

13. A 67-year-old male presents to your clinic complaining of diminished urinary stream and urinary dribbling. His past medical history is significant for UTIs and frequent catheterizations. Which diagnostic modality is the best option for the suspected cause of his symptoms?
    A. Retrograde urethrogram
    B. Urine analysis
    C. PSA
    D. CT scan

14. Which one of the following is a common long-term complication of vesicoureteral reflux?
    A. Renal scarring and dysfunction
    B. Painless bleeding
    C. Malignancy
    D. Urethral prolapse

15. Which of the following symptoms occurs in 80% of patients with bladder cancer at presentation?
    A. Painless gross hematuria
    B. Microscopic hematuria
    C. Urinary frequency
    D. Dysuria

▶ ANSWERS AND EXPLANATIONS TO SECTION A PRETEST

1. **D.** Paraphimosis should be treated urgently to prevent serious complication.
2. **C.** Inability to maintain an erection best describes erectile dysfunction.
3. **A.** Vesicoureteral reflux occurs in 75% of patients with epispadias.
4. **C.** Erectile dysfunction may also indicate the presence of cardiovascular disease.
5. **C.** Poor personal hygiene is important to address in patient education following the diagnosis of phimosis.

6. **C.** Presence of HPV infection is one of the biggest risk factors for the development of penile cancer. Lack of circumcision is a risk factor. No associated risk with tinea cruris or chlamydia.

7. **A.** Surgical correction is recommended for hypospadias.

8. **B.** Peyronie disease is an organic etiology of erectile dysfunction.

9. **C.** Stage I/II penile cancer has a 5-year survival rate of 85%. Survival rate drops to 59% for advanced-stage cancer.

10. **C.** Metoprolol is a reversible cause of erectile dysfunction.

11. **B.** The tunica albuginea is the fascial layer surrounding the male genitalia. The vas deferens is the tubular structure that transmits sperm. The epidermis is the skin layer. The seminal vesicles are a pair of glands that open into the vas deferens near to its junction with the urethra and secrete many of the components of semen.

12. **B.** Urology referral is the best initial management for Peyronie disease.

13. **B.** Consult urology for bedside Foley. Placing a Foley at the bedside could potentially make an injury worse and would be contraindicated. Placing a condom catheter or monitoring the patient are both forms of conservative management and could potentially result in missed diagnosis.

14. **A.** Biopsy would be prudent given the length of time the lesion has been present, along with appearance and hx of HPV.

15. **D.** Penile cancer is associated with HPV-16 and HPV-18. Squamous cell carcinoma is the most common type of carcinoma, and lesions typically grow slowly. The mean age of diagnosis is 60 years old.

16. **D.** Phimosis is a congenital narrowing of the opening of the foreskin so that it cannot be retracted. The other options are all commonly seen in penile fractures or other injuries.

17. **A.** Amputation is appropriate for a thick tumor. The other treatment options listed are appropriate for thinner tumors.

18. **C.** Hematuria, bloody meatus, and urinary retention are all signs of a urethral injury. Pyuria, or purulence in the urine, is a sign of infection. Although infection may eventually occur in patients with trauma to the urethra, it would not be an initial presenting sign.

19. **A.** Prompt surgical intervention is proven to reduce long-term complications. Placement of a Foley catheter at bedside could worsen any existing injury. Conservative management almost always results in long-term disability. Antibiotic therapy may be necessary, although this would be adjunctive to definitive surgical repair.

▶ ANSWERS AND EXPLANATIONS TO SECTION B PRETEST

1. **D.** Urinalysis helps to rule out causes of lower urinary tract symptoms that are not related to BPH.

2. **D.** Age, a family history of prostate cancer in a first-degree relative, and ethnicity all increase a patient's risk of developing prostate cancer.

3. **B.** Because they often cause orthostatic hypotension, nonspecific α-blockers can be difficult for patients to tolerate.

4. **A.** A tender, boggy prostate is indicative of acute bacterial prostatitis.

5. **C.** The PDE5 inhibitor tadalafil is indicated for both lower urinary tract symptoms likely secondary to BPH and erectile dysfunction.

6. **C.** Discuss the risks vs. benefits of screening and weigh the patient's preference in the decision to screen for this patient.

7. **A.** Foley catheter placement should be completed for a patient in urinary retention secondary to prostatic obstruction.

8. **B.** Refer this patient to urology to discuss TRUS-guided biopsy.

9. **A.** Overdiagnosis of prostate cancer in men who would have never been affected by the cancer is a risk of prostate cancer screening.

10. **D.** Prostate massage should not be performed as part of the physical examination in acute bacterial prostatitis.

11. **C.** Repeat PSA testing in 4 weeks for this patient.

12. **C.** Fluoroquinolone is considered first-line therapy for chronic bacterial prostatitis.

13. **C.** Checking a postvoid residual volume is the most appropriate next step in the management for this patient.

▶ ANSWERS AND EXPLANATIONS TO SECTION C PRETEST

1. **A.** Age 12–24 months is the most appropriate time to perform an orchiopexy in a child affected with cryptorchidism.

2. **C.** Overcoming the cremasteric reflex by holding tension on the testis in the scrotum for ~1 minute is the treatment of choice for a retractile testis.

3. **A.** Urinalysis with culture should be your initial first test in this patient to rule out an infection as the cause of the pain and swelling. A complete blood count should only be considered if the patient is systemically unwell. An ultrasound of the scrotum is an imaging study that should be considered if there is a sudden onset of pain with concern of testicular

torsion or if there is a mass or nodule concerning for testicular cancer. A Gram stain would be helpful if there was a urethral discharge present or concern of an exposure to a sexually transmitted infection.

4. **A.** Males aged 10 to 20 years are most at risk for testicular torsion.

5. **B.** A diagnosis of bilateral cryptorchidism cannot be made until female congenital hyperplasia is ruled out.

6. **C.** Surgical exploration is indicated for this patient.

7. **C.** Sterility is most frequently associated with an untreated bilateral undescended testis.

8. **C.** Best practices for manual detorsion advise that the testis should be rotated 720°.

9. **D.** All adolescent boys who present for abdominal pain and vomiting have their testicles examined because testicular torsion has been diagnosed in boys who do not initially complain of abdominal pain, undiagnosed testicular torsion can result in infertility, and they might be embarrassed to tell their parents or a stranger that their testicles hurt.

10. **A.** Varicocele is the most common cause of male infertility that can be corrected surgically.

11. **C.** Testicular cancer is most consistent with this patient's findings.

12. **D.** Acute-onset unilateral testicular pain and swelling that comes and goes is most concerning for intermittent testicular torsion.

13. **B.** Seminoma is the most likely type of cancer in this patient.

14. **C.** Obtain an immediate scrotal ultrasound and CT of the abdomen and pelvis for this patient.

15. **C.** Observation is the most appropriate next step in this patient, as most noncommunicating types resolve by age 12 months.

16. **D.** Testicular torsion can be a serious medical condition due to the potential loss of a testicle without prompt surgical intervention. Mumps is due to a viral infection affecting both the parotid glands and the testes that are typically self-limiting. Acute epididymitis is inflammation of the epididymis with patients responding well to nonemergent management. A hydrocele is a collection of peritoneal fluid between the layers of the tunica vaginalis and does not require any emergent intervention.

17. **C.** Acute epididymitis is suspected in a sexually active patient with testicular pain and swelling with tenderness over the epididymis. Testicular torsion often presents with an acute onset of moderate-to-severe testicular pain and seen more frequently in neonates and postpubertal boys than adults. Testicular cancer is generally painless and should not present with acute symptoms. Fournier gangrene is a necrotizing fasciitis of the perineum, which often involves the

scrotum and often has systemic findings such as fever and the patient appearing sick.

18. **A.** Ceftriaxone 250 mg IM in a single dose plus doxycycline 100 mg orally twice a day for 10 days is recommended by the CDC for treating acute epididymitis due to a sexually transmitted infection caused by chlamydia or gonorrhea. Levofloxacin is recommended for treating acute epididymitis caused by enteric organisms. Metronidazole is recommended in the treatment of the sexually transmitted pathogen trichomoniasis.

19. **B.** *C. trachomatis* would be the most likely pathogen in a patient aged <35 years. *E. coli* and *P. aeruginosa* are typically found in men aged >35 years. Cytomegalovirus cases are rare in the United States, except in immunocompromised patients.

▶ ANSWERS AND EXPLANATIONS TO SECTION D PRETEST

1. **A.** Stress incontinence is characterized by leakage of urine during activities that increase intra-abdominal pressure, such as sneezing, coughing, or physical exercise.

2. **D.** Transitional cell carcinoma is the most common type of bladder cancer.

3. **C.** Menstrual changes and dysmenorrhea are not associated with incontinence in women.

4. **B.** Struvite stones form in the presence of an upper UTI with a urease-producing organism.

5. **B.** Mixed incontinence is a combination of stress and urge incontinence.

6. **D.** CVA tenderness is associated with urolithiasis.

7. **C.** Lifestyle changes and complementary therapies including pelvic floor exercises, weight loss, and bladder training are the first-line treatments for stress incontinence.

8. **B.** Increase fluid intake for patients with recurrent calcium oxalate stones.

9. **A.** Women with a history of multiple pregnancies are at higher risk for bladder prolapse. Infections and malignancies are less likely to contribute to this condition.

10. **A.** Vesicoureteral reflux frequently occurs in children often due to ureteral abnormalities, congenital in nature, that allow urine to leave the bladder backup through the ureters. Bladder prolapse and BPH affect older patients with the incidence increasing with age. Similarly, interstitial cystitis is less common in children.

11. **A.** Since this patient is an asymptomatic child, the initial treatment is a conservative trial of hormone cream and sitz baths. If that does not improve the condition, or the patient is symptomatic, surgical

excision may be necessary. On occasion, topical antibiotics may be prescribed, but oral antibiotics would not be an initial treatment for this patient. Placing a stent in the urethra is not indicated for urethral prolapse.

12. **C.** Smoking history is most strongly associated with a risk of bladder cancer.

13. **A.** Because of the patient's symptoms and past medical history involving UTIs and frequent catheterizations, we are suspicious of urethral stricture. While the other options may be helpful and will probably be ordered during the course of treatment to rule in/out other conditions, a RUG would be the best option to evaluate the patency of the urethra.

14. **A.** Owing to the urine moving up the ureters in VUR, bacteria are more likely to cause infection in the upper urinary tract, which over time can cause scarring and thus renal dysfunction. Painless bleeding, malignancies, and urethral prolapses are not common complications.

15. **A.** Painless gross hematuria occurs in 80% of patients with bladder cancer at presentation.

CHAPTER
111

Hypospadias, Epispadias, Paraphimosis, and Phimosis

Natalie Schirato, MPAS, PA-C

▶ GENERAL FEATURES

- Hypospadias:
  - Congenital abnormality of the penis and anterior urethra that results in the urethral meatus being located on the ventral surface of the penis, proximal to its normal location at the tip of the glans
  - May also be associated with ventral chordee, which is shortening and curving of the penis
  - Incidence is ~1 in 300 live male births.
  - May be associated with other anomalies such as inguinal hernias, undescended testes (cryptorchidism), or upper tract anomalies
- Epispadias:
  - Congenital abnormality of the penis that results in a urethral opening located on the dorsal surface of the penis
  - 90% of cases are associated with bladder exstrophy.
  - 75% of patients will also have vesicoureteral reflux.
- Paraphimosis:
  - Condition in which the foreskin cannot be advanced back over the glans once retracted
  - Frequently occurs when foreskin is left retracted after urinary catheter placement/management or during routine bathing
  - Emergency requiring immediate treatment; if left untreated, can result in infection and ischemia of the glans penis
- Phimosis:
  - Condition characterized by inability to retract the prepuce/foreskin from the glans penis
  - May be congenital or acquired, typically due to poor hygiene and/or chronic infection
  - Physiologic phimosis is often present at birth, although 90% of foreskins are retractable by age 3.

▶ CLINICAL ASSESSMENT

- Hypospadias:
  - Patients may report a family history of hypospadias or other genital abnormalities.
  - Condition is typically asymptomatic.
  - The physical examination in a patient with hypospadias should focus on the meatal location, glans configuration, skin coverage, and whether there is any penile curvature.
- Epispadias:
  - Condition is mainly asymptomatic, but some patients may have urinary incontinence.
  - Typically diagnosed at birth by physical examination
  - Examination reveals urethral meatus located on the dorsum of penis.
- Paraphimosis:
  - Patients will be uncircumcised.
  - Patients may report pain and/or drainage and ulceration.
  - Symptoms of urinary obstruction may be present.
  - Physical examination will reveal retracted foreskin, edema of glans penis, and a phimotic/constrictive ring.
- Phimosis:
  - Patients may describe recurrent balanitis, painful erections, or ballooning of foreskin with voiding.
  - Physical examination will reveal foreskin that is unable to be retracted easily or at all and may also present with balanitis.

▶ DIAGNOSIS

- Hypospadias: clinical diagnosis is based on history and physical examination; additional testing is not needed unless disorders of sex development or other abnormalities are suspected.
- Epispadias, paraphimosis, and phimosis: clinical diagnosis is based on history and physical examination; additional diagnostic testing is typically not required.

TREATMENT

- Hypospadias:
  - Routine circumcision is contraindicated.
  - Definitive treatment is surgical correction/repair.
- Epispadias: surgical correction with the goal of ventrally located urethral meatus in a straight penis.
- Paraphimosis:
  - Immediate treatment is indicated.
  - Manual reduction should be attempted first and may require preemptive analgesics.
  - If manual reduction is not successful, a dorsal surgical incision should be performed under local anesthesia without delay in treatment.
  - Elective circumcision should be considered after manual reduction.
- Phimosis:
  - Minor phimosis may be treated with improvement of hygiene or topical betamethasone to soften foreskin.
  - May require circumcision

CHAPTER 112

Erectile Dysfunction

Nathan Bates, MMS, PA-C

GENERAL FEATURES

- Erectile dysfunction (ED) is the inability to achieve or maintain an erection sufficient for satisfactory sexual response.
- Etiologies for ED are classified as either organic or psychogenic; however, they often manifest in combination.
  - Organic: hypertension, diabetes, dyslipidemia, smoking, hypogonadism, hypothyroidism, stroke, spinal cord injury, Peyronie disease, or drug-induced
  - Psychogenic: strained relationships, stress, anxiety, depression, or history of abuse
- Affects ~30 million men in the United States; incidence increase with age

CLINICAL ASSESSMENT

- Timing of onset and progression provides diagnostic clues; acute onset is suggestive of a psychogenic cause, whereas a gradual onset suggests progression of underlying diseases, such as diabetes or hypertension.
- Patients typically report difficulty achieving or maintaining an erection sufficient to fulfill sexual activities.
- Sexually induced penile pain or curvature that may indicate Peyronie disease (localized fibrotic disorder of the tunica albuginea resulting in penile deformity and sexual dysfunction)
- Validated surveys such as the Sexual Health Inventory for Men (SHIM) or International Index of Erectile Function 5-item questionnaire can help assess ED and response to treatment.
- Physical examination should focus on organ systems frequently responsible for ED to include cardiovascular, neurologic, psychological, endocrine, and genitourinary.
  - Findings such as obesity, hypertension, decreased perfusion, neurologic deficits, mood aberrations, thinning of skin or hair, penile plaques, or deformity can help identify an underlying etiology.
- Reviewing patient's medications is imperative to identify reversible medication-related causes of ED, such as the use of antidepressant or antihypertensive agents.

DIAGNOSIS

- ED is a clinical diagnosis based on the patient's inability to achieve or maintain an erection.
- The American Urological Association (AUA) recommends selective diagnostic testing, including fasting blood glucose level, lipid panel, thyroid-stimulating hormone, or total testosterone levels, to evaluate contributing comorbidities.
- Peyronie disease is diagnosed clinically based on the presence of a subcutaneous penile plaque or abnormal curvature; if diagnosis is unclear, ultrasound may be used with or without an intracavernosal injection.

TREATMENT

- The AUA recommends shared decision-making with goal-directed therapy of the available treatment options, including PDE5 inhibitors, vacuum devices, intracavernosal injections, or penile prosthesis.
  - PDE5 inhibitors such as sildenafil or tadalafil remain a popular first choice based on ease of use, effectiveness, and safety profile.
  - However, they are contraindicated in men taking nitrates either regularly or intermittently.
- Additional considerations include routine psychosocial therapy, increased exercise, weight reduction, smoking cessation, discontinuation of harmful medication, and strict management of comorbidities.
- If Peyronie disease is identified, referral to urology is recommended to pursue intralesional injections or surgery.

Penile Carcinoma

Nicole Dettmann, DSc, MPH, PA-C
Stephanie Maclary, RN, MHS, PA-C

▶ GENERAL FEATURES

- Squamous cell carcinoma accounts for 95% of all penile cancers.
- Carcinoma of the penis is rare in industrialized countries, including the United States.
- Mean age at diagnosis is 60 years, and rates increase with advancing age.
- Risk factors include phimosis, balanitis, penile trauma, lack of neonatal circumcision, HIV infection, human papillomavirus subtypes 16 and 18, smoking/chewing tobacco, and poor hygiene.

▶ CLINICAL ASSESSMENT

- Penile carcinoma typically presents with a skin abnormality or palpable lesion on the penis. The majority occur on the glans, in the coronal sulcus, or on the prepuce.
- Slow-growing lesions often result in delay in seeking medical attention and diagnosis; 25% of penile lesions are misdiagnosed as benign.
- Inguinal adenopathy is present in 30%–60% of cases at the time of diagnosis.
- Penile carcinoma should be suspected in men who present with a penile mass or ulcer, especially in those who have not been circumcised.

▶ DIAGNOSIS

- Biopsy is required for diagnostic confirmation.
- Benign-appearing lesions that do not resolve after 4–6 weeks of antibiotic, antifungal, or steroid therapy, or that progress at any time during treatment, should be biopsied using punch, excision, or incisional biopsy techniques.
- Biopsy of penile lesions should not be delayed in suspicious-appearing lesions or with a penile lesion with associated lymphadenopathy.

- The presence of other physical symptoms (eg, weight loss, confusion, cough, or bone pain) may indicate distant metastatic disease or associated metabolic abnormalities, such as hypercalcemia, and should prompt full laboratory and imaging evaluation.
- The tumor-node-metastases (TNM) system is used to define prognostic stage groups and establish the appropriate treatment plan.

▶ TREATMENT

- The 5-year survival rates for men with penile carcinoma are 85% for early disease (stage I/II) and 59% for advanced-stage cancers.
- Excision of the primary tumor as treatment depends on whether the lesion can be adequately excised with negative margins with limited excision and still preserve penile form or function or both.
  - For bulky-stage T2 to T4 primary tumors, primary tumor control essentially requires amputation to achieve tumor-free margins.
- Alternative organ-preserving strategies should be reserved for men with small, low-stage primary penile tumors.
- Choice of treatment approach depends upon the provider expertise and patient preference.
  - Available options include topical therapy (fluorouracil and imiquimod), laser ablation, total glans resurfacing (TGS), Mohs micrographic surgery (MMS), and penile radiation therapy (RT; external beam or interstitial brachytherapy).
- Characteristics of the primary tumor (eg, grade, stage, lymphovascular invasion, perineural invasion) as well as the presence or absence of palpable inguinal nodes determines the need for additional surgical staging and subsequent treatment of the regional lymph nodes.
- **Patients** with locally advanced disease (eg, unresectable primary tumor and/or bulky lymphadenopathy, recurrent or metastatic disease) should be treated initially with systemic or multimodal therapy rather than surgery or RT alone.

CHAPTER 114

Traumatic Disorders of the Male Reproductive System

Ryan Olivero, MMS, PA-C

GENERAL FEATURES

- Severe trauma to the male genitalia is rare, comprising <0.25% of total trauma activations in the United States.
- It can result in devastating long-term morbidity and can lead to permanent loss of function and disability.
- Firearm injuries and stab wounds account for >90% of all penetrating traumas.
- Blunt trauma most often occurs while riding motorcycles or bicycles, or while playing sports.
- Sexual injuries such as penile fracture are also common.
- The tunica albuginea is the fascial layer composed of collagen and elastin that surrounds both the penis and the testicles.
- In blunt traumas, the intracavernosal or intratesticular pressure exceeds the strength of the surrounding tunica albuginea, resulting in fracture or tear.

CLINICAL ASSESSMENT

- Blunt injuries will most often present with severe pain, ecchymosis, and swelling.
- Penile injuries may have a classic "eggplant deformity," which results in swelling and ecchymosis; patients may also note the presence of a "snap-pop" sensation.
- Other symptoms may include hematuria, dysuria, and urinary retention, and blood may be present at the penile meatus.
- Urethral injuries are common.

DIAGNOSIS

- Diagnosis is often clinical based on history and physical examination.
- Imaging studies may also help isolate the exact location of injury, which can assist in the intraoperative repair.

- Ultrasound is the fastest and most cost-effective form of imaging, though accuracy is operator dependent.
- CT and MRI are more accurate, though more expensive and time-consuming.
- The American Urological Association recommends intraoperative cystoscopy be performed to rule out urethral injury, which can occur in 15%–20% of patients with penile injury.

TREATMENT

- Mild injuries with negative imaging studies require no intervention.
- Moderate-to-severe injuries will likely require prompt surgical intervention/exploration or cystoscopy.
- Cystoscopy is the modality of choice to evaluate urethral injuries.
- Urinary catheter placement, if indicated, should take place under cystoscopy guidance to avoid further damage to the penis or the urethra.
- During open surgical exploration, the tunica is repaired in a primary manner with absorbable suture.
- Surgical exploration and repair of the tunica and any urethral injuries within 8 hours of injury significantly reduces but does not eliminate chronic complications.
  - Hemostasis should be achieved, and any hematomas evacuated.
  - The vas deferens should be inspected and repaired if possible.
- Chronic complications include, but are not limited to, erectile dysfunction, curvature of the penis, painful erections, reduced penile length, chronic pain, infertility, swelling, poor self-image, and anxiety.

CHAPTER
115

Benign Prostatic Hyperplasia

Matthew Steidl, MPAS

▶ GENERAL FEATURES

- Benign prostatic hyperplasia (BPH) is a proliferation of smooth muscle and epithelial cells within the prostatic transition zone that leads to prostatic enlargement and potential obstruction of the urethra at the level of the bladder neck.
- BPH is very common and becomes increasing prevalent after age 40 years, with autopsy proven the presence in 60% of men at age 60 years and 80% of men at age 80 years.
- Some studies indicate a genetic component to the risk of developing BPH, but additional risk factors are not well understood.

▶ CLINICAL ASSESSMENT

- BPH with obstruction often leads to the development of bothersome lower urinary tract symptoms (LUTS).
- LUTS are subdivided into:
  - Obstructive symptoms: urinary hesitancy, straining to void, weak stream, intermittency of the urine stream, postvoid dribbling, prolonged voiding, and incomplete bladder emptying
  - Irritative symptoms: urinary frequency, urgency, nocturia, and urge incontinence
- History may also include medications contributing to symptoms, such as sympathomimetic drugs, opioids, antihistamines, muscle relaxants, tricyclic antidepressants, antispasmodics, and diuretics.
- Digital rectal examination (DRE) should be performed to rule out prostate nodules, induration, or masses that may indicate the presence of prostate cancer.
- Unfortunately, a DRE is unreliable in estimating prostate size, and prostatic size on DRE correlates poorly with symptoms.

▶ DIAGNOSIS

- The American Urological Association Symptom Index (AUA-SI), a seven-question validated, self-administered questionnaire, should be used to objectively quantify the patient's symptom burden and monitor patient response to therapy.
- Urinalysis may help rule out other causes of LUTS, such as glucosuria, proteinuria, hematuria, and infection.
- Measurement of a postvoid residual bladder volume with a bladder scanning device is optional but helpful in ruling out significant urinary retention.
- Prostate-specific antigen (PSA) testing may be considered in patients with a life expectancy of >10 years if there is concern for prostate cancer, and the results would change management.
- Prostate imaging and/or cystoscopy may be indicated for patients who fail to improve or when other causes of symptoms are suspected.

▶ TREATMENT

- Observation and behavioral changes may be sufficient for men with mild-to-moderate symptoms.
- Medical management includes:
  - α-blockers: relax the smooth muscle of the prostate
  - 5-α-reductase inhibitors: block the conversion of testosterone to dihydrotestosterone, causing a reduction in prostate size
  - Phosphodiesterase-5 inhibitor tadalafil is approved for the treatment of both BPH and erectile dysfunction with minimal adverse effects.
- A well-designed, randomized, double-blind, placebo-controlled trial of saw palmetto for BPH did not improve symptoms when compared to placebo.
- Patients who fail medical therapy should be referred to a urology provider for further diagnostic workup and consideration of surgical therapy.
- Transurethral resection of the prostate remains the gold standard of minimally invasive surgical therapy.

CHAPTER 116

Prostate Cancer

Teresa Sanders, MPAS, PA-C

▶ GENERAL FEATURES

- Prostate cancer is one of the most prevalent cancers in men, with ~192 000 new cases and 33 000 deaths annually.
- For US men, the average lifetime risk of developing prostate cancer is ~12%.
- Risk factors for developing prostate cancer include:
  - Age >50 years
  - Family history (in first-degree relative or female relatives with *BRCA*-associated breast cancer)
  - African American ancestry
  - Diet high in animal fat and low in vegetables
- Prostate-specific antigen (PSA) screening:
  - Guidelines differ among professional organizations; discussions regarding risks vs. benefits of prostate cancer screening should begin at age 50 (or age 40-45 in high-risk men).
  - Benefits:
    - May identify aggressive prostate cancer early, when curative treatment is more likely
    - May reduce the risk of death from prostate cancer
  - Risks:
    - May lead to an unnecessary invasive biopsy with potential risks, including infection, pain, hematuria, and difficulty urinating
    - May lead to over-diagnosis of prostate cancer that would never become life-limiting or symptomatic
- For patients desiring screening, PSA levels should be checked every 2 years until age 69. Prostate cancer screening is not recommended in men who are ≥70 years.

▶ CLINICAL ASSESSMENT

- Early localized disease is typically asymptomatic.
- Advanced localized disease can cause lower urinary tract symptoms, such as urinary hesitancy, weak stream, straining to urinate, prolonged urination, incomplete bladder emptying, dribbling, urinary frequency, urgency, urge incontinence, nocturia, hematuria, or hematospermia.
- Metastatic disease may cause additional symptoms, such as fatigue, unintentional weight loss, back pain, pelvic pain, or other areas of bone pain.
- History may include family history of prostate cancer or *BRCA*-associated breast cancer in blood relatives.
- Digital rectal examination findings may be normal or may reveal a hardened and/or asymmetric prostate with discrete nodules or areas of induration.

▶ DIAGNOSIS

- Definitive diagnosis is made by prostate biopsy.
- If prostate cancer is suspected, refer to urology to determine appropriateness of a transrectal ultrasound (TRUS)–guided biopsy and/or other diagnostic testing.
- Laboratory findings may reveal elevated PSA: typically ≥4.0 ng/mL; adjust for patients on a 5-α-reductase inhibitor (finasteride/dutasteride).
- In more advanced/metastatic disease, laboratory workup may reveal anemia, renal dysfunction from urinary outflow obstruction, or elevated alkaline phosphatase if bone metastases are present.

▶ TREATMENT

- Initial treatment options include:
  - Observation for patients with low-risk disease
  - Surgical intervention by radical prostatectomy, with or without pelvic lymph node dissection
  - Radiation therapy including brachytherapy or external beam radiation, typically in combination with 18–36 months of androgen-deprivation therapy (ie, leuprolide injections)
- If prostate cancer metastasizes or recurs after definitive treatment, lifelong androgen-deprivation therapy is indicated, with or without hormonal therapies or IV chemotherapy, at the direction of a medical oncologist.

CHAPTER 117

Prostatitis

Natalie Schirato, MPAS, PA-C

▶ GENERAL FEATURES

- Prostatitis is an infectious or inflammatory condition of the prostate that may be acute or chronic.
- Acute and chronic bacterial prostatitis typically results from ascending bacteria (most commonly Gram-negative pathogens, specifically *Escherichia coli*) in the urinary tract.

- *Neisseria gonorrhoeae* and *Chlamydia trachomatis* should be considered in patients aged <35 years.
  - In nosocomial infections, *Pseudomonas aeruginosa* and enterococci should be considered.
- Chronic abacterial prostatitis, also known as *chronic pelvic pain syndrome*, has a poorly understood etiology; it may initially have an infectious cause and likely involves functional or structural pathology.
- Asymptomatic prostatitis is an inflammatory condition with causes similar to chronic abacterial prostatitis; patients are asymptomatic, and diagnosis is typically made incidentally after prostate biopsy.

▶ CLINICAL ASSESSMENT

- Acute bacterial prostatitis:
  - Patients may report a combination of fever, chills, low back pain, malaise, myalgias, perineal pain, prostatodynia, urinary frequency, urinary urgency, dysuria, nocturia, weak stream, hesitancy, incomplete bladder emptying, and dysuria.
  - Physical examination may reveal a tender, hot, nodular, boggy prostate on digital rectal examination (DRE), with or without suprapubic abdominal tenderness; avoid prostate massage when acute bacterial prostatitis is suspected.
- Chronic bacterial prostatitis:
  - Patients often lack systemic symptoms, but may experience perineal pain, prostatodynia, hematospermia, intermittent dysuria, intermittent urinary frequency, and intermittent incomplete bladder emptying.
  - Physical examination may be a normal between acute episodes. Prostate may be nodular, tender, or even normal on DRE.
- Chronic abacterial prostatitis:
  - Patients may present with pelvic pain (perineal, suprapubic, rectal, urethral, or scrotal), urinary frequency, dysuria, incomplete bladder emptying, painful ejaculation, hematospermia, or erectile dysfunction.
  - Physical examination may reveal a tight anal sphincter and a mildly tender or normal prostate on DRE.
- Physical examination in patients with asymptomatic prostatitis usually reveals a normal prostate on DRE.

▶ DIAGNOSIS

- Urinalysis in patients with acute bacterial prostatitis may reveal white blood cells and bacteria; these may also be present in chronic bacterial prostatitis but tend to be lower in number.

- Urine culture may identify the causative organism, most often *E. coli*; urine culture may be negative in patients with chronic bacterial prostatitis and will be negative in patients with chronic abacterial prostatitis and asymptomatic prostatitis.
- Prostate-specific antigen (PSA) may be elevated but should not be used to diagnose prostatitis.
- Transrectal ultrasonography or CT scan of the pelvis is not recommended for the diagnosis of prostatitis but can be used to diagnose prostatic calculi or prostatic abscess, an uncommon complication of acute bacterial prostatitis.
- Prostate biopsy specimen histology will show incidental inflammation in patients with chronic prostatitis and asymptomatic prostatitis, but prostate biopsy should not be used for diagnosis.

▶ TREATMENT

- Urethral or suprapubic catheterization may be required in patients with obstruction and urinary retention secondary to prostatitis, warranting a urology consultation.
- Acute bacterial prostatitis:
  - First-line therapy should be directed at Gram-negative organisms (may include fluoroquinolones, trimethoprim-sulfamethoxazole, or ampicillin plus gentamicin) and tailored based on culture results when available.
  - Prolonged treatment (up to 6 weeks) may be required based on severity and patient response.
  - α-blockers may also be used to relieve urinary obstruction.
  - Supportive care may include fluids, analgesics, and antipyretics.
- Chronic bacterial prostatitis:
  - First-line therapy is a fluoroquinolone for 4–6 weeks.
  - Second-line therapy is trimethoprim-sulfamethoxazole for 4–6 weeks.
  - Analgesics, α-blockers, and sitz baths may help alleviate symptoms.
  - Transurethral resection of the prostate should be considered if prostatic calculi are involved.
- Chronic abacterial prostatitis:
  - Treatment is challenging and often trial and error for alleviation of symptoms.
  - Antibiotics are not recommended.
  - α-Blockers are controversial, and studies have shown little benefit; anti-inflammatories and sitz baths may be helpful.
- No treatment is indicated for asymptomatic prostatitis.

CHAPTER 118

Cryptorchidism

Ryan Clancy, MSHS, MA, PA-C, DFAAPA

▶ GENERAL FEATURES

- One of the most common genitourinary conditions in infants defined by one or both testicles failing to descend into the hemiscrotum
- Occurs in 2%–8% of newborns; occurs unilaterally in two-thirds and bilaterally in one-third of those affected
- Risk factors that have been suggested include family history of cryptorchidism, premature birth, low birth weight, Down syndrome, maternal smoking, maternal gestational diabetes, maternal alcohol use, and maternal analgesic use.
- Left untreated, half of all cases of undescended testicles may spontaneously descend within the first 3 months of the infant's life.
- Without treatment, patients are at an increased lifetime risk of testicular germ cell cancer (1% risk), inguinal hernias, and testicular torsion in the nondescended side.

▶ CLINICAL ASSESSMENT

- Gestational history may reveal the presence of risk factors, and family history may reveal parent of sibling with history of cryptorchidism.
- Diagnosis is typically made by physical examination:
  - Approximately 70% of undescended testicle cases are palpable in the inguinal canal or upper scrotum.
  - Defect may be found in the abdominal cavity, abdominal wall, or inguinal canal.
- Presence of additional abnormalities such as hypospadias or micropenis should raise suspicion for disorders of sexual development (DSD).

▶ DIAGNOSIS

- Referral to a surgical specialist should be made for diagnostic confirmation and treatment of the disorder.
- Use of ultrasound and other imaging studies is not recommended before referral to a specialist.
- Additional hormone blood tests and/or genetic testing may be useful in diagnosing DSD.

▶ TREATMENT

- Surgical repair of an undescended testicle is usually performed by a urologist during the patient's first 6–12 months of life and reduces the risk of complications and infertility.
- Orchiopexy is the standard surgical treatment of cryptorchidism and is utilized to reposition the testis within the scrotal sac.
- Hormonal therapy is discouraged as response rates are very low.

CHAPTER 119

Testicular Torsion

Bart Gillum, DSc, MHS, PA-C

▶ GENERAL FEATURES

- Testicular torsion is a urologic emergency occurring when the testicle twists within the scrotum, partially or completely obstructing testicular venous return and/or arterial flow and potentially leading to testicular ischemia.

- Bimodal age distribution: neonatal and during adolescence but can occur at any age
- "Bell-clapper" deformity, in which the testis is inadequately fixed to the tunica vaginalis within the anterior scrotum, is a common anatomic predisposition to torsion.

▶ CLINICAL ASSESSMENT

- Often presents with acute onset of testicular pain and swelling, nausea and vomiting, and lower abdominal or inguinal pain; young children may present only with lower abdominal pain and nausea/vomiting.
- Often occurs during REM sleep due to cremasteric contraction, waking the patient from sleep
- May be associated with trauma or strenuous activity
- Intermittent testicular torsion may cause acute pain with rapid resolution.
- Physical examination findings include:
  - Exquisitely tender testis
  - High-riding testicle with long axis oriented horizontally as opposed to vertically
  - Absence of cremasteric reflex
  - Testicular swelling/firmness
  - Tender mass superior to the testicle

▶ DIAGNOSIS

- Rapid diagnosis is vital; permanent ischemic changes can occur in 4–8 hours.

- Primarily a clinical diagnosis based on history and physical examination.
- Obtain a color Doppler ultrasound to evaluate testicular blood flow.

▶ TREATMENT

- Requires emergent surgery to save the affected testis. Includes de-torsion of the affected testis and fixation of both the testes to prevent future torsion of the contralateral testis
- Treatment within 4–6 hours of onset is associated with nearly 100% testicular viability, which decreases to almost 0% at 24 hours.
- If operative care is not immediately available, manual detorsion should be attempted.
  - Involves grasping the testicle and rotating it toward the thigh two full turns after appropriate pain medication
  - If pain does not resolve, try rotating the testicle in the opposite as up to one-third of torsions occur laterally instead of medially.
- Even after successful manual reduction restores blood flow, surgical exploration and fixation of both the testes is required to prevent future torsion.

CHAPTER

120

Hydrocele, Varicocele, and Testicular Cancer

Travis Layne, DMSc, MPAS, PA-C

▶ GENERAL FEATURES

- Hydrocele:
  - Refers to a collection of fluid in the scrotum; the most common cause of painless scrotal swelling
  - Communicating, noncommunicating, and reactive types:
    - Communicating implies a connection to the peritoneum via a patent processus vaginalis; diurnal variation in size; more common in children.
    - Noncommunicating types are more common in adults. Not usually variable in size.
    - Reactive can cause an acquired hydrocele due to injury, infection, or inflammatory etiologies. Testicular torsion can also present this way.

- Varicocele:
  - Cystic scrotal mass composed of varicose veins due to primary or secondary venous reflux.
  - Common condition with 10%–15% prevalence in the adult male population
  - Most commonly occurs on the left side (85%-95%) as the left spermatic vein enters the left renal vein at a 90° angle
  - Common cause of surgically correctable male infertility
- Testicular cancer:
  - Most common neoplasm in men aged 20–35 years
  - Usually presents with a painless testicular mass or nodule

- A 5-year survival is 90% with treatment.
- Major risk factors include cryptorchidism (40-fold increased risk) and family history.
- Most commonly occurs in the right testicle (also most common side for cryptorchidism)
- Germinal cell tumors (GCTs) account for 97% of testicular cancers and are usually malignant.
  - Two subtypes:
    - Seminoma (SGCT):
      - Most common in males aged 30–40 years
      - Lack tumor markers
      - Sensitive to radiation
      - Slow growing with stepwise spread
    - Nonseminomas (NSGCT):
      - Embryonal cell carcinoma, teratoma, and yolk sac
      - Most common in boys age <10 years
      - Choriocarcinoma has the worst prognosis.
      - Associated with increased tumor markers and radiation resistance
- Non-GCTs account for only 3% of testicular cancers.
  - Can spread hematogenously and cause pulmonary symptoms
  - Leydig cell tumors can be benign and can secrete androgen/estrogen, causing precocious puberty in children and gynecomastia and loss of libido in adults.
  - Sertoli cell tumors are also often benign. Can also secrete sexual hormones.
  - Other potential nongerminal types include gonadoblastoma and lymphoma.

CLINICAL ASSESSMENT

- Hydrocele:
  - Patient may present with an uncomfortable scrotal fullness or a painless scrotal mass found on self-examination.
  - Physical examination reveals a uniform collection of fluid upon inspection/palpation of the scrotum.
  - The mass will transilluminate when a light source is applied (differentiating it from nontransilluminating causes, such as varicocele or other solid mass).
  - Communicating-type hydrocele is made worse with Valsalva maneuver.
- Varicocele:
  - Often characterized by an irregular, palpable scrotal mass classically described as a "bag of worms"
    - Usually superior to the testicle
    - Worsens when the patient is upright or during a Valsalva maneuver
  - Usually painless but can cause a dull ache or heaviness
  - Atrophy of the testicle is possible because of cell death from increased scrotal pressure.

- Testicular cancer:
  - Patients typically experience a painless testicular nodule, solid mass, or enlargement of the testicle.
  - Dull aching or testicular heaviness may be present.
  - Hydroceles are present in 10% of cases.
  - Acute testicular pain (due to acute hemorrhage) occurs in a small percentage of patients.
  - Metastatic disease can present with back pain, cough, or lower extremity edema due to retroperitoneal spread, pulmonary metastases, or vena cava obstruction.
  - Physical examination may also reveal supraclavicular adenopathy, abdominal mass, or gynecomastia.

DIAGNOSIS

- Hydrocele:
  - Scrotal ultrasound confirms diagnosis and helps distinguish hydrocele from hernia or other solid mass/tumor.
  - Duplex ultrasound study may be useful if testicular torsion is suspected.
- Varicocele:
  - If not obvious by history and physical examination, an ultrasound can be used to confirm or to rule out other causes.
  - Sudden-onset left-sided varicocele in an older patient should raise suspicion for possible renal cell carcinoma, especially if not decompressing in the recumbent position, and warrants additional workup.
  - Unilateral right varicoceles are uncommon and warrant CT of the abdomen with contrast to rule out underlying retroperitoneal malignancy or venous thrombosis.
- Testicular cancer:
  - Scrotal ultrasound can differentiate intratesticular and extratesticular masses.
  - Useful labs include α-fetoprotein, β-hCG, and LDH.
    - β-hCG often elevated in nonseminomas (particularly choriocarcinomas).
    - α-Fetoprotein is usually also elevated in nonseminomas (with the exception of choriocarcinoma in the case of this tumor marker).
    - LDH may be elevated with either tumor type.
  - Diagnosis is made by biopsy and/or radical inguinal orchiectomy (with histologic diagnosis), followed by staging.
  - Obtaining CT scans of the chest, abdomen, and pelvis aid in disease staging.

TREATMENT

- Hydrocele:
  - Many noncommunicating hydroceles will resolve spontaneously within the first year of life; if not, eventual surgical repair may be needed.

- Communicating hydroceles typically require surgical repair.
- Reactive hydroceles will often resolve with primary treatment of the underlying etiology, and additional treatment is rarely necessary.
- Varicocele:
  - Observation is appropriate for most patients in the absence of intolerable symptoms, infertility, or concerning underlying etiology.
  - Surgery is required in some and involves either spermatic vein ligation or varicocelectomy.
- Testicular cancer:
  - Varies by tumor type and stage:

- Low-grade (stage 1) nonseminoma limited to the testes: orchiectomy with retroperitoneal lymph node dissection
- Low-grade seminoma: orchiectomy and radiation
- High-grade seminoma: debulking chemotherapy, orchiectomy, and radiation
  - Postoperative active surveillance is followed up every 2–6 months for the first 2 years and every 4–6 months in the third year.
- Surveillance includes a combination of tumor markers, chest x-ray, and abdominal/pelvic CT scans depending on the tumor type.
- 80% of relapses occur in the first 2 years.

CHAPTER 121

Epididymitis and Orchitis

Shaun Lynch, MS, MMSc, PA-C

▶ GENERAL FEATURES

- Epididymitis:
  - Acute inflammation of the epididymis, sometimes accompanied by inflammation of the testis (epididymo-orchitis), with symptoms occurring for <6 weeks
  - Most cases of acute epididymitis and epididymo-orchitis are due to infectious etiology.
    - In men aged <35 years, most cases are typically due to a sexually transmitted pathogen such as *Neisseria gonorrhoeae* or *Chlamydia trachomatis.*
    - In men aged >35 years, most cases are caused by *Escherichia coli* or other Gram-negative coliform bacteria and typically occur in patients with urologic abnormalities (eg, benign prostatic hyperplasia), indwelling catheters, or recent urologic procedures.
  - Less common noninfectious causes are due to local trauma or a retrograde flow of urine into the epididymis, causing chemical irritation.
- Orchitis:
  - Inflammation of the testes is usually due to infection; most cases are caused by viruses, most commonly the mumps virus.
  - Bacterial orchitis often results from infectious spread from the epididymis to the testis.

▶ CLINICAL ASSESSMENT

- Epididymitis:
  - History:
    - Acute onset of scrotal pain that is often unilateral and may extend into the groin; bilateral scrotal pain should raise the suspicion for other etiologies.
    - Patients may also report scrotal swelling on the affected side or involving the entire scrotum.
    - Urinary symptoms (such as dysuria, frequency, urgency, or urethral discharge) may be reported in serious bacterial infections or disseminated disease.
    - Associated fever, chills, and nausea may be reported in severe cases.
    - Other contributing factors may include recent unprotected sexual intercourse.
  - Physical examination:
    - Swelling, induration, and marked tenderness of a portion or of all the epididymis
    - Erythema, swelling, and tenderness of the scrotum can also be noted with the presence of a reactive hydrocele.
    - The spermatic cord may also be swollen and tender, and an inflammatory nodule may be felt as well.
    - Pain may be relieved by testicular elevation (Prehn sign).

- Cremasteric reflex is typically intact (stroking or pinching medial thigh causes contraction of cremaster muscle).
- Fever and tachycardia are uncommon in acute epididymitis and warrant admission and inpatient evaluation.
- Urethral discharge or crusting around the meatus in suspected cases of *N. gonorrhoeae* or *C. trachomatis*
- Orchitis:
  - Frequently occurs unilaterally but can spread bilaterally
  - Presents with testicular pain and edema and scrotal erythema
  - Systemic symptoms may include fever, malaise, headache, and myalgias.
  - In patients with mumps, symptoms or orchitis usually manifest 4–7 days after parotitis.
  - Testicular examination reveals tenderness, enlargement, and induration of the testis with erythema and edema of the scrotal skin.

▶ DIAGNOSIS

- Epididymitis:
  - Diagnosis is typically clinical based on history and physical examination.
  - The Centers for Disease Control and Prevention (CDC) recommends one of the following diagnostic tests be used to assist in diagnosing suspected cases of acute epididymitis:
    - Gram or methylene blue or gentian violet stain of urethral secretions demonstrating ≥2 white blood cells (WBCs) per oil immersion field
    - Positive leukocyte esterase test on first-void urine
    - Microscopic examination of sediment from a spun first-void urine demonstrating ≥10 WBC per high-power field
  - The CDC recommends urine as the preferred source for nucleic acid amplification testing for gonorrhea and chlamydia.
  - Radionuclide scanning is considered the most accurate approach for diagnosis, but it is not readily available in most settings.
  - Ultrasound scan of the scrotum including Doppler flow can confirm or rule out alternative diagnoses or complications, such as abscesses, tumors, or testicular torsion.

- Orchitis:
  - Typically a clinical diagnosis based on history and physical examination
  - Mumps can be confirmed by serum immunofluorescence antibody testing.

▶ TREATMENT

- Epididymitis:
  - Supportive measures:
    - Analgesia is often required, typically acetaminophen or nonsteroidal anti-inflammatory drugs are helpful.
    - Ice packs, rest from athletic activity, warm to hot water baths, and scrotal elevation are helpful adjuncts to decrease inflammation and pain.
  - Antibiotic therapy:
    - If gonorrhea and/or chlamydia are suspected pathogens, treatment based on CDC guidelines should include a single dose of ceftriaxone 250 mg intramuscular injection plus doxycycline 100 mg orally twice daily for 10 days.
    - If enteric pathogens are suspected or confirmed (eg, *E. coli*), a quinolone such as ofloxacin 300 mg by mouth twice daily for 10 days or levofloxacin 500 mg by mouth once daily for 10 days can be used.
  - Complete resolution of symptoms may take up to 6 weeks.
  - Treatment of nonbacterial epididymitis is conservative utilizing the supportive measures outlined earlier without antibiotic therapy and usually progresses to a chronic condition.
  - Referral should be considered to an urologist with persistent symptoms such as pain and swelling or signs of infection despite antibiotic therapy.
- Orchitis:
  - Typically self-limited and resolves over the course of 7–10 days
  - Managed with supportive care that includes rest, over-the-counter analgesia, ice or heat, and scrotal elevation to minimize pain
  - Bacterial orchitis is treated with antibiotic coverage targeting pathogens causing acute epididymitis.

Urinary Tract Infections and Pyelonephritis

Sarah Neguse, PA-C

A 27-year-old woman with a sulfa allergy presents to the emergency department with sudden onset of left-sided flank pain, fever, chills, and vomiting. For the past 3 days, she reports dysuria and increased urinary frequency. A dipstick urinalysis reveals leukocyte esterase, trace hematuria, and nitrites.

▶ GENERAL FEATURES

- Urinary tract infections (UTIs) typically involve urethritis (inflammation/infection of the urethra), cystitis (infection of the urinary bladder), and/or pyelonephritis (infection of the kidney).
- Infections generally begin in the lower urinary tract and ascend to one or both kidneys via the ureters.
- If not treated properly, it can cause permanent kidney damage or bacteremia, leading to sepsis.
- Most common causative agents are Gram-negative bacteria, especially *Escherichia coli*; other less common pathogens include *Proteus*, *Klebsiella*, *Pseudomonas*, *Enterococci*, and *Staphylococci*.
- Risk factors for UTIs and pyelonephritis include immunosuppression, foreign body in urinary tract (such as a calculus or catheter), anatomic or functional urinary abnormality, sexual intercourse, pregnancy, and diabetes.
- Two categories:
  - Acute uncomplicated:
    - Mild-to-moderate illness in a patient without underlying disease
    - Majority of acute uncomplicated cases occur in healthy women aged 18–40 years.
  - Acute complicated:
    - Patient has an underlying condition that increases risk of therapy failing.

- Diabetes, pregnancy, renal transplant, acute kidney injury, chronic kidney disease, functional or anatomic urinary tract abnormality

▶ CLINICAL ASSESSMENT

- Urethritis and cystitis typically present with dysuria, urinary frequency, and/or urinary urgency. Patients may report changes in urine color (including hematuria), turbidity, or odor.
- Patients with pyelonephritis may report flank or back pain, fever, chills, nausea, or vomiting, with or without preceding symptoms of UTI.
- Young children may present with fever and/or abdominal pain.
- Less common, patients may present in sepsis or acute renal failure.
- Physical examination may be unremarkable in the setting of urethritis and cystitis or may be notable for fever and/or suprapubic tenderness.
- Physical examination in the setting of pyelonephritis may be notable for fever, abdominal tenderness, and/or costovertebral angle (CVA) tenderness to percussion.

▶ DIAGNOSIS

- Clean-catch, mid-stream urine sample for urinalysis and culture with antimicrobial susceptibility is the preferred initial test.
- Dipstick urinalysis may show signs of bacteriuria (nitrites, leukocyte esterase, visible bacteria), pyuria (increased white blood cells), and/or varying degrees of hematuria.
- Culture may reveal >100 000 CFU/mL bacterial colony count of the offending organism.
- Microscopic urinalysis may show white blood cell casts in pyelonephritis.

- Imaging is not routinely required for diagnosis but may be useful in complicated cases or when obstruction is suspected; obstructive hydronephrosis (found on ultrasound or CT scan) in the setting of UTI often requires intervention.

▶ TREATMENT

- Outpatient management is acceptable for mild-to-moderate illness in patients who can be stabilized with rehydration and antibiotics and have adequate follow-up.
- Admission should be considered for patients with complications, urinary tract obstruction, or signs of sepsis.
- Empiric antibiotic therapy should begin in suspected or confirmed disease before urine culture sensitivity results based on local resistance patterns.
- Nitrofurantoin is an acceptable first-line agent for uncomplicated cystitis (though it is not appropriate for pyelonephritis).

- Treatment options for pyelonephritis include an oral fluoroquinolone for 5–7 days, oral sulfamethoxazole/trimethoprim 160/800 mg daily for 7–10 days. If susceptibility is not yet known, an initial dose of a long-acting parenteral antibiotic such as ceftriaxone may be administered in conjunction with the oral antibiotic.

Case Conclusion

This patient presents with classic symptoms of acute pyelonephritis (sudden-onset flank pain, fever, nausea, and vomiting accompanied by symptoms suggestive of cystitis). Urinalysis was consistent with pyelonephritis. Although urine culture must be obtained, empiric treatment with a 7-day course of ciprofloxacin can be initiated for this acute, uncomplicated case.

CHAPTER 123

Urinary Incontinence and Overactive Bladder

Amy M. Klingler, MS, PA-C, DFAAPA

▶ GENERAL FEATURES

- Risk factors for women: parity, obesity, urinary urgency and frequency, functional or cognitive impairment limiting access to toilet, and family history
- Risk factors for men: benign prostatic hypertrophy (BPH), bladder outlet obstruction, functional and cognitive impairment, neurologic disorders, and history of prostatectomy
- Neurogenic bladder is commonly associated with a large postvoid residual (PVR) urine volume and urinary incontinence.
- Types of urinary incontinence:
  - Overflow incontinence: leakage of urine associated with urinary retention and bladder distention
  - Urge incontinence: involuntary loss of urine associated with a sudden involuntary bladder contraction, causing the abrupt need (or urge) to void. More common in women than men
    - Overactive bladder (OAB) involves urinary urgency with or without incontinence. Associated with urinary frequency and nocturia. Urge incontinence and OAB with incontinence can be used interchangeably.

  - Stress incontinence: involuntary leakage of urine with activity such as physical activity, coughing, or sneezing
  - Mixed incontinence: involves a combination of both urge and stress incontinence
  - Functional incontinence: the involuntary loss of urine due to a physical or mental impairment preventing the recognition of the need to urinate

▶ CLINICAL ASSESSMENT

- Review risk factors and obtain a detailed history.
- Review for medications associated with incontinence and OAB: antidepressants, diuretics, bronchodilators, and antihistamines.
- Physical examination includes functional assessment and evaluation of cognition.
- Perform a rectal examination to assess neurologic deficit, constipation, and bulbocavernosus reflex in all patients and the prostate in men.
- Obtain PVR to rule out incomplete voiding secondary to neurogenic bladder or outflow obstruction.
- In women, document estrogen status and perform a vaginal examination to assess pelvic floor strength and rule out cystocele, rectocele, or enterocele.

DIAGNOSIS

- Diagnosis is based on patient history and physical examination; further testing can rule out other treatable causes of incontinence.
- Laboratory tests should include urinalysis with culture, if indicated; urine cytology if tumor is suspected; glucose, BUN, and creatinine to rule out diabetes and evaluate kidney function.
- Imaging with ultrasound or CT can rule out a pelvic mass.

TREATMENT

- Treatment is directed at the type and cause of incontinence.
- First-line treatments for women with urinary incontinence or OAB may include lifestyle changes and complementary therapies, such as weight loss, pelvic floor strengthening, bladder training, and treatment of vaginal atrophy in women and BPH in men.

- For women who fail conservative treatments or who prefer to use medications: antimuscarinic drugs such as tolterodine, oxybutynin, darifenacin solifenacin, fesoterodine, or trospium can be effective.
  - These medications can have dose-dependent side effects, such as dry mouth, tachycardia, drowsiness, decrease in cognitive function, inhibition of gut motility, and constipation.
  - For patients who fail treatment with antimuscarinics, the β-3 adrenoreceptor agonist mirabegron may be effective.
- In men, an α-blocker (terazosin, doxazosin, tamsulosin, alfuzosin, silodosin) alone or combination with an α-reductase inhibitor (finasteride, dutasteride) can reduce OAB and lower urinary tract symptoms. Men can also be treated with antimuscarinics.
- For refractory OAB, sacral neuromodulation or cystoscopy-guided botulinum toxin injection into the detrusor muscle may be effective.

CHAPTER
124

Urolithiasis and Nephrolithiasis

Melissa Johnson Chung, MMS, PA-C

GENERAL FEATURES

- Urolithiasis is stones formed or located anywhere in the urinary system, including the kidneys and bladder.
- Five major types of stones are calcium oxalate, calcium phosphate, struvite, uric acid, and cystine; 80% of patients form calcium stones.
- Epidemiology:
  - Male-to-female ratio is 2:1.
  - Increased incidence in white patients
  - Increased incidence in areas of high humidity and elevated temperatures
  - Southeastern United States is considered the "stone belt."
- Risk factors:
  - Previous history of stone formation, family history of stones, hypertension, obesity, diabetes, gout, and history of gastric bypass or bariatric surgery
  - Dietary factors include low fluid intake; low calcium intake; high intake of oxalate, animal protein, or sodium; and high intake of vitamin C (men only).
- Noncalcium stones:
  - Cystine stones:
    - Genetic predisposition: cystinuria should be suspected in patients presenting with their first stone during childhood or adolescence.
    - Pathognomonic hexagonal crystals on urinalysis

- Uric acid stones:
  - Radiolucent
  - Urinary pH of 5.5 or less
  - Associated conditions: gout, chronic diarrhea, diabetes, myeloproliferative disorders, malignancies, excessive purine ingestion, abrupt and dramatic weight loss
- Struvite stones:
  - Form in the presence of an upper urinary tract infection with a urease-producing organism
  - Alkaline urinary pH (typically >7)
  - "Coffin-lid" crystals in the urine sediment
  - Can grow rapidly and develop into staghorn calculi

CLINICAL ASSESSMENT

- History:
  - Classic presentation:
    - Acute severe unilateral flank pain
    - Nausea with or without vomiting
    - Hematuria
  - Pain:
    - Dull ache to severe colic
    - Typically paroxysmal
    - Pain waxes and wanes
    - Severe pain usually lasts 20–60 minutes

- May radiate to the lower abdomen, groin, ipsilateral testicle or labium, or tip of penis
- Physical examination findings:
  - Classic patient with urolithiasis is writhing in pain and constantly moving, trying to find a comfortable position.
  - The patient may have costovertebral angle tenderness.
  - Abdominal examination typically is unremarkable.

▶ DIAGNOSIS

- Differential diagnosis:
  - Pyelonephritis, renal cell carcinoma, ectopic pregnancy, ovarian torsion or cyst rupture, acute abdominal aneurysm, acute intestinal obstruction, pancreatitis, diverticulitis, appendicitis, biliary colic, cholecystitis, acute mesenteric ischemia, herpes zoster, and mechanical back pain
- Diagnosis:
  - Urinalysis:
    - Detection of microscopic or gross hematuria (70%-90% of patients)
    - Assessment of urinary pH
  - The gold standard is noncontrast helical CT, which can detect both stones and evidence of obstruction. Stone density can help determine stone type.
  - Additional diagnostic studies:
    - Abdominal radiograph: will only identify sufficiently large, radiopaque stones
    - Abdominal ultrasound: procedure of choice for patients who should avoid radiation
    - IV pyelogram: no longer the procedure of choice because of potential contrast reactions, lower sensitivity, and higher radiation exposure compared with noncontrast helical CT

▶ TREATMENT

- Acute management:
  - Conservative treatment:
    - Hydration
    - Pain management using NSAIDs or opioids
    - Straining urine
    - Patients can be managed at home if they are able to take oral medications and fluids.
  - Stone passage:
    - Stones of 5 mm or smaller diameter frequently pass spontaneously.
    - Stones of 10 mm or greater diameter and proximal ureteral stones are unlikely to pass spontaneously.
  - Medical expulsive therapy:
    - α-Blockers and calcium channel blockers have been shown to facilitate the passage of stones <10 mm in diameter.

- Most providers prescribe tamsulosin 0.4 mg daily and reimage in 4 weeks.
  - Surgical options:
    - Shock wave lithotripsy
    - Ureteroscopic lithotripsy
    - Percutaneous nephrolithotomy
    - Laparoscopic stone removal
    - Open surgical stone removal
  - Urology consultation:
    - Urgent for patients with urosepsis, acute renal failure, anuria, or unyielding pain, nausea, or vomiting
    - Outpatient for patients with stones 10 mm or greater in diameter or patients with smaller stones who have failed to pass the stone after a trial of conservative management with or without expulsive therapy
- Subsequent management:
  - Focused history of the patient's dietary habits, supplements, medications, and family history
  - Stone composition analysis (if available)
  - Laboratory testing:
    - Assessment of renal function and calcium levels
    - Intact parathyroid hormone (PTH) level if calcium is elevated or high normal
    - Primary hyperparathyroidism is associated with urolithiasis/nephrolithiasis.
  - Two 24-hour urine collections:
    - 1–2 months after stone event or intervention
    - Patients should maintain their usual diet, fluid intake, and physical activities before collection.
  - Long-term dietary modifications (calcium stones):
    - Increase the intake of fluid, dietary calcium, and potassium.
    - Decrease the intake of oxalate, animal protein, sucrose, fructose, sodium, supplemental calcium, and supplemental vitamin C (men).
  - Monitor for the formation of new stones with abdominal radiograph or ultrasound at 1 year, then every 2–4 years if negative.
- Treatment of noncalcium stones:
  - Cystine stones:
    - Urinary alkalization with potassium citrate
    - Increase fluid intake
    - Reduction in sodium and protein intake
  - Uric acid stones:
    - Urinary alkalization with potassium citrate
    - Increase fluid intake
    - Reduce uric acid production by reducing purine intake or using a xanthine oxidase inhibitor such as allopurinol
  - Struvite stones: surgical therapy is required to treat struvite stones in almost all cases.

Bladder Prolapse, Vesicoureteral Reflux, and Urethral Prolapse and Stricture

Lauren Stanford, MPAS

▶ GENERAL FEATURES

- Bladder prolapse:
  - Cystocele occurs when the bladder pushes against the wall of the vagina and commonly affects older females.
  - Risk factors include pregnancy, childbirth, and increases in intra-abdominal pressure.
- Vesicoureteral reflux (VUR):
  - Occurs when urine passes from the bladder ureter or renal pelvis
  - Commonly due to congenital anomalies of the ureterovesical junction
  - It may occur if bladder outlet obstruction or dysfunctional voiding increases bladder pressure significantly.
  - Bacteria that travel up the ureter can contribute to upper urinary tract infections (UTIs) and subsequent scarring, sometimes leading to renal dysfunction.
- Urethral prolapse:
  - Occurs when the urethra falls and is apparent at the urethral meatus
  - It is a rare condition, more common in young girls and postmenopausal women.
  - The exact cause is unknown.
- Urethral stricture: narrowing of the urethra, often due to scarring from trauma, ischemia, or inflammation; more common in males

▶ CLINICAL ASSESSMENT

- Bladder prolapse:
  - Many patients are asymptomatic.
  - May cause a sensation of pelvic or vaginal fullness or pressure; patients sometimes feel that their organs are "falling out."
  - May also report dyspareunia and/or stress urinary incontinence
  - Physical examination is notable for visible or palpable bulge/prolapsing tissue to or past the vaginal opening on pelvic examination, often worsening with Valsalva or coughing.
- VUR:
  - Children with VUR may present with frequent UTIs.
  - The child may have fever, abdominal pain, dysuria, urgency, and urinary incontinence.
  - Patients with VUR may have a history of fetal hydronephrosis.

- Urethral prolapse:
  - Prepubertal girls with urethral prolapse are frequently asymptomatic.
  - The most common presentation is vaginal bleeding.
  - Postmenopausal women are commonly symptomatic with vaginal bleeding and voiding symptoms, such as urinary frequency or urgency.
- Urethral stricture:
  - Patients with urethral strictures may be asymptomatic or have pain due to urinary retention.
  - Obstructive voiding symptoms, such as a diminished stream, urinary dribbling, and incomplete bladder emptying, and UTIs, are common.

▶ DIAGNOSIS

- Bladder prolapse: clinical diagnosis not requiring additional tests or imaging
- VUR:
  - Voiding cystourethrography (VCUG) findings graded from mild to severe (grades I-V).
  - Ultrasound of the kidneys, ureters, and bladder may be obtained as well as a radioisotope scan.
  - Urinalysis and urine culture may reveal recurrent infection.
- Urethral prolapse:
  - Easy to diagnose by physical examination
  - It appears as a doughnut-shaped protrusion at the urethral meatus; the tissue is often tender and ulcerated.
  - It should be distinguished from other conditions by visualizing a central opening in the tissue and appropriately identifying the urethral meatus.
- Urethral stricture:
  - Diagnosis relies on history, physical examination, and imaging.
  - The preferred imaging technique is retrograde urethrogram (RUG). Images can identify the severity and location of the stricture.
  - An ultrasound scan may be useful, as well as endoscopy with a flexible or rigid cystourethroscopy.

▶ TREATMENT

- Bladder prolapse:
  - Mild cases may be treated with pelvic floor muscle exercises (such as Kegel exercises).
  - Pessaries may be inserted into the vagina to support the bladder.

- Moderate-to-severe cases that are unresponsive to conservative treatment may require reconstructive or obliterative surgery.
- VUR:
  - If mild to moderate, VUR may spontaneously resolve.
  - Active infection must be treated, and antibiotic prophylaxis with trimethoprim/sulfamethoxazole, nitrofurantoin, or cephalexin, may be considered.
  - Severe reflux is treated with anticholinergic drugs and surgery in persistent cases.

- Urethral prolapse:
  - Asymptomatic urethral prolapse is treated with sitz baths and topical hormones.
  - Occasionally, topical antibiotics or steroids may be applied.
  - Symptomatic urethral prolapse is treated by surgical excision.
- Urethral stricture: surgical intervention is recommended for patients with severe symptoms, which may include dilating the urethra, releasing or excising scar tissue, or placing permanent urethral stents.

CHAPTER 126

Bladder Cancer

Natalie Schirato, MPAS, PA-C

▶ GENERAL FEATURES

- Defined as a primary malignancy in the urinary bladder; can be transitional cell carcinoma (90%), squamous cell carcinoma (8%), or adenocarcinoma (2%)
- Second-most common urologic malignancy
- Classified as superficial (70%-80%) or invasive (20%) at presentation
- Incidence increases with age (median age of diagnosis is 73 years); more common in males and more common in Caucasian than Asian or African American patients.
- Smoking is the highest risk factor; other risk factors include occupational exposure to carcinogens, history of radiation to the pelvis, history of chronic urinary tract infections (UTIs), history of chronic indwelling urinary catheter, high-fat diet, and history of schistosomiasis.

▶ CLINICAL ASSESSMENT

- About 80% of patients present with painless gross hematuria.
- About 30% of patients present with irritative voiding symptoms (frequency, urgency, dysuria).
- A secondary UTI may be present in up to 30% of patients.
- Physical examination is often unremarkable, but patients may have an abdominal or pelvic mass in advanced disease.
- Patients with advanced disease may also have flank pain, bone pain, or lower extremity edema.

▶ DIAGNOSIS

- Urinalysis may be notable for microscopic (3+ red blood cells per high-power field) or gross hematuria.

The incidence of bladder cancer in patients with microscopic or gross hematuria is 2% and 20%, respectively.
- Urine culture to rule out UTI as cause of symptoms. However, concurrent infection may occur, and level of suspicion should remain high in patients with persistent hematuria following complete treatment of UTI.
- Urine cytology should be performed in any adult patient with hematuria and can be done with voided urine or bladder washing.
  - Cytology is more sensitive in high-grade tumors.
  - Fluorescence in situ hybridization (FISH) may improve accuracy.
- Other urine tumor markers have been used, but none have been found to be sensitive enough to rule out bladder cancer.
- Cystoscopy with biopsy or transurethral resection of bladder tumor (TURBT) is the gold standard for diagnosis and must be performed for hematuria evaluation in all adult patients.
- Ultrasonography can be used to evaluate upper tracts, but small urothelial tumors may be missed.
- CT of the abdomen and pelvis with and without contrast is a more sensitive study for evaluating the kidneys, ureters, and intra-abdominal/pelvic lymph nodes; the upper tracts need to be evaluated in any adult with hematuria, and this test is preferred to ultrasonography.
- No serum testing is specific for bladder cancer, but workup may include complete blood count, alkaline phosphatase, kidney function studies or liver function studies as a part of a metastatic workup, or baseline before various treatments for bladder cancer.

▶ TREATMENT

- For nonmuscle invasive lesions:
  - Cystoscopy with TURBT can facilitate both diagnosis and treatment. All visible lesions must be completely resected, which may be sufficient treatment. Lesions are sent to pathology, and if there is no evidence of muscle invasion, management involves surveillance cystoscopies every 3 months for the first year, every 6 months for the second year, and annually thereafter.
  - Intravesical therapy, the instillation of immunotherapeutic or chemotherapeutic agents via catheter, can be indicated in cases of rapid tumor recurrence, presence of carcinoma in situ, or progression to higher grade disease on subsequent biopsies.
- Muscle invasive bladder cancer is typically treated with radical cystectomy or radiation with chemotherapy, based on patient factors such as comorbidities and patient preference.
- Smoking cessation is strongly encouraged in all incidence of bladder cancer because of the high recurrence rate.
- Prognosis of noninvasive bladder cancer is generally good, with a 5-year survival rate of 82%–100%. Cancer grade, depth of invasion, the presence of carcinoma in situ, and nodal involvement are all important prognostic factors, with survival rates decreasing as stage increases.

Section A Pretest: Esophageal Disorders

1. A 72-year-old patient with a history of renal transplant presents for evaluation of retrosternal pain and dysphagia to solids. Which of the following is the most appropriate next step in the management of this patient?
   A. Barium esophagram
   B. Ganciclovir for 14–21 days
   C. EGD with biopsy
   D. Liquid budesonide for 4–8 weeks
   E. Acyclovir for 3–6 weeks

2. Which of the following symptoms of gastroesophageal reflux disease (GERD) is considered atypical?
   A. Heartburn
   B. Regurgitation
   C. Dysphagia
   D. Wheezing
   E. Waterbrash

3. A 32-year-old patient is evaluated for gradually progressive dysphagia to solids and weight loss. EGD reveals esophageal candidiasis but is otherwise unremarkable. Which of the following should be ordered next for the management of this patient?
   A. Fluticasone for 14–21 days
   B. Valacyclovir for 14–21 days and evaluation for diabetes mellitus
   C. Famciclovir for 14–21 days and assessment of HIV status
   D. Fluconazole for 14–21 days and assessment of HIV status

4. Which of the following is the most common cause of benign esophageal strictures?
   A. Mechanical trauma
   B. Immunosuppressive diseases such as scleroderma
   C. Barrett esophagus
   D. GERD

5. A 44-year-old patient presents for evaluation of retrosternal discomfort, unrelated to exertion, frequent belching, and occasional pain after swallowing. She has no other symptoms, and her medical history is otherwise unremarkable. Which of the following is the best option for the management of this patient?
   A. EGD with biopsy
   B. Ranitidine 150 mg at bedtime
   C. Omeprazole 40 mg at bedtime

   D. Rabeprazole 20 mg before breakfast
   E. Weight loss and lifting the head of her bed 6 in

6. A 62-year-old patient with a history of osteoporosis, hypertension, hyperlipidemia, and osteoarthritis presents for evaluation of noncardiac retrosternal burning and odynophagia. Which of her medications would you temporarily discontinue given a presumptive diagnosis of medication-induced esophagitis?
   A. Vitamin D
   B. Teriparatide
   C. Naproxen
   D. Lisinopril
   E. Atorvastatin

7. Which of the following is the treatment of choice for a patient who presents with nausea, coffee ground emesis, and mild epigastric pain?
   A. Viscous lidocaine
   B. Protonix 40 mg and ondansetron 4 mg
   C. Morphine 2 mg and aspirin 500 mg/sodium bicarbonate
   D. Trial of low residue diet

8. A 14-year-old patient with a history of eczema presents for evaluation of intermittent dysphagia for 1 year. A recent barium esophagram suggests esophageal rings. Which of the following should be done next in the management of this patient?
   A. Refer for EGD and biopsy
   B. 4- to 8-week trial of liquid budesonide
   C. 8-week course of a PPI
   D. Begin an elimination diet

9. Which of the following is NOT likely to be seen on imaging in a patient with Boerhaave syndrome?
   A. Hydropneumothorax
   B. Extravasation of contrast
   C. Pleural effusion
   D. Zenker diverticulum

10. What is the preferred diagnostic study in patients with symptoms suggestive of achalasia?
    A. Esophageal 24-hour pH monitoring
    B. Barium esophagram
    C. Upper endoscopy
    D. Esophageal manometry

11. Which of the following diagnostic findings is *most* suggestive of diffuse esophageal spasm?
    A. "Bird's-beak" appearance on barium esophagram
    B. An isolated connective tissue ring at the gastroesophageal junction on endoscopy
    C. Esophageal manometry results showing >20% premature, uncoordinated contractions
    D. Esophageal biopsy with >15 eosinophils per high-power field

12. Which finding represents an atypical presentation of esophageal stricture?
    A. Dysphagia
    B. Odynophagia
    C. Aspiration asthma
    D. Gagging when swallowing

13. Which of the following is the diagnostic gold standard for GERD?
    A. Barium esophagram
    B. Endoscopy with biopsy
    C. Esophageal manometry
    D. 24-hour esophageal pH monitoring
    E. Chest radiograph

14. An esophageal stricture caused by dysmotility is best diagnosed by which of the following?
    A. Barium swallow
    B. Manometry
    C. Endoscopy
    D. Balloon dilatation

Section B Pretest: Food Allergies and Sensitivities

1. Where does most lactose digestion occur?
   A. Greater curvature of the stomach
   B. Mid-jejunum
   C. Terminal ileum
   D. Ascending colon

2. Which type of an immunoglobulin is responsible for the tree nut allergy?
   A. IgA
   B. IgE
   C. IgM
   D. IgG

3. Which of the following is the gold standard confirmatory test of lactose intolerance?
   A. Hydrogen breath testing
   B. Serology glucose testing
   C. Intestinal small bowel biopsy via endoscopy
   D. Strong clinical correlation with dietary triggers

4. Which of the following medications should be given to patients with a known food allergy to carry at all times in case of an anaphylactic reaction?
   A. Epinephrine autoinjector
   B. Prednisone autoinjector
   C. Benadryl autoinjector
   D. Zyrtec autoinjector

5. When providing patient education regarding lactose-containing foods, research suggests that most people are able to consume how many grams of lactose at a time with minor symptoms?
   A. 2
   B. 6
   C. 12
   D. 60

6. A 3-month-old Asian full-term male infant is brought to the clinic by his mother after she notes he has had "continuous watery diarrhea." The stooling occurs within 30 minutes of breastfeeding. The infant is well developed though has physical examination findings concerning for dehydration and is underweight. He has been hospitalized twice before for diarrhea and dehydration. What are your next steps?
   A. Recommend presenting to hospital to be treated for volume depleting diarrhea.
   B. Request pediatric gastroenterology consultation.
   C. Request registered dietician consultation.
   D. All of the above.

7. What is the most common way used to manage tree nut allergies?
   A. Oral food challenge
   B. Oral immunotherapy
   C. Complete avoidance of trigger food
   D. Partial avoidance of trigger food

8. A 13-year-old female was brought to the clinic by her mother on account of a 7-month history of abdominal cramps, bloating, and diarrhea that occur usually about 2 hours after ingesting cow's milk. What is her most likely diagnosis?
   A. Celiac disease
   B. Giardiasis
   C. Primary lactase deficiency
   D. Irritable bowel syndrome

9. Which of the following should be part of the patient counseling for a patient with confirmed tree nut allergy?
   A. There is no cross-reactivity between tree nuts and peanuts.
   B. Restaurant meals pose limited potential harm.
   C. Highlighting the importance of reading food labels.
   D. Previous allergic reaction predicts the next one.

Section C Pretest: Gastric Disorders

1. Which of the following can be identified on endoscopy in a patient with a hiatal hernia?
   A. Size of the hernia
   B. Reflux esophagitis
   C. Cause of the hernia
   D. Esophageal dysmotility

2. What is the radiographic test of choice in infants with suspected pyloric stenosis?
   A. Contrasted upper GI series
   B. Ultrasound
   C. CT
   D. MRI

3. Which of the following is used to evaluate a patient for a hiatal hernia?
   A. Barium esophagography
   B. Abdominal CT scan
   C. MRI enterography
   D. Pill endoscopy

4. Which of the following has the highest risk of developing pyloric stenosis?
   A. Second born
   B. Maternal smoking
   C. Female
   D. Penicillin antibiotic use during pregnancy

5. Which of the following is a risk factor associated with development of a hiatal hernia?
   A. Smoking
   B. Alcohol use
   C. Exercise
   D. Previous abdominal surgery

6. Which of the following disorders is associated with antiparietal and anti-intrinsic factor antibodies with marked diffuse atrophy of parietal and chief cells, achlorhydria, and possible development of pernicious anemia?
   A. Plummer-Vinson syndrome
   B. Zollinger-Ellison syndrome
   C. Autoimmune metaplastic atrophic gastritis
   D. Primary sclerosing cholangitis
   E. Autoimmune hepatitis

7. Which of the following symptoms best describes toxicity to anticholinergics?
   A. Salivation, lacrimation, confusion, bradycardia, urinary incontinence
   B. Dry mouth, mydriasis, tachydysrhythmia, urinary retention
   C. Respiratory depression, lethargy, miosis
   D. Seizures, respiratory failure, pancreatitis, visual damage, tachypnea

8. Which of the following is the preferred treatment for an object lodged in the distal esophagus?
   A. Barium swallow
   B. Endoscopy
   C. Surgery
   D. Laryngoscopy

9. Which of the following emesis descriptions is associated with pyloric stenosis?
   A. Bilious
   B. Bloody
   C. Projectile
   D. Effortless

10. A 5-year-old patient arrives for evaluation. The mother reports the child accidentally drank an unknown amount of children's liquid acetaminophen. Which of the following is considered a treatment for an acetaminophen overdose?
    A. Naloxone
    B. *N*-Acetylcysteine
    C. Atropine
    D. Flumazenil

11. Which of the following substances is known to present with metabolic acidosis?
    A. Acetaminophen
    B. Methanol
    C. Amitriptyline
    D. Diphenhydramine

12. Which of the laboratory findings are associated with pyloric stenosis?
    A. Hyperchloremia
    B. Hyponatremia
    C. Hyperglycemia
    D. Hypokalemia

13. A 28-year-old male is brought to the emergency department for a reduced level of consciousness and lethargy. Friends report the patient was found in a college dormitory and initially appeared to be sleeping, but they were unable to wake the patient. You note vitals with a blood pressure of 95/56, heart rate is 45 bpm, respiration rate is 6 breaths per minute, and oxygen at 89%. On examination, the patient is lethargic, alert only to painful stimulus, shallow breaths. Examination of the eyes reveals miosis. Which of the following is the most appropriate initial step to take for this patient?
    A. Naloxone should be given empirically, and treatment should not be delayed for toxicology results.
    B. Order toxicology screen to better determine the possible toxic substance.
    C. Naloxone should not be given as this is not an opiate overdose.
    D. Seek advice from poison control to help determine the toxic substance and guidance on treatment.

Section D Pretest: Hepatobiliary Disease

1. Which of the following is NOT a symptom of choledocholithiasis?
   A. Jaundice
   B. Melena
   C. Tea-colored urine
   D. Pruritus
   E. RUQ abdominal pain

2. The likelihood of developing chronic hepatitis B is higher in which of the following patients?
   A. Male with multiple sexual partners
   B. The wife whose husband has chronic hepatitis B
   C. Children born to hepatitis B–positive mothers in the United States
   D. Asian born children

3. Which of the following is NOT a complication of choledocholithiasis?
   A. Acute pancreatitis
   B. Ascending cholangitis
   C. Acute hepatitis
   D. Acute cholecystitis

4. In the United States, what percentage of gallstones are composed of cholesterol?
   A. 60
   B. 70
   C. 80
   D. 90

5. A 46-year-old woman with primary biliary cirrhosis presents to clinic for her annual physical examination. She informs you she is planning a visit to South America soon. You recommend good handwashing and which vaccine before her trip?
   A. Hepatitis A
   B. MMR
   C. Pneumococcal
   D. Shingles

6. Charcot triad is strongly indicative of which of the following?
   A. Cholangitis
   B. Pancreatitis
   C. Cholelithiasis
   D. Choledocholithiasis

7. For a 65-year-old male with elevated AST and ALT on routine examination, which of the following tests should be included in the initial evaluation of this patient?
   A. Serum ceruloplasmin
   B. Ferritin
   C. Liver biopsy
   D. ANA
   E. HCV antibody

8. Which of the following is most likely to cause progression to more advanced liver disease such as cirrhosis or hepatocellular cancer?
   A. Patient with hepatitis C who takes acetaminophen off and on for muscle aches
   B. Patient with hepatitis C who has unprotected sex
   C. Patient with a family history of cirrhosis
   D. Patient with hepatitis C who continues to drink alcohol
   E. Infant born to a hepatitis C–positive mother

9. A positive hepatitis B surface antigen and negative hepatitis B surface antibody indicates which of the following?
   A. Hepatitis B infection
   B. Immunity from hepatitis B
   C. Cannot tell from these results
   D. Acute hepatitis B infection

10. What physical examination findings are characteristic of acute cholangitis?
    A. RUQ pain, fever, and jaundice
    B. RUQ pain, jaundice, and dizziness
    C. Jaundice, fever, and hypertension
    D. Fever, RUQ pain, and positive Murphy sign

11. What CT finding is most suggestive of cirrhosis?
    A. Superior mesenteric vein thrombus
    B. Dilatation of the common bile duct
    C. Renal cortical atrophy
    D. Nodular hepatic parenchyma

12. A 23-year-old female with a history of primary sclerosing cholangitis presents to the emergency department with recent onset of fever, chills, and abdominal pain. Her labs reveal an elevation of her baseline bilirubin to 10 as well as a leukocytosis with left shift. What intervention would provide diagnostic and therapeutic benefit?
    A. MRI/MRCP of the abdomen
    B. Initiation of IV piperacillin/tazobactam
    C. EGD
    D. Endoscopic retrograde cholangiopancreatography (ERCP)

13. An 85-year-old male presents with a 3-month history of jaundice and new-onset abdominal pain and fever. He reports noted weight loss of 30 pounds in the last 6 months. Labs reveal a bilirubin level of 8 and a mild elevation to transaminases, amylase, and lipase. What finding on ERCP provides the most likely explanation of his clinical history?
    A. Malignant biliary stricture
    B. Nonobstructive cholelithiasis
    C. Common bile duct injury
    D. Biliary atresia

14. Which of the following is a complication of cirrhosis?
    A. Thrombocytosis
    B. Secondary bacterial peritonitis
    C. Esophageal varices
    D. Vascular dementia

15. What physical examination finding and lab result appropriately correspond to a diagnosis of hepatic encephalopathy?
    A. Asterixis, elevated ammonia level
    B. Sarcopenia, low albumin
    C. Flapping tremor, low ammonia level
    D. Delirium, low sodium

16. Which of the following is the gold standard for diagnosing common bile duct obstruction?
    A. Transabdominal ultrasound
    B. HIDA scan
    C. Total bilirubin
    D. ERCP/MRCP
    E. Abdominal CT

17. What laboratory results suggest an acute infection with hepatitis B without prior vaccination?
    A. Positive hepatitis B surface antigen, negative antibody
    B. Positive hepatitis B surface antigen, positive antibody
    C. Negative hepatitis B surface antigen, negative antibody
    D. None of the above

18. You are caring for a 35-year-old man with fulminant liver failure in the ICU awaiting transplantation. What scoring system is used for risk stratification of patients listed for liver transplant?
    A. Murray
    B. SOFA
    C. MELD
    D. H-score

Section E Pretest: Intestinal Disorders

1. A late sign of intussusception is which of the following?
   A. Vomiting
   B. Abdominal pain
   C. Fever
   D. Dance sign
   E. Bloody stools

2. Small bowel obstruction may be the initial presentation of which of the following conditions?
   A. Pregnancy
   B. Crohn disease
   C. Cholecystitis
   D. Appendicitis
   E. Whipple disease

3. The highest risk associated with pneumatic reduction is which of the following?
   A. Tension pneumothorax
   B. Tension pneumoperitoneum
   C. Pneumoperitoneum
   D. Failure of intervention
   E. Transmural necrosis

4. Beyond abdominal pain, the classic triad of appendicitis includes which of the following?
   A. Indigestion, nausea, and vomiting
   B. Anorexia, nausea, and bowel changes
   C. Nausea, vomiting, and anorexia
   D. Diarrhea, nausea, and vomiting

5. Which of the following is NOT a common finding in a patient with a suspected small bowel obstruction?
   A. Abdominal distention
   B. Tympany to percussion
   C. History of several days of severe diarrhea
   D. Air-fluid levels on imaging
   E. Feculent emesis

6. What is the most common cause of secondary intussusception in children?
   A. Malignancy
   B. Lymph node hypertrophy
   C. Meckel diverticulum
   D. Crohn disease
   E. Cystic fibrosis

7. If a small bowel obstruction is caused by a hernia, which is the most appropriate initial management of it?
   A. Immediate surgical intervention
   B. Nasogastric tube decompression
   C. Air-contrast barium enema

   D. Reduction of the hernia
   E. Bowel rest

8. If an intussusception recurs after pneumatic reduction, which of the following is the next best step?
   A. Hydrostatic reduction
   B. Nasogastric tube placement
   C. Rectal tube placement
   D. Exploratory laparotomy
   E. Repeat pneumatic reduction

9. In which of the following populations does appendicitis most commonly occur?
   A. Younger than age 10 years
   B. 10- to 19-year-olds
   C. 20- to 30-year-olds
   D. Older than age 30 years

10. What is the common cause of an anal fissure?
    A. Local anal trauma
    B. Ulcerative colitis
    C. Crohn disease
    D. Food intolerances

11. Antibiotics for appendicitis should cover for which of the following?
    A. Anaerobes, enterococci, and Gram-positive intestinal flora
    B. Enterococci, Gram-positive intestinal flora, and parasites
    C. Gram-negative intestinal flora, enterococci, and *E. coli*
    D. Anaerobes, enterococci, and Gram-negative intestinal flora

12. Which of the following is NOT a common clinical feature of an anal fissure?
    A. The typical location is midline.
    B. An associated distal tag often occurs with chronic disease.
    C. Most fissures occur proximal to the dentate (aka: pectinate) line.
    D. Symptoms include anal pain and bleeding.

13. You are seeing a patient after routine screening colonoscopy, who was found to have diverticular disease. Your counseling for this patient includes which of the following?
    A. Diverticulosis does not always cause symptoms.
    B. Colonoscopies will be required every 3 years for monitoring.

C. The majority of patients with diverticulosis will develop acute diverticulitis.

D. The patient should be started on a daily probiotic for colon health.

14. Which type of obstruction is always a surgical emergency?
    A. Caused by adhesive disease
    B. Caused by a reducible hernia
    C. Caused by inflammatory bowel disease
    D. Caused by a closed-loop configuration
    E. One that is partial in nature

15. A 76-year-old male presents to your office with a 2-day history of intermittent left lower quadrant abdominal pain. Which of the following features from the patient's history, physical examination, and laboratory evaluation is most suggestive of colonic perforation?
    A. Hematochezia
    B. Rebound tenderness
    C. Fever
    D. Leukocytosis

16. Which of the following is NOT one of the four subtypes of IBS?
    A. Diarrhea
    B. Psychogenic
    C. Constipation
    D. Mixed

17. A 60-year-old female presenting to the emergency department reports a history of intermittent hematochezia. She has not sought medical advice since she had history of hemorrhoids. She now has left-sided abdominal pain and chills. Vital signs include temperature of 101.8 °F, pulse 90 beats per minute, and blood pressure 118/86 mm Hg. Abdominal examination reveals hypoactive bowel sounds, distension, and mild tenderness. There is no guarding or rebound tenderness. Laboratory studies are unremarkable. Which of the following is the most appropriate next step?
    A. CT scan of the abdomen
    B. IV ceftriaxone
    C. Emergent surgery
    D. Colonoscopy

18. A patient presents with anal pain and bleeding for 2 weeks. On examination, there is a small skin tag in the posterior midline where the patient localizes the pain. What medical management would be appropriate for this patient?
    A. Hydrocortisone suppositories
    B. Topical nifedipine 2–4 times daily for 1–2 months
    C. External hemorrhoidectomy
    D. Oral opioids for pain management

19. Which of the following is the treatment of choice for patients with celiac disease?
    A. Splanchnic antispasmodics
    B. Corticosteroids
    C. Antidiarrheal medications
    D. Gluten-free diet

20. Which of the following statements regarding hemorrhoids is false?
    A. Prevention and conservative management of hemorrhoids includes stool softeners and increased fiber.
    B. Excision of a thrombosed hemorrhoid will provide immediate relief to patients who present within 72 hours of onset of severe pain.
    C. Internal hemorrhoids arise proximal to the dentate line and are typically not painful.
    D. Most patients with hemorrhoidal disease will require surgical intervention.

21. Which of the following is NOT usually found on physical exam in acute appendicitis?
    A. Positive straight leg raise
    B. Abdominal rebound tenderness
    C. Psoas and obturator signs
    D. RLQ tenderness over McBurney point

22. Which of the following are red flags of a potential organic cause for abdominal pain and diarrhea?
    A. Evidence of GI bleeding
    B. Anorexia/weight loss
    C. Fever
    D. Nocturnal symptoms
    E. All of the above

23. What lifestyle measures are advised for prevention of hemorrhoids and anal fissures?
    A. High-fiber diet with possible fiber supplementation
    B. Straining avoidance and having a bowel movement as soon as you feel the urge
    C. Exercising regularly and staying hydrated with water
    D. All of the above

24. Risk factors for colorectal cancer include which one of the following?
    A. IBS
    B. Low dietary fiber intake
    C. Low red meat intake
    D. Chronic aspirin therapy

25. What high-risk group would a pelvic examination be recommended due to the possibility of a malignancy presenting with recent onset of lower abdominal pain and bowel changes?
    A. Postmenopausal
    B. <25 years old
    C. Anyone with IBS symptoms
    D. All of the above

26. Which of the following is a complication of diverticular disease that is most likely to require surgical intervention?
    A. Acute diverticulitis
    B. Diverticular bleeding
    C. Colorectal cancer
    D. Fistula formation

27. Which of the following diagnostic tests is considered the preferred initial diagnostic study of choice for celiac disease?
    A. Anti–endomysial antibodies (EMA)
    B. Anti–tissue transglutaminase antibodies (tTG-IgA)
    C. Upper endoscopy with biopsy
    D. Colonoscopy with biopsy

28. Which of the following is true regarding management of irritable bowel syndrome?
    A. Increase intake of high fructose beverages
    B. Highly fermentable fiber is best in IBS-D–type patients
    C. Avoid cruciferous vegetables in all types of IBS patients
    D. Osmotic laxatives are contraindicated in IBS-C–type patients

29. Which of the following diagnostic tests is considered confirmatory and ultimately diagnostic for celiac disease?
    A. Anti-EMA
    B. Anti-tTG-IgA
    C. Upper endoscopy with biopsy
    D. Improvement of symptoms with a gluten-free diet

30. A 57-year-old African American male presents with new-onset constipation and painless bright red blood per rectum. Several small internal hemorrhoids are visualized with anoscopy. He denies any prior history of colon cancer screening. Which of the following evaluations would be the most appropriate next step?
    A. Colonoscopy
    B. Barium enema
    C. Serum CEA level
    D. Treatment of internal hemorrhoids followed by hs-gFOBT

31. Which of the following extraintestinal symptoms is commonly found in patients with celiac disease?
    A. Dermatitis herpetiformis
    B. Poikilocytosis
    C. Nausea and vomiting
    D. Weight gain

32. A 40-year-old woman presents to your office with newly diagnosed metastatic colon cancer. Her mother had colon cancer at age 45, and one of her mother's sisters was diagnosed with endometrial cancer at age

38. Which of the following conditions is the most likely cause of her colon cancer?
    A. Lynch syndrome
    B. Familial adenomatous polyposis
    C. Turcot syndrome
    D. Peutz-Jeghers syndrome

33. Which of the following is true of celiac disease?
    A. There is a slight male predominance.
    B. It is rare to be diagnosed after the age of 5 years.
    C. There is an increased incidence in individuals with autoimmune conditions.
    D. The prognosis is poor, and mortality is high.

34. Which of the following colon polyp histologies is most concerning for an increased risk of colorectal cancer?
    A. Tubular
    B. Hyperplastic
    C. Villous
    D. Inflammatory

35. What is the most common cause of large bowel obstruction?
    A. Hernia
    B. Malignancy
    C. Hematoma
    D. Inflammatory bowel disease
    E. Diverticular disease

36. A 60-year-old female asks about colon cancer screening and a colonoscopy is advised. The patient is hesitant because her older sister "had a terrible time with all the laxatives" and because she does not want to take time off work for the procedure. Which of the following colonoscopy alternatives is recommended by the U.S. Preventive Services Task Force for CRC screening?
    A. hs-gFOBT every 3 years
    B. FIT every 3 years
    C. FIT-DNA every 10 years
    D. FIT annually

37. You have been called to evaluate a patient who was admitted to the medical service with a large bowel obstruction. The CT done on admission the day prior shows what appears to be a mass in the sigmoid colon. The patient is currently stable and has actually passed a small amount of liquid stool since being admitted. How should you advise this patient on the "next step" in treatment?
    A. Recommend GI for stenting
    B. Recommend surgical resection and possible ostomy
    C. Recommend palliative care consult
    D. Recommend expectant management
    E. Recommend endoscopic decompression

38. Which of the following is a risk factor for acute mesenteric ischemia?
    A. Age <50 years
    B. Abdominal pain lasting <1 hour
    C. Abdominal pain consistent with examination findings
    D. History of cardiovascular disease

39. A 28-year-old female with no past medical history presents with a 2-day history of nonbloody diarrhea. Furthermore, she reports loss of appetite and stomach cramping. She is not on any medications and has had no recent travel. She further denies fever, nausea, vomiting, or weight loss. She works at a day care center where other children and staff have had similar symptoms. What is the first-line treatment for her symptoms?
    A. Fluids and loperamide
    B. Opioids
    C. Octreotide
    D. Clonidine

40. Which of the following is NOT a risk factor for mesenteric venous thrombosis?
    A. Pancreatitis
    B. Hypercoagulable state
    C. Portal hypertension
    D. Inflammatory bowel disease

41. A 35-year-old male presents with voluminous stools for the past 2 years. He denies fever, weight loss, and hematochezia. He notes the diarrhea improves with fasting. What is the most likely cause of his symptoms?
    A. Carcinoid tumor
    B. Celiac disease
    C. Ulcerative colitis
    D. Lactose intolerance

42. You assume care for a patient who has been diagnosed with a large bowel obstruction secondary to fecal impaction. How should you manage this patient?
    A. Surgical consultation
    B. Oral prokinetic agents
    C. Gastroenterology consultation
    D. Manual disimpaction
    E. Colonic lavage

43. A 16-year-old, otherwise healthy male presents with abdominal pain, fever, and bloody diarrhea for 3 days. The symptoms started shortly after eating food at a cookout. Other people who attended the cookout have similar symptoms. Which of the following should not be a part of his treatment plan?
    A. Fluids
    B. Bland diet
    C. Loperamide
    D. Bismuth subsalicylate

44. Which of the following is NOT part of the classic triad for chronic mesenteric ischemia?
    A. Postprandial pain
    B. Fever
    C. Abdominal bruit
    D. Weight loss

45. A 50-year-old male with hypertension recently diagnosed with type 2 diabetes is started on medication management. Shortly after starting medication, he develops new-onset diarrhea. He denies fever, chills, weight loss, or blood in the stool. No other household contacts have symptoms. What medication most likely caused the diarrhea? Symptoms?
    A. Metoprolol
    B. Acetaminophen
    C. Insulin
    D. Metformin

Section F Pretest: Pancreatitis

1. Which is the most common cause of acute pancreatitis in the United States?
   A. Alcohol abuse
   B. High cholesterol
   C. Gallstones
   D. Genetics

2. Elevated phenylalanine levels with no genetic abnormality related to phenylalanine hydroxylase is most likely related to which cofactor?
   A. Tetrahydrobiopterin
   B. Iron
   C. Guanosine triphosphate
   D. GTP cyclohydrolase I

3. Patients who present with acute pancreatitis will often complain of what type of pain?
   A. Generalized, cramping, periumbilical pain
   B. Generalized aching pain in the left upper quadrant cramping
   C. Steady, deep epigastric pain with radiation to the back
   D. Gnawing burning epigastric pain with radiation to the left upper quadrant

4. The amino acid phenylalanine is converted to tyrosine by which of the following hepatic enzymes?
   A. Tetrahydrobiopterin
   B. Phenylalanine hydroxylase
   C. Pectinase
   D. Alkaline phosphatase

5. A patient with a history of alcohol abuse presents with nausea and vomiting and epigastric back pain that radiates to his back. Which of the following laboratory tests would most likely be elevated 8–14 days after initial presentation?
   A. Serum amylase
   B. Serum lipase
   C. Serum triglycerides
   D. Serum lactate

6. When should an infant be screened for PKU?
   A. After the first feeding
   B. After the child has past the meconium
   C. 24–72 hours after birth
   D. At the first wellness visit

7. Which of the following is a known side effect of a patient having very high triglyceride levels?
   A. Cholecystitis
   B. Pancreatitis
   C. Hypercalcemia
   D. Renal failure

8. A 6-month-old child whose family recently immigrated from Albania presents to your clinic with irritability, loss of interest in surroundings, and chronic rashes. Parents are unsure if the child had any newborn screening. A serum level of phenylalanine above what level would be concerning for PKU?
   A. 4 mg/dL
   B. 10 mg/dL
   C. 20 mg/dL
   D. 40 mg/dL

9. Which of the following is commonly used to define pancreatitis severity?
   A. Atlanta criteria
   B. Chicago criteria
   C. Memphis criteria
   D. Seattle criteria

▶ ANSWERS AND EXPLANATIONS TO SECTION A PRETEST

1. **C.** This patient is at risk for infectious esophagitis, most likely with HSV. EGD with biopsy is indicated for identification of causative pathogen and to rule out malignancy or other condition. Barium esophagram may demonstrate large ulcers, but will not identify the causative pathogen. Medical therapy is not indicated without definitive identification of the underlying cause.

2. **D.** Atypical symptoms of GERD are those that are extraesophageal, particularly of the pulmonary tree including wheezing, cough, asthma exacerbation, and hoarseness. Typical symptoms of GERD are those which relate to the esophagus, including heartburn, regurgitation, dysphagia, and waterbrash.

3. **D.** Most cases of infectious esophagitis occur in patients who are immunocompromised. Although diabetes mellitus can increase risk for esophageal candidiasis, it is crucial to determine this patient's HIV status. Fluticasone is used for EoE. Valacyclovir and famciclovir are used for HSV.

4. **D.** GERD is the most common cause of benign esophageal strictures.

5. **D.** The most likely diagnosis is reflux esophagitis. Once-daily, prescription-strength H2RA or PPI therapy for 8 weeks are reasonable choices, along with appropriate lifestyle and dietary adjustments. EGD is not yet indicated given her lack of warning signs and presumptive diagnosis of reflux esophagitis (vs. infective or EoE). Ranitidine is no longer available in the United States. PPIs should be given 30–60 minutes before breakfast. We do not know that she is overweight or experiencing nocturnal symptoms, so those measures alone may not improve her symptoms.

6. **C.** Many oral medications can cause injury to the esophageal mucosa with extended contact. Patients should be advised to be upright when taking medication, if possible, and swallow a moderate volume of liquid to help propel the medication into the stomach. NSAIDs are known to cause esophageal injury due to disruption of the cytoprotective layer of the mucosa. Vitamin D, lisinopril, and atorvastatin are less likely to cause injury. Teriparatide is given subcutaneously.

7. **B.** Treatment with PPI and antiemetic is the best choice. The first choice is incorrect because viscous lidocaine (often part of a compounded "GI cocktail") will only mask symptoms. Morphine does not treat the tear, and aspirin/bicarbonate will delay healing via COX enzyme inhibition. A low residue diet may also make the tear worse.

8. **A.** The diagnosis of EoE requires a biopsy demonstrating at least 15 eosinophils per high-power field. The other options are reasonable after the diagnosis has been established.

9. **D.** A Zenker diverticulum is an upper esophageal outpouching and is unassociated with distal esophageal tears. It is most commonly associated with regurgitation of undigested food. Hydropneumothorax, extravasation of contrast, and pleural effusions are all common findings on imaging associated with esophageal tears.

10. **D.** Esophageal manometry is the gold standard diagnostic test for achalasia and reveals absence of normal peristalsis and elevated LES pressure. Esophageal 24-hour pH monitoring is the diagnostic test of choice for GERD. Barium esophagram that reveals the esophageal dilation and bird's-beak sign is not a sensitive test for achalasia and may be normal in up to one-third of patients. Upper endoscopy is used to rule out pseudoachalasia or occult carcinoma.

11. **C.** Esophageal manometry is the gold standard diagnostic test for motility disorders and shows the occurrence of >20% premature, uncoordinated contractions in DES in the setting of a normal LES response. Barium esophagram is neither sensitive nor specific for DES, and few patients with DES have a "corkscrew appearance" on evaluation. A bird's-beak appearance is a classic finding for achalasia. Schatzki ring is an isolated thin mucosal connective tissue ring located at the gastroesophageal junction, which causes episodic, intermittent, non-progressive dysphagia for solids. Esophageal biopsy with >15 eosinophils per high-power field is associated with EoE, a chronic inflammatory condition associated with food or environmental allergies that is characterized by esophageal dysfunction and eosinophilic infiltrate.

12. **C.** Aspiration asthma and chronic coughing are atypical presentations of esophageal strictures. Dysphagia, odynophagia, and gagging when swallowing are common presentations.

13. **D.** For typical uncomplicated GERD symptoms, the diagnosis is presumed, and empiric therapy initiated. The diagnostic gold standard for GERD is 24-hour esophageal pH monitoring, which is utilized when symptoms are refractory to medications, in situations when the diagnosis of GERD is in question, and before surgery. Endoscopy with biopsy is reserved for patients with atypical or red flag symptoms suspicious for malignancy, long-standing GERD, and symptoms unresponsive to medication. Esophageal manometry may be performed in GERD patients before surgery and reveals decreased lower esophageal sphincter tone. Barium esophagram and chest radiograph are not utilized in the diagnosis of GERD.

14. **B.** Manometry is indicated in esophageal dysfunction that is secondary to dysmotility. Dilatation techniques are used to treat esophageal strictures.

▶ ANSWERS AND EXPLANATIONS TO SECTION B PRETEST

1. **B.** Most lactase phlorizin is expressed in the mid-jejunum in the brush borders of the intestinal villi. Those with symptomatic lactase deficiency have increased amounts of lactose reaching the large intestine, creating symptoms of diarrhea, flatus, abdominal bloating, nausea, and abdominal distress.

2. **B.** IgE is responsible for the tree nut allergy.

3. **C.** While the gold standard is to obtain a small bowel biopsy to confirm lactose intolerance, this is a highly invasive and a costly test in routine clinical practice for such a mild disease. Hydrogen breath testing for lactose intolerance is minimally invasive, inexpensive, patient preferred, and highly sensitive and specific.

4. **A.** An epinephrine autoinjector should be given to patients with a known food allergy to carry at all times in case of an anaphylactic reaction.

5. **C.** Most adolescents and adults with lactose intolerance can ingest at least 12 g of lactose in a single dose (equivalent to 1 cup of milk) with only minor symptoms reported. Most people with lactose intolerance can enjoy some milk products without symptoms.

6. **D.** Owing to the life-threatening condition of volume depleting diarrhea, resuscitation and stabilization should be first priority. Congenital lactase deficiency is rare, it should though be considered in this clinical context. Careful history and additional diagnostics should be obtained by specialty care team members to establish diagnosis and therapy plan.

7. **C.** Complete avoidance of trigger food is the most common way used to manage tree nut allergies.

8. **C.** Primary lactase deficiency is a physiologic decline of lactase production within the small intestine. This typically does not occur before age 6. In humans, the incidence rises as the population ages.

9. **C.** Highlighting the importance of reading food labels should be part of the patient counseling for a patient with confirmed tree nut allergy.

▶ ANSWERS AND EXPLANATIONS TO SECTION C PRETEST

1. **B.** Reflux esophagitis can be identified on endoscopy in a patient with a hiatal hernia.

2. **B.** Ultrasound is the radiographic test of choice in infants with suspected pyloric stenosis.

3. **A.** Barium esophagography is used to evaluate a patient for a hiatal hernia.

4. **B.** Maternal smoking has the highest risk of developing pyloric stenosis.

5. **D.** Previous abdominal surgery is a risk factor associated with development of a hiatal hernia.

6. **C.** Autoimmune metaplastic atrophic gastritis is a rare condition, and similar to other autoimmune disorders, is more common in females, and strongly associated with other autoimmune conditions. It is associated with antiparietal and anti-intrinsic factor antibodies with marked diffuse atrophy of parietal and chief cells, achlorhydria, and possible development of pernicious anemia. The condition may progress to intestinal dysplasia and adenocarcinoma.

7. **B.** Anticholinergic toxicity may result in dry flushed (red) skin, dry mucous membranes, hyperthermia, mydriasis, delirium, decreased peristalsis, urinary retention, wide-complex tachydysrhythmia, and seizures. While salivation, lacrimation, confusion, bradycardia, and urinary incontinence are considered cholinergic effects, respiratory depression, lethargy, and miosis are more consistent with opiates. Seizures, respiratory failure, pancreatitis, visual damage, tachypnea can be seen in methanol toxicity.

8. **B.** Endoscopy is the preferred method for visualization and retrieval of a retrained ingested foreign body.

9. **C.** Projectile emesis is associated with pyloric stenosis.

10. **B.** *N*-Acetylcysteine acts as a substitute for glutathione in the metabolism and elimination of acetaminophen. Naloxone is used in opiate overdoses. Atropine is used for cholinergic toxicity (eg, organophosphates), and flumazenil is used for benzodiazepine toxicity.

11. **B.** The mnemonic MUDPILES is often used to recall states of anion gap metabolic acidosis. Methanol, metformin, uremia, DKA, paraldehyde, propylene glycol, isoniazid, iron, lactic acidosis, ethylene glycol, salicylates.

12. **D.** Hypokalemia is associated with pyloric stenosis.

13. **A.** Although the substance may not be known, naloxone can be given empirically based on suspicion derived from the differential diagnosis. This should not be delayed while awaiting results of a drug screen. Additionally, drug screens can give results that are not consistent with the actual toxicity occurring in the patient.

▶ ANSWERS AND EXPLANATIONS TO SECTION D PRETEST

1. **B.** Jaundice, tea-colored urine, pruritus, and RUQ abdominal pain are all symptoms of choledocholithiasis. Clay-colored stool, not melena, is also a symptom.

2. **D.** Chronic hepatitis B infections are more common in Asian countries when patients are infected at a younger age. Acute infection is more likely with multiple sexual contacts and rare with a monogamous relationship.

3. **C.** Acute pancreatitis, ascending cholangitis, and acute cholecystitis are all possible complications of choledocholithiasis.

4. **C.** In the United States, 80% of gallstones are cholesterol.

5. **A.** Hepatitis A is spread via the fecal-oral route and does not cause chronic hepatitis. However, patients with underlying cirrhosis are at higher risk of severe hepatitis due to the disease and should be vaccinated before international travel.

6. **A.** Charcot triad (fever, RUQ tenderness, and jaundice) is strongly indicative of cholangitis, a stone that obstructs the common bile duct, leading to infection.

7. **E.** The CDC recommends one time screening for hepatitis C antibody should be performed in all adults aged 18 years and older. Evaluation for liver transaminase elevations in adult patients should include evaluation for hepatitis C even if there are no obvious risk factors. Serum ceruloplasmin is associated with Wilson disease and usually presents in younger patients. ANA can be performed if suspected autoimmune causes and a liver biopsy would not be included in an initial evaluation.

8. **D.** Patients with chronic hepatitis C should be counseled to avoid alcohol as studies have shown a strong correlation between alcohol use and progression of liver disease in hepatitis C–positive patients. Patients should avoid high regular doses of hepatotoxic drugs, such as acetaminophen. The risk of sexual transmission of HCV in a monogamous relationship is very low as is the vertical transmission from mother to baby is about 5% according to the Society for Maternal-Fetal Medicine (https://www.contemporaryobgyn.net/authors/society-maternal-fetal-medicine-smfm).

9. **A.** The patient is infected, but without the hepatitis B core antibody and hepatitis B antigen/antibody we cannot tell if it is an acute or a chronic infection.

10. **A.** RUQ pain, fever, and jaundice are characteristics of acute cholangitis.

11. **D.** Nodular hepatic parenchyma on CT is most suggestive of cirrhosis.

12. **D.** ERCP would provide diagnostic and therapeutic benefit to this patient.

13. **A.** Malignant biliary stricture found on ERCP provides the most likely explanation of his clinical history.

14. **C.** Esophageal varices is a complication of cirrhosis.

15. **A.** Asterixis and an elevated ammonia level are the physical examination findings and lab results appropriately correspond to a diagnosis of hepatic encephalopathy.

16. **D.** Cholangiography (ERCP or MRCP) is the gold standard for diagnosing common bile duct obstruction. The other tests may be performed as part of the evaluation.

17. **A.** A positive hepatitis B surface antigen and a negative antibody suggest an acute infection with hepatitis B without prior vaccination.

18. **C.** The MELD score uses dialysis, creatinine, bilirubin, INR, and sodium to predict 3-month survival in hepatic failure.

▶ ANSWERS AND EXPLANATIONS TO SECTION E PRETEST

1. **E.** Bloody stools are a late sign of intussusception.
2. **A.** Small bowel obstruction may be the initial presentation of pregnancy.
3. **B.** Tension pneumoperitoneum is the highest risk associated with pneumatic reduction.
4. **C.** Beyond abdominal pain, the classic triad of appendicitis includes nausea, vomiting, and anorexia.
5. **C.** History of several days of severe diarrhea is not a common finding in a patient with a suspected small bowel obstruction.
6. **C.** Meckel diverticulum is the most common cause of secondary intussusception in children.
7. **D.** Reduction of the hernia is the most appropriate initial management if a small bowel obstruction is caused by a hernia.
8. **E.** Repeat pneumatic reduction is the next best step if an intussusception recurs after pneumatic reduction.
9. **B.** Appendicitis most commonly occurs in 10- to 19-year-olds.
10. **A.** Local anal trauma is the common cause of an anal fissure.
11. **D.** Antibiotics for appendicitis should cover anaerobes, enterococci, and Gram-negative intestinal flora.
12. **C.** Most anal fissures occur proximal to the dentate line.
13. **A.** Diverticulosis in itself is asymptomatic. Only a small minority of patients will go on to develop diverticulitis or diverticular bleeding. There is no treatment or surveillance required for diverticular disease unless complications occur.
14. **E.** Partial obstruction is always a surgical emergency.
15. **B.** Rebound tenderness would raise concern for peritonitis caused by bowel perforation. Hematochezia is associated with diverticular bleeding, whereas fever and leukocytosis can occur in uncomplicated diverticulitis.
16. **B.** Psychogenic is not a subtype of IBS.
17. **A.** The patient is presenting with signs of diverticulitis. The most appropriate test would be a CT scan of the abdomen, which would show evidence of diverticular disease and inflammation. Antibiotics are indicated in most cases of diverticulitis, but the first-line therapy is metronidazole and ciprofloxacin. Emergent surgery is not indicated for this patient, and colonoscopy is not done when diverticulitis is suspected because of the risk of bowel perforation.
18. **B.** Topical nifedipine 2–4 times daily for 1–2 months is appropriate medical management for a patient with anal pain and bleeding for 2 weeks.
19. **D.** A diet completely free of gluten (found in wheat, barely, and rye) effectively treats celiac disease and allows for the mucosal lining of the small intestine to heal.
20. **D.** Most patients with hemorrhoidal disease will require surgical intervention is not true regarding hemorrhoids.
21. **A.** Examination does not commonly reveal a positive straight leg raise test in appendicitis.
22. **E.** Evidence of GI bleeding, anorexia/weight loss, fever, and nocturnal symptoms are all red flags of a potential organic cause for abdominal pain and diarrhea.
23. **D.** Lifestyle measures for prevention of hemorrhoids and anal fissures include a high-fiber diet with possible fiber supplementation, straining avoidance and having a bowel movement as soon as you feel the urge, and exercising regularly and staying hydrated with water.
24. **B.** Low dietary fiber intake is a risk factor for colorectal cancer.
25. **A.** In postmenopausal women, a pelvic examination be recommended due to the possibility of a malignancy presenting with recent onset of lower abdominal pain and bowel changes.
26. **D.** Diverticulitis and diverticular bleeding can often be managed conservatively. Colorectal cancer is not a complication of diverticulosis. Patients with fistula formation with other organs may require surgical management.
27. **B.** tTG-IgA is highly sensitive, highly specific, and more cost-effective than other serologic tests available and should be considered before endoscopy in most patients.
28. **C.** Regarding management of IBS, all types of IBS patients should avoid cruciferous vegetables.
29. **C.** The diagnosis of celiac disease is confirmed by the presence of villous atrophy and increased intraepithelial lymphocytes on biopsy samples of the small intestine.
30. **A.** Colonoscopy is the most appropriate next step for this patient.
31. **A.** Dermatitis herpetiformis is a characteristic skin rash that is commonly associated with celiac disease.
32. **A.** Lynch syndrome is the likely cause of this patient's colon cancer.
33. **C.** There is an increased incidence of celiac disease in individuals with autoimmune conditions.
34. **C.** A villous colon polyp is most concerning for an increased risk of colorectal cancer.
35. **B.** Malignancy is the most common cause of large bowel obstruction.
36. **D.** FIT annually is a colonoscopy alternative for this patient.
37. **B.** Recommend surgical resection and possible ostomy for this patient.
38. **D.** History of cardiovascular disease is a risk factor for AMI.
39. **A.** Loperamide and fluids are the first-line treatment for diarrhea caused by viral gastroenteritis. Opioids have a limited indication for chronic diarrhea.

Octreotide and clonidine are used in secretory diarrhea.

40. **D.** Inflammatory bowel disease is not a risk factor for mesenteric venous thrombosis.

41. **D.** The history given suggests an osmotic diarrhea with the change in stool volume with fasting. Celiac disease would be associated with weight loss. Ulcerative colitis usually has fever and hematochezia. The volume of stool would not change with fasting with a carcinoid tumor.

42. **D.** Manage a patient who has been diagnosed with a large bowel obstruction secondary to fecal impaction with manual disimpaction.

43. **C.** Loperamide should be avoided with those with bloody acute diarrhea. Fluids and a bland diet are encouraged. Bismuth subsalicylate is not explicitly contraindicated.

44. **B.** Fever is not part of the classic triad for CMI.

45. **D.** Metformin is a drug used in diabetes that can cause diarrhea. Insulin does not usually cause diarrhea. Antihypertensives such as angiotensin II receptor blockers may cause diarrhea, but not β-blockers. NSAIDs, not acetaminophen, cause diarrhea.

▶ ANSWERS AND EXPLANATIONS TO SECTION F PRETEST

1. **C.** Gallstones most likely caused this patient's acute pancreatitis.

2. **A.** Elevated phenylalanine levels with no genetic abnormality related to phenylalanine hydroxylase is most likely related to tetrahydrobiopterin.

3. **C.** Patients who present with acute pancreatitis will often complain of steady, deep epigastric pain with radiation to the back.

4. **B.** Phenylalanine hydroxylase converts phenylalanine to tyrosine.

5. **B.** Serum lipase would most likely be elevated 8–14 days after this initial presentation.

6. **C.** An infant be screened for PKU 24–72 hours after birth.

7. **B.** Pancreatitis is a known side effect of very high triglyceride levels.

8. **B.** A serum level of phenylalanine >10 mg/dL is concerning for PKU.

9. **A.** The Atlanta criteria are used to define pancreatitis severity.

CHAPTER

127

Esophagitis

Daniel Provencher, MS, PA-C

A 54-year-old patient presents to your family medicine clinic for evaluation of nonexertional chest pain. He was seen 2 days ago in the emergency department with similar complaints and, after a negative cardiac evaluation, was diagnosed with "reflux" and advised to follow up with you. What is the most likely cause of his symptoms?

▶ GENERAL FEATURES

- Esophagitis is inflammation of the esophageal mucosa.
- Caused by direct irritation or an immune-mediated inflammatory response
- Most common cause: abnormal reflux of acidic gastric fluid
- Contributing factors: obesity, pregnancy, and presence of a hiatal hernia
- Smoking and alcohol use; medications including anticholinergics, calcium channel blockers, and opioids; and high-fat foods, chocolate, caffeine, and peppermint all decrease lower esophageal sphincter (LES) pressure and allow for increased reflux.
- Eosinophilic esophagitis (EoE) most commonly diagnosed in patients younger than 30 years
- Consider if a history of atopic disorders such as eczema, asthma, allergic rhinitis
- Incidence increasing over the past several decades
- More commonly identified in Caucasians and males
- Infectious esophagitis usually due to herpes simplex virus (HSV), cytomegalovirus (CMV), and *Candida albicans*
- Consider primarily in immunocompromised patients
- Medication-induced or "pill" esophagitis due to direct contact or alteration of the cytoprotective layer of the squamous esophageal mucosa
- Typically associated with bisphosphonates (eg, alendronate), antibiotics (eg, tetracycline), and NSAIDs. Larger tablet size and smaller volume of swallowed liquid increase risk

▶ CLINICAL ASSESSMENT

- Typical complaint: noncardiac retrosternal discomfort
- Additional symptoms include heartburn, dysphagia, and odynophagia.
- Symptoms may be worse when lying flat and after large meals.
- Patients may also complain of indigestion, sore throat, regurgitation, or frequent belching.
- However, some patients are asymptomatic.
- Children with EoE: failure to thrive, feeding difficulties, vomiting, or difficulty swallowing
- Older patients: chest or upper abdominal pain, dysphagia, or intermittent solid food impactions
- HSV and CMV: significant pain, especially while swallowing, due to esophageal ulcerations
- Fungal esophagitis: odynophagia and dysphagia
- Additional symptoms of infectious esophagitis are fever, nausea, and abdominal pain.
- Consider medication-induced esophagitis if retrosternal pain, odynophagia (often severe), or dysphagia after ingesting substances or medications known to damage the esophagus.

▶ DIAGNOSIS

- Often a clinical diagnosis based on history
- Upper endoscopy (EGD) with biopsy required for the diagnosis of EoE and infectious esophagitis
- Also indicated if symptoms not responding to treatment or with warning signs: weight loss, hematemesis, iron deficiency anemia, severe pain, dysphagia, etc.
- Diagnostic criteria for EoE: esophageal biopsy demonstrating ≥15 eosinophils per high-power field, symptoms consistent with esophageal dysfunction, exclusion of other conditions, which may produce these findings
- Endoscopic and radiographic studies in patients with EoE may demonstrate esophageal rings ("feline esophagus"), strictures, or linear furrows.

- Barium esophagram usually unnecessary before EGD in patients with dysphagia, unless concern for anatomic abnormality (Zenker diverticulum)

▶ TREATMENT

- Treatment of reflux esophagitis is multidimensional.
- Lose weight if overweight or obese
- Raise the head of the bed at least 6 in and avoid eating within 2–3 hours of bedtime if nocturnal symptoms.
- Minimize foods that trigger symptoms, along with factors that decrease LES pressure (smoking, alcohol, certain medications, fatty foods, etc.).
- Medical management: antacids, antisecretory agents, and surfactants, either singly or in combination
- Antacids work quickly to neutralize gastric acid, but limited duration of action, best suited for mild or occasional symptoms.
- Antisecretory medications include histamine-2 receptor antagonists (H2RAs) such as famotidine and nizatidine and proton-pump inhibitors (PPIs) such as omeprazole and pantoprazole.
- PPIs more potent and more expensive than H2RAs; concern about potential side effects (eg, *Clostridioides difficile* infection), especially with long-term daily use
- 8-week course of once-daily, prescription-strength H2RA or PPI is recommended initially.
- If symptoms persist, consider additional evaluation, a trial of twice-daily medication or combination therapy.
- The surfactant sucralfate occasionally used, especially with reflux esophagitis during pregnancy
- Topical corticosteroids recommended as first-line management for EoE

- Examples include inhaled (no spacer) then swallowed fluticasone, or liquid viscous budesonide for 4–8 weeks.
- Additional treatment options: PPIs, elimination diets (typically avoidance of common allergenic foods including milk, eggs, wheat, nuts, shellfish, and wheat), and dilation of known strictures
- Treatment for infectious esophagitis directed against causative pathogen
- HSV is treated with acyclovir, valacyclovir, or famciclovir for 14–21 days in patients with immune suppression.
- CMV treated with ganciclovir for 3–6 weeks
- Therapeutic options for *Candida*: 14–21-day course of fluconazole, voriconazole, or posaconazole
- Discontinue suspected irritants, if possible, in medication-induced esophagitis
- Most patients will heal within 14 days.
- Consider antisecretory agents and endoscopic evaluation for refractory cases

Case Conclusion

Based on the patient's symptoms and negative cardiac evaluation, we diagnosed this patient clinically with reflux esophagitis. EGD was not indicated because he did not exhibit any warning signs. We treated him empirically with pantoprazole 40 mg every morning and encouraged gradual weight loss and avoidance of potential trigger foods. His symptoms improved, and we discontinued his PPI after he completed an 8-week course.

CHAPTER
128

Mallory-Weiss Tear and Boerhaave Syndrome

Ryan Olivero, MMS, PA-C

▶ GENERAL FEATURES

- Partial- or full-thickness tears of the esophagus are common complications among patients presenting with prolonged nausea, vomiting, or retching.
- Two main classifications:
  - Mallory-Weiss syndrome is the less severe and most common of the two, consisting of a partial esophageal tear (the inner mucosal layer only) and subsequent nonvariceal bleeding.

- Boerhaave syndrome, although relatively rare, is the most serious of the two. It results in a full-thickness tear of all esophageal layers.
- Both are most common in the distal esophagus, near the gastroesophageal junction.
- Risk factors include nausea, vomiting, retching, trauma to the chest or abdomen, severe or prolonged hiccups, intense coughing, heavy lifting or straining, gastritis, hiatal hernia, seizure or convulsions, chest compressions, or recent instrumentation.

- Patients with chronic emesis are most at risk including alcoholics and bulimics, or those with underlying esophageal pathology (stricture, ulcer, mass, esophagitis).
- Complications of a partial tear are usually minor and mostly include bleeding as manifested by frank hematemesis, coffee ground emesis, melena, or pain.
- Complications of a complete tear are serious and life-threatening resulting from severe chemical burn and gross contamination. These would include hydropneumothorax, sepsis, respiratory failure, multiorgan failure, empyema, or death.

CLINICAL ASSESSMENT

- Patients with a partial tear may be asymptomatic or most commonly will present with upper abdominal or atypical chest pain, followed by a bout of nausea or vomiting. Most will have some form of upper gastrointestinal bleeding noted such as coffee ground emesis or nasogastric (NG) tube output, bloody NG output, or melena. Frank hematochezia is less likely, though possible in the case of a brisk bleed.
- Complete tears are promptly symptomatic, often presenting with severe chest pain, shortness of breath, hypotension, or other signs of sepsis, bleeding, or subcutaneous emphysema.

DIAGNOSIS

- Patients present with mild chest or abdominal pain and coffee grounds emesis or NG output, followed by bouts of nausea or vomiting or retching. The clinician can then add a diagnosis of Mallory-Weiss tear to the differential diagnosis.
- If symptoms are severe or fail to resolve, the patient can be referred to the gastroenterology service for an esophagogastroduodenoscopy (EGD). Here the images would confirm partial-thickness tear of the distal esophagus.
- Severe symptoms can indicate a complete tear and require emergent investigation.
  - Begin with a plain chest and abdominal radiograph, which may show pneumomediastinum, hydrothorax, or pneumothorax with or without mediastinal shift.
  - Often chest computed tomography (CT) scan is the fastest and safest next step depending on the availability. This will most often again show pneumomediastinum, hydropneumothorax or plain pneumothorax, pleural effusion, and pneumomediastinum and may or may not show an esophageal tear depending on the size and severity.
  - Barium esophagram if available would show extravasation of contrast, clearly confirming the diagnosis.

- EGD would not be indicated because it could further worsen an existing tear and extravasation of gastric contents.

TREATMENT

- Mallory-Weiss tear:
  - For most mild-to-moderate cases, conservative management should result in healing.
  - The patient ideally should be kept nothing by mouth (NPO) or on clear liquids if in an outpatient setting.
  - The underlying cause of nausea and vomiting should be treated, and the patient started on antiemetic therapy such as ondansetron (Zofran). Metoclopramide (Reglan) should be avoided because it may increase esophageal and gastric motility, worsening the tear, especially in the setting of a hiatal hernia, paraesophageal hernia, gastric volvulus, or small bowel obstruction.
  - Proton-pump inhibitor (PPI) therapy such as protonix or omeprazole should be initiated once or twice daily, intravenous (IV) or NPO, depending on the severity.
  - Complete blood count (CBC) should be obtained, and if indicated, transfusion may be necessary.
- Boerhaave syndrome:
  - Treatment depends on the severity of the tear, and availability and experience of consulting physicians.
  - Emergent laboratory studies such as CBC, electrolytes, lactic acid, hepatic and renal panels, coagulation profile, and blood typing should be obtained, and all abnormalities corrected as able.
  - A small complete tear can be treated with conservative management. Supportive care, antibiotics, and PPIs may be sufficient. These patients can be identified by having no signs of sepsis, a small amount of free mediastinal air on imaging, and a negative esophagram (indicating a small tear may have already closed).
  - Moderate-to-severe tears must be treated urgently and definitively. In the early setting, the patient should be made NPO, started on an IV PPI, given broad-spectrum IV antibiotic coverage, fluid resuscitated, and transferred to the intensive care unit (ICU).
  - In the presence of pneumothorax, a chest tube with Pleur-evac (Atrium) must be placed and hooked to continuous wall suction of 20 mm Hg.
  - If the patient is stable or is not a good surgical candidate, esophageal stenting is an emerging treatment choice as it spares the patient surgery.
  - If the patient is unstable or has a large tear, emergent surgical repair with thoracotomy is indicated. This may require transfer to a tertiary care center.

Esophageal Motility Disorders

Danielle Kruger, PA-C, MS Ed

A 45-year-old white female with no significant past medical history presents with complaint of progressive dysphagia for solids and liquids associated with mild substernal chest pain for 6 months. She also reports regurgitation of undigested food with coughing, particularly while lying down at night. She has lost 8 lb in the past 4 months. She denies heartburn, abdominal pain, hematemesis, or melena. She denies history of smoking, alcohol use, or recreational drugs. Vital signs are stable, and physical examination is noncontributory. Barium esophagram reveals a dilated lower esophagus with a "bird's-beak" sign.

▶ GENERAL FEATURES

- Achalasia:
  - Primary esophageal motility disorder characterized by failure of lower esophageal sphincter (LES) to relax in response to swallowing and absence of peristalsis in the lower two-thirds of the esophagus
    - Caused by progressive degeneration of inhibitory ganglion cells of the myenteric (ie, Auerbach) plexus in the esophageal wall
    - Obstructive nature of LES leads to stasis of ingested food causing dilation of the distal esophagus (proximal to the LES) and may be associated with the development of an epiphrenic diverticulum.
  - No gender predilection and is usually diagnosed in patients aged 25–60 years.
  - Increases the risk for development of esophageal cancer, typically squamous cell type
- Diffuse esophageal spasm (DES):
  - Esophageal contractions are of normal or increased amplitude but are uncoordinated, simultaneous, or rapidly propagated.
    - Caused by dysfunction of the inhibitory neurons
  - Hypercontractile esophagus (HC) (ie, "jackhammer or nutcracker esophagus") and esophageal contractions are coordinated, but the amplitude is excessive (>2 standard deviations from normal).
    - HC may be caused by excessive excitation and/or smooth muscle hypertrophy.
  - More commonly seen in patients with anxiety and depression
  - Underlying conditions such as gastroesophageal reflux disease (GERD), diabetes mellitus, scleroderma, and chronic alcohol consumption may cause secondary esophageal motility disorders.

▶ CLINICAL ASSESSMENT

- Achalasia:
  - Presents with insidious onset of progressive dysphagia for solids and liquids, regurgitation of undigested food, and/or saliva with resultant risk of aspiration, malnutrition, or dehydration.
  - May experience hiccups, cough, and weight loss
  - May employ specific maneuvers (ie, pacing, eating slowly, extending the neck, moving shoulders) to aid esophageal emptying
  - Some patients experience substernal chest pain and heartburn, which may lead to misdiagnosis of GERD.
- DES:
  - Patients may be asymptomatic or experience intermittent, nonprogressive dysphagia for both solids and liquids.
  - May have noncardiac chest pain, usually described as squeezing retrosternal pain that radiates to back; it may be provoked by hot or cold liquids or food, reflux, or alcohol use and may occur with exercise
    - This chest pain can mimic the pain of angina.
  - Symptoms last a few minutes to hours and occur spontaneously or during meals.
  - Other symptoms include regurgitation, heartburn, and globus sensation (ie, food stuck in the esophagus).

▶ DIAGNOSIS

- Achalasia:
  - Esophageal manometry is gold standard diagnostic test; positive findings include incomplete relaxation of the LES and the absence of peristalsis in the distal esophagus.
  - Barium esophagram supports diagnosis in patients with equivocal manometry results. Positive findings include dilation of the proximal esophagus, tapering of the distal esophagus at the LES into a classic "bird's-beak" appearance, and distal aperistalsis with delayed emptying of barium.
  - Upper endoscopy allows for assessment of the gastroesophageal junction and gastric cardia as needed and may be used to rule out conditions, causing pseudoachalasia or occult carcinoma.
- DES:
  - Manometry is gold standard diagnostic and should be combined with upper endoscopy and barium esophagram to rule out other abnormalities.

- DES is defined as the occurrence premature and uncoordinated contractions in ≥20% of swallows in the setting of normal LES response.
- HC is defined as at least 2 liquid swallows with a distal contractile integer (DCI) >8000 mm Hg/s/cm over 10 swallows in the setting of normal LES response.
- Barium esophagram may reveal multiple simultaneous contractions, causing "corkscrew" or "rosary-bead" appearance in DES; HC has a normal esophagram.
- Upper endoscopy is often performed to exclude structural abnormality.

▶ TREATMENT

- Achalasia:
  - The goal of treatment is symptom relief by eliminating LES outflow resistance.
  - Initial therapy includes either graded pneumatic dilation of the LES or surgical treatment with Heller myotomy and partial fundoplication or peroral endoscopic myotomy (POEM).
  - Botulinum toxin therapy and/or oral nitrates and/or calcium channel blockers can be considered in patients who are not the good candidates for more definitive therapy.

- DES:
  - Manage underlying associated conditions: proton-pump inhibitors for patients with GERD and tricyclic antidepressants for associated psychiatric illnesses have been shown to alter pain sensation in the esophagus.
  - Calcium channel blockers are the first-line treatment to reduce amplitude of esophageal contractions.
  - Phosphodiesterase inhibitors (sildenafil) and botulinum toxin injection may also be used to decrease contractions.
  - Surgical myotomy is an option for refractory DES.

Case Conclusion

In the case presented, the most likely diagnosis is achalasia. Progressive dysphagia to solids and liquids, regurgitation, and the classic barium esophagram findings indicated support for the diagnosis of achalasia. GERD would not cause progressive dysphagia unless peptic strictures or other complications develop, and heartburn is the most common presentation. Diffuse esophageal spasm presents as an intermittent dysphagia to solids and liquids, is not associated with heartburn, and has a "corkscrew esophagus" finding on barium esophagram. Adenocarcinoma of the esophagus presents with progressive dysphagia and weight loss, but often occurs in the setting of older men with long-standing history of GERD and Barrett esophagus. Hiatal hernia (usually the sliding type) precipitates GERD symptoms and is not associated with esophageal narrowing or obstruction.

CHAPTER 130

Gastroesophageal Reflux Disease

Danielle Kruger, PA-C, MS Ed

A 45-year-old obese white male with no significant past medical history complains of a 4-month history of substernal chest discomfort and burning with regurgitation that is worse after eating and at night. Symptoms are aggravated by a large meal and lying down and improved with the use of antacids. There is no relation to exertion. He denies smoking, alcohol, and illicit drug use. He denies any cough, difficulty breathing, palpitations, dysphagia, abdominal pain, weight loss, and diaphoresis. Vital signs are normal, and his physical examination is unremarkable. What is the most likely diagnosis?

▶ GENERAL FEATURES

- Gastroesophageal reflux diseases (GERD) occurs when the amount of gastric acid (or duodenal, pancreatic, and biliary secretions) that refluxes into the esophagus exceeds the normal limit, causing symptoms with or without associated erosive esophagitis.

- The incidence of GERD is equal among gender, but the presence of esophagitis is more common among males.
- There is increased prevalence with increasing age (>40 years old) and in smokers.
- GERD most often results from altered or incompetent lower esophageal sphincter (LES) tone.
  - Transient relaxation of the LES is the most common cause of GERD and may be worsened by:
    - Foods: fatty, acidic or spicy food, chocolate, peppermint, alcohol, onion, caffeine, and citrus
    - Medications: calcium channel blockers, anticholinergics, nitrates, β-blockers, Demerol, progesterone, and nicotine
  - GERD may also be precipitated by increased intra-abdominal pressure (ie, pregnancy, obesity, tight-fitting clothing) that may overcome LES pressure and when the LES is displaced into the thorax (ie, hiatal hernia) and exposed to decreased thoracic pressure.

- Poor esophageal motility and delayed gastric emptying (ie, gastroparesis) may also cause GERD.
  - Gastroparesis may be idiopathic or caused by diabetes mellitus, hypothyroidism, surgery, viral infection, medications, radiation, scleroderma, and neurologic disease (eg, Parkinson disease).
- Barrett esophagus is a premalignant condition occurring with long-standing GERD where normal healthy esophageal squamous epithelium is replaced with metaplastic columnar cells (ie, *specialized intestinal metaplasia* [SIM] *in the esophagus*).
  - The risk for esophageal adenocarcinoma is greatly increased with Barrett metaplasia.
  - The condition is most common among middle-aged white males with chronic GERD and with the use of oral bisphosphonate therapy.

▶ CLINICAL ASSESSMENT

- Typical symptoms of GERD relate to the esophagus.
  - Heartburn (pyrosis) is the most common symptom of GERD; it is described as retrosternal squeezing or burning discomfort that occurs after meals and is relieved by antacids.
  - It can last minutes to hours and is provoked by the supine position or bending over.
  - Reflux is the most common cause of noncardiac chest pain and can mimic angina.
  - Other symptoms include regurgitation, halitosis, waterbrash (reflex salivary hypersecretion), or a sour taste in the mouth.
  - Dysphagia or odynophagia may result from mucosal damage, stricture development, or motility disorder. Patients may present with a globus sensation in the retrosternal area (ie, "food gets stuck").
- Atypical symptoms of GERD are extraesophageal manifestations.
  - Respiratory complications include chronic cough, wheezing, asthma exacerbation, aspiration, and pneumonitis.
  - Other manifestations include sore throat, hoarseness (vocal cord exposure to reflux), and tooth enamel decay.

▶ DIAGNOSIS

- In patients with typical symptoms of uncomplicated GERD, the diagnosis can be presumed, and empiric therapy started with close follow-up.
- Patients with noncardiac chest pain suspected to be due to GERD should have cardiac causes excluded before gastrointestinal (GI) evaluation.
- Endoscopy and routine biopsies, barium esophagram, and testing for *Helicobacter pylori* infection are not recommended in the presence of typical GERD symptoms.
- The gold standard test for GERD is 24-hour esophageal pH monitoring and is indicated when symptoms are refractory to medications, in situations where the diagnosis of GERD is in question and before surgery.

- Patients with atypical or red flag symptoms (eg, evidence of GI bleeding, iron deficiency anemia, weight loss, dysphagia, family history of GI cancer), long-standing GERD symptoms (eg, >5 years), particularly in those aged 50 years or older; patients with abnormal imaging; or patients with symptoms that are recurrent or unresponsive to medication should have endoscopic evaluation.
  - Endoscopy is used to evaluate esophageal anatomy, determine the severity of esophagitis, and evaluate through biopsy the presence of Barrett esophagus or malignancy and to exclude other disorders.
  - Esophageal manometry is recommended for preoperative evaluation and may reveal decreased LES tone. Nuclear medicine gastric-emptying studies can be performed to evaluate for gastroparesis.

▶ TREATMENT

- Goals of treatment are to control symptoms, heal esophagitis, and prevent recurrence or complications.
- All patients should be educated on lifestyle modifications: eat small meals, wait 3 hours after meal before lying down, and elevate head of bed 6–8 in; lose weight (if overweight), eliminate foods that trigger reflux (listed earlier), avoid tight-fitting clothes, and abstain from smoking and alcohol.
- Antacids are effective for mild symptoms and may be taken after each meal and at bedtime.
  - H_2 receptor antagonists are the first-line agents for mild-to-moderate GERD symptoms and may be used as maintenance therapy.
  - Proton-pump inhibitors (PPIs) are the first-line medications for moderate-to-severe GERD symptoms, erosive esophagitis, or if symptoms are unresponsive to H_2 receptor antagonists.
  - Prokinetic agents may be used to improve motility of the esophagus and stomach.
- Surgery is indicated for patients with GERD for symptoms not completely controlled by PPIs, in the presence of Barrett esophagus, and for extraesophageal manifestations of GERD; Nissen fundoplication is the most common antireflux procedure.

Case Conclusion

In the case presented, the most likely diagnosis is GERD. The typical features of GERD are postprandial heartburn worsened meals, bending or lying supine, regurgitation, dysphagia, and water brash. PUD presents with gnawing or burning epigastric pain that is most commonly caused by either NSAID use or *Helicobacter pylori* infection. Adenocarcinoma of the esophagus is a complication of long-standing GERD and Barrett esophagus and presents with progressive dysphagia to solids, weight loss, and, possibly, other alarm symptoms. Achalasia presents as progressive dysphagia to solids and liquids along with regurgitation and weight loss. Biliary colic usually presents as right upper quadrant pain that occurs after fatty meals.

Esophageal Strictures

K. Alexis Moore, MPH, PA-C

GENERAL FEATURES

- Most common type of benign esophageal stricture (70% of cases) is a peptic stricture, which is associated with gastroesophageal reflux disease (GERD), but 25% of patients with benign esophageal strictures may not experience or report GERD or heartburn symptoms.
- Other causes of esophageal strictures include cancer of the esophagus, scarring secondary to radiation therapy, and dysmotility disorders.
- Environments that are conducive to peptic stricture formation are those that result from a dysfunctional lower esophageal sphincter, leading to reduced lower sphincter tone. Dysfunctions of motility and hiatal hernias may also give rise to peptic stricture formation.
- Proximal vs. distal esophageal strictures:
  - Proximal result from malignancy, radiation, infections, or medication-induced "pill esophagitis" from drugs such as NSAIDs or ferrous sulfate.
  - Distal narrowing is associated with peptic strictures, GERD, Zollinger-Ellinson syndrome, and collagen vascular diseases, such as scleroderma.
- Esophageal strictures are thought to be more common in older adults, white males, and individuals who have a longer duration of reflux symptoms.
- More recent studies suggest African Americans and Hispanics share a similar predominance.
- Consider other causes of dysphagia:
  - Achalasia
  - Schatzki ring
  - Barrett esophagus

CLINICAL ASSESSMENT

- Patients most commonly complain of progressive dysphagia for solid food.
- Symptoms related to benign strictures are insidious and progressive over a period of months to years.
  - Rapid development of symptoms may indicate the presence of malignant stricture.
- Other symptoms can range from sensation of food sticking in throat or chest, coughing or gagging when swallowing, drooling, to unexpected weight loss.
- Atypical presentations are seen as aspiration asthma from poor swallowing of liquids and chronic coughing.
- Physical examination is usually unremarkable.

DIAGNOSIS

- Barium swallow is indicated as first test in the case of caustic ingestion or when a patient has had radiation to the neck/thorax.
- Manometry should be performed if dysmotitity is suspected.
- Endoscopy is indicated for all others.

TREATMENT

- Mechanical dilatation is indicated in simple strictures and balloon in complex (strictures that are long or tortuous in configuration).
- Acid control with proton-pump inhibitors.

CHAPTER
132
Lactose Intolerance

Victoria Louwagie, PA-C

▶ GENERAL FEATURES

- Lactose digestion occurs in the small intestine by an enzyme called *lactase* on the brush border of the intestinal villi.
- When the enzyme is absent or deficient, unabsorbed lactose attracts fluids into the bowel, thus increasing volume and liquidity of bowel contents.
- The lactose also passes into the large intestine where fermentation occurs, causing a variety of complaints.
- Congenital lactase deficiency:
  - Autosomal recessive, extremely rare
  - Symptoms include severe watery stools, life-threatening dehydration, metabolic alkalosis, and growth delay since first intake of any mammalian milk.
- Primary lactase deficiency:
  - Physiologic decline of lactase production
  - Typically does not occur before age 6 years, and the incidence rises as the population ages
  - Very common
  - In Asians, Africans, Alaskan natives, and Native Americans, genetic lactase deficiency develops in virtually 100% of the population by adulthood. In African Americans, incidence is over 70%. In Caucasian Americans, the incidence is 30% to 60%.
- Acquired or secondary lactase deficiency:
  - Brought on by intestinal injury
  - Frequently seen in clinical practice
  - Most commonly caused by viral or bacterial infections, inflammatory bowel disease, celiac disease, radiation exposure, or medications

▶ CLINICAL ASSESSMENT

- Gastrointestinal complaints and severity vary but can include:
  - Diarrhea, gassy abdominal distention, bloating, flatus, abdominal pain and distress, vomiting, nausea, and borborygmi related to milk product consumption
- Systemic symptoms of headache, vertigo, fatigue, memory impairment, or arrhythmia are more consistent with a possible cow's milk allergy rather than lactose intolerance.

▶ DIAGNOSIS

- Assessing clinical correlation of ingestion with symptoms:
  - Food journaling can identify triggering foods, though not always accurate.
  - A limited trial of avoiding dairy may improve symptoms, thus inferencing lactose intolerance.
  - To confirm diagnosis, testing should be offered, especially if long-term dietary lactose avoidance or restriction is being considered.
- Gold standard testing requires intestinal biopsy; this is a costly and invasive test for such a mild condition.
- Hydrogen breath testing:
  - Lactose hydrogen breath testing (lactose HBT) is noninvasive, reliable, and inexpensive.
    - Sensitivity is as high as 76% to 100% with excellent specificity of 90% to 100%.
    - Can be completed in a clinic setting or a take-home test
      - Patients follow a carbohydrate restricted diet and to fast the day of testing.
      - Baseline breath samples of hydrogen and methane are collected.
      - For adults, 25 g of lactose is then ingested.
      - Breath samples are then collected and analyzed every 30 minutes for 4 hours.
      - Results are positive when hydrogen particles increase >20 parts per million over the baseline value.
    - Symptoms are typically recorded during testing and possibly up to 8 hours after testing.

◗ TREATMENT

- Alimentary restriction:
  - Symptoms are alleviated when dietary lactose is restricted or avoided.
  - Consider oral calcium or vitamin/multivitamin supplementation if restricting lactose.
  - Most adolescents and adults with lactose intolerance can ingest at least 12 g of lactose in a single dose (equivalent to 1 cup of milk), with only minor symptoms reported.
  - Identifying low-lactose foods and high-lactose foods is important for patient education and prevention of symptoms:
    - Lactose-free foods contain no lactose.
    - Low-lactose foods contain 1 g or less of lactose per serving.
    - High-lactose foods contain 2 g or more of lactose per serving.
  - Following up with a registered dietician may be helpful.
- Drug therapy:
  - Dietary supplementation of lactase from nonhuman source 5–30 minutes before a meal is another approach to therapy.
  - These are commonly purchased over the counter in either tablets or drops.

CHAPTER 133

Tree Nut Allergy

Ziemowit Mazur, EdM, MS, PA-C

◗ GENERAL FEATURES

- Tree nut allergy, along with peanut and seed allergies, represents the most common food allergies in adults and children and tends to persist over time; tolerance can be developed; however, it is rare.
- Tree nuts include cashews, pistachios, almonds, and hazelnut, but notably not peanuts, which are legumes; however, there is known cross-reactivity between tree nuts, peanuts, and seeds.
- Anaphylactic reaction to tree nuts can be life-threating and can be characterized by cough, dyspnea, pruritis, nausea, and abdominal pain.

◗ CLINICAL ASSESSMENT

- Allergy to tree nuts can be through primary or secondary sensitization; most reactions are immunoglobulin E (IgE) mediated, with reactions ranging from isolated and mild to anaphylactic reaction.
- There is an association between tree nut allergy and atopic disease (asthma, allergic rhinitis, and atopic dermatitis).
- Most commonly, the first tree nut exposure and allergic reaction occurs between the ages of 1 and 2 years.

◗ DIAGNOSIS

- Detailed history is the key to diagnosing a tree nut allergy.
- Development of typical and reproducible allergic signs and symptoms (eg, swelling of face, lips, or throat; wheezing; nausea; urticaria; cough) immediately after tree nut ingestion plus positive tree nut IgE antibody skin-prick test establish the diagnosis.
- If history and/or IgE testing is equivocal, a double-blind, placebo-controlled oral food challenges constitutes gold standard of being able to establish a food allergy.

◗ TREATMENT

- Complete, lifelong avoidance of tree nuts is the primary management strategy.
- Patient education about food cross-reactivity, reading food labels, ordering meals at restaurants, and cooking meals at home is important to empower the patient.
- The severity of the previous reaction does not predict the next reaction; thus, prescribing epinephrine autoinjector for patients to have with them at all times along with a written anaphylaxis emergency action plan is advised.

CHAPTER
134

Hiatal Hernia

Brian Peacock, MMS

▶ GENERAL FEATURES

- A hiatal hernia is caused by laxity of the hiatus at the diaphragm that allows abdominal contents to herniate into the thoracic cavity.
- Risk factors include increased age, previous abdominal or gastroesophageal surgery, and obesity.
- More common in females, advancing age, and patients who have had gastroesophageal surgery.
- Four types:
  - Type 1 is a sliding hiatal hernia, typically minimally to asymptomatic.
  - Types 2–4 are considered paraesophageal hernias, gastric fundus, and potentially abdominal contents remain in the thoracic cavity.
- Potential complications include gastric ulcerations/bleeding, gastric volvulus, intestinal obstruction, and respiratory compromise.

▶ CLINICAL ASSESSMENT

- Patients may complain of dysphagia, regurgitation, shortness of breath, or epigastric pain.
- The severity of symptoms is dependent on the contents and orientation of the herniated tissue.

- Misdiagnosis can lead to progression of symptoms and gastric bleeding and/or gastric volvulus.
- Physical examination is typically normal.

▶ DIAGNOSIS

- Patient's history typically supports the diagnosis.
- Barium esophagography identifies the portion and extends of the esophagus or stomach herniated into the chest.
- Endoscopic evaluation with EGD identifies the external compression of the stomach and allows for identification of ulcerations and/or chronic reflux.
- Complete blood count may be obtained to evaluate anemia secondary to bleeding ulcerations.

▶ TREATMENT

- Therapy is aimed at managing symptoms by eating smaller meals and taking antireflux medications (such as antacids and proton-pump inhibitors) and minimizing risks for gastric ulcerations/bleeding, gastric volvulus, intestinal obstruction, and respiratory compromise with an organized weight loss program.
- Surgery may be required in patients who remain symptomatic despite these measures.

Pyloric Stenosis

Kristopher Maday, MS, PA-C, DFAAPA

GENERAL FEATURES

- Epidemiology:
  - Higher male-to-female ratio (4-6:1)
  - One and a half times higher incidence in first-born children
  - Highest incidence in Caucasian infants
- Risk factors:
  - Up to 2 times increased risk in mothers who smoke
  - Up to 4 times increased risk in bottle-feeding in the first 4 months
  - Increased risk if given macrolide antibiotics age <2 weeks old

CLINICAL ASSESSMENT

- History and physical examination:
  - Postprandial, nonbilious, projectile vomiting after feeding
  - Ravenous feeding after vomiting
  - Palpable epigastric mass
  - May be dehydrated or emaciated
- Differential diagnosis of vomiting in infancy:
  - Physiologic reflux/GERD
  - Obstruction
  - Congenital atresias, malrotation, Hirschsprung disease, intussusception
  - Necrotizing fasciitis
  - Increased intracranial pressure
  - Metabolic disorders
  - Adrenal crisis
  - Dietary intolerance
  - Toxic ingestion

DIAGNOSIS

- Laboratory findings:
  - Hypochloremic metabolic alkalosis

- Hypokalemia
- Increased BUN and creatinine if severe
- Radiography:
  - Ultrasound is test of choice:
    - "Target sign" on short-axis view
    - Measurements:
      - Remember "π-lorus"
      - Pyloric thickness >3 mm
      - Pyloric diameter >14 mm
      - Pyloric channel length >16 mm
  - Contrasted upper gastrointestinal series:
    - Used if ultrasound is inconclusive
    - Classic findings:
      - "String sign" from elongated channel
      - "Beak sign" from tapered point at pylorus
      - "Shoulder sign" from prepyloric barium collection

TREATMENT

- Surgery is curative in the majority of infants but must correct metabolic derangement.
  - In some cases, surgery can be performed same day of diagnosis if infant is healthy enough.
- Procedure:
  - Ramstedt pyloromyotomy: longitudinal incision of pylorus with dissection to the submucosa
- Postoperative considerations:
  - Feeding:
    - May be resumed a few hours after surgery
    - Regurgitation is common.
  - Monitor for breathing problems and apnea.
  - Mucosal perforation are rare but should be considered if an infant not improving.

Gastritis and Peptic Ulcer Disease

Danielle Kruger, PA-C, MS Ed

A 35-year-old athletic male with a past medical history of knee surgery presents with a 2-month history of epigastric pain described as dull, aching, and burning along with indigestion, nausea, and anorexia. He has tried over-the-counter antacids for the last 2 weeks with only mild relief. The pain is made better by eating and recurs a few hours after meals and is also worse at night. He denies any fever, chills, weight loss, dysphagia, chest pain, heartburn, hematemesis, or melena. Physical examination reveals epigastric pain to deep palpation, otherwise is normal. Stool guaiac test is negative. A urease breath test is negative. Patient reports the use of nonsteroidal anti-inflammatory drugs (NSAIDs) daily for joint pain. He denies smoking, alcohol, and illicit drug use. What is the most likely diagnosis?

▶ GENERAL FEATURES

- Acute gastritis involves inflammatory changes and/or cell damage to the gastric mucosa; inflammation may involve the entire gastric mucosa or just sections.
  - Gastritis is most common among patients older than 60 years, and there is no gender predilection.
  - *Gastropathy* is defined as mucosal injury without histopathologic evidence of inflammation.
- *Peptic ulcer disease* (PUD) is defined as a discrete mucosal defect in the gastrointestinal tract exposed to acid and pepsin that extends through the muscularis mucosa.
- Risk factors, etiologies, and clinical presentations of acute gastritis vs. PUD are indistinguishable.
- *Helicobacter pylori* infection and use of NSAIDs are the most common causes of gastritis and PUD in the United States.
- Other etiologies of acute gastritis and PUD include:
  - Reactive (chemical) gastropathy from exposure to an irritant (eg, aspirin/NSAIDs via prostaglandin inhibition, alcohol, glucocorticosteroids, bile and/or pancreatic fluid reflux, iron salts, bisphosphonates, radiation therapy, corrosive ingestion)
  - Vascular gastropathy is the result of portal hypertension.
  - Stress (ischemic) gastropathy is caused by ischemia and breakdown of the protective layer of gastric mucosa in critically ill patients (massive burns, head injury, increased intracranial pressure, hypovolemia, sepsis, severe trauma, and cocaine abuse).
  - Infectious gastritis is associated with *H. pylori* infection and other bacterial, viral, parasitic, or fungal infections.

- Chronic *H. pylori* infection can also lead to atrophic gastritis, metaplasia, and increased risk of gastric cancer.
- Gastrinoma (ie, Zollinger-Ellison syndrome) is a gastrin-secreting neuroendocrine tumor usually located in the pancreas, duodenum, or other ectopic tissue that increases basal acid secretion.
  - Associated with multiple endocrine neoplasia (MEN) type 1
  - Peptic ulcers may be diffuse through gastrointestinal tract; malabsorptive diarrhea occurs due to acid inactivation of lipase in the duodenum.
  - Labs reveal increased serum gastrin level.
  - Treatment is proton-pump inhibitors (PPIs) and surgical removal of the tumor.
- Other causes include autoimmune and granulomatous disease (eg, Crohn disease, sarcoidosis).
- Smoking is an independent risk factor for PUD, and prevalence is doubled in smokers.
- Chronic atrophic gastritis is most commonly caused by long-term inflammation from *H. pylori* infection but may also be caused by long-term use of aspirin or NSAIDs, bile reflux, radiation, and granulomatous gastritis.

▶ CLINICAL ASSESSMENT

- May often be asymptomatic, particularly in older adults on NSAIDs
- When symptomatic, patients may complain of burning, aching, or gnawing abdominal pain localized to the epigastric region or left upper quadrant (LUQ).
- Other manifestations include dyspepsia, anorexia, nausea, vomiting, bloating, abdominal fullness, and reported frequent use of antacids.
- Screen patients for alarm symptoms:
  - Anemia, hematemesis, melena, positive stool occult blood, and/or pallor suggest bleeding.
  - Anorexia, weight loss, early satiety, progressive dysphagia, upper gastrointestinal bleeding (UGIB) symptoms, and family history of gastrointestinal cancer may suggest malignancy.
  - Posterior penetrating peptic ulcers may present with pain radiating to the back.
- Location of ulcers may be suggested by presentation:
  - Duodenal ulcers often have pain relieved by food intake, and painful bouts occur 2–5 hours after meals; nocturnal pain is more common.
  - Gastric ulcers typically have pain exacerbated by eating.

- Complications of PUD include:
  - UGIB is most common complication of PUD.
  - Gastric outlet obstruction may present as early satiety, bloating, nausea, recurrent vomiting, and abdominal pain shortly after eating.
  - Gastric perforation has a classic triad of sudden onset of abdominal pain, tachycardia, and abdominal rigidity.

▶ DIAGNOSIS

- All patients suspected to have PUD, mucosal-associated lymphoid tissue (MALT) lymphoma, or gastric cancer should undergo testing for *H. pylori* infection.
- There are multiple modalities to diagnose (Dx) *H. pylori* infection and to confirm eradication (Er) post-therapy.
  - Endoscopy with biopsy (Dx) is the gold standard for *H. pylori* diagnosis.
  - Rapid urease breath test (Dx/Er): noninvasive method of choice when endoscopy is not indicated
  - Stool antigen test (Dx/Er)
  - Serology (Dx): remains positive for up to 3 years postinfection; may be used for initial diagnosis only if the patient has received no prior treatment for *H. pylori*; cannot confirm eradication
- Patients older than 55 years, those with alarm symptoms, chronic or persistent symptoms refractory to medication, or symptoms of complications should be referred for prompt upper endoscopy.
- A complete blood cell count can be used to evaluate acute or chronic blood loss.

- Serum gastrin levels are ordered if gastrinoma is suspected.

▶ TREATMENT

- Goals of treatment are pain relief, protection of the gastric mucosa to promote healing, and eradication of *H. pylori* infection if present.
- Remove causative agents.
- First-line therapy for *H. pylori* eradication is triple therapy with a PPI plus clarithromycin and amoxicillin for 10–14 days; metronidazole can be substituted for amoxicillin in penicillin allergy.
- For *H. pylori*–negative patients, PPIs are most effective; misoprostol (Cytotec) is a prostaglandin E1 analog and approved for the treatment and prevention of NSAID-induced PUD.
- Surgical management in PUD is indicated for complications. Most require highly selective vagotomy.

Case Conclusion

The case described is most likely PUD with hallmark symptoms of epigastric pain and relief with antacids. This is likely a duodenal ulcer that occurs more commonly in young patients, is associated with offensive factors (eg, NSAIDs, *H. pylori*, alcohol), has pain relief with food intake, and nocturnal pain is more common. Gastric ulcers are one-third as common as duodenal ulcers and have a risk for malignancy (and should be biopsied) and higher likelihood of complications.

CHAPTER

137

Foreign Body and Toxic Ingestion

Bryan Nelson, DMSc

▶ GENERAL FEATURES

- Toxic ingestions are categorized as unintentional or intentional events, and a comprehensive history must be obtained to determine events surrounding the toxic exposure.
  - Poisonings occur most commonly in children aged <6 years, with the highest incidence found between the ages of 1 and 2 years; in 2018, nearly all exposures in children aged <6 years were considered unintentional.
    - Most common reported substances in children were cosmetics and personal care products, followed by household cleaners, and analgesics.

- Analgesics are implicated in the majority of pediatric toxic exposure fatalities.
- In adults, during 2018, the percentage of unintentional exposures was about 60%.
  - A higher incidence of intentional exposures is in teens and adults.
  - Most common reported substance were analgesics, followed by sedatives and hypnotics, and antidepressants.
  - Opiates are implicated in the majority of overdose fatalities in the United States.

- With intentional exposures or ingestions, the first priority is to stabilize any immediate medical threats to the patient, followed by a required mental health evaluation. Intentional events are associated with more severe outcomes.
- Difficulty results when the substance is not known, and the suspected drug class must be inferred based on the patient's clinical features, referred to as a *toxidrome*.
- Swallowed foreign bodies create a danger of airway compromise and mucosal injury. They are most common among children and patients with mental illness. Objects can become lodged in the upper GI tract.
  - If an object passes beyond the pylorus, it will typically pass without complication. Objects with sharp edges or an irregular shape can become lodged or damage the mucosa.
  - Chemical erosion can also occur, for example, with button batteries.

CLINICAL ASSESSMENT

- For toxic ingestion, gather as much information from emergency medical services, family, friends, and the patient to determine the possible toxic substance.
  - The route, dose amount, time since ingestion, and intent must be determined.
  - Patients may present alert, and in stable condition, yet as the substance is absorbed or metabolized, they may deteriorate rapidly.
  - Physical examination includes evaluation for odors, mental status changes, cyanosis, temperature, blood pressure, burns around the mouth, hypersalivation, respiratory status, arrhythmias, pupil size, gait, reflexes, tremors, urinary retention, dry or moist skin, and signs of drug abuse.
- Examples of toxidromes:
  - Anticholinergics (eg, diphenhydramine, TCAs):
    - Found in several hundred compounds
    - May result in dry flushed (red) skin, dry mucous membranes, hyperthermia, mydriasis, delirium, decreased peristalsis, urinary retention, wide-complex tachydysrhythmia, and seizures
  - Opiates (eg, hydrocodone, oxycodone):
    - Many acetaminophen combinations exist, must check for concurrent toxicity
    - May result in miosis, lethargy, respiratory depression, orthostatic hypotension, bradycardia, urticaria, nausea, vomiting, decreased GI motility, and urinary retention
- For ingested foreign bodies, evaluation should be made for airway compromise, dysphagia, choking, and vomiting.
- Plain films may be able to visualize radiopaque objects.
- CT can be used to assess the foreign body and visualize mucosal damage.

DIAGNOSIS

- If the substance remains unknown, consider evidence based on toxidrome.
- Diagnostic tests include CBC, CMP, EKG, cardiac monitoring, consider ABG, and urine drug screen.
- Blood levels of toxins can be obtained (eg, salicylate, iron, ethanol), although may not correlate with the true toxicity.
- It is important to maintain a broad differential diagnosis, including neurologic, cardiovascular, and metabolic, infectious etiologies.

TREATMENT

- Prevention is a key goal. Parents and caregivers should be educated on methods to restrict children from accessing hazardous chemicals or medications in the household.
- Use of proper labeling, storage, and organization of hazardous materials and medications can help reduce the risk.
- If a substance is known, a clinician can call poison control (800-222-1222) with questions regarding management and treatment guidelines.
- Priorities include the management of cardiac arrhythmias, airway support, fluids, elimination techniques, and decontamination of skin, eyes, and clothing.
  - Correction of laboratory abnormalities and potential acid/base disturbances. Several substances may present with metabolic acidosis.
  - Examples include metformin, methanol, iron, and salicylates.
- Treatment is directed at the substance whether known or suspected based on the clinical toxidrome; antidotes are available and can be administered based on the substance.
- Thiamine, dextrose, and naloxone can be given empirically; naloxone is a mainstay of treatment for opiate overdose.
- *N*-Acetylcysteine is used for acetaminophen overdose, and administration is based on the Rumack-Matthew nomogram.
- Elimination techniques include activated charcoal, orogastric lavage, whole bowel irrigation, urinary alkalinization, and hemodialysis.
- Stable patients can be discharged after a period of observation if an unintentional exposure is determined to be a known substance, with a known dose, which has been determined to be a nontoxic level of exposure.
- If a swallowed object becomes lodged in the upper GI tract (eg, esophagus), an urgent endoscopy is indicated. Surgery is indicated for more distal objects.
- If a nonthreatening object has passed beyond the pylorus, then expectant management is appropriate.

CHAPTER

138

Cholelithiasis and Choledocholithiasis

Jill Gore, PA-C

▶ GENERAL FEATURES

- Stones in the gallbladder (cholelithiasis) usually develop insidiously, and patients may remain asymptomatic for years.
- Stones are composed of two main substances: cholesterol and calcium bilirubinate. In patients in the United States, 80% of gallstones are cholesterol.
- In the United States, the prevalence of cholelithiasis is about 5.5% for men and 8.6% for women. This rate is higher in people over age 60 years and Hispanics.
- Common risk factors for the development of cholelithiasis include obesity, rapid weight loss, and insulin resistance.
- Choledocholithiasis, which develops in about 15% of patients with cholelithiasis, occurs when stones migrate from the gallbladder into one of the bile ducts (usually the common bile duct). The resulting gallbladder wall tension leads to a characteristic pain known as *biliary colic*.
- Complications result from migration of gallstones and obstruction in various biliary ducts.
  - Cystic duct obstruction leads to inflammation of the gallbladder, known as *acute cholecystitis*.
  - A stone that obstructs the common bile duct may lead to ascending cholangitis; blockage and stagnation of bile leads to infection and ascension of bacteria throughout the biliary tree and into the liver.
  - Obstruction of the pancreatic duct triggers pancreatic enzyme production within the pancreas and leads to acute pancreatitis.

▶ CLINICAL ASSESSMENT

- Commonly, patients are asymptomatic, and cholelithiasis may be an incidental finding.
- Choledocholithiasis may cause:
  - Intense spasmodic and intermittent right upper quadrant (RUQ) abdominal pain that can radiate to the back or right shoulder

- Postprandial pain, commonly after the patient eats fatty or greasy foods
- If obstruction is present, the patient may complain of fever, clay-colored stool, tea-colored urine, jaundice, nausea and vomiting, pruritus, and symptoms specific to pancreatitis.
- On examination, the patient may appear jaundiced, and RUQ tenderness may be present with palpation; a positive Murphy sign may be elicited.
- Charcot triad (fever, RUQ tenderness, and jaundice) is strongly indicative of cholangitis.

▶ DIAGNOSIS

- Cholelithiasis:
  - Ultrasound is the preferred modality and may show stones in the gallbladder with subsequent dilation of the duct or gallbladder wall thickening. Computed tomography (CT) has no advantage over ultrasound.
  - Hepatobiliary (HIDA) scan can assess for gallbladder function and aid in diagnosing obstruction.
- Choledocholithiasis:
  - Cholangiography is the gold standard for determining common bile duct obstruction.
  - Endoscopic retrograde cholangiopancreatography (ERCP) is the most common diagnostic modality because it is highly sensitive and specific, and stones can be extracted during the procedure.
  - Magnetic resonance cholangiopancreatography (MRCP) is the most accurate noninvasive test, with a high sensitivity and specificity.
- Cholelithiasis:
  - Other imaging that may be performed includes transabdominal or endoscopic ultrasound, abdominal CT, and HIDA scan.
  - The patient's total bilirubin may be increased; direct hyperbilirubinemia indicates obstruction.

- The patient's AST, ALT, alkaline phosphatase, and GGT (γ-glutamyl transferase) likely will be elevated.
- If infection is present, leukocytosis and positive blood cultures may be noted.
- If the pancreatic duct is obstructed, elevated levels of amylase and lipase will be seen.

▶ TREATMENT

- Asymptomatic cholelithiasis requires no immediate intervention; nonsteroidal anti-inflammatory drugs may be administered for intermittent pain; a low-fat diet may be beneficial.
- Broad-coverage antibacterials are prescribed for suspected biliary tract infection. Options include piperacillin-tazobactam, ampicillin-sulbactam, levofloxacin, and ciprofloxacin.
- Laparoscopic cholecystectomy is the treatment of choice for symptomatic cholelithiasis, cholecystitis, and cholecystectomy with stone extraction from duct should be performed in choledocholithiasis.

CHAPTER

139

Chronic Hepatitis

Julie Kinzel, MEd, PA-C, DFAAPA

▶ GENERAL FEATURES

- Chronic hepatitis is inflammation of the liver lasting at least 6 months.
- Common causes of chronic hepatitis include: chronic viral hepatitis B (HB), hepatitis C, autoimmune hepatitis, nonalcoholic fatty liver disease (NAFLD), and chronic alcohol abuse.
- Primary biliary cholangitis may be a cause and is more common in women than men and affects the bile ducts in the liver.
- Primary sclerosing cholangitis is an immune-mediated inflammatory condition affecting the bile ducts, causing fibrosis and leading to cirrhosis and hepatocellular cancer (HCC).
- NAFLD is commonly associated with disorders, including obesity, type 2 diabetes, and lipid abnormalities; nonalcoholic steatohepatitis (NASH) is a more advanced form and has greater inflammation, fibrosis, and potential for progression to cirrhosis.
- The pathophysiology of chronic liver injury occurs due to:
  - Hepatocyte inflammation
  - Activation of Kupfer cells
  - Infiltration of lymphocytes
  - Increased resistance of blood flow within the sinusoid lumen
  - Cell injury or scarring leading to bridging fibrosis

▶ CLINICAL ASSESSMENT

- Many patients are asymptomatic, they should be asked about risk factors and a review of symptoms for chronic hepatitis, including:
  - Recalling an episode of flulike symptoms or jaundice
  - Alcohol use, intravenous drug user (IVDU) recent or in the past at any time, intranasal cocaine use
  - History of acute hepatitis
  - Alterations in stool or urine color due to poor metabolism of bilirubin
  - Fatigue, weight changes, skin rashes
- Patients should be asked about medication use: isoniazid, propylthiouracil, nitrofurantoin, minocycline, fibrates, statins, hydralazine, and methyldopa may cause hepatitis.
- Physical examination may reveal jaundice, spider angiomas, palmar erythema, lower extremity edema, or hepatosplenomegaly.
  - Patients with ascites can present with abdominal distention or fluid wave.
  - Right upper quadrant tenderness may be present.
  - Lower extremities should be evaluated for edema related to chronic liver disease.

▶ DIAGNOSIS

- Laboratory evaluation should include evaluation of chronic viral hepatitis, autoimmune hepatitis, NAFLD, and NASH.
- Medication-induced hepatitis and alcohol-related hepatitis should be evaluated on each patient.
- Cholestatic injury should be considered a cause of chronic hepatitis in disproportionate elevation of alkaline phosphatase level compared with the AST and ALT.
- Lab tests findings include:
  - ALT generally higher than ALT.
  - Alk Phos, bilirubin: may be normal or near normal but should be ordered to rule out other etiologies
  - Low serum albumin, low platelet count, and prolonged PT suggest cirrhosis.

- Hepatitis serologies should be ordered, including HB surface antigen, HB core antibody, HB surface antibody, hepatitis C antibody with a confirmatory PCR test if positive.
  - Iron panel to rule out possible hemochromatosis.
- Further imaging with ultrasound, MRI, or CT may identify NAFLD; a liver biopsy is required for NASH.
- Ultrasound imaging of the liver should be included to evaluate the liver parenchyma.

▶ TREATMENT

- Patient education on reducing or avoiding any hepatotoxic medications and abstinence from alcohol

- Vaccinations for hepatitis A and HB are recommended.
- Avoid sharing toothbrushes, razors, or needles with others in the household.
- Evaluate for direct-acting antiviral therapies for the treatment of chronic hepatitis C.
- Ultrasound surveillance for HCC (with or without α-fetoprotein testing) every 6 months is recommended for patients with cirrhosis.
- Patients with ongoing risk for HCV infection (eg, intravenous drug use or men who have sex with men or those who have unprotected sex) should be counseled about risk reduction and test for HCV RNA annually and whenever they develop elevated ALT, AST, or bilirubin.

CHAPTER 140

Cholangitis

Jennifer Vonderau, MMS, PA-C

▶ GENERAL FEATURES

- Acute cholangitis is inflammation and infection of the biliary tree.
- The most common causes of acute cholangitis are cholelithiasis or hepatolithiasis; iatrogenic injury following endoscopic procedure or prior biliary surgery; autoimmune conditions such as primary sclerosing cholangitis, biliary atresia (a pediatric condition), and primary biliary cirrhosis; and biliary cysts or malignancy.
- Failure to treat may result in biliary strictures, cholestasis, intrahepatic abscess, liver failure, and sepsis.

▶ CLINICAL ASSESSMENT

- Charcot triad describes cholangitis with symptoms of fever, jaundice, and right upper quadrant pain.
- Reynolds pentad describes acute ascending cholangitis with those symptoms of Charcot triad as well as shock and altered mental status.
- Many patients, especially older patients or those with more severe presenting symptoms, may have signs and symptoms of systemic inflammatory response syndrome or sepsis.
- Physical examination may reveal fever, tachycardia, scleral icterus (often evident with bilirubin level >3), jaundice (often evident with bilirubin level >6), and abdominal tenderness with or without peritoneal signs.

▶ DIAGNOSIS

- Appropriate lab testing includes:
  - CBC: leukocytosis with left shift
  - CMP: elevated bilirubin, alkaline phosphatase (ALKP), and γ-glutamyl transferase (GGT)

- Blood cultures
- Serum amylase and lipase: potential elevation if there is a related pancreatitis
- MRI/MRCP (magnetic resonance cholangiopancreatography) is imaging modality of choice to confirm the diagnosis.
- Endoscopic retrograde cholangiopancreatography (ERCP) provides most accurate diagnosis and offers therapeutic benefit.
  - Findings include obstructive biliary stones and sludge (thickened bile). Brushings taken during ERCP may sample strictures and masses for potential malignancy.
- Common infective organisms include *Escherichia coli*, *Klebsiella*, *Enterococcus*, and *Bacteroides*.

▶ TREATMENT

- Antibiotic regimen is indicated while awaiting final cultures; options include those that treat GI pathogens and abdominal anaerobes, such as piperacillin/tazobactam, ciprofloxacin, or levofloxacin with metronidazole, ceftazidime, or meropenem.
- Acute cholangitis caused by biliary strictures or obstruction requires ERCP for possible stent placement and/or stone retrieval.
- Percutaneous transhepatic biliary drainage is commonly used for multiple intrahepatic biliary strictures or severe biliary injury.
- Surgery may be indicated for severe biliary injury or obstruction causing cholangitis, or in the case of malignancy or neoplastic mass. The type of surgery required depends on the location and size of the mass as well as prognosis.
- Bactrim is considered an appropriate prophylactic agent for recurrent cholangitis not caused by an iatrogenic source.

Cirrhosis and Esophageal Varices

Jennifer Vonderau, MMS, PA-C

▶ GENERAL FEATURES

- Liver cirrhosis is the final stage of liver disease, in which scar tissue replaces healthy liver tissue. It is an irreversible condition.
- Fibrosis is a precursor to cirrhosis.
- Most common causes include nonalcoholic fatty liver disease (NAFLD) or nonalcoholic steatohepatitis (NASH), alcohol use, and hepatitis C virus.
- Impaired hepatocyte function may cause elevated ammonia levels, leading to recurrent hepatic encephalopathy, a state of delirium characterized by flapping tremor (asterixis).

▶ CLINICAL ASSESSMENT

- May be incidentally found on imaging or through investigation following abnormal labs, or may be diagnosed following clinical presentation
- Clinical changes may be insidious and chronic, or they may present as a severe acute event.
- Clinical features may include ascites and peripheral edema, GI bleed (hematemesis or melena), spontaneous bacterial peritonitis (SBP), and altered mental status known as *hepatic encephalopathy*.
- Most esophageal varices are found on screening upper endoscopy, as recommended for all cirrhotic patients. Esophageal varices are graded according to severity.
- Physical examination may demonstrate a variety of atypia, including:
  - Altered mentation and possible asterixis
  - Positive fluid wave and ascites
  - Abdominal pain to palpation
  - Splenomegaly
  - Peripheral edema
  - Telangiectasia
  - Sarcopenia or other muscle wasting

▶ DIAGNOSIS

- Lab changes may include elevation of PT-INR, elevated bilirubin, decreased albumin, mild elevation to transaminases, decreased sodium, and increased creatinine.

- High ammonia level suggests hepatic encephalopathy in the setting of cirrhosis and mental status changes.
- Abdominal CT of the abdomen/ pelvis with contrast or MRI with contrast may demonstrate nodularity of the hepatic parenchyma, portal hypertension, thrombosis, splenomegaly, or ascites.
- MRI is modality of choice to screen for hepatocellular carcinoma, and there is increased risk in the cirrhotic patient.
- Upper endoscopy is the best modality to assess esophageal varices.
- Diagnostic paracentesis may be performed in the setting of ascites and abdominal pain to diagnose SBP. A predominantly neutrophilic leukocytosis on fluid analysis is suggestive of SBP, and a positive fluid culture is diagnostic.
- Liver biopsy is the gold standard for diagnosis of cirrhosis.

▶ TREATMENT

- There is no treatment to improve liver function.
- Medical therapies manage sequela and complications of the disease. Offending toxins must be discontinued and/or causative condition treated.
- Esophageal varices can often be managed with routine screening endoscopy. Varices may be banded to prevent acute bleed. In cases of severe GI bleed, a balloon stent may be placed.
- Hepatic encephalopathy is preventable with routine use of lactulose and/or rifaximin.
- Ciprofloxacin is routinely used for SBP prophylaxis.
- Management of portal hypertension with nonselective β-blocker (ie, nadolol) can help prevent worsening of esophageal varices and ascites.
- Transjugular intrahepatic portosystemic shunt (TIPS) procedure may improve symptoms of ascites and esophageal varices.
- MELD score is a calculation of sodium, PT-INR, bilirubin, and creatinine, and a score >15 provides indication for liver transplant.

CHAPTER 142

Acute Hepatitis

Erin Niles, PA-C

GENERAL FEATURES

- Acute hepatitis occurs when the liver becomes acutely inflamed due to viral infection or toxic ingestion.
- Less common causes of acute hepatitis include pregnancy-related liver disease, ischemia, heatstroke, and autoimmune disease.
- Inflammation results in hepatocyte damage and release of liver enzymes and accumulation of toxic metabolites, including bilirubin and ammonia.
- Although some patients have only mild symptoms including fatigue, gastrointestinal upset, and jaundice, others progress into fulminant liver failure with complications such as coagulopathy and encephalopathy.
- Management depends on the etiology of acute hepatitis and ranges from supportive care, N-acetylcysteine infusion, antivirals, and, in severe cases of fulminant liver failure, evaluation for liver transplantation.

CLINICAL ASSESSMENT

- A detailed history should be taken to include recent travel, exposure, ingestion of alcohol, acetaminophen, or other medications, drug, or supplement use, as well as family history and vaccination status.
- Patients may complain of abdominal pain, nausea, vomiting, and anorexia and report a viral prodrome/flu-like illness preceding these symptoms.

- Physical examination may reveal jaundice, scleral icterus, and hepatosplenomegaly.

DIAGNOSIS

- Laboratory tests should be ordered, including a viral hepatitis panel, measurements of liver enzymes (AST/ALT, alkaline phosphatase, and GGT), PT/INR, ammonia, bilirubin, and a toxicology workup as indicated (eg, acetaminophen level).
- Abnormal laboratory values may include elevated alkaline phosphatase, γ-glutamyl transferase (GGT), AST/ALT, bilirubin, PT/INR, and ammonia levels.
- An abdominal ultrasound can be considered to assess for intrahepatic and extrahepatic causes of cholestasis, as well as to assess hepatic vasculature.

TREATMENT

- For mild cases, supportive care is sufficient.
- For severe viral infections, antivirals may be indicated.
- For toxin-induced acute hepatitis, discontinuation of the causative agent is warranted.
- For acute hepatitis resulting in hepatic failure, referral to a transplant center is recommended.

SECTION E

Intestinal Disorders

CHAPTER 143

Intussusception

Brennan Bowker, MHS, PA-C

GENERAL FEATURES

- Intussusception occurs when peristalsis brings a segment of proximal bowel into a more distal segment, thus invaginating on itself. The bowel lumen becomes obstructed from this, as can the vessels leading to ischemia and necrosis.

- Most common cause of bowel obstruction in children younger than 2 years and is most frequently seen in children between the ages of 6 months and 3 years.
- Estimated to occur in 1–4 per 1000 live births, with a male predominance of about 3:1.

- Less common in adults and, when present, is typically not idiopathic

▶ CLINICAL ASSESSMENT

- Can be divided into primary and secondary:
  - Primary intussusception is the name given to idiopathic cases.
    - Often seen following upper respiratory illnesses; thought to be due to hypertrophied Peyer patches (lymphatic nodules) within the wall of the bowel
    - Adenoviruses and rotaviruses are often identified in as many as 50% of cases.
    - Seen more frequently than secondary intussusception
  - Secondary intussusception occurs as a result of an identifiable lead point.
    - Lead points are recognized in 2% to 8% of children presenting with intussusception.
    - Lead points are typically benign and can include Meckel diverticulum, hemangiomas, carcinoid tumors, foreign bodies, ectopic pancreatic tissue, and lipomas; the most common lead point is a Meckel diverticulum.
    - Malignant lead points are less common in children but increase with age. Malignant lead points may include lymphomas and small bowel tumors.
    - Systemic diseases including Crohn disease, celiac disease, and cystic fibrosis have all been associated with intussusception as well.
- Most cases of intussusception are ileocolic, although ileoileocolic and ileoileo intussusception is also seen.
- Patient history:
  - Children present with sudden onset of intermittent, crampy, abdominal pain. Episodes of pain often come in waves lasting 15–20 minutes.
  - Oftentimes, the child cannot be consoled and may draw his or her knees to the chest.
  - The pain may be associated with vomiting, which is often initially nonbilious but may progress to bilious.
  - Child may be normal between episodes, and the episodes may go as quickly as they come.
  - As the patient worsens, they may develop lethargy, which can be confused with a variety of central nervous system processes.
  - Bowel function may or may not be present. Early on in the process, stools are often normal appearing. As the intussusception evolves, the child may cease to have bowel function passing little to no flatus and having no bowel movements.
    - The classic "currant jelly stool" is often a late sign and indicative of bowel ischemia, though less than half of patient with intussusception have this pathognomonic finding.
  - Classic triad of pain, bloody "currant jelly" stools, and vomiting is present in <20% of cases.

- The positive predictive value of a child with pain, vomiting, and a palpable mass in the abdomen is ~90%; if the child has bloody stools in addition, the positive predictive value approaches 100%.
- Physical examination:
  - Vital signs may be normal early on in the course of the disease, although, as the process progresses, the patient may show signs of shock, including fever, hypotension, and tachycardia.
  - If examined in between episodes, the abdominal examination may very well be benign and minimally helpful for determining a diagnosis.
  - Auscultation of the abdomen may reveal peristaltic rushes.
  - Palpation may reveal a sausage-shaped abdominal mass. If the child is thin, visualization of the abdomen may reveal the mass or an emptiness of the right lower quadrant.
  - Dance sign is the flat appearance or emptiness upon palpation of the right lower quadrant, which occurs when the intussusception is drawn cephalad. This may or may not be present.
  - Rectal examination, especially late in the process, may reveal blood or bloody mucus. If prolapse of the intussusception occurs, this will be noted and is a particularly ominous sign. The provider must take caution in not confusing prolapse of the intussusception with rectal prolapse.

▶ DIAGNOSIS

- Although not diagnostic, standard labs should be obtained for a patient presenting with sudden onset of abdominal pain. These labs should include at least a complete blood count and electrolytes.
- Abdominal x-ray may note the presence of a mass or show an obstructive bowel gas pattern. In the case of a perforation from intussusception, the plain abdominal radiograph may be useful in detecting free air.
- Preferred diagnostic modality is ultrasound. With an experienced sonographer, the sensitivity and specificity of this test can approach 100%. It can also guide subsequent therapeutic interventions.
  - Characteristic finding is the "target sign" in the transverse plane; this is seen because of the mesenteric fat and bowel wall telescope within the intussusception. In the longitudinal plane, this may be seen as the "pseudo-kidney sign."
- Computed tomography and magnetic resonance imaging are not routinely used, although both are capable of diagnosing intussusception.

▶ TREATMENT

- Placement of a nasogastric tube for gastric decompression and initiation of bowel rest.

- Resuscitation of fluids and correction of any electrolyte abnormalities.
  - In a small number of cases, may reduce spontaneously with supportive care only and may not require any further intervention.
- If process does not resolve spontaneously, the management can be either operative or nonoperative.
- In the absence of contraindications such as free air, peritonitis, or unstable vital signs, it is reasonable to attempt nonoperative treatment.
  - Nonoperative management includes attempting reduction via hydrostatic or pneumatic pressure.
    - Historically, the use of a barium enema under fluoroscopic guidance has been the nonoperative treatment of choice, but because of the risk of barium peritonitis, most have changed to using air- or water-soluble contrast.
    - Pneumatic reduction is safer, quicker, and cleaner than using barium or water-soluble contrast. The risk of perforation is low (~0.8%), and reduction with either method (hydrostatic or pneumatic) can be achieved ~85% of the time.
    - With pneumatic reduction, there is a risk of tension pneumoperitoneum, which requires immediate decompression and exploration in the operating room.
    - In cases where reduction is not achieved, if the patient is stable, a second attempt at reduction 30 minutes to 24 hours later is reasonable; this is often done in the operating room as a second

failure requires exploration (will reduce ~50% of the time upon second attempt).
- Operative intervention should occur when unable to reduce by pneumatic pressure, if the patient is unstable, with evidence of peritonitis, or free air, or if a malignant lead point is suspected.
  - In adults, almost all cases of intussusception will require operative intervention.
  - A traditional midline or right lower quadrant incision can be utilized. The bowel should be inspected for viability and for the presence of a lead point. If the segment of intussusception is long or a lead point identified, a small bowel resection should be performed.
  - Operative intervention can start with laparoscopic exploration. Depending on the findings, conversion to open may be necessary, although newer data are showing good success with laparoscopic technique.
- Prognosis:
  - The prognosis for a child with intussusception who is diagnosed and treated early is excellent. If left untreated, however, the condition is almost always fatal.
  - In the case of nonoperative management, the recurrence rate is ~10% to 15%.
  - Recurrence rates after operative reduction can be as high as 10% but are usually lower.
  - When an intussusception recurs, the provider should raise concern for an occult neoplasm as the lead point.

CHAPTER 144

Small Bowel Obstruction

Brennan Bowker, MHS, PA-C

▶ GENERAL FEATURES

- Small bowel obstructions (SBOs) are caused by a mechanical blockage of the bowel, and, although the nomenclature varies, some can be classified as partial, complete, or closed loop.
  - In partial obstruction, the bowel is partially blocked, and fluid/air can continue to pass.
  - Complete obstruction can be further classified to "high grade" if it is radiographically severe and has a single point of obstruction (transition point).
  - When the bowel lumen is occluded on two ends, this "closed loop" is nearly always a surgical emergency.
- In individuals who have had prior abdominal surgery, the most common cause of obstruction is adhesions, which account for nearly 70% of all SBOs.

- In the patient who has never had abdominal surgery, tumor/malignancy should be high on the differential, although most obstructions in patients without prior abdominal surgeries are due to hernias.
- About 20% of obstructions are caused by tumors that are typically of metastatic origin; they can also be a primary tumor, such as a gastrointestinal stromal tumor (GIST).
- Hernias are a fairly common cause of obstruction and can be seen with any hernia but are especially common with femoral, obturator, and parastomal types.
- Internal hernias, whether congenital or iatrogenic (such as left in Roux-en-Y-gastric bypass procedures or in the case of ileal conduits), can also be a source of obstruction.

- Less commonly, obstruction can be a result of Crohn disease, gallstones (ileus), volvulus, or intussusception; in some cases, SBO may be the first presentation of inflammatory bowel disease.
- Bezoars are rare but can cause a mechanical obstruction as well.

▶ CLINICAL ASSESSMENT

- History:
  - Patients frequently present with obstipation (lack of flatus and bowel movements), nausea, and vomiting.
  - Most complain of complete inability to take anything by mouth.
  - Abdominal pain can be severe and is often described as crampy.
  - If the obstruction is proximal, the nausea and vomiting can be severe; at times, vomitus may be feculent.
  - Some patients may report severe nausea, vomiting, and distention but may have recently had a bowel movement or diarrhea; the patient can evacuate distal to the obstruction initially when symptomatic.
- Physical examination:
  - Note vital signs, taking careful attention of any fevers, tachycardia, hypotension, and/or oliguria.
  - Inspect the abdomen for any scars; often, the abdomen is distended, especially when the obstruction is distal in the alimentary canal, and asking the patient if this is the normal appearance of their abdomen is a useful tool in distinguishing distention for newer clinicians.
  - May be diffusely tender or have localized tenderness; percussion often reveals tympany; however, if the loops of bowel are fluid filled, percussion may exhibit dullness.
  - Bowel sounds are typically hyperactive in the early phases of the disease process, but transition to hypoactive as the obstruction progresses.
  - Always check for the presence of any hernias, a physical examination finding that can be missed but may lead to the diagnosis if found.
  - Rectal examination is always necessary to check for fecal occult blood and the presence of stool in the vault.

▶ DIAGNOSIS

- Check labs including a CBC and BMP; ABG and lactate are sometimes helpful in determining the degree of dehydration and assessing acidosis, although the bicarbonate measured by the BMP is usually enough of a marker for this.
- The provider may or may not send blood cultures depending on the condition of the patient; the decision to send cultures should be determined on a case-by-case basis.

- Labs are not diagnostic but will help the provider assess and manage any metabolic derangements associated with the obstruction and can help guide resuscitation efforts.
- Abdominal x-ray can be helpful and will assess for free air.
  - It may show evidence of aspiration if the patient has been vomiting.
  - It may also help rule out (or in) presence of volvulus, show air fluid levels, a distended stomach, and a paucity of gas in the colon or rectum.
  - Fluid-filled bowel loops can provide a deceptively normal-appearing radiograph, so caution must be taken with this.
- Computed tomography provides better images but requires oral contrast for best results, costs more than a plain radiograph, and has a higher associated dose of radiation.
  - Typically, the diagnostic modality of choice when SBO is suspected
  - Able to show partial vs. complete vs. closed-loop obstruction and the approximate transition point of the obstruction
  - Much more sensitive for noting the presence of ischemia and/or perforation. Can also visualize the lung bases and give a diagnosis of aspiration pneumonia if this is a concern
  - The best study is completed with both PO and IV contrast when the patient condition allows.
  - If the patient does have an obstruction and undergoes a CT with PO contrast, plain abdominal x-ray(s) in the following day(s) can help show the evolution of the disease by noting the progression of the contrast within the digestive tract.

▶ TREATMENT

- Nonoperative management is successful in 65% to 80% of cases.
- SBOs can frequently be managed with conservative measures:
  - Bowel rest:
    - Patients with bowel obstructions should be kept NPO until bowel function has returned.
    - A nasogastric tube (NGT) may or may not be placed.
  - Nasogastric decompression:
    - Provides relief of nausea and vomiting while reducing the risk of aspiration
    - Recent research notes that NGT decompression has little effect on outcomes (need for operative intervention) and should be placed for comfort.
  - Resuscitation and optimization of electrolytes:
    - Replace electrolytes as necessary, especially potassium and magnesium.

- Monitor urine output closely, especially in the case of high NGT output.
- Pain and nausea control as needed with IV anti-emetics and analgesics:
  - Pain control can present many challenges in these patients.
  - Narcotics should be used carefully as they are well known to affect motility of the gastrointestinal tract.
- Operative intervention may be necessary in patients who fail nonoperative interventions as well as in the cases of bowel compromise or ischemia.
  - Closed-loop obstruction almost always requires operative intervention.
  - If the patient fails to progress with conservative management or if there is any evidence of bowel compromise, the decision should be made to operate.

- Additionally, operative intervention is always required emergently if there is any evidence of free air on initial or subsequent imaging.
- With the increasing popularity of laparoscopic surgery, many surgeons will attempt to proceed laparoscopically and convert to an open procedure if they are unable to obtain adequate visualization.
- Prognosis:
  - When treated appropriately, the morbidity and mortality of SBOs is relatively low, although data vary on the exact numbers.
  - SBOs managed nonoperatively have a higher rate of recurrence than do those that are managed operatively.
  - Even when managed operatively, obstructions due to adhesions can recur, and there is little, if anything, that can be done to prevent this.
  - In the case of bowel strangulation, if left untreated, the mortality rate is 100%.

CHAPTER 145

Acute Appendicitis

Timothy Hirsch, MS, PA-C

A 17-year-old male presents to the emergency department for evaluation of abdominal pain. He states he has had 2 days of decreased appetite, occasional nausea with vomiting, and pain that was intermittent and around his belly button. Today, the pain became more constant and intense, prompting mom to bring him in for further evaluation. He has not had any previous abdominal surgeries, no recent illnesses, and no chronic medical problems.

GENERAL FEATURES

- Appendicitis is the most common surgical abdominal emergency.
- Most commonly presents in the second and third decades, with highest incidence among 10–19 years old
- Develops from obstruction of the appendiceal lumen, increasing lumen pressure and leading to vascular compromise, bacterial invasion, inflammation, and tissue necrosis
- Mortality is <1% but increases to 3% if the appendix is ruptured and approaches 15% in the elderly.
- Delayed diagnosis and rupture is more common in the extremely young and the elderly, leading to higher mortality in these populations.
- Appendicitis is the most common extrauterine surgical emergency in pregnancy.

CLINICAL ASSESSMENT

- Right lower quadrant (RLQ) abdominal pain is most reliable symptom of acute appendicitis.
- Migration of periumbilical pain to the RLQ occurs in 50% to 60% of confirmed cases.
- The classic triad of symptoms in appendicitis includes abdominal pain, anorexia, and nausea and vomiting, with 60% of patients presenting with some combination of these symptoms.
- Atypical presentations can occur due to anatomic variability in location of the appendix, including indigestion, flatulence, bowel changes, diarrhea, and malaise.
- Examination commonly reveals generalized abdominal tenderness, RLQ tenderness, McBurney point tenderness, Rovsing sign, psoas sign, obturator sign, digital rectal examination tenderness, and abdominal-rebound tenderness.
  - In children, rebound tenderness is the most reliable sign on physical examination.
- Fever is typically a late and unreliable finding and rarely exceeds 39 °C (102.2 °F) unless rupture or other complications occur.

DIAGNOSIS

- Diagnosis is primarily clinical in addition to a proper history and physical examination.

- A complete blood count may show leukocytosis which is sensitive but not specific for appendicitis.
- Urinalysis is important to rule out other diagnoses, including ureterolithiasis and urinary tract infection.
  - Pyuria and hematuria can occur when an inflamed appendix overlies a ureter.
- Pregnancy test should be performed on fertile females.
- Ultrasound is operator dependent and is significantly better in institutions where it is routinely used.
- CT is 98% sensitive and 95% specific for appendicitis.
- Magnetic resonance imaging (MRI) is useful for pregnant patients; however, it is more costly, time-consuming, and availability is limited in many institutions.

▶ TREATMENT

- Prompt surgical intervention is considered the most appropriate therapy for early appendicitis.
- Ruptured appendicitis with localized abscess may be treated with antibiotics and percutaneous drainage, followed by delayed appendectomy.

- Leading to surgery, patients should have nothing by mouth and should have IV access, antibiotics, and analgesia.
  - Antibiotics should cover anaerobes, enterococci, and Gram-negative intestinal flora as preoperative treatment decreases the incidence of postoperative wound infection and abscess formation.
  - Several antibiotic regimes have been recommended, including piperacillin/tazobactam 3.375 g IV or ampicillin/sulbactam 3 g IV.

Case Conclusion

The patient was diagnosed with acute appendicitis after he was noted to have a WBC count of 24 500 and CT findings consistent with appendicitis. He was given Zosyn before surgery, underwent successful appendectomy, and was discharged from the hospital the following day.

CHAPTER 146

Diverticular Disease

Johanna D'Addario, PA-C

▶ GENERAL FEATURES

- Colonic diverticular disease is a condition in which intestinal mucosal layers protrude through the smooth muscle layer of the colon (ie, false diverticuli).
  - Results from increased pressure within the bowel
  - Associated with low-fiber diet, constipation, and obesity
  - More common with advanced age, but incidence has increased in younger population
- Diverticulosis commonly occurs in the sigmoid colon due to decreased diameter and higher intraluminal pressure; however, more than half of diverticular bleeds occur in the ascending colon.
- Diverticular bleeding occurs from vasa recta arteries, at the weak point where they penetrate the bowel wall.
  - Most common cause of hematochezia
- Diverticulitis is localized inflammation of a diverticulum:
  - Increased pressure or luminal obstruction leads to distension, ischemia, and microperforation of tissue
  - Occurs in 10% of cases of diverticulosis
  - Can progress to macroperforation, abscess, fistulae, and peritonitis
  - Multiple episodes may lead to colonic scarring and strictures.

▶ CLINICAL ASSESSMENT

- Diverticulosis in itself is asymptomatic.
- Diverticular bleeding presents with painless hematochezia, bloating, cramping, or urge to defecate.
- Acute diverticulitis presents with fever and cramping abdominal pain:
  - Pain is usually located in the left lower quadrant.
  - Diarrhea, constipation, nausea, or vomiting may occur.
  - If right sided, diverticulitis can mimic acute appendicitis.
  - Physical examination may reveal normal or decreased bowel sounds, abdominal distension, and tenderness to palpation.
  - Abdominal guarding and rebound tenderness are signs of acute peritonitis.

▶ DIAGNOSIS

- Laboratory studies are nonspecific; leukocytosis with left shift may indicate diverticulitis, but is not always present.
- Colonoscopy is used to diagnose diverticulosis and diverticular bleeding, but should not be performed when diverticulitis is suspected owing to risk of perforation.

- In patients with gastrointestinal bleeding of unknown source, tagged red blood cell scan or CT angiography may reveal source of bleeding.
- CT scan is imaging method of choice for acute diverticulitis:
  - CT findings include presence of diverticuli, colonic wall thickening, and pericolic soft-tissue changes.
  - Complications visible on CT include abscesses, fistulae, bowel obstruction, or perforation.
- Abdominal flat plate can also be used to evaluate for bowel obstruction or perforation.

▶ TREATMENT

- Dietary fiber may reduce incidence of disease but may not reduce symptoms in the presence of diverticular disease.
- Diverticular bleeding is usually self-limited but may require localized therapy or surgical intervention.
  - Endoscopic treatment options include epinephrine injection, clipping, or band ligation.
  - Intra-arterial vasopressin infusion during angiography
  - If significant hemorrhage occurs, blood transfusion may be necessary.
- Treatment of acute diverticulitis includes bowel rest, hydration, and oral or intravenous antibiotics (ciprofloxacin, metronidazole for 14 days).
  - In certain cases of uncomplicated diverticulitis, antibiotics may not change patient outcomes, and patients may be managed without antibiotic therapy.
  - Percutaneous drainage or surgical intervention in cases of abscess formation or peritonitis
  - Elective surgical resection may be considered following recurrent episodes.
  - Surgical intervention may also be required in the case of fistula formation.
- Patients should undergo colonoscopy after symptoms of acute diverticulitis have resolved completely, usually after 6–8 weeks, to evaluate the severity of diverticular disease.

CHAPTER
147

Common Causes of Anal Pain

Victoria Louwagie, PA-C
Jonathan Baker, PA-C

▶ GENERAL FEATURES

- Anal fissures and hemorrhoids are benign, common causes of anal pain in the United States and often associated with anal bleeding.
- Diagnosis is made through visual (including anoscopy when available) and digital anorectal examination.
- Prevention strategies including home treatment options for mild disease can reduce need for medical or surgical management.
- If disease is atypical or severe, consultative services are recommended.
- Rectal bleeding should never be assumed to be from a hemorrhoid or anal fissure without comprehensive clinical evaluation.

▶ CLINICAL ASSESSMENT

- Anal fissure:
  - Painful longitudinal tear in the anoderm of the anal canal does not extend proximal the dentate line.
  - Pain is present at rest but exacerbated by defecation and ambulation.
  - Anal fissures can also present as painful hematochezia.
  - Anal fissures should be suspected based on history of anal pain.
  - Visualizing the fissure on physical examination is not required to establish the diagnosis at initial examination.
  - The diagnosis can be confirmed on physical examination by directly visualizing the fissure or reproducing the patient's presenting complaint by gentle digital palpation on the midline anal verge.
  - Acute anal fissures appear as a superficial laceration.
  - Chronic anal fissures typically have raised edges exposing horizontally oriented fibers the internal anal sphincter muscle, which are attributed to chronic inflammation and fibrosis.
  - Skin tag formation at the distal end of fissures is common, especially with chronic disease.
  - The majority of fissures are primary in nature, caused by local trauma associated with anal spasm or high anal pressure; most commonly, primary fissures are located in the posterior midline.
  - Fissures located other than the midlines are atypical and often secondary to another disease process (eg, Crohn disease) and should be referred to gastroenterology or colorectal surgery.
- Hemorrhoids:
  - Normal vascular structures in the anal canal that can become symptomatic
  - Nearly three out of four adults have symptomatic hemorrhoidal disease from time to time.

- Patients may complain of painless hematochezia associated with bowel movements, although hemorrhoids can also be a spontaneous bleeding source.
- It is rare to have blood loss anemia from hemorrhoidal bleeding.
- Other associated symptoms include sensation of fullness in the perianal area due to prolapse of internal hemorrhoids, irritation or itching of perianal skin, mucus discharge or wetness, or mild fecal incontinence.
- Risk factors include advanced age, straining during bowel movements, chronic constipation or diarrhea, obesity, pregnancy, low-fiber diet, and regular heavy lifting.
- External hemorrhoids are distal to the dentate line and present with pain, irritation due to somatic innervation.
    - External hemorrhoids can become thrombosed when pooling blood forms a thrombus.
    - Typical symptoms are severe pain, inflammation, and/or a firm palpable lump around the anus.
    - External thrombosis will often present as a bluish lump. The thrombus may extrude, resulting in an ulcerated tag.
- Internal hemorrhoids are proximal to the dentate line.
    - The general practitioner should be familiar with the grading scale of hemorrhoids.
    - Without somatic innervation, internal hemorrhoids are typically not painful and more commonly present with bleeding or mucous discharge.
- Prevention for both hemorrhoids and fissures include high-fiber diet with possible fiber supplementation, straining avoidance, having a bowel movement as soon as you feel the urge, exercising regularly, and staying hydrated with water.

▶ TREATMENT

- Conservative management includes preventive measures listed earlier as well as inducing soft, formed stools with bulk.

- Over-the-counter (OTC) stool softeners (eg, docusate) or gentle laxatives (eg, polyethylene glycol 3350) should be recommended.
- A high-fiber diet and OTC fiber supplements aim to achieve 25–35 g of fiber/day to bulk stools.
- For pain relief, sitz baths, topical analgesics, and oral pain relievers (such as acetaminophen, aspirin, or ibuprofen) are useful; oral opioids should be avoided.
- Fissure:
    - Medical treatment includes compounded topical nifedipine or diltiazem applied 2–4 times daily to facilitate localized vasodilation; topical nitroglycerin is commercially available, but headache is a common side effect.
        - Patients should be re-evaluated after 1 month; if the patient remains symptomatic, therapy is continued.
        - At the end of the second month, if still symptomatic and/or fissure is still present, the provider should refer patient to gastroenterology or colorectal surgery for evaluation of underlying etiology (eg, occult Crohn disease) or consideration of additional medical therapy or surgical options.
- Hemorrhoids:
    - Medical management includes OTC hemorrhoid topicals, topical steroids, steroid suppositories, and witch hazel pads.
        - If symptoms worsen, noninvasive procedures such as rubber band ligation, sclerotherapy, or coagulation therapy can be considered.
        - Excision of a thrombosed hemorrhoid will provide immediate relief to patients who present within 72 hours of onset of severe pain. Incision within 48 hours of symptoms onset can relieve pain may be incomplete and allow reaccumulation of blood.
        - Only a minority of patients with hemorrhoids will require hemorrhoidectomy or hemorrhoid stapling.

CHAPTER
148

Irritable Bowel Syndrome

Travis Layne, DMSc, MPAS, PA-C

▶ GENERAL FEATURES

- Chronic functional disorder characterized by idiopathic chronic abdominal pain (>3 months) with alterations in bowel habits
- Not explained by an organic cause such as the presence of structural or biochemical abnormalities

- Can be classified as mild, moderate, or severe. Four subtypes exist including constipation predominant, diarrhea predominant, mixed, and unsubtyped. These are represented by the acronyms IBS-C, IBS-D, IBS-M, and unsubtyped IBS, respectively.
- There is a strong association with noncardiac chest pain and functional dyspepsia.

- Symptoms usually begin in late teens or early 20s.
- Up to 10% of adults have symptoms compatible with IBS.
- Up to 75% of patients with IBS are women.
- Over half of patients have underlying depression, anxiety, or somatization.

CLINICAL ASSESSMENT

- Abdominal pain is intermittent, crampy, and in the lower abdomen.
- These "alarm symptoms" (red flags) should be recognized that suggest organic disease:
  - Evidence of GI bleeding
  - Anorexia/weight loss
  - Fever
  - Nocturnal symptoms
  - Family history of GI cancer, IBD, or celiac disease
  - Persistent diarrhea causing dehydration
  - Severe constipation or fecal impaction
  - Acute onset in someone over 45 years old
- Examination is focused on ruling out organic disease.
- Checking for thyroid abnormalities, lymph node enlargement, abdominal masses/hernias, local muscle injury, and perianal disease is important when ruling out organic causes.
- Typically, a physical examination is normal other than lower abdominal tenderness.
- A digital rectal examination should be performed in patients with constipation.
- In postmenopausal women with recent-onset constipation and lower abdominal pain, a pelvic examination is indicated to screen for gynecologic malignancy.
- Labs should include CBC, TSH, serologies for celiac disease, and fecal occult blood testing.
- CRP and fecal calprotectin level to screen for IBD in diarrhea-prominent patients.
- Stool for culture and ova/parasites in at-risk populations.
- Indications for colonoscopy in this setting include age >50 years, positive fecal occult blood test (FOBT) or rectal bleeding, and family history of colon cancer.

DIAGNOSIS

- The diagnosis is established in the presence of compatible symptoms and the judicious use of tests to exclude organic disease.
- Rome IV criteria is used as a diagnostic criterion:
  - Recurrent pain at least 1 day per week for at least 3 months.
  - Two of three of the following accompany the abdominal pain:
    - Pain improved or worsened with defecation

- Change in stool frequency
- Change in stool form (appearance)

TREATMENT

- Reassurance, education, and support are the most important interventions.
  - Discussion of the mind-gut interaction can explain that visceral motility and sensitivity can be exacerbated by environmental, social, or psychological factors.
  - Transparency to the patient that this is a chronic condition characterized by waxing and waning of symptoms
- Lifestyle changes of smoking cessation and a low-fat/unprocessed food diet
- Adequate sleep and moderate exercise is beneficial.
- Avoid beverages containing sorbitol or fructose.
- Avoid cruciferous vegetables like collard greens, cabbage, and broccoli.
- Poorly fermentable soluble fiber (psyllium, oatmeal) improves global symptoms in many patients and is recommended.
- Pharmacologic therapy is not needed in 75% of patients when education, reassurance, and dietary interventions are used.
- Drug therapy is targeted at the dominant symptom.
- Anticholinergic/antispasmodics like dicyclomine can be used for acute episodes of pain or bloating. Antidiarrheals like loperamide and diphenoxylate hydrochloride-atropine sulfate can reduce stool frequency and urgency. It can be used prophylactically when diarrhea is anticipated.
- Eluxadoline is a newer agent for IBS-D; it is an opioid antagonist used to decrease abdominal pain and improve stool consistency.
- Prokinetics, bulk-forming laxatives, and saline or osmotic laxatives can be used for constipation-prone patients.
- Tricyclic antidepressants, such as amitriptyline hydrochloride and nortriptyline hydrochloride, prescribed at low doses, are beneficial in patients with and without diagnosed depression and anxiety because their benefit derives more from pain reduction than depression.
- Selective serotonin reuptake inhibitors (SSRIs) citalopram and fluoxetine, which are commonly used for depression, were effective in patients with IBS in regard to pain and bloating.
- Lubiprostone is used to treat constipation-prone patients. It enhances intestinal fluid and motility through its effect on the intestinal chloride activator. Linaclotide is also used to increase motility and intestinal fluid through its effect on intestinal chloride.
- Cognitive behavioral therapy (CBT) appears to be beneficial in some patients.

Celiac Disease

Tyler D. Sommer, MPAS, PA-C

A 21-year-old female presents to the primary care clinic with concerns of diarrhea, bloating, flatulence, fatigue, and weakness. She reports that these symptoms have been progressively worsening over the past 6–9 months and she has also noticed a recent unintentional weight loss of 15 pounds. What should you consider?

▶ GENERAL FEATURES

- Also known as gluten-sensitive enteropathy or celiac sprue, celiac disease is a chronic digestive condition that has a global prevalence of ~1%.
- This immune disorder is characterized by the inability of the body to tolerate gliadin, a portion of the gluten protein that is found in wheat, rye, and barley.
- Gliadin is absorbed into the lamina propria of the small intestine and is often bounded by tissue transglutaminase (tTG).
- Two human leukocyte antigens (HLA-DQ2 and HLA-DQ8) bind gliadin and present it to helper T cells, which mediate an inflammatory response and production of antibodies against gliadin and tTG.
- This inflammatory response results in intestinal epithelial invasion by lymphocytes and destruction of the absorptive surface of the small intestine, manifested by atrophic mucosa and blunting of intestinal villi.
- There is a slight female predominance and a bimodal distribution of age at diagnosis, including waves at age 8–12 months and 20–40 years.
- First- and second-degree relatives of patients with celiac disease are at increased risk of being diagnosed with celiac disease, suggesting a genetic basis for the condition.
- There is also an increased incidence in individuals who have Down syndrome, Turner syndrome, autoimmune thyroiditis, type 1 diabetes, and other autoimmune conditions.

▶ CLINICAL ASSESSMENT

- Classic symptoms are considered gastrointestinal (GI) manifestations, generally including diarrhea, steatorrhea, bloating, flatulence, signs of malabsorption, weight loss, and nutritional or vitamin deficiencies.
- The majority of patients, however, complain of few or only minor GI symptoms.
- Extraintestinal manifestations are also common and can include neurologic symptoms, dermatologic signs (dermatitis herpetiformis), amenorrhea, infertility, osteopenia, and anemia (often related to nutritional deficiencies).
- Unless the patient has signs of neurologic dysfunction, the dermatitis herpetiformis rash, or signs of malnutrition, physical examination findings are generally normal.

▶ DIAGNOSIS

- For patients who are considered low risk or have only minor symptoms, diagnostic evaluation can initially begin with serologic testing.
- The serologic test with the most clinical value is IgA antibodies against tissue transglutaminase (tTG-IgA), which is highly sensitive and specific.
- Other serologic tests may be used to support the diagnosis, including:
  - Antiendomysial antibodies (EMAs), antigliadin antibodies (IgA or IgG), and anti-deamidated gliadin peptide (second-generation gliadin antibody test).
- Patients with positive serologic testing should undergo upper endoscopy (EGD) with multiple small bowel biopsies assessing for characteristic mucosal atrophy and blunting of intestinal villi.
- For patients who are considered high risk for celiac disease, serologic testing and biopsy of the small intestine should both be performed, regardless of serologic results.
- The diagnosis is confirmed by the presence of villous atrophy and increased intraepithelial lymphocytes of the small intestine.
- Testing should ideally be performed while the patient is still consuming gluten-containing foods.

▶ TREATMENT

- A completely gluten-free diet is essential to treatment of this chronic condition, and prognosis is generally excellent.
- It generally takes 4–8 weeks of a strict gluten-free diet before they start to notice a significant improvement in their symptoms.
- Because it is often difficult for a layperson to accurately determine which foods are free of gluten, a referral to a dietitian can be helpful.
- Periodic follow-up, especially in the early stages of treatment, should be performed by a clinician with knowledge of celiac disease and gluten-free foods.
- Patients should also be tested for different nutritional deficiencies, including deficiencies of vitamin A, vitamin D, vitamin E, vitamin B12, folic acid, iron, and so on.
- Patients seem to have a very slight increased risk of lymphoma and GI cancer, particularly if left untreated.

Case Conclusion

Because of her chronic GI symptoms and clinical signs of malabsorption, this patient should undergo diagnostic testing for evaluation of celiac disease.

Colorectal Polyps and Cancer

Lisa Dickerson, MD

▶ GENERAL FEATURES

- Colorectal cancer (CRC) is a malignant neoplasm of the colon or rectum, almost always adenocarcinoma that develops from the columnar glandular epithelium (mucosal lining) of the large intestine.
- It is the third most common cancer diagnosed in both men and women in the United States and the second most common cause of cancer deaths when men and women are combined.
- Risk factors include advancing age, family history of polyps and CRC in first-degree relatives, tobacco use, heavy alcohol use, diabetes and obesity, low-fiber diet, and high red/processed meat consumption; inflammatory bowel disease (IBD) also confers increased risk.
- Most CRC arises from adenomatous polyps and sessile serrated polyps; adenomatous polyps are the precursor for about 80% of CRC, with stepwise progression from benign to dysplastic to carcinoma in situ to invasive cancer over many years; progression is associated with accumulating acquired gene mutations.
- Adenomatous polyps are classified by histologic features (tubular, tubulovillous, and villous) and the degree of dysplasia (low grade or high grade).
  - Polyp features most worrisome for CRC development include large size (≥10 mm), the number of polyps (>2), villous histology, and high-grade dysplasia.
- Hereditary syndromes account for ~5% of CRC and are classified as those with polyposis (eg, familial adenomatous polyposis [FAP] or those without polyposis such as Lynch syndrome [LS], also known as hereditary nonpolyposis CRC).
  - FAP results from a mutation in the tumor-suppressor gene *APC* and is autosomal dominant.
  - LS is caused by a mutation in DNA mismatch repair genes and is also autosomal dominant.
  - Other cancers associated with LS include endometrial, ovarian, stomach, small bowel, and bile duct.
- Mortality from CRC can be largely prevented by utilizing evidence-based screening strategies.

▶ CLINICAL ASSESSMENT

- Polyps and early stages of CRC are often asymptomatic. Left-sided CRC may cause bright red blood per rectum (BRBPR) or hematochezia, abdominal pain, and change in bowel habits such as diarrhea, constipation, and/or narrowing of stool.
- Right-sided cancers more frequently present with iron deficiency anemia and occult blood in the stool.
- Nonspecific constitutional symptoms include anorexia, unintentional weight loss, and fatigue.

▶ DIAGNOSIS

- Diagnosis of CRC is via colonoscopy.
- The US Preventive Services Task Force (USPSTF) recommends screening for CRC in average-risk individuals starting at age 50 and continuing until age 75. The American Cancer Society recommends screening start at age 45.
  - Stool-based screening options are quick, noninvasive, less expensive, and may be done at home.
    - Methods include three high-sensitivity guaiac-based fecal occult blood tests (hs-gFOBT) annually, a single fecal immunochemical test (FIT) annually, and a single multitargeted stool DNA with FIT (FIT-DNA, Cologuard) every 3 years.
    - Positive stool–based screening results must be followed up with colonoscopy.
  - High-quality colonoscopy is the preferred visual screening modality; advantages of colonoscopy include a 10-year interval between normal examinations and the ability to detect and remove precancerous polyps.
- Patients with IBD for >8 years should receive surveillance colonoscopies with random biopsies for dysplasia every 1–2 years.
- Patients who have undergone endoscopic removal of adenomatous polyps should have more frequent colonoscopies; recommended surveillance postresection depends on the size, histology, and number of polyps and generally ranges between 3 and 5 years.
- Lab tests should include a serum carcinoembryonic antigen (CEA) level.
  - CEA is a tumor marker that is not particularly sensitive or specific for CRC and thus is not helpful as a screening test but should be obtained preoperatively in patients with known CRC.
- Clinical staging includes imaging of the chest, abdomen, and pelvis, usually with a CT (or MRI for rectal cancer).
- CRC staging is based on the American Joint Committee on Cancer (AJCC) TNM system based on the depth of the primary Tumor through the layers of the colorectal wall, the spread to nearby lymph Nodes, and the spread to distant sites (Metastasis); metastases are most common to the liver and lungs.

▶ TREATMENT

- Surgical resection is curative for early-stage tumors with removal of the involved segment, along with associated mesentery and draining lymph nodes; use of postoperative adjuvant chemotherapy (generally a 6-month course of oxaliplatin-based therapy) is recommended with node involvement.
- A solitary metastatic lesion may be surgically removed. Palliative chemotherapy and/or surgery to alleviate bowel obstructions may be used with extensive metastatic disease.

- A 5-year survival is ~90% to 95% for early-stage disease and drops to <10% for metastatic disease.
- Cancers within 6 in from the anal verge are classified as rectal cancers.
  - Surgery is more challenging in this location.
  - Preoperative chemotherapy and radiation therapy may be used to shrink tumors before surgery.
- Close surveillance after CRC treatment includes regular physical evaluation, colonoscopy, CT scanning, and serum CEA levels.

CHAPTER 151

Large Bowel Obstruction

Brennan Bowker, MHS, PA-C

▶ GENERAL FEATURES

- Large bowel obstruction (LBO) can occur from a number of different pathologies, but, by definition, they are typically considered closed-loop obstructions because the ileocecal valve prevents retrograde flow.
- If left untreated, it can lead to mucosal edema and ischemia, which may result in perforation or ischemia of the affected colon.
- While the colon can perforate at the site of the obstruction or any point proximal, the thin-walled cecum is at highest risk of perforation due to LBO pathology.
- Colorectal cancer is the number one cause and must be considered until proven otherwise.
- Other causes include diverticular stricture/diverticulitis, volvulus, constipation/fecal impaction, extraluminal compression from a mass or collection, and Ogilvie syndrome or colonic pseudo-obstruction.
- Less commonly, LBO can be caused by intussusception, hernia, inflammatory bowel disease, and foreign body.

▶ CLINICAL ASSESSMENT

- History:
  - Depending on etiology, the clinical presentation of a patient with an LBO can vary
  - While the pathophysiology of LBO is often insidious in nature, its presentation is quite frequently acute.
  - In general, patients will present with colicky abdominal pain, obstipation, and distention, which, at times, can be rather impressive. Nausea and/or vomiting may or may not be present. When vomiting is present, it is often a late sign of obstruction.
  - In the case of diverticulitis, patients may present with pain, distention, obstipation, and fever. Fever

can also occur if the patient has perforated and developed peritonitis.
  - Patients who develop LBO due to malignancy will often report a change in bowel habits, noting small caliber stools or periods of alternating constipation and diarrhea. These patients also may notice blood in the stool or toilet after defecation.
  - In the case of volvulus, patients will not report the same insidious signs as those with malignancy; rather, they will typically present with acute onset of pain and distention.
  - When interviewing patients with suspected bowel obstruction, it is especially important to obtain a history of bowel habits, the date and results of their last colonoscopy, and family history.
- Physical examination:
  - Frequent vital sign checks are important to monitor for hypotension, tachycardia, and/or pyrexia.
  - Abdominal examination should include:
    - Inspection for the presence of any scars or hernias
    - Evaluation of distension and tympanitic percussion
    - Rebound tenderness or guarding resulting from possible perforation or peritonitis
    - Location of tenderness in the region of the cecum as this could indicate impending perforation
    - Bowel sounds are not a particularly useful diagnostic tool because they may be hyperactive or hypoactive and are, therefore, nonspecific.
  - Digital rectal examination must be performed and often reveals an empty rectal vault. Occult blood testing should be performed as well and may be positive depending upon the etiology of the obstruction. Rectal examination may also note the presence of a mass.

DIAGNOSIS

- A full laboratory panel including complete blood count and comprehensive metabolic panel. Although these studies are not specific to LBO, they will help guide resuscitative efforts and may offer insight to potential infectious etiology.
- Occult blood testing should be done with the digital rectal examination and is often positive if the LBO is caused by malignancy or bowel compromise is present.
- If there is concern for malignancy, tumor markers can be sent, including CEA and CA 19-9, but results of the tumor makers should not influence management if perforation is imminent; additionally, these studies may not result immediately and should be used to help guide further treatment.
- The diagnostic modality of choice for diagnosing an LBO is computed tomography (CT) scan, preferably with intravenous and oral contrast.
- Plain radiographs can be helpful in determining the presence of free air and may detect a volvulus; however, there is limited utility in determining bowel compromise.

TREATMENT

- Treatment depends on etiology and acuity of the situation.
- Patients must be resuscitated with intravenous fluids.
  - If concern for infection or perforation, intravenous, broad-spectrum antibiotics should be initiated.
  - Analgesics and antiemetics should also be implemented as necessary.
- When LBO is caused by a sigmoid volvulus, endoscopic decompression can be attempted, but if ineffective, surgical resection must be performed.
- For cases of malignancy and diverticular obstruction, initial treatment is frequently surgical and may involve resection and/or colostomy formation.
- Patients who have a diverticular or malignant obstruction can possibly undergo endoscopic stenting; however, this is not widely popular and can only be done in patients who have no signs of ischemia or peritonitis.
- In cases where perforation has occurred or there is grave concern for impending perforation, the patient should be immediately taken to the operating room for exploration and decompression. In some cases, it may be necessary to bring up a decompressive colostomy to prevent perforation and perform a definitive operation at a later time.
- Obstructions caused by fecal impaction often can be resolved with manual and/or endoscopic disimpaction in conjunction with an aggressive bowel regimen. It is important to note that these patients can develop stercoral colitis and manual disimpaction can result in perforation.
- Prognosis:
  - LBOs are often associated with a high degree of morbidity and mortality.
  - Delays in diagnosis/treatment can worsen prognosis; thus, it is prudent to act swiftly.
  - Prognosis also varies depending upon the etiology of the obstruction.
  - Benign causes of LBO such as volvulus, fecal impaction, and diverticular disease often offer excellent outcomes after intervention.

CHAPTER
152

Infectious and Noninfectious Diarrhea

Frank Giannelli, PhD, PA-C

A 28-year old female with no past medical history presents with a 2-day history of nonbloody diarrhea. Furthermore, she reports loss of appetite and stomach cramping. She is not on any medications and has had no recent travel. She further denies fever, nausea, vomiting, or weight loss. She works at a day care center where other children and staff have had similar symptoms.

GENERAL FEATURES

- Diarrhea is defined as >stools (increased stool frequency) per day or liquid stools.
- Important to distinguish acute (<2 weeks) vs. chronic (>4 weeks) diarrhea to help differentiate the underlying cause
- Acute diarrhea is most commonly caused by infection; can be further differentiated as noninflammatory (no blood or pus) or inflammatory (blood or pus, commonly with fever).
- Most common cause of noninflammatory diarrhea is a virus: common viral causes include norovirus, adenovirus, and rotavirus; other less common causes include bacterial and protozoal causes.

- Bacterial causes include infection from *Staphylococcus aureus*, *Clostridium perfringens*, *Vibrio cholerae*, and *Bacillus cereus*.
- Protozoal causes include infection from *Giardia lamblia* and *Cryptosporidium*.
- Common causes of inflammatory diarrhea include toxin-producing bacteria, including *Escherichia coli*, *Clostridioides difficile*, *Shigella*, *Salmonella*, *Campylobacter jejuni*, and *Listeria monocytogenes*.
  - Viral causes such as cytomegalovirus and protozoal causes such as *Entamoeba histolytica* are less common in inflammatory diarrhea.
- The differential for chronic diarrhea is broad and can be categorized into osmotic, secretory, inflammatory, medications, malabsorption, motility disorders, chronic infections, and factitious.

▶ CLINICAL ASSESSMENT

- Most patients present with abdominal pain and cramping.
- A review of systems should include questions such as asking if the patient has fever, blood, or pus in the stool.
- Additionally, a detailed medication, surgical, diet, and travel history are required.

▶ DIAGNOSIS

- Acute diarrhea is differentiated into noninflammatory (no blood or pus) or inflammatory (blood, pus, fever).
  - Noninflammatory diarrhea typically does not require workup.
  - The workup for inflammatory diarrhea includes sending stool samples for fecal leukocytes, culture, *C. difficile* testing, and ova and parasite testing.
- Chronic diarrhea (>4 weeks) requires a detailed history to point to most likely cause. Additional tests include fecal leukocytes, stool occult blood testing, colonoscopy (with biopsy), stool weight, and stool osmotic gap.
  - Osmotic diarrhea, such as that caused by lactose intolerance, may show a stool osmotic gap and will stop with fasting.
  - Secretory diarrhea should be suspected with large amounts of diarrhea that do not stop with fasting. Causes include tumors, Zollinger-Ellison syndrome, carcinoid tumor, and factious causes, such as laxative abuse.
  - Inflammatory diarrhea is associated with fever, hematochezia, ulcerative colitis, Crohn disease, and malignancy.
  - Common medication causes of diarrhea include nonsteroidal anti-inflammatories, selective serotonin reuptake inhibitors, and metformin.
  - Malabsorptive diarrhea is associated with weight loss and high fecal fat content (steatorrhea);

pancreatic disorders and celiac disease can cause this type of diarrhea.
  - Diarrhea related to motility disorders may be caused by hyperthyroidism, irritable bowel syndrome, diabetes mellitus, and surgical injury.
  - Infectious causes of chronic diarrhea are most commonly caused by parasites such as *G. lamblia* and *Strongyloides* or chronic bacterial infections such as *C. difficile*.

▶ TREATMENT

- For all causes of diarrhea, rehydration, along with loperamide or bismuth sulfate, is the first-line treatment.
- Treatment for acute diarrhea depends on the suspected cause:
  - Noninflammatory diarrhea usually managed symptomatically with fluids, antipyretic medications, and antidiarrheal medications such as loperamide.
  - Inflammatory diarrhea is empirically treated with an antibiotic, such as ciprofloxacin or other fluoroquinolones, in severe cases such as when patients are dehydrated, immunocompromised, or hospitalized. Treatment is otherwise targeted for the underlying cause.
    - Loperamide should not be given to patients with bloody diarrhea.
- Treatment for chronic diarrhea is targeted to the underlying cause.
  - For food- or medication-based diarrhea, eliminate the underlying cause.
  - For functional diarrhea, such as IBS-D, loperamide is the mainstay of therapy. Other drugs such as anticholinergics and tricyclic antidepressants may have a role in therapy.
  - The approach to treating Crohn disease and ulcerative colitis ranges from medical management to surgical resection of diseased bowel.
    - Treatment of acute episodes includes the use of 5-aminosalicylic acid and corticosteroids.
    - Maintenance therapy in moderate/severe cases includes immunomodulating drugs and biologic therapies.
    - Surgery is reserved for severe disease or disease not responding to medication therapy.
  - Bile acid binders, such as cholestyramine, may be used bilious diarrhea.
  - Pancreatic enzyme replacement may be used in the case of steatorrhea.

Case Conclusion

The most likely cause of our patient's diarrhea is viral. A strong detailed history can often point to the most likely and common causes before undergoing an extensive workup.

Ischemic Bowel Disease

Travis Layne, DMSc, MPAS, PA-C

▶ GENERAL FEATURES

- Caused by a reduction in intestinal blood flow most commonly as a result of occlusion, vasospasm, or hypoperfusion of the mesenteric circulation.
- Categorized as acute or chronic and episodic or constant.
- Divided into AMI, CMI, and colonic ischemia. AMI can be further subdivided by the potential etiologies of arterial embolism/thrombosis, venous thrombosis, and a variety of nonocclusive causes.
- Acute mesenteric ischemia (AMI):
  - Can be further divided into arterial versus venous, embolic versus thrombotic, and occlusive versus nonocclusive.
  - AMI is a medical and surgical emergency; mortality rate exceeds 50%.
  - Classic presentation is abdominal pain out of proportion to physical exam findings.
  - Consider the diagnosis in patients age >50 years who present with sudden onset of severe abdominal pain lasting greater than 2 hours, especially if they have a history of cardiovascular disease.
  - The most common cause is SMA embolism accounting for 50% of the cases, most frequently due to a dislodged thrombus originating from the left atrium, left ventricle, or cardiac valves.
  - Risk factors of mesenteric venous thrombosis (MVT) include hypercoagulable states, pancreatitis, intra-abdominal sepsis, cirrhosis, and portal hypertension.
  - Over half of MVT patients have a personal or family history of deep venous thrombosis or pulmonary embolism
  - Nonocclusive ischemia results from intense mesenteric vasoconstriction. Suspect in patients with patients with diffuse atherosclerotic disease with hypotensive states, in the setting of vasoconstrictive agents, and in patients with vasculitis.
  - Chronic mesenteric ischemia (CMI):
    - Result of atherosclerotic narrowing of generally at least two of three major splanchnic vessels (celiac, SMA, or IMA).
    - If only one vessel is involved, collateral circulation usually prevents symptoms from occurring.
  - Colonic ischemia:
    - Also referred to as ischemic colitis, the most frequent form of mesenteric ischemia, accounting for 75% of all intestinal ischemia and affecting primarily the elderly (90% of patients are age >60 years).
    - Colonic ischemia is rarely life threatening and usually resolves with only supportive care.

- The majority of cases resolve within 2 weeks.
- Many cases are misdiagnosed as inflammatory bowel disease or infectious colitis especially in patients age <50 years.
- Similar to AMI, the pathogenesis centers around reduction in blood flow resulting in a low flow state.
- The most common areas affected are the splenic flexure and left colon.
- In elderly, risk factors include hypotension, CHF, and dehydration. In those less than 50 years of age, pathologic states such as vasculitis (such as systemic lupus), hypercoagulable states, sickle cell crisis, and infectious hemorrhagic colitis can be the cause.

▶ CLINICAL ASSESSMENT

- AMI-arterial emboli/thrombosis:
  - On exam, the abdomen may be soft with minimal to no tenderness; distention is often the first sign.
  - Peritoneal signs may come later if infarction or gangrene occur.
  - Associated nausea, vomiting, and transient diarrhea may be present.
  - Occult blood in the stool is found in >50% of cases.
  - Obtain a CBC (leukocytosis in 75%) but may be normal in early ischemia; elevation of lactic acid and liver function studies are late findings.
  - No single biomarker has been proven to diagnose or exclude AMI.
- AMI-mesenteric venous thrombosis:
  - Presentation can be acute, subacute, or chronic.
  - Nausea, vomiting, and diarrhea are common.
  - Fever, abdominal distention/tenderness, and hypotension can occur.
  - Guarding and rebound tenderness are late findings.
- AMI-nonocclusive mesenteric ischemia (NOMI):
  - Presentation is similar to other forms of AMI.
  - Patients are usually elderly given the comorbidities associated with this type of AMI.
  - These predisposing factors such as an MI, CHF, septic shock would influence the clinical presentation of these patients.
- CMI:
  - CMI is a clinical diagnosis; the classic diagnostic triad is postprandial abdominal pain (abdominal angina), weight loss, and an abdominal bruit.
  - The pain is typically recurrent, dull, crampy, epigastric, and periumbilical lasting up to 30 minutes after meals and lasting up to 3 hours.
  - Food fear causes patients to lose weight.

- Abdomen is usually soft without tenderness and includes the classic pain out of proportion to exam findings that is also found in AMI.
- Nausea, vomiting, and early satiety are common associated symptoms.
- Colonic ischemia:
  - Typically, sudden onset of LLQ crampy pain followed by hematochezia within 24 hours.
  - Physical exam reveals mild to moderate abdominal tenderness over most often the left side of the abdomen from the splenic flexure to the sigmoid colon.
  - Usually do not appear acutely ill (in contrast to the patient with AMI).
  - Rectal bleeding is usually not massive and rarely requires a transfusion.

▶ DIAGNOSIS

- AMI:
  - Initial evaluation should include radiographic imaging to exclude other causes of acute abdominal pain such as perforation or obstruction; plain films have been used early in the presentation to rule out these other potential causes of the pain.
  - Regarding AMI due to an arterial embolus/thrombus or nonocclusive source, mesenteric angiography is the gold standard; it is used both for diagnostic and therapeutic purposes.
  - CT with contrast demonstrates some utility with overall sensitivity of 80% detecting arterial AMI.
    - Findings may be either more specific or nonspecific.
    - This is the gold standard of diagnostic imaging when considering MVT.
  - Findings include a dilated superior mesenteric vein with a clot or filling defect.
- CMI:
  - Difficult to diagnose due to vagueness of complaints, no exam findings, and lack of an accurate noninvasive test.
  - The average duration of symptoms prior to diagnosis is 1 year.
  - Although CMI is primarily diagnosed on clinical grounds, angiography is the test of choice and typically reveals stenosis or occlusion of at least two vessels.
- Colonic ischemia:
  - Usually established on the basis of clinical history, physical exam, and endoscopic or radiologic studies.
  - Diagnostic modalities include flexible sigmoidoscopy/colonoscopy, abdominal plain films, and CT scan.
  - Colonoscopy with biopsy makes the definitive diagnosis.
  - Thumbprinting on plain films may be seen in 25% of patients. This represents submucosal hemorrhage and edema.

- CT scans can show wall thickening, mucosal hemorrhage, and pericolic fat stranding.
- In contrast to AMI and CMI, angiography is usually not necessary for diagnosis.
- Stool cultures should be considered if an infectious diarrhea is suspected.

▶ TREATMENT

- AMI:
  - Regardless of the cause, the goal is to restore intestinal blood flow as rapidly as possible.
  - Initial management includes hemodynamic resuscitation and correction of precipitating causes.
  - Patients with peritoneal signs or suspicion of gangrene and/or perforation require an emergent laparotomy whether from an arterial, venous, or nonocclusive source.
  - In AMI patients who are stable with no peritoneal signs and the cause is suspected to be an arterial source, immediate angiography should be performed.
  - In the setting of MVT, if laparotomy is not indicated as mentioned above, conservative management can be attempted with anticoagulation.
  - Catheter-directed thrombolysis has been performed in some cases.
  - Most patients with MVT will have already undergone mesenteric angiography to confirm adequacy of arterial flow.
  - In addition to hemodynamic resuscitation, treatment of NOMI includes an intra-arterial infusion of papaverine, a smooth muscle dilator, which reverses vasoconstriction.
  - Addressing the predisposing factors including decreased cardiac output, hypotension and use of vasoconstrictive drugs is also paramount in treatment of NOMI.
- CMI:
  - The gold standard is open surgical revascularization using aortomesenteric grafting.
  - Endovascular therapy with angioplasty and stenting may be effective but has a higher rate of recurrence of symptoms.
- Colonic ischemia:
  - Bowel rest
  - Monitor with serial abdominal exams and labs as indicated.
  - Although randomized controlled studies are lacking to support reduced morbidity and mortality, broad-spectrum intravenous antibiotics are recommended.
  - Discontinue any vasoconstricting drugs such as digitalis, vasopressin, and diuretics.
  - Marked colon distention is treated with rectal tubes and NG tube decompression if necessary.
  - If suspect peritonitis due to perforation, massive bleeding, toxic megacolon, or recurrent sepsis, then surgery is recommended.

Inflammatory Bowel Disease: Crohn Disease and Ulcerative Colitis

Brian Peacock, MMS

GENERAL FEATURES

- Inflammatory bowel disease (IBD) is a diagnosis that describes either Crohn disease (CD) or ulcerative colitis (UC).
- Specific etiology is unknown but is thought to be a combination of an industrialized environment, immune factors, and genomic predisposition.
- CD involves segmental transmural inflammation of the gastrointestinal (GI) tract anywhere from the mouth to the anus.
  - Patients manage intermittent flares throughout their life.
- UC is circumferential confluent inflammation confined to the mucosa of the colon and rectum.
  - Inflammation starts distally in the rectum and progresses proximally through the colon.
  - Patients have an increased risk for the development of colon adenocarcinoma.

CLINICAL ASSESSMENT

- IBD should be on the differential for patients with concerns for a colitis (bloody stools, mucous stools, abdominal pain, diarrhea, tenesmus), especially if they are in their first four decades of life.
- UC typically presents with blood and mucous in the stools, diarrhea, tenesmus, and fecal incontinence/anal leakage.
  - Patients can have weight loss and abdominal pain depending on the severity of disease.
  - Missed diagnosis can lead to rapid dehydration and malnourishment.
- The presentation of CD is dependent on the location and severity of the disease.
  - CD can present with cramping/abdominal pain, nonbloody diarrhea, and/or symptoms of an abscess/fistula or bowel obstruction.

- CD is more likely to have extraintestinal manifestations: arthritis, uveitis, erythema nodosum, pyoderma gangrenosum, and osteoporosis.
- Misdiagnosis of CD can lead to perforation of GI tract and abscess or fistula formation or structuring of the GI tract and development of an obstruction.

DIAGNOSIS

- In all patients suspected of IBD, infectious colitis should be ruled out.
- Physical examination should look for signs of extraintestinal manifestations.
- Endoscopic evaluation with colonoscopy is the gold standard for diagnosis.
  - UC is classically identified by edema, confluent erythema, and loss of vascular markings starting in the rectum.
  - CD is classically identified by "skip lesions" and a "cobblestone" appearance to the mucosa.
- Order basic labs to evaluate anemia, infection, and systemic inflammation levels for baseline and trending.
- CT scan can be used if there are concerns for complications associated with IBD.
- Upper endoscopy and pill endoscopy can be utilized to evaluate Crohn-like symptoms from the mouth to the ileum.

TREATMENT

- Goals of therapy are generally aimed at managing the inflammatory process.
- Aminosalicylates are typically first line for maintenance therapy of mild-to-moderate disease; immunomodulators and biologics are additional agents used when patients fail aminosalicylate therapy.
- Steroids can used to help manage acute flares.
- Medically refractory IBD requires surgical intervention.
  - UC is cured with a total colectomy.

Toxic Megacolon

Melodie Kolmetz, MPAS, PA-C

▶ GENERAL FEATURES

- Toxic megacolon is a rare but potentially deadly complication of colonic inflammation.
- Nonobstructive dilation of the colon (total or segmental) with associated systemic toxicity
- Most commonly a complication of inflammatory bowel disease, but can be seen in other conditions that lead to inflammation of the colon, including inflammatory, ischemic, infectious, radiation-induced processes
- The risk of toxic megacolon is increased proportionally with the severity of colitis.
- Rapid tapering or discontinuation of immunomodulators such as steroids, sulfasalazine, and 5-ASA can precipitate development of toxic megacolon.

▶ CLINICAL ASSESSMENT

- Careful history is crucial, focusing on recent travel, antibiotic use, chemotherapy, immunosuppression, and history of inflammatory bowel disease.
- Abdominal complaints may include diarrhea, abdominal pain, rectal bleeding, tenesmus, vomiting, and fever.
- Systemic inflammation/toxicity drives tachycardia and fever.
- Examine for abdominal distension or decreased bowel sounds, rebound tenderness, abdominal rigidity, or peritoneal irritation concerning for perforation.
- Patients with inflammatory colitis may be on high-dose steroids, which can mask the physical examination findings.

▶ DIAGNOSIS

- Diagnostic criteria include:
  - Radiographic evidence of colonic dilation, classically >6 cm (with loss of haustration) in the transverse colon on plain abdominal radiographs; imaging can also show the presence of intraluminal soft-tissue masses known as pseudopolyps and segmental parietal thinning.
  - Any three of the following: fever, tachycardia, leukocytosis, or anemia

  - Any one of the following: dehydration, altered mental status, electrolyte abnormality, or hypotension
- A complete blood count with differential may be elevated, but in patients on immunosuppression, this is not reliable.
- An electrolyte panel may show electrolyte disturbances owing to ongoing GI fluid and salt loss.
- CT scan of the abdomen may help identify localized or contained perforation. It can also be helpful if the diagnosis is unclear.
- Direct examination via flexible sigmoidoscopy or colonoscopy should generally be avoided, given the risk of perforation with those procedures.

▶ TREATMENT

- Goals of treatment include reduction of colonic distension, correction of fluid and electrolyte disturbances, and treatment of systemic inflammatory response.
- Initial resuscitation of fluid and electrolytes is necessary.
- Blood transfusion may be indicated.
- Broad-spectrum antibiotic coverage and IV steroids are indicated.
- Medications that can affect colonic motility, such as narcotics, anticholinergic agents, and antidiarrheal medications, should be stopped.
- A nasogastric tube should be placed for bowel rest. Some evidence shows that patient movement and positioning (prone or knee to chest position) can be helpful.
- Frequent monitoring with physical examination, laboratory testing, and radiographic exams is crucial; free intraperitoneal air on abdominal radiographs is concerning for perforation.
- Early surgical consult is critical as these patients can decompensate rapidly and require urgent operative intervention for subtotal colectomy.
  - Indications for urgent surgical intervention include perforation, massive hemorrhage, increasing toxicity, and worsening colonic dilatation.
  - Colectomy may also be indicated if there is no improvement after 24–48 hours of maximum medical therapy.

Hernias

Kate Woodard, PA-C

▶ GENERAL FEATURES

- Hernias are defined as a protrusion of an organ, vessel, or other component through an abnormal opening or hole in the tissue.
- Most often diagnosed in the groin and abdominal wall, with inguinal hernias representing the most frequently seen groin hernia
- Inguinal hernias occur in the inguinal canal, either due to a congenital defect or due to acquired defect.
  - Indirect inguinal hernias are most often congenital, whereas direct inguinal hernias are acquired.
- Risk of developing a hernia increases with advanced age, male sex, conditions that increase abdominal pressure including excessive heavy lifting, chronic cough and constipation, history of smoking, abdominal wall injury or prior hernia repair, and family history of hernia.
- Femoral hernias are more common in female patients.

▶ CLINICAL ASSESSMENT

- Often asymptomatic when small
- Typical presentation of a bulge, pressure, or pain in the affected area
  - Should resolve completely when the patient is supine if the hernia is not incarcerated or strangulated
  - Incarcerated hernias: unable to be reduced back into the cavity from which it protrudes
  - Strangulated hernia: has blood flow reduced due to incarceration, and this represents a surgical emergency
  - Patients with incarcerated or strangulated hernias may present with a bowel obstruction.
- Patients with femoral hernias are more likely to present with strangulated hernias than are patients with inguinal or abdominal wall hernias, and the mass is typically below the inguinal canal.

▶ DIAGNOSIS

- Most often clinical with adequate history and physical examination
- Most notable with the patient standing and the examiner seated
  - The use of Valsalva maneuver or coughing may also reveal an occult hernia.
- In evaluating a male patient for inguinal hernia, the examiner should insert the dominant index finger gently into the inguinal canal of the affected side.
  - Indirect inguinal hernias protrude through the open internal inguinal ring and will be palpable at the tip of the examiners finger when inserted into the inguinal canal.
  - Direct inguinal hernias occur within Hesselbach triangle, superior to the inguinal ligament.
- Ultrasound may be useful if the diagnosis is not clear on physical examination; more advanced imaging modalities are not typically needed.

▶ TREATMENT

- Patients presenting with a strangulated hernia or with bowel obstruction due to incarcerated or strangulated hernia should undergo surgical repair immediately.
- Incarcerated hernias should be watched closely for progression to strangulation, and patients should be offered surgical repair.
- Femoral hernias should be repaired promptly owing to their high risk of strangulation.
- In asymptomatic inguinal or abdominal wall hernias, elective surgical repair and watchful waiting are both appropriate options.
- Surgical repair of any of these hernias may be performed via a laparoscopic or open approach.

CHAPTER
157

Acute Pancreatitis

Paul "PJ" Koltnow, MS, MSPAS, PA-C

▶ GENERAL FEATURES

- Acute pancreatitis is an inflammatory process of the pancreas.
  - Ranges from mild to severe as determined by the absence or presence of organ failure
    - Mild acute pancreatitis: not associated with organ failure and has no local or systemic complications
    - Moderate acute pancreatitis: characterized by transient organ failure (resolves in <48 hours) and/or local or systemic complications without persistent organ failure (organ failure of >48 hours duration)
    - Severe acute pancreatitis: characterized by persistent organ failure that may involve one or many organs
- The most common cause of acute pancreatitis is gallstones.
- Other common causes of acute pancreatitis include:
  - Heavy alcohol use
  - Hypertriglyceridemia (>1000 mg/dL)
  - Post–endoscopic retrograde cholangiopancreatography (ERCP)
  - Medications
  - Genetics
  - Hypercalcemia

▶ CLINICAL ASSESSMENT

- Acute pancreatitis usually presents with sudden and persistent epigastric abdominal pain that may extend to the back; it is often described as constant in duration and boring in character.
- Nausea and vomiting occur in 90% of patients.
- There may be pain to the epigastrium on physical examination.
  - The level of pain will vary with the severity of acute pancreatitis.

- Mild acute pancreatitis will likely present with minimal tenderness to palpitation to the epigastrium, whereas severe acute pancreatitis will present with more severe pain.

▶ DIAGNOSIS

- Pancreatic enzymes (serum amylase and serum lipase) are digestive enzymes of the pancreas, which are typically elevated 3 times the normal level during acute pancreatitis:
  - Serum amylase levels will rise 6–12 hours after the onset of acute pancreatitis and will return to normal levels in 3–5 days.
  - Serum lipase will rise within 4–8 hours after the onset of acute pancreatitis, will peak at 24 hours, and return to normal within 8–14 days; levels >3 times the norm are sensitive (82%-100%) for acute pancreatitis.
    - Serum lipase results are more useful for detecting acute pancreatitis in patients who present >24 hours after onset of symptoms.
    - Serum lipase is also more sensitive for detecting those with acute pancreatitis secondary to alcohol.
- Abdominal ultrasound can be used to visualize gallstones in the gallbladder or bile duct as well as to possibly detect an enlarged and hypoechoic pancreas.
- Severity of disease should be established by clinical examination to focus on fluid loss, organ failure, or inflammatory response.
  - Obtain a complete metabolic panel, serum calcium, complete blood count, serum triglycerides, and lactate.
- The Atlanta Criteria is commonly used to define disease severity.

▶ TREATMENT

- Patients who present with acute pancreatitis should be hospitalized for initial evaluation, classification of disease severity, and management of the disease.
- Fluid replacement is given unless cardiovascular, renal, or other related comorbid factors preclude it.
- Pain control with intravenous opioids.
- Close monitoring for first 24–48 hours for complications and/or organ failure.
- Nutritional support is vital as patients will be NPO initially.
- If the acute pancreatitis was caused by gallstones, all patients should have a cholecystectomy after the patient recovers from the initial illness.
- Any underlying predisposing condition needs to be addressed to minimize further reoccurrences.

CHAPTER
158

G6P Deficiency

Jamie Saunders, MSc, FHEA, PA-R

▶ GENERAL FEATURES

- Rare inherited disorder in which a person is missing the enzyme glucose-6-phosphate (G6P) dehydrogenase
  - Enzyme necessary for breaking down certain carbohydrates
  - Without this, exposure to specific carbohydrates will cause hemolysis.
  - Episodes often prompted by consumption of legumes such as fava beans; certain medications such as antimalarial drugs, NSAIDs, and sulfonamides; or by infection.
- X-linked, males > females
- More common in people with heritage from Africa, Asia, Middle East, or Mediterranean

▶ CLINICAL ASSESSMENT

- Neonatal jaundice in an at-risk population should alert the provider to evaluate for this deficiency.
- Darkening of urine, yellowing of skin or sclera, rapid onset of back pain, or shortness of breath following consumption of legumes, certain medications, or following infections suggests likelihood of G6P deficiency.
- Often, this disorder is asymptomatic in the absence of inciting events.
- Physical examination findings following ingestion of inciting food or medication may include:
  - Jaundice or pallor
  - Tachypnea and/or tachycardia
  - Hepatosplenomegaly
  - Confusion
  - Fatigue
  - Fever

▶ DIAGNOSIS

- Suggested by history and physical examination and confirmed by quantitative serum G6D activity test (Beutler test)
- Complete blood count revealing low hemoglobin and hematocrit and low reticulocyte counts and urine hemosiderin are suggestive of hemolysis.
- Screening should be performed in newborns who are at risk based on heritage or family history.

▶ TREATMENT

- Largely focused on prevention by avoidance of legumes and inciting medications
- Newborn jaundice related to G6P deficiency treated with lamp phototherapy, in rare cases exchange transfusion is necessary.
- Acute hemolysis in an adult should be treated by discontinuation of inciting medication or food or treatment of infection if still present.
  - If severe, intravenous fluid replacement or blood transfusion may help.

Phenylketonuria

Bart Gillum, DSc, MHS, PA-C

▌ GENERAL FEATURES

- Inherited as an autosomal-recessive condition
- Inborn error of amino acid metabolism effecting phenylalanine (Phe).
- Prevalence is ~1 in 10 000 live births.
- Results from mutations in the phenylalanine hydroxylase (*PAH*) gene
- Without this functional liver enzyme, ingested Phe cannot be converted to tyrosine.
- Rarely, PAH is present and functions normally, but tetrahydrobiopterin (BH4), an important cofactor in this metabolic process, is deficient.
- Toxic levels of Phe in blood and developing brain lead to progressive intellectual impairment.
- Mild phenotype includes only nontoxic increase in blood Phe concentrations without intellectual disability.
- Early diagnosis and intervention can mitigate development of severe mental disability.

▌ CLINICAL ASSESSMENT

- Newborn infants are asymptomatic before ingesting breast milk or standard infant formula.
- Undiagnosed infants develop symptoms insidiously throughout infancy.
- Symptoms include irreversible intellectual disability, seizures, autism, behavioral abnormalities, motor dysfunction, and eczematous rash.
- Signs and symptoms can vary from mild to severe.
- Severity of disease is related to specific PAH genetic mutation.
- Discontinuation of dietary management in adolescents or adults can lead to depression, social isolation, or subtle deficits in cognitive neuropsychological function.

- Mild impairment in cognitive function is seen in patients with even good dietary control.

▌ DIAGNOSIS

- PKU screening test is given 24–72 hours after birth, after infant has ingested protein.
- Traditionally, screening test checks for elevated Phe in blood.
- Normal is <4 mg/dL.
- 10–20 mg/dL is considered mild PKU.
- >20 mg/dL is considered classic PKU, usually indicates complete deficiency of PAH.
- Screening test is followed by molecular testing to determine specific PAH mutations.
- Although not normally performed, white matter lesions can be seen on MRI, severity of which is related to dietary control.

▌ TREATMENT

- Mainstay of treatment is dietary restriction with Phe-free proteins.
- Breast milk should be no >25% of feedings, alternated with Phe-free formula.
- Treatment should be initiated within 1 week of birth.
- Dietary restriction is indicated for all infants with Phe concentrations >7–10 mg/dL and should continue throughout life.
- Higher blood Phe level averages correlate with lower IQ.
- For mild PKU associated with low BH4, synthetic BH4 (sapropterin) can be prescribed.
- Management of this complex condition requires an interdisciplinary team of pediatricians, metabolic specialists, nutritionists, and psychologists.

Section A Pretest: Acute Kidney Injury

1. A 37-year-old woman presents to the ED with a 3-day history of vomiting and diarrhea. On physical examination, she looks pale, diaphoretic, and "sick." Her BP is 120/80 sitting but drops to 90/58 standing. She has tachycardia, and a pinch test shows skin tenting. STAT labs show a SCr of 2.3 mg/dL and an elevated RBC count. She is treated with 2 L 1/2 NS IV. Repeat examination shows better skin turgor, and the orthostatic changes are resolved. STAT labs show an SCr of 1.2 mg/dL with a normal RBC count. What is her diagnosis?

    A. Prerenal AKI
    B. Postrenal AKI
    C. Intrarenal AKI
    D. This is not AKI

2. A 62-year-old surgical PA developed tachycardia during surgery, stepped back from the operating room table, and passed out. He was revived and transported to the ED. His cardiologist recently increased his lisinopril dose for albuminuria. In the ED, his SCr was 2.1 mg/dL, K was 6.8 mEq/dL, and his EKG showed tachycardia with peaked T waves. Past medical history (PMH): cardiac cath with one vessel stent, prior smoker, CKD. What is the immediate treatment?

    A. IV fluids
    B. Stopping the lisinopril

    C. IV calcium carbonate
    D. Oral sodium polystyrene sulfate (Kayexalate)

3. What is the most likely cause of an AKI in a 68-year-old man?

    A. Atorvastatin
    B. Prostate
    C. Nephrolithiasis
    D. Dehydration

4. A 58-year-old woman who presents to the ED with chest pain that developed while she was shoveling snow. EKG shows ST elevation. PMH: DM, hypertension (HTN), CKD 3a, all well controlled. She is taken to the cath lab and stented. She is discharged at 24 hours without issues and presents to her primary care office where, per KDIGO guidelines, a follow-up SCr is done: 2.7 mg/dL (historical 1.9 mg/dL). What is the most likely cause of her AKI?

    A. Cholesterol embolization
    B. Postrenal AKI
    C. Contrast nephropathy
    D. β-Blocker–induced hypotension

Section B Pretest: Chronic Kidney Disease

1. What is the most predictive factor in who will progress to kidney failure?

    A. Age
    B. HTN
    C. Male gender
    D. Urine albumin-to-creatinine ratio (UACR)

2. A 24-year-old college student went to a kidney screening run by the NKF. She was told that she had albumin in her urine (she states "microalbuminuria") and was referred to your office. She is

concerned about CKD. What can you tell her about the microalbuminuria?

    A. She is more likely to develop kidney failure because she is female.
    B. She has CKD because she had microalbuminuria.
    C. You cannot tell anything and need to repeat the lab.
    D. You are not quite sure if the collection was done right.

3. A patient presents to the ED complaining of sudden-onset low back pain that feels like "a horse kicked me in my back." He denies recent trauma. He is urinating frank red blood. Physical exam shows an uncomfortable male who is no longer in pain. Patient is concerned with the bloody urination. PMH is positive for HTN, controlled with diet. Family history is significant for HTN in all maternal family members and four of his five siblings. The fifth sibling had a kidney transplant at age 15. Meds include NSAIDs PRN. What confirmatory test is needed?

   A. UACR
   B. Kidney ultrasound
   C. UPEP/SPEP
   D. Renal angiogram

Section C Pretest: Congenital and Structural Kidney Disease

1. Which chromosome is affected in ADPKD1?

   A. Chromosome 4
   B. Chromosome 6
   C. Chromosome 13
   D. Chromosome 16

2. Your 50-year-old patient has a history of HTN and recently completed treatment for her third UTI of the year. She comes to your office for repeat urinalysis (UA) after treatment and is found to have persistent hematuria. PE reveals palpable kidneys bilaterally and elevated BP. Upon further questioning, the patient reports her father died of end-stage kidney disease at age 65. What test would confirm your suspected diagnosis of this patient?

   A. CBC
   B. IV pyelogram
   C. Microscopic UA
   D. MRI

3. Which of the following meets the diagnostic criteria for polycystic kidney disease (PKD)?

   A. 1 cyst in each kidney 21–45 years
   B. 2 cysts in one kidney 15–39 years
   C. 3 cysts in one kidney 15–39 years
   D. 4 cysts in one kidney at 75 years

4. Horseshoe kidneys are more common in which of the following populations?

   A. Male patients
   B. Female patients
   C. White patients
   D. Black/AA patients

5. Which of the following should be included in the management plan for a patient with PKD?

   A. Aggressive BP control with diuretics
   B. Avoidance of acetaminophen
   C. Avoidance of ibuprofen
   D. Fluid restriction

6. Which of the following is most likely to be associated with a finding of horseshoe kidneys?

   A. Cystic fibrosis
   B. Autosomal PKD
   C. Turner syndrome
   D. IgA nephropathy

7. A patient with an established diagnosis of PKD presents to the ED with "the worst headache he has ever had in his whole life." You are concerned that he has which of the following?

   A. Intracranial cyst
   B. Migraine headache
   C. Meningitis
   D. Ruptured intracranial berry aneurysm

Section D Pretest: End-Stage Renal Disease

1. What lab finding is most compatible with end-stage renal disease (ESRD)?

   A. Potassium level 3.3
   B. Sodium level 147
   C. Estimated GFR of 12
   D. Phosphate level 1.1

2. A patient with a history of HTN presents to the ED with a BP of 196/102 and complaint of nausea. Physical exam reveals crackles on pulmonary examination and 2+ pitting edema. Lab testing is significant for a BUN of 113 and creatinine of 3.72. What treatment is most indicated for management of this patient's disease process?

   A. Thoracentesis
   B. Hemodialysis
   C. Hydration with IV fluids
   D. Initiation of an angiotensin-converting enzyme inhibitor (ACEi) such as lisinopril

3. A patient with a known history of type 2 diabetes mellitus is at increased risk for developing chronic kidney disease and ESRD. What test is best to assess for early detection of kidney dysfunction?

   A. Basic metabolic panel
   B. CBC
   C. Serum albumin
   D. Urine microalbumin

4. A patient requiring hemodialysis has questions regarding an appropriate diet to manage his disease process. What dietary changes are suggested for patients with ESRD?

   A. Low potassium, low phosphorus
   B. Low potassium, high phosphorus
   C. High potassium, low phosphorus
   D. High potassium, high phosphorus

Section E Pretest: Fluid and Electrolyte Disorders

1. What is the primary underlying pathophysiology that produces symptoms of hyponatremia?

   A. Fluid shifts in the brain causing cerebral edema
   B. Cerebral vasodilation resulting from the presence of pathogens in the bloodstream
   C. Embolic effects of clots produced from low sodium levels
   D. Low serum sodium may induce a biochemical cascade resulting in elevated ethanol in the blood producing neurologic symptoms

2. Which acid-base disturbance can be seen with excessive administration of lactated Ringer solution?

   A. Metabolic acidosis
   B. Metabolic alkalosis
   C. Respiratory acidosis
   D. Respiratory alkalosis

3. A concerned family member brings in her elderly mother for complaints of weakness, decreased thirst, and irritability. On examination, you find patient is hypotensive with tachycardia. What would you expect to see on the patient's labs?

   A. Serum sodium of 177 mEq/L and decreased urine sodium
   B. Serum sodium of 155 mEq/L and BUN/creatinine ratio 30
   C. Serum sodium of 200 mEq/L and increased urinary sodium
   D. Serum sodium of 135 mEq/L and BUN/creatinine ratio 19

4. You are performing your rounds on one of your patients who was admitted for weakness and confusion. Her labs come back with a sodium level of 148 mEq/L. The patient has been able to tolerate liquids and food orally. What would be the first line of treatment?

   A. Replace free water orally.
   B. Stop all sodium intake.
   C. Replace potassium with oral supplement.
   D. Continue to hold free water replacement.

5. A patient with a new diagnosis of non-Hodgkin lymphoma is deemed an appropriate candidate for chemotherapy. In the initial phase of chemotherapy, what electrolyte abnormality should this patient be monitored for?

   A. Hyponatremia
   B. Hypermagnesemia
   C. Hypocalcemia
   D. Hyperphosphatemia
   E. Hypophosphatemia

6. Risk factors for hypernatremia include which of the following?

   A. Old age
   B. Children
   C. DM
   D. All of the above

7. What is the most important complication to avoid while treating hyponatremia?

   A. Severe dehydration resulting from fluid restriction
   B. Osmotic demyelination syndrome causing potentially permanent neurologic deficits
   C. Gait abnormalities from fluid shifts causing cerebral edema
   D. Disruption of bone metabolism resulting in osteoporosis

8. The most common type of hypernatremia is which of the following?

   A. Euvolemic hypernatremia
   B. Hypovolemic hypernatremia
   C. Hypervolemic hypernatremia
   D. Euvolemic hypercalcemia

9. Which of the following is false regarding hypovolemia?

   A. Hypovolemia results in tissue hypoperfusion, whereas dehydration results in desiccated cells.
   B. Hypovolemia is typically caused by not drinking enough water.
   C. Pregnant females and children can be severely hypovolemic while temporarily compensating with a normal BP.

10. Euvolemic hypotonic hyponatremia is often found in patients taking which class of medications?

    A. Aminoglycosides
    B. β-Blockers
    C. NSAIDs
    D. Diuretics

11. Signs of hypovolemia do NOT include which of the following?

    A. Sunken eyes, extended capillary refill time, altered mental state, weak peripheral pulses
    B. Dry mucous membranes, sunken eyes, extended capillary refill time, weak peripheral pulses
    C. Hypotension, tachycardia, altered mental state, tachypnea
    D. JVD, peripheral edema, crackles in the lung bases on auscultation

12. When treating acute hyponatremia with severe CNS symptoms or seizure, you should raise serum sodium by which of the following?

    A. 8–10 mEq/L in 4–6 hours or to >120–125 mEq/L using hypertonic saline
    B. 5–15 mEq/L in 6–12 hours or to >125–130 mEq/L using hypertonic saline
    C. 1–3 mEq/L in 6–12 hours or to >125–135 mEq/L using hypertonic saline
    D. 8–10 mEq/L in 12–24 hours or to >120–125 mEq/L using hypertonic saline

13. Which of the following statements is false regarding hypovolemia treatment?

    A. Fluid resuscitation is the mainstay therapy. Crystalloids are used for nonhemorrhagic hypovolemia, and blood products are used for hemorrhagic hypovolemia.
    B. An initial 30 mL/kg bolus of crystalloid is safe for most patients. In patients with heart failure and kidney disease, smaller boluses with frequent reassessment of response is advisable.
    C. If the patient does not respond to a fluid bolus, the clinician should give several more liters of fluid in rapid succession until patient begins to cough up pink frothy sputum.

14. Which of the following conditions can cause an increased anion gap metabolic acidosis?

    A. Lactic acidosis
    B. Diarrhea
    C. Renal tubular acidosis
    D. Hyperaldosteronism

15. A patient's original clinical data included JVP 2 cm H_2O, capillary refill 6 seconds, HR 122, and MAP 61. The clinician will recognize the best overall improvement from which of the following sets of data?

    A. JVP 4 cm H_2O, capillary refill 6 seconds, HR 110, MAP 62
    B. JVP 6 cm H_2O, capillary refill 3 seconds, HR 88, MAP 68
    C. JVP 10 cm H_2O, capillary refill 5 seconds, HR 88, MAP 90

16. Hypervolemic-hypotonic hyponatremia is NOT often a result of which of the following conditions?

    A. Heart failure
    B. Liver disease
    C. Hypothyroidism
    D. Nephrotic syndrome

17. A 51-year-old man presents to the ED with a 3-day history of shortness of breath, fevers, and cough. He reports a recent upper respiratory illness 2 weeks ago that never fully resolved. Vital signs show BP 136/84, HR 106, RR 26, O₂ 93% on room air, and temperature 102.3 °F. Physical exam reveals decreased breath sounds in the right lower lobe with scattered rhonchi. Due to the patient's hypoxemia on pulse oximetry, an ABG is ordered and shows 7.45/34/72/24/+1. Based on this presentation, what acid-base disturbance does this patient have?

    A. Metabolic acidosis
    B. Metabolic alkalosis
    C. Respiratory acidosis
    D. Respiratory alkalosis

18. A 45-year-old patient presents with tingling of the lips, fingers, and toes and abdominal pain for the past week. Assuming there is an electrolyte disorder to blame for this patient's symptoms, what is the most likely diagnosis?

    A. Hyponatremia
    B. Hypocalcemia
    C. Hypophosphatemia
    D. Hyperphosphatemia
    E. Hypercalcemia

19. A 27-year-old man with history of IV drug use is brought into the ED by EMS for what is presumed to be an overdose. A battery of labs has been drawn including an ABG, which shows 7.20/65/80/23/−1. What acute acid-base disturbance does this patient have?

    A. Metabolic acidosis
    B. Metabolic alkalosis
    C. Respiratory acidosis
    D. Respiratory alkalosis

20. Which of the following conditions is most likely to precipitate hypokalemia?

    A. Insulin overdose
    B. Metabolic acidosis
    C. Poor oral intake
    D. Hypermagnesemia

Section F Pretest: Glomerular Disease

1. A 30-year-old woman presents with significant peripheral edema, SOB, and fatigue. Lab evaluation shows hypoalbuminemia, hyperlipidemia, and hypocalcemia. Her UA reveals 4+ proteinuria with bland sediment. What is the best diagnostic study to order to confirm the etiology of her symptoms?

    A. Renal biopsy
    B. CT scan of the kidneys and urinary tract
    C. Cystoscopy
    D. Urine culture and sensitivity

2. A previously healthy child presents with significant periorbital and sacral edema. She denies a sore throat, abdominal or joint pain. Her UA appears frothy and reveals 3+ proteinuria and trace hematuria on the dipstick. Her vital signs are within normal limits. Labs are pending. Which of the following is the most likely cause of her presentation?

    A. Minimal change disease
    B. Membranous nephropathy
    C. Goodpasture syndrome
    D. Amyloidosis
    E. Poststreptococcal nephritis

3. A 60-year-old man with a known cancer diagnosis is admitted to the hospital with nephrotic syndrome. He is placed on a loop diuretic and fluid restriction. On day 3, he develops increasing edema in his right leg and mild shortness of breath. Labs done earlier in the day revealed worsening hypoalbuminemia. What is the probable cause of his increasing edema?

    A. Increased loss of fluid from the intravascular space
    B. Formation of a thrombus in the lower extremity
    C. Inadequate dosing of the loop diuretics
    D. Development of CHF

4. An 8-year-old boy is brought to the ED by his worried parents. The child is complaining of abdominal pain and sore knees. The parents deny any recent URI or GI infections. On examination, you note a rash on his buttocks and posterior thighs. UA reveals hematuria, pyuria, and 1+ proteinuria. Microscopy shows many dysmorphic RBCs and RBC casts. What is the most likely diagnosis?

    A. Minimal change disease
    B. Membranous nephropathy
    C. IgA vasculitis
    D. Goodpasture syndrome

5. A young boy presents to your clinic complaining of dark-colored urine. He reports that his throat hurt last week. On serologic and urologic workup, you diagnosis the patient with a glomerulonephritis. What is the most likely cause of his glomerulonephritis?

    A. Antineutrophil cytoplasmic antibody–associated vasculitis

    B. Immune mediated (postinfectious)

    C. Goodpasture syndrome

    D. Systemic lupus erythematosus

6. A previously healthy 30-year-old man complains of visible blood in his urine for the past 24 hours. He denies recent trauma, dysuria, fevers, or flank pain. His history is significant for a recent diarrheal illness that has resolved. UA microscopy reveals many RBCs along with RBC casts and a few WBCs. What is the most likely diagnosis at this point in the evaluation?

    A. UTI

    B. IgA nephropathy

    C. Anti-GBM antibody disease

    D. Minimal change disease

    E. Membranous nephropathy

Section G Pretest: Renal Malignancies

1. Which of the following patients has the highest likelihood of developing renal cell carcinoma?

    A. Male, 60yo, smoker

    B. Female, 75yo, nonsmoker

    C. Male, 23yo, underweight

    D. Female, 29yo, immunosuppressed

2. Which of the following is the most common presentation of a Wilms tumor?

    A. Abdominal pain with flexing of the knees and intermittent bouts of inconsolable crying

    B. Painless gross hematuria that is often unnoticed until toilet training

    C. A painless abdominal mass discovered by the caregivers incidentally

    D. Nocturnal awakenings, bone pain, unexplained weight loss, and anemia

3. Which of the following is the classic triad of renal cell carcinoma?

    A. Nausea, flank pain, anemia

    B. Palpable flank mass, anemia, hematuria

    C. Hematuria, flank pain, palpable flank mass

    D. Nausea, anemia, hematuria

4. Which of the following imaging studies is indicated as a first-line evaluation method for an abdominal mass in a toddler?

    A. Plain film abdominal x-ray

    B. Ultrasound

    C. CT with contrast

    D. MRI

5. Which of the following is associated with the highest risk for renal cell carcinoma?

    A. Alcohol use disorder

    B. Chronic malnourishment

    C. Obesity

    D. Tobacco use

6. A 2-year-old is suspected to have a Wilms tumor. Which of the following would be appropriate patient education for the family?

    A. Avoid trying to feel the mass and activities that could be associated with trauma to the abdomen.

    B. Your child will need a bone marrow biopsy to determine if the cancer has spread.

    C. This type of disease has a better prognosis if diagnosed after age 3 years.

    D. A simple urine test is able to give us a diagnosis 90% of the time.

7. What are the current screening guidelines for early detection of renal cell carcinoma in asymptomatic patients?

    A. CT of the abdomen without contrast every 3 years

    B. There is no current screening guideline

    C. Renal ultrasound every 5 years

    D. MRI of the abdomen every 3 years

Section H Pretest: Renal Vascular Disease

1. A 45-year-old man presents for follow-up after starting lisinopril (Zestril) 10 mg PO daily for stage 2 HTN 2 weeks ago. PMH is significant for obesity, dyslipidemia, and tobacco abuse. He reports taking his medication as prescribed and denies headache, chest pain, leg swelling, or changes in urine output. Today, his BP is 150/94 mm Hg in his left arm and 152/90 mm Hg in his right arm. Heart is regular rate and rhythm. Peripheral pulses are full and equal. His SCr is 1.8 mg/dL today and was 1.2 mg/dL 2 weeks ago. Which of the following is the most appropriate next step in his evaluation?
   A. Abdominal ultrasound
   B. Decrease lisinopril (Zestril) dose
   C. Renal angiography
   D. Start amlodipine (Norvasc)

2. A 58-year-old man presents to the ED with acute onset of shortness of breath and a cough productive of pink frothy sputum. PMH is significant for a 15-year history of HTN previously well controlled with hydrochlorothiazide and tobacco abuse. His BP is 180/102 mm Hg in his left arm and 178/104 mm Hg in his right arm. He is tachycardic, tachypneic, and hypoxic. S1 and S2 are distinct. Rales are auscultated in bilateral lung fields. Chest radiograph reveals diffuse patchy infiltrates, cephalization, and increased vascular markings. ECG reveals sinus tachycardia and nonspecific ST segment and T wave changes. Chemistry panel reveals elevated BUN and creatinine and low potassium. Which of the following is the most likely underlying cause of his presentation?
   A. Acute mitral regurgitation
   B. Interstitial pneumonitis
   C. Myocardial ischemia
   D. Renal artery stenosis (RAS)

3. Which of the following is an uncommon but important complication of the use of gadolinium contrast in magnetic resonance imaging (MRI)?
   A. Mesenteric artery ischemia
   B. Nephrogenic systemic fibrosis
   C. Secondary hyperparathyroidism
   D. Toxic epidermal necrolysis

4. Which of the following is most likely to be affected by fibromuscular dysplasia (FMD)?
   A. Bone marrow
   B. Cerebral arteries
   C. Lymph nodes
   D. Pulmonary veins

5. Which of the following treatment modalities is most likely to be curative in a patient with RAS secondary to FMD?
   A. Angioplasty
   B. Angiotensin-receptor blockade (ARB)
   C. Renal artery bypass
   D. Renal denervation

▶ ANSWERS AND EXPLANATIONS TO SECTION A PRETEST

1. **D.** While many of us might call this prerenal AKI due to dehydration, by definition, this is not AKI. The SCr is better than it was when she presented in the ED. This particular group of patients are missed due to strict definitions of AKI dependent on SCr and urine output.

2. **A.** Although he does have changes on his ECG, meaning that he should be covered for cardiac irritability, the placement of an IV is the immediate treatment. Calcium carbonate does not lower the serum (extracellular) potassium in the body but instead will stabilize the heart muscle. It is given IV and thus the IV is placed before the medication. In real life, the IV fluid dropped Bill's potassium to 5.6 mEq/dL and a normal cardiac rhythm. Sodium polystyrene sulfate is often given in the ED, although it is not Food and Drug Administration approved for emergent use. Stopping the lisinopril will keep this from happening again, but it is not the immediate treatment.

3. **B.** In this age group, prostate issues (postrenal AKI) are the most common issue. Often, males will not notice a decrease in urination, but if questioned carefully, they will admit getting up at night or not drinking fluids after dinner to decrease nocturia.

4. **C.** She was at risk for CIN due to her PMH. KDIGO encourages precatherization IV fluids to decrease the risk of CIN and postcatherization SCr (at 48-72 hours) to look for AKI. Often, the SCr is done at the hospital upon discharge and misses the diagnosis. Postrenal AKI is less likely as there is nothing in the vignette to suggest it. Cholesterol emboli can occur after catherization but present with a "lacy, purple" pattern on areas distal to the kidneys, often the feet and legs. Although

patients are often given β-blockers post cath, there is nothing in the vignette to suggest that is the issue.

▶ ANSWERS AND EXPLANATIONS TO SECTION B PRETEST

1. **D.** UACR, including the amount of albumin, is the most predictive factor. Although males/older patients and those with HTN are more likely to progress, one cannot state equivocally that any of these factors are predictive.

2. **C.** CKD is diagnosed by either a drop in GFR or albuminuria for 3 months. You need to repeat the screening test at 12 weeks. Men are more likely to develop kidney failure; however, women are more likely to develop CKD.

3. **B.** He has autosomal-dominant polycystic disease (ADPKD), and the incredible pain with urinating blood is diagnostic for a cyst popping. The clue is in the personal and family history of HTN. His whole maternal side and siblings have ADPKD, which presents differently, at different ages and in different manners even within the same family. The diagnostic test of choice is an ultrasound because it is cheap, quick, easy to do, and rules out the other likely diagnosis, nephrolithiasis. The UACR is to rule out CKD, the UPEP/SPEP to is rule out multiple myeloma (unlikely given the presentation and age), and the renal angiogram is to rule out RAS. RAS is unlikely to present with pain; it is unusually painless, there is no hematuria and presents as an increasing SCr after starting an ACEi/ARB.

▶ ANSWERS AND EXPLANATIONS TO SECTION C PRETEST

1. **D.** ADPKD2 is chromosome 4, ARPKD is chromosome 6, and chromosome 13 is not affected in PKD.

2. **D.** MRI is preferred to ultrasound for patient with positive FHx and symptoms. CBC and UA would not be confirmatory tests. IV pyelogram not commonly used being replaced by improved imaging methods, like MRI or CT.

3. **C.** The diagnostic criteria are characterized by the number of cysts by age range:
   3+ cysts unilateral or bilateral ages 15–39 years
   2+ cysts in each kidney 40–59 years
   4+ cysts in each kidney at ≥60 years

4. **A.** Horseshoe kidneys are more common in male patients.

5. **C.** NSAIDs should be avoided in PKD. High fluid intake encouraged. ACEi or ARB is first-line treatment for HTN, acetaminophen can be taken.

6. **C.** Turner syndrome is most likely to be associated with a finding of horseshoe kidneys.

7. **D.** Intracranial berry aneurysm is a known extrarenal complication of PKD.

▶ ANSWERS AND EXPLANATIONS TO SECTION D PRETEST

1. **C.** An estimated GFR of 12 is most compatible with ESRD.

2. **B.** Hemodialysis is most indicated for the management of this patient's disease process.

3. **D.** Urine microalbumin is best to assess for early detection of kidney dysfunction.

4. **A.** A low-potassium, low-phosphorus diet is recommended for patients with ESRD.

▶ ANSWERS AND EXPLANATIONS TO SECTION E PRETEST

1. **A.** Fluid shifts in the brain causing cerebral edema is the primary underlying pathophysiology that produces symptoms of hyponatremia.

2. **B.** Metabolic alkalosis can be seen with excessive administration of lactated Ringer solution.

3. **B.** You would expect to see serum sodium of 155 mEq/L and BUN/creatinine ratio 30 on this patient's labs.

4. **A.** Replace free water orally would be the first line of treatment.

5. **D.** This patient is at high risk for tumor lysis syndrome, which commonly presents with hyperphosphatemia.

6. **D.** Risk factors for hypernatremia include old age, children, and DM.

7. **B.** Avoid osmotic demyelination syndrome causing potentially permanent neurologic deficits while treating hyponatremia.

8. **B.** The most common type of hypernatremia is hypovolemic hypernatremia.

9. **B.** Hypovolemia is typically caused by not drinking enough water is not true.

10. **D.** Euvolemic-hypotonic hyponatremia is often found in patients taking diuretics.

11. **D.** This constellation of exam findings is often present in volume overload.

12. **A.** When treating acute hyponatremia with severe CNS symptoms or seizure, you should raise serum sodium by 8–10 mEq/L in 4–6 hours or to >120–125 mEq/L using hypertonic saline.

13. **C.** If the patient does not respond to a fluid bolus, the clinician should give several more liters of fluid in rapid succession until patient begins to cough up pink frothy sputum is not true regarding hypovolemia.

14. **A.** Lactic acidosis can cause an increased anion gap metabolic acidosis.

15. **B.** In this patient, the clinician will recognize the best overall improvement from JVP 6 cm H_2O, capillary refill 3 seconds, HR 88, MAP 68.
16. **C.** Hypervolemic-hypotonic hyponatremia is not often a result of hypothyroidism.
17. **D.** Based on this presentation, this patient has respiratory alkalosis.
18. **B.** This patient presents with perioral and acral paresthesia and abdominal cramping consistent with hypocalcemia.
19. **C.** This patient has respiratory acidosis.
20. **A.** Insulin overdose is most likely to precipitate hypokalemia.

ANSWERS AND EXPLANATIONS TO SECTION F PRETEST

1. **A.** The best diagnostic study to order to confirm the etiology of her symptoms is renal biopsy.
2. **A.** Minimal change disease is the most likely cause of her presentation.
3. **B.** Formation of a thrombus in the lower extremity is the probable cause of his increasing edema.
4. **C.** IgA vasculitis is the most likely diagnosis.
5. **B.** The most likely cause of his glomerulonephritis is immune mediated (postinfectious). Owing to the patient's recent infection, this is the most likely cause of his glomerulonephritis. His age would also make the other diagnoses much less likely.
6. **B.** IgA nephropathy is the most likely diagnosis at this point in the evaluation.

ANSWERS AND EXPLANATIONS TO SECTION G PRETEST

1. **A.** A 60-year-old male smoker has the highest likelihood of developing renal cell carcinoma of this group.
2. **C.** Wilms tumors do not metastasize to the bone, so bone pain would be a very unusual presentation. Although hematuria can be seen with a Wilms tumor, it more commonly presents as a painless abdominal mass with hematuria as an incidental finding as part of the workup for the abdominal mass. If the child does present with a painful abdomen, it is usually not associated with symptoms similar to intussusception.
3. **C.** Hematuria, flank pain, and palpable flank mass is the classical triad of renal cell carcinoma.
4. **B.** Given its quick, noninvasive, nonionizing and ability to adapt to a squirmy child, abdominal ultrasound with Doppler is typically the first imaging studies ordered for pediatric patients needing soft-tissue or organ evaluation. In the case of a Wilms tumor, ultrasound with Doppler is used to determine structure, location, and blood flow. Longer and more involved studies that might require sedation, such as CT or MRI, are usually reserved for follow-up studies once initial information has been gathered, so a more focused study can be planned.
5. **D.** Tobacco use is associated with the highest risk for renal cell carcinoma.
6. **A.** As the most favorable outcomes are if the mass is removed while still encapsulated, avoiding excessive palpation of the already fragile tissue can help prevent rupture of the capsule and potential spread of the tumor. Wilms tumors do not metastasize to the bone, so bone marrow biopsy would not be indicated. The best prognoses are in children under the age of 2 years with favorable histology. Urine catecholamines can be used to detect neuroblastomas, but not nephroblastomas.
7. **B.** There is no current screening guideline for early detection of renal cell carcinoma in asymptomatic patients.

ANSWERS AND EXPLANATIONS TO SECTION H PRETEST

1. **A.** Abdominal ultrasound is the most appropriate next step in his evaluation.
2. **D.** RAS is the most likely underlying cause of his presentation.
3. **B.** Nephrogenic systemic fibrosis is an uncommon but important complication of the use of gadolinium contrast in MRA.
4. **B.** The cerebral arteries are most likely to be affected by FMD.
5. **A.** Angioplasty is most likely to be curative in a patient with RAS secondary to FMD.

CHAPTER

160

Acute Kidney Injury

Kim Zuber, PA-C, MS
Jane Davis, DNP

▶ GENERAL FEATURES

- Acute kidney injury (AKI) was previously known as acute renal failure (ARF); terminology discontinued in 2010.
- Occurs in >25% of all hospitalized patients and associated with increased morbidity and mortality
- Defined as an increase in serum creatinine and/or a decrease in hourly urine output
- Risk factors include:
  - Older age
  - Comorbidities (CKD, diabetes, hypertension [HTN], cardiovascular disease)
  - Previous episodes of AKI
  - Sepsis
  - Hypotension
- Etiology:
  - Prerenal: typically caused by decreased renal perfusion
    - Examples include:
      - Hypovolemia
      - Hemorrhage
      - Systemic vasodilation (eg, sepsis)
      - Cardiogenic shock or cardiorenal syndrome
      - Hepatorenal syndrome
  - Intrarenal: caused by processes within the kidney
    - Examples include:
      - Interstitial nephritis (AIN)
      - Acute tubular necrosis (ATN)
      - Glomerular nephritis (GN)
      - Nephrotoxic medication
  - Postrenal: caused by obstructed drainage of urine distal to the kidneys
    - Examples include:
      - Renal calculi
      - Cancer or tumors
      - Neurogenic bladder

▶ CLINICAL ASSESSMENT

- History may include evidence of an underlying insult, such as nephrotoxic medications, contrast exposure, and/or hypovolemia/dehydration.

- Severe symptomatic disease may present as fatigue, confusion, anorexia, nausea, vomiting, and sudden weight gain.
- Patients may report oliguria or anuria.
- Severe uremia may cause confusion, anemia, or abnormal bleeding.
- Physical examination findings are nonspecific and may reflect underlying cause.
- Signs of volume overload such as peripheral edema and crackles on lung auscultation may be present.

▶ DIAGNOSIS

- Labs are typically notable for elevated BUN and serum creatinine (an increase in ≥0.3 mg/dL over 48 hours or an increase in ≥1.5 times baseline within the past 7 days is diagnostic).
- Hourly urine output is often decreased (<0.5 mL/kg/h for 6 hours is diagnostic).
- Labs may reveal electrolyte abnormalities, notably hyperkalemia.
- Imaging is often nondiagnostic, although CT or renal ultrasound may reveal mechanical obstruction and/or hydronephrosis in obstructive nephropathy.

▶ TREATMENT

- Identification, removal, and/or correction of the underlying cause
- Treatment often involves:
  - Achieving euvolemia
  - Optimizing renal perfusion
  - Avoiding nephrotoxic agents
  - Ensuring renal and bladder drainage
- Dialysis may be indicated in severe AKI. Indications for dialysis include:
  - Severe volume overload
  - Acidemia
  - Severe electrolyte disturbances
  - Severe/symptomatic uremia
- Patients with AKI are at increased risk of repeat episodes of AKI, renal failure, and CKD.

CHAPTER
161

Chronic Kidney Disease

Kim Zuber, PA-C, MS
Jane Davis, DNP

▶ GENERAL FEATURES

- Chronic kidney disease (CKD) is a gradually progressive decline in kidney function for ≥3 months.
- The most common cause is diabetes mellitus, followed by hypertension (HTN).
- Other causes include glomerulonephritis, inherited conditions (polycystic kidney disease), auto-immune disorders (IEs: lupus, Sjögren syndrome, etc), medications (NSAIDs, lithium, intravenous [IV] dye), and congenital.
- More common in people aged >65 years or those with a history of previous kidney injury (AKI)
- More common in women than men, although men are more likely to progress to kidney failure
- More common in Black, Latinx, and Asian populations

▶ CLINICAL ASSESSMENT

- The most common presentation is asymptomatic, and the diagnosis is found on routine labs.
- Risk factors trigger the testing: a history of low birth weight, premature delivery and childhood enuresis, diabetes, HTN, age, race, previous history of AKI, obesity
- Higher risk medications include NSAIDs, lithium, PPIs, IV contrast, and some herbals (star fruit, turmeric, etc).
- Symptoms (although less common) include: pedal edema, SOB, confusion ("uremic brain"), paroxysmal nocturnal dyspnea (PND), HTN, "foamy" urine (protein in the urine causes the foaming), periorbital edema, fatigue
- A urinary albumin-to-creatinine ratio (UACR) >30 mg/dL is pathognomonic for CKD and will appear before the serum creatinine (SCr) increases.
- SCr will be elevated, although the CKD-EPI calculation needs to be used to correct for normal age-related nephron loss.

- CBC will show anemia, Fe stores will be low, hyperkalemia may be present as kidneys unable to excrete K, and metabolic acidosis (low serum bicarb) is common.
- Edema can be massive with muscle wasting present.

▶ DIAGNOSIS

- CKD is defined as signs of kidney damage or estimated glomerular filtration rate (eGFR) <60 mL/min/1.73 m² for 3 months or more.
  - + Albuminuria >30 mg/dL or electrolyte disorders
  - + Structural abnormalities including transplant
- Based on history, physical examination, and/or laboratory findings
- UACR is most predictive indicator of disease progression.

▶ TREATMENT

- Lifestyle modification can slow progression: increased physical activity, reduced sodium diet, plant-based protein (vs. animal-based), and weight management are advised.
- Cessation of nephrotoxic medications; most commonly NSAIDs
- Management of underlying medical conditions, including diabetes
- HTN management:
  - First-line agents include angiotensin-converting enzyme inhibitor (ACEi) or angiotensin-receptor blocker (ARB), followed by a diuretic and/or calcium channel blocker.
  - Thiazide diuretics lose effectiveness below a GFR <30 mL/min and a loop diuretic must be used.
- In CKD patients not on dialysis, statins are recommended.

- Diabetes management:
  - Metformin is first line for GFR >30 mL/min.
  - SGLT2 inhibitors are second line (GFR >30 mL/min) owing to renoprotective qualities (even in the nondiabetic with albuminuria).
- Anemia: patients will often need supplemental iron; IV iron is used if oral supplementation fails.
- The National Kidney Foundation (NKF) suggests follow-up for CKD: stage 3A every 6 months, stage 3B every 3 months, stage 4 every 2 months, and stage 5 every 4–6 weeks for labs + PE.
- Complications:
  - Most CKD patients will die of cardiovascular disease (CVD); thus, CVD treatment (statins, BP control, low NaCl diet) is paramount.

- There is an increased incidence of atrial fibrillation in CKD patients, along with increased CVD. Direct-acting oral anticoagulants (DOACs) are the preferred choice in CKD.
- Metabolic acidosis (defined as a bicarb <22 mg/dL) develops in stage 3b and, if not corrected, will increase progression to end-stage kidney disease (ESKD) treatment of metabolic acidosis.
- Activated vitamin D supplementation is often warranted as the kidneys are responsible for conversion of vitamin D from an inactivated form to an activated form.
- If hepatitis C is present, treatment with direct-acting antiviral (DAA) medications will slow progression to ESKD.

SECTION C   Congenital and Structural Kidney Disease

CHAPTER 162   Horseshoe Kidney

Molly Band, PA-C

▶ GENERAL FEATURES

- Horseshoe kidney is the most common fusion anomaly of the kidney and occurs in ~1 in 400 people.
- Males are affected more frequently than females.
- The anatomy consists of two distinct kidneys that are connected by an isthmus crossing the midline of the body (thus the term "horseshoe").
- The majority of patients are asymptomatic.

▶ CLINICAL ASSESSMENT

- Prenatal, often occurring between weeks 7 and 9 of development
- Associated with congenital anomalies of the kidney and urinary tract (CAKUT) (hydronephrosis, vesicoureteral reflux, ureteropelvic junction obstruction, duplication of the ureters, hypospadias)
- Associated with other congenital anomalies (Edward syndrome, Turner syndrome, trisomy 18, trisomy 9)
- Patients are predisposed to higher-than-normal rates of nephrolithiasis and urinary tract infections.
- Associated with higher-than-normal rates of malignancies (transitional cell carcinoma, Wilms tumor, and carcinoid tumor)

▶ DIAGNOSIS

- Incidental finding on abdominal/pelvic imaging; often during the prenatal ultrasound
- Can be identified on most abdominal imaging modalities, including ultrasound, CT, MRI, and, occasionally, on plain abdominal films

▶ TREATMENT

- Treatment is based on complications:
  - Stone disease: consideration for metabolic evaluation, medical expulsion therapy, or surgical intervention if needed
  - Infection: standard treatment for UTI with antibiotics followed by consideration for voiding cystourethrogram (VCUG) if febrile urinary tract infection for evaluation of vesicoureteral reflux
  - Hydronephrosis: consideration for nuclear medicine studies to evaluate for ureteropelvic junction obstruction

Polycystic Kidney Disease

Nicole Dettmann, DSc, MPH, PA-C
Stephanie Maclary, RN, MHS, PA-C

▶ GENERAL FEATURES

- Polycystic kidney disease (PKD) is an inherited disorder in which cysts develop within the kidneys, causing enlargement and loss of function over time.
- Varies in severity:
  - Can be asymptomatic
  - Can cause serious complications, including hypertension and renal failure
  - 50% of PKD patients require dialysis by age 60 years.
- Two types of PKD: autosomal-dominant PKD (ADPKD) and autosomal-recessive PKD (ARPKD)
- Two identifiable genes account for ADPKD:
  - *ADPKD1* on chromosome 16 affects ~78% of patients with ADPKD.
    - Typical age of onset is 54 years.
    - Male gender is associated with more rapid progression.
  - *ADPKD2* on chromosome 4 affects ~14% of patients with ADPKD.
    - Less severe phenotype
    - Typical age of onset is 74 years, and renal failure typically develops late in diagnosis.
- ARPKD has an early onset in infancy or childhood and is associated with a short life expectancy that rarely surpasses childhood' patients present with pulmonary insufficiency and progressive renal failure with bilateral renal and hepatic cysts.
- The remainder of this chapter focuses on ADPKD.

▶ CLINICAL ASSESSMENT

- Most patients are asymptomatic in early stage; symptoms progress with age.
- Patients may present with hypertension, hematuria, proteinuria, or renal impairment, which is typically detected by routine laboratory examinations.
- The diagnosis is often made during initial workup for new-onset hypertension, hematuria, renal calculi, or recurrent urinary tract infections (UTIs) or as an incidental finding during imaging studies.
- Flank pain or abdominal pain due to renal hemorrhage, calculi, or UTI is the most common symptom; may also present with symptoms secondary to cysts in other organs, such as the liver, pancreas, spleen, epididymis, testes, or ovaries.

- Patients may have early onset of hypertension, frequent UTIs and/or frequent kidney stones, large kidneys palpable on examination, microscopic or gross hematuria and/or proteinuria, and/or family history of PKD.
- Extrarenal complications include heart valve defects, left ventricular hypertrophy, increased colonic diverticuli, and cerebral berry aneurysm.

▶ DIAGNOSIS

- Patients may have an elevated serum creatinine and reduced GFR consistent with decreased renal function.
- Microscopic or gross hematuria may be present on urinalysis. Proteinuria occurs in ~25% of patients.
- Ultrasound (US) is often sufficient for diagnosis in at-risk patients; CT or MRI may be useful if US is not definitive, especially in younger patients.
- Diagnostic criteria is characterized by the number of cysts and age range:
  - 3+ cysts unilateral or bilateral ages 15–39 years
  - 2+ cysts in each kidney 40–59 years
  - 4+ cysts in each kidney at ≥60 years
- Genetic testing should be considered in patients with equivocal imaging results and a need for definitive diagnosis or in patients with atypical presentations; genetic counseling may also be considered during prenatal genetic consultations as there is 50% chance of offspring inheriting PKD.

▶ TREATMENT

- Treatment is aimed at addressing complications of the disease.
- Patients with large kidneys should be counseled to avoid contact sports due to risk of kidney rupture.
- Aggressive treatment of UTIs, kidney stones, and hypertension
- Avoid nephrotoxic drugs including NSAIDs.
- Patients at high risk for progression may be benefited from tolvaptan, a short-acting vasopressin V2-receptor (V2R) that completely blocks vasopressin action on cyst production and slows kidney function decline for those at risk for rapid progression.
- Patients with ADPKD who progress to end-stage kidney disease are commonly treated with hemodialysis or kidney transplant.

CHAPTER

164

End-Stage Renal Disease

Jennifer Vonderau, MMS, PA-C

▶ GENERAL FEATURES

- End-stage renal disease (ESRD) is defined as the final stage of kidney dysfunction during which patients require renal replacement therapy, such as dialysis.
- Chronic kidney disease (CKD) is often the precursor to ESRD, and it is classified in stages by GFR: stage 5 CKD is defined as a GFR <15; ESRD is distinguished from stage 5 CKD by the requirement of dialysis.
- No specific GFR or serum creatinine measurement indicates a need for dialysis; dialysis is initiated based on the presence of symptoms related to renal dysfunction or profound, potentially dangerous electrolyte disturbances (such as hyperkalemia).
- Common indications for dialysis include metabolic acidosis, hyperkalemia, uremia, and significant volume retention, especially in patients with oliguria or anuria.
- Once patients have progressed to ESRD, the use of dialysis is often indefinite unless renal transplantation is utilized.
- Dialysis modalities include in-center hemodialysis (typically 3 days per week), nightly home hemodialysis, or nightly peritoneal dialysis.
- Hemodialysis requires venous access via a central venous access line or a surgically created arteriovenous fistula; peritoneal dialysis utilizes a surgically placed peritoneal dialysis catheter.

▶ CLINICAL ASSESSMENT

- The most common etiologies of CKD and ESRD in the United States include hypertension, diabetes mellitus, focal sclerosing glomerulosclerosis (FSGS), nephrotic syndromes, polycystic kidney disease, and drug toxicities.
- Patients with CKD presenting at the stage of ESRD commonly have symptoms of volume overload, including shortness of breath and peripheral edema.

- Patients who present with profound metabolic disturbance may have arrhythmias and other EKG changes, as well as weakness and nausea.
- Physical examination may reveal hypertension, tachycardia, tachypnea, pulmonary crackles, jugular venous distension, and peripheral edema.

▶ DIAGNOSIS

- Elevated urine microalbumin is often the first laboratory marker of development of CKD.
- Basic metabolic panel will typically reveal an elevated creatinine, reduced GFR <20, and elevated BUN.
- Electrolyte abnormalities, especially hyperkalemia and hypercalcemia, may be present.
- Phosphorus levels may be elevated.
- Ultrasound or CT scan may reveal enlarged polycystic kidneys or atrophic kidney(s) depending on the underlying cause of renal disease.

▶ TREATMENT

- Dialysis is the mainstay of treatment and acts as a temporizing measure, as ESRD is typically irreversible.
- Hemodialysis is far more commonly utilized than peritoneal dialysis, although survival outcomes are similar.
- Patients with ESRD may require erythropoietin to manage anemia of CKD.
- Patients with ESRD often require phosphate binders and vitamin D to help facilitate phosphate and calcium balance and prevent bone disease; occasionally, parathyroidectomy will be required to suppress release of parathyroid hormone.
- A low potassium and low phosphorus diet is recommended for ESRD patients.
- Kidney transplant is the only definitive treatment of ESRD. Kidney transplant evaluation is indicated when GFR <20.

- Kidney transplant provides on average 10–12 years of kidney function, with a range of 0 to 20+ years.
  - Wait times for a deceased donor kidney transplant is 5 years on average.

- Living donor kidney transplant expedites the possibility of transplant but requires a compatible donor.

SECTION E — *Fluid and Electrolyte Disorders*

CHAPTER 165 — Hyponatremia

Timothy Hirsch, MS, PA-C

▶ GENERAL FEATURES

- Hyponatremia is the most common electrolyte disturbance and is defined as a serum sodium concentration <135 mEq/L.
- A dysfunction of water balance, typically due to a failure to excrete water or due to excessive water intake
- No sex or age prevalence
- Many patients will have multiple factors contributing to a single underlying cause.
- Classified based on serum osmolality:
  - Hypertonic hyponatremia (serum osmolality >295 mOsm/kg)
  - Isotonic hyponatremia (serum osmolality of 280-295 mOsm/kg)
  - Hypotonic hyponatremia (serum osmolality <280 mOsm/kg):
    - Hypotonic hyponatremia is further classified based on volume status:
      - Hypovolemic
      - Euvolemic
      - Hypervolemic

▶ CLINICAL ASSESSMENT

- Neurologic symptoms result from fluid shifts due to a serum-brain osmolality gradient causing cerebral edema.
- Symptoms vary depending on the severity and acuity of the disease:
  - Mild symptoms are often vague and include nausea, malaise, and headache.
  - In severe cases, disorientation followed by seizure, coma, and respiratory arrest can result in death.

- History may reveal features of underlying cause:
  - Fluid losses in hypovolemic patients due to GI losses (vomiting or diarrhea), renal losses (diuretics), and dermal losses (sweating, burns)
  - Euvolemic patients with low solute intake ("tea-and-toast" diet), hypothyroidism, and water intoxication, syndrome of inappropriate antidiuretic hormone (SIADH)
  - Hypervolemic patients with heart failure, cirrhosis, CKD, and nephrotic syndrome
- Physical examination findings may depend on volume status:
  - Hypovolemic patients may display low skin turgor, dry mucous membranes, tachycardia, low jugular venous pressure, or orthostatic hypotension.
  - Hypervolemic patients may display peripheral edema, ascites, or crackles on lung auscultation.

▶ DIAGNOSIS

- Direct measurement of serum sodium levels is diagnostic for hyponatremia (Na$^+$ <135 mEq/L).
- Direct measurement of serum osmolality distinguishes between hypertonic/isotonic/hypotonic hyponatremia.
- Urine sodium and urine osmolality levels can help distinguish between the underlying cause of hypotonic hyponatremia.
- Additional testing is directed at evaluating the underlying cause of disease.
- Differential diagnosis of hyponatremia:
  - Hypertonic hyponatremia (serum osmolality >295 mOsm/kg):
    - Hyperglycemia can falsely lower lab-measured sodium.

- In a patient with severe hyperglycemia, correct sodium accordingly by adding 1.6 mEq/L sodium for each 100 mg/dL of glucose above normal.
  - Iatrogenic causes: mannitol, sorbitol, glycerol, maltose
  - Radiocontrast agents
- Isotonic hyponatremia (serum osmolality 280-295 mOsm/kg):
  - Likely laboratory error due to:
    - Hyperproteinemia
    - Hyperlipidemia (chylomicrons, triglycerides, cholesterol)
- Hypotonic hyponatremia (serum osmolality <280 mOsm/kg):
  - Further divided based on volume status of the patient:
    - Hypovolemia:
      - Urine sodium level <20 mEq/L
        - Extrarenal loss from dehydration, diarrhea, or vomiting
      - Urine sodium level >20 mEq/L
        - Renal loss from diuretics, selective serotonin reuptake inhibitors, nephropathies, mineralocorticoid deficiency, or cerebral sodium-wasting syndrome
    - Euvolemic:
      - SIADH:
        - Diagnosis of exclusion
        - Hyperosmolar urine compared with plasma (urine osmolality >100 mOsm/kg H_2O)
      - Hypothyroidism
      - Postoperative hyponatremia
      - Beer potomania
      - Psychogenic polydipsia
      - Medications (most commonly diuretics)
      - Extreme exercise
      - Adrenocorticotropin deficiency
    - Hypervolemic:
      - Heart failure
      - Nephrotic syndrome
      - Kidney disease
      - Liver disease

▶ TREATMENT

- Treatment depends on cause, chronicity, and severity of hyponatremia guided by laboratory and urine sodium and urine osmolality values.
- Mild hyponatremia and asymptomatic moderate hyponatremia can be treated in an outpatient setting and will vary depending on the cause (eg, medications, CHF, cirrhosis, SIADH).
- Symptomatic hyponatremia and severe hyponatremia (<120 mEq/L) require hospitalization and close monitoring during correction.
- Acute hyponatremia with severe central nervous system symptoms or seizure:
  - Immediately raise serum sodium by 8–10 mEq/L in 4–6 hours, or to >120 mEq/L using hypertonic saline.
  - Consider intensive care unit admission and expert consultation.
- Avoid too-rapid or overcorrection as this can lead to osmotic demyelination syndrome (central pontine myelinolysis) characterized by severe neurologic symptoms, seizure, coma, and death.
  - Patients with hyponatremia for >48 hours should correct sodium no >8–10 mEq/L per day.
  - Check serial serum sodium levels every 4–6 hours.
- For patients with hypovolemic hyponatremia:
  - Correct underlying cause; sodium typically improves with volume replacement.
  - Consider isotonic crystalloid fluids for volume replacement.
- For patients with chronic euvolemic or hypervolemic hyponatremia:
  - Water restriction to <1 L/day
  - High dietary salt intake
  - 0.9% sodium chloride solution with loop diuretic for faster correction
  - Chronic hyponatremia that does not correct with water restriction may benefit from demeclocycline or vasopressin antagonists.

CHAPTER
166

Hypernatremia

Timothy Hirsch, MS, PA-C

▶ GENERAL FEATURES

- Hypernatremia is defined as a serum sodium concentration level >145 mEq/L.

- Typically results from a combined water and sodium loss, with water loss exceeding sodium loss; may also result from a net sodium gain

- Hypernatremia may exist with:
  - Hypovolemia (most common): decreased total body water and total body sodium
  - Euvolemia: no change in total body water; increase in total body sodium
  - Hypervolemia (rare): increase in total body water and increase in total body sodium
- Associated with increased mortality and morbidity
- Risk factors: extremes of age, diabetes mellitus, surgery, diuretic therapy, intubation, altered mental status, and prior brain surgery
  - Older adults at increased risk due to decreased thirst mechanism and impaired renal function.
  - Diarrhea and vomiting most common cause in infants.

CLINICAL ASSESSMENT

- Patients may present with lethargy, weakness, irritability or agitation, confusion, profound alterations in mental status, and seizure.
- History may be notable for an underlying mechanism of volume loss, such as diarrhea.
- Examination findings may be consistent with volume expansion or loss, including tachycardia, hypotension, dry mucous membranes, changes in skin temperature or turgor, fever, and muscle weakness.
- Urinalysis along with urine sodium and urinary osmolality
- Special tests can include:
  - Water deprivation with diabetes insipidus:
    - Urine osmolality does not increase when hypernatremic.
  - Antidiuretic hormone stimulation in nephrogenic diabetes insipidus:
    - Urine osmolality does not increase after stimulation.

DIAGNOSIS

- Hypernatremia is confirmed by a direct serum measurement:
  - Serum sodium >145 mEq/L is diagnostic.
  - Serum sodium 150–170 mEq/L is often related to dehydration and hypovolemia.
  - Serum sodium 170–190 mEq/L is often related to diabetes insipidus.
  - Serum sodium >190 mEq/L is typically related to salt ingestion/poisoning.

- Chemistry panel may be notable for concurrent electrolyte abnormalities or elevated BUN/creatinine.
- Urine sodium and osmolality can be useful to distinguish underlying etiology:
  - In hypovolemic patients:
    - If urinary osmolality >600 mOsm/kg or urinary sodium <20 mEq/L:
      - Consider burns, insensible losses (skin/respiration), and gastrointestinal loss.
    - If urinary osmolality 300–600 mOsm/kg or urinary sodium >20 mEq/L:
      - Consider mannitol use, diuretics, hyperglycemia, and history of enteral feeding.
  - In euvolemic patients:
    - Urinary osmolality <300 mOsm/kg and low plasma osmolality along with urinary sodium >20 mEq/L:
      - Consider diabetes insipidus (nephrogenic vs. central) depending on history.
  - In hypervolemic patients:
    - Urinary sodium >20 mEq/L:
      - Consider primary hyperaldosteronism, especially in setting of hypertension and hypokalemia.
      - Consider iatrogenic causes: enteral feedings, dialysis, or recent administration of hypertonic saline or sodium bicarbonate.

TREATMENT

- Rapid correction of hypernatremia can cause seizure, cerebral/pulmonary edema, and death.
- Rate of sodium correction depends on chronicity:
  - Acute hypernatremia (<48-hour duration): correct sodium by 1 mmol/L/h for the first 6–8 hours.
  - Chronic hypernatremia (>48-hour duration): correct sodium by 8–10 mmol/day.
  - Monitor sodium levels every 4–6 hours.
- Hourly fluid replacement is based on the calculated free water deficit plus any anticipated insensible losses.
- Treat hypovolemic patients with isotonic fluids to replace volume before addressing hyponatremia.
- In euvolemic patients:
  - Consider vasopressin to treat central diabetes insipidus.
  - Consider chlorothiazide to treat nephrogenic diabetes insipidus.
- In hypervolemic patients:
  - Administer replacement fluid with diuretics.
  - Stop causative medications when possible.

Hypovolemia

Rebecca Dodd, DMSc, PA-C

A 55-year-old male with a previous medical history of hypertension presented to the ED with a 5-day history of nausea, vomiting, and diarrhea, with altered mental status. His vital signs are notable for a heart rate of 122 bpm and a blood pressure (BP) of 88/47(61) mm Hg. Physical examination is notable for dry mucous membranes and capillary refill of 4 seconds in the hands and feet bilaterally.

▶ GENERAL FEATURES

- Hypovolemia is the loss of sodium and water, or blood loss alone, from the extracellular space; if not corrected, it can result in hypovolemic shock.
- Hypovolemic shock is characterized by hypovolemia with inadequate tissue perfusion/oxygenation and can result in death.
- Types and etiologies:
  - Hemorrhagic: bleeding events, bleeding diathesis, and trauma
  - Nonhemorrhagic: gastrointestinal (GI), renal, skin, fever, endocrine, over-diuresis, and third-space losses
- Dehydration results primarily from pure water loss from the intracellular space, creating desiccated cells; patients with dehydration are always hypernatremic with increased serum osmolality.

▶ CLINICAL ASSESSMENT

- Hypovolemia: symptoms include headache, confusion, weakness, fatigue, and thirst.
  - Physical examination may be notable for increased skin turgor and dry mucous membranes.
  - Oliguria may be present.
- Hypovolemic shock: initial response is tachycardia to increase cardiac output and tissue perfusion.
  - Hypotension (systolic BP <100 mm Hg), tachypnea, slow capillary refill, weak peripheral pulses, low or absent jugular venous distention, diaphoresis, pallor, cyanosis, chest pain, agitation, and altered mental state

▶ DIAGNOSIS

- Laboratory abnormalities may include hyponatremia, contraction alkalosis, or elevated lactic acid level.
- Metabolic acidosis may be present if volume loss is due to significant GI losses.

▶ TREATMENT

- Nonhemorrhagic hypovolemia: for patients unable to take adequate fluid by mouth, IV crystalloid fluid resuscitation is the mainstay treatment of hypovolemia not associated with bleeding.
  - No general consensus exists on resuscitative volume; initial fluid resuscitation is typically given in a series of boluses with frequent reassessment of hypovolemia and response to treatment, especially in patients with CHF and CKD.
  - Balanced crystalloids (lactated Ringer) are typically preferred.
  - Encourage PO intake of fluids when appropriate.
- Hemorrhagic shock: blood products, such as packed red blood cells and fresh-frozen plasma, are the preferred agent of volume resuscitation in the hemorrhaging patient.
- Massive transfusions should employ a balanced transfusion strategy.
- Source of bleeding must be investigated and controlled.
- Any coagulopathy should be addressed, if possible.

Case Conclusion

The patient received a 30-mL/kg bolus (2 L) of lactated Ringer solution over 3 hours. By hour 2, his MAP had increased to 64, his heart rate had declined to 95, and respiratory rate 12. His IV rate was decreased, and he was taking oral fluids successfully. By hour 3, he was no longer confused, and his lactic acid had declined from 3.9 to 2.2 and capillary refill had returned to normal. He was admitted for 24 hours for monitoring, and he was released home in stable condition.

Acid-Base Disorders

Kristopher Maday, MS, PA-C, DFAAPA

▶ GENERAL FEATURES

- Henderson-Hasselbach equation: $pH = pK_a + log(HCO_3^-/CO_2)$
  - Serum bicarbonate (HCO_3^-) is calculated from a measured serum pH and carbon dioxide (CO_2).
  - This can be simplified to:
    - $pH = HCO_3^-/CO_2$
    - Acidity = bicarbonate/carbon dioxide
    - A = B/CD
- Standard arterial blood gases (ABG) reporting and results:
  - $pH/CO_2/O_2/HCO_3^-/base (\pm)$
  - 7.35-7.45/35-45 mm Hg/80-100 mm Hg/22-26 mg/dL/0
- Steps to interpret ABG:
  - Look at the pH:
    - If <7.35 = acidemia/acidosis present
    - If >7.45 = alkalemia/alkalosis present
  - Determine if respiratory or metabolic: look at the CO_2 and HCO_3^-
    - Respiratory:
      - Acidosis = low pH, high CO_2
      - Alkalosis = high pH, low CO_2
    - Metabolic:
      - Acidosis = low pH, low HCO_3^-
      - Alkalosis = high pH, high HCO_3^-
    - Mixed:
      - Two or more of these conditions may be present simultaneously.
      - May contribute additive or opposing effects on pH
      - Consider calculating "delta gap" (DG) to identify concurrent metabolic disorders.
  - Determine if the condition is acute or chronic, if there is compensation, and if it is adequate:
    - Timeline of the disease will be evident by the patient presentation:
      - Acute <2 days
      - Chronic >2 days
      - Kidneys can take up to 2 days to fully compensate.
    - Metabolic compensation for respiratory acidosis:
      - Acute = 1 mEq/L increase in HCO_3^- for every 10 mm Hg increase in CO_2
      - Chronic = 3 mEq/L increase in HCO_3^- for every 10 mm Hg increase in CO_2
    - Metabolic compensation for respiratory alkalosis:
      - Acute = 2 mEq/L decrease in HCO_3^- for every 10 mm Hg decrease in CO_2
      - Chronic = 4 mEq/L decrease in HCO_3^- for every 10 mm Hg decrease in CO_2
    - Respiratory compensation for metabolic acidosis:
      - Winter formula: expected $CO_2 = 8 + (1.5 \times HCO_3^-) \pm 2$
    - Respiratory compensation for metabolic alkalosis:
      - Expected $CO_2 = 20 + (0.7 \times HCO_3^-) \pm 5$
  - If metabolic acidosis is present, calculate the anion gap (AG) to determine if it is a high anion gap (HAGMA) or normal gap (NAGMA):
    - $AG = Na^+ - (Cl^- + HCO_3^-)$
      - Normal = <12
  - If HAGMA, calculate DG to determine if multiple metabolic conditions are present:
    - $DG = (AG - 12)/(24 - HCO_3^-)$
      - <0.4 = hyperchloremic NAGMA
      - 0.4-1.0 = HAGMA and NAGMA
      - 1.0-2.0 = uncomplicated HAGMA
      - >2.0 = HAGMA with metabolic alkalosis

▶ CLINICAL ASSESSMENT

- Respiratory acidosis:
  - Physiology: decreased pH and increased $PaCO_2$ typically due to decreased minute ventilation (tidal volume × respiratory rate)
  - Causes:
    - Normal lungs:
      - CNS depression: medications/drugs, head trauma, central sleep apnea, obesity hypoventilation syndrome
      - Neuromuscular impairment: Guillain-Barre syndrome, myasthenia gravis, amyotrophic lateral sclerosis (ALS)
      - Thoracic/lung expansion restriction: pneumothorax, pleural effusions, rib fractures/flail chest
    - Abnormal lungs:
      - Obstruction: asthma (late), foreign-body aspiration, COPD
      - Alveoli: ARDS, interstitial lung disease, severe pneumonia
      - Perfusion defects: cardiac arrest, PTE (massive)
- Respiratory alkalosis:
  - Physiology: increased pH and reduced $PaCO_2$ typically due to increased minute ventilation (hyperventilation), often as a result of increased respiratory demand or as physiologic compensation for metabolic acidosis
  - Causes:
    - Cardiac (congenital/cyanotic heart disease, heart failure)
    - Hypoxemia (pneumonia, PE)

- Anemia
- Medications (oral contraceptive pills, aspirin)
- Pregnancy
- Iatrogenic (mechanical ventilation)
- Asthma (early)
- Neurologic (CNS tumors, stroke, meningoencephalitis)
- Stress (fever, anxiety disorders, pain)
- Metabolic acidosis:
  - Physiology: decreased pH with decreased HCO_3^-
  - Causes:
    - HAGMA:
      - Carbon monoxide, cyanide poisoning
      - Aminoglycosides
      - Theophylline, toluene poisoning
      - Methanol
      - Uremia
      - Diabetic ketoacidosis
      - Propylene glycol toxicity
      - Inborn errors of metabolism
      - Lactic acidosis
      - Ethylene glycol poisoning, ethanol
      - Salicylates
    - NAGMA:

- Ureteric diversion
- Small bowel fistulae
- Excessive saline: high chloride content in saline solutions
- GI losses (diarrhea, high-output ostomy)
- Carbonic anhydrase inhibitors
- Renal tubular acidosis
- Adrenal insufficiency
- Pancreatic fistulae
- Metabolic alkalosis:
  - Physiology:
    - Increased pH with increased HCO_3^-, often due to:
      - Loss of hydrogen ions (H^+)
      - Volume depletion with retention of HCO_3^-
      - Physiologic compensation for respiratory alkalosis
  - Causes:
    - Contraction (dehydration/hypovolemia, diuresis)
    - Licorice ingestion (glycyrrhizic acid)
    - Endocrine disorders (hyperaldosteronism)
    - Loss of H^+ from the stomach (vomiting, excessive NG tube suction)
    - Ringer solution (lactate converted to HCO_3^-)
    - Hypercapnia (leading to physiologic compensation)

CHAPTER 169

Hypokalemia and Hyperkalemia

Brendan Riordan, MPAS, PA-C

▶ GENERAL FEATURES

- Potassium is a common cation that humans take in primarily through ingestion; it is essential for proper cardiac, muscular, and neurologic functions.
- Potassium is stored intracellularly in the body, and excess is excreted via the kidneys; intracellular and extracellular concentrations of potassium are tightly regulated by sodium-potassium pumps.
- Since only the extracellular concentration of potassium can be measured, normal values range from 3.5 to 5.5 mEq/L.
- Hypokalemia:
  - Etiology:
    - Decreased oral intake, increased intracellular shift (increased insulin, β-agonist therapy, alkalemia), and extracorporeal losses (urinary, GI, sweat)
    - Extracorporeal losses are by far the most common; decreased intake alone will generally not cause hypokalemia, though it may exacerbate hypokalemia induced by other mechanisms.

- Hyperkalemia:
  - Etiology:
    - Increased potassium release from cells (pseudohyperkalemia, metabolic acidosis, low insulin availability/hyperglycemia, and tissue breakdown) and/or reduced urinary potassium secretion (aldosterone depletion or resistance, decreased sodium/water delivery to potassium-secretory sites, and acute or chronic kidney disease)
    - Increased oral intake of potassium is unlikely to cause hyperkalemia unless it is an acute, excessive, and accompanying one of the above conditions.

▶ CLINICAL ASSESSMENT

- Hypokalemia:
  - Generally asymptomatic until extracellular levels fall below 3.0 mEq/L.
  - Symptoms may include muscle cramps and weakness; patients may present with rhabdomyolysis and/or electrocardiographic changes.

- Potassium levels <2.5 mEq/L may result in severe symptoms and may be life-threatening.
- Severe hypokalemia may result in ascending paralysis and respiratory distress/failure.
- Hyperkalemia:
  - Clinical manifestations of hyperkalemia depend on severity and acuity.
  - The presentation of hyperkalemia may include ascending muscle weakness or paralysis, metabolic acidosis, and ECG changes.
  - ECG changes may include peaked T waves, PR segment/QRS lengthening, Brugada sign, bundle branch blocks, idioventricular rhythms, and sine wave rhythm.

▌DIAGNOSIS

- Hypokalemia:
  - Physical examination may be notable for muscle weakness or flaccidity, decreased bowel sounds due to ileus, and irregular cardiac rhythm due to arrhythmias.
  - ECG changes may include decreased T wave amplitude, development of U waves, QT prolongation.
- Hyperkalemia:
  - ECG changes are not sensitive or specific for hyperkalemia; suspicion should be confirmed by measurement of serum potassium levels.
  - Severe leukocytosis or hemolysis can result in misdiagnosis of hyperkalemia (pseudohyperkalemia).

▌TREATMENT

- Hypokalemia:
  - Treatment typically entails administration of exogenous potassium in order to prevent life-threatening cardiac and neuromuscular conditions.
  - Potassium chloride can be given either orally or intravenously.
  - Hypomagnesemia may contribute to excess potassium excretion; magnesium should also be replaced to ensure normalization of potassium levels.
  - Etiology of should be investigated and corrected.
- Hyperkalemia:
  - Management decisions can be divided into three patient categories: hyperkalemic emergency, prompt correction, and slow correction.
  - "Hyperkalemic emergency" refers to a patient with any of the above clinical signs or symptoms, severe hyperkalemia (K$^+$ >6.5 mEq/L).
  - Moderate hyperkalemia (>5.5 mEq/L) in the presence of significant renal dysfunction requires immediate treatment.
  - Patients with hyperkalemic emergencies should be treated with intravenous calcium (for cardiac membrane stabilization), intravenous insulin (to redistribute potassium intracellularly), and one or more therapies to remove potassium from the body (diuresis, GI cation exchanger, or hemodialysis).
  - Patients should be placed on continuous telemetry monitoring and receive frequent measurements of serum potassium levels.
  - Reversible causes should be worked up and treated.

CHAPTER

170

Calcium, Phosphate, and Magnesium Disorders

Jeremy Amayo, MMSc, PA-C

▌GENERAL FEATURES

- Hypocalcemia:
  - Defined as a total serum calcium concentration <8.5 mg/dL
    - The most common causes of hypocalcemia include hypoparathyroidism, vitamin D deficiency, and malnutrition.
    - Other causes of hypocalcemia include acute pancreatitis, hypomagnesemia, pseudohypoparathyroidism, large volume blood transfusion, and DiGeorge syndrome (in infants).

- Hypercalcemia:
  - Defined as a total serum calcium concentration >10.2 mg/dL
    - The most common causes are hyperparathyroidism and malignancy.
    - Other causes include excess calcium supplementation, hyperthyroidism, thiazide diuretics, Paget disease, sarcoidosis, milk-alkali syndrome, and multiple endocrine neoplasia (MEN) type 1.
- Hypophosphatemia:
  - Defined as a serum phosphate concentration <2.5 mg/dL

- Most common causes are hyperparathyroidism and poor intake/absorption.
- Other causes include increased insulin secretion, refeeding syndrome, hungry bone syndrome, chronic diarrhea, vitamin D deficiency, Fanconi syndrome, and medications (acetazolamide, tenofovir, intravenous [IV] iron, antacids, niacin, and phosphate binders).
- Hyperphosphatemia:
  - Defined as a serum phosphate concentration >4.5 mg/dL
    - The most common causes of hyperphosphatemia are acute phosphate loads (eg, tumor lysis syndrome, rhabdomyolysis), severe acidemia, kidney disease, and hypoparathyroidism.
    - Other causes of hypophosphatemia include vitamin D toxicity, medications (bisphosphonates, fibroblast growth factor receptor inhibitors), and familial tumoral calcinosis (rare).
- Hypomagnesemia:
  - Quite common in the inpatient setting with an incidence of 12% among hospitalized patients and an incidence of 65% among patients admitted to an intensive care unit
  - Defined as a serum magnesium concentration <1.8 mg/dL, though this varies by laboratory
  - Most common causes of hypomagnesemia include gastrointestinal losses (vomiting, diarrhea) and renal losses, often secondary to medications (loop and thiazide diuretics, alcohol, aminoglycosides, amphotericin, isotonic fluid administration).
  - Other causes include osmotic diuresis, pentamidine, calcineurin inhibitors, and chemotherapeutic agents like cisplatin.
- Hypermagnesemia:
- Defined as a serum magnesium concentration >2.6 mg/dL
- Most common causes are high-dose magnesium administration or magnesium administration to patients with renal failure.

▶ CLINICAL ASSESSMENT

- Hypocalcemia:
  - May present with abdominal muscle cramps, muscular tetany, perioral and acral paresthesias, convulsions, and dyspnea
  - Severe manifestations include cardiac arrhythmias, laryngospasm, and bronchospasm.
  - Patients may also demonstrate facial spasms elicited by tapping the facial nerve (known as Chvostek sign) and/or carpal spasm after arterial occlusion using a blood pressure cuff (known as Trousseau sign). These findings are typically only seen in severe hypocalcemia.
- Hypercalcemia:
  - Often asymptomatic, though patients may present with bone fractures due to osteopenia, nephrolithiasis,

constipation, anorexia, weakness, fatigue, and/or altered mental status
  - The constellation of symptoms associated with hypercalcemia is often recited as "stones, bones, abdominal groans, and psychiatric overtones," which alludes to the renal, skeletal, gastrointestinal, and neurologic phenomena associated with the disease.
- Hypophosphatemia:
  - Can affect multiple organ systems; however, overt symptoms are rare unless serum phosphate concentration is significantly low (<2 mg/dL)
  - Patients with severe hypophosphatemia may present with the following:
    - Neurologic: can range from paresthesias and irritability to delirium, seizure, and coma
    - Cardiovascular: ventricular arrhythmias or symptoms of acute heart failure
    - Pulmonary: depression of diaphragmatic contractility, leading to hypoventilation and hypercapnia
    - Musculoskeletal: patients may present with proximal myopathy or rhabdomyolysis, particularly if there is an underlying history of alcohol abuse.
    - Hematologic: patients may present with hemolysis (due to fragile red blood cell membranes), immunosuppression (due to impaired granulocyte chemotaxis), and gingival bleeding (due to platelet dysfunction and thrombocytopenia).
- Hyperphosphatemia:
  - Presentation ultimately depends on the underlying cause.
  - May be incidentally discovered in the clinical context of acute or chronic kidney disease, rhabdomyolysis, severe acidemia, or in patients with lymphoma or certain leukemias undergoing chemotherapy
  - Patients are usually asymptomatic unless concurrent hypocalcemia exists.
- Hypomagnesemia: may present with hyperactive reflexes, tetany, paresthesias, numbness, confusion, irritability, arrhythmias, and seizure.
- Hypermagnesemia:
  - Patients with symptomatic hypermagnesemia often present with signs and symptoms of neuromuscular toxicity, including diminished deep tendon reflexes, weakness, and, in severe cases, flaccid quadriplegia and apnea.
  - Hypermagnesemia can also lead to hypocalcemia through inhibition of parathyroid hormone secretion.

▶ DIAGNOSIS

- Hypocalcemia:
  - In patients with a low total calcium level, ordering an ionized calcium level may be helpful in diagnosing true hypocalcemia requiring treatment. Patients with low total calcium but a normal ionized calcium do not typically require calcium supplementation.

- Total calcium should be corrected for albumin level.
- Serum magnesium, parathyroid hormone, 25-OH vitamin D, and 1,25-OH vitamin D levels may be useful to diagnose concomitant or underlying conditions.
- ECG may demonstrate a prolonged QT interval.
- Hypercalcemia:
  - Measured with serum total calcium and/or ionized calcium levels
  - Total calcium should be corrected for albumin level.
  - Check phosphate, parathyroid hormone, parathyroid hormone–related peptide (PTHrP), 25-OH vitamin D, and 1,25-OH vitamin D levels.
  - ECG may demonstrate a shortened QT interval.
- Hypophosphatemia:
  - The cause is usually apparent after a thorough history and physical examination.
  - For cases that are not clear, calculating a fractional excretion of phosphorus (FEPO4) can help differentiate renal from nonrenal causes (FEPO4 <5% suggests a nonrenal mechanism).
- Hyperphosphatemia:
  - Serum phosphate levels are adequate to make the initial diagnosis.
  - Additional testing should focus on detecting concurrent conditions (such as other electrolyte disorders) or causative conditions (such as renal failure or parathyroid disease).
- Hypomagnesemia:
  - Diagnosis should be confirmed by direct laboratory measurement.
  - Additional workup should focus on determining the underlying etiology.
  - Labs may be notable for concurrent hypocalcemia and hypokalemia.
  - ECG findings are usually nonspecific, but may include prolonged QT interval, peaked T waves, and ST-segment depression.
- Hypermagnesemia:
  - Diagnosis should be confirmed by direct laboratory measurement.
  - ECG findings are nonspecific and may include flattened P waves, prolonged PR interval, widened QRS, peaked T waves, and prolonged QT interval.

▶ TREATMENT

- Hypocalcemia:
  - Treatment involves both calcium replacement therapy and treatment of the underlying cause.
  - Patients can be given both IV and oral calcium supplementation, though oral calcium supplementation usually requires concomitant administration of oral vitamin D.

- Hypomagnesemia should also be corrected, if present.
- Hypercalcemia:
  - Patients with hypercalcemia should be given IV isotonic fluids followed by furosemide to maximize calcium excretion.
    - Avoid thiazide diuretics in patients with hypercalcemia as they increase tubular reabsorption of calcium and render efforts to improve renal calcium excretion ineffective.
  - Refractory cases of hypercalcemia can be treated with calcitonin, bisphosphonates, glucocorticoids, and calcimimetics such as cinacalcet.
  - Patients with severe, life-threatening cases of hypercalcemia should be evaluated for urgent hemodialysis.
- Hypophosphatemia:
  - Many causes of hypophosphatemia will correct spontaneously once the underlying cause is resolved (eg, resolution of DKA or cessation of vomiting/diarrhea).
  - For severe, symptomatic, or persistent hypophosphatemia, patients should be given oral or IV phosphate replacement therapy.
- Hyperphosphatemia:
  - Acute hyperphosphatemia can be life-threatening, particularly if it is associated with hypocalcemia.
    - If renal function is preserved or the patient has mild, nonoliguric kidney injury, hyperphosphatemia usually resolves in <24 hours. Phosphate excretion can be increased in these patients by administering isotonic fluid.
    - If renal function is impaired or there is significant hypocalcemia, the patient should be evaluated for urgent hemodialysis.
  - Chronic hyperphosphatemia, which occurs in patients with chronic kidney disease or familial tumoral calcinosis, can be managed with a low-phosphate diet and enteral phosphate binders like calcium acetate.
- Hypomagnesemia: nearly every cause can be successfully treated with IV or oral magnesium supplementation; further therapies are rarely indicated.
- Hypermagnesemia:
  - Prevention is effective; most cases can be avoided by limiting excessive magnesium administration, especially in patients with renal failure.
  - Isotonic fluids and/or furosemide can be used to increase renal excretion of magnesium and lower serum magnesium levels.
  - For refractory cases or patients presenting with severe neuromuscular symptoms, urgent hemodialysis should be considered.

CHAPTER
171

Glomerulonephritis

Heather White, MPAS

▶ GENERAL FEATURES

- Glomerulonephritis (GN) is a collection of renal conditions characterized by immune-mediated damage to portions of the nephron.
- Manifestations include nephrotic syndromes, characterized by severe proteinuria and edema, or nephritic syndromes, characterized by hematuria and hypertension.
- Acute forms of GN can be divided into those caused by primary renal conditions and those caused by secondary illnesses.
- Four types of primary (idiopathic) GN include:
  - Focal segmental glomerulosclerosis
  - Membranoproliferative GN
  - Membranous nephropathy
  - Minimal change disease
- Secondary causes include:
  - Postinfectious causes, such as poststreptococcal or viral infections
  - HIV nephropathy
  - Hepatitis B or C
  - Autoimmune diseases such as systemic lupus erythematosus, Goodpasture syndrome (rare), or IgA nephropathy
  - Vasculitis, such as granulomatosis with polyangiitis or microscopic polyangiitis

▶ CLINICAL ASSESSMENT

- Presentation may include vague constitutional symptoms in addition to:
  - Peripheral or periorbital edema
  - Hematuria (microscopic or gross)
  - Frothy urine
  - Decreased urine output
- Patients with poststreptococcal GN may report dark or "coca-cola"–colored urine.

- Patients with granulomatosis with polyangiitis may report symptoms of sinusitis and shortness of breath.
- Patients with Goodpasture syndrome may also have pulmonary symptoms, including persistent cough and hemoptysis.
- Patients with lupus may also report rashes or arthralgia.

▶ DIAGNOSIS

- Basic metabolic panel may be notable for elevated creatinine and decreased glomerular filtration rate (GFR); blood urea nitrogen (BUN) may or may not be elevated.
- Urinalysis will reveal microscopic hematuria and proteinuria.
- Serologic tests including a C-reactive protein (CRP), erythrocyte sedimentation rate (ESR), c-ANCA, p-ANCA, antinuclear antibody (ANA), C3 and C4 complement levels, and an anti–glomerular basement membrane antibody may be abnormal depending on underlying etiology.
- A serum immunoelectrophoresis panel (SIEP) may be abnormal in the case of multiple myeloma.
- When a diagnosis is not clear from laboratory workup alone, a renal biopsy can be performed for a definitive diagnosis.

▶ TREATMENT

- Treatment depends on the underlying cause of disease.
- May include steroids and other immunosuppressants such as cyclosporine, tacrolimus, cyclophosphamide, mycophenolate mofetil, bortezomib, and rituximab
- Patients with postinfectious GN often eventually recover after treatment of infection.
- If renal function continues to decline despite therapy, or if renal impairment is too severe at presentation, dialysis may be required for treatment.

Nephrotic and Nephritic Syndromes

Kathy Clift, MSPAS, PA-C

▶ **GENERAL FEATURES**

- Nephrotic syndrome:
  - Renal disorder characterized by heavy proteinuria (>3.5 g in 24 hours), hypoalbuminemia (<3 g/dL), and peripheral edema
  - Pathophysiology:
    - Glomerular injury results in increased permeability to large proteins (primarily albumin but can include immunoglobulins, transferrin, antithrombin III).
    - Hypoalbuminemia leads to an alteration in oncotic pressure and a shift of fluid out of the intravascular space into extravascular spaces; loss of vascular volume induces water and salt retention, which further contributes to the edema.
    - Loss of immunoglobulins increases risk of infection.
    - Loss of antithrombin III, protein C, and protein S increases risk of deep vein thrombosis, renal vein thrombosis, and pulmonary embolism; thrombosis more likely to occur when albumin levels <2 g.
    - Loss of proteins triggers reactive protein synthesis of lipids in the liver.
  - Etiology:
    - Classified as primary (confined to kidney) or due to secondary causes (DM, SLE, amyloidosis, HIV, infections, malignancy, medications such as NSAIDs and lithium)
    - Categorized by appearance on microscopy:
      - Minimal change disease (MCD): most common in children
      - Membranous nephropathy:
        - Most likely to have thrombosis
        - More common in adults than children
      - Focal segmental glomerulosclerosis:
        - More common in Black and Hispanic patients
        - Associated with several conditions including sickle cell disease
  - DM most common secondary cause in adults and children.
- Nephritic syndrome:
  - Immune-mediated inflammatory reaction with deposition/formation of immune complexes in the glomerulus
  - Immune complexes compromise blood flow and filtration, leading to a significant reduction in GFR.
  - Hallmark is glomerular hematuria, oliguria, and hypertension (HTN) with variable proteinuria.
  - Etiology: can be primary or from secondary causes
  - Most common etiologies:
    - IgA nephropathy (Berger disease): most common cause worldwide
      - Typically occurs after an URI/GI infection or exercise
      - May be associated with celiac disease, cirrhosis, HIV
    - Anti–glomerular basement membrane (anti-GBM) antibody disease:
      - Associated with lung hemorrhage (Goodpasture syndrome)
      - High risk for rapidly progressive glomerulonephritis and renal failure
    - Postinfectious: most commonly poststreptococcal (PSGN)
    - Connective tissue disorders such as SLE
    - Systemic vasculitis
      - Henoch-Schönlein purpura (IgA vasculitis)
      - Granulomatosis with polyangiitis (formerly known as Wegener's disease)

▶ **CLINICAL ASSESSMENT**

- Nephrotic syndrome:
  - History: fatigue, major periorbital, sacral, or pedal edema; "foamy" urine (from proteinuria), acute weight gain from fluid retention, nonspecific symptoms may include SOB, weakness, anorexia
  - PE: significant periorbital, sacral, pedal edema; may have crackles on lung auscultation and/or findings consistent with pleural effusion, elevated JVP, ascites, HTN
- Nephritic syndrome:
  - History: acute onset of edema, oliguria, hematuria (often described as tea or cola colored); may report recent infection, symptoms of systemic diseases (eg, fevers, joint pain, rashes)
  - Physical examination: periorbital and pedal edema (typically less pronounced than nephrotic syndrome); gross hematuria, and HTN (can be severe); may have crackles/rales on lung auscultation (from fluid overload), ascites, arthritis, hemoptysis if associated lung hemorrhage

▶ DIAGNOSIS

- Nephrotic syndrome:
  - Urinalysis (UA): dipstick 2+ or greater proteinuria, may have hematuria; microscopy may show nonactive or bland urinary sediment; may have lipiduria with the presence of fat droplets or fatty casts
  - A 24-hour UA protein >3.5 g or a spot urine protein-to-creatinine ratio >3 to 3.5.
  - Serum creatinine and BUN are typically not elevated at presentation.
  - Lipid panel may show elevated LDL and triglycerides.
  - Hypocalcemia may be present (correct for low albumin), and vitamin D levels may be low.
  - Renal biopsy is typically needed for diagnosis (usually not required in children), as most cases are caused by MCD and in patients with known systemic disorders (eg, DM, SLE).
- Nephritic syndrome:
  - UA:
    - Dipstick typically positive for proteinuria and hematuria; may have leukocytes.
    - Microscopy typically shows active sediment with dysmorphic RBCs, RBC casts, WBCs (may have granular or WBC casts).
  - AKI is common at presentation.
  - A 24-hour urine protein is typically in 1–2 g range (though may be in the nephrotic range).
  - Elevated ESR/C-reactive protein, decreased complement levels
  - Additional workup may be warranted to determine etiology (eg, antistreptolysin O [ASO] titer for strep, anti-GM antibodies).
  - Renal biopsy may be needed for definitive dx if unclear from history and diagnostics.

▶ TREATMENT

- Nephrotic syndrome:
  - Nephrology consult is warranted.
  - Treat underlying cause and stop offending agents/medications, if possible.
  - MCD is typically responsive to corticosteroids, although relapses are common.
  - Salt restriction and loop diuretics to manage edema.
  - ACE inhibitor or ARB can control HTN and reduce proteinuria.
  - Dietary modification and statins for hyperlipidemia.
  - Monitor for infections and avoid nephrotoxic medications.
  - Patients are considered hypercoagulable—management of thrombosis should they occur.
  - Prognosis depends on the underlying cause of disease.
- Nephritic syndrome:
  - Nephrology consultation is warranted.
    - Treatment should address underlying etiology and may include antibiotics, steroids, immunosuppressive medication, or plasmapheresis.
    - Medical management of HTN
    - Management of volume overload: loop diuretics, restricted dietary salt and fluid intake
    - Prognosis is typically good in PSGN, IgA vasculitis, and most cases of IgA nephropathy; subset of patients will have rapidly progressive glomerulonephritis, which can lead to renal failure.

SECTION G　　*Renal Malignancies*

CHAPTER 173　　# Renal Cell Carcinoma

Victoria Louwagie, PA-C
Becky Ness, MPAS, PA-C

▶ GENERAL FEATURES

- Renal cell carcinomas (RCCs) account for 80% to 85% of primary renal neoplasms and about 2% of all cancers worldwide.
- Originates within the renal cortex

- Epidemiology:
  - 2:1 male-to-female predominance
  - Median age at diagnosis is 64, with greatest incidence in the sixth to eighth decades of life.
  - At presentation:
    - 65%, present with localized disease

- 17% regional lymph node involvement
- 16% metastatic disease
- 3% unstaged
- Risk factors:
  - Smoking (greatest correlation of disease manifestation)
  - Hypertension
  - Obesity
  - Chronic kidney disease: chronic decreased eGFR increases risk of kidney cancer:
    - Dialysis dependent with acquired cystic disease = 30-fold greater risk than the general population
  - Occupational exposure:
    - Cadmium
    - Asbestos
    - Petroleum byproducts
- Staging has a direct correlation with morbidity:
  - Stage I: 90% 5-year survival rate
  - Stage II: 75% to 95% 5-year survival rate
  - Stage III: 59% to 70% 5-year survival rate with nephrectomy: location and degree of extrarenal involvement impacts survival
  - Stage IV: survival is typically ~12 months; treatment with vascular endothelial growth factor (VEGF) antagonist results in survival averaging 28–29 months.

CLINICAL ASSESSMENT

- Many patients are asymptomatic during early stages, and disease is discovered incidentally.
- Symptoms include:
  - Classic triad (present in 9% of patients): hematuria, flank pain, palpable abdominal mass:
    - Hematuria indicates tumor invasion into the collecting system.
    - Palpable mass (abdominal or flank) best felt in thin adults: associated with lower pole tumors and is nontender/firm/moves with respiration and homogeneous
  - Unintentional weight loss
  - Scrotal varices (about 11% of patients): occur when tumor has obstructed gonadal vein at entry to renal vein; typically left sided, abnormal vessels do not empty when patient is supine
  - Inferior vena cava involvement can result in a variety of clinical presentations, including:
    - Lower extremity edema
    - Ascites
    - Pulmonary emboli
    - Hepatic dysfunction
  - Paraneoplastic syndromes
  - Anemia can precede diagnosis by months.
    - Is disproportionately severe
    - Can be normocytic or microcytic
    - Iron studies resemble those seen with anemia of chronic disease.
  - Fever (up to 20%): usually intermittent and associated with other constitutional complaints (night sweats, fatigue, anorexia, unintentional weight loss)

- Hypercalcemia (up to 15%): usually in advanced disease
- Erythrocytosis: usually in advanced disease and suspected to be due to constitutive erythropoietin production
- Secondary amyloidosis
- Symptoms at common sites for metastatic disease:
  - Lung (45%): cough, dyspnea, hemoptysis
  - Bone (30%): pain, spinal cord compression, pathologic fx
  - Lymph nodes (22%): lymphadenopathy
  - Liver (20%)
  - Adrenal/brain (9% each): headache, neurologic changes

DIAGNOSIS

- Imaging:
  - Abdominal/pelvic CT with and without iodinated contrast is the preferred imaging modality; typical findings include:
    - Solid renal mass
    - Lesions with thickend/irregular walls or septa
    - Contrast-enhancing lesions
  - Ultrasound can be used if CT is unavailable or contraindicated.
  - MRI if prior studies inconclusive or iodinated contrast cannot be used.
- Histopathologic review:
  - Full or partial nephrectomy: provides tissue for histologic review and is potentially curative
  - Biopsy of metastatic site (used less often; useful in patients who are not surgical candidates)

TREATMENT

- Localized:
  - Surgery is curative for the majority without metastatic disease (stages I-III).
    - Radical vs. partial nephrectomy based on the extent of disease as well as patient specific factors (age, comorbidities)
- Advanced or metastatic:
  - Clear cell RCC:
    - If not controlled by local/regional treatments:
      - Systemic therapy
      - Immunotherapy + systemic therapy
      - Antiangiogenic for those not eligible for immunotherapy
  - Non–clear cell carcinoma: varies and is tailored to the specific histologic subtype as well as the pathologic and molecular features of each tumor
  - Brain metastases:
    - Surgical resection and/or radiation therapy (RT) (stereotactic radiosurgery preferred)
    - Systemic therapy follows surgical/RT:
      - VEGF inhibitors
      - Immunotherapy

CHAPTER 174

Wilms Tumor

Tanya Fernandez, MS, PA-C, IBCLC

▶ GENERAL FEATURES

- Wilms tumor (nephroblastoma) is the most common pediatric renal malignancy.
- Peak age for diagnosis is 2- to 3-years-old, and 95% are diagnosed before age 10.
- Linked to genetic mutations in the *WT1* gene, especially Wilms Tumor, Aniridia, Genitourinary Abnormalities, Range of Developmental Delays (WAGR) syndrome (50% incidence of Wilms tumor) and Denys-Drash syndrome (90% incidence); Beckwith-Wiedemann syndrome is less commonly associated (5%-10% incidence).

▶ CLINICAL ASSESSMENT

- Presents with a painless and fixed palpable mass in the abdomen that rarely crosses the midline
- May be accompanied by hypertension, hematuria, abdominal vein distension, as well as constitutional symptoms including weight loss, pallor, and fatigue, which are typically secondary to subcapsular hemorrhage

▶ DIAGNOSIS

- When Wilms tumor is suspected, excessive or forceful palpation should be avoided to prevent capsular rupture.
- Abdominal ultrasound with Doppler is typically the first imaging study ordered and is used to determine, structure, location, and blood flow; subsequent CT or MRI can aid in localization, visualization of the lymph nodes, and detection of metastases.
- Complete blood count with a differential may reveal anemia or polycythemia, due to bleeding into the tumor or increased erythropoietin secretion, respectively.
- Urinalysis may show gross or microscopic hematuria.
- Confirmatory diagnosis and prognosis are based on histology of the tumor specimen; biopsy is not typically performed before surgical investigation.

▶ TREATMENT

- Prognosis is based on age, stage, histology, and the presence of molecular and genetic markers.
- Staging is based on the anatomic involvement.
  - Stage I: tumor is completely within the pseudocapsule.
  - Stage II: tumor extending beyond the kidney and capsule but is completely resectable
  - Stages III and IV: localized remnants of tumor following resection or hematogenous spread
  - Stage V: bilateral kidney involvement; has the most unfavorable survival rate
- Treatment may be composed of nephrectomy alone (very low-risk stage I or II tumors), nephrectomy and chemotherapy with or without radiation (stages II-IV), or presurgical chemotherapy followed by surgical resection of the tumor loci (stage V) in an effort to preserve nephrons and renal parenchyma.

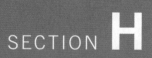

SECTION **H**

Renal Vascular Disease

CHAPTER 175

Renal Vascular Disease

Stephanie Hull, EdS, MMS, PA-C

▶ GENERAL FEATURES

- Renal vascular disease includes abnormalities of the renal arteries or veins and may lead to kidney damage, kidney failure, and hypertension.
- Renal vascular hypertension is blood pressure elevation due to activation of the renin-angiotensin system in the setting of occlusive renal artery disease.
- Renal artery stenosis (RAS) is most commonly due to atherosclerotic occlusive disease (80%-90% of patients).

- Fibromuscular dysplasia (FMD; 10%-15% of patients), a less common but important cause of RAS, typically affects young women; FMD also affects other medium-sized arteries, such as the cerebral, carotid, and coronary arteries.

▶ CLINICAL ASSESSMENT

- Renal vascular hypertension most commonly occurs in patients aged ≥45 years with a history of atherosclerotic disease but should also be considered in the following clinical contexts:
  - Acute onset of severe hypertension in patients aged <30 years or >55 years
  - Abrupt acceleration of previously stable hypertension
  - Severe hypertension (blood pressure >160/100 mm Hg) or hypertension refractory to optimal medical management (three of more antihypertensives)
  - Pulmonary edema associated with poorly controlled hypertension
  - Acute kidney injury upon starting ACE inhibitor, angiotensin-receptor blocker, or renin inhibitor therapy (persistent elevation in serum creatinine of ≥50%)
- Hypertensive retinopathy on funduscopic examination may be present.
- A systolic-diastolic bruit near the epigastrium is more common in FMD.

▶ DIAGNOSIS

- Retrospective diagnosis revealed after blood pressure improvement following correction of RAS.

- Serum creatinine and blood urea nitrogen (BUN) will be elevated in significant disease.
- Hypokalemia may be seen in bilateral RAS.
- Ultrasound may reveal asymmetric kidneys (if one renal artery is disproportionally affected) or bilateral small hyperechoic kidneys (if both renal arteries are affected).
- CT angiography and MRA may also be utilized but require intravenous contrast agents; CT angiography or magnetic resonance imaging (MRA) should only be performed if a corrective procedure for RAS would be performed.
- Renal angiography is considered the gold standard for diagnosis but is invasive and only performed after positive screening with ultrasound, CT, or MRA.
- FMD has a characteristic "string-of-beads" appearance on renal angiography.

▶ TREATMENT

- All patients should receive counseling for lifestyle modification:
  - Weight reduction
  - Reduce dietary sodium
  - Increase physical activity
  - Moderation of alcohol
- Pharmacologic management of hypertension with an ACE inhibitor or angiotensin-receptor blocker is preferred if no contraindications exist.
- Revascularization for RAS due to atherosclerotic disease remains controversial, and evidence has not revealed measurable benefits.
- Percutaneous transluminal angioplasty is often curative in FMD.

Section A Pretest: Anemias

1. A patient with iron deficiency anemia would most likely have which of the following lab results?
   A. Hb 11, MCV 105, platelets 250, ferritin 150, normal reticulocyte count
   B. Hb 11, MCV 90, platelets 250, ferritin 90, normal reticulocyte count
   C. Hb 9, MCV 74, platelets 500, ferritin 2, low reticulocyte count
   D. Hb 6, MCV 74, platelets 10, ferritin 100, low reticulocyte count

2. What supplementation is recommended in patients with chronic hemolytic anemia?
   A. Vitamin B12
   B. Folate
   C. Iron
   D. None

3. Findings of bone marrow cellularity of <25%, ANC <500/µL, and platelet count <20 000/µL indicate which of the following?
   A. Moderate aplastic anemia (AA)
   B. Severe aplastic anemia (AA)
   C. Very severe aplastic anemia (AA)

4. Which of the following is appropriate counseling for a patient starting iron therapy?
   A. Your oral iron supplement may cause upset stomach and/or constipation.
   B. Administration of IV iron is associated with a risk of anaphylaxis.
   C. You should premedicate with diphenhydramine before taking your oral iron supplements.
   D. Both A and B.

5. Folate deficiency is uncommon in patients from developed countries. Which of the following conditions would NOT predispose a patient to folate deficiency anemia?
   A. Type 1 diabetes mellitus treated with insulin
   B. Chronic alcohol abuse
   C. Rheumatoid arthritis treated with methotrexate
   D. Celiac disease

6. Which of the following laboratory evaluations would you expect to be abnormal in a patient with anemia of chronic disease?
   A. MCV
   B. Peripheral blood smear
   C. Serum iron
   D. Serum creatinine

7. Which of the following is an appropriate next step for evaluation of unexplained iron deficiency anemia?
   A. Bone marrow biopsy
   B. PET scan
   C. Colonoscopy and EGD
   D. Pap smear

8. In the evaluation of a patient with macrocytic anemia in whom you suspect vitamin B12 or folate deficiency, a normal methylmalonic acid (MMA) level and elevated homocysteine level is most indicative of which of the following:
   A. Vitamin B12 deficiency
   B. Folate deficiency
   C. Both vitamin B12 and folate deficiency
   D. Neither vitamin B12 nor folate deficiency

9. Which of the following patterns of iron studies are most consistent with a diagnosis of anemia of chronic disease?
   A. Low serum iron, elevated transferrin, and normal or elevated ferritin
   B. Low serum iron, elevated transferrin, and low or normal ferritin
   C. High serum iron, low transferrin, and normal or elevated ferritin
   D. Low serum iron, low transferrin, and normal or elevated ferritin

10. A 9-year-old Caucasian boy presents with episodic history of fatigue, jaundice, and right upper quadrant (RUQ) pain. He is currently experiencing fatigue and jaundice but is otherwise asymptomatic. Initial laboratory testing reveals anemia and reticulocytosis; peripheral smear demonstrates spherocytes. He is not on any medications, and past medical history is otherwise unremarkable. Which of the following is the most likely diagnosis?
    A. Sickle cell anemia
    B. Hereditary spherocytosis
    C. Autoimmune hemolytic anemia (AIHA)
    D. G6PD deficiency

11. What treatment is recommended for a 25-year-old female with findings consistent with severe aplastic anemia (AA) and a matched HSC donor is?
    A. Observation and supportive care
    B. IST
    C. Referral to transplant center for immediate HCT

12. A 40-year-old Greek male with HIV was started on dapsone for *pneumocystis* pneumonia prophylaxis. Recent laboratory evaluation demonstrated anemia, reticulocytosis, and elevated indirect bilirubin. Which finding on peripheral smear would be consistent with the most likely cause of hemolytic anemia?

    A. Schistoctyes
    B. Sickle cells
    C. Heinz bodies
    D. Elliptocytes

13. A 68-year-old male with non-Hodgkin lymphoma presents with anemia, reticulocytosis, and elevated indirect bilirubin. He is found to have positive IgG on Coombs testing. His Hb is 9.0 g/dL, and he is clinically stable. What is the best next step in treating his hemolytic anemia?

    A. RBC transfusion
    B. Splenectomy
    C. Eculizumab
    D. Corticosteroids

14. Which of the following clinical laboratory findings is least consistent with a diagnosis of aplastic anemia?

    A. Hemoglobin <10 g/dL
    B. Neutrophil count <1.5 × 10⁹/L
    C. Platelet count 150 to 450 × 10⁹/L
    D. Hypocellular bone marrow without dysplasia or fibrosis

15. What is the most appropriate treatment for patients with pernicious anemia?

    A. Oral vitamin B12 supplementation
    B. Parenteral vitamin B12 supplementation
    C. Oral folate supplementation
    D. No supplementation is required in patients with pernicious anemia

16. What study is required to establish the diagnosis of aplastic anemia (AA)?

    A. Ultrasound
    B. Bone marrow biopsy
    C. MRI
    D. Skin biopsy

17. Which of the following laboratory parameters would you expect to be normal in a patient with hemolytic anemia?

    A. Haptoglobin
    B. Indirect bilirubin
    C. Direct bilirubin
    D. Reticulocyte count

18. The recommended treatment for an 85-year-old male with findings of moderate aplastic anemia (AA) plus COPD, diabetes, and dementia is?

    A. Observation and supportive care
    B. IST
    C. Referral to transplant center for immediate HCT

Section B Pretest: Coagulation Disorders

1. Which of the following should be considered in determining the length of anticoagulation for a newly diagnosed DVT?

    A. Patient's family history of VTE
    B. Presence of a provoking event such as a recent surgery
    C. Presence of an unresolved/persistent risk factor such as malignancy
    D. All of the above

2. For which of the following would you consider warfarin instead of a DOAC as first-line therapy?

    A. Patient with confirmed prothrombin mutation and history of unprovoked DVT
    B. Patient with confirmed factor V Leiden heterozygosity and no history of DVT

    C. Patient with triple positive antiphospholipid antibody syndrome and recurrent PE
    D. Patient with history of three provoked distal DVTs

3. For which of the following patients would thrombophilia testing be warranted?

    A. Patient with acute DVT following knee replacement surgery
    B. Patient with no history of DVT but with a grandmother with history of PE
    C. Patient with recurrent provoked DVT in the setting of mild provoking risk factors such as long-distance car rides
    D. Patient with acute DVT and newly diagnosed renal cell carcinoma

Section C Pretest: Hemochromatosis

1. Which of the following would be the best test to solidify a working diagnosis of hemochromatosis?

   A. Renal ultrasound
   B. Gene mutation testing
   C. CT of the abdomen/pelvis
   D. HbA1c

2. What is the best treatment for hemochromatosis?

   A. Iron chelation therapy
   B. Metformin
   C. Liver transplant
   D. Therapeutic phlebotomy

3. Your patient with hemochromatosis is getting weekly therapeutic phlebotomy. He is tired of coming in for blood draws every week. What is your goal lab that is needed in order to reduce his therapeutic phlebotomy down to maintenance frequency (every 3 months)?

   A. Serum ferritin <50 ng/mL
   B. Negative *HFE* gene testing
   C. Hb >12 g/dL
   D. TIBC (total iron binding capacity) above 450 µg/dL

4. You have a patient with a new diagnosis of hereditary hemochromatosis. What dietary recommendations should you give him?

   A. Avoid dairy and gluten-containing products
   B. Take a multivitamin with iron
   C. Avoid vitamin C supplements
   D. Introduce more raw shellfish into diet

Section D Pretest: Hemoglobinopathies

1. A 10-year-old boy with sickle cell anemia presents to your office to establish care after recently moving to town. Which of the following would NOT be part of your initial laboratory evaluation?

   A. CBC
   B. Blood culture
   C. Reticulocyte count
   D. Renal function tests

2. Which country does NOT have a known increased risk for thalassemia disorders?

   A. Africa
   B. China
   C. Europe
   D. Middle East

3. When counseling the patient and his family about the complications and course of sickle cell anemia, which of the following should be included in your guidance?

   A. Priapism is common and will always resolve spontaneously with conservative management at home.

   B. A fever does not warrant medical evaluation unless the fever is very high or lasts longer than 3 days.
   C. The patient should receive annual influenza vaccination.
   D. The patient may participate in all activities without limitations.

4. What is the most common symptom of a thalassemia disorder?

   A. Hemolytic anemia
   B. Splenomegaly
   C. Increased bleeding
   D. Jaundice

5. Which of the following is false regarding the pathophysiology of sickle cell anemia?

   A. It is an autosomal-recessive inherited condition.
   B. It leads to chronic anemia due to blood loss.
   C. Sickling of RBCs causes damage to vascular endothelium.
   D. Sickled RBCs can occlude peripheral blood vessels, leading to ischemia and pain.

6. Which thalassemia disorder is incompatible with life?
   A. β-Thalassemia trait
   B. Hb H disease
   C. Hemoglobin Barts
   D. α-Thalassemia trait

7. Sickle cell disease is often diagnosed by family history and newborn screening. However, which of the following is one of the first manifestations of the disease in childhood?
   A. Dactylitis
   B. Hypoxia
   C. Pain
   D. Priapism

8. In a patient suspected of thalassemia disorder, what is the first laboratory test to be considered?
   A. Prothrombin time (PT)
   B. CBC
   C. Iron studies
   D. Hb electrophoresis

9. You are counseling a patient about the risks and benefits of receiving regular blood transfusions. For patients with sickle cell anemia who receive therapeutic blood transfusions, what additional treatment must be considered?
   A. Supplemental oxygen to prevent hypoxia during transfusions
   B. Antibiotic prophylaxis with oral penicillin
   C. Antiviral medication to prevent transfusion-related infections
   D. Iron chelation therapy to prevent hemosiderosis

10. Which of the following is the most specific laboratory finding in β-thalassemia disorders?
    A. Microcytic anemia
    B. Normal red blood cell distribution (RDW)
    C. Increased Hb A2
    D. Schistocytes

Section E Pretest: Neoplasms, Premalignancies, and Malignancies

1. Which finding is pathognomonic in acute myeloid leukemia (AML)?
   A. Smudge cell
   B. Auer rod
   C. Philadelphia chromosome
   D. Howell-Jolly body

2. A mutation in which of the following genes is commonly associated with polycythemia vera (PV)?
   A. JAK1
   B. JAK2
   C. BRCA1
   D. BRCA2

3. Which of the following is a risk factor for acute lymphoblastic leukemia (ALL)?
   A. Advanced paternal age
   B. Trisomy 18
   C. Decreased birth weight
   D. Frequent febrile infection

4. Which of the following is NOT an indication for treatment in a patient with chronic lymphocytic leukemia (CLL)?
   A. Worsening anemia or thrombocytopenia
   B. Acute infection
   C. Symptomatic or enlarging lymphadenopathy
   D. Massive, progressive, or symptomatic splenomegaly

5. Which of the following is NOT a prognostic factor in acute myeloid leukemia (AML)?
   A. Age
   B. Performance status
   C. Karyotype/cytogenetics
   D. WBC count at the time of diagnosis

6. Which of the following is NOT a phase of chronic myeloid leukemia (CML)?
   A. Chronic phase
   B. Accelerated phase
   C. Acute phase
   D. Blast crisis

7. Which of the following is NOT a risk factor for acute myeloid leukemia (AML)?
   A. Trisomy 21
   B. Exposure to certain chemicals
   C. Previous chemotherapy
   D. History of preexistent hematologic disorder

8. Which of the following is NOT a common objective finding in chronic myeloid leukemia (CML) or chronic lymphocytic leukemia (CLL)?
   A. Lymphocytosis
   B. Hepatosplenomegaly
   C. Lymphadenopathy
   D. Multiple ecchymoses on extremities

9. Which of the following is a major WHO criterion for diagnosing polycythemia vera (PV)?

    A. Elevated HgB (>16.5 g/dL) and elevated HCT (>49% in men or >48% in women)
    B. Hypercellular bone marrow
    C. Identification of a mutation in the *JAK2* gene
    D. All of the above

10. What is the only known risk factor for chronic myeloid leukemia (CML)?

    A. Exposure to asbestos
    B. Exposure to ionizing radiation
    C. Radon exposure
    D. Exposure to arsenic in drinking water

11. Which of the following meets SLiM-CRAB criteria in a patient with >10% clonal plasma cells on a bone marrow biopsy?

    A. Hb of 11.0 g/dL
    B. κ free light chain 10 mg/dL, λ free light chain 1.0 mg/dL, free light chain ratio 10
    C. One focal lesion on MRI, 4 mm in diameter
    D. Bony lytic lesions identified on an x-ray; biopsy proven to contain clonal plasma cells

12. Which of the following treatments is initially utilized in the treatment plan for patients with polycythemia vera (PV)?

    A. Therapeutic phlebotomy
    B. Hydroxyurea administration
    C. Ruxolitinib administration
    D. Lestaurtinib administration

13. You suspect multiple myeloma (MM) in a patient and plan to refer him to hematology as an outpatient. What tests should be performed and resulted before allowing him to return home, assuming his pain is well controlled and there is no concern for spinal cord impingement?

    A. No further tests are needed; he can go home and follow up with hematology in their first available appointment
    B. CBC with differential and CMP to evaluate for anemia, acute kidney injury, and hypercalcemia
    C. SPEP, UPEP, and quantitative immunoglobulin heavy and free light chains
    D. PET-CT

14. Which percentage of blasts is diagnostic for acute leukemia?

    A. >5%
    B. >10%
    C. >15%
    D. >20%

15. You are completing the outpatient evaluation for a 76-year-old female complaining of low back pain >2 years. Of the following, which set of values would make the diagnosis of MM based on the IMWG criteria?

    A. Hb 12.0 g/dL, calcium 9.5 mg/dL, creatinine 0.9 mg/dL (eGFR >60 mL/min), skeletal survey showed osteopenia.
    B. PET-CT with uptake corresponding to lytic lesions. Biopsy of a lytic lesion demonstrates clonal plasma cells. Bone marrow biopsy shows 50% clonal plasma cells.
    C. Bone marrow biopsy shows 5% clonal plasma cells. CT skeletal survey shows one lytic lesion with associated compression fracture of the L1 vertebral body. No other lytic lesions are identified. Biopsy of the lesion demonstrates clonal plasma cells. CBC and CMP are normal.
    D. Normal CMP, microcytic anemia, ferritin of 9 g/dL, hemoccult positive, no monoclonal protein identified on serum protein electrophoresis.

16. A 69-year-old male presents to his primary care provider with a recently new diagnosis of myelodysplastic syndrome. He wishes to inquire about anything that may have contributed to his condition. Which of the following is NOT a known risk factor for the development of myelodysplastic syndrome?

    A. Increased age
    B. Tobacco smoking
    C. Ionizing radiation
    D. Previous chemotherapy
    E. Diet

17. Which of the following is a pathognomonic finding in chronic myeloid leukemia (CML)?

    A. Smudge cell
    B. Auer rod
    C. Philadelphia chromosome
    D. Howell-Jolly body

18. What percentage of patients will progress from myelodysplastic syndrome to acute myeloid leukemia (AML)?

    A. 10%
    B. 25%
    C. 33%
    D. 45%
    E. 50%

19. Which of the following components of the CBC are elevated in patients with polycythemia vera (PV)?

    A. WBCs
    B. RBCs
    C. Platelets
    D. All of the above

Section F Pretest: Thrombotic Disorders

1. Which of the following clinical findings is due to obstruction of the microvasculature in thrombotic thrombocytopenic purpura (TTP)?
   A. Confusion
   B. Fever
   C. Hemoptysis
   D. Purpura

2. Which of the following is the most common vector for the bacteria associated with this condition?
   A. Airborne
   B. Bloodborne
   C. Fecal-oral route
   D. None of the above

3. Which of the following is the primary cause of immune thrombocytopenic purpura (ITP)?
   A. Accelerated platelet clearance
   B. Bone marrow failure
   C. Decreased platelet production
   D. Splenic sequestration

4. Which of the following age groups is HUS most commonly seen in?
   A. Infants
   B. Children
   C. Adolescent
   D. Seniors

5. Easy bruising in ITP is associated with which of the following laboratory findings?
   A. Bleeding time >7 minutes
   B. Fibrinogen level > 400 mg/dL
   C. Platelet count <50 000/μL
   D. Reticulocyte count <1%

6. A child presents with fever and bloody diarrhea for the past 5 days. After work-up, a hemolytic anemia is diagnosed. Which of the following features would be most indicative that extravascular red cell destruction is occuring in this patient?
   A. Hemoglobinemia
   B. Decreased haptoglobin
   C. Splenomegaly
   D. Hemoglobinuria

7. A 30-year-old female presents with mild fatigue and heavier menses than usual over the past 3 months. Her last menstrual period was 7 days ago. Urine pregnancy test is negative. Mild conjunctival pallor is noted. Abdomen is soft and nontender. No abnormal findings are noted on pelvic and bimanual examination. Diffuse petechia and purpura are noted on skin examination. Laboratory studies reveal a mild normocytic, normochromic anemia, and thrombocytopenia (platelet count 20 000/μL). Which of the following is the most appropriate initial treatment?
   A. Blood transfusion
   B. Fostamatinib
   C. Platelet transfusion
   D. Prednisone

8. Which of the following platelet counts best correlates with the diagnosis of HUS?
   A. $70 \times 10^3/\mu L$
   B. $170 \times 10^3/\mu L$
   C. $270 \times 10^3/\mu L$
   D. $370 \times 10^3/\mu L$

9. Which of the following vaccinations is recommended before therapeutic splenectomy for ITP?
   A. Diphtheria
   B. Hepatitis B
   C. Pneumococcal
   D. Varicella

10. Which of the following laboratory findings is expected in TTP?
    A. High partial thromboplastin time (PTT)
    B. Low lactate dehydrogenase (LDH)
    C. Positive direct antiglobulin test
    D. Schistocytes on peripheral blood smear

Section G Pretest: Transfusion Reactions

1. Which of the following is the most common cause of acute hemolytic transfusion reactions?

    A. ABO incompatibility
    B. Transfusion-associated circulatory overload
    C. Anamnestic response
    D. Hyperkalemia

2. Fatal hemolytic transfusion reactions often result from which of the following?

    A. Elevated LDH
    B. Multiorgan failure
    C. Hyperkalemia
    D. Spherocytosis

3. Which of the following is the most frequent preventable cause of fatal transfusion reactions?

    A. Monitoring the volume of IV fluids
    B. Bacterial contamination
    C. Patient misidentification
    D. Mechanical hemolysis

4. Disseminated intravascular coagulation (DIC) may be treated with which of the following?

    A. Calcium gluconate
    B. Aggressive hydration
    C. Dialysis
    D. Blood components

5. A 57-year-old female calls the clinic and reports having brown urine, decreased urination, and fever 7 days after receiving a transfusion. This hemolytic reaction is most likely associated with which of the following?

    A. Intravascular hemolysis
    B. Extravascular hemolysis
    C. Bacterial contamination
    D. DIC

▶ ANSWERS AND EXPLANATIONS TO SECTION A PRETEST

1. **C.** A patient with iron deficiency anemia would most likely have Hb 9, MCV 74, platelets 500, ferritin 2, and low reticulocyte count.

2. **B.** In patients with chronic hemolysis, the ongoing need to produce new RBCs can use up the body's stores of folate, resulting in folate deficiency. Oral folate supplementation is recommended.

3. **B.** Bone marrow cellularity of <25%, ANC <500/µL, and platelet count <20 000/µL indicates severe AA.

4. **D.** When counseling a patient starting iron therapy, explain that oral iron supplement may cause upset stomach and/or constipation and that administration of IV iron is associated with a risk of anaphylaxis.

5. **A.** Neither type 1 diabetes mellitus nor insulin is associated with increased risk for folate deficiency. Chronic alcohol abuse is associated with reduced dietary folate intake as well as malabsorption and decreased liver uptake and storage of folate. Methotrexate inhibits enzymes critical to folate synthesis and is associated with folate deficiency. Celiac disease can cause folate deficiency through malabsorption.

6. **C.** Serum iron levels are typically low in patients with anemia of chronic disease due to disordered iron homeostasis. Anemia of chronic disease is typically normocytic and not associated with any specific abnormalities on peripheral smear. An abnormal serum creatinine, particularly if elevated, should prompt an evaluation for anemia of chronic kidney disease as the most appropriate diagnosis.

7. **C.** Colonoscopy and EGD are appropriate next steps for evaluation of unexplained iron deficiency anemia.

8. **B.** While both vitamin B12 and folate are required for metabolism of homocysteine, metabolism of MMA only requires vitamin B12. A normal MMA level and elevated homocysteine suggest adequate supply of vitamin B12 but inadequate folate for homocysteine metabolism.

9. **D.** Both iron deficiency anemia and anemia of chronic disease can present with low serum iron. Transferrin is typically high in patients with iron deficiency anemia due to inadequate iron supply and low in patients with anemia of chronic disease because there are adequate iron stores that are not readily available. Similarly, ferritin levels are low in iron deficiency anemia due to inadequate iron supply but are typically normal or elevated in patients with anemia of chronic disease as the iron is present but sequestered in cells. Ferritin may also be elevated in patients with anemia of chronic disease because of its role as an acute-phase reactant reflecting inflammation associated with the underlying condition.

10. **B.** Anemia and reticulocytosis in the absence of bleeding suggest the presence of hemolysis. The patient's

age and episodic history of clinical features of hemolysis, accompanied by the presence of spherocytes on
peripheral smear, suggest a diagnosis of hereditary
spherocytosis. The patient does not fit the typical
demographic for sickle cell anemia, nor is there evidence of sickle cells on peripheral smear. There are
no risk factors for AIHA or G6PD deficiency present.

11. **C.** Referral to a transplant center for immediate HCT
is the recommended treatment for a 25-year-old female with findings consistent with severe AA and a
matched HSC donor.

12. **C.** Exposure to dapsone in a patient of Mediterranean
descent followed by laboratory evidence of hemolysis
suggests a diagnosis of G6PD deficiency, which can be
associated with Heinz bodies on peripheral smear. Bite
cells can also be seen on peripheral smear in patients
with G6PD deficiency. Schistocytes are more commonly seen in mechanical or microangiopathic causes
of hemolysis, sickle cells in sickle cell anemia, and el-
liptocytes in conditions with inherited abnormalities in
the RBC membrane such as hereditary elliptocytosis.

13. **D.** A patient with known hematologic malignancy
accompanied by evidence of hemolysis and positive
IgG on Coombs testing suggests a diagnosis of warm
AIHA, for which frontline therapy is corticosteroids.
The patient is hemodynamically stable with an Hb
above the typical transfusion threshold and does not
require RBC transfusion. Splenectomy can be utilized in warm AIHA but is not considered frontline
therapy. Eculizumab is used to treat paroxysmal nocturnal hemoglobinuria and does not have a role in
the treatment of warm AIHA.

14. **C.** Aplastic anemia is associated with pancytopenia
with involvement of 2 or more lineages in the peripheral blood smear, such as low platelet count ($<50 \times 10^9$/L).

15. **B.** Pernicious anemia is an autoimmune condition in
which patients have autoantibodies to intrinsic factor, which impairs absorption of oral B12 by the gastric mucosa. The most effective way to correct B12
deficiency in these patients is with parenteral supplementation of vitamin B12.

16. **B.** Bone marrow biopsy is required to establish the
diagnosis of AA.

17. **C.** Direct bilirubin is usually normal in a patient presenting with hemolysis, whereas indirect bilirubin is elevated due to breakdown of RBCs into unconjugated
bilirubin. Haptoglobin is often decreased; free Hb released from RBC breakdown binds circulating haptoglobin. Reticulocyte count is typically elevated as the
bone marrow produces new RBCs to compensate for
the peripheral destruction of RBCs resulting in anemia.

18. **A.** Observation and supportive care is the recommended treatment for an 85-year-old male with
findings of moderate AA plus COPD, diabetes, and
dementia.

ANSWERS AND EXPLANATIONS TO SECTION B PRETEST

1. **D.** When determining the length of anticoagulation
for a newly diagnosed DVT, consider the patient's
family history of VTE, the presence of a provoking
event such as a recent surgery, and the presence of an
unresolved/persistent risk factor such as malignancy.

2. **C.** For the patient with triple positive antiphospholipid antibody syndrome and recurrent PE, warfarin
instead of a DOAC is first-line therapy.

3. **C.** Thrombophilia testing is warranted for the patient with recurrent provoked DVT in the setting of
mild provoking risk factors such as long-distance car
rides.

ANSWERS AND EXPLANATIONS TO SECTION C PRETEST

1. **B.** The most common cause of hemochromatosis is
hereditary hemochromatosis and so screening for
gene mutation is a good step in evaluation. A renal
ultrasound may be ordered if kidney function is altered but, in this case, is not the next step to confirm
a diagnosis of hemochromatosis. Typically, MRI, not
CT, is used to quantify iron deposition. An HbA1c
would be helpful to monitor diabetes but would
not be ordered to confirm a working diagnosis of
hemochromatosis.

2. **D.** Therapeutic phlebotomy is the preferred treatment for hemochromatosis. Iron chelation therapy is
a good answer but is not first line and is only utilized
if the patient is anemic or has other reason to not tolerate phlebotomy. Metformin may help treat diabetes but is not effective at treating hemochromatosis.
A liver transplant would not treat hemochromatosis
but may be necessary if the patient developed liver
failure.

3. **A.** In this condition, therapeutic phlebotomy is utilized to get to a goal of iron depletion with a ferritin
<50 ng/mL. The patient can then be transitioned to
maintenance level therapeutic phlebotomy of every 3
months to maintain a goal ferritin level between 20
and 50 ng/dL. The patient has hemochromatosis, and
the *HFE* gene testing will not change. The patient
needs to maintain normal Hb in order to use phlebotomy as hemochromatosis treatment. Hb is not
a measure of control of hemochromatosis. A TIBC
above 450 µg/dL usually means that there is a low
level of iron in the blood. This is not used to measure
control of hemochromatosis.

4. **C.** Dairy and gluten-containing products should not
affect hemochromatosis. Dietary recommendations
for patients with hemochromatosis include avoiding
iron supplements and multivitamins containing iron,
raw shellfish, vitamin C supplements, and alcohol.

ANSWERS AND EXPLANATIONS TO SECTION D PRETEST

1. **B.** Blood cultures should be drawn in patients with sickle cell anemia who are presenting with fever or other signs of infection. Routine laboratory tests include CBC, reticulocyte count, and renal and liver function tests.

2. **B.** Patients originating from Africa, the Middle East, India, Southeast Asia, Melanesia, and around the Mediterranean basin have an increased likelihood of thalassemia disorders.

3. **C.** In addition to routine childhood vaccinations, patients with sickle cell anemia should be immunized against pneumococcus and seasonal influenza.

4. **A.** Patients with thalassemia disorders can present commonly with hemolytic anemia, splenomegaly, and jaundice. However, many can present with asymptomatic hemolytic anemia. They can also have other symptoms depending on the type and severity of their disease. Increased bleeding is not a typical symptom.

5. **B.** Sickle cell disease is associated with hemolytic anemia, not anemia due to blood loss.

6. **C.** Hemoglobin Barts, also called hydrops fetalis, is a deletion of all four α-globin genes and is not compatible with life.

7. **A.** Dactylitis is one of the first signs of sickle cell anemia in young children. Hypoxia, pain, and priapism are presenting signs and symptoms of an acute sickle cell crisis.

8. **B.** Initial evaluation of suspected thalassemia syndromes can include CBC and iron studies. However, the first step would be a CBC to identify anemia before proceeding to iron studies. Hb electrophoresis is used after iron deficiency is ruled out.

9. **D.** Patients receiving chronic transfusions may require iron chelation therapy to prevent hemosiderosis.

10. **C.** Hb electrophoresis commonly shows an increased Hb A2 in β-thalassemia. In addition, thalassemia disorders can present with microcytic anemia and a normal RDW. Schistocytes are commonly seen in DIC.

ANSWERS AND EXPLANATIONS TO SECTION E PRETEST

1. **B.** An Auer rod is pathognomonic for AML. Smudge cells are commonly seen with CLL, Philadelphia chromosome with CML, and Howell-Jolly bodies with sickle cell anemia.

2. **B.** *JAK2* mutation is the most common cause for PV.

3. **A.** Advanced paternal age, maternal fetal loss, increased birth weight, and trisomy 21 are all risk factors for ALL.

4. **B.** Indications for treatment of CLL include worsening lymphadenopathy, splenomegaly, anemia, or thrombocytopenia; weight loss, extreme fatigue, fever, night sweats, and rapidly progressive lymphocytosis.

5. **D.** Advanced age, poor performance status, and certain cytogenetic abnormalities are all poor prognostic factors.

6. **C.** Chronic phase, accelerated phase, and blast crisis are all phases of CML.

7. **A.** Trisomy 21 is a risk factor for ALL, but not for AML.

8. **D.** Lymphocytosis, hepatosplenomegaly, and lymphadenopathy are all common findings in CML and CLL. Multiple ecchymotic areas are common in acute leukemia, such as AML and ALL.

9. **D.** All answers are correct because according to the WHO criteria, all of them are needed to make the diagnosis of PV.

10. **B.** Exposure to ionizing radiation is the only known risk factor for CML. Exposure to asbestos is known to cause mesothelioma, radon exposure is known to cause lung cancer, and exposure to arsenic in drinking water is known to cause bladder cancer.

11. **D.** An Hb of 11.0 g/dL is now low enough to classify as myeloma, and if lower would need to have additional workup to rule out other causes of anemia. Answers B and C are incorrect because SLiM-CRAB criteria include free light chain ratio of at least 100 and requires >1 focal lesion on MRI which must be at least 5 mm in diameter, respectively.

12. **A.** Therapeutic phlebotomy is the main treatment for decreasing RBC volume in PV.

13. **B.** A patient cannot be discharged from the emergency department without first evaluating for anemia, hypercalcemia, and AKI. These would be potential reasons to admit a patient or perform a higher level of care. The protein studies are important and could be ordered but results can take 1–7 days to obtain and usually will not change your acute management plan. PET-CT is typically reserved for outpatient ordering by a specialist.

14. **D.** According to the WHO, >20% blasts in the circulating blood or the bone marrow is diagnostic for acute leukemia.

15. **B.** This answer meets the >10% clonal plasmacytosis of the bone marrow with at least one bone lesion related to the plasma cell disorder (confirmed by biopsy). Answer A is incorrect because osteopenia itself does not make a diagnosis of MM. Answer C is representative of a solitary plasmacytoma since the bone marrow biopsy demonstrated <10% clonal plasma cells. D is representative of iron deficiency anemia secondary to blood loss; MM is ruled out with no clonal plasma cell disorder by serum protein electrophoresis.

16. **E.** Diet is not a known risk factor for the development of myelodysplastic syndrome.
17. **C.** The Philadelphia chromosome is pathognomonic for CML. Smudge cells are commonly seen with CLL, Auer rods with AML, and Howell-Jolly bodies with sickle cell disease.
18. **C.** One-third (33%) of patients will progress from myelodysplastic syndrome to AML.
19. **D.** PV due to a *JAK2* mutation results in an increase of all cell lines, not just RBCs.

▶ ANSWERS AND EXPLANATIONS TO SECTION F PRETEST

1. **A.** Confusion is due to obstruction of the microvasculature in TTP.
2. **C.** *E. coli O157:H7* is colonized in the intestines of cattle. When meat is contaminated with bacteria and ingested by a host, there is a chance of infection.
3. **A.** Accelerated platelet clearance is the primary cause of ITP.
4. **B.** HUS can affect anyone, but most often it is children.
5. **C.** Easy bruising in ITP is associated with a platelet count <50 000/μL.
6. **C.** Extravascular hemolysis is the breakdown of RBCs in the reticuloendothelial system, such as the spleen and liver. Patients with extravascular hemolysis can present with splenomegaly secondary to splenic hypertrophy and jaundice. Extravascular hemolysis is more common with RBC membrane disorders (eg., hereditary spherocytosis) but some forms of hemolytic anemia may include both intra- and extravascular hemolysis.
7. **D.** Prednisone is the most appropriate initial treatment for this patient.
8. **A.** A low platelet count is key for diagnosing HUS.
9. **C.** The pneumococcal vaccine is recommended before therapeutic splenectomy for ITP.
10. **D.** Schistocytes on peripheral blood smear are expected in TTP.

▶ ANSWERS AND EXPLANATIONS TO SECTION G PRETEST

1. **A.** Acute hemolysis is caused by recipient antibody destroying donor red cells. Transfusion associated circulatory overload is a nonimmune transfusion reaction not associated with hemolysis. Anamnestic response is seen with delayed hemolytic transfusion reactions. Hyperkalemia is a symptom in some transfusion reactions, not a cause.
2. **B.** Multiorgan failure can result from a severe inflammatory response. Elevated LDH is a symptom of hemolytic transfusion reactions, but not the cause of death. Hyperkalemia is a symptom of hemolytic transfusion reactions, but not the cause of death. Spherocytes can be observed on the peripheral smear, but are not the cause of death.
3. **C.** Patient misidentification is the most common preventable cause of fatal transfusion reactions. Transfusion-associated circulatory overload is a common cause of fatal transfusion reactions, but it is not the most common preventable cause. Bacterial contamination is a common cause of fatal transfusion reactions, but it is not the most common preventable cause.
4. **D.** Blood components (platelets, plasma, cryoprecipitate, and coagulation factors) are used to raise platelet counts and coagulation factor levels (especially fibrinogen) with this coagulopathy. Calcium gluconate is used to treat hyperkalemia, not DIC. Aggressive hydration is to support renal output, not DIC. Dialysis may be necessary with renal failure associated with free Hb.
5. **B.** Extravascular hemolysis is associated with delayed hemolytic transfusion reactions. This is a delayed hemolytic transfusion reaction 7 days after transfusion. Intravascular hemolysis is associated with acute hemolytic transfusion reactions. This is a delayed hemolytic transfusion reaction 7 days after transfusion. Bacterial contamination would have more acute, severe symptoms of high fever, hypotension, and shock. These minor symptoms are associated with delayed hemolysis. DIC would have more severe, acute symptoms including mucosal bleeding and bruising due to coagulopathy, shortness of breath, and hypotension.

Iron Deficiency Anemia

Cassiopeia Frank, MMSc

▶ GENERAL FEATURES

- Iron deficiency anemia is characterized by low hemoglobin/hematocrit with hypochromasia and microcytosis with low reticulocyte count.
- Platelets may be elevated.
- Iron studies demonstrate low iron, low transferrin saturation, and low ferritin.
- Etiology of iron deficiency is variable but can include decreased iron intake, poor absorption, or blood loss.
- Decreased intake is generally due to dietary restrictions.
- Poor absorption can occur in the setting of gastric bypass surgery or other GI surgery impacting absorption.
- Chronic blood loss can occur from menorrhagia or occult or frank GI bleeding.
- Symptoms may include those characteristic of anemia such as dyspnea, fatigue, and decreased concentration.
- Symptoms may also be more specific to iron deficiency including brittle hair or nails and pica.

▶ CLINICAL ASSESSMENT

- Complete a thorough history including evaluation of dietary intake, surgical history, family history, and assessment of possible bleeding sources such as GI bleeding and menorrhagia.
- Physical examination includes evaluation of heart rate and respiratory rate, which may be elevated with severe anemia, as well as skin and mucosal changes (pallor, jaundice).
- An abdominal examination may also reveal signs of other causes of anemia (hepatomegaly, splenomegaly) or indications of GI pathology, including mass or tenderness.
- Consideration of alternative causes of anemia should be included in a patient with other symptoms, abnormalities in other cell lines, or family history of other forms of anemia.

▶ DIAGNOSIS

- A full laboratory evaluation for iron deficiency anemia should be completed at presentation and include CBC, reticulocytes, and iron studies (including iron, iron-binding capacity, iron saturation, and ferritin).
- Erythrocyte sedimentation rate and C-reactive protein can also be helpful in detecting overall inflammation for context as the ferritin value can be misleading when evaluated alone.
- Anemia with microcytosis, hypochromasia, and corresponding low iron studies is consistent with iron deficiency anemia.
- Evaluation for the underlying etiology of iron deficiency may also include accompanying diagnosis of menorrhagia or source of GI bleeding.
- Unexplained anemia is an indication for GI evaluation including colonoscopy and upper endoscopy.

▶ TREATMENT

- Initial management includes oral iron supplements, which should be taken as tolerated.
- Increasing dietary iron content is also encouraged.
- In patients who cannot tolerate oral iron supplementation due to constipation or other side effects, or those with impaired absorption due to history of bypass or other pathology, IV iron should be considered.
- IV iron comes in multiple forms and can be given in a wide range of dosages; all forms of IV iron carry risk of anaphylactic infusion reaction, and the patient should be appropriately counseled, premedicated, and monitored.
- Monitoring of response to oral or IV iron should be conducted at 3- to 12-month intervals with repeat labs and symptom assessment.

CHAPTER 177

Anemia of Chronic Disease, Vitamin B12, and Folate Deficiency

Amber Koehler, MPAS, PA-C

▶ GENERAL FEATURES

- Anemia of chronic disease results from abnormalities in iron homeostasis due to chronic inflammation, resulting in decreased production of red blood cells (RBCs); if related to malignancy or infection, direct cellular destruction of RBCs can also occur.
- Anemia of chronic disease is typically normocytic, whereas anemia due to vitamin B12 or folate deficiency is typically macrocytic.
- Anemia of chronic disease is generally a diagnosis of exclusion; laboratory tests can confirm deficiencies in vitamin B12 or folate.
- Folate deficiency is uncommon in developed countries but can be seen in high-risk populations.
- B12 deficiency is typically related to either inadequate oral intake or malabsorption syndromes.

▶ CLINICAL ASSESSMENT

- Patients may present with symptoms related to anemia, including fatigue, shortness of breath, and conjunctival pallor, but may be asymptomatic.
- Malignancy, infections, or inflammatory conditions can be associated with anemia of chronic disease; it can also be seen in obesity, diabetes mellitus, and heart failure, among other conditions.
- Patients who follow vegan or vegetarian diets or those from developing countries are at increased risk for vitamin B12 and folate deficiency due to inadequate dietary intake, as are patients with chronic alcohol abuse; conditions that impact absorption such as gastritis, malabsorption syndromes, celiac disease, inflammatory bowel disease, small bowel bacterial overgrowth, or history of gastric bypass surgery also increase the risk for vitamin B12 or folate deficiency.
- Neurologic symptoms such as symmetric paresthesias or numbness as well as gait abnormalities and weakness are classic symptoms associated with B12 deficiency, as is glossitis (inflammation and soreness of the tongue).
- Neuropsychiatric symptoms such as depression, irritability, insomnia, cognitive slowing, forgetfulness, and dementia, among others, can be seen in both vitamin B12 and folate deficiency.
- Certain medications such as methotrexate, sulfamethoxazole, and phenytoin can be associated with folate deficiency.

▶ DIAGNOSIS

- Initial laboratory evaluation should include a CBC to confirm the presence of anemia and to determine mean corpuscular volume (MCV).

- Iron studies can be useful for further evaluation of suspected anemia of chronic disease. Typical findings include low serum iron, low transferrin and transferrin saturation, and normal or increased ferritin levels. In contrast, iron deficiency anemia is marked by increased transferrin and decreased ferritin levels.
- Additional markers of inflammation such as C-reactive protein (CRP) and erythrocyte sedimentation rate (ESR) may be elevated in patients with chronic inflammatory conditions, resulting in anemia of chronic disease.
- Peripheral blood smear may demonstrate hypersegmented neutrophils in patients with vitamin B12 or folate deficiency.
- Methylmalonic acid (MMA) and homocysteine levels can be helpful if you suspect vitamin B12 or folate deficiency.
  - In B12 deficiency, MMA is elevated because vitamin B12 is an essential cofactor in the metabolism of MMA.
  - Both vitamin B12 and folate are required for the metabolism of homocysteine; elevated homocysteine levels can be seen in both vitamin B12 and folate deficiency.
  - A normal MMA but elevated homocysteine level suggests folate deficiency.
- In patients with B12 deficiency without an obvious cause, consider testing for autoantibodies to intrinsic factor (IF), which are present in an autoimmune condition that impairs vitamin B12 absorption called pernicious anemia.

▶ TREATMENT

- The mainstay of treatment for anemia of chronic disease is treatment of the underlying condition. Iron supplementation and transfusions are typically not indicated.
- Patients with anemia due to vitamin B12 deficiency without significant symptoms can be managed with oral supplementation; patients with vitamin B12 deficiency presenting with severe anemia or significant neurologic or neuropsychiatric symptoms, or those with pernicious anemia, should be treated with parenteral vitamin B12.
- Folate deficiency anemia is typically treated with oral supplementation, though intravenous folic acid is available for patients requiring more rapid correction or those who cannot take oral medications.

CHAPTER 178

Hemolytic Anemia

Amber Koehler, MPAS, PA-C

▶ GENERAL FEATURES

- Hemolytic anemia should be suspected in patients presenting with anemia and reticulocytosis without evidence of bleeding.
- Causes of hemolytic anemia can be categorized into inherited vs. acquired, intrinsic vs. extrinsic to the red blood cell (RBC), immune mediated vs. non–immune mediated, and intravascular vs. extravascular.
  - Causes of hemolysis intrinsic to the RBC are typically inherited; causes extrinsic to the RBC are typically acquired.
- Hemolytic anemia causes premature destruction of RBCs and can present as acute or chronic and compensated or uncompensated.

▶ CLINICAL ASSESSMENT

- Assess for findings related to anemia, including fatigue, shortness of breath, and conjunctival pallor.
- Jaundice and scleral icterus may be present due to breakdown of RBCs into unconjugated bilirubin.
- Hematuria can occur if levels of intravascular hemolysis overwhelm the kidney's ability to reabsorb free hemoglobin.
- Petechiae and purpura may occur if hemolysis is due to thrombotic thrombocytopenic purpura (TTP), hemolytic uremic syndrome (HUS), disseminated intravascular coagulation (DIC), or HELLP (Hemolysis, Elevated Liver enzymes, Low Platelets).
- Assess recent infectious history for potential causes of hemolysis:
  - Mononucleosis and mycoplasma pneumonia are associated with cold autoimmune hemolytic anemia (AIHA).
  - Malaria, *Babesiosis*, and *Bartonella* can cause parasitic infections of RBCs.
- Ensure a complete medication history:
  - Dapsone, sulfamethoxazole, and methylene blue can cause oxidative stress and subsequent hemolysis in G6PD deficiency.
  - Valproic acid and immunosuppressive therapies such as cyclosporine or tacrolimus can cause microangiopathic hemolytic anemia (MAHA).
  - Antibiotics including penicillin and cephalosporins can cause AIHA.
- Suspect hereditary spherocytosis in children presenting with episodic history of anemia and jaundice.
- Consider other aspects of the history:
  - Sickle cell anemia is more common in African American patients.
  - Hemolysis after exposure to a new medication in African American or Mediterranean patients suggests G6PD deficiency.
  - Presence of hematologic malignancy:
    - Chronic lymphocytic leukemia (CLL) and non-Hodgkin Lymphoma (NHL) are associated with warm AIHA.
    - Lymphoplasmacytic lymphoma/Waldenstrom macroglobulinemia is associated with cold AIHA.
  - Mechanical heart valves and splenomegaly can cause mechanical hemolysis.

▶ DIAGNOSIS

- Typical laboratory findings include:
  - Anemia
    - Thrombocytopenia may also be present if hemolysis is due to TTP, HUS, DIC, or HELLP.
  - Reticulocytosis due to increased production of RBCs
  - Elevated indirect bilirubin and LDH due to RBC breakdown
    - Direct bilirubin is usually normal.
  - Decreased haptoglobin; free hemoglobin released by RBC breakdown binds circulating haptoglobin.
- Peripheral smear can provide clues to the cause of hemolysis:
  - Schistocytes suggest intravascular hemolysis, including mechanical and microangiopathic causes.
  - Sickle cells suggest sickle cell anemia.
  - Bite cells and Heinz bodies can be seen in G6PD deficiency.
  - Spherocytes suggest the presence of RBC membrane defects, including hereditary spherocytosis.
- Additional testing may include:
  - Hemoglobin electrophoresis to confirm hemoglobinopathy
  - Coombs testing to confirm AIHA
    - IgG is positive in warm AIHA and negative in cold AIHA.
    - Complement is positive in cold AIHA.
  - Osmotic fragility testing to confirm inherited defects in the RBC membrane

▶ TREATMENT

- Always stabilize the patient first: in acute, uncompensated hemolysis, transfuse if necessary.
- Blood products should be warmed before transfusion for patients with cold AIHA.

- Next steps in treatment depend on the cause of hemolysis:
  - Frontline therapy of warm AIHA is corticosteroids; patients with cold AIHA should avoid exposure to cold.
  - In hemolytic anemia due to medications and/or G6PD deficiency, discontinue the offending agent.
    - Patients with G6PD deficiency should avoid oxidative agents and fava beans.

- Paroxysmal nocturnal hemoglobinuria (PNH) is treated with eculizumab.
  - Splenectomy is the treatment of choice for hereditary spherocytosis.
- Folate supplementation is recommended in patients with chronic hemolysis.

CHAPTER 179

Aplastic Anemia

Natasha McKee, MMSc, PA-C

▶ GENERAL FEATURES

- Aplastic anemia (AA) is a life-threatening form of bone marrow failure.
  - Characterized by ancytopenia secondary to bone marrow hypoplasia or aplasia
  - Usually due to immune injury of multipotent hematopoietic stem cells (HSCs)
- Left untreated, AA has a high mortality rate.
- Rare, with incidence of ~2 per million in Western countries and 2–3 times higher in Asia
  - Incidence in males and female is similar.
  - Approximately half of cases occur in the first three decades of life.
- Often considered idiopathic, though certain drugs, radiation, toxins, viral infections, and inherited genetic disorders are known causes

▶ CLINICAL ASSESSMENT

- Patients complain of easy bruising or bleeding; this may include frequent nosebleeds, bleeding gums, or menorrhagia.
- New petechiae or pallor of the skin may be noted secondary to thrombocytopenia.
- Frequent or recurring infections, often bacterial, including pneumonia, urinary tract infections, or sepsis due to neutropenia
- General fatigue due to anemia
- Liver, spleen, or lymph node enlargement is generally not present.
- Short stature, microcephaly, development delay, or nail dystrophy may be present (more commonly in children) and be representative of an inherited disorder.

▶ DIAGNOSIS

- CBC reveals pancytopenia.
  - Reticulocytopenia is present, and peripheral blood smear reveals normocytic red blood cells.

- No abnormal cells would be seen that would be indicative of a blood disorder.
- Serum chemistries, liver and renal function tests, and vitamin B12 and folate levels should be performed to exclude other causes of anemia.
- Bone marrow biopsy is required to establish the diagnosis and rule out other causes of pancytopenia.
- AA is defined as pancytopenia with hypocellular bone marrow in the absence of an abnormal infiltrate or marrow fibrosis; bone marrow findings of AA include:
  - Profound decrease in all cellular elements
  - Residual HSCs that are morphologically normal, and hematopoiesis is not megaloblastic.
  - Infiltration of the bone marrow with malignant cells or fibrosis is not present.
- Diagnostic criteria:
  - Severe AA (sAA): bone marrow cellularity <25% and at least two of the following:
    - Absolute neutrophil count (ANC) <500/μL
    - Platelet count <20 000/μL
    - Reticulocyte count <20 000/μL
  - Very severe AA (vsAA): includes above criteria plus ANC <200/μL
  - Non-sAA: hypocellular bone marrow without blood cytopenia criteria as described above
- Further testing may be ordered to detect the presence of coexistent disorders or an inherited genetic abnormality. Megaloblastic anemia, infiltrative disorders (ie, myelodysplastic syndrome, primary myelofibrosis, large granular lymphocytosis), hypersplenism, and reversible causes such as drugs, toxins, viral infections, and radiation exposure must be ruled out.

▶ TREATMENT

- Referral to hematology is necessary; in addition, these patients often need to be referred to a transplant center.
- Management depends on the underlying cause and severity of disease.

- Initial supportive care includes transfusions and prophylaxis (antibiotic, antiviral, and antifungal); transfusions should be used with caution to minimize sensitization to donor antigens.
- Reversible causes (drug, radiation, or viral infection) should be removed or treated; further treatment may be required even while waiting for spontaneous resolution.
- Treatment of vsAA and sAA is based on age, availability of an HSC donor, and clinical status.
- For patients aged <20 years, an HSC transplant (HCT) is the recommended treatment and should be performed as soon as a matched donor is identified.

- Between the ages of 20 and 50 years, HCT is generally the preferred treatment for those in good health with a matched donor available.
- For those aged >50 years, the upper age limit for recommending HCT continues to increase as a result of advances in therapy and improved outcomes, though increasing age correlates with increasing toxicities of treatment.
- Graft-versus-host disease (GVHD) may occur as a result of HCT and is a high cause of morbidity and mortality and may lead to a more quality of life.
- Immunosuppressive therapy (IST) is the alternative treatment to HCT and is associated with lower survival rates.

SECTION B *Coagulation Disorders*

CHAPTER 180 Coagulation Disorders

Cassiopeia Frank, MMSc

▶ GENERAL FEATURES

- Venous thrombosis (DVT) and venous thromboembolism (VTE) can be initially categorized into "provoked" events for which a mild, moderate, or strong risk factor was present, or "unprovoked" where no risk factor is identified; in addition to provoking events, underlying persistent risk factors contribute to the acute event.
- Transient provoking risk factors include surgery, trauma, immobility, and exogenous hormone use, such as oral contraceptive pills.
- Underlying risk factors, which require consideration, include persistent but modifiable risk factors such as underlying malignancy or obesity as well as nonmodifiable risk factors such as acquired or hereditary thrombophilia and family history of VTE.
- Acquired thrombophilia includes antiphospholipid antibody syndrome, which can develop at any time and may or may not present with family history of VTE.
- Hereditary thrombophilias may be accompanied by positive family history and most commonly include factor V Leiden mutation, prothrombin 20210 mutation, antithrombin deficiency, and protein S or C deficiency.

- Distal and superficial thrombosis is typically managed with serial monitoring or 3 months of anticoagulation and, in most cases, does not require consideration of longer term therapy or thrombophilia evaluation.

▶ CLINICAL ASSESSMENT

- Thorough history is essential in determining the constellation of factors contributing to the development of acute or recurrent VTE.
  - A meticulous assessment of both transient and persistent risk factors should be collected for each event.
  - Further, an overall assessment of history of other provoking events and the occurrence of VTE should be evaluated (prior pregnancies, surgeries, etc.) as well as a thorough family history.
- Imaging should be obtained with each event and ideally whenever discontinuing anticoagulation to establish a new baseline and avoid misdiagnosis of recurrence.
- Consideration of acquired or inherited thrombophilia should be considered in the setting of unprovoked VTE or recurrent VTE.
- In some cases, consideration of thrombophilia testing is warranted with a provoked DVT in a patient with

VTE in an unusual location, strong family history, or persistent nonmodifiable risk factors.

- For provoked DVT with no family or personal history of VTE, thrombophilia is not recommended.
- A decision to pursue thrombophilia testing should only be made when it will change decision-making and when the ordering provider is able to appropriately interpret results.

▶ DIAGNOSIS

- Testing for acquired thrombophilia should include antiphospholipid antibody testing.
  - These include cardiolipin antibodies, β-2 glycoprotein antibodies, and lupus anticoagulant.
  - To confirm antiphospholipid syndrome, at least one of these must be persistently elevated on two samples collected at least 12 weeks apart.
- Testing for inherited thrombophilia includes factor V and factor II mutation testing, protein S and protein C activity and antigen levels, and antithrombin III levels.
- Age-appropriate malignancy screening is recommended to rule out malignancy as a provoking factor.

▶ TREATMENT

- Long-term anticoagulation is recommended for unprovoked VTE and should be considered in individuals with provoked DVT with persistent risk factors.
- Long-term anticoagulation should be considered for individuals with history of VTE and an acquired or hereditary thrombophilia; risk assessment should be discussed with the patient based on their specific thrombophilia and bleeding risks.
- Direct oral anticoagulants are recommended in most cases as first-line therapy. Exceptions include triple positive antiphospholipid syndrome (elevation in all three antiphospholipid antibodies) for which a vitamin K antagonist should be considered.
- Annual CBC and renal function assessment should be collected for patients on long-term anticoagulation to monitor for occult blood loss, changes in platelets, or need for change in drug or dosing with changes in renal function.

SECTION **C**   *Hemochromatosis*

CHAPTER **181**

Hemochromatosis

Sonya Peters, PA-C

A 59-year-old white male presented to primary care with concerns of an elevated blood sugar. At a recent health screening at a local grocery store, his blood sugar was found to be 276 mg/dL. He had fasted for 12 hours before this test was performed. His BMI is 20. He has no significant past medical history. He reports body weakness and has noticed his skin is "more tan" than it used to be at this time of year. He feels well. He denies a family history of diabetes but reports a brother with cirrhosis and alcoholism who died at age 52 years. He is not aware of other family members with liver disease. The patient denies alcohol use. On examination, he was found to have hepatomegaly. An abdominal ultrasound reveals cirrhosis. His labs revealed a markedly elevated ferritin and transferrin saturation. What other tests should you order to solidify your working diagnosis?

▶ GENERAL FEATURES

- Hemochromatosis is characterized by iron overload and deposition into organs.
- Most commonly attributed to hereditary hemochromatosis:
  - C282Y mutation on the "high Fe" or HFE hemochromatosis gene is the primary cause.
  - Also linked to mutations in the *HJV, HAMP, TFR2,* and *SLC40A1* genes
- Secondary causes of iron overload include:
  - Parenteral overload of iron
  - Iron-loading anemias (thalassemia major/intermedia, sideroblastic anemia, inherited anemias)
  - Gestational alloimmune liver disease
  - Dysmetabolic iron overload syndrome
  - Chronic liver disease

- Risk factors:
  - Family history of hemochromatosis in a first-degree relative
  - Northern European ethnicity
  - Male sex
- Generally asymptomatic at presentation; identification of abnormal liver function tests or screening due to family history are common.
- Symptoms usually present between the ages of 50–60 years in men and after age 60 years in women (when iron is no longer lost through menstruation).
- Iron can deposit in any organ, although deposition generally occurs first in the liver, because blood containing iron absorbed from the gastrointestinal tract passes through the liver first before other organs; cirrhosis is a common result.
- Individuals are also at an elevated risk for diabetes mellitus, cardiomyopathy, and hypogonadism due to iron deposition.
- If treated before organ damage, life expectancy is normal.

CLINICAL ASSESSMENT

- Individuals may be found to have multiple symptoms along with laboratory abnormalities, including:
  - Liver function abnormalities
  - Weakness and lethargy
  - Skin hyperpigmentation
  - Diabetes mellitus
  - Arthralgia
  - Impotence in males
  - ECG abnormalities

DIAGNOSIS

- Clinical diagnosis of iron overload is based on transferrin saturation >45% or an elevated ferritin level >150 ng/mL in women and >200 ng/mL in men.
- If either test meets these thresholds, next steps in evaluation would include:
  - Gene mutation testing
  - MRI of the liver with the addition of any organs that may be affected based on labs and symptoms (eg, heart, pancreas)
  - Liver biopsy can be helpful in assessing the extent of fibrosis and presence of cirrhosis as well as other causes of liver disease that may be contributing to liver injury.
- Increased ferritin levels can be caused by any inflammatory state, so individuals with isolated increased ferritin level may need testing to rule out the following conditions:
  - Alcoholic liver disease
  - Nonalcoholic liver disease
  - Hemolysis
  - Ineffective erythropoiesis
  - Chronic liver disease

- Screening for hemochromatosis is recommended for all first-degree relatives of patients who have hereditary hemochromatosis.

TREATMENT

- Phlebotomy is the treatment of choice for individuals with iron overload, given in two phases:
  - Initial treatment:
    - Initiated upon diagnosis
    - Used to achieve an iron depleted state (ferritin <50 ng/mL)
    - Typically done weekly unless the patient becomes anemia
  - Maintenance treatment:
    - Initiated once iron depleted state achieved
    - Typically done once every 3–4 months unless patient becomes anemic
    - Target ferritin level is 20–50 ng/mL
    - Typically done weekly unless the patient becomes anemia
- Iron chelation therapy is reserved for patients who cannot undergo phlebotomy due to conditions like anemia.
- Routine laboratory tests to screen for condition worsening are recommended every 6–12 months and include a CBC, liver function tests, and iron studies.
- Given increased risk of hepatocellular carcinoma, it is recommended that patients have a liver ultrasound and α-fetoprotein completed every 6 months.
- Patients who have hereditary hemochromatosis should avoid:
  - Iron supplements
  - Multivitamins containing iron
  - Vitamin C supplements
  - Alcohol
  - Raw shellfish
- Liver transplant is utilized if liver failure develops.

Case Conclusion

This is a classic example of hemochromatosis. The patient is between the ages of 50 and 60 years, male, and white (potentially of Northern European decent). He was mostly asymptomatic until he became diabetic. He had noticed weakness and skin hyperpigmentation, which are signs of hemochromatosis. His diabetes was more suspect to underlying disorder because he had no family history of diabetes, and he was not overweight. He has a first-degree relative who died of liver disease at a young age. Although his brother did have a history of alcohol use/abuse, death at the age of 52 years of cirrhosis may arise suspicion to an underlying disorder contributing to the damage from the alcohol abuse. Finally, the markedly elevated ferritin and transferrin saturation leads further to the suspicion of hemochromatosis.

CHAPTER 182

Sickle Cell Disease

Johanna D'Addario, PA-C

▶ GENERAL FEATURES

- Sickle cell disease is an autosomal-recessive inherited condition most commonly diagnosed in families of African descent.
- Homozygous sickle cell anemia is characterized by the genotype Hb SS.
- Hb SS disease leads to chronic, intrinsic hemolytic anemia due to sickling of RBCs in hypoxemic or acidotic states.
- Sickled RBCs cause endothelial damage, and vaso-occlusion of small blood vessels by sickled RBCs leads to pain, inflammation, tissue ischemia, and necrosis.
- Acute splenic sequestration of RBCs can lead to acute decreases in hemoglobin, hypovolemia, hypoxia, and, potentially, death.
- Functional asplenia causes increased risk of bacterial infections, including pneumonia, meningitis, osteomyelitis, and sepsis.
- Other complications include stroke, retinopathy, acute chest syndrome, pulmonary hypertension, cholelithiasis, splenic infarction, renal disease, priapism, and avascular necrosis.
- Evolving research has shown that climate factors (temperature, humidity, wind, air quality) may be related to increased acute pain episodes and hospitalizations.
- Although life expectancy has improved for patients with sickle cell anemia, patients are known to have a shortened life span due to complications of the disease.

▶ CLINICAL ASSESSMENT

- Family history is the key to diagnosis and can be diagnosed by newborn screening.
- Often asymptomatic in infancy due to the presence of fetal hemoglobin (Hb F).
- Dactylitis is one of the first manifestations of disease in young children.

- Physical examination findings include systolic murmur, hepatosplenomegaly, jaundice or pallor, and delayed growth.
- Symptoms of vaso-occlusive crisis include severe musculoskeletal, abdominal, and/or back pain; fever or priapism may also be present.
- Acute chest syndrome presents with hypoxia, fever, tachycardia, and abnormal lung sounds.
- Long-term complications of sickle cell disease affect multiple organ systems and include cognitive impairment, retinopathy, chronic lung disease, pulmonary hypertension, avascular necrosis, renal failure, and cholelithiasis.

▶ DIAGNOSIS

- Sickle cell disease can be identified during prenatal testing or newborn screening, which can allow for early diagnosis and intervention to prevent complications.
- Sickle cell anemia manifests as chronic hemolytic anemia with normal to high MCV, reticulocytosis, and leukocytosis.
- Serum haptoglobin is low or absent, with elevated bilirubin and lactate dehydrogenase:
  - Peripheral blood smear reveals sickled RBCs, target cells, and Howell-Jolly bodies.
  - Additional evaluation depends on the clinical picture:
    - Chest radiograph reveals pulmonary infiltrate(s) in acute chest syndrome.
    - MRI or bone scan can be used if osteomyelitis is suspected.
    - Brain imaging to evaluate for stroke in patients with neurologic symptoms
    - Patients presenting with fever should be thoroughly evaluated for infection, including blood cultures.

▶ TREATMENT

- Ideally, patients are managed in a sickle cell disease program for chronic disease management and to prevent acute conditions related to sickle cell disease.
- Once the diagnosis of sickle cell anemia is established, patients should be closely managed with regular screenings including:
  - CBC, reticulocyte count, renal and liver function tests, urinalysis
  - Pulmonary function tests
  - Neurophysiologic testing
  - Transcranial Doppler
  - Retinal examinations
  - Echocardiogram
- Prevention of pain crises is achieved by adequate hydration and avoidance of smoking, high altitude, infection, and hypoxia.
- Oral hydroxyurea is used to prevent acute sickle cell crises, acute chest syndrome, and stroke.
- Patients receiving chronic transfusions may require iron chelation therapy to prevent hemosiderosis.
- Antibiotic prophylaxis against *Streptococcus pneumoniae* sepsis with oral penicillin 62.5–250 mg twice daily is given to young children until at least age 5.
- Immunizations against pneumococcus and influenza are necessary, in addition to routine childhood vaccinations.
- Address psychosocial issues, including delayed growth and puberty, activity limitations (avoidance of dehydration, cold temperatures, smoking, alcohol, and drug use), contraception and family planning, impact of chronic disease, and awareness of decreased life span
- Genetic counseling should be provided to all patients with sickle cell anemia and sickle cell trait.
- Women with sickle cell disease who become pregnant are at high risk of preterm labor, low birth weight, or other complications and should be managed by a high-risk obstetrician.
- Hematopoietic stem cell transplantation may be considered in patients with significant complications but carries significant associated risks.
- Management of acute complications:
  - Treatment of pain crises including supplemental oxygen, analgesics, and fluids NSAIDs, acetaminophen, or opioids can alleviate pain.
  - Severe pain requiring hospitalization is treated with parenteral analgesics or patient-controlled analgesia.
  - Broad-spectrum antibiotics should be initiated promptly if signs of infection are present.
  - Acute chest syndrome is treated with oxygen, incentive spirometry, and antibiotics including coverage for atypical organisms.
  - Urology consultation should be obtained for prolonged priapism that does not respond to hydration and analgesics.
  - Blood transfusions may be used in select patients with acute chest syndrome, splenic sequestration, aplastic crisis, abnormal transcranial Doppler studies, and before surgical procedures.

CHAPTER
183

Thalassemias

Brittany Strelow, MS, PA-C

▶ GENERAL FEATURES

- Congenital disorders of hemoglobin production
  - α- or β-globin chain is produced in inadequate amounts.
- Most common monogenic disease worldwide
- Two main types, classified according to globin chains:
  - α:
    - Hemoglobin Barts (hydrops fetalis):
      - Deletion of all four α-globin genes
      - Most severe form of α-thalassemia
      - Incompatible with life
- Hemoglobin H disease:
  - Deletion of three of four α-globin genes
  - Moderately severe form of α-thalassemia
  - Results in chronic hemolytic anemia
- α-Thalassemia trait:
  - Deletion of one to two α-globin genes
  - Associated with red blood cell microcytosis
  - No clinical significance
  - Detected typically on routine blood count

- β:
  - Transfusion-dependent β-thalassemia:
    - Often associated with deletion of both β-globin genes
    - Severe form of β-thalassemia
    - Management with blood transfusions and iron chelation
    - Age of presentation: 6–12 months
  - Nontransfusion-dependent β-thalassemia:
    - A less severe form of β-thalassemia
    - Does not require regular blood transfusions
    - Age of presentation: 2–4 years
  - β-Thalassemia trait: little or no clinical significance
- Risk factors: patients originating from Africa, the Middle East, India, Southeast Asia, Melanesia, and around the Mediterranean basin

CLINICAL ASSESSMENT

- Individuals with β and α can have variable presentations:
  - Many are found incidentally on routine examinations.
  - However, some α disorders may be found after a pregnancy loss.
  - In β-thalassemia, newborns are typically asymptomatic; yet, many are found within the first year of life.
- Possible signs and symptoms:
  - Asymptomatic microcytic hypochromic anemia
  - Iron overload
  - Hepatosplenomegaly
  - Cholelithiasis/hyperbilirubinemia
  - Skeletal changes:
    - Facial deformity
    - Changes in body habitus
    - Osteopenia/osteoporosis
    - Bony masses
    - Pain
  - Growth impairment
  - Endocrine/metabolic abnormalities:
    - Hypogonadism
    - Hypothyroidism
    - Insulin resistance and diabetes
  - Heart failure and arrhythmias
  - Pulmonary abnormalities and pulmonary hypertension
  - Thrombosis
  - Leg ulcers

DIAGNOSIS

- Perform CBC, iron studies, and hemoglobin electrophoresis:
  - CBC shows microcytic red blood cell indices with or without anemia.
  - Iron studies:
  - Hemoglobin electrophoresis
    - After iron deficiency is ruled out
    - Hemoglobin A2 level elevated
- May consider genetic testing:
  - Does not impact patient management
  - Required only when the patient is considering pregnancy.
    - If found to have or be a carrier for a significant hemoglobinopathy, the partner or other sperm donor should be tested.
    - If both parents have the thalassemia trait, offspring could be born with one of the more severe thalassemia syndromes; referral to a genetic counselor.
- Newborn screening panel: screening panels may vary from state to state.

TREATMENT

- Minor thalassemia syndromes:
  - α- and β-thalassemia traits
  - Treatment is not required.
- More severe forms of thalassemia may require:
  - Blood transfusions, especially when experiencing a drop in hemoglobin concentration, such as during infections, pregnancy, or surgery
  - Iron chelation
  - Splenectomy
  - Folate
- Avoid iron supplementation as these patients are at risk for iron overload.
- Perioperative precautions:
  - Thalassemia trait: none
  - More severe forms of thalassemia: preoperative hematology consult

CHAPTER

184

Acute Leukemias

Jill Gore, PA-C

A 72-year-old male presents to his primary care provider's office with a 2-week history of progressive dyspnea and fatigue. He has a 10 pack-year history of smoking but quit over 20 years ago. He has felt intermittently sweaty but has not taken his temperature. He has soreness in his left upper abdomen and is easily satiated. Subsequently, he has lost about 10 lb in the past month. You notice multiple ecchymotic areas on his extremities. A CBC is performed and reveals the following abnormalities: WBC: 78 000 with 28% myeloblasts, Hgb: 10.8, Hct: 31.1, Plt: 81 000. What is the most likely diagnosis?

▶ GENERAL FEATURES

- Acute lymphoblastic leukemia (ALL) and acute myeloid leukemia (AML) are malignant disorders of the bone marrow, resulting in excessive, uncontrolled production of immature WBCs.
- Most cases of ALL have an idiopathic cause.
  - Increased incidence in children with advanced paternal age and maternal fetal loss
  - Increased birth weight may be a risk factor. Despite this, ALL is not considered to be a familial disease.
  - Trisomy 21 predisposes patients to an increased risk of ALL by 10- to 20-fold.
- AML has been associated with environmental factors, including exposure to chemicals, radiation, tobacco, chemotherapy, and retroviruses.
  - It can also be preceded by another hematologic disorder, such as myelodysplastic syndrome (MDS).
  - Inherited genetic abnormalities are rarely associated with AML.
- ALL is the most common childhood malignancy, with a peak incidence between the ages of 2 and 5 years.
  - ALL accounts for 74% of childhood leukemia, but only 20% of adult leukemia.
  - Unlike childhood ALL, which is curable, adult ALL carries a poor prognosis.

- AML is more common in adults, with a median age of 65 years at presentation.
- Identifying genetic mutations, including chromosomal translocations, deletions, and inversions, is important in determining treatment and clinical outcomes in patients diagnosed with acute leukemia. In addition to age, certain karyotypes (also referred to as "cytogenetics") are known to carry a favorable, intermediate, or unfavorable prognosis.
- According to the National Cancer Institute (NCI), the remission rate for children with ALL is ~98%.
  - Children with ALL have an 85% likelihood of cure; this rate decreases in adolescents.
  - In adults, prognosis is poor, with a cure rate of about 40%.
- Advanced age and poor performance status are the main prognostic predictors in AML.
  - Patients aged >60 years have a median survival of <1 year.
  - Patients aged <60 years typically achieve a complete remission; however, relapse is common, and a 5-year survival is <50%.

▶ CLINICAL ASSESSMENT

- Symptoms are present for only a short time, typically days to weeks, and are related to pancytopenia.
  - Neutropenia may lead to bacterial or fungal infection, such as cellulitis, pneumonia, or perirectal infection. Excessive blast production may produce symptoms of gum hypertrophy and, more often in children, bone pain.
  - Patients frequently complain of easy bruising and prolonged bleeding. Gingival bleeding, epistaxis, or menorrhagia may be noted.
  - Signs of anemia are common and include fatigue, dizziness, palpitations, and dyspnea.

- On examination, patients appear pale and fatigued and may have petechiae, purpura, gum hypertrophy, hepatosplenomegaly, and lymphadenopathy.
  - Fever, focal infection, and dyspnea may be present.
  - Bone tenderness may be elicited, especially in the sternum, tibia, and femur.

▶ DIAGNOSIS

- CBC count reveals the hallmark finding of pancytopenia with circulating blasts.
- Bone marrow biopsy confirms the diagnosis and reveals a hypercellular marrow with either excess lymphoblasts, as in ALL, or excess myeloblasts, as in AML.
- According to the World Health Organization (WHO), >20% blasts on bone marrow or in peripheral blood is diagnostic of acute leukemia.
- An Auer rod may be seen on peripheral smear and is pathognomonic of AML.
- Lumbar puncture is required for patients who have ALL to evaluate for the presence of meningeal leukemia/central nervous system (CNS) involvement.

▶ TREATMENT

- Acute leukemia can progress rapidly, over weeks to months. Without prompt diagnosis and treatment, acute leukemia can be fatal.
- ALL:
  - Combination chemotherapy is divided into the following phases: induction, consolidation, CNS treatment, and maintenance. Total treatment time is 2–3 years.

- Leukemic involvement of the CNS is uncommon, but craniospinal radiotherapy is standard protocol.
- Allogeneic stem cell transplant is reserved for select patients with high-risk disease.
- AML:
  - Treatment with combination chemotherapy is divided into two phases: induction and consolidation.
    - The goal of induction chemotherapy is to achieve a remission, defined as <5% blasts in the bone marrow.
    - Because nearly all patients have residual disease and the risk of relapse is high with induction chemotherapy alone, consolidation chemotherapy is part of the standard treatment regimen.
    - The goal of this phase is to eliminate undetectable malignant cells, improve survival, and prevent relapse.
    - Allogeneic stem cell transplant provides the highest probability of remission and cure and the lowest risk of recurrence.

Case Conclusion

The patient most likely has AML as evidenced by an acute onset of symptoms, including dyspnea, fatigue, possible fever, and weight loss; concern for splenomegaly and his noticeable ecchymoses; and pancytopenia. He will need an urgent referral to a hematologist for further evaluation and treatment.

CHAPTER
185 Chronic Leukemias

Jill Gore, PA-C

A 56-year-old male presents to his primary care provider for his annual examination. He works at a nuclear power plant and states that his job has been more stressful than usual. He is overweight and has a history of hypertension, gastrointestinal reflux disease (GERD), and type 2 diabetes mellitus. Current medications include atenolol, omeprazole, and metformin. He occasionally drinks beer and has never smoked. He mentions that he has been having some discomfort in his left upper abdomen and jokes that his boss has probably caused him to develop an ulcer. Otherwise, he has felt fine. Routine blood work is performed, and his white blood cell (WBC) count is markedly elevated at 81 000. What is his most likely diagnosis?

▶ GENERAL FEATURES

- Chronic myeloid leukemia (CML) is a myeloproliferative disorder characterized by overproduction of mature, but abnormal, myeloid WBCs.
- Chronic lymphocytic leukemia (CLL) is a clonal malignancy of B cells, leading to an accumulation of lymphocytes that are immunoincompetent and are unable to adequately respond to presenting infections.
- CLL is considered to be identical to non-Hodgkin lymphoma, except that the latter manifests primarily in lymph nodes as opposed to in blood.

- CML and CLL follow an indolent course. Patients rarely notice symptoms of their illness, and the malignancy is frequently an incidental finding on routine complete blood cell (CBC) count.
- Both disorders affect middle-aged to older adults: most patients are diagnosed with CML between the ages of 50 and 60 years; the median age of diagnosis of CLL is 70 years.
- In developed countries, CLL is the most common form of leukemia in adults, comprising 25% to 35% of leukemias in the United States.
- CML is one of only a few cancers known to be linked to a specific gene mutation, the reciprocal translocation on the long arms of chromosomes 9 and 22 known as the Philadelphia chromosome (sometimes referred to as *BCR-ABL1*).
- Exposure to ionizing radiation is the only known risk factor for CML; genetic factors, not environmental or occupational exposures, contribute to the risk for developing CLL.
- Patients with CML present at various stages of the disease and transition between various stages:
  - Chronic phase: patients have a gradual rise in WBC count.
    - In peripheral blood, blasts composed <15% of the WBC count.
    - Splenomegaly, weight loss, and B symptoms (fever, night sweats, and weight loss) may be present.
    - 85% of patients are initially diagnosed with CML in this phase.
  - Accelerated phase: patients with previously controlled disease develop worsening blood counts:
    - 10% to 20% of peripheral blood is composed of blasts.
    - Organomegaly develops, and a new chromosomal abnormality may be acquired.
  - Blast crisis: patients have signs and symptoms of acute leukemia, including bone pain and B symptoms; an increased number of blasts are found in the peripheral blood and bone marrow, with >20% blasts being diagnostic for this phase.

▶ CLINICAL ASSESSMENT

- Patients frequently are asymptomatic; leukocytosis is an incidental finding on a CBC count.
- Symptoms, if present, include fatigue, weight loss, night sweats, low-grade fever, recurring infections, abdominal fullness, early satiety, and lymphadenopathy.
- Physical examination findings may include hepatosplenomegaly, sternal tenderness, and, most commonly, lymphadenopathy.

▶ DIAGNOSIS

- CML: patients will have an elevated WBC count on CBC count:
  - Anemia and thrombocytopenia may be present.
  - Confirmation of diagnosis is made by bone marrow biopsy.
  - Hypercellularity with expansion of the myeloid cell line will be noted.
  - The Philadelphia chromosome, which is pathognomonic for CML, will be present in 95% of patients.
- CLL: patients will have a high WBC count on CBC count:
  - Peripheral blood flow cytometry will confirm the diagnosis.
  - Bone marrow biopsy is not required to diagnose CLL; if performed, >30% lymphocytes will be present.
  - Ultrasound of the liver and spleen may be performed.
  - If the patient has had frequent infections, immunoglobulin testing may be indicated.

▶ TREATMENT

- CLL:
  - Patients who are asymptomatic do not require treatment and can be observed with frequent CBC counts and clinical examinations.
  - Treatment is indicated for patients who have "active disease": this includes worsening anemia or thrombocytopenia; development of symptomatic, enlarging lymph nodes; development of massive, progressive, symptomatic splenomegaly; rapidly progressive lymphocytosis; or complaints of fever, weight loss, extreme fatigue, or night sweats.
  - When indicated, there are several treatment options, based on patient and tumor characteristics, but it typically includes a combination of medications.
- CML:
  - Since 2001, tyrosine kinase inhibitors have been indicated as the first-line treatment for CML (e.g., imatinib, dasatinib, nilotinib, bosutinib, and ponatinib).
  - The only known curative therapy is an allogeneic stem cell transplant.

Case Conclusion

The patient likely has CML, and splenomegaly may be the underlying cause of his left upper quadrant abdominal discomfort. He should be referred to a hematologist for further evaluation and treatment.

Hodgkin and Non-Hodgkin Lymphoma

Jamie Saunders, MSc, FHEA, PA-R

GENERAL FEATURES

- Lymphomas are a group of blood cancers caused by malignant lymphocytes that accumulate in the lymph nodes (LNs) and lymphoid tissues.
  - Lymphomas are subdivided into Hodgkin lymphoma (HL) or non-Hodgkin lymphoma (nHL).
  - Typically, patients present with painless lymphadenopathy and constitutional symptoms, such as fever, night sweats, and weight loss.
- HL is a B-cell cancer that mainly affects young males in their early to mid-20s. It has been historically associated with painful lymphadenopathy following alcohol use, as well as intractable itching.
- nHLs can be either B cell, T cell, or NK cell in origin and are further subdivided in to high-grade or low-grade lymphomas, which predicts disease severity and treatment options; they typically affect older adults in their 60s and 70s.
- High-grade nHLs are rapidly progressive, life-threatening lymphomas that always require treatment to avoid death.
  - The most common type of nHL is diffuse large B-cell lymphoma (DLBCL).
- Low-grade nHLs are usually indolent and well-tolerated conditions, which only occasionally require treatment if causing systemic issues; the most common low-grade nHL is follicular lymphoma (FL).
- In a small number of patients, a low-grade nHL can progress to a high-grade nHL and is historically associated with a poor prognostic outcome.

CLINICAL ASSESSMENT

- Persistent (>4 weeks), painless, rubbery, nontender lymphadenopathy (LN >1 cm)
- Associated with constitutional ("B" symptoms); fever, night sweats, weight loss (and intractable itch can be present)
- Assess cervical, axillary, and inguinal LNs:
  - HL typically presents with enlarging cervical lymphadenopathy.
- Exclude recent or incurrent viral illness as potential differentials for lymphadenopathy.
- Blood tests are not usually helpful diagnosing or excluding lymphoma, but may indicate an alternative diagnosis, such as a current viral infection or an autoimmune disease.
- Lymphomas can present with secondary immune thrombocytopenic purpura (ITP) or autoimmune hemolytic anemia (AIHA).

- Full blood count, renal/liver/bone profiles, current virology status (HIV, hepatitis B, hepatitis C, CMV, EBV), LDH (*can be normal even in advanced-stage disease*) and CRP should be first-line blood tests.

DIAGNOSIS

- Based on the presence or absence of the Reed-Sternberg cell
- Excision LN biopsy is the gold standard diagnostic method.
  - HL: Reed-Sternberg cells present, on a background of inflammatory (reactive) of differing cells, CD15/CD30 positive B cells
  - nHL: no Reed-Sternberg cells present, CD20-positive B cells in DLBCL
- PET-CT for staging of disease severity
- Ann Arbor staging (stages I-IV)

TREATMENT

- Management varies based on the subtype, age, diagnostic and prognostic factors, and staging:
  - For NHL, consider the Ann Arbor stage at presentation, the International Prognostic Index (IPI) risk score, and presence/absence of B symptoms.
- Sperm cryopreservation for males, referral to fertility clinic for females for egg harvesting.
- Treatment depends on the subtype but includes conventional chemotherapy, immunotherapy, and checkpoint inhibitors.
- HL:
  - First-line treatment options: ABVD chemotherapy (overall survival 82%-90%) or escBEACOPP chemotherapy (overall survival 95%); however, escBEACOPP comes at the cost of infertility and an increased risk of secondary acute myeloid leukemia later in life.
  - Second-line treatment options include brentuximab vedotin (anti-CD30 monoclonal antibody) or pembrolizumab/nivolumab (anti-programmed death 1 [PD-1] pathway antibodies).
  - Autologous hematopoietic stem cell transplantation can be considered in refractory/relapsed cases, as can CAR-T cell therapy.
- nHL:
  - DLBCL; rituximab (anti-CD20 monoclonal antibody) + CHOP chemotherapy, with around a 60% to 70% overall survival in all comers
  - FL:
    - In asymptomatic patients, with no significant cytopenia(s) and no local compression of organs, a

"watch-and-wait" strategy can be implemented where no treatment is administered, and the patient is monitored regularly.

- If treatment is indicated, then range of treatment options available including monoradiotherapy and chemoradiotherapy; regimens include rituximab + various chemotherapy options (eg, CHOP, bendamustine, CVP).
- Autologous hematopoietic stem cell transplantation can be considered in refractory/relapsed cases.

CHAPTER 187

Multiple Myeloma

Amie Fonder, MS, PA-C

▶ GENERAL FEATURES

- Multiple myeloma (MM) is a disorder that involves neoplastic proliferation of plasma cells:
  - Malignant plasma cells produce antibodies called monoclonal or "M" proteins.
  - Serum and urine protein electrophoresis identify specific M protein.
  - Heavy-chain immunoglobulins include IgG, IgA, IgM, IgD, and IgE.
  - Light-chain immunoglobulins include κ and λ.
- MM can lead to organ system damage (eg, pathologic fractures, bone lytic lesions, renal insufficiency or renal failure, and anemia).
- Median age at diagnosis is around 66 years, and non-Hispanic Black persons are more commonly affected.
- A 5-year survival rate in the United States is >50%.

▶ CLINICAL ASSESSMENT

- Nonspecific presentation is common, with arthralgia and fatigue as more frequent presenting symptoms.
- Suspect MM with otherwise unexplained pathologic fracture, bone pain, anemia, renal insufficiency, hypercalcemia, fatigue/generalized weakness, or unexplained weight loss.
- MM evolves from an asymptomatic precancerous condition:
  - Monoclonal gammopathy of undetermined significance (MGUS)
  - Smoldering multiple myeloma (SMM)

▶ DIAGNOSIS

- MM diagnosis can be incidental in asymptomatic patients, or patients may have symptoms.
- International Myeloma Working Group (IMWG) criteria are used for diagnosis (**SLiM-CRAB** mnemonic).
- Diagnostic definition: clonal bone marrow plasma cells >10% or biopsy-proven bony or extramedullary plasmacytoma and any one or more myeloma defining events:
  - Sixty percent monoclonal plasma cells in the bone marrow
  - Free Light chain ratio >100 or <0.10 (involved free light chain should be >10 mg/dL)
  - MRI studies reveal >1 focal lesions, each at least 5 mm in size
  - Calcium >11 or >1 mg/dL higher than the upper limit of normal
  - Renal insufficiency: creatinine clearance <40 mL/min or serum creatinine >2 mg/dL
  - Anemia: hemoglobin <10 or 2 mg/dL below the lower limit of normal
  - Bone lesions: one or more osteolytic lesions on skeletal radiography, CT, or PET-CT imaging

▶ TREATMENT

- Treatment is similar for all MM patients, but the genetic studies of the cancerous plasma cells are helpful in stratifying risk for disease resistance and relapse:
  - Age, comorbidities, frailty, and patient preference factor into type of therapy chosen
- Types of therapies:
  - Chemotherapy and immunotherapy
  - Radiation can be used for palliative pain control.
  - Autologous stem cell transplant is still a mainstay of therapy in patients who are eligible.
- MM is a treatable, but not curable, "relapsing-remitting" malignancy.
- Treatment of myeloma defining events is also important:
  - Hypercalcemia: use of hydration and bisphosphonates
  - Bone fractures/large lytic lesions: may require surgical fixation or vertebroplasty
  - AKI: hydration and usual management based on severity of renal insufficiency
  - Anemia: blood transfusions as needed

Myelodysplastic Syndrome

Jamie Saunders, MSc, FHEA, PA-R

▶ GENERAL FEATURES

- Myelodysplastic syndrome (MDS) is a heterogeneous family of clonal hematopoietic stem cell disorder characterized by ineffective/dysplastic hematopoiesis.
  - Leads to anemia, thrombocytopenia, and/or leukopenia
- One-third of patients progress to acute myeloid leukemia (AML).
- Elderly patients are most commonly affected, with median age of onset between 70 and 75 years.
  - Onset in patients of Asian descent may occur at a younger age.
- Cause is unknown, but environmental exposures (eg, radiation, chemotherapy) have been associated:
  - Previous exposure to chemotherapy (particularly alkylating agents and purine analogues), radiotherapy, ionizing radiation, tobacco smoking, and benzene exposure increase risk.
- Different types exist based on cell lineage:
  - Refractory cytopenias with unilineage dysplasia (RCUD):
    - Refractory anemia (RA), refractory neutropenia (RN), refractory thrombocytopenia (RT), refractory anemia with ring sideroblasts (RARS)
  - Refractory cytopenias with multilineage dysplasia (RCMD):
    - More than one cell lineage is affected.
  - Refractory anemia with excess blasts 1 (RAEB-1) (5%-9% blasts in the bone marrow)
  - Refractory anemia with excess blasts 2 (RAEB-2) (10%-19% blasts in the bone marrow)

▶ CLINICAL ASSESSMENT

- Consider MDS in patients with CBC abnormalities and symptomatic cytopenias.
- Presentation may include signs and symptoms of bone marrow failure.
  - Anemia (typically macrocytic) resulting in shortness of breath, fatigue, chest pains, and headache
  - Thrombocytopenia resulting in bleeding and bruising symptoms (eg, petechiae, epistaxis, gum bleeding)
  - Leukopenia: predominantly neutropenic, resulting in recurrent and abnormal infections (eg, oral thrush, other fungal infections)
- Monitor for signs and symptoms of progression to AML, such as worsening cytopenias, worsening of constitutional symptoms (fevers, night sweats, weight loss), or increase in peripheral blast percentage on blood film.
- Rule out other causes of anemia (eg, hemolytic anemia, vitamin B12 deficiency, folate deficiency, anemia of renal disease).

▶ DIAGNOSIS

- Diagnosis supported by diagnostic testing:
  - CBC with differential and reticulocyte count, bone marrow aspirate with biopsy, serum erythropoietin levels, and cytogenetic/molecular testing
- Peripheral blood tests show the presence of a cytopenia(s):
  - Typically a macrocytic anemia and/or thrombocytopenia
- Peripheral blood film shows the presence of dysplastic features:
  - Granulocytes: left-shift, pseudo-Pelger cells, hypogranular cells
  - Platelets: giant platelets
  - Red cells: anisocytosis, teardrop cells, basophilic stippling
- Bone marrow examination reveals >10% of cells in a cell lineage as demonstrating dysplastic features based on morphology.
- Absence of Auer rods and <20% of white cell blasts in the bone marrow, as the presence of these features defines AML.

▶ TREATMENT

- Based on risk stratification using the Revised International Prognostic Scoring System (IPSS-R) for MDSs
- Patients in the high-risk category have a high chance of progression to AML, which is associated with poor outcomes.
  - Treatment options should aim to include allogeneic hematopoietic stem cell transplantation (HSCT), if the patient is deemed clinically fit for transplant, and the use of hypomethylating agents such as azacitidine.
  - Consider HLA typing with HSCT or platelet management.
- Patients in low-risk categories have a lesser risk of long-term progression to AML and, as such, confer a longer survival chance, with around 50% of patients dying of other causes.
- Treatment includes management of the cytopenia itself, for example, blood transfusions or erythropoietin-stimulating agents (eg, EPO).

CHAPTER
189

Polycythemia Vera

Joshua Shepherd, MMS, PA-C
Bill Engle, DD, MS

▶ GENERAL FEATURES

- Polycythemia vera is a neoplastic clonal myeloproliferative neoplasm that is commonly associated with a peripheral blood pancytosis (elevated WBC, RBC, and platelet counts).
- It typically occurs in patients aged >60 years with some measure of familial predisposition.
- A recently discovered genetic mutation in the *JAK2* gene is detected in the vast number of cases; the *JAK2* gene codes for the *JAK2* protein, which is a tyrosine kinase enzyme that is involved in the regulation of cellular division.
- In the case of polycythemia vera, the mutation in the *JAK2* protein causes the unregulated cellular growth of the myeloid cell lines and thus leading to the characteristically elevated WBC, RBC, and platelet counts.

▶ CLINICAL ASSESSMENT

- History of mild headaches and fatigue over several years
- Hypertension due to the hyperviscosity of the blood
- Weight loss
- General weakness
- Pruritis
- Palpable splenomegaly

▶ DIAGNOSIS

- Diagnosis requires meeting the following WHO criteria:
  - Elevated HgB (>16.5 g/dL) and elevated HCT (>49% in men or >48% in women)
  - Hypercellular bone marrow
  - Identification of a mutation in the *JAK2* gene
- Other minor criteria include low serum erythropoietin with normal oxygen saturation.
- The peripheral blood pancytosis (elevated WBC, RBC, and platelet counts) coupled with the elevated HgB/HCT with normal oxygen saturation should warrant a bone marrow collection.
- Bone marrows are typically hypercellular with panmyelosis with larger clusters of normoblasts and enlarged megakaryocytes with lobulate nuclei.

▶ TREATMENT

- Three options: therapeutic phlebotomy, myelosuppressive therapy, and molecular therapy
- Initially, polycythemia vera patients undergo therapeutic phlebotomies to lower the plasma hematocrit levels, which, in turn, lowers the hyperviscosity of the blood, leading to a lowering of the patient's blood pressure.
- Therapeutic phlebotomies should be performed often enough to maintain a hematocrit level within the medical reference limits.
- In addition to routine therapeutic phlebotomies, high-risk patients are treated with an alkylating agent such as hydroxyurea.
- Interferon-γ can be utilized in place of hydroxyurea in younger patients, and busulfan can be substituted for hydroxyurea in older patients with known resistance to hydroxyurea.
- Molecular therapy options include the use of JAK inhibitors like ruxolitinib and lestaurtinib.

CHAPTER

190

Hemolytic Uremic Syndrome

Joshua Shepherd, MMS, PA-C
Bill Engle, DD, MS

▶ GENERAL FEATURES

- Hemolytic uremic syndrome (HUS) is a form of microangiopathic hemolytic anemia associated with low platelet counts and rapid onset to acute renal failure, especially in children.
- Most HUS cases are caused by a Shiga toxin–producing bacterial infection; *Escherichia coli* serotype *0157:H7* and some toxin-producing strains of *Shigella* have been associated.
- Consumption of contaminated food and water and undercooked ground beef are the most common means of infection; once ingested, the hemorrhagic *E. coli* and/ or *Shigella* serotypes release Shiga toxins that are absorbed from the GI into the plasma.
- Shiga toxins have an affinity for endothelial cells in the glomerulus and brain; once inside the endothelial cells, these toxins induce prothrombic changes in the kidneys that result in blockages in the microvasculature of the glomeruli that ultimately result in acute renal failure.
- Obstructions in the kidneys can cause the activation of platelets and the formation of thrombi, which can cause a hemolytic anemia as characterized by a decreased hemoglobin, hematocrit, and haptoglobin.
- Atypical HUS can occur in patients without coexisting infection or underlying diseases.
- Atypical HUS is a type of thrombotic microangiopathy, which is usually caused by uncontrolled activation of the complement system and is characterized by a triad of nonimmune microangiopathic hemolytic anemia, thrombocytopenia, and organ damage (e.g., brain, kidneys).

▶ CLINICAL ASSESSMENT

- Abdominal cramping, vomiting, bloody diarrhea
- Decreased levels of hemoglobin, hematocrit, and platelet counts
- Normal PT and aPTT (helps differentiate from DIC)
- Decreased levels of haptoglobin levels (which indicate intravascular hemolysis)
- Elevated BUN (uremia)
- Positive stool cultures for *E. coli* serotype *0157:H7* or *Shigella*

▶ DIAGNOSIS

- Detection of *E. coli 0157:H7* or other Shiga toxin–producing bacteria in the stool cultures
- Low platelet count
- Elevated BUN and creatinine levels
- Normal PT and aPTT

▶ TREATMENT

- Supportive care
- Blood transfusion
- Platelet transfusion
- IV fluid and electrolyte management
- Kidney dialysis
- Plasma exchange
- Kidney transplant in severe cases

Idiopathic Thrombocytopenic

Stephanie Hull, EdS, MMS, PA-C

> An 8-year-old male is evaluated for a 3-day history of a rash on his lower legs. He has also had epistaxis that his mother attributes to a recent cold. He is afebrile. Diffuse petechiae are noted on the bilateral lower extremities. No lymphadenopathy is noted. Complete blood count is normal, except for platelet count of 20 000/μL. No abnormal cells are noted on the peripheral blood smear. PT/INR and PTT are normal. What is the most appropriate treatment?

▶ GENERAL FEATURES

- Thrombocytopenia (platelet count <150 000/μL) results from decreased platelet production (bone marrow), increased platelet destruction, and/or platelet sequestration (spleen).
- Immune (idiopathic) thrombocytopenic purpura (ITP) results from immune-mediated platelet destruction (impaired platelet production may also occur).
  - The spleen produces IgG autoantibodies against GPIIb/IIIa, which bind platelets and accelerates their clearance from circulation.
  - The resultant thrombocytopenia leads to mucocutaneous bleeding.
- Acute ITP (recovery within 3-6 months without treatment) is most common in children and is most often preceded by a viral upper respiratory tract infection or vaccination.
- Chronic ITP (lasts >6 months and usually requires treatment) is more common in adults, is insidious in onset, and is most commonly idiopathic but may be secondary to other conditions.
- Secondary ITP may be due to connective tissue disease (eg, systemic lupus erythematosus), lymphoproliferative disease (eg, lymphoma), medications, alcohol, chronic liver disease, thyroid disease, autoimmune hemolytic anemia, antiphospholipid antibody syndrome, and infections (eg, HIV, HCV, COVID-19).

▶ CLINICAL ASSESSMENT

- History may include recent viral upper respiratory tract infection, vaccination, easy bruising, epistaxis, gingival bleeding, and menorrhagia.
- Physical examination findings may include petechiae, purpura, ecchymosis, and hematomas.
  - Easy bruising is usually associated with platelet counts <50 000/μL.
  - Petechiae, purpura, ecchymosis, and other significant bleeding are usually associated with platelet counts <20 000/μL.

- Intracranial hemorrhage, retinal hemorrhages, wet purpura (blood-filled blisters on the oral mucosa), hemoptysis, hematuria, and gastrointestinal bleeding are rare but suggest life-threatening bleeding.
- Consider secondary thrombocytopenia (see "General Features").

▶ DIAGNOSIS

- Diagnosis requires isolated thrombocytopenia with clinical findings of mucosal bleeding tendency without other clinically apparent cause.
- Laboratory findings include low platelet count, no abnormal cells on peripheral blood smear, increased bleeding time, and normal PT/INR, PTT, fibrinogen, and D-dimer.
- Iron deficiency anemia may be present in gastrointestinal bleeding or menorrhagia.
- Consider and rule out secondary thrombocytopenia (see "General Features").
- Consider diagnostic testing for *Helicobacter pylori* as current infection can impair response to ITP treatment.
- Serologic testing for antibodies is generally not indicated.
- Bone marrow examination is reserved for patients with red and/or white blood cell abnormalities or who do not respond to initial therapy.

▶ TREATMENT

- All patients with ITP should be evaluated and managed by a hematologist.
- Recovery is typically spontaneous, and the risk of serious bleeding is low in children; therefore, watchful waiting is the most appropriate treatment.
- Oral corticosteroids and intravenous immunoglobulin (IVIG) are considered first-line therapy in newly diagnosed adult patients with platelet counts of <30 000/μL. Most patients respond to initial treatment with oral corticosteroids, typically within 1 week; however, many will relapse following reduction of corticosteroid dose. Response to IVIG usually occurs within 36 hours.
- Kinase inhibitors (eg, fostamatinib), monoclonal antibodies (eg, rituximab) anti–D immunoglobulin, thrombopoietin receptor agonists (eg, eltrombopag), and splenectomy (laparoscopic preferred) may be considered in relapsed or persistent ITP; pneumococcal, *Haemophilus influenzae* type b, and meningococcal vaccination should be administered at least 2 weeks before therapeutic splenectomy.
- Secondary thrombocytopenia due to HIV or HCV infection typically resolves with treatment of HIV or HCV.

- The risk of fatal hemorrhage from ITP is low in general, but the incidence of major hemorrhagic complications and ITP-related death are higher in elderly patients.
- Admit patients with major hemorrhage or severe thrombocytopenia associated with bleeding; consider platelet transfusions for active bleeding.

Case Conclusion

Watchful waiting is appropriate for this patient.

CHAPTER 192

Thrombotic Thrombocytopenic Purpura

Stephanie Hull, EdS, MMS, PA-C

A 32-year-old female presents with a severe headache, abdominal pain, and nausea. Physical examination is significant for temperature 100 °F, diffuse abdominal tenderness to palpation, and diffuse petechiae on all extremities. Complete blood count reveals anemia and thrombocytopenia. What other laboratory findings support a diagnosis of thrombotic thrombocytopenic purpura (TTP)?

▶ GENERAL FEATURES

- TTP is a rare life-threatening condition classically characterized by the pentad of microangiopathic hemolytic anemia, thrombocytopenia, renal failure, neurologic findings, and fever.
- TTP is most commonly an acquired condition in which autoantibodies against plasma metalloprotease ADAMTS-13 (also known as von Willebrand factor [vWF] cleaving protease) leads to accumulation of ultra-large vWF multimers. These multimers bridge and aggregate platelets in the absence of hemostatic triggers, leading to microvasculature obstruction. Clinical findings are due to obstruction of vessels in multiple organ systems (eg, neurologic, gastrointestinal, renal) and bleeding from thrombocytopenia (eg, petechiae, purpura).
- Acquired TTP is typically idiopathic but may be precipitated by infections, drugs, pregnancy, and autoimmune disorders.
- Acquired TTP appears to be more common in women, patients with HIV infection, and pregnancy.
- Hereditary TTP is often diagnosed in childhood.

▶ CLINICAL ASSESSMENT

- Clinical findings are related to obstruction of the microvasculature (eg, headache, altered mental status, paresis, seizures, coma due to occlusion of cerebral vasculature) and bleeding due to thrombocytopenia (eg, petechiae, purpura, epistaxis, hemoptysis and gastrointestinal bleeding).
- History may include abdominal pain, nausea, vomiting, fatigue, headache, confusion, and fever.
- Physical examination findings may include fever (temperature above 102 °F suggests infection, not TTP), altered mental status, focal neurologic deficits, petechiae, and purpura.

▶ DIAGNOSIS

- Fever, neurologic findings, and renal failure are not reliably seen in TTP; therefore, the diagnosis can be made if microangiopathic hemolytic anemia (low hemoglobin, low hematocrit, high reticulocyte count, and schistocytes on peripheral blood smear) and thrombocytopenia (platelet count $<50\,000/\mu L$) are present.
- Other laboratory findings supportive of TTP include high lactate dehydrogenase, high indirect bilirubin, low haptoglobin, and negative direct antiglobulin test.
- Decreased activity of ADAMTS-13, ADAMTS-13 inhibitor, and *ADAMTS-13* gene mutations may also be identified on laboratory analysis.
- High serum blood urea nitrogen (BUN) and creatinine, microscopic hematuria, and albuminuria may be seen with renal impairment.
- Prothrombin time/international normalized ratio (PT/INR), partial thromboplastin time (PTT), and fibrinogen are normal. These studies should be ordered to exclude disseminated intravascular coagulopathy (DIC).

▶ TREATMENT

- All patients with TTP should be evaluated and managed by a hematologist.
- Mortality without treatment is >90%. Hospital admission is required for appropriate management.

- Therapeutic plasma exchange (TPE) is first-line therapy for TTP and is associated with a high survival rate. TPE is continued until the platelet count returns to normal and signs of hemolysis have resolved for 2 days or more.
- Hemodialysis may be required for severe renal impairment.
- Red blood cell transfusions may be necessary for clinically significant anemia. Platelet transfusions are generally not recommended.
- The use of corticosteroids is controversial but generally not recommended.
- Discontinue drugs that may have precipitated the microangiopathic hemolytic anemia associated with TTP (eg, clopidogrel, ticlopidine, cyclosporine).

- Caplacizumab, an anti-vWF antibody that blocks the interaction between vWF and platelets, may have a role in TTP management.
- TPE, rituximab, intravenous immunoglobulin (IVIG), vincristine, cyclophosphamide, corticosteroids, and splenectomy may be considered in TTP relapse or cases refractory to initial management.

Case Conclusion

A normal PT supports a diagnosis of TTP in this patient.

CHAPTER 193

Thrombocytosis

Jamie Saunders, MSc, FHEA, PA-R

▶ GENERAL FEATURES

- Thrombocytosis is defined as a platelet count of >450 $\times 10^9$/L.
- Most often secondary to another condition, such as infection, chronic inflammation, or malignancy
- Less commonly may result from a primary hematologic cause such as a myeloproliferative neoplasm, myelodysplastic syndrome, or genetic disorders.
- Laboratory finding of thrombocytosis is often incidental, with minimal to no clinical signs or symptoms.
- No evidence that platelet count is associated with an increased risk of thrombotic or bleeding complications in secondary causes, unless the patient has a prior medical history of arterial disease.
- Patients who present with a prior medical history of thrombosis and/or hemorrhage (due to ineffective platelet aggregation) and primary/hematologic cause should be considered, particularly in the context of a portal vein thrombosis.
- Primary/hematologic causes are due to a clonal proliferation disorder:
  - Essential thrombocythemia (ET): most cases are asymptomatic (~40%-50%), with the remainder reporting vasomotor symptoms (headache, dizziness, paresthesia, and erythromelalgia) and/or report a thrombosis/bleeding history.
  - Polycythemia vera (PV): most patients will have a raised hemoglobin (Hb) and/or hematocrit (Hct) on full blood count and/or elevated red cell mass.
    - Decreased iron and erythropoietin levels are usually found in PV.

- However, ~15% of patients may present with a marked thrombocytosis as the only sign.
- Primary myelofibrosis (PMF): patients usually present with constitutional symptoms (tiredness, fever, night sweats, weight loss), and physical examination reveals splenomegaly; usually associated with other cytopenias, such as anemia, and a leucoerythroblastic blood smear with dacrocytes, but can present with marked thrombocytosis.
- Chronic myeloid leukemia (CML): usually asymptomatic and diagnosed after finding a significantly raised white blood cell (WBC) count, but can present with a severely raised platelet count.

▶ CLINICAL ASSESSMENT

- Distinguish if presentation is related to primary or secondary thrombocytosis:
  - Most cases are secondary (also called *reactive*), without an underlying primary hematologic cause.
- Differential diagnosis for secondary causes includes acute or chronic infections, inflammatory conditions, iron deficiency, malignancy, hemolysis, hypersplenism, and postoperative and other acute-phase responses.
- In chronic infection or inflammatory conditions, there may be an accompanying anemia of chronic disease.
- Presence of constitutional symptoms (night sweats, fevers, or weight loss), particularly with hepatomegaly/splenomegaly, is suggestive of a primary/hematologic cause for the thrombocytosis.

▶ DIAGNOSIS

- Exclude secondary causes based on clinical history.
- Conduct physical examination along with laboratory investigations such as:
  - Repeat full blood count to confirm persistent thrombocytosis, peripheral blood smear, C-reactive protein, iron studies, and erythrocyte sedimentation rate.
- Peripheral blood smear can identify reactive picture vs. a clonal neoplastic cause and potentially suggest other conditions (eg, the presence of dacrocytes suggests bone marrow fibrosis).
- When suspecting a primary/hematologic cause, perform molecular testing for MPN-associated mutations: *JAK2 V617F*, *CALR exon 9*, and *MPL 515L/K*.
- Bone marrow examination (aspirate and trephine) with cytogenetic analysis can confirm the diagnosis.

▶ TREATMENT

- In secondary causes, treat the underlying cause (eg, iron deficiency, infection).

- Patients with confirmed ET should be risk stratified based on thrombotic risk:
  - High risk would include ET-related thrombosis/hemorrhage in the past, age >60 years, and/or a platelet count of >1500×10^9/L.
  - Low risk is anyone not in the high-risk group.
- Low-dose aspirin (eg, 75 mg once daily) should be offered to all patients with a confirmed diagnosis of ET, except those with a platelet count of >1500×10^9/L where bleeding risk outweighs thrombosis risk.
- Patients with low-risk disease should be actively monitored, but usually, there is no indication for cytoreductive therapy.
- Patients with high-risk disease should be offered cytoreductive therapy (eg, hydroxycarbamide, anagrelide, and/or pegylated interferon), with the treatment aim to bring the platelet count to within the normal reference range and control symptom burden.
- Standard anticoagulation treatment and duration, as per other patient populations, should be offered where a thrombotic event has occurred.

SECTION **G**   *Transfusion Reactions*

CHAPTER **194**

Transfusion Reactions

Michelle Brown, PhD

▶ GENERAL FEATURES

- Transfusion reactions can be classified into two broad categories:
  - Common immune causes are related to antibodies, antigens, and complement.
  - Common nonimmune causes are related to volume, bacteria, hyperkalemia, hypothermia, coagulopathy of massive transfusion, and mechanical injury of red blood cells.
- Hemolytic transfusion reactions are categorized into acute and delayed reactions:
  - Acute hemolytic reactions often occur within 24 hours of transfusion, and most are related to ABO incompatibility.
  - Delayed hemolytic reactions present 24 hours to 30 days after transfusion.

- Delayed reactions are usually caused by an anamnestic response of the immune system, which was previously exposed to an antigen.
- The immune systems recognized the foreign antigen and increases antibody production.
- Hemolysis with delayed reactions is mostly extravascular, whereas hemolysis with acute reactions is intravascular.
- In hemolytic transfusion reactions, recipient antibody destroys donor red blood cells.
- Hemolytic transfusion reactions can be life-threatening; it is the fourth leading cause of transfusion-related fatalities behind (1) transfusion-associated circulatory overload, (2) transfusion-related acute lung injury, and (3) bacterial contamination.
- Hemolytic transfusion reactions can result in a systemic inflammatory response syndrome with vasodilation,

hypotension, increased capillary permeability, and disseminated intravascular coagulation; these symptoms can progress to shock, multiorgan failure, and death.

▶ CLINICAL ASSESSMENT

- The classic diagnostic triad for acute hemolytic transfusion reactions is fever, flank pain, and red or brown urine.
- Additional symptoms include hypotension, respiratory distress, anxiety, and oliguria. Flank pain and oliguria are due to renal involvement.
- Immediately upon noting these signs and symptoms, the transfusion should be stopped and the unit(s) and tubing that were transfused sent to the blood bank with a fresh blood sample for a transfusion reaction investigation.
- Ensure the patient has intravenous access.
- Perform a clerical check to confirm identification between the patient and the unit being transfused; misidentification of the patient is the most frequent preventable cause of lethal hemolysis.

▶ DIAGNOSIS

- A transfusion reaction investigation in the blood bank includes visual inspection of the new blood sample for plasma free hemoglobin, repeat ABO testing, and a direct antiglobulin test to see if patient antibody is attached to donor cells.
  - In the case of a suspected hemolytic transfusion reaction, additional testing is performed.

- The antibody screen and crossmatches will be repeated on both the pre- and post-transfusion reaction specimens.
- Hemolysis should be evaluated with the following labs: ↑bilirubin, ↓haptoglobin, and ↑lactate dehydrogenase.
- On a peripheral smear, there will likely be signs of immune hemolysis: keratocytes, bite cells, and spherocytes.
- Urinalysis will likely demonstrate hemoglobinuria.
- Coagulation studies should be performed to monitor for disseminated intravascular coagulation, and a basic metabolic panel should be performed to assess for renal failure.

▶ TREATMENT

- Management is primarily supportive with acute hemolytic transfusion reactions.
- Aggressive hydration with normal saline is recommended to maintain urine output of 1 mg/kg/hr to reduce the impact of free hemoglobin on the kidneys; diuretics may also be used to achieve desired urinary output.
- Electrolyte abnormalities such as hyperkalemia need to be monitored and corrected.
- Dialysis may be required.
- With disseminated intravascular coagulation and severe bleeding, component therapy with fresh-frozen plasma, cryoprecipitate, platelets, and coagulation factors may be required.

Section A Pretest: Bacterial Diseases

1. A 35-year-old male presents with a 5-hour history of progressively worsening, generalized, intensely painful muscle spasms. History indicates the patient sustained a puncture wound to the foot from broken glass 1 week ago. He denies being vaccinated in >10 years. Physical examination reveals spastic paralysis with an abnormally appearing grin and a markedly arched back. Which of the following additional physical examination findings would be most expected with this presentation?

    A. Generalized urticaria
    B. Heart rate of 135 beats per minute
    C. Positive Homan sign
    D. Positive Kernig sign

2. Which of the following is inconsistent with a diagnosis of botulism?

    A. Diarrhea
    B. Bradycardia
    C. Respiratory failure
    D. Flaccid paralysis

3. A 35-year-old male presents to the emergency department with rapidly worsening trismus and diffuse muscle cramps. Generalized tetanus is quickly diagnosed by the physician assistant. Which of the following is the most probable mode of transmission of this infection?

    A. IV drug use
    B. Unprotected sexual intercourse
    C. Ingestion of undercooked meat
    D. Ingestion of contaminated water

4. A patient with evidence of carditis is being evaluated; you suspect acute rheumatic fever. Which of the following is most inconsistent with major diagnostic criteria for that condition?

    A. Arthritis
    B. Chorea
    C. Erythema marginatum
    D. Prolonged QT

5. The hallmark symptom of generalized tetanus is which of the following?

    A. Fever
    B. Dysphagia
    C. Flaccid paralysis
    D. Trismus

6. A 20-year-old female presents to the emergency department with a 1-day history of worsening blurry vision, descending symmetrical weakness, difficulty breathing, and constipation after eating home-canned vegetables. She is afebrile, normotensive, and bradycardic at 59 beats per minute. Oxygen saturation is 90% on room air. Botulism is suspected. Which of the following interventions should be performed first?

    A. Electrocardiogram
    B. Intubation and mechanical ventilation
    C. Computed tomography (CT) of the head
    D. Anaerobic serum cultures for *Clostridium botulinum*

7. What is the mechanism of tetanospasmin?

    A. Blocks presynaptic acetylcholine receptors
    B. Blocks GABA in motor neurons
    C. Blocks skeletal muscle calcium channels
    D. Prevents chloride channel closure

8. Which of the following is the most common cause of death from botulism?

    A. Dehydration
    B. Cardiac dysrhythmias
    C. Respiratory failure
    D. Disseminated infection

9. What is the most common site of gonococcal infection in women in the United States?

    A. Urethra
    B. Knee joint
    C. Liver capsule
    D. Cervix

10. Untreated chlamydia infections can lead to which of the following sequelae?

    A. Future ectopic pregnancy
    B. Septic joint
    C. Rheumatic heart disease
    D. Uterine fibroids

Section B Pretest: Fungal Diseases

1. A 41-year-old woman presents to clinic with her fourth episode of vulvovaginal itching, vaginal discharge, and erythema this year. She reports no recent antibiotic or glucocorticoid use. Microscopy in office shows budding yeast with pseudohyphae. Lab testing to screen for which of the following should be considered?

   A. Viral hepatitis
   B. Anemia
   C. HIV
   D. Vitamin D deficiency

2. A 35-year-old transgender woman presents to clinic with painful white patches in her mouth, difficulty swallowing, and loss of sense of taste for 3 weeks. She says he was diagnosed with HIV 5 years ago but never started treatment. She has no medication allergies. You suspect her CD4 count is very low, and you want to start her on prophylaxis for *Pneumocystis jirovecii* while you obtain labs and refer her to an HIV specialist. Which of the following medications would you use?

   A. Fluconazole
   B. Dapsone plus trimethoprim (TMP)
   C. Doxycycline
   D. Trimethoprim/sulfamethoxazole (TMP/SMX)

3. A 25-year-old man with HIV is currently being treated for pulmonary histoplasmosis. He most likely reports which of the following in his social history?

   A. Work on a sheep farm the previous summer
   B. Spelunking 3 weeks ago
   C. New pet turtle purchased 1 month ago
   D. Drinking unfiltered river water while camping 2 months ago

4. A 53-year-old man with HIV infection is suspected of having sarcoidosis based on findings from his ophthalmologist. A chest CT is ordered and shows bilateral reticular opacities. He is started on immunosuppressive therapy and develops fever, chills, cough, and weight loss. Which of the following organisms is most likely responsible for his symptoms?

   A. *Cryptococcus neoformans*
   B. *P. jirovecii*
   C. *Histoplasma capsulatum*
   D. *Mycobacterium tuberculosis*

5. A 50-year-old man with HIV disease and a CD4 cell count of 83 presents to clinic with a generalized headache for 1 month. His temperature is 99.6 °F; other vital signs are within normal limits. His cranial nerve examination and strength are normal. His gait is unsteady. You are concerned about an opportunistic infection and send him to the hospital for evaluation and treatment. After discharge, you review his hospital records. Which of the following would you expect to see as initial treatment for his diagnosis?

   A. Liposomal amphotericin B and flucytosine
   B. Oral fluconazole
   C. IV Trimethoprim/sulfamethoxazole (TMP/SMX)
   D. Oral itraconazole

Section C Pretest: Mycobacterial Diseases

1. A college student spends a semester studying in Haiti working in a health care facility. One month after she returns, she develops a cough with hemoptysis, fever, and fatigue. After taking the student's history, a blood test and chest x-ray are taken, and it is confirmed that she has active TB. Combination therapy is recommended minimally for what period of time?

   A. 1 month
   B. 2 months
   C. 4 months
   D. 6 months

2. Which of the following patients are at increased risk for developing nontuberculous mycobacterial (NTM) disease?

   A. 34-year-old with a past medical history of cardiac amyloidosis
   B. 46-year-old with a past medical history of osteoporosis
   C. 40-year-old with a past medical history of hypertension
   D. 23-year-old with a past medical history of bronchiectasis

3. An immigrant from Pakistan has a history of having the BCG vaccine. He develops a dry cough, fever, and night sweats. What is the first recommended test for him given his vaccination record?

   A. T-Spot TB
   B. Chest x-ray
   C. Mantoux test (PPD)
   D. CT scan of the chest

4. A patient with GOLD B stage II chronic obstructive pulmonary disease (COPD) presents with a 1-week history of dyspnea on exertion, wheezing, and productive cough. Chest radiograph is unremarkable, and this is the patient's second COPD exacerbation in the past year. What is the most appropriate next step?

   A. Treat the patient for COPD exacerbation with oral steroids and antibiotics, if indicated.
   B. Treat the patient for both COPD exacerbation and nontuberculous mycobacteria (NTM) disease.
   C. Initiate a workup for nontuberculous mycobacteria (NTM) disease including acid-fast bacilli sputum culture and high-resolution CT.
   D. Begin a three-drug regimen for noncavitary NTM disease.

5. A 29-year-old patient presents to the emergency department with hemoptysis. He was recently released from prison 6 weeks ago, and he reports a cough and night sweats for about the past month. On examination, he is cachectic and pale. Vitals reveal fever and tachypnea. There is a consolidation of the right upper lung field on chest x-ray. Blood and sputum samples were obtained for culture. Which of the following is the most likely diagnosis?

   A. Pulmonary TB
   B. Influenza
   C. Pertussis
   D. Pneumonia

6. A 44-year-old patient with HIV/AIDS presents with hypotension and fever. Blood cultures result positive for *Mycobacterium abscessus*. What is the most likely diagnosis?

   A. Pulmonary NTM infection
   B. *Mycobacterium avium* complex
   C. Disseminated mycobacterial disease
   D. Disseminated candidiasis

7. Which of the following chest x-ray findings are the most consistent with tuberculosis (TB)?

   A. Patchy infiltrates bilaterally
   B. Consolidation in the apex of a lung
   C. Solid mass in a lower lung field
   D. Honeycomb appearance bilaterally

8. A 3-year-old child is treated 3 times with three separate antibiotics in a 1-month period for streptococcal pharyngitis. All three streptococcal tests were negative, but the patient was treated empirically due to high-grade fevers and significant lymphadenopathy. On physical examination, the patient has unilateral cervical lymphadenopathy with a violaceous skin lesion overlying the anterior cervical lymph nodes. What is the most likely diagnosis?

   A. Epstein-Barr virus (EBV) infection
   B. Nontuberculous mycobacteria (NTM) disease
   C. Ludwig angina
   D. Streptococcal pharyngitis

9. A health care worker who works in infectious disease has her annual PPD placed. Forty-eight hours later, she goes back to her PCP who measures the induration to be 7 mm. For health care workers, what measurement is consistent with a positive MST?

   A. <5 mm
   B. 5-9 mm
   C. 10-14 mm
   D. >15 mm

10. A patient is diagnosed with cavitary pulmonary NTM disease. Which of the following is an appropriate drug regimen for this patient?

   A. Rifampin, isoniazid, pyrazinamide, and ethambutol
   B. Azithromycin monotherapy
   C. Azithromycin and clarithromycin combination therapy until sputum cultures are clear for 1 year
   D. Azithromycin, ethambutol, and rifampin

Section D Pretest: Other Infectious Diseases

1. While hospitalized with malaria, a 40-year-old man develops acute-onset seizures over the course of 1 hour, ultimately resulting in coma. After ruling out other causes, his neurologic symptoms are attributed to cerebrovascular occlusion by the infectious agent implicated in his hospitalization. Which of the following is the most likely causative organism?

    A. *Plasmodium falciparum*
    B. *Plasmodium vivax*
    C. *Plasmodium malariae*
    D. *Plasmodium ovale*
    E. *Plasmodium knowlesi*

2. Which of the following is a common presentation of secondary syphilis?

    A. Gummas
    B. Tabes dorsalis
    C. Painless genital ulcer
    D. Condyloma lata

3. Upon returning to Florida from a medical mission trip, a 25-year-old man discloses to his primary care provider that he fell ill to malaria while in Brazil. Although he admits his noncompliance to taking his prescribed prophylaxis, he states that he faithfully completed his treatment, including a medication to prevent "the symptoms from coming back." Which medication is indicated to prevent such a relapse?

    A. Mefloquine
    B. Doxycycline
    C. Chloroquine
    D. Primaquine

4. What retinal changes are likely to be noted with fundoscopic examination of a patient with retinochoroiditis?

    A. Dot hemorrhages
    B. Foggy, white lesions
    C. Punctate exudates
    D. Tiny, yellowish drusen

5. Which of the following is the definitive host for *Toxoplasma gondii*?

    A. Cat
    B. Horse
    C. Pig
    D. Sheep

6. Which of the following medications is the best option for treatment of early localized Lyme disease?

    A. Erythromycin
    B. Ceftriaxone
    C. Doxycycline
    D. Ciprofloxacin

7. A 26-year-old pregnant woman presents to a prenatal clinic in a high state of anxiety. She explains that she is concerned for the life of her baby, as her previous pregnancy ended with a stillbirth caused by toxoplasmosis. Which of the following would be the most accurate advice to give her?

    A. She has significant risk, as both acute and chronic forms can be transplacentally transmitted.
    B. There is currently no risk, as only acute toxoplasmosis can be transplacentally transmitted.
    C. Her risk is the same as her previous pregnancy, as she has the same chance of acquiring acute infection.
    D. Her risk is higher than in her previous pregnancy, as her chronic infection may become acute.

8. Malaria is transmitted through which of the following?

    A. *Anopheles* mosquito
    B. Deer tick
    C. *Aedes* mosquito
    D. *Culex* mosquito

9. Which of the following is a common complication of reactivated toxoplasmosis in the immunocompromised patient?

    A. Pneumonitis
    B. Elevated liver enzymes
    C. Encephalitis
    D. Hyperkalemia

10. A 42-year old male with suspected sexually transmitted infection presents with sores around the penis. A positive result on which of the following tests would be most inconsistent with a diagnosis of syphilis?

    A. Tzanck Smear
    B. FTA-ABS
    C. RPR
    D. VDRL

11. A patient with G6PD deficiency is at increased risk to develop which of the following from antimalarial use?

    A. Hemolytic anemia
    B. Aseptic meningitis
    C. Acute chest syndrome
    D. Disseminated intravascular coagulation

12. A 28-year-old man presents to urgent care with concern of a genital lesion that he first noticed 4 days ago. He reports unprotected sex with multiple male and female partners in the last 3 months. Laboratory testing is positive for VDRL and FTA-ABS. What is the preferred treatment for this patient?

    A. Ceftriaxone 250 mg IM
    B. Penicillin G benzathine 2.4 million units IM as a single dose
    C. Penicillin G benzathine 2.4 million units IM once weekly for 3 weeks
    D. Azithromycin 1 g PO

13. Which of the following best describes the characteristic rash seen with Lyme disease?

    A. Annular, erythematous rash with central clearing
    B. Erythematous papular rash with vesicles
    C. Rash rarely occurs in Lyme disease
    D. Erythematous rash with satellite lesions

14. What is the name of an acute febrile reaction that may occur during the first 24 hours after initiation of treatment for syphilis?

    A. Jarisch-Herxheimer
    B. Treponema pallidum
    C. TORCH syndrome
    D. Gummas

15. Which of the following statements is true regarding Lyme disease?

    A. Most infections occur in the fall and winter.
    B. Incidence of infection is higher if the tick is attached longer than 72 hours.
    C. Dogs and horses represent the largest reservoir for *Borrelia burgdorferi*.
    D. Most patients are seropositive early in the stages of Lyme disease.

16. Which of the following is the most curable sexually transmitted infection in the United States?

    A. Chancroid
    B. Chlamydia
    C. Syphilis
    D. Trichomoniasis

Section E Pretest: Prenatal Transmission of Infection

1. Which of the following statements is most accurate about herpes simplex infection in pregnancy?

   A. Patients should be screened with HSV serology at the initial prenatal visit.
   B. Patients should have mucosal PCR swabs performed at the initial prenatal visit.
   C. Patients with a history of recurrent genital herpes should receive antiviral therapy.
   D. Patients with genital HSV 2 are at higher risk of transmission to the fetus.

2. Which of the following is the recommended screening test in pregnancy for hepatitis B?

   A. HBsAg
   B. HBsAb
   C. Anti-HBc
   D. Anti-HBs

3. Which of the following is the best next step in managing a pregnant patient with a positive RPR test?

   A. Begin treatment with benzathine penicillin.
   B. Begin treatment with a broad-spectrum cephalosporin.
   C. Order a treponemal antibody test.
   D. Refer to maternal-fetal medicine.

4. A 42-year-old G2P1 presents at 25 weeks' gestation with clinical evidence of varicella zoster. Review of her chart reveals she was varicella nonimmune. Which of the following is the most appropriate management of the patient?

   A. Administer varicella vaccine.
   B. Initiate acyclovir therapy.
   C. Prescribe gabapentin to help alleviate pain.
   D. Begin an oral prednisone protocol with tapering.

Section F Pretest: Sepsis and Systemic Inflammatory Response Syndrome

1. An 84-year-old woman with an indwelling Foley catheter is sent from her long-term care facility because of fever. Which of the following findings is consistent with systemic inflammatory response syndrome (SIRS) criteria?

   A. Temperature of 36.2 °C
   B. Heart rate of 94 beats per minute
   C. Respiratory rate of 18 breaths per minute
   D. Lactic acid of 4 mg/dL

2. Which of the following is considered the vasopressor of choice in septic shock?

   A. Dopamine
   B. Norepinephrine
   C. Phenylephrine
   D. Vasopressin

3. Which of the following is NOT an example of hemodynamic monitoring after IV fluid administration?

   A. Capillary refill time
   B. Cardiac output monitoring
   C. Glasgow Coma Scale
   D. Bedside ultrasound of inferior vena cava

4. Which of the following components is currently recommended for treatment of severe sepsis and septic shock?

   A. IV colloid fluids 20 mL/kg with broad-spectrum antibiotics
   B. IV crystalloid fluids 30 mL/kg with oral antibiotics
   C. IV crystalloid fluids 30 mL/kg with IV antibiotics
   D. IV antibiotics with stress-dose steroids

5. A 68-year-old female presenting with left flank pain, dysuria, and fever states that the symptoms have been present for about 1 week. On arrival, you note her vital signs to include a regular heart rate at 110 beats per minute, a temperature of 38.2 °C, a respiratory rate of 20 breaths per minute with an oxygen saturation of 94% on room air, and a blood pressure of 102/70. She has left CVA tenderness and suprapubic abdominal tenderness to palpation. Capillary refill is <2 seconds in bilateral upper extremities. She is alert and oriented. At this point, how would you classify this patient?

   A. SIRS
   B. Sepsis
   C. Severe sepsis
   D. Septic shock

Section G Pretest: Viral Diseases

1. A 17-year-old girl presents to the urgent care center with a 5-day history of fever up to 100.3 °F (37.9 °C), sore throat, mild nausea, swollen lymph nodes, and fatigue. Physical examination reveals pharyngeal erythema, 2+ tonsillar swelling with mild exudate, and palpable tender anterior and posterior cervical lymph nodes. The remainder of the examination is normal. A rapid strep test and Monospot are ordered and both are negative. Which drug is most appropriate to prescribe?

   A. Acetaminophen
   B. Oseltamivir
   C. Penicillin
   D. Prednisone

2. Erythema infectiosum is caused by which agent?

   A. *Haemophilus influenzae*
   B. Herpes simplex
   C. Parvovirus B19
   D. *Staphylococcus aureus*

3. A 20-year-old college football player presents to your clinic with a 10-day history of fatigue, fever, and pharyngitis. His Monospot is positive, with a white blood cell count of 18 000 cells/mm^3 and 16% atypical lymphocytes seen on differential. His erythrocyte sedimentation rate is 48 mm/hr; AST, 45 U/L; and ALT, 58 U/L. His abdomen has mild left upper quadrant tenderness but is not distended, and he has no palpable splenomegaly. His coach wants to know when he can return to practice. Which is the correct response?

   A. 1 week from the visit
   B. 4 weeks from onset of acute symptoms
   C. As soon as the fever is gone
   D. When his laboratory work returns to normal

4. A full-term infant is born to a 36-year-old female who had no prenatal care. The infant failed the infant hearing screen, and on examination, the baby has a low birth weight for her age, appears to have bilateral cataracts and an irregular heartbeat. On ultrasound, a ventricular septal defect is seen. Which of the following diseases most likely is the cause of these complications?

   A. Hepatitis B
   B. Rubella
   C. HIV
   D. Tetanus

5. A 17-year-old male presents to the clinic for a follow-up visit, 3 days after being seen for a complaint of sore throat. He now has a 7-day history of sore throat, with new symptoms of fatigue and subjective fever. His parents report a history of exposure to mono through a close friend in the week before the onset of symptoms. The patient has no prior history of mono. Physical examination shows nonerythematous pharynx and tonsils without exudate or swelling, and no lymph node enlargement on palpation. A rapid strep test was negative at his initial visit, and the culture showed no growth. His vital signs are temperature 99.1 °F, heart rate 84, and respiratory rate 14. Which of the following laboratory findings would most likely confirm the suspected diagnosis of mononucleosis?

   A. CBC with manual differential showing a while blood cell count of 12 500 cells/mm^3 with few atypical lymphocytes present
   B. Positive Monospot test in clinic
   C. Negative rapid strep test
   D. Comprehensive metabolic panel with no results outside the normal range

6. Which of the following is pathognomonic for rabies infection?

   A. Aerophobia
   B. Myoedema
   C. Opisthotonos
   D. Asymmetric flaccid paralysis

7. A 21-year-old male who works for the local EMS service presents with a 2-day history of fever, fatigue, and pharyngitis. He has no prior history of mono. He has been exposed to multiple ill patients recently due to his occupation. His temperature in the clinic is 100.8 °F, and on examination, he has 2+ tonsils with erythema and swollen, tender cervical lymph nodes in the anterior chain. A rapid strep test is performed and is positive. You next step would be:

   A. Symptomatic treatment with OTC medication and rest
   B. Throat culture for confirmation of rapid strep
   C. Initiate oral antibiotic therapy
   D. Monospot testing in clinic
   E. Initiate oral antiviral therapy

8. A 17-year-old boy presents with fever, headache, and pain with eating. He also states he has noticed his scrotum appears larger than normal on one side. On physical examination, he has a mild fever and swollen and painful parotid glands. There is unilateral swelling of the right testicular with pain on palpation. Which of the following complications does he have relating to his diagnosis?

   A. Epididymitis
   B. Testicular torsion
   C. Orchitis
   D. Lipoma

9. Which antibody type is most useful in diagnosing an acute infection of erythema infectiosum?

   A. IgA
   B. IgE
   C. IgG
   D. IgM

10. A 6-month-old presents to the clinic with high fever, cough, and rash on her face and trunk for the past 2 days. The father states the rash has spread. On examination, the child has a fever of 104.5 °F and has injected conjunctiva bilaterally. A maculopapular rash is seen on the child's face, upper extremities, and trunk. Bluish white spots are visible on the soft palate of the child's mouth and buccal mucosa. Which of the following is the most likely diagnosis?
    A. Hand-foot-mouth disease (HFMD)
    B. Erythema infectiosum
    C. Rubella
    D. Rubeola

11. Which of the following patient is at highest risk for complication from erythema infectiosum infection?
    A. 15-year-old woman with hypertension
    B. 25-year-old pregnant woman
    C. 40-year-old man with diabetes
    D. 7-year-old male child

12. An unvaccinated 24-year-old male presents with unilateral swelling of the right side of his neck. On examination, he has a low-grade fever, tenderness to the parotid gland, and lymphadenopathy of the submandibular glands. Which of the following is the most likely cause of his symptoms and signs?
    A. Mumps virus
    B. Coxsackievirus
    C. Rubivirus
    D. Coronavirus

13. Which of the following is the best test to diagnose acute HIV?
    A. Fourth-generation ELISA
    B. HIV1/HIV2 discrimination assay
    C. HIV PCR
    D. HIV Western blot

14. According to the CDC, at what ages is the MMR vaccine recommended?
    A. At birth, 2 months, and 4 months
    B. 1 year and 18 months
    C. 2, 4, and 6 months
    D. 1 year and 4-6 years

15. The virus that causes acute infectious mononucleosis is a HHV best known as:
    A. CMV
    B. HSV-1
    C. VZV
    D. EBV
    E. Roseola

16. Which of the following viruses targets epithelial, monocyte, and lymphocyte cells and spreads through close contact, transplant, and blood transfusion? Additionally, in immunocompromised hosts, this virus can cause esophagitis, retinitis, and colitis.
    A. CMV
    B. Parvovirus B19
    C. Toxoplasmosis
    D. Varicella zoster

17. In a patient co-infected with HIV and HBV, you will include which of the following medications in their treatment regimen?
    A. Abacavir
    B. Emtricitabine
    C. Lamivudine
    D. Tenofovir

18. A 54-year-old male comes to the hospital with diarrhea, abdominal pain, and fever. Past medical history is significant for a renal allograft, and he is on immunosuppression therapy. He is diagnosed with CMV colitis. Which of the following medications is most likely to be used to treat his infection?
    A. IV acyclovir
    B. IV ganciclovir
    C. IV oseltamivir
    D. Oral prednisone

19. Which animal is the predominate source of rabies in the United States?
    A. Dog
    B. Bat
    C. Raccoon
    D. Opossum

20. A patient being treated for CMV disease of the esophagus was recently transitioned from ganciclovir to a second-line drug due to viral drug resistance. The patient goes on to develop an acute kidney injury and genital ulceration from this second-line drug. Which of the following medications best fits this second-line drug?
    A. Acyclovir
    B. Cyclophosphamide
    C. Foscarnet
    D. Valganciclovir

21. Your new patient is a 54-year-old female with no prior HIV test. Regarding HIV, where will you include the test?
    A. On her new patient labs if she requests it
    B. On her new patient labs informing her is among the routine tests
    C. Only if she has ever engaged in risky behaviors
    D. Only if she has engaged in recent risk behavior

22. Which of the following is the most common manifestation of CMV disease in the immunocompromised population?

    A. Meningitis
    B. Vasculitis
    C. Colitis
    D. Pancreatitis

23. Your patient is a 34-year-old man who has sex with men found to be HIV infected. Which of the following vaccines NOT indicated for an uninfected man who has sex with men should he receive?

    A. Hepatitis B
    B. HPV
    C. Pneumococcus
    D. Tdap

24. Which of the following is the best test to diagnose a patient with symptoms consistent with genital HSV infection?

    A. Viral culture
    B. HSV serology
    C. Direct fluorescence assay (DFA)
    D. Tzanck smear

25. Which class of antiretroviral medication is included in all currently recommended combinations used in a patient with newly diagnosed HIV?

    A. Entry inhibitor
    B. Integrase inhibitor
    C. Maturation inhibitor
    D. Protease inhibitor

26. A newborn is diagnosed with CMV disease. Which of the following is this newborn at high risk for?

    A. Congenital hearing loss
    B. Congenital cardiac valvular defect
    C. Pancreatic insufficiency
    D. Secondary hematologic malignancy

27. A young girl is brought in by her mother for a well-child visit. Her mother inquires about the HPV. What is the recommended age to begin Gardasil?

    A. 8-9 years old
    B. 4-6 years old
    C. 15-16 years old
    D. 11-12 years old

28. Which of the following is indicative that someone with erythema infectiosum is no longer contagious?

    A. Appearance of rash
    B. Resolution of fever
    C. Seronegative IgM antibodies
    D. Serum detection of IgG antibodies

29. A 21-year-old male presents to the clinic after noticing some raised bumps on his penis. He is sexually active, though he does not usually wear a condom. On examination, there are multiple flesh colored, small lesions around the head of the penis and along the shaft. Which of the following is the most likely diagnosis?

    A. Syphilis
    B. Chancroid
    C. Genital warts
    D. Chlamydia

30. Which of the following is the most common sexually transmitted disease in the United States?

    A. Chancroid
    B. Syphilis
    C. HPV
    D. Gonorrhea

31. Which of the following is the recommended patient applied treatment for genital warts?

    A. Imiquimod 3.75% cream
    B. Penicillin 2.5 million units IM
    C. Ceftriaxone 250 mg IM
    D. Trichloroacetic acid

32. Erythema infectiosum is transmitted most commonly by which route?

    A. Blood
    B. Contact
    C. Respiratory droplet
    D. Semen

33. When is a woman recommended to have her initial Pap smear?

    A. When she becomes sexually active
    B. Menarche
    C. When she becomes pregnant
    D. Age 21 years

34. An 8-year-old year old boy is brought to the emergency department with worsening fever, chills, and tachypnea. He was diagnosed with influenza A 2 days ago. He has multilobar consolidations on chest radiographs with an elevated white blood cell count. Which of the following is the most likely etiology of this secondary infection?

    A. *B. pertussis*
    B. *C. diphtheriae*
    C. Methicillin-resistant *Staphylococcus aureus*
    D. *Legionella pneumoniae*

35. Which of the following is the most likely to be the cause of a nonpruritic truncal rash that appeared after defervescence from temperatures as high as 41 °C?

    A. Erythema infectiosum
    B. HFMD
    C. Roseola
    D. Scarlet fever

36. Which of the following syndromes could occur after using aspirin for the treatment of fever in a child with influenza?

   A. Acute rheumatic fever
   B. HFMD
   C. Kawasaki disease
   D. Reye syndrome

37. A rosy-red, macular rash is described as appearing abruptly on the chest, neck, and face of a toddler with a 3-day history of fever. A key history component that would differentiate roseola from other rashes is which of the following?

   A. Cephalocaudal direction of the rash progression
   B. Appearance of the rash after the fever broke
   C. Rash preceded by a herald path
   D. Rash associated with strawberry tongue

38. An unvaccinated pregnant woman with a history of asthma presents to the emergency department with a 1-day history of acute onset of fever, chills, cough, and dyspnea. A nasal swab was performed, and the reverse transcription polymerase chain reaction (RT-PCR) test is positive for influenza A. Which of the following is the best treatment?

   A. Baloxavir marboxil
   B. Dexamethasone
   C. Oseltamivir
   D. Zanamivir

39. Which of the following skin eruptions typically starts on the trunk and spreads to the neck and face?

   A. Erythema infectiosum
   B. Measles
   C. Roseola
   D. Rubeola

40. The most common causative organism for exanthem subitum is which of the following?

   A. Hantavirus
   B. HHV-6
   C. HHV-7
   D. HPV

41. Which of the following is a key differentiating factor between roseola and a drug allergy?

   A. Drug allergy rash is not blanchable and is associated with petechiae, but roseola is blanchable.
   B. Rash of roseola occurs immediately after fever breaks, but drug allergy rash occurs before the fever breaks.
   C. Drug allergy rash persists for 4–7 days, but roseola typically clears within 48 hours of onset.
   D. Rash of roseola is pruritic with a sandpapery feel, but the drug allergy rash is macular and nonpruritic.

42. Of the following, which viral family does varicella zoster belong to?

   A. Poxvirus
   B. Parvovirus
   C. Herpesvirus
   D. Retrovirus

43. A 2-year-old has been diagnosed with a roseola rash. Which of the following would be appropriate patient education for the family?

   A. Avoid contact with any women who are potentially pregnant.
   B. Child is no longer contagious and can resume normal activities as tolerated.
   C. Give the child diphenhydramine and apply wet-to-dry wraps on the child's rash.
   D. Keep the child out of daycare until the rash resolves completely.

44. Which of the following is the most appropriate treatment in a patient with HFMD?

   A. Antiviral therapy
   B. Supportive care
   C. Antibiotic therapy
   D. Immunoglobulin

45. How long is an individual considered contagious after VZV rash manifests?

   A. 3 days after onset
   B. 5 days after onset
   C. Until all lesions have crusted over
   D. They are not contagious once a rash appears

46. How is HFMD usually diagnosed?

   A. Clinically based on signs and symptoms
   B. CBC indicating lymphocytosis
   C. Punch biopsy of the skin rash
   D. Tzanck smear of the vesicle

47. Of the following, which best describes the rash of chickenpox?

   A. Yellow-brown crusted papular rash
   B. Vesicular rash that does not spare the hands and feet
   C. Erythematous scaly maculopapular rash
   D. Papulovesicular rash starting on the face or trunk

48. A 3-year-old boy is brought in for evaluation due to 2 days of fever, drooling, and vesicles noted only on the palms of his hands and soles of his feet. The parent reports a decreased appetite but denies any cough or congestion. He is up to date on immunizations. What is the most likely cause?

   A. Parvovirus B19
   B. HHV-6
   C. Coxsackievirus A16
   D. Respiratory syncytial virus

49. Of the following, which diagnostic modality is the most sensitive in detecting VZV viral antigen?
    A. DFA
    B. PCR
    C. Tzanck smear
    D. Viral culture

50. Which of the following statements is TRUE regarding the epidemiology of HFMD?
    A. Most cases of HFMD occur in older adults.
    B. The disease is more prevalent in winter months.
    C. Outbreaks can occur in daycare centers, summer camps, schools, and hospital wards.
    D. Transmission cannot occur with contact of respiratory secretions.

ANSWERS AND EXPLANATIONS TO SECTION A PRETEST

1. **B.** Additional physical examination findings in this patient would include a heart rate of 135 beats per minute.
2. **A.** Diarrhea is the least likely finding in a patient with botulism.
3. **A.** The most probable mode of transmission of this infection is IV drug use.
4. **D.** Major criteria for rheumatic fever include polyarthritis, carditis, chorea, erythema marginatum, or subcutaneous nodules.
5. **D.** The hallmark symptom of generalized tetanus is trismus.
6. **B.** Intubation and mechanical ventilation should be performed first for this patient.
7. **B.** Tetanospasmin blocks GABA in motor neurons.
8. **C.** Respiratory failure is the most common cause of death from botulism.
9. **D.** The cervix is the most common site of gonococcal infection in women in the United States.
10. **A.** Untreated chlamydia infections can lead to future ectopic pregnancy.

ANSWERS AND EXPLANATIONS TO SECTION B PRETEST

1. **C.** HIV is a risk factor for recurrent candidal vulvovaginitis. Other risk factors include uncontrolled diabetes mellitus, use of oral or intrauterine contraception, long-term glucocorticoid use, immunosuppression after transplant, or malignancy.
2. **D.** The recommended regimen for *P. jirovecii* in immunosuppressed individuals is TMP/SMX DS 1 tablet PO every day or 3 days per week.

3. **B.** *H. capsulatum* is a soil-based fungus found in bird and bat droppings. Exploring a cave would expose the patient to bat droppings. Exposure to sheep and turtles can place an individual at risk for a number of infections; however, *H. capsulatum* is not one of them. *H. capsulatum* is transmitted via inhalation of spores. Drinking unfiltered river water would put an individual at risk for *Giardia lamblia*.
4. **C.** The presentation of *H. capsulatum* can resemble sarcoidosis. It is important to rule out *H. capsulatum* before initiating therapy for sarcoidosis.
5. **A.** This patient has cryptococcal meningitis. Initial treatment is liposomal amphotericin B and flucytosine. After 2 weeks, if his condition improves, he can be transitioned to oral fluconazole for consolidation and maintenance therapy. TMP/SMX is used for the treatment of *P. jirovecii* pneumonia. Oral itraconazole can be used for the treatment of mild, nonmeningeal histoplasmosis.

ANSWERS AND EXPLANATIONS TO SECTION C PRETEST

1. **D.** It is recommended that combination therapy be used for 6–9 months.
2. **C.** Patients with preexisting pulmonary disease, advanced age, and immunocompromise are at increased risk of NTM disease.
3. **A.** Due to his having had the BCG vaccine, the interferon-gamma release assays are the recommended first-line diagnostic.
4. **A.** This patient is at increased risk for NTM disease, but there is little to no evidence that this is anything more than a standard COPD exacerbation. A diagnostic workup for (and treatment of) NTM is not indicated at this time.
5. **A.** Pulmonary TB is the most likely diagnosis in this patient.
6. **C.** This patient presents with evidence of disseminated mycobacterial disease via positive blood cultures. There may be coexisting pulmonary disease, but there is certainly now mycobacterial seeding elsewhere, qualifying the patient for a diagnosis of disseminated disease.
7. **B.** Because the bacteria that cause TB are aerobic in nature, a typical chest x-ray finding is a consolidation in the upper lung fields and is usually unilateral.
8. **B.** This patient is likely to have NTM disease based on unilateral lymphadenopathy and a violaceous skin lesion overlying the swelling.
9. **C.** Any induration of at least 10 mm is considered positive for health care workers.
10. **D.** This is the standard three-drug regimen for NTM disease.

▶ **ANSWERS AND EXPLANATIONS TO SECTION D PRETEST**

1. **A.** *P. falciparum* is the most likely causative organism in this patient.

2. **D.** Condyloma lata is an example of secondary syphilis. Gummas and tabes dorsalis are examples of tertiary syphilis, and a genital ulcer is the common presentation of primary syphilis.

3. **D.** Primaquine is indicated to prevent a relapse of malaria.

4. **B.** Retinal lesions appear as focal, white lesions with an overlying inflammation that causes a foggy appearance.

5. **A.** Although undercooked meats may be contaminated with *T. gondii*, the definitive host is the cat.

6. **C.** Doxycycline is the best option for treatment of early localized Lyme disease.

7. **B.** Chronic toxoplasmosis cannot be transmitted transplacentally.

8. **A.** Malaria is transmitted through the *Anopheles* mosquito.

9. **C.** Although symptoms vary significantly, the site of infection that is typically involved is the central nervous system.

10. **A.** The definitive method for diagnosing syphilis is visualizing Treponema pallidum bacterium via darkfield microscopy. More commonly, screening is done with nontreponemal tests: rapid plasma reagin (RPR) and venereal disease research laboratory (VDRL) tests. If a screening test is positive, then a treponemal test (eg., FTA-ABS, TP-PA, various EIAs, chemiluminescence immunoassays, immunoblots, etc.) can confirm the diagnosis.

11. **A.** A patient with G6PD deficiency may develop hemolytic anemia from antimalarial use.

12. **B.** One dose of penicillin G benzathine 2.4 million units IM is the preferred treatment for primary, secondary, and early latent phase syphilis. Penicillin G benzathine 2.4 million units IM once weekly for 3 weeks is the preferred treatment for tertiary syphilis, late latent syphilis, and syphilis of unknown duration. Limited clinical trials suggest that ceftriaxone (1-2 g IM or IV for 10-14 days) may be effective for the treatment of primary and secondary syphilis; ceftriaxone 250 mg IM is likely a suboptimal dose. Azithromycin use in syphilis has been associated with high treatment failures and macrolide resistance.

13. **A.** The characteristic rash seen with Lyme disease is described as an annular, erythematous rash with central clearing.

14. **A.** The Jarisch-Herxheimer reaction is an acute febrile reaction typically associated with headache, myalgia, and other symptoms that may occur within the first 24 hours after the initiation of any therapy for syphilis.

15. **B.** Incidence of infection with Lyme disease is higher if the tick is attached longer than 72 hours.

16. **D.** Trichomoniasis is one of the most common STIs in the United States and is also the most curable.

▶ **ANSWERS AND EXPLANATIONS TO SECTION E PRETEST**

1. **C.** Patients with a history of genital HSV infections should receive antiviral therapy beginning at 36 weeks' gestation. There is no recommendation to screen for HSV using serology or mucosal swabs. Patients with genital HSV 1 are more likely to transmit the virus than those with HSV 2.

2. **A.** If HBsAg is positive, the patient should undergo further testing to determine if the infection is active or chronic as well as obtaining a viral load in the third trimester. If the patient has an acute infection, the anti-HBc and anti-HBs will be positive; if there is chronic infection, the anti-HBc and anti-HBs will be positive as well. However, the IgM anti-HBc will be positive in acute infections and negative in chronic infections.

3. **C.** A patient with a positive RPR should have a confirmatory treponemal antibody test, such as the FTA-ABS test. If the FTA-ABS is positive, treatment with benzathine penicillin G is recommended. Patients should be referred to maternal-fetal medicine once a diagnosis has been confirmed and treatment initiated.

4. **B.** Initiate acyclovir (or another approved antiviral medication). The varicella virus vaccine is contraindicated in pregnancy, but varicella-zoster immunoglobulin (VZIG) is recommended to help prevent morbidity and mortality. Gabapentin was listed as a category C medication during pregnancy, and it should only be used if the benefits outweigh the risks. Although oral prednisone can be used as an adjunct therapy in adults with zoster, it is not recommended routinely in pregnant women with VZV infection.

▶ **ANSWERS AND EXPLANATIONS TO SECTION F PRETEST**

1. **B.** Heart rate >90 beats per minute is one of SIRS criteria. The temperature and respiratory rate values are within normal limits. Lactic acid is not part of SIRS criteria.

2. **B.** Norepinephrine is considered the vasopressor of choice according to 2017 Surviving Sepsis Campaign guidelines.

3. **C.** Each of the other examinations is an example of hemodynamic monitoring. Glasgow Coma Scale is an example of mental status monitoring.

4. **C.** IV crystalloids 30 mL/kg with broad-spectrum IV antibiotics are currently recommended in severe sepsis and septic shock. IV colloids, oral antibiotics, and stress-dose steroids are not routine recommended.

5. **B.** The patient has 2/4 SIRS criteria with a suspected source of infection. Evaluation should include CBC, metabolic panel, urinalysis, lactate, and blood cultures, as well as other items on the differential diagnosis. SIRS is the case when there is no known or suspected source of infection. Severe sepsis requires a sign of end-organ dysfunction, hypoperfusion, or hypotension. Septic shock requires persistent hypotension after adequate IV fluid administration.

▶ ANSWERS AND EXPLANATIONS TO SECTION G PRETEST

1. **A.** Administer acetaminophen and symptomatic care. None of the patient's clinical findings provide an indication for antibiotics, antivirals, or corticosteroids. The negative Monospot early in the course of illness may be a false negative owing to low sensitivity; repeat the test in 7–10 days.

2. **C.** Erythema infectiosum is caused by parvovirus B19.

3. **B.** Four weeks from symptom onset is a good general guideline for return to practice. For the competitive athlete, repeating the examination and laboratory work is recommended before clearing the patient to return to full contact activity. Although palpable splenomegaly may indicate an increased likelihood of a spontaneous or traumatic splenic rupture, the absence of palpable splenomegaly should not be used as a measure of when a patient can return to play.

4. **B.** Congenital rubella syndrome causes birth defects and complications such as deafness, cataracts, heart defects, and low birth weight, along with other conditions such as glaucoma, mental retardation, blindness, and even death.

5. **B.** The duration of symptoms and the subjective history are consistent with a diagnosis of mono. Although a Monospot test can have low sensitivity, especially depending on when a patient is tested in the course of their illness, it has high specificity, meaning the positive test is the best confirmation of the diagnosis in this scenario.

6. **A.** Aerophobia is pathognomonic for rabies infection.

7. **C.** Initiate oral antibiotic therapy. The patient has symptoms of acute streptococcal pharyngitis, confirmed by rapid testing in clinic. Treatment with oral antibiotics is indicated. While it is possible for the patient to have acute infection with mono concurrently, the best course of action with just 2 days of symptoms is to address the acute strep. Even if the patient was known to have mono, antiviral therapy would not be indicated. A throat culture is unnecessary.

8. **C.** Orchitis is a complication of the mumps virus and presents with painful, unilateral swelling of the testicle along with other symptoms and signs of mumps.

9. **D.** IgM is most useful in diagnosing an acute infection of erythema infectiosum.

10. **D.** The prodrome of fever, cough, and conjunctivitis along with the pathognomonic Koplik spots makes measles the most likely cause of her rash.

11. **B.** A 25-year-old pregnant woman is at highest risk for complication from erythema infectiosum infection.

12. **A.** The mumps virus typically causes swelling of the parotid gland that can be unilateral or bilateral, as well as fever, lymphadenopathy, and malaise.

13. **C.** During the acute phase, even the highly sensitive fourth-generation ELISA may be negative, but the virus itself can be detected by PCR.

14. **D.** The CDC recommends that the MMR vaccine be given at 12–18 months with a booster at 4–6 years.

15. **D.** While all of the above are HHV and can cause some symptoms similar to mono, initial infection with the EBV typically results in the classic triad of fever, pharyngitis, and lymphadenopathy that is the hallmark of mono.

16. **A.** CMV targets epithelial, monocyte, and lymphocyte cells; spreads through close contact, transplant, and blood transfusion; and, in immunocompromised hosts, can cause esophagitis, retinitis, and colitis.

17. **D.** Abacavir has no effect on HBV, and both emtricitabine and lamivudine are somewhat effective but without tenofovir resistance of the HBV will develop.

18. **B.** IV ganciclovir is most likely to be used to treat his CMV colitis.

19. **B.** Bats are the predominate source of rabies in the United States.

20. **C.** Foscarnet best fits this second-line drug.

21. **B.** Recommendations from DHHS and the USPHSTF are that all adolescents and adults be screened at least once for HIV using and opt-out strategy; informing the patient the test will be run as a part of routine screening and allowing them the option of requesting it not be done.

22. **C.** Colitis is the most common manifestation of CMV disease in the immunocompromised population.

23. **C.** Defects in the cellular immunity put people with HIV at increased risk for infection with *S. pneumoniae*. The other vaccines listed are appropriate for both HIV positive and negative men who have sex with men.

24. **A.** A viral culture should be performed by obtaining a swab from the base of an ulcer. HSV serology will not provide the information necessary to diagnose a symptomatic infection. DFA and Tzanck smear are less sensitive and specific than viral culture.

25. **B.** Integrase inhibitors used in combination with one or two nucleoside or nucleotide inhibitors have demonstrated efficacy and are both well tolerated and available in single or two tablet regimens that aid in adherence.

26. **A.** This newborn with CMV is at high risk for congenital hearing loss.
27. **D.** It is recommended by the CDC to have girls and boys vaccinated for HPV between 11 and 12 years old.
28. **A.** The appearance of rash is indicative that someone with erythema infectiosum is no longer contagious.
29. **C.** Genital warts are commonly found on the penis and can present as described above or as single or multiple keratotic plaques.
30. **C.** HPV is the most common STI in the United States, almost 80% of sexually active persons will become infected with it during their lifetime.
31. **A.** Imiquimod 3.75% cream is one of the treatment options for genital warts that can be applied by the patient.
32. **C.** Erythema infectiosum is transmitted most commonly by respiratory droplets.
33. **D.** According to the American College of Gynecologists, it is recommended that all women have a Pap smear when they turn 21, regardless of when they begin menstruating or become sexually active.
34. **C.** Secondary bacterial co-infection (eg, pneumonia or bacteremia), most commonly due to *S. pneumoniae* or *S. aureus*, may occur in children with or without high-risk conditions and can be particularly severe and rapidly fatal.
35. **C.** The classic description of roseola is a high fever that resolves with simultaneous appearance of a truncal rash. Erythema infectiosum, also known as fifth disease, is caused by parvovirus and classically presents as a slapped cheek appearance. HFMD, typically caused by enterovirus, presents with a pustular rash on the hands and feet with an enanthem in the posterior oropharynx. Scarlet fever is the classic sandpapery rash that is associated with strep pharyngitis, which is associated with *Streptococcus pyogenes*.
36. **D.** Reye syndrome is characterized by encephalopathy and fatty degeneration of the liver, usually after influenza or varicella. Salicylates seem to be the most important inducing factor of the syndrome in pediatric patients affected by certain viral infections. Beginning in 1980s, warnings were issued about the use of salicylates in children with those viral infections because of the risk of Reye syndrome.
37. **B.** Roseola is classically associated with a rash that appears after the high fevers break. Measles is associated with a cephalocaudal rash progression, whereas scarlet fever is associated with a strawberry tongue. Pityriasis rosea may present with a truncal herald patch followed by smaller oval rose-colored lesions.
38. **C.** Oseltamivir is generally preferred to inhaled zanamivir for the treatment of pregnant patients, assuming that prevalence of oseltamivir resistance is low among circulating influenza viruses. Oseltamivir is the drug of choice because of its systemic absorption and the greater clinical experience using this drug in pregnancy. Zanamivir is relatively contraindicated in patients with asthma or COPD. Safety data on baloxavir marboxil use in pregnancy are limited, so this is not the best choice. Dexamethasone is a steroid and not the first choice in treatment but could be added on as adjunct therapy.
39. **C.** The only skin eruption on the list that starts on the trunk is roseola. Measles and rubeola both start at the head and spread inferiorly, clearing in the same pattern. Erythema infectiosum typically starts with a slapped cheek appearance and then may present with a lacy rash on the trunk.
40. **B.** HHV-6 is the most common cause of roseola, also known as sixth disease or exanthema subitum. Other viruses have been implicated in roseola; however, much less commonly than HHV-6.
41. **C.** As drug allergy rash is associated with hypersensitivity reaction, it typically has some pruritic properties and may take longer to resolve than roseola. Drug allergy reactions can vary in their presentation from maculopapular and blanchable to petechial/purpuric, so this is not a reliable differentiating factor. A drug allergy eruption can occur in variable time periods after the initiation of the medication, so it may or may not occur before the fever breaks.
42. **C.** Varicella zoster belongs to the Herpesvirus family.
43. **B.** Roseola is a self-limited viral illness that in most cases does not require any treatment, as by the time the rash appears, the child is no longer viremic. Parvovirus infection carries a small risk for women in the first half of pregnancy, as it has been associated with fetal demise, fetal anemia, and hydrops fetalis.
44. **B.** Supportive care is advised to treat the symptoms of the disease since it is self-limited. No specific antiviral therapy is available for the treatment of enteroviruses. Antibiotics or immunoglobulin have no role in the treatment of HFMD.
45. **B.** An individual is considered contagious after VZV rash manifests until all lesions have crusted over.
46. **A.** HFMD is usually a clinical diagnosis based on the typical presentation of the disease. A CBC indicating lymphocytosis is not specific for HFMD. A punch biopsy of the skin is not usually performed in patients with HFMD. A Tzanck smear is typically performed for a rapid diagnosis of HSV infections.
47. **D.** A papulovesicular rash starting on the face or trunk describes the rash of chickenpox.
48. **C.** This patient has a typical presentation of HFMD caused by coxsackievirus A16. Parvovirus B19 causes erythema infectiosum ("fifth disease"), resulting in fever and upper respiratory symptoms

with an erythematous "slapped-cheek" rash on the face. HHV-6 causes the disease roseola infantum, manifesting with high fever and a maculopapular exanthem on the chest and abdomen. Respiratory syncytial virus causes upper respiratory symptoms, such as congestion and cough.

49. **B.** PCR is the most sensitive diagnostic modality in detecting VZV viral antigen.

50. **C.** HFMD is very contagious with outbreaks occurring in people within close proximity such as daycare centers, summer camps, schools, and hospital wards. The disease is more prevalent in infants and children, with cases occurring more in the summer months. Transmission can occur by contact with respiratory and oral secretions.

PART IX Infectious Disease

SECTION A Bacterial Diseases

CHAPTER 195 Tetanus

David Gelbart, DO, MMS, MS, PA-C

▶ GENERAL FEATURES

- Tetanus is a disorder of the nervous system that results in uncontrollable muscle spasm caused by inoculation of the bacteria *Clostridium tetani*:
  - Bacteria found in soil and animal feces (flora of the mammalian gut)
  - Gram-positive, spore-forming anaerobe produces the neurotoxin, tetanospasmin (tetanus toxin).
  - Once in human tissue, bacteria travel up axons (retrograde) to spinal cord and brainstem.
  - Toxin blocks GABA (an inhibitory neurotransmitter) in motor neurons, resulting in intense, diffuse spastic paralysis.
- Extremely rare in developed countries because of widespread vaccination.
  - In the United States, overall annual incidence is 0.10 cases per million.
  - Worldwide: annual incidence is 0.5–1.0 million.
  - Afflicted patients will be un-immunized or under-immunized.
- It is a reportable disease to health departments in all US states and territories.
  - Information is sent to the CDC for disease surveillance.

▶ CLINICAL ASSESSMENT

- Can present as one of four patterns:
  - Generalized pattern is most common and most severe.
    - Hallmark symptom is trismus (lockjaw).
    - Intensely painful muscle spasm:
      - Risus sardonicus (smile or grin resulting from intense facial muscle spasm)
      - Opisthotonus (backward arching or the neck and back resulting from extensor muscle spasm)
    - Other clinical features include rigid abdomen, bone fractures, fever, tachycardia, diaphoresis, hypertension, headache, and laryngospasm (dysphagia and apnea).
  - Local tetanus: localized to one body region such as an extremity; may evolve into generalized tetanus
  - Cephalic tetanus: localized to cranial nerves (especially CN VII); focal deficits may mimic cerebrovascular accidents.
  - Neonatal tetanus: occurs in infants within 24 days of birth:
    - Due to contamination of the umbilical cord/stump
    - Trismus → poor feeding
- Incubation period is variable (2-38 days):
  - Mean incubation period is 7–10 days postexposure.
  - Inoculation sites more distal to the CNS will take longer.

▶ DIAGNOSIS

- Diagnosis is made clinically:
  - History of soft-tissue injury allowing bacteria access through the broken skin:
    - Wounds, IV or subcutaneous drug abuse (especially heroin)
    - Cutting of umbilical cord with unsterile instrumentation (neonatal tetanus)
  - Physical examination findings as noted above.

▶ TREATMENT

- Management is largely supportive: airway management, benzodiazepines for muscle cramps, anticoagulants for DVT prophylaxis
- Magnesium sulfate to control autonomic dysfunction:
  - Loading dose 40 mg/kg IV infusion over 30 minutes, then 2 g/hr continuously for patients >45kg or 1.5 g/hr continuously for patients weighing <45 kg
- Human tetanus immunoglobulin (HTIG) to neutralize unbound toxin
- Wound debridement to eradicate spores at inoculation site
- Antibiotics:
  - Metronidazole (first line) 500 mg IV every 6–8 hours for 7–10 days

- Penicillin G (second line) 2–4 million units IV every 4–6 hours for 7–10 days
- Tetanus toxoid vaccine (part of DTap, Tdap, Td booster):
  - Infection does not confer immunity, so infected patients require vaccination.

- Td generally given every 10 years.
- Should be administered to women during every pregnancy

CHAPTER 196

Botulism

David Gelbart, DO, MMS, MS, PA-C
Joel Hamm, MD, MPH

GENERAL FEATURES

- Botulism is a rare but potentially life-threatening syndrome involving cranial nerve palsies and descending flaccid paralysis that usually occurs via foodborne illness.
- Paralytic syndrome caused primarily by *Clostridium botulinum* neurotoxin:
  - Heat-stable, spore-forming, Gram-positive obligate anaerobic bacillus
  - Found worldwide in soil, ocean, and freshwater sediment
  - Multiple heat-stabile botulinum toxins are implicated in human disease:
    - Toxin binds and blocks cholinergic presynaptic receptors → inhibiting release of multiple neurotransmitters.
    - Toxin type A causes majority of cases in the United States.
- Several types of botulism exist, including foodborne, infant (intestinal), wound, and inhalation.
- Clinical botulism occurs from ingesting environmental or foodborne spores:
  - Home-canned foods, raw honey, home-fermented products including alcohol
  - Contaminated foods contain preformed toxin that causes illness.
  - Infants, and occasionally adults, may ingest spores, which colonize the gut and subsequently release toxin.
- *C. botulinum* can also contaminate open wounds and is associated with injection drug use and, rarely, intranasal cocaine use.
- Reportable disease (>100 cases reported per year in the United States)
- Potential bioterrorism agent

CLINICAL ASSESSMENT

- Infant botulism occurs in the first year of life (symptoms may last >1 month).
- Median incubation period for foodborne botulism (most common type) is 1 day but may be as long as 10 days.
- Acute-onset descending motor weakness/paralysis with neurologic deficits (usually bilateral) including cranial neuropathies and blurry vision
- Diaphragm paralysis, respiratory distress → acute respiratory failure (most common cause of death)
- Mydriasis, nystagmus
- Bradycardia
- Urinary retention
- Constipation
- Dysphagia, feeding difficulty (in infants), xerostomia
- Typically afebrile unless concurrent wound infection

DIAGNOSIS

- Diagnosis is made clinically and confirmed by the presence of botulinum toxin in blood, stool, wound, vomitus, or implicated food; obtained by anaerobic culture of *C. botulinum*.

TREATMENT

- Supportive measures in an intensive care setting
- Early intubation and mechanical ventilation (may require respiratory support for several months)
- Early administration of antitoxin per consultation with state health department for acquisition and dosing
- Early administration of botulinum immunoglobulin (BIG) for patients aged <12 months
- Catheterization for urinary retention as needed
- Contaminated wound debridement as needed

Chlamydia and Gonorrhea

Bart Gillum, DSc, MHS, PA-C

▶ GENERAL FEATURES

- Gonorrhea and chlamydia are bacterial infections that can cause sexually transmitted infections (STIs).
- Infections can occur anywhere in the male or female lower genitourinary (GU) tract.
- Other sites of infection include the pharynx, rectum, or conjunctiva.
- If untreated, infection can lead to pelvic inflammatory disease (PID), ectopic pregnancy, and infertility in women and epididymitis or proctitis in men.
- Gonorrhea:
  - Caused by the Gram-negative coccus *Neisseria gonorrhoeae*
  - Common cause of urethritis in men and cervicitis in women
  - If untreated, serious complications can occur, such as disseminated gonococcal infection.
  - Men can develop upper GU tract infections, including epididymitis or prostatitis.
  - Upper GU infections in women are more common, given higher incidence of asymptomatic infections.
  - Rarely, *N. gonorrhoeae* infects the capsule surrounding the liver, causing a perihepatitis (Fitz-Hough-Curtis syndrome) associated with right upper quadrant tenderness and fever.
  - Gonorrhea conjunctivitis is more common in newborns due to perinatal infection; in adults, this is usually through autoinoculation from a genital source.
  - Rarely, gonorrheal infections can become disseminated, causing arthralgia, septic joint, tenosynovitis, or skin lesions.
  - *N. gonorrhoeae* associated with antibiotic resistance and this issue is rapidly emerging globally.
- Chlamydia:
  - Caused by *Chlamydia trachomatis*, a Gram-negative, obligate intracellular bacterium
  - Incubation period and symptoms, if present, may occur several weeks after exposure.
  - Often asymptomatic in both women and men, which can contribute to disease transmission during sexual contact
  - Untreated cervicitis can lead to PID or perihepatitis.
  - Associated with ectopic pregnancy due to fallopian tube scarring
  - Upper GU infections in men, usually from asymptomatic urethral infection, include epididymitis or prostatitis.
  - Individuals who participate in receptive anal intercourse can develop proctitis.
  - Lymphogranuloma venereum is a genital ulcer disease caused by certain serotypes of chlamydia, which induce a lymphoproliferative reaction; these are rare in temperate climates, except for limited outbreaks among MSM.

▶ CLINICAL ASSESSMENT

- Chlamydia and gonorrhea screening recommendations:
  - Women: annually if sexually active and age <25 or >25 years and high risk
  - Men: consider for young sexually active men in areas with high prevalence of disease.
    - MSW: at least annually, screen all sights of contact (urethra, rectum, posterior pharynx).
- Women:
  - Usually develop symptoms within 10 days of exposure
  - Mucopurulent cervical discharge, pruritis, irritative voiding symptoms, occasionally asymptomatic
  - Lower abdominal pain, pelvic pain, dyspareunia, and abnormal uterine bleeding are concerning for PID.
- Men:
  - Usually develop them within 2–8 days of exposure
  - Irritative voiding symptoms, mucopurulent penile discharge, testicular pain, occasionally asymptomatic
  - Epididymitis and prostatitis in men aged <35 years who are at high risk should be treated, empirically for both gonorrhea and chlamydia.
  - Proctitis is more common in MSW, causing broad spectrum of symptoms including mucopurulent discharge, proctalgia, tenesmus, constipation, or hematochezia.

▶ DIAGNOSIS

- Diagnosis is largely clinical, based on symptoms and risk factors.
- Laboratory confirmation using nucleic acid amplification tests (NAATs):
  - In women, vaginal swab or endocervical specimen (if speculum examination is done) is preferred to first-void urine.
  - In men, use first-void urine.
- Rectal and oropharyngeal samples may be collected.
- With gonorrhea, a culture is reserved for treatment failure or in cases of sexual assault.

▶ TREATMENT

- Owing to high rates of co-infection in urethritis, concurrent treatment for gonorrhea and chlamydia is recommended.
- Gonococcal urethritis/cervicitis:
  - Ceftriaxone 250 mg intramuscularly in a single dose (plus azithromycin 1 g orally [PO] in a single dose)
  - In cases of PID, epididymitis, or proctitis, a prolonged course of doxycycline (100 mg PO BID for 10 days) is recommended with the ceftriaxone.

- Disseminated gonococcal infection requires prolonged treatment in consultation with an infectious disease specialist.
- Chlamydia urethritis/cervicitis:
  - Azithromycin 1 g PO in single dose or doxycycline 100 mg PO BID for 7 days.
  - If pregnant, use azithromycin.
  - A test of cure (repeat testing 3-4 weeks after completing therapy) for pregnant patients or if suspected nonadherence/reinfection.
  - Treatment cures >90% of infections, but reinfection occurs in one of five people within a year.

CHAPTER 198

Diphtheria

Alicia Quella, PhD, PA-C

> An 8-year-old boy was brought to a hospital in India with fever, productive cough, and dyspnea with odynophagia for 5 days. He was finding it extremely difficult to eat and drink and had labored noisy breathing. His voice had also changed with slight hoarseness in character for 2 days. The child was repeatedly coughing and expectorating yellow-colored sputum. On physical examination he has marked edema of the neck, a "bull's-neck appearance" with a distinct collar of swelling. Oral examination reveals a membrane formation involving the pharyngeal walls, tonsils, and uvula. Which infection should you consider?

▶ GENERAL FEATURES

- Diphtheria is a vaccine-preventable, bacterial toxin–mediated infectious disease, caused by toxin-producing *Corynebacterium diphtheriae.*
- This disease primarily manifests as an upper respiratory tract illness that may result in death, but it may also present as mild infections in nonrespiratory sites, such as the skin (eg, cutaneous diphtheria).
- Diphtheria spreads through close contact or droplet infection from a case or carrier.
- Diphtheria is rare in the United States but is endemic primarily in developing regions of Africa, Asia, and South America.
- In 2020, Brazil, the Dominican Republic, Haiti, and the Bolivarian Republic of Venezuela had reported confirmed cases of diphtheria.
- Diphtheria toxoid is available in the following combination vaccines: diphtheria and tetanus toxoids and acellular pertussis vaccine (DTaP); diphtheria and tetanus toxoids and pertussis vaccine (DTP); diphtheria

and tetanus toxoid (DT); tetanus toxoid, reduced diphtheria toxoid, and acellular pertussis vaccine (Tdap); and tetanus and diphtheria toxoid (Td).
- The Centers for Disease Control and Prevention (CDC) recommends five-dose series of DTaP at 2, 4, 6, 15–18 months, and 4–6 years old.

▶ CLINICAL ASSESSMENT

- Infection may lead to respiratory disease, myocarditis, cutaneous disease, or an asymptomatic carrier state.
- The word *diphtheria* comes from the Greek word for *leather*, which refers to the tough pharyngeal membrane that is the clinical hallmark of infection.
- Patients present with sore throat, malaise, cervical lymphadenopathy, and low-grade fever 2–5 days after infection.
  - Mild pharyngeal erythema typically progresses to areas of white exudate; these coalesce to form an adherent gray pseudomembrane that bleeds with scraping.
- Diphtheria should be suspected in the setting of adherent pharyngeal, palatal, or nasal membranes; systemic toxicity; hoarseness; stridor; palatal paralysis; and/or serosanguineous nasal discharge.

▶ DIAGNOSIS

- Swab the back of the throat, nose, open sore, or ulcer, and test it for the bacteria that cause diphtheria.
- Isolation of *C. diphtheriae* from any site plus confirmation of toxin production by Elek test or by another validated test capable of confirming toxin production

▶ TREATMENT

- Even with treatment, about 1 in 10 people with respiratory diphtheria will die.
- Diphtheria antitoxin plus antibiotics are mainstays of treatment.
- Diphtheria antitoxin to stop the toxin made by the bacteria from damaging the body. This treatment is very important for respiratory diphtheria infections, but it is rarely used for diphtheria skin infections.
- Antibiotics (eg, erythromycin or procaine penicillin G)
- Close monitoring for respiratory compromise is warranted, and aggressive supportive care may require early respiratory and airway management.

Case Conclusion

The patient's clinical presentation, as well as recent travel and vaccination histories, is highly suspicious for diphtheria. The diagnosis is typically made clinically because prompt treatment with antitoxin and antibiotic therapy is warranted. Consider the diagnosis of diphtheria in patients with a compatible syndrome, most commonly presenting with fever and sore throat plus the observation of a whitish membrane on the tonsils, palate, or pharynx. Diagnosis would be confirmed with culture of the affected site.

CHAPTER 199

Rheumatic Fever

Michael Stephens, DMS, PA-C

▶ GENERAL FEATURES

- Rheumatic fever (ARF) is a multisystem disease that results from an autoimmune response after an upper respiratory tract infection with group A *Streptococcus* (GAS) 2–6 weeks earlier.
- Relatively uncommon in the United States
- Clinical manifestations include polyarthritis, carditis, chorea, erythema marginatum, and subcutaneous nodules over extensor surfaces.
- Most often affects children aged 5–14 years
- Most sequelae resolve completely, except for valvular heart damage in the form of rheumatic heart disease.
- Mitral valve is most often affected, causing mitral regurgitation.

▶ CLINICAL ASSESSMENT

- Fever: generally >39 °C
- Polyarthritis (60%): inflammatory arthropathy, typically of large joints, showing a migratory pattern
- Carditis (40%-50%): including tachycardia, new murmur, pericarditis, cardiomegaly, and heart failure; ~60% progress to rheumatic heart disease
- Sydenham chorea: includes tongue, mouth, and upper extremities; most definitive and often sole manifestation
- Erythema marginatum: evanescent rash that begins as pink macules that clear in the center, leaving a serpiginous margin
- Subcutaneous nodules: small, painless nodules over bony prominences on extensor surfaces

- Less common features include:
  - Abdominal pain
  - Epistaxis
  - Hematuria (microscopic)
  - Increased liver enzymes
  - Proteinuria
  - Pulmonary infiltrates
  - Pyuria

▶ DIAGNOSIS

- Revised Jones criteria: combination of typical clinical features in the presence of a document precipitating GAS infection.
  - Major criteria include polyarthritis, carditis, chorea, erythema marginatum, or subcutaneous nodules.
  - Minor criteria include fever, polyarthralgia, prolonged QT, or elevated ESR.
  - Confirmation of antecedent GAS infection includes increase or rising antistreptolysin O titer or streptococcal antibodies (anti-DNAase B), positive throat culture, or positive rapid antigen test.
  - Diagnosed when two major criteria or one major plus two minor criteria are met.
  - Recurrent ARF can be diagnosed when two major or one major plus two minor or three minor criteria are met.
- Echocardiography should be done to assess the possibility and severity of any carditis.
- Additional labs that aid in diagnosis include ESR, CRP, and CBC.

▶ TREATMENT

- Major goals of therapy are supportive care, including bed rest until temperature, ESR, pulse, and ECG have returned to baseline, along with eradication of GAS infection.
- All patients should receive penicillin as:
  - 500 mg PO twice daily (250 mg for children weighing <27 kg) for 10 days, or
  - Amoxicillin 50 mg/kg (maximum 1000 mg) PO daily for 10 days, or
  - A single dose of 1.2 million units of IM benzathine penicillin G (600 000 units <27 kg)
  - Alternative regimens include cephalexin and azithromycin.
- Joint involvement is highly responsive to salicylates and other NSAIDs.

- Preferred medications for the management of chorea include carbamazepine or sodium valproate.
- Prednisone or prednisolone may reduce inflammation in congestive heart failure.
  - 1–2 mg/kg/day (maximum 80 mg)
- Prevention:
  - Primary prevention includes timely and complete treatment of GAS infections.
  - Secondary prevention should begin with prophylactic benzathine penicillin G 1.2 million units IM monthly; this should be continued for 5 years, or until age 21 in rheumatic fever without carditis, for 10 years, or until age 21 with carditis, or for 10 years, or until age 40 with valvular disease.

CHAPTER 200

Salmonellosis

Alicia Quella, PhD, PA-C

▶ GENERAL FEATURES

- Salmonellosis is an infection caused by bacteria (Gram-negative bacillus) from the genus *Salmonella*.
- Salmonella infection can be typhoidal (*Salmonella typhi* or *Salmonella paratyphi*) or nontyphoidal (*Salmonella enteritidis*, *Salmonella newport*, and *Salmonella typhimurium*).
- Typhoid or enteric fever, *S. typhi*, presents as systemic illness with fever, abdominal pain, malaise, diarrhea/constipation, and occasional rash (rose spots) and is typically found in low-resource countries and in travelers from endemic areas.
- Infection is common in areas that are overcrowded and have poor access to sanitation.
  - Humans are the only reservoir for the typhoidal type, and it is transmitted by ingestion of food and water contaminated with human feces.
  - Incubation period is several days to weeks.
  - Vaccine is available for *S. typhi* four doses of oral live, weakened vaccine.
- The nontyphoidal type, *S. enteritidis*, is often localized to the gastrointestinal (GI) tract and is found worldwide.
- It is the leading cause of foodborne illness in the United States and is usually caused by eating raw or undercooked meat, raw produce, poultry, eggs, or egg products.

- Some pets, particularly birds and reptiles, can carry and transmit *Salmonella* bacteria.
- Incubation period is 12–48 hours.
- Infections can range from no symptoms to mild gastroenteritis (vomiting and diarrhea) or to severe invasive infections (especially in infants, elderly, and immunocompromised patients).
- Nontyphoidal salmonella infections outside the GI tract can be seen in the extremes of age and immunocompromised patients (bacteremia, meningitis in neonates, osteomyelitis in children with hemoglobinopathies, particularly sickle cell disease, or endocarditis with atherosclerotic disease).

▶ CLINICAL ASSESSMENT

- Consider typhoid fever in patients with fever and abdominal pain for >3 days with accompanying GI symptoms that have travelled from or visiting from endemic areas (South and Southeast Asia, China, and Africa).
  - Hepatosplenomegaly, intestinal bleeding, and perforation may occur, leading to secondary bacteremia and peritonitis.
- Consider the nontyphoidal type in patients with acute diarrhea (sometime bloody), particularly when accompanied by abdominal cramping and fever or in the setting of a community outbreak.

▶ DIAGNOSIS

- In the typhoidal type, patients frequently exhibit anemia, abnormal liver function tests, elevated C-reactive protein, and either leukopenia or leukocytosis.
  - Blood cultures are most likely to be positive early in the illness, and stool cultures are commonly positive after the second week of illness; bone marrow biopsy is the most sensitive screening test (90%) but is performed only in complicated cases.
  - Chronic carriage is defined as excretion of the organism in stool or urine >12 months after acute infection. Rates of chronic carriage after *S. typhi* infection range from 1% to 6%.
- Nontyphoidal type:
  - The definitive diagnosis requires isolation of this pathogen in stool cultures. May need to rule out other infections: *Escherichia coli O157:H7*, Shiga toxin testing, stool leukocytes, parasites, or *Clostridium difficile*.
  - The median duration of excretion following infection is ~5 weeks, but routine follow-up stool cultures are not recommended after uncomplicated gastroenteritis.

▶ TREATMENT

- Adequate hydration and electrolyte replacement with gastroenteritis, preferably by the oral route, with solutions that contain water, salt, and sugar (oral rehydration solution)

- Typhoid fever: multidrug-resistant strains are prevalent worldwide, and therapy should be based on results of susceptibility testing.
  - First-line therapy is a fluoroquinolone, azithromycin, or a third-generation cephalosporin in adults, adolescents, and children.
  - First-line therapy is a third-generation cephalosporin or ampicillin in infants.
  - Add dexamethasone in septic shock.
- Nontyphoidal type: illness is generally self-limited, so antibiotic treatment for immunocompetent individuals between the ages of 12 months and 50 years is not usually indicated; antimicrobial therapy does not shorten the duration of illness and can increase the risk of extended asymptomatic carriage of salmonella.
  - Antibiotic treatment is indicated for those with severe disease and those at the extremes of age with a higher risk of complications (eg, bacteremia, focal infection, or persisting symptoms) and for preemptive treatment in immunocompromised patients.
  - Given the prevalence of antimicrobial resistance, local antibiotic resistance patterns must be considered when choosing antibiotic therapy.
    - First-line therapy includes fluoroquinolones or a third-generation cephalosporin in adults and adolescents.
    - First-line therapy is third-generation cephalosporins or ampicillin in infants aged <12 months and children.

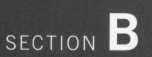

SECTION **B**   *Fungal Diseases*

CHAPTER **201**   # Candidiasis, Cryptococcosis, Histoplasmosis, and Pneumocystis

Amanda Miller, MPH, MPAS, PA-C, AAHIVS

▶ GENERAL FEATURES

- Candidiasis:
  - Normal human flora but can be opportunistic
  - *Candida albicans* is most common cause of symptomatic infection.
  - Risk factors for infection include recent antibiotic use, inhaled corticosteroid use, dentures, oral and intrauterine contraceptives, pregnancy,

immunosuppression (HIV with CD4 cell count <200, chemotherapy, solid organ or hematopoietic cell transplant recipients), diabetes mellitus, IV catheterization, trauma, and IV drug use.
  - Vulvovaginitis is the most common form of mucosal candidiasis.
  - Esophageal candidiasis is most common in individuals with HIV and is an AIDS-defining condition.

- Oral candidiasis can be an initial sign of HIV in individuals who have never been diagnosed and are late in the disease process.
- Cryptococcosis:
  - *Cryptococcus neoformans* is a yeast-like fungus found in soil across the globe; exposure is through bird droppings, particularly pigeons and chickens. Transmitted via inhalation.
  - Most often affects individuals who are immunocompromised
    - Most common non–candidal fungal infection among individuals with HIV (CD4 cell count <100)
    - Uncommon in children
- Histoplasmosis:
  - *Histoplasma capsulatum* is a dimorphic soil-based fungus, found in bird and bat droppings. Transmitted via inhalation of spores.
  - Individuals with HIV and a CD4 cell count <150 or are immunosuppressed for other reasons are at higher risk of disseminated disease.
  - Can be a new infection, reinfection, or reactivation
- Pneumocystis:
  - *Pneumocystis jirovecii* (formerly *Pneumocystis carinii*) is a ubiquitous fungus transmitted via inhalation.
  - Individuals with HIV and a CD4 cell count <200 and other individuals who are immunosuppressed are at risk.

▶ CLINICAL ASSESSMENT

- Candidiasis:
  - Oropharyngeal candidiasis (thrush) and esophageal candidiasis:
    - Oropharyngeal disease may cause loss of sense of taste, "cotton mouth," and pain with swallowing (odynophagia).
    - White plaques on the buccal mucosa, palate, tongue, and oropharynx that, if scraped, reveal a red, inflamed mucosa that may bleed.
    - Patients with esophageal disease have retrosternal pain on swallowing; may not have thrush.
  - Vulvovaginitis: vulvar itching, erythema and white, cottage cheese–like vaginal discharge
  - Invasive candidiasis:
    - Focal invasive infections of the urinary tract, lung, liver, spleen, eyes, joints, meninges, and heart are possible.
      - Mild fever, characteristic eye lesions, and clusters of pustules on an erythematous base; multisystem organ failure possible.
- Cryptococcosis:
  - Immunocompetent individuals often have mild pulmonary disease that resolves. Severe respiratory disease or progression to disseminated disease is more common in individuals who are immunosuppressed.

- Symptoms include productive cough, hemoptysis, dyspnea, fever, night sweats, malaise, and weight loss.
- Symptoms of cryptococcal meningitis include fever and headache. Patients typically do not have traditional "meningeal" signs; may have other neurologic symptoms such as seizure, stroke, confusion, and behavioral change; cryptococcomas are rare.
- Chest x-ray may show noncalcified nodules, lobar infiltrates, hilar adenopathy, and pleural effusion.
- Histoplasmosis:
  - May go undetected since patients may be asymptomatic or have mild symptoms
  - Pulmonary disease, chronic meningitis, fibrosing mediastinitis, pericarditis, endocarditis, erythema nodosum, arthralgia, and indolent disseminated disease
    - Symptoms of pulmonary infection include fever, chills, headache, myalgia, cough, and chest pain beginning 2 to 4 weeks after exposure to spores. Lung examination may have rales.
    - Signs and symptoms of disseminated disease include fever, chills, weight loss, hepatosplenomegaly, lymphadenopathy, pulmonary infiltrates, focal CNS lesions, adrenal insufficiency, altered mental status, oral and GI tract ulcerations, pancytopenia, and elevated liver function tests (LFTs).
  - Chest x-ray may be normal or show hilar and mediastinal lymphadenopathy, diffuse reticulonodular infiltrates.
    - Findings may resemble reactivation TB.
  - Presentation may be similar to sarcoidosis, so it is important to rule out histoplasmosis before starting immunosuppressive therapy.
- Pneumocystis:
  - Gradual onset of nonproductive cough, dyspnea, and fever
  - Lung examination may be normal.
  - Patients have normal O_2 saturation at rest and desaturation with physical activity.
  - Chest x-ray may be normal or have diffuse interstitial or alveolar infiltrates; nodules, masses, blebs; absence of pleural effusions.
  - Spontaneous pneumothorax possible.

▶ DIAGNOSIS

- Candidiasis:
  - Diagnosis of oropharyngeal and vulvovaginal disease can be clinical.
    - Budding yeast with pseudohyphae on KOH.
  - Esophageal candidiasis is diagnosed by visualization of white plaques on EGD and confirmation with biopsy culture.
  - Diagnosis of invasive candidiasis can be made by culture of skin pustules.

- Cryptococcosis:
  - Culture of blood, sputum, skin, or CSF
    - MRI or CT should be performed before LP or if there is concern for cryptococcoma.
    - CSF shows mild increase in protein, low-normal glucose, and pleocytosis with lymphocytes.
    - CSF cryptococcal antigen is the diagnostic test of choice for cryptococcal meningoencephalitis.
- Histoplasmosis:
  - Culture of tissue and blood is gold standard.
  - Antigen testing of urine, serum, or fluids from bronchoalveolar lavage provides rapid results.
  - CSF shows lymphocytic pleocystosis, elevated protein, and low glucose.
- Pneumocystis:
  - Dye-based staining, fluorescent staining, or PCR of respiratory specimens
  - Elevated LDH is common, but not specific.
  - Elevated β-D-glucan can indicate infection with *Pneumocystis* but can also be elevated in other fungal infections.

▶ TREATMENT

- Candidiasis:
  - Oropharyngeal and esophageal:
    - Duration is 7–14 days.
    - Mild thrush can be treated with local topical therapy.
    - For recurrent thrush, moderate-to-severe disease, or individuals with suspected esophageal disease, oral fluconazole is recommended.
    - Oral azole therapy is recommended for all esophageal disease.
  - Vulvovaginitis:
    - Oral and topical antimycotic treatments are both effective for uncomplicated infection.
    - Topical therapy is preferred for individuals who are pregnant.
  - Invasive candidiasis:
    - Caspofungin, micafungin, anidulafungin, and fluconazole are used most commonly; liposomal amphotericin B is used less often because of toxicity and tolerability issues.

- Oral step-down therapy with fluconazole can be considered after 5 to 7 days in stable patients with negative blood cultures.
- Remove the catheter in non-neutropenic patients where a central venous catheter is the suspected source of infection.
- Cryptococcosis:
  - Mild-to-moderate pulmonary disease or nonmeningeal disease can be treated with high-dose oral fluconazole for 6 to 12 months.
  - Cryptococcal meningitis and severe pulmonary disease are treated with liposomal amphotericin B plus flucytosine; after patient has shown improvement and been on treatment for >2 weeks, patient can be transitioned to oral fluconazole for consolidation and maintenance therapy.
- Histoplasmosis:
  - Mild, nonmeningeal disease is treated with oral itraconazole.
  - Liposomal amphotericin B is the preferred initial therapy for moderate-to-severe disseminated disease and meningeal disease; patients can be transitioned to oral itraconazole after 1 to 2 weeks if they are afebrile and otherwise stable.
- Pneumocystis:
  - IV or PO trimethoprim/sulfamethoxazole (TMP/SMX)
  - Alternatives include dapsone plus TMP, atovaquone, clindamycin plus primaquine, and pentamidine.
  - Duration of antibiotic treatment is 21 days.
  - Corticosteroids added in PaO_2 <70 mm Hg or A-a gradient >35 mm Hg.
  - Prophylaxis is recommended for individuals with HIV and a CD4 cell count <200, cancer, stem cell transplant recipients, solid organ transplant recipients, and some individuals on long-term glucocorticoids.
    - TMP/SMX 160 mg/800 mg 1 tablet daily or 1 tablet 3 times a week.
    - Alternatives: atovaquone, dapsone
    - Aerosolized pentamidine is a less favorable alternative.

CHAPTER
202 Tuberculosis

Alyssa Abebe, PA-C

▶ GENERAL FEATURES

- Pulmonary TB is a clinical syndrome of the respiratory system caused by *Mycobacterium tuberculosis*:
  - Pathogen is spread via aerosolized droplets through the air from person to person.
- TB most often affects the lungs but can infect other organ systems (eg, skin, brain, kidneys, spine).
- Two TB-related conditions exist: latent TB infection (LTBI) and TB disease.
- Risk factors for developing TB:
  - Conditions that cause immunocompromise (eg, HIV, diabetes, cancer, organ transplant, substance use disorder, use of immunosuppressant drugs)
  - Close contact with someone with infectious TB disease
  - Travel to regions or working/living in facilities at high risk for TB
  - IV drug use or homelessness
- Though TB can be found in all countries, those with the highest prevalence include China, India, Bangladesh, Pakistan, South Africa, Indonesia, Philippines, and Nigeria.
- The TB vaccine (bacille Calmette-Guérin [BCG]) is used in countries where TB is common and only given to select people at the discretion of a TB specialist.

▶ CLINICAL ASSESSMENT

- Suspect TB in patients presenting with fever, cough, fatigue, night sweats, weight loss, or hemoptysis:
  - Patients with LTBI are asymptomatic, are not infectious, and cannot spread TB infection to others.
  - Initial symptom may be mild and insidious.

▶ DIAGNOSIS

- Identification of *M. tuberculosis* in a respiratory sample in a symptomatic person confirms pulmonary TB.
- Laboratory tests used for diagnosis include:
  - Acid-fast bacillus smear microscopy
  - Nucleic acid amplification test (NAAT)
  - Liquid and solid mycobacterial culture
- Mantoux tuberculin skin (MTS) test will be positive if a patient has been exposed to TB; it does not determine acute or latent infection; recommended for patients aged <5 years
  - Induration of 0–5 mm is a negative test.
  - For those with risk factors: induration between 5 and 15 mm is positive.
  - >15 mm for those without risk factors is positive.
  - Positive MST testing requires further testing.
- Serum tests: interferon γ release assays (T-Spot®TB and QuantiFERON®TB-Gold In-Tube) detects acute and latent TB; recommended for those who received BCG vaccine.
- Sputum culture for acid-fast bacilli confirms TB and obtained through bronchoscopy or induction.
- Chest x-ray can show consolidation or cavities in the upper lung fields along with ipsilateral hilar enlargement.

▶ TREATMENT

- TB is reportable disease, and co-management with local health department is required; directly observed therapy (DOT) used in some cases.
- Airborne infection isolation and infection control measures for hospitalized patients with suspected TB or with AFB-positive sputum.

- Individuals with multidrug-resistant TB and special populations (eg, concurrent HIV, pregnancy, children) should be referred to a specialist.
- For LTBI: combination therapy or monotherapy is recommended:
  - Isoniazid and rifapentine therapy for 3 months
  - Rifampin monotherapy for 4 months
  - Isoniazid and rifampin for 3 months
  - Isoniazid for 6 months
- For active TB: 10 drugs are currently approved for treatment.
- First-line therapies for treatment have an induction phase (2 months) and a continuation phase (4-7 months) and include combinations of:
  - Isoniazid
  - Rifampin
  - Ethambutol
  - Pyrazinamide
- Side effects should be reported to a health care provider and include orange color to bodily fluids (rifampin or rifapentine), changes in vision, easy bruising, neuropathy, anorexia, jaundice, fatigue, abdominal pain, or tenderness.
- Liver function tests should be ordered to monitor for any liver toxicity.

CHAPTER 203

Atypical Mycobacterial Disease

Jeremy Amayo, MMSc, PA-C

▶ GENERAL FEATURES

- Nontuberculous mycobacteria (NTM), or atypical mycobacteria, are mycobacterial species other than *Mycobacterium tuberculosis* (tuberculosis) and *Mycobacterium leprae* (leprosy).
  - Over 180 species in the genus *Mycobacterium* have been isolated from animals, food, water, soil, and even human skin.
  - The most common species causing human disease in the United States include:
    - Slowly growing species like *Mycobacterium avium complex* (MAC) and *Mycobacterium kansasii*.
    - Rapidly growing species in the *Mycobacterium abscessus* group (*M. abscessus*, *Mycobacterium massiliense*, and *Mycobacterium bolletii*)
- Despite the ubiquitous nature of NTM in the environment, NTM disease is relatively rare.
- Infection acquired from environmental exposures (eg, inhalation, contaminated water contact with open skin) or iatrogenic causes like trauma or surgery
- Four main clinical diseases:
  - Chronic pulmonary disease is the most common.
  - Skin, soft-tissue, and bone infections
  - Disseminated disease (usually in immunocompromised patients)
  - Lymphadenitis (usually in children)

- Risk factors include:
  - Advanced age
  - Preexisting lung disease
  - Immunocompromise (eg, HIV infection, transplantation, use of TNF-α inhibitor drugs)

▶ CLINICAL ASSESSMENT

- Pulmonary NTM disease typically occurs in the context of some preexisting pulmonary disease, most notably previous tuberculosis, bronchiectasis (including cystic fibrosis), chronic obstructive pulmonary disease, and any of the pneumoconioses (eg, silicosis, berylliosis, asbestosis).
- Patients with primary pulmonary NTM disease present with fever, chills, malaise, fatigue, weight loss, dyspnea, cough, hemoptysis, and chest pain.
- NTM is particularly difficult to diagnose because its clinical manifestations mirror those of the underlying pulmonary diseases that put patients at risk for infection.
- It can also be difficult to differentiate true infection from transient infection, or lab sample contamination; this sometimes necessitates careful assessment of at-risk patients over a period of weeks to months.
- Patients with HIV and very low CD4 cell counts (<100 cells/μL) are at risk for disseminated NTM disease, which presents with fever, nausea, vomiting,

cardiovascular collapse, and multiple organ dysfunction/failure in addition to the symptoms seen in primary pulmonary NTM.

- Young children, typically age <5 years, present with unilateral, nontender cervical lymphadenitis and violaceous skin patches over areas of swelling.

▶ DIAGNOSIS

- Requires consideration of clinical features, radiographic findings, and microbial laboratory testing
  - Important to rule out TB
- Radiographic (chest x-ray or high-resolution computed tomography) findings are highly variable but include nodular or reticulonodular infiltrates, cavitary lung lesions, dilated airways (bronchiectasis), dense consolidations, and pleural thickening; pleural effusions are uncommon.
- Clinical criteria suggesting a diagnosis of pulmonary NTM disease include:
  - Symptoms consistent with NTM infection or nodular/cavitary opacities on chest x-ray or multifocal bronchiectasis and lung nodules high-resolution computed tomography
  - An unrevealing, thorough workup to exclude other, more likely, pulmonary diagnoses
- Definitive diagnosis requires microbiologic confirmation:
  - Positive culture results from at least two separate expectorated sputum samples or two separate acid-fast bacilli (AFB) smears and cultures
  - Or a positive culture result from at least one bronchial wash or lavage sample
  - Or a transbronchial/excisional lung biopsy with histopathologic features consistent with mycobacterial disease
- Patients who are suspected of having NTM clinically but have a negative microbiologic workup should be followed and retested over time until the diagnosis is confirmed or definitively excluded.
- Diagnosis of disseminated NTM disease in individuals with HIV/AIDS is usually made through positive blood cultures or, unfortunately, through postmortem histopathology studies.
- Children with suspected NTM lymphadenitis can be screened with tuberculin skin testing and subsequently evaluated with sputum culture or lymphoid tissue biopsy.
- Any patient undergoing a workup for NTM infection should also be evaluated for *M. tuberculosis*.

▶ TREATMENT

- The specific therapy for NTM infection is dependent on the species of the infecting organism. Members of MAC are the most common; these organisms are slow growing and can be difficult to eradicate.
- Antimycobacterial agents are only moderately effective, difficult for patients to tolerate, and require prolonged durations of therapy; not all patients diagnosed with pulmonary NTM disease require treatment.
- Patients who should initiate immediate therapy for NTM infection include:
  - Cavitary lung disease (associated with rapid progression and significant parenchymal destruction)
  - Noncavitary disease but severe symptoms
  - Noncavitary disease and low body mass index, advanced age, or multilobar pulmonary involvement
- Patients who present with asymptomatic, noncavitary NTM infections can be either started on antimycobacterial therapy or monitored with serial sputum cultures and chest imaging.
- Patients with noncavitary NTM disease who require therapy should be treated with a three-times-weekly regimen of azithromycin, rifampin, and ethambutol.
- Patients with cavitary NTM disease should be treated with a daily regimen of azithromycin, rifampin, and ethambutol.
- All patients started on antimycobacterial therapy should continue treatment until quarterly sputum cultures are consistently negative for 1 year; most patients will require therapy for 15–20 months.
- Patients should be evaluated for drug toxicity every 4–6 weeks for the duration of antimycobacterial therapy:
  - Complete blood count, renal function (blood urea nitrogen and creatinine), liver enzymes, and an assessment of visual acuity
- Alternative medication regimens do exist for patients who are intolerant of the standard therapies or have mycobacterial strains that are resistant to therapy.

CHAPTER
204

Malaria

David Gelbart, DO, MMS, MS, PA-C

▶ GENERAL FEATURES

- Malaria is a vector-borne, parasitic infection of erythrocytes caused by species of *Plasmodium* (protozoa).
  - *Plasmodium falciparum* (most virulent), *Plasmodium vivax*, *Plasmodium malariae*, *Plasmodium ovale*, *Plasmodium knowlesi*
- Vector of transmission: *Anopheles* mosquito
- Geographical distribution: Africa, Asia, South America, Central American, and the Caribbean
- Estimated annual cases: 1500–2000 in the United States, 214 million worldwide in 2015
  - *Falciparum* malaria: greatest prevalence in continental Africa
  - *Vivax* malaria: greatest prevalence in South and Central America
- Genetic traits may confer protection against malaria.
  - Hemoglobin S, β-thalassemia, G6PD deficiency
  - Lack of duffy antigen protects against *P. vivax*.
- Reportable to state health department.

▶ CLINICAL ASSESSMENT

- Asymptomatic for up to 1 month during incubation period (range: 1 week to 1 month)
- Initial symptoms: nonspecific; similar to influenza-like illness
- Cyclical fever pattern every 48 or 72 hours depending on the species
  - May lead to febrile seizures in children
  - *P. falciparum* has unpredictable, irregular fever pattern.
  - Fever with a positive travel history to areas with high malaria risk should alert clinical suspicion.
- Hemolytic anemia → jaundice, pallor
- Splenomegaly, hepatomegaly
- Nephrotic syndrome (*P. malariae*)

- Severe symptoms include:
  - "Blackwater fever" = acute renal failure plus hemoglobinuria (most often *P. falciparum*)
  - Cerebral malaria = neurologic symptoms secondary to CNS blood vessel occlusion (*P. falciparum*)
    - Delirium, decreased consciousness, seizures, coma → death
  - Shock, coagulopathy, and/or DIC
    - Thrombocytopenia, petechia
  - ARDS, metabolic acidosis
  - Liver failure, hypoglycemia

▶ DIAGNOSIS

- Blood smear (Giemsa or Wright stain): gold standard; collect serial samples 12–24 and 48 hours after initial sample
- Serology: detects past exposure

▶ TREATMENT

- Based on plasmodial sensitivity to chloroquine
- Targets stages of protozoal life cycle
- Treatment is started within first day of fever onset when malaria is suspected.
- Prophylaxis for those who travel to areas with known malaria transmission
- Primaquine 30 mg orally once daily for 2 weeks:
  - *P. vivax* and *P. ovale* form hypnozoites that remain dormant in liver:
    - Causes relapses of disease (usually 2-3 years postinfection)
    - Primaquine eradicates dormant hypnozoites and prevents relapses.
  - Also used prophylactically: 30 mg orally once daily starting 1–2 days pre-exposure through 1 week postexposure
  - Contraindicated in pregnancy

- Chloroquine 600 mg orally once, then 300 mg orally at 6, 24, and 48 hours:
  - Drug of choice for active erythrocytic form
  - Also used prophylactically: 300 mg orally once weekly starting 1–2 weeks pre-exposure through 4 weeks postexposure
  - Not effective against *P. falciparum*
- Artemisinin-based combination therapy:
  - Regimens of choice for severe and *falciparum* malaria
  - Also kills gametocytes = ↓ transmission of disease
- Other prophylactic agents:
  - Atovaquone/proguanil 250 mg/100 mg orally starting 1–2 days pre-exposure through 1 week postexposure
    - Also used as treatment for uncomplicated malaria: 1000 mg/400 mg orally once daily for 3 days
  - Mefloquine 250 mg orally once weekly starting 2–3 weeks pre-exposure through 4 weeks postexposure
    - Also used as single-dose treatment: 1.25 g orally

- Doxycycline 100 mg orally once daily starting 1–2 days pre-exposure through 4 weeks postexposure
  - Contraindicated in pregnancy and in children
  - Phototoxic reactions can occur: consider in those who anticipate prolonged sun exposure
- Special populations:
  - Pregnant first trimester: 7 days quinine + clindamycin
  - Infants <5 kg: ACT at same mg/kg target dose as children weighing 5 kg
  - Concurrent HIV infection: if on SMZ/TMP, do not use artesunate plus sulfadoxine/pyrimethamine; if on efavirenz or zidovudine, avoid artesunate plus zidovudine
  - Antimalarials can precipitate hemolytic anemia in patients with G6PD deficiency, so screen prior to starting therapy.
- Prevention:
  - Insecticides: permethrin, DDT
  - Bed nets

CHAPTER 205

Toxoplasmosis

Gina Brown, MPAS

A 25-year-old female with no history of chronic disease complains of general malaise and muscle aches for the past 3 weeks. Physical examination is normal, except for bilateral, nontender cervical and occipital lymphadenopathy. She reports no change to her social history, except for adopting a stray kitten 1 month ago. Assuming the patient has toxoplasmosis, what would be the preferred treatment?

▶ GENERAL FEATURES

- Parasitic infection disease caused by the protozoa *Toxoplasma gondii* that intracellularly infects body tissues and fluids
- Cats serve as the definitive host and transmit the protozoa through its feces; humans consume water or food that has been directly contaminated via cat feces, or they consume poorly cooked meat from previously infected mammals.
- *T. gondii* can also be transmitted transplacentally (but only when the mother is acutely infected when pregnant, or just before pregnancy) or, rarely, through organ transplantation.

- Infections can be acute (active), chronic (inactive), or reactivated.
- Found worldwide but most common in tropical areas of Latin America and in Africa
  - Global prevalence ranges widely from 10% to 80%, with lower prevalence seen in the United States.
  - Foodborne toxoplasmosis is the second leading cause of death and fourth leading cause of hospitalization from foodborne illness in the United States.

▶ CLINICAL ASSESSMENT

- Clinical findings are divided into four groups: acute infection in the immunocompetent patient, congenital infection, retinochoroiditis, and reactivated infection in the immunocompromised patient.
- Acute infection in an immunocompetent patient is usually asymptomatic but can present with general malaise and nonspecific muscle aches or mono-like symptoms that continue for weeks to months; nontender cervical or occipital lymphadenopathy is the most common finding in immunocompetent patients.
- Congenital infection may result in spontaneous abortion or stillbirth. Infants born with congenital infection

may quickly present with symptoms, such as hydrocephalus or microcephaly, or initially be asymptomatic and develop symptoms later in life.

- Symptoms include neurologic and ophthalmic disorders such as visual impairments, seizures, and mental disabilities.
- There are no pathognomonic findings for congenital toxoplasmosis.

- Retinochoroiditis can present in patients of all immune states and result from direct infection, either acute or reactivated, or from congenital infection.

- Patients may complain of eye pain, photophobia, and visual changes.
- Fundoscopic examination may reveal white retinal lesions that appear foggy due to overlying inflammation in the vitreous fluid ("headlight-in-fog" lesion).

- Reactivated infection in the immunocompromised patient can be life-threatening.

- CNS symptoms from encephalitis are the most common, including hemiparesis and speech abnormalities.
- Pneumonia and multiorgan involvement are also possible.

▶ DIAGNOSIS

- Immunocompetent patients can be tested for *Toxoplasma*-specific IgG or IgM antibodies.
- Congenital infection is determined through polymerase chain reaction (PCR) of amniotic fluid after the mother is diagnosed with acute infection.
- If the patient is immunocompromised, PCR should be performed in addition to antibody testing to increase accuracy.

- Retinochoroiditis can be diagnosed through fundoscopic examination; if necessary, a PCR of vitreous fluid can aide in the diagnosis.

▶ TREATMENT

- Treatment of immunocompetent patients with symptoms of lymphadenopathy or malaise, or mild cases of retinochoroiditis, is not indicated.
- The combination of pyrimethamine, folinic acid (leucovorin), and sulfadiazine is standard treatment for the following patients:

- Severe or persistent cases of retinochoroiditis
- Pregnant women with acute infections after 18 weeks of gestational age
- Congenitally infected newborns
- Immunocompromised patients who are symptomatic and have positive antibody titers for *T. gondii*
- Immunocompromised patients who have completed treatment for reactivated infection may continue as maintenance therapy.

- Prevention is through thoroughly cooking meat and good hygiene; care should be taken to avoid contamination from cat feces.

Case Conclusion

This is an immunocompetent patient with mild symptoms, so specific treatment is not indicated, and symptomatic care will suffice.

CHAPTER
206

Syphilis

Joshua Merson, MS-HPEd, PA-C
Mimoza Shehu, MPAS, PA-C

▶ GENERAL FEATURES

- Systemic illness caused by the spirochete *Treponema pallidum*
- Most often sexually transmitted through direct contact with active lesion; can be vertically transmitted resulting in congenital infection
- Known as "the great imitator" because of varied presentation and may resemble other diseases
- Organism forms a primary chancre at inoculation site, travels to the regional lymph nodes, and can spread.

- Increasing rate of syphilis in the past decade is attributed to increased cases of men having sex with men (MSM); ~90% of syphilis cases occur in men, and 80% of those are MSM.

- Incidence highest among Black men, regardless of sexual orientation.

- There are higher rates of co-infection with other HIV among MSM with syphilis.

CLINICAL ASSESSMENT

- Clinical diagnosis involves a pertinent history, physical examination, and serologic evidence.
- Incubation period after exposure is usually 3 weeks but can range from 3 days to 3 months.
- Primary syphilis is the early local infection, which may present as a painless genital ulcer called a chancre that spontaneously heals in 3–4 weeks.
- Secondary syphilis may occur weeks to months later if primary syphilis is left untreated.
  - Characterized by a diffuse maculopapular rash commonly in the palms and soles, condyloma lata (highly contagious wart-like lesions found in mucous/moist areas), or systemic signs and symptoms.
- If left untreated, secondary syphilis may become dormant (latent), which is characterized by an asymptomatic patient with reactive treponemal and nontreponemal tests.
  - Latent syphilis is categorized as early or late depending on when the patient was exposed.
  - Early latent syphilis refers to the infection occurring within 12 months of exposure.
  - If the time of exposure is unknown, or >12 months prior, the patient has late latent syphilis.
- Tertiary syphilis may occur anywhere from 1 to 20 years after initial infection, and only in ~15% of untreated patients, characterized by gummas (small, noncancerous granulomas) or cardiovascular manifestations.
- Neurosyphilis may occur at any stage of syphilis, leading to CNS manifestations including headache, meningitis, dementia, vision/hearing loss, Argyll-Robertson pupil, and tabes dorsalis.
- Signs of congenital syphilis secondary to acquisition of spirochete in the uterus before birth may include Hutchinson teeth, saddle-nose deformity, and TORCH syndrome.

DIAGNOSIS

- Serologic tests provide a likely diagnosis and include nontreponemal- and treponemal-specific tests.
  - One test alone is insufficient for diagnosis as serologic testing can be associated with false-positive results.
  - False negatives may also occur because serologic testing relies on a humoral response to infection.
- Two types of serologic tests:
  - Nontreponemal tests are nonspecific and used for initial screening and monitoring of therapy.
    - Include rapid plasma regain (RPR), Venereal Disease Research Laboratory (VDRL), chemiluminescence immunoassay, and toluidine red unheated serum test (TRUST).
  - Treponemal tests are traditionally used as confirmatory tests when nontreponemal tests are reactive.
    - Include fluorescent treponemal antibody absorption (FTA-ABS), microhemagglutination test for antibodies to *T. pallidum* (MHA-TP), chemiluminescence immunoassay, and *T. pallidum* enzyme immunoassay (TP-EIA)

TREATMENT

- Penicillin G is the treatment of choice for all stages.
- Penicillin formulation, dose, and duration of treatment vary by stage and clinical presentation:
  - Primary, secondary, and early latent phase syphilis:
    - Adults and pregnant patients: penicillin G benzathine IM 2.4 million units as a single dose
    - Infants and children: penicillin G benzathine 50 000 U/kg IM (to maximum of 2.4 million units) as a single dose
  - Tertiary or late latent phase: penicillin G 2.4 million units IM, once weekly for 3 weeks
  - Neurosyphilis: aqueous crystalline penicillin G (18-24 million units per day, administered as 3-4 million units IV every 4 hours or 24 million units daily as a continuous infusion for 10-14 days); or procaine penicillin G (2.4 million units IM once daily) plus probenecid (500 mg orally 4 times a day for 10-14 days)
  - Penicillin desensitization should occur in all patients with a known penicillin allergy.
- Jarisch-Herxheimer reaction may occur within 24 hours after initiation of any therapy for syphilis.
- All patients with primary or secondary syphilis should also be tested for HIV infection.
- Perform clinical and serologic evaluation at 6 and 12 months after treatment with serologic response compared with the titer at the time of treatment; failure of nontreponemal test titers to decline 4-fold within 6–12 months after therapy for primary or secondary syphilis may indicate treatment failure.

Lyme Disease

Travis Layne, DMSc, MPAS, PA-C

▶ GENERAL FEATURES

- The most common tick-borne disease in the United States and Europe
- Caused by spirochetes of the *Borrelia burgdorferi*
  - Mice and deer comprise the largest reservoir of *B. burgdorferi*.
- True incidence is unknown owing to lack of a standardized serologic test, nonspecific clinical manifestations, and low sensitivity of serology testing in early disease.
- Most infections occur from April to September while the ticks are in the nymph phase.
- Incidence of infection is significantly higher when the tick is attached for >72 hours.
- A history of brushing the tick off the skin (tick was not attached and feeding) and removing the tick on the same day of exposure decreases the infection risk.

▶ CLINICAL ASSESSMENT

- Divided into three stages, based on early and late manifestations and whether disease is localized or disseminated
  - Stage 1: 7–10 days postexposure: localized infection characterized by erythema migrans (classic EM is the "bull's-eye" appearance of the rash around the bite area) commonly seen in the groin, thigh, or axilla.
    - Classic EM is an expanding, annular, erythematous rash with central clearing seen in 90% of patients with Lyme disease.
    - A viral-like illness may accompany this stage with myalgias, arthralgias, headache, and fatigue.
    - Fever may or may not be present.
  - Stage 2: early disseminated infection, meaning the patient has become bacteremic.
    - This phase can last from 1 to 12 weeks.
    - The presentation ranges from continuation of the viral-like illness and secondary skin lesions (smaller than in stage 1) to rheumatologic, cardiac, and neurologic manifestations.
    - This can include large joint arthritis, myopericarditis, heart block, and aseptic meningitis.
    - The most common peripheral nervous system presentation is a facial palsy (cranial nerve VII neuropathy).
  - Stage 3: late persistent infection phase.
    - It can occur months to years after the initial infection and classically presents as monoarticular or oligoarticular arthritis of large weight-bearing joints.
    - It can also include the neurologic and skin disease.
    - Late Lyme disease can present with subacute encephalitis, although this is rare.
    - The cutaneous late manifestation is called acrodermatitis chronica atrophicans that presents as bluish red discoloration of the extremities with swelling; this is rarely seen in the United States and more commonly in Europe.
    - Asymptomatic disease can occur but is very rare.

▶ DIAGNOSIS

- Based on both clinical manifestations and laboratory findings:
  - US Surveillance Case Definition specifies a person with exposure to a potential tick habitat (within the 30 days just before developing erythema migrans) with (1) erythema migrans diagnosed by a clinician or (2) at least one late manifestation of the disease and (3) laboratory confirmation as fulfilling the criteria for Lyme disease.
- Nonspecific lab abnormalities can be seen particularly early in the disease, including elevated ESR, mildly elevated liver enzymes, anemia, and leukocytosis.
- Late disease requires objective evidence of clinical manifestations, such as recurrent arthritis, aseptic meningitis, facial palsy, or atrioventricular conduction defects with or without pericarditis.
- Patients with nonspecific symptoms not specific for Lyme disease should not have serologic testing.
- Two-tier serologic testing is standard for diagnosis in patients without the classic EM presentation:
  - Tier 1: Obtain an enzyme immunoassay or immunofluorescence assay; if negative, no further testing needed and consider an alternative diagnosis.
  - Tier 2: If immunoassay positive or equivocal result, then obtain a confirmatory Immunoblot test based on the duration of symptoms.
    - IgM and IgG if signs and symptoms <30 days
    - IgG only if signs and symptoms >30 days
  - Of note, most patients are seronegative in early disease.

▶ TREATMENT

- According to the CDC, doxycycline 100 mg BID for 10–14 days is usually preferred in early disease such as when EM is present.

- For early disseminated disease (stage 2), extend the duration of doxycycline to 21 days for neurologic and cardiac manifestations and 28 days for rheumatologic involvement.
- Amoxicillin and cefuroxime are alternatives if any contraindication to using doxycycline exists.
- Macrolides can be used if any contraindications to doxycycline and coexisting penicillin allergy.
  - Lower efficacy rate noted with this class, so close monitoring to ensure symptoms resolve is paramount.

- In late or severe disease, can use intravenous ceftriaxone. Reasons would include second- or third-degree heart block, syncope, dyspnea, chest pain, and CNS disease (other than facial nerve palsy).
- Generally, any patient with symptomatic CNS or cardiac disease should be admitted.

CHAPTER
208

Helminth Infestations

Judy Truscott, MPAS

A 3-year-old boy is brought into a primary care office by his mother for concern that he has been putting his hands into the back of his pants and scratching. His mother has tried to stop the scratching and is concerned that this is a new habit or that she needs to be more careful about hygiene when wiping the child after a bowel movement. She also expresses worry that maybe the child is not cleaned well after bowel movements at day care. When she looked a little closer to make sure that there was not a rash around his anus, she noticed what she thought might be small white threads. What is likely to be causing this child's pruritus? What is the recommended method to best prevent secondary infections in this patient?

▶ GENERAL FEATURES

- Pinworms (*Enterobius vermicularis*) are small white worms that cause the most common nematode infection in the United States.
- This infestation, or enterobiasis, occurs with the highest incidence in preschool- or school-age children and their caregivers.
- Transmission:
  - Transmission occurs by ingestion of the egg.
  - Ingestion via the fecal oral route is common, but surface contamination can occur as eggs may survive indoors for 2–3 weeks.
  - After ingestion, it takes up to 2 months for the adult female pinworm to mature and lay eggs; traveling from the colon to the anus, the adult female lays eggs at night in the perianal area.

- Hookworm (*Necator americanus*) infection is another helminth infestation in the United States but is very rarely seen; it had been much more common in the United States in the early 1900s before indoor plumbing and widespread footwear use.
- The differential diagnosis list for pruritus ani is extensive, but more narrowly focused in children than adults; in a child, consider atopic dermatitis, contact dermatitis, and perianal streptococcal dermatitis as other common causes.

▶ CLINICAL ASSESSMENT

- Most infections are asymptomatic, but perianal pruritus is the most common clinical complaint.
  - The patient may also complain of disturbed sleep, anxiousness, or irritability.
  - Secondary bacterial infections related to scratching may occur.
- On physical examination:
  - Signs of excoriation can be noted in the perianal area. Because of excoriation and the intense pruritus, secondary bacterial infections can occur.
- White thread-like worms may be visible around the anus but may not be noted on clinical examination because these are best visualized within 3 hours of the patient going to sleep.

▶ DIAGNOSIS

- The diagnosis is straightforward once the history is described, particularly of nighttime perianal itching.

- The definitive diagnosis is made by detection of worms or eggs in the perianal area:
  - Tape test:
    - After the patient has awoken, the adhesive side of transparent tape is adhered to the perianal skin.
    - When viewed microscopically, eggs may be visible; once the patient has washed the area, eggs may no longer be present.
    - It is recommended that the tape test is done on 3 consecutive days to ensure accuracy.
  - Because intense pruritis may cause the patient to scratch their perianal skin, a sample collected from under a patient's nails may also yield eggs.
  - Stool samples are not recommended for pinworms or eggs as they are not typically seen in stool.

▶ TREATMENT

- Antihelmintic treatment:
  - Given as two dose treatments, the first dose is given at the time of diagnosis and the second 2 weeks later if infection persists.
  - Options are:
    - Albendazole
    - Mebendazole
    - Pyrantel pamoate is an over-the-counter treatment but is not as effective in killing the eggs, and treatment must be repeated.
  - Contraindications: all three are contraindicated for use in age <1 year; additionally, all three are pregnancy category C, although mebendazole is safe for us in breastfeeding.
- Prophylactic treatment in a setting of outbreak can help to reduce the spread. Additionally, if more than one family member is infected, the entire family should be treated.
- Supportive treatment:
  - Nails should be trimmed so that there is less chance of trauma to skin and, therefore, less chance of a secondary infection.
  - Proper handwashing, washing sheets, undergarments, and pajamas in the morning can help prevent transmission of eggs.
  - Siblings should not co-bathe if one is infected as the bath water might become contaminated with eggs; showering is recommended.

Case Conclusion

This child has pinworms. Keeping his nails short will lessen trauma to perianal skin and help prevent secondary infection.

CHAPTER 209

Trichomoniasis

Alyssa Abebe, PA-C

▶ GENERAL FEATURES

- Trichomoniasis is the most common curable sexually transmitted infection (STI) in the United States.
- Caused by the urogenital protozoan *Trichomonas vaginalis*
- More common in women and in the older population
- Can cause preterm labor, premature rupture of membranes, and low birth weight
- Infection can increase the risk of contracting other STIs such as HIV due to genital inflammation.
- Condoms can prevent the infection.

▶ CLINICAL ASSESSMENT

- Up to 70% of patients are asymptomatic.
- Symptoms can begin 5–28 days after sexual contact with an infected individual.

- Common symptoms in women include pruritis and/or burning of the genitals, dysuria, vaginal discharge that can be clear and white or yellow greenish with a foul, fishy odor.
  - On examination, vaginal erythema and red macular cervical lesions can be visible also known as a "strawberry cervix."
- Men may present with penile discharge, dysuria, pruritis, penile irritation, or no symptoms.
- Dyspareunia may also be present in men and women.

▶ DIAGNOSIS

- Nucleic acid amplification testing is a preferred diagnostic test.
  - Alternative diagnostics include immune chromatography assay test, nucleic acid probe testing, or culture (eg, vaginal secretions in women; urethral swab, urine, or semen in men).

- Microscopic examination of wet mount preparation of vaginal or urethral secretions mixed with normal saline can be used to visualize the protozoan.

▶ TREATMENT

- Nonpregnant patients:
  - Metronidazole 2 g orally in a single dose
  - Tinidazole 2 g orally in a single dose
  - Metronidazole 500 mg orally twice daily for 7 days
- Pregnant patients:
  - Consider metronidazole 2 g orally as a single dose.
  - During lactation, withhold breastfeeding during and for a short period after treatment (12-24 hours after metronidazole, 72 hours after tinidazole).
- Avoid alcohol consumption with medication.
- Treat sexual partners.
- Abstinence should be practiced for 1 week following treatment and with resolution of symptoms.

CHAPTER 210

Rocky Mountain Spotted Fever

Shaun Lynch, MS, MMSc, PA-C

A 33-year-old man presents to the primary care clinic with low-grade fever, headache, and erythematous maculopapular rash on his hands, wrist, feet, and ankles. He reports camping in the woods of Western North Carolina over the past weekend. What is the most likely diagnosis?

▶ GENERAL FEATURES

- Rocky Mountain spotted fever (RMSF) is a potentially life-threatening tick-borne illness caused by the intracellular bacterium *Rickettsia rickettsii*.
- RMSF occurs primarily through tick bites from American dog tick (most common vector), Brown dog ticks, and Rocky Mountain wood tick, with most cases occurring between May and August.
- Although RMSF has been reported in all areas within the continental United States, the highest number of cases occur in:
  - Arkansas
  - Missouri
  - North Carolina
  - Oklahoma
  - Tennessee
- Most cases of RMSF occur between May and September.
- Symptoms usually arise between 2 and 14 days after exposure.
- RMSF can be a rapidly progressive disease without prompt recognition and treatment.

▶ CLINICAL ASSESSMENT

- The classic symptoms of RMSF occurring in a person with a history of a tick bite include:
  - Fever
  - Headache
  - Rash
- Early signs include fever, headache, myalgias, malaise, and gastrointestinal symptoms, such as abdominal pain, nausea, and vomiting.
- Most patients develop a rash between 3 and 5 days of feeling ill, beginning as small blanching macules that later become petechial over time.
- The rash typically begins on the wrist and ankles and spreads to the trunk, often sparing the face.
- Progression of the illness may lead to altered mental status, respiratory or renal failure, or multiorgan system damage.

▶ DIAGNOSIS

- Gold standard for diagnosis is serology:
  - Serologic testing includes the indirect immunofluorescence antibody (IFA) assay for immunoglobulin G (IgG) against the *R. rickettsii* antigen.
  - The IgG IFA assays should demonstrate a 4-fold increase in IgG when performed 2–4 weeks apart.
- Laboratory findings that may be present include thrombocytopenia.
- Skin biopsy of the rash can be obtained with direct immunofluorescence testing in certain laboratories.
- Treatment should not be withheld for RMSF with a negative test result when clinical manifestations of the disease are suggestive of RMSF.
- A polymerase chain reaction (PCR) amplification test can be performed from the blood or skin biopsy of the rash, but a negative result does not rule out the diagnosis.

▶ TREATMENT

- Doxycycline is first-line treatment for suspected RMSF and all other tick-borne rickettsial diseases in patients of all ages.

- Adults: should receive 100 mg of doxycycline for 7 days
- Children under 45 kg: should receive 2.2 mg/kg body weight twice a day for 5–7 days
- Start treatment immediately to minimize life-threatening complications such as encephalitis, pulmonary edema, adult respiratory distress syndrome, coagulopathy, cardiac arrhythmias, and skin necrosis.

- Post-tick bite antibiotic prophylaxis or treatment of asymptomatic individuals is not recommended.

Case Conclusion

This patient has RMSF, a tick-borne illness causing a prodrome of fever and headache for several days before the onset of the characteristic rash.

Prenatal Transmission of Infection

Prenatal Transmission of Infectious Pathogens

Elyse Watkins, DHSc, PA-C, DFAAPA

A 22-year-old G1 presents to the labor and delivery department in active labor. The patient has had no prior prenatal care and is ~39 weeks by her last menstrual period (LMP). She admits to regular intravenous drug use and works in the sex industry. What interventions should be initiated at this time?

▶ GENERAL FEATURES

- Vertical transmission of infectious pathogens from mother to fetus can lead to serious consequences for a developing fetus.
- Morbidity and mortality are highest during the antepartum period, but peripartum and postpartum transmission can occur.
  - Transmission through the placenta is the most common route during the antepartum period.
- The initial prenatal laboratory panel includes screening for rubella, HIV, hepatitis B, *Treponema pallidum*, and varicella zoster virus (VZV).
- It is not recommended to routinely screen for herpes simplex virus (HSV), parvovirus, toxoplasmosis, or cytomegalovirus (CMV).
- Patients who are considered at risk should be screened for hepatitis C with a hepatitis C antibody test.
  - Hepatitis C is associated with low birth weight and fetal growth restriction.
  - There is no treatment recommendation for hepatitis C in pregnancy.

- The TORCH screen assesses a panel of pathogens associated with harm:
  - *Toxoplasma gondii*, other (*T. pallidum*, parvovirus B19, HIV, VZV, *Listeria monocytogenes*, Zika virus, hepatitis B and C, and severe acute respiratory syndrome coronavirus 2 [SARS-CoV-2]), rubella, CMV, and HSV 1 and HSV 2.
- TORCH pathogens are usually associated with hepatosplenomegaly, risk of prematurity, and fetal demise.
  - All patients with suspected or confirmed TORCH infections should be referred to a maternal-fetal medicine specialist.
- Other pathogens linked to teratogenic effects in pregnancy:
  - Coxsackievirus appears to slightly increase the risk of miscarriage and stillbirth.
  - Toxoplasmosis is associated with miscarriage, fetal anemia, hydrocephalus, chorioretinitis and blindness, developmental delay, intracranial calcifications, and seizures.
  - *Treponema* infections are associated with chorioretinitis, glaucoma, sensorineural hearing loss, hydrocephalus, and musculoskeletal deformities.
  - Zika virus is associated with microcephaly and other neurologic disorders.
  - Rubella is associated with fetal cardiac anomalies, such as patent ductus arteriosus and other septal defects, pulmonary artery stenosis, hydrocephalus, chorioretinitis, microcephaly, microphthalmia, hearing loss, and cataracts.

- Risk of rubella infection is greatest when exposure occurs during the first trimester.
- CMV is associated with central nervous system anomalies, including microcephaly, ventricular dilation, hypoplastic corpus callosum, and calcifications. Other sequelae include fetal ascites, pericardial effusion, and hydrops.
- VZV is associated with intrauterine growth restriction, microcephaly, hepatic lesions, and limb deformities; in the gravid patient, infection carries significant risk of pneumonia and is associated with significant mortality.
- HSV 1 and HSV 2 are associated with a triad of fetal findings that include dermatologic, neurologic, and ophthalmologic anomalies:
  - Derm: skin lesions, scarring, and pigmentation issues
  - Neuro: microcephaly, hydranencephaly, and calcifications
  - Eyes: chorioretinitis, optic atrophy, and chorioretinitis
- Infants born to mothers with hepatitis B and did not receive antiviral therapy are likely to develop chronic hepatitis B infection, with resultant cirrhosis, hepatic failure, and hepatic malignancy.
- Parvovirus B19 is linked to hydrops, severe anemia, heart failure, maternal mirror syndrome (maternal edema, proteinuria, and hypertension in the presence of hydrops), and fetal demise.
- A detailed medical history includes questions about possible exposure to known microbial teratogens, and all patients should be asked about possible Zika exposure at each trimester.
- Risk factors for toxoplasmosis include ingesting undercooked meat and fish, cleaning a cat litter box, or coming into contact with an infected feline's feces.

▶ CLINICAL ASSESSMENT

- Hepatitis B:
  - The US Preventive Services Task Force supports screening all pregnant patients for hepatitis B with HBsAg serology at the first prenatal visit.
  - Patients who had a negative test in a prior pregnancy should still be screened with each subsequent pregnancy.
  - Patients with risk factors should also be screened upon admission for delivery
- HIV:
  - The American College of Obstetricians and Gynecologists (ACOG) recommends opt-out HIV testing prepregnancy, at the initial prenatal visit, and in the third trimester in patients who are at risk of contracting the virus using the antibody-antigen test.
  - In patients who present in labor with no prior testing or an unknown HIV status, rapid HIV testing is recommended.

- HSV:
  - A primary HSV outbreak during pregnancy poses a higher risk for transmission to the fetus than a recurrent outbreak.
    - Genital HSV 1 infections are associated with a higher risk of transmission to the newborn than genital HSV 2.
  - Patients who present with a genital lesion and do not have a history of HSV should receive a viral culture and polymerase chain reaction (PCR) testing.
  - Patients with suspected HSV infection who have not had confirmatory testing may undergo serologic testing.
  - The ACOG does not support routing screening in pregnant patients without a history of HSV.
- Syphilis:
  - Screening for syphilis is recommended for all pregnant patients as early as possible with RPR or VDRL.
    - If either is positive, confirmation with a specific treponemal antibody test is done.
      - Two tests available are the fluorescent treponemal antibody absorption and *T. pallidum* particle agglutinization test.
    - A new testing option is with an automated treponemal antibody testing followed by VDRL or RPR. This is referred to as reverse screening.
      - Automated enzyme-linked immunosorbent assays (EIAs) and chemiluminescence immunoassays (CIAs) are better than older testing options for detecting primary syphilis.
  - Screening again early in the third trimester and at delivery is recommended for patients considered at high risk or live in a high syphilis prevalence region.
  - Fetal ultrasound findings may include polyhydramnios, hepatomegaly, ascites, and placentomegaly; abnormal flow of the middle cerebral artery may also be seen.

▶ DIAGNOSIS

- Hepatitis B:
  - Confirmation of acute or chronic hepatitis B infection is made through evaluation of results from a hepatitis B panel, including HBV DNA viral load. Other labs include a complete blood count, liver enzyme panel, and international normalized ratio.
- HIV:
  - Diagnosis is confirmed with HIV antigen/antibody testing.
  - If acute infection is suspected, plasma HIV RNA may be ordered.
- HSV:
  - Confirmatory diagnosis of genital herpes is through HSV PCR.
  - Serologic testing may be appropriate in patients suspected of having HSV.
    - The presence of HSV 1 antibodies could indicate prior orolabial or genital infection.

- The presence of HSV 2 antibodies is almost always indicative of prior genital infection.
- Syphilis:
  - The diagnosis of syphilis is through positive treponemal antibody testing. Direct visualization of the organism cannot be achieved using standard microscopes.
  - A reactive test does not differentiate between current or past infection.
  - If a treponemal immunoassay is reactive and the nontreponemal antibody test is negative, it could be a false positive that commonly occurs in pregnancy.
    - A different treponemal antibody test should be performed, such as the *T. pallidum* particle agglutination test for confirmation.

▶ TREATMENT

- Hepatitis B:
  - If prenatal HBV DNA is >200 000 IU/mL, antiviral therapy is recommended. Tenofovir is the recommended antiviral during pregnancy.
  - Patients who are at risk of contracting hepatitis B during pregnancy may be given the hepatitis B vaccine.
  - Neonates born to hepatitis B–positive mothers should receive hepatitis B vaccination and hepatitis immunoglobulin, regardless of birth weight within 12 hours of birth.
- HIV:
  - The goal of treatment of HIV in pregnancy is to reduce perinatal transmission of the virus to the newborn by viral suppression with antiretroviral therapies (ARTs).
  - Earlier suppression with ART is associated with a decreased risk of perinatal transmission.
  - There are various ART regimens available, and decisions on which regimen to use is based upon several factors, including drug resistance, drug-drug interactions, comorbidities, and adverse effects.
  - Other factors that influence ART choice includes whether or not the patient has used ART previously, if they did not tolerate an ART regimen in the past, and if they are restarting an ART regimen.
  - HIV RNA levels are monitored periodically throughout pregnancy to ensure adequate viral suppression.
  - Patients who are HIV positive should be offered elective cesarean delivery at 38 weeks' gestation.
  - Zidovudine is used during the intrapartum management of HIV.
    - Patients who are undergoing cesarean delivery should receive zidovudine intravenously 3 hours before surgery.
  - Postpartum management of HIV-positive patients involves the continued use of ART, comprehensive multidisciplinary support, and patient education.

- Patients in the United States are advised against breastfeeding.
- Contraception counseling should occur during the prenatal period in anticipation of instituting an acceptable form of contraception postpartum.
- Infants born to HIV-positive mothers receive immediate postpartum ART and are continued on an age-appropriate ART regimen.
- HSV:
  - Oral acyclovir or valacyclovir can be used for primary and recurrent outbreaks.
  - Intravenous acyclovir can be used in severe HSV disease.
  - Patients with recurrent HSV infections should be considered for chronic suppressive therapy with acyclovir beginning at 36 weeks.
  - When active genital lesions are present, or when prodromal symptoms are present during labor, patients should be offered cesarean delivery, regardless of the duration of rupture of membranes.
  - Breastfeeding should be encouraged.
    - Antiviral therapy is considered safe during lactation.
- Syphilis:
  - Long-acting intramuscular benzathine penicillin G is the only recommended treatment for syphilis.
  - Early infection is treated with one intramuscular injection of 2.4 million units of benzathine penicillin G; a second dose may be considered within 10 days of initial injection.
  - Syphilis of unknown duration or late syphilis should be treated with 3 weekly injections of 2.4 million units benzathine penicillin G in each dose.
  - If patients have a history of an IgE-mediated hypersensitivity reaction to penicillin, referral for desensitization is recommended.
  - Nontreponemal antibody titers are followed over the course of treatment to verify response.
  - Of note, some patients may experience a Jarisch-Herxheimer reaction characterized by fever, myalgias, fetal heart rate abnormalities, and possible preterm labor because of large amounts of lipopolysaccharides released from dying spirochetes.
  - Patients should be encouraged to breastfeed postpartum.

Case Conclusion

For this patient, perform a rapid HIV test and begin intravenous zidovudine if positive. Elective cesarean delivery should be offered to all patients at 38 weeks' gestation; if delivery is not imminent, risks, benefits, and alternatives of vaginal vs. cesarean delivery should be offered.

Sepsis and Systemic Inflammatory Response Syndrome

CHAPTER

212

Sepsis and Systemic Inflammatory Response Syndrome

Ryan Hunton, MSc, PA-C

> A 74-year-old male presents to the emergency department from a long-term care facility with cough and shortness of breath. Nursing home staff also noted confusion last night that worsened this morning. He was noted to have a temperature of 101.2 °F. On initial evaluation, he has a heart rate of 104 beats per minute, blood pressure of 85/40 mm Hg, oxygen saturation of 87% on room air with mild respiratory distress, and respiratory rate at 24 breaths per minute. Crackles are noted on auscultation of the posterior right lung. He was arousable to voice with a Glasgow Coma Scale score of 11. What is the next most appropriate step in the management for this patient?

▶ GENERAL FEATURES

- Sepsis is a life-threatening organ dysfunction caused by a dysregulated response to infection.
- Sepsis now understood to involve early activation of both pro-inflammatory and anti-inflammatory responses.
  - Normal response to localized infection includes activation of neutrophils and monocytes, release of inflammatory mediators, local vasodilation, increased endothelial permeability, and activation of coagulation pathways.
  - Sepsis results from an exaggerated systemic inflammatory response.
- Septic shock is a severe subset in which circulatory, cellular, and metabolic abnormalities are associated with a higher risk of mortality than with sepsis alone.
  - Most common type of distributive shock: impaired distribution of blood flow secondary to excessive vasodilation leads to inadequate tissue perfusion and results in end-organ dysfunction.
  - Inadequate tissue perfusion manifested by physical examination and laboratory signs (eg, decreased capillary refill time or increased creatinine).

- Bacterial infections are the most common cause of sepsis; however, it can also be caused by viral, fungal, or parasitic infections.
- Early identification and appropriate management in the initial hours improve outcomes in patients with severe sepsis or septic shock.
- Recommendations continue to evolve frequently.
- Epidemiology:
  - Incidence rate of sepsis increases with mortality rate decreasing.
    - Related to increasing elderly population, invasive procedures, and use of immunosuppressive agents
    - Also thought to be related to increased clinical awareness, more screening, decreased diagnostic thresholds, and more diligent coding
- Gram-positive bacteria are now more common as a source of sepsis in the United States.
- Risk factors for sepsis:
  - Advanced age
  - Comorbidities (eg, alcoholism, cirrhosis, diabetes mellitus, cardiopulmonary disease, malignancy)
  - Immunosuppression
  - Major surgery, trauma, or burns
  - Invasive procedures (eg, catheters, intravascular devices, hemodialysis or peritoneal dialysis, endotracheal tubes)
  - Prolonged hospitalization
  - Previous antibiotic treatment

▶ CLINICAL ASSESSMENT

- Patients have fever, tachypnea, tachycardia, and hypotension.
- May present with localizing symptoms of infectious disease; the most common sources of infection are the lung, abdomen, urinary tract, and soft tissue.
- Symptoms include:

- Constitutional: fever, chills, or generalized weakness
- Pulmonary: cough, shortness of breath, or pleuritic chest pain
- Gastrointestinal: vomiting, diarrhea, or abdominal pain
- Genitourinary: dysuria, hematuria, urinary frequency, urgency, or flank pain
- Dermatologic: skin redness, purpura, swelling, or warmth
- Patients may also present with a nonspecific sign of end-organ damage:
  - Altered mental status as evidenced by Glasgow Coma Scale
  - Respiratory distress requiring ventilator support
  - Lightheadedness with an MAP of <65 mm Hg
  - Oliguria or anuria with <0.5 mL/kg/hr urine output or <500 mL in 24 hours

DIAGNOSIS

- Acute care settings currently use a combination of systemic inflammatory response syndrome (SIRS) criteria and sequential (sepsis-related) organ failure assessment (SOFA) score to identify sepsis.
- SIRS criteria have been criticized for not being specific enough, and SOFA criteria have been criticized for not being sensitive enough.
- SIRS criteria:
  - SIRS criteria are positive if a patient has two of the following four diagnostic signs:
    - Temperature >38 °C (100.4 °F) or <36 °C (96.8 °F)
    - Heart rate >90 beats per minute
    - Respirations >20 or $Paco_2$ <32 mm Hg
    - White blood cell count >12 000 cells/mm^3 or <4000 cells/mm^3, or >10% immature white blood cell bands
  - Sepsis: SIRS criteria in a patient with a known or suspected infectious source
  - Severe sepsis: sepsis with signs of new organ dysfunction, hypoperfusion, or hypotension
  - Septic shock: hypotension (systolic blood pressure <90 mm Hg or reduction of 40 mm Hg from baseline) despite adequate intravenous (IV) fluid resuscitation
  - SIRS criteria might also be positive with noninfectious disorders like diabetic ketoacidosis, pancreatitis, congestive heart failure exacerbation, chronic obstructive pulmonary disease exacerbation, and trauma, or with mild infectious disorders.
  - Multiple organ dysfunction syndrome (MODS): development of physiologic dysfunction of two or more organs or organ systems. It varies from mild degree of organ dysfunction to irreversible organ failure.

- SOFA score:
  - SOFA score serves as a proxy for organ dysfunction. It includes markers for organ dysfunction in several systems: respiratory (Pao_2/FIo_2), coagulation (platelets), hepatobiliary (bilirubin), renal (creatinine), cardiovascular (MAP), and central nervous (Glasgow Coma Scale) systems.
  - Sepsis: acute increase in ≥2 points in SOFA with a suspected or documented infection
  - Septic shock: sepsis plus a lactate >2 mmol/L with persistent hypotension, despite adequate fluid resuscitation and requiring vasopressor therapy
  - "Severe sepsis" was removed from the lexicon.
  - For acute care settings, a quick SOFA (qSOFA) score was recommended, where two of the following clinical criteria define a positive score:
    - Respiratory rate of ≥22/min
    - Altered mentation
    - Systolic blood pressure of ≤100 mm Hg
- Evaluation for suspected focal infection, clinically occult infection, or complications of sepsis typically involves lactate, two sets of blood cultures, complete blood count with differential, comprehensive metabolic panel, urinalysis with urine culture, chest x-ray, and coagulation studies.
- Depending on presentation, evaluation might also involve arterial or venous blood gas, lumbar puncture, radiograph of extremity, or computed tomography of the abdomen, pelvis, or head.

TREATMENT

- Ensure the patient's airway is intact and provide supplemental oxygen as needed.
- Establish IV access and place patient on cardiac monitor.
- Broad-spectrum antimicrobials:
  - Administer within 1 hour of diagnosis. Obtain necessary cultures before antibiotic administration, but do not delay therapy for this purpose.
  - Antibiotics often include both Gram-negative coverage (eg, β-lactam or later generation cephalosporins) and Gram-positive coverage (eg, vancomycin).
  - Patient severity, patient risk, likely microorganism, local resistance patterns, and previous cultures should be considered in antibiotic selection.
  - De-escalation with discontinuation of combination therapy is recommended within the first few days in response to clinical improvement or infection resolution.
  - Sustained systemic antimicrobial prophylaxis not recommended for patients with severe inflammatory states of noninfectious etiology (eg, pancreatitis or burns).
  - Antimicrobial duration is typically 7–10 days for most serious infections associated with sepsis and septic shock.

- IV fluids and vasopressors:
  - The 2017 guidelines recommend that sepsis-induced hypoperfusion (ie, severe sepsis or septic shock) is resuscitated with ≥30 mL/kg of IV crystalloid fluids within the first 3 hours with frequent reassessment of hemodynamic status.
  - Hemodynamic status can be assessed through lactic acid measurement, capillary refill time, cardiac output monitoring, or bedside ultrasound of the inferior vena cava.
  - Vasopressors are used if patient has refractory shock (MAP <65 mm Hg after adequate fluid administration).
  - Norepinephrine is the vasopressor of choice; arterial line placement should be considered.
  - Stress-dose steroids are only recommended if adequate fluid resuscitation and vasopressor therapy are not able to restore hemodynamic stability.

- Source control:
  - Specific anatomic diagnosis of infection requiring emergent source control should occur as rapidly as possible.
  - Examples of source control include removal of intravascular access devices, intrauterine catheter devices, and nasogastric tubes.

Case Conclusion

Based on the patient's presentation, you ensured his airway was intact, started him oxygen by nasal cannula at 4 L/min, obtained IV access with two large-bore IVs, and placed him on a cardiac monitor. You considered septic shock in your differential and quickly started an IV bolus of crystalloid fluids and provided broad-spectrum antibiotic coverage. After a chest x-ray showed a right-sided lower lobe pneumonia, you admitted him to the intensive care unit for continued management.

SECTION **G**   *Viral Diseases*

CHAPTER
213

Infectious Mononucleosis

Joel Schwartzkopf, MPAS, MBA

▶ GENERAL FEATURES

- Infectious mononucleosis is a viral disease that classically presents with the triad of fever, lymphadenopathy, and pharyngitis.
- Most acute infections are caused by the Epstein-Barr virus (EBV).
- Most adults in the United States are positive for antibodies to EBV, and most patients gain exposure in early childhood without ever showing acute symptoms.
- Single exposure to EBV confers lifelong immunity.
- Typical acute presentation involves a patient in mid- to late adolescence; acute infection is rare in patients aged >30 years.
- Direct salivary contact with an acutely infected patient is the chief mechanism of transmission for EBV, and patients will actively shed the virus for months after acute infection.
- Incubation period is typically 1–2 months.

▶ CLINICAL ASSESSMENT

- Acute symptomatic phase lasts 2–4 weeks.
- Fever is typically low grade; chills, sweats, myalgia, and arthralgia are rare.
- Classically, the patient has palpable posterior cervical lymph nodes but may be diffuse.
- Patients usually have notable pharyngitis and tonsillar swelling; tonsillar exudates and palatal petechiae can mimic the appearance of an acute streptococcal infection.
- Fatigue is one of the most common symptoms, and though it generally is limited to the acute phase, it may persist for weeks or even months after other symptoms resolve.
- Splenomegaly is also common and, in a few patients, may be the presenting symptom.

- Nausea, vomiting, rash, and headache are frequent, with other symptoms such as oral hairy leukoplakia, facial edema, jaundice, and hepatomegaly occurring in a minority of patients.

▶ DIAGNOSIS

- A thorough history and physical examination are important for accurate clinical diagnosis.
- Laboratory testing includes the rapid Monospot test, which detects the presence of heterophile antibodies and is highly specific for EBV. Sensitivity is decreased early in the illness but improves after the first week of acute infection and peaks at 2–5 weeks.
- EBV-specific antibody testing is available but generally should be reserved for patients with chronic or persistent symptoms in which the diagnosis of mononucleosis is uncertain.
- Obtain a complete blood cell count with manual differential.
  - Lymphocytes may be elevated with atypical lymphocytes normally >10%.
  - Total leukocytosis with elevated white blood cells up to 20 000 cells/mm³ is common.
  - Thrombocytopenia is sometimes seen.
- Erythrocyte sedimentation rate, AST, and ALT typically will be elevated in patients with EBV.
- Owing to the similar presenting symptoms, rapid testing for group A *Streptococcus* and a throat culture may be performed. Antibiotics should be initiated only if indicated.

▶ TREATMENT

- Acute mononucleosis is a self-limited viral illness that will typically resolve without intervention.
- Serious complications may include airway compromise and spontaneous or traumatic rupture of the spleen.
- In cases of suspected splenic rupture, imaging, admission, and/or consult with a general surgeon are appropriate, though most cases are managed nonoperatively.
- Actively ill patients should refrain from any activity that would place them at risk for splenic rupture. Four weeks from acute onset generally is considered an appropriate waiting period before returning to sports.
- In more severe cases, admission for IV hydration and monitoring is appropriate.
- Use of antiviral medication is not beneficial. Corticosteroids are ineffective and may limit the natural immune response to infection, though they may be indicated in patients with airway swelling.
- Patients with mononucleosis who receive β-lactam antibiotics for treatment of suspected bacterial infection frequently develop a diffuse but benign maculopapular rash. Clinicians who suspect *Streptococcus* should use appropriate laboratory testing before initiating treatment.

CHAPTER
214

Measles, Mumps, and Rubella

Alyssa Abebe, PA-C

▶ GENERAL FEATURES

- Measles (rubeola):
  - Measles is a paramyxoviral infection and is highly contagious, spread via respiratory droplets.
  - The vaccine-preventable illness causes fever and rash.
  - Measles is endemic throughout the world, particularly in Europe, Africa, and most of Asia, although it is largely eradicated from the Americas.
- Mumps:
  - Mumps is a paramyxoviral infection spread via respiratory droplets.
  - The mild vaccine-preventable illness characteristically causes parotitis and orchitis (which can cause infertility in biologic males).
  - Leading cause of pancreatitis in children
  - Mumps is endemic throughout the world. In the United States, several hundred cases are reported annually, most occurring in college students with high vaccination coverage.
- Rubella (German measles):
  - Rubella is caused by the *Rubivirus*.
  - The mild vaccine-preventable illness causes fever and rash.

- Rubella titer is done at beginning of pregnancy to determine serostatus.
- Exposure during the first- and second-trimesters pregnancy can cause congenital rubella, which can present as cataracts, glaucoma, congenital heart defects, deafness, psychomotor retardation, and fatality.
- Rubella is endemic throughout the world; the illness was largely eradicated from the Americas by 2010, and incidence has remained low.
- MMR vaccine is routinely given at 12–15 months of age, with a booster between the ages of 4 and 6 years.

CLINICAL ASSESSMENT

- Measles:
  - High fever (104–105 °F) and malaise present 7–10 days before the rash and may persist throughout illness.
  - Prodrome of cough, coryza, and conjunctivitis
  - Koplik spots (blue-white dots surrounded by an erythematous base) on the mucous membranes is pathognomonic and appear ~2 days before rash.
  - Erythematous maculopapular rash begins on the face (typically behind ears first) and spreads to trunk and upper and lower extremities and fades in same pattern within 3–4 days.
- Mumps:
  - Parotid tenderness either unilaterally or bilaterally
  - Lymphadenopathy of the submaxillary and sublingual glands
  - Fever and malaise are minimal, though high fever and neck stiffness indicate meningeal complications.
  - Testicular swelling and tenderness indicate orchitis (typically unilateral).
  - Upper abdominal pain with nausea and vomiting can indicate pancreatitis.
- Rubella:
  - Fever, malaise, adenitis, and coryza can present 1 week before rash.
  - Polyarthritis can found in adults.
  - Posterior cervical and postauricular lymphadenopathy is common 5–10 days before rash.
  - Maculopapular rash is found on the face, trunk, and extremities and spreads rapidly within 2 days of onset and recedes quickly.

DIAGNOSIS

- Measles:
  - Diagnosed clinically
  - Leukopenia may be present due to secondary bacterial complications.
  - Virus can be cultured from nasal washings.
- Mumps:
  - Diagnosed clinically when there are known outbreaks.
  - PCR testing can be done to confirm via saliva or CSF.
- Rubella:
  - Can be hard to distinguish from other viral exanthemas
  - Clinical diagnosis is made during outbreaks; can use serology to confirm.
  - Leukopenia can be present.
  - Congenital rubella is confirmed through isolating the virus and confirmed with IgM rubella antibody.

TREATMENT

- Measles:
  - Symptomatic treatment, fever can be treated with acetaminophen.
  - Isolation for 1 week following the rash is recommended.
  - Vitamin A treatment for 2 consecutive days has been linked to reduced rates of morbidity and mortality.
- Mumps:
  - Generally, lasts <2 weeks
  - Symptomatic treatment for uncomplicated cases
  - Isolation until swelling and fever subsides
  - Meningitis treated with appropriate antibiotics
  - Orchitis treated with suspension and ice
- Rubella:
  - Typically, a mild illness that lasts 3–5 days.
  - Symptomatic treatment with acetaminophen
  - Congenital rubella treatment is aimed at the complications.

Rabies

David Gelbart, DO, MMS, MS, PA-C

GENERAL FEATURES

- Rabies is a neurotropic infection caused by single-stranded RNA viruses of the Rhabdoviridae family and is virtually always fatal.
- The virus is carried by all mammals (usually in saliva) and infects humans through direct inoculation (bite or scratch).
  - Virions then bind nACh receptors in local muscle tissue to amplify before retrograde transport via peripheral nerves to dorsal root ganglia and ultimately to the brain and salivary glands.
  - Incubation period is generally 1–3 months but can range from days to years.
- Found in every US State except Hawaii and worldwide with exceptions, including Antarctica and island countries such as Japan and New Zealand.
- Dog bites are implicated in 99% of cases worldwide.
  - Estimated worldwide incidence is 59 000 annually.
  - Bats are the predominate vector in regions where animals are generally vaccinated.
- Vast majority of human rabies cases occur in Asia and Africa.

CLINICAL ASSESSMENT

- Encephalitic or paralytic rabies follow nonspecific viral prodrome during the first week of infection after animal bite or scratch.
- Paresthesias and dysesthesias radiating proximally from wound are classic.
- Affected muscle tissue may mound to percussion (myoedema).
- Aerophobia is pathognomonic.
- Encephalitic form is most common:
  - Classic clinical picture of hydrophobia → spasm (facial, oropharyngeal, opisthotonos) → paralysis → coma → death (2° to pulmonary arrest and vascular collapse)
  - Autonomic instability: dysrhythmias, diaphoresis, temperature dysregulation, ↑ salivation/lacrimation, mydriasis, orthostasis

- Neuropsychiatric: aggression, agitation, altered mental status, visual/auditory hallucinations, delirium
- Paralytic form presents similarly to Guillain-Barré syndrome: progressive ascending flaccid paralysis (symmetric or asymmetric) → loss of reflexes → respiratory collapse → death
- Either form may present with nuchal rigidity.

DIAGNOSIS

- Diagnosis is primarily made based on history and physical examination.
- Diagnostic testing is not confirmatory before the onset of clinical symptoms.
- Viral RNA may be detected by reverse transcriptase PCR or direct fluorescent antibodies.
  - Consult with the CDC before obtaining human samples.
- Negri bodies, when present on postmortem histologic examination, are pathognomonic.

TREATMENT

- Treatment in symptomatic patients is palliative; preventive efforts focus on animal control and vaccination efforts.
  - Pre-exposure prophylaxis is recommended for high-risk persons: veterinarians, spelunkers, certain lab technicians
    - Vaccination schedule varies based on risk category.
- Thorough wound cleansing
- Supportive treatment: benzodiazepines for spasms and cramps; opioid analgesics; haloperidol as needed for neuropsychiatric symptoms as above; scopolamine for hypersalivation
- Postexposure prophylaxis with rabies vaccine and immunoglobulin per immediate consult with animal control/public health officials

Cytomegalovirus

Kevin Michael O'Hara, MMSc, MS, PA-C

A 57-year-old female comes to the emergency department with complaints of nausea, right lower quadrant abdominal pain (rated 4/10), and moderate volume diarrhea for the past 48 hours. This patient is 145 days status post conventional allogeneic stem cell transplant for acute myelogenous leukemia. Vital signs are oral temperature of 101.1 °F, blood pressure 102/60 mm Hg, 110 beats per minute, and respirations 18 breaths per minute. The abdomen is diffusely tender without guarding, peritoneal signs, or organomegaly. *Clostridium difficile* and a broad gastrointestinal infectious PCR panel are negative. The white blood cell count is normal. A CT scan shows colitis, and antibacterial agents are started. The next day, a diagnostic colonoscopy shows diffuse inflammation with several ulcerative lesions. Biopsy of the lesions was sent for pathology, which included stains for adenovirus and cytomegalovirus (CMV). Which empiric antiviral medication would be indicated at this time?

GENERAL FEATURES

- CMV is a member of the herpesvirus family.
- Following primary infection, which may or may not be symptomatic, the virus enters a latent stage and infects the human host for life.
- There is no cure or vaccine for CMV, and over 50% of the US general population is infected.
- Transmission primarily occurs through body fluid exposure, including saliva and breast milk.
- When CMV infection produces abnormal signs and symptoms, it is referred to as CMV disease. The primary risk factor for CMV disease is a compromised immune system. People may develop CMV disease following primary infection, reinfection with a different CMV strain, or reactivation of a previous infection.

CLINICAL ASSESSMENT

- A mononucleosis like syndrome is the most common CMV presentation in immunocompetent patients.
  - Presents with lymphocytosis and abnormal lymphocytes; almost always self-limiting without complications
- Other presentations include disseminated infection and a diverse range of tissue-invasive disease presentations.
  - Retinitis and colitis are the most common.
  - This type of CMV disease almost always occurs in a patient with a significantly compromised immune system.

- Congenital CMV infection causes permanent disabilities in >5000 children each year in the United States. The likelihood of congenital infection and disability is highest for infants whose mothers were CMV seronegative before conception and who acquire infection during pregnancy. About 10% of infants with congenital CMV infection will have health problems at birth. And a small percentage of those infants will have long-term health consequences, such as hearing and vision loss, and intellectual disabilities (Rawlinson).

DIAGNOSIS

- The diagnosis of CMV is challenging. The gold standard for diagnosis of tissue-invasive disease is histology that is aided by immunohistochemistry (Kotton).
  - This special lab study is necessary because CMV PCR of the tissue or of the blood can lead to false positives.
  - The types of cells CMV infects are activated in inflammation of any kind. The use of CMV serology is limited, given a positive test for CMV IgG indicates that a person was infected with CMV at some time during their life but does not indicate when. The sensitivity of IgM varies based on the type of CMV disease but, in no circumstance, approaches 100% and its use is limited.
- Diagnosis of disseminated disease, such as CMV mononucleosis, can be assisted by CMV DNA PCR of the blood.
  - Tissue-invasive disease may have detectable CMV PCR in the blood, but the positive and negative predictive values vary based on the type of CMV disease and none approach 100%.
  - CMV PCR can be obtained from CSF in the event a rare CMV meningoencephalitis is suspected.

TREATMENT

- Anti-CMV drug therapy is used in the treatment of CMV disease, and preemptive treatment or prophylaxis in those at high risk.
- For example, you may employ preemptive treatment in a patient without obvious CMV disease that has detectable CMV in the blood and with significant immune compromise (Kotton).
- CMV disease is almost always treated in immunocompromised patients. However, in those with a competent immune system, especially with a mild CMV mononucleosis, often only supportive care is rendered.

- CMV drug resistance is possible, and there are tests available to help detect if this is occurring.
- Ganciclovir (IV) and its prodrug valganciclovir are widely used for first-line treatment and prevention of CMV disease.
- Foscarnet, common second-line treatment, is only available in an IV formulation. This drug causes many adverse reactions, including headache, genital ulcers, nausea, fatigue, nephrotoxicity, and electrolyte disturbances; close patient monitoring is essential.
- Cidofovir is also only available IV. The half-life of this drug is long and typically dosed weekly based on current renal function. Its role in CNS infection is limited by poor penetration. One of the more noteworthy adverse effects is nephrotoxicity.
- Letermovir is a newer drug currently only approved in the prophylaxis of CMV disease in transplant patients, and its role may expand as more data become available.

Case Conclusion

Given the presence of ulcerations on colonoscopy and the patient's immune compromise, a strong suspicion for CMV arose and IV ganciclovir started. Eventually, the histology and immunohistochemistry of the biopsied lesion confirmed CMV disease.

CHAPTER 217

HIV Infection

Susan LeLacheur, DrPH, PA-C

▶ GENERAL FEATURES

- HIV virus is a bloodborne pathogen transmitted via sexual intercourse, shared IV drug paraphernalia, or mother-to-child during birth or breastfeeding.
- HIV-1 and HIV-2 are distinct retroviruses.
- Risk factors for development include unprotected sexual intercourse, including anal-receptive intercourse, large number of sexual partners, history of STIs, sharing IV drug paraphernalia, mucosal contact with infected blood or needlestick, and maternal HIV infection.
- Rate and progression to AIDS and death are determined by the viral load.
- Three classifications of HIV infections, according to the CDC:
  - Category A: asymptomatic, with no history of AIDS-defining illness
  - Category B: HIV infection with symptoms consistent with HIV infection
  - Category C: HIV infection with AIDS-defining illness
- Acute HIV infection mimics other common conditions and can present with a wide range of nonspecific symptoms (fever, chills, malaise, headache, nausea, myalgias as well as those listed above) or can be asymptomatic.
  - No physical findings are specific for HIV; however, with acute seroconversion, a patient typically presents with a flulike illness (fever, malaise, generalized rash) and that generalized lymphadenopathy is a common presenting symptom of infection.
- Diagnosing acute HIV allows the patient to begin treatment as early as possible, which will both significantly improve his or her own prognosis and help to prevent transmission to others.
- Routine opt-out screening for HIV is recommended at least once for all adult and adolescent patients. Those at higher risk should be both screened more regularly. Opt-out means that the patient is informed a routine test will be done unless he or she specifically requests otherwise.
- Pre-exposure prophylaxis should be recommended for anyone at ongoing HIV risk.
- Recommendations regarding HIV prevention, screening, diagnosis, and treatment are updated regularly and can be found at https://aidsinfo.nih.gov/.

▶ CLINICAL ASSESSMENT

- A complete and nonjudgmental social and sexual history will help to identify risk for HIV exposure but should not circumvent standard HIV screening for all patients, regardless of risk.
- Acute HIV infection can lead to an abrupt drop in the CD4 cell count; hence, a complete physical examination should include sites of manifestations of immune dysfunction. Oral or vaginal candidiasis, aphthous ulcers, and folliculitis or seborrheic dermatitis are common findings in initial or early HIV disease.

- Depression is a common reason for poor adherence to HIV therapy as well as a normal reaction to an HIV diagnosis. Screening for anxiety and depression is an important part of the baseline evaluation of a person with HIV.
- Further evaluation of a patient found to be HIV infected should include testing for STIs, hepatitis A and C, tuberculosis screening, and routine chemistries including liver enzymes and CBC.
- Reference range of 500–2000 cells/μL; after seroconversion, CD4 counts continue to fall; in the United States, CD4 count <200 cells/μL is AIDS defining.
- Any patient with newly diagnosed HIV infection should be tested for the following: TB, CMV, syphilis, gonorrhea, chlamydia, hepatitis (A, B, and C), and anti-*Toxoplasma* antibody.
  - Also should check serum chemistries, BUN/creatinine, fasting lipids, and thyroid function
  - In addition, patients should be screened for DM, osteoporosis, and colon cancer.
  - Once infection is controlled, viral load should be checked every 6–12 months.

▶ DIAGNOSIS

- Fourth-generation ELISA, recommended for initial screening, includes both antibody and p24 antigen components and can diagnose HIV early in the infection (2-4 weeks) but may miss acute HIV. For this reason, an HIV viral PCR should be ordered if acute HIV is suspected.
- HIV ELISA is confirmed with a discrimination assay, which will distinguish between HIV1 and the less common HIV2.
- Initial evaluation of HIV disease must include HIV PCR (viral load), CD4, and specific testing to guide therapy, including HLA-B*5701, hepatitis B antibody and antigen, and creatinine.
- Routine screening for cervical dysplasia and high-risk HPV is important in females with HIV, and evaluation for HPV in other genital sites should be considered for all.

▶ TREATMENT

- Treatment depends on the stage of disease and presence/absence of opportunistic infections.
  - Use HAART to treat; leads to gradual recovery or CD4 T cells and helps promote immune response.
  - Treatment guidelines are age specific.
  - The majority of ART-naive patients are treated with an integrase component with a nucleoside backbone (tenofovir DF or AF plus emtricitabine).
  - Suppression is defined as HIV-RNA level below the lower limit of detection and should be seen between 8 and 24 weeks of HAART.
  - Nonoccupational postexposure prophylaxis: tenofovir DF plus raltegravir or dolutegravir
- Initial treatment with a recommended antiretroviral combination should begin as soon as possible.
- Combinations of one or two nucleoside (or nucleotide) reverse transcriptase inhibitors with an integrase inhibitor are available in one or two tablet formulations. These medications are very well tolerated and highly effective.
- Because all the recommended HIV regimens include medications that are at least partially effective against hepatitis B virus (HBV), it is important to fully treat HBV if treating HIV in anyone co-infected with chronic HBV.
  - In HIV/HBV co-infection, a combination including tenofovir alafenamide or disoproxil is indicated.
  - Patients should be advised not to stop treatment as a rebound of HBV can occur.
  - Lamivudine and emtricitabine are partially effective against HBV but should not be used without tenofovir in a co-infected patient.
- Patients should be re-evaluated soon after starting ART to assure full adherence and to assess for side effects. Most side effects will be transient and may include headache, nausea, and fatigue.
- Patients should receive all routine vaccines as well as pneumococcal and meningococcal (MenACWY) vaccines.

CHAPTER
218

Erythema Infectiosum

Brian Robinson, MS, MPAS, M(ASCP)CM, PA-C

▶ GENERAL FEATURES

- Erythema infectiosum is caused by parvovirus B19. It is also known as fifth disease, one of the six classic childhood exanthems.

- Commonly affects children aged 5–15 years and less commonly adults. It is more common in the spring and summer months.
- Transmission most common via respiratory droplet but can also occur via blood.

- Symptoms are mild and may include rash, runny nose, fever, joint pain, and headache. Occasionally, rash is the only symptom.
- A patient is contagious 5–15 days after exposure and infection onset. Once rash and joint pain occur, the patient is likely no longer contagious and can return to school or work.
- Those at highest risk for complications include pregnant patients, immunocompromised patients, and those with sickle cell disease.
- There is no vaccine or preventative medication for parvovirus B19.

▶ CLINICAL ASSESSMENT

- Classic presentation is a mild fever with the characteristic "slapped-cheek" rash that appears on the face as erythema, progressing to papules that coalesce to form plaques on the cheeks sparing the nose and the perioral area, which persists for 5–7 days. It may also appear on the limbs and trunk. At the presentation of the rash, the patient typically feels back to normal. This presentation is more common in children than adults. Immunocompromised patients may demonstrate atypical symptoms and have no rash or joint pain.

- Possible complications in pregnancy include hydrops fetalis, intrauterine death, and miscarriage. The highest risk of fetal death is in <20 weeks' gestations. Fetal death occurs in ~10% of cases.
- Possible complications in patients with sickle cell disease include aplastic anemia.

▶ DIAGNOSIS

- Lab work is typically not performed because of the self-limited nature of infection.
- Presence of serum parvovirus B19 IgM antibodies confirms the presence of acute infection. These are detectable within 7–10 days of infection and up to 3 months postinfection.
- Serum parvovirus B19 IgG antibody testing can be performed to determine prenatal immunity to infection.

▶ TREATMENT

- The disease is typically self-limiting, and treatment is usually centered around symptom control.
- Aplastic crisis is treated with blood transfusion throughout the course of infection.
- Infection during pregnancy needs close follow-up with obstetrics for serial fetal ultrasounds.

CHAPTER 219

Herpes Simplex Virus

Amanda Miller, MPH, MPAS, PA-C, AAHIVS

▶ GENERAL FEATURES

- Herpes simplex virus 1 (HSV-1) and herpes simplex 2 (HSV-2) are common viruses that can cause mucocutaneous and CNS infection.
  - HSV-1 generally causes symptoms on the oral mucosa and lips (herpes labialis). HSV-2 generally causes symptoms in the genital region (herpes genitalis); however, either can cause symptoms in other regions of the body.
  - Herpes genitalis is a common sexually transmitted infection (STI).
    - In the United States, the estimated prevalence of HSV-1 is 47.8% and HSV-2 is 11.9% among individuals aged 14–49 years.
  - HSV can also cause herpes keratitis, eczema herpeticum, and herpes encephalitis.
- HSV is spread through skin-to-skin contact, mucosal contact, or contact with herpetic lesions.

- HSV establishes a lifelong latent infection in the dorsal root ganglia after cutaneous or mucosal exposure.
- A substantial number of individuals with HSV are asymptomatic; however, they may still transmit the virus through cutaneous or mucosal shedding.
- Some individuals with mucocutaneous HSV infection experience recurrent infections that are triggered by illness, stress, physical trauma to the affected area of the body, and sunlight.
  - Frequency and severity of recurrences are variable from person to person.
  - 50% to 90% of individuals with herpes genitalis experience recurrence.
  - 20% to 40% of individuals with herpes labialis experience recurrence.
- Immunocompromise increases risk for recurrent infection, severe symptoms, and longer duration of illness.
- Genital HSV infection in individuals who are pregnant poses a high risk of transmission to the infant during delivery.

▶ CLINICAL ASSESSMENT

- Herpes labialis and herpes genitalis:
  - Symptoms of primary oral or genital infection vary and may be asymptomatic.
    - Typically painful vesicular lesions that ulcerate on the mucosa or skin
    - Systemic symptoms such as fever, malaise, headache, and lymphadenopathy are common with primary infection.
  - Genital infection can present with dysuria secondary to painful ulcerations. In severe cases, sacral radiculitis can lead to urinary retention.
  - Symptoms of oral and genital infections can last from 5 to 18 days.
  - You cannot distinguish between HSV-1 and HSV-2 on clinical examination.
- HSV can cause proctitis, ocular infections, encephalitis, neonatal chorioretinitis, Bell palsy, and aseptic meningitis.
- Eczema herpeticum can occur in individuals with atopic dermatitis or those with burns.
- Individuals with HSV keratitis present with blurred vision, red eye, and eye pain.
  - Dendritic lesions of the cornea are characteristic.
  - Risk of permanent vision loss
- HSV encephalitis presents with acute neurologic symptoms, such as altered mental status, hemiparesis, speech difficulties, or seizures.
  - Possibility for high morbidity and mortality

▶ DIAGNOSIS

- Clinical diagnosis for herpes labialis and herpes genitalis should be confirmed with laboratory testing through identification of HSV DNA by PCR or viral culture of a sample taken from the base of the ulcer.
  - Other tests such as direct fluorescence antibody assay and Tzanck smear are less sensitive and specific than PCR or culture.
  - Syphilis testing should be performed when an oral or genital ulcer is present.
  - Presence of genital HSV can increase the risk of HIV acquisition 3-fold, so HIV testing should be performed as well.
- Antibody testing can provide information about past symptoms that were never evaluated, help determine susceptibility of sexual partners, or identify asymptomatic infection in individuals who are pregnant.
  - HSV serology is not recommended for asymptomatic individuals as part of routine screening for STIs.
- Diagnosis of eczema herpeticum is made by viral culture or direct fluorescence antigen testing.
- Ocular infection is a clinical diagnosis.
- Suspected meningitis and encephalitis should be evaluated by lumbar puncture.

- Presence of HSV DNA in CSF by PCR is gold standard for diagnosis of CNS infection.
- CSF may show lymphocyte-predominant pleocytosis and normal glucose.

▶ TREATMENT

- Herpes genitalis:
  - First episode:
    - Acyclovir 400 mg TID, or valacyclovir 1000 mg BID, or famciclovir 250 mg TID for 7–10 days
  - Recurrent episodic therapy:
    - Acyclovir 400 mg TID or 800 mg BID for 5 days, or acyclovir 800 mg TID for 2 days, or valacyclovir 500 mg BID for 3 days, or valacyclovir 1000 mg QD for 5 days, or famciclovir 125 mg BID for 5 days, or famciclovir 1 g BID for 1 day, or famciclovir 500 mg once followed by 250 mg BID for 2 days
  - Recurrent suppressive therapy:
    - Acyclovir 400 mg BID, or valacyclovir 500 mg QD, or famciclovir 250 mg BID
  - Topical antiviral therapy is less effective than oral therapy and, therefore, not recommended.
  - Supportive therapy may include oral analgesics and sitz baths.
- Herpes labialis:
  - First episode:
    - Acyclovir 400 mg TID, or valacyclovir 1000 mg BID, or famciclovir 500 mg TID for 7–10 days
  - Recurrent episodic therapy:
    - Acyclovir 200 mg for 5 days or 400 mg TID for 5 days, or valacyclovir 2000 mg BID for 1 day, or famciclovir 1500 mg once
  - Recurrent suppressive therapy:
    - Acyclovir 400 mg BID or valacyclovir 500 mg QD
- Treatment recommendations for individuals who are pregnant, immunocompromised, and neonates are available through the CDC.
- Patients with herpes genitalis or herpes labialis should be counseled on the risk of transmission to others, safe sex practices including the use of barrier methods; possible impact on pregnancy and delivery, and increased risk of HIV and other STI when an ulcer is present.
- Ocular infections:
  - Patients with suspected ocular infection should have an urgent evaluation by an Ophthalmologist.
  - Avoid use of topical glucocorticoids in suspected herpes keratitis.
  - Topical and oral antiviral options are available based on patient preference.
- CNS infections:
  - Initiate treatment with IV acyclovir while awaiting CSF results.
  - Oral valacyclovir is not recommended.

Human Papillomavirus

Alyssa Abebe, PA-C

▶ GENERAL FEATURES

- HPV is the most common sexually transmitted infection in the United States
  - Most sexually active persons (80%) will become infected during their lifetime.
- Spread through oral, vaginal, and anal sex; a person can be asymptomatic and spread the virus
  - Condom use and limiting the number of sexual partners can decrease the risk of infection.
- >200 HPV types:
  - Most infect cutaneous epithelium (nonmucosal) and cause skin warts on hands or feet
  - Around 40 types infect mucosal epithelium causing genital warts and can lead to cancers (eg, genital/anal and oropharyngeal cancers)
- Affects men and women, with highest prevalence in women aged 20–25 years
  - HPV-related cervical cancer is the second most common cancer in women worldwide.
- Two vaccines (Cervarix and Gardasil) available to protect against the most common strains that cause cervical cancer and/or genital warts:
  - Cervarix is recommended for girls starting at ages 11–12 years.
  - Gardasil is also protective against the strains that cause genital warts and is recommended for either boys or girls aged 11–12 years.

▶ CLINICAL ASSESSMENT

- For women, the most common areas affected by HPV include the vulva, vagina, and cervix.
- For men, the most common areas affected include urethra, penis, and scrotum.
- For both sexes, HPV can infect the oropharynx, perianal, and anal areas.
- HPV can be asymptomatic.
- Genital warts (condylomata acuminate) are caused by strain 6 or 11 and are a clinical diagnosis.
  - Appear as small, soft, fleshy growths that are smooth or rough with finger-like projections
  - Can also appear in groups or as a keratotic plaque with a rough, pigmented surface, especially on the penis and vulva
- HPV types 16 and 18 are the most common strains causing cervical cancer (70%-85% of cases), anal cancers (almost 90% of cases), and vaginal, penile, and oropharyngeal cancers.

- 10 other strains are carcinogenic, including 31, 33, 35, and 45.
- HPV-related cancers can present with normal findings.
- Early carcinomas may appear as an erosion with friability.
- Later stages present with ulcerated lesions or a mass with or without bleeding.
- Metastatic disease can present with bowel and/or bladder obstruction due to the extension of a mass.

▶ DIAGNOSIS

- Identification of warts is generally done clinically, but confirmation via biopsy is warranted in some situations such as:
  - Immunocompromised patient
  - Suspicion of squamous cell carcinoma or Bowen disease
  - Lesions that do not improve with treatment
  - Lesions that have sudden growth, color change, or appear atypical
- Diagnosis of HPV is related to screening for the oncogenic strains with Pap smears for women.
  - Women aged 21–65 years should have a Pap smear every 3 years if initial and subsequent Pap smears are normal.
  - If a Pap smear reveals abnormal cells, a repeat Pap with or without an HPV test may be recommended with follow-up testing every 1–3 years.
  - Colposcopy with biopsy and endometrial sampling may be done after an abnormal Pap smear based on the specific abnormalities.
- Currently, there is no approved test to diagnose HPV in the mouth or throat.
- HPV screening is not recommended for men or those under 30 years.

▶ TREATMENT

- There is no treatment for HPV, it generally resolves on its own within 6–9 months.
- Treatment is available for genital warts and precancerous lesions.
  - Genital warts can resolve spontaneously within a year.
  - Medical treatment is aimed at the removal of the wart and symptom relief and can take up to 3 months.

- Creams, gels, ointments, or other therapies can be applied by the patient or by a provider.
  - Patient applied: imiquimod 3.75% or 5% cream, or podofilox 0.5% gel or solution, or sinecatechins 15% ointment can be used.
  - Provider applied: cryotherapy or cryoprobe, or surgical removal, or trichloroacetic acid or bichloroacetic acid 80% to 90% solution
- HPV-related cancers should be treated by oncologists and require prompt referral.

CHAPTER 221

Influenza

Alicia Quella, PhD, PA-C

GENERAL FEATURES

- Influenza is an illness caused by infection with influenza type A or B viruses, which are RNA viruses in the Orthomyxoviridae family. Influenza causes seasonal epidemics of acute febrile respiratory illness with duration of up to 2 weeks.
- The natural reservoir for all influenza A subtypes is waterfowl, with certain subtypes transmissible among humans, pigs, and other mammals.
- Standard influenza nomenclature includes the virus type (A, B, or C), geographical origin, strain number, year of isolation, and virus subtype.
- Outbreaks of influenza occur almost exclusively during the winter months in the Northern and Southern hemispheres but can occur sporadically, year-round in tropical areas.
  - Influenza is transmissible by three routes: contact exposure, droplet spray exposure, and airborne exposure.
- Influenza A viruses have caused pandemics of varying severity within the past century:
  - The 1918-1919 H1N1 pandemic caused at least 500 000 deaths in the United States and >40 million worldwide.
  - The 2009 H1N1 pandemic was associated with substantially less mortality than in 1918 but was associated with significant morbidity (pneumonia and sepsis) and mortality when compared to seasonal influenza.
- According to the CDC, people at risk of complications (such as pneumonia) and death from influenza include:
  - People 65 years and older
  - People of any age with certain chronic medical conditions (such as asthma, diabetes, obesity, heart disease, immunocompromise, or certain disabilities)
  - Pregnant women
  - Children with neurologic conditions
  - Children age <5 years, but especially age <2 years
  - The Advisory Committee Immunization Practices recommends annual influenza vaccination for everyone 6 months and older with any licensed, influenza vaccine that is appropriate for the recipient's age and health status with no preference expressed for any one vaccine over another:
    - Inactivated influenza vaccine (IIV)
    - Recombinant influenza vaccine (RIV)
    - Live attenuated nasal spray influenza vaccine (LAIV4)

CLINICAL ASSESSMENT

- Illness is found more commonly in children aged <18 years, and they are more than twice as likely to develop a symptomatic influenza infection than adults aged ≥65 years.
  - Classic symptoms are characterized by abrupt onset of fever, myalgias, headache, cough, sore throat, and nasal drainage after a 1- to 4-day incubation period.
    - The average duration of influenza virus shedding in immunocompetent patients is for 5 days (starts 1-2 days before symptoms manifest).
    - Elderly patients, especially in long-term care facilities, may presents with no fever but have confusion, lethargy, and anorexia.
  - Complications of influenza: bacterial pneumonia, ear infections, sinus infections, and worsening of chronic medical conditions, such as congestive heart failure, asthma, or diabetes
    - Rapidly progressive cough, dyspnea, and cyanosis may occur after typical onset and could be caused by influenza pneumonia or secondary bacterial pneumonia (staphylococcal or pneumococcal co-infection).

DIAGNOSIS

- Swab the back of the throat or nose to detect influenza viruses in respiratory specimens:
  - Rapid influenza diagnostic tests (RIDTs) detect virus antigens and result in 15 minutes. RIDTs are not as sensitive as other tests. (A negative test does not

exclude diagnosis of influenza, and clinicians should consider a follow-up rapid molecular assay.)

- Rapid molecular assays detect influenza virus nucleic acids and have a high sensitivity and specificity, results take 15–30 minutes.
- Reverse transcription polymerase chain reaction (RT-PCR) detects the presence of influenza viral RNA or nucleic acids with very high sensitivity and specificity. Some molecular assays are able to detect infections with influenza A and B viruses, results take from 45 minutes to hours depending on setting.
- Viral culture results do not yield timely results to inform clinical management but are essential for influenza surveillance.
- Consider multiplex assays in hospitalized patients for simultaneous detection of influenza viruses, SARS-CoV-2, and other common respiratory viruses (adenovirus, coronaviruses, metapneumovirus, parainfluenza viruses, respiratory syncytial viruses, rhinovirus/enterovirus), results take from 45 minutes to hours depending on setting.
- Chest radiographs if primary influenza pneumonia is suspected and may demonstrate bilateral reticular or reticulonodular opacities with or without superimposed consolidation.

▶ TREATMENT

- Compared with the common cold, influenza infection can cause a more severe illness, with a mortality rate of about 0.1% of people infected with the virus.
- Antivirals as soon as possible (ideally within 48 hours) for patients at risk of severe disease, hospitalized patients, and anyone with severe illness
  - Oral or enterically administered oseltamivir is recommended.
- For outpatients or uncomplicated influenza (depending upon approved age groups and contraindications):
  - Oral oseltamivir
  - Inhaled zanamivir
  - Intravenous peramivir
  - Oral baloxavir
- Chemoprophylaxis with antivirals for control of influenza outbreaks in institutional settings is recommended (ie, oral oseltamivir for people aged ≥1 year).
- Early respiratory and airway management is important.

CHAPTER 222

Roseola Infantum

Tanya Fernandez, MS, PA-C, IBCLC

▶ GENERAL FEATURES

- Roseola (aka sixth disease, exanthem subitum or pseudorubella) is an acute, benign childhood infection that characteristically presents with a high fever and rash.
- The rash is macular or maculopapular.
- Commonly caused by human herpesvirus 6 (HHV-6) and less frequently by HHV-7
- Other viruses (eg, coxsackievirus A and B, echovirus, adenovirus, parainfluenza virus) have also been associated with roseola.
- 90% of roseola cases occur in children younger than 2 years of age.
- Roseola can be confused with other childhood exanthems such as rubella, rubeola, and erythema infectiosum, although each of these have their own classic presentations that typically include a low-grade fever and a rash that starts on the face and spreads distally.
- Other febrile illnesses associated with rash include scarlet fever, hand-foot-mouth disease, and drug allergies.

▶ CLINICAL ASSESSMENT

- Classically presents with 3–5 days of high fever (usually above 40 °C), abrupt defervescence, and simultaneous eruption of the rash
- Most children are well-appearing and active, but occasionally, the high fever can cause irritability and other sequelae, such as seizures, aseptic meningitis, and thrombocytopenia purpura.
- The virus's ability to cross the blood-brain barrier, in conjunction with the high fevers, can lead to seizures in upward of 15% of patients with roseola.
- Other symptoms that may present with roseola include:
  - Cervical, postauricular, and/or occipital lymphadenopathy, 67%
  - Nagayama spots (macules or ulcers on the uvula or palate), 65%
  - Cough, 62%
  - Rhinorrhea, 61%
  - Edematous eyelids, 30%

- Palpebral conjunctivitis, 25%
- Vomiting, 21%
- Diarrhea, varies between 21% and 68%.

▶ DIAGNOSIS

- Diagnosis is made clinically by the presence of distinctive rash that appears after high fevers defervesce.
- Rash is typically 2–5 mm rose pink to red macules or papules sometimes surrounded by a halo of pale skin. It is nonpruritic and starts on the trunk and spreads to the face and extremities.
- Laboratory testing is generally unnecessary.
- If laboratory testing is done as a means of working up a fever source, especially if the child presents before the onset of the rash, findings might include:
  - CBC with neutropenia and mild atypical lymphocytosis

- Less commonly, **thrombocytopenia may be present.**
- **Urinalysis reveals sterile pyuria.**
- Like other herpes viruses, HHV-6 lies dormant in the host, with unpredictable shedding throughout the life span.

▶ TREATMENT

- Roseola is a self-limited viral illness that typically resolves without sequelae.
- Treatment is supportive, such as hydration and fever control.
- Antiviral medications are not recommended in otherwise healthy patient with primary infection.
- By the time the rash appears, the child is no longer viremic.
- The rash will usually resolve without any interventions within 24–48 hours.

CHAPTER 223

Varicella-Zoster Virus

Nathan Bates, MMS, PA-C

A 64-year-old man presents to an urgent care with a painful rash. He first noticed it on the back of his right shoulder 2 days ago. The rash is now spreading down the posterior aspect of his arm. He describes it as burning and painful to touch, with new "bumps" appearing daily. He denies any new soaps, lotions, detergents, allergies, or recent illnesses. Vaccination history is unknown, but he had chickenpox as a child. Physical examination is significant for a maculopapular rash, with scattered vesicles on the right posterior shoulder extending down the arm in a dermatomal distribution pattern. Which of the following is the best next step in care?

▶ GENERAL FEATURES

- Infection with varicella-zoster virus (VZV) can manifest as primary varicella zoster (chickenpox) and herpes zoster (shingles) upon viral reactivation.
- VZV belongs to the Human Herpesvirus family, specifically type 3, and is transmitted via respiratory droplets or direct contact with skin lesions. It is considered highly contagious.
- Upon initial exposure, VZV invades epithelial and T cells, then shed new virus in the skin to target keratinocytes and resulting in chickenpox rash.
- Despite resolution of symptoms, a latent infection is established in the dorsal root or cranial nerve ganglia

and may later reactivate due to stress or a weakened immune system, resulting in shingles.
- VZV infections are typically self-limiting; however, they can be severe in high-risk populations and also target the brain, eyes, lungs, liver, pancreas, or bone.
- Incidence rate of chickenpox infection is <1% annually due to routine vaccination, whereas the lifetime risk of developing shingles is 20% to 30%, with the majority of cases occurring in individuals older than 50 years.

▶ CLINICAL ASSESSMENT

- The rash of VZV infections may be confused with impetigo, contact dermatitis, insect bites, papular urticaria, candidal infection, dermatitis herpetiformis, or drug eruptions.
- Chickenpox presents with a pruritic, maculopapular rash that transitions into vesicles with surrounding erythema. This has been described colloquially as "dew drops on a rose petal."
  - Rash originates on the face or trunk and extends distally (sparing the hands and feet).
  - Multiple stages of rash is a characteristic feature as new lesions continually appear and crust over within 4–7 days.

- Prodromal symptoms such as fever, headache, malaise, or abdominal pain occur 1–2 days before rash.
- Superimposed bacterial skin infections may occur secondary to intense pruritus.
- Shingles presents with a painful maculopapular and vesicular rash in a dermatomal distribution pattern, most commonly thoracic or cervical, and does not cross midline.
  - Prodromal symptoms include pain, burning, and paresthesia of the skin.
  - Rash resolves within 4 weeks.
  - Pain may persist for months as post-herpetic neuralgia occurs in up to 20% of individuals.
  - Other complications include Ramsay Hunt syndrome and herpes zoster ophthalmicus.

▶ DIAGNOSIS

- Diagnosis of VZV infections is generally based on clinical findings.
- Additional testing is reserved for atypical, disseminated, or visceral disease.
  - PCR is highly sensitive and specific and can be used with various samples (lesion swabs, CSF, biopsy tissue, corneal swab, bronchoalveolar lavage fluid, etc).
  - Direct fluorescence antibody assay (DFA) may be used on skin lesions but is less sensitive than PCR.
  - New testing options have reduced utility of Tzanck smear and viral cultures.
- Lower diagnostic thresholds are reasonable for high-risk populations, such as pregnant women, newborns, or immunocompromised (HIV/AIDS, bone or solid organ transplant, cancer, etc).
- Serologic antibody (IgG) titers can assess VZV susceptibility, but are not used for diagnosis.

▶ TREATMENT

- Chickenpox management is supportive with use of oral antihistamines, acetaminophen, frequent bathing, wet compress, calamine lotion, oatmeal baths, and avoidance of scratching lesions.
  - Aspirin should be avoided due to increased risk of Reye syndrome.
  - Antivirals are reserved for high-risk populations or disseminated infection.
- Shingles management is also mainly supportive; however, oral antivirals such as acyclovir are recommended within 72 hours of symptoms to reduce viral shedding and hasten healing of lesions.
  - There is no role for glucocorticoids, gabapentin, or tricyclic antidepressants in uncomplicated infections; however, may be utilized for post-herpetic neuralgia.
  - If a complicated infection ensues, IV antiviral therapy is warranted.
- Individuals are considered contagious until all lesions have crusted and, therefore, need to exercise caution by avoiding pregnant women, immunosuppressed, or individuals who are naïve to VZV.
- Vaccination is the mainstay for preventing VZV infections.
  - Chickenpox: two-dose series at age 12–15 months and 4–6 years
  - Shingles: two dose series at age 50, separated by 2–6 months

Case Conclusion

Based on the patient presentation, the best next step in care is to start him on oral antiviral therapy. Although shingles management is mainly supportive, oral antivirals such as acyclovir are recommended within 72 hours of symptoms to reduce viral shedding and hasten healing of lesions.

CHAPTER
224

Hand, Foot, and Mouth Disease

Shaun Lynch, MS, MMSc, PA-C

A 2-year-old girl is brought to the office by her mother for a sick visit for a skin rash. She has refused to eat much over the past 2 days with the mother reporting a subjective fever. The mother describes the rash as blisters on the hands and feet of her daughter with other children in her daycare with similar symptoms. What is most likely found on examination of the oropharynx in this patient?

▶ GENERAL FEATURES

- Highly contagious enteroviral infectious disease most commonly occurring in infants and children
- Transmitted easily through person-to-person contact, inhalation of infected air droplets, or contact with contaminated surfaces

- Disease spread noted in settings such as daycare centers, summer camps, and schools
  - Most contagious during the first week of illness
- Typically caused by coxsackievirus A16 or enterovirus 71
- Hand, foot, and mouth disease (HFMD) usually occurs in the summer and early autumn months, although cases can be seen throughout the year.

▶ CLINICAL ASSESSMENT

- Rash is a hallmark finding of the disease.
  - Exanthem involves nonpruritic vesicles arising from macules or macule-papules on the palms of the hands and soles of the feet.
  - Less commonly, the rash may appear on the knees, elbows, buttocks, and genital area.
- Mouth sores may develop that begin as small red spots and evolve into vesicles distributed over the buccal mucosa and tongue.
- Patients often experience a fever, malaise, sore throat, or mouth pain and eating or drinking less.
- Prodromal symptoms are usually absent but, if present, include fever, abdominal pain, vomiting, and diarrhea lasting between 12 and 36 hours.

▶ DIAGNOSIS

- Diagnosis usually made clinically, based on the characteristic rash and mouth sores.

- Herpangina is considered in cases of high fever and painful oral papulovesicular lesions on the tonsils, soft palate, and uvula without the skin rash.
- Although not commonly done, throat, stool, or vesicular fluid samples can be obtained for culture or nucleic acid amplification testing in cases of severe illness or uncertainty in diagnosis.

▶ TREATMENT

- Spontaneous resolution without treatment in 5–10 days is common.
- Management is supportive, such as hydration and over-the-counter medications to manage pain and fever.
- Hand hygiene is important to prevent the spread of HFMD.
- Parents can consider sending children back to school or daycare once afebrile for 24 hours and without any open blisters.

Case Conclusion

Examination of this child's oropharynx will likely reveal vesicles surrounded by a thin halo of erythema on tongue and buccal mucosa, caused by HFMD.

Section A Pretest: Compartment Syndrome

1. A 19-year-old male has developed compartment syndrome secondary to a left-sided closed tibial shaft fracture. Which of the following will he most likely demonstrate first?

   A. Pain
   B. Palor
   C. Paresthesia
   D. Pulselessness

2. What is the definitive treatment for a patient whose clinical findings are consistent with compartment syndrome?

   A. Emergent fasciotomy
   B. Hyperbaric oxygen therapy
   C. Ice therapy
   D. Observation

Section B Pretest: Infectious Disorders

1. Which of the following statements is true with regards to the management of a patient with suspected septic arthritis?

   A. Drainage of the infected joint requires operative arthrotomy.
   B. Empiric antibiotics should be initiated once specimens for synovial fluid and blood cultures have been obtained.
   C. Initiation of antibiotic regimen should occur once synovial fluid culture and susceptibility data have resulted.
   D. Most cases of septic arthritis can be successfully treated with a course of oral antibiotics.

2. What is the most common organism causing osteomyelitis in adults?

   A. *Enterobacter*
   B. *Haemophilus influenzae*
   C. *Streptococcus aureus*
   D. *Streptococcus*

3. A 35-year-old man who injects heroin IV presents to the emergency department with acute, atraumatic right wrist pain and fever. He denies injecting substances into the affected limb. He is febrile with an erythematous, edematous right wrist, which he is unable to flex or extend due to pain. Septic arthritis is suspected. Given this patient's history, which of the following organisms should be considered as the infective pathogen?

   A. *Escherichia coli*
   B. *Eikenella corrodens*
   C. *Neisseria gonorrhoeae*
   D. *Pseudomonas aeruginosa*

4. Which of the following is the most common mechanism of infection for septic arthritis?

   A. Extension of infection from surrounding soft tissues
   B. Hematogenous seeding of the synovial membrane
   C. Iatrogenic direct inoculation of the affected joint, such as joint injection
   D. Traumatic direct inoculation of the affected joint, such as animal bites

5. The recurrence rate of chronic osteomyelitis in adults is which of the following?

   A. 10%
   B. 30%
   C. 50%
   D. 66%

6. A 55-year-old generally healthy woman seeks care for a 4-day history of left ankle pain and swelling. She has not experienced trauma to the joint, and she denies fever. Her examination reveals a left ankle that is warm to the touch with decreased range of motion and a limping gait. Joint fluid analysis reveals: WBC 120 000 cells/μL (90% neutrophils), Gram-negative bacilli, and absence of crystals. Culture results are pending. Which of the following is the best initial pharmacologic intervention for this patient?

   A. Intra-articular glucocorticoid injection
   B. Oral colchicine
   C. Oral corticosteroid
   D. Parenteral ceftriaxone

7. A 68-year-old woman with diabetes and osteoarthritis (OA) status post remote right total knee replacement seeks emergency department care for a 2-day history of atraumatic pain and swelling of her right knee with associated fever. On physical examination, her right knee is warm to the touch with a moderate effusion, and she cannot flex or extend her knee actively nor passively due to pain. Which diagnostic study can definitively establish this patient's most likely diagnosis?

   A. Blood cultures
   B. CT of the right knee
   C. Synovial fluid crystal analysis
   D. Synovial fluid culture

Section C Pretest: Inflammatory and Autoimmune Disorders

1. Which of the following is a second-line agent used in the treatment of gout?

   A. Allupurinol
   B. Febuxostat
   C. Probenecid
   D. Pegloticase

2. Which of the following are risk factors for ankylosing spondylitis (AS)?

   A. Presence of *HLA-B27* gene
   B. Male gender
   C. Age of onset <40 years
   D. All of the above

3. Which of the following is a common finding on knee radiographs of patients with calcium pyrophosphate dihydrate (CPPD) disease?

   A. Chondrocalcinosis
   B. Subluxation of the fibula
   C. Dislocation of the patella
   D. Joint destruction

4. A patient's plain radiographs of the bilateral sacroiliac (SI) joints show findings of moderate sacroiliitis. She trials the recommended initial treatments for AS including physical therapy, occupational therapy, and scheduled ibuprofen 800 mg TID for 4 weeks. She continues to complain of severe pain in the low back and SI joint region. What is the best next step in management?

   A. Perform office-based SI joint cortisone injections.
   B. Trial Celebrex 200 mg BID and discontinue ibuprofen 800 mg TID.
   C. Refer patient to rheumatology for consideration of treatment with biologic medications.
   D. Refer patient to orthopedic surgery for consideration of SI joint fusion.

5. A patient has been successfully treated for an acute gout flare. Which of the following dietary restrictions should be included in post-treatment patient education?

   A. Increased seafood consumption
   B. Decreased alcohol consumption
   C. Increased fruit juice consumption
   D. Decreased legume consumption

6. Which of the following is NOT an extra-articular manifestation of AS?

   A. Peripheral arthritis
   B. Enthesitis
   C. Atopic dermatitis
   D. Acute anterior uveitis

7. Polymyalgia rheumatica most commonly affects which of the following age ranges?

   A. 20-30 years old
   B. 35-45 years old
   C. 45-55 years old
   D. 60-70 years old

8. A 38-year-old woman presents to clinic with a 2-year history of all-over achy body pain, headaches, and difficulty sleeping. To date, her workup has been negative for any objective findings. Which of the following symptoms is particularly important in narrowing the differential diagnosis for this patient?

    A. Significant level of fatigue
    B. Presence of depression
    C. Stiffness on waking
    D. Episodes of diarrhea

9. What laboratory finding is both specific and sensitive for rheumatoid arthritis (RA)?

    A. Elevated anti–cyclic-citrullinated peptide antibody (anti-CCP)
    B. Elevated anti–double-stranded DNA (anti-dsDNA)
    C. Elevated erythrocyte sedimentation rate (ESR)
    D. Elevated rheumatoid factor (RF)
    E. Elevated C-reactive protein (CRP)

10. A 48-year-old woman presents to the clinic with widespread chronic body aches, difficulty sleeping, and near-daily headaches. Physical examination shows 12 of 18 tender points along specific locations in the trapezius, knee, and elbow. Laboratory studies include a normal ESR, normal CRP, and negative rheumatoid factors and antinuclear antibody (ANA). Which of the following treatment approaches would likely benefit this patient?

    A. Corticosteroid joint injections
    B. A moderate exercise program
    C. Increasing dietary sodium
    D. Bedrest

11. When assessing a patient with polymyalgia rheumatica, which of the following joints is usually unaffected?

    A. Ankle
    B. Hip
    C. Shoulder
    D. Wrist

12. A 45-year-old female presents with a 6-month history of bilateral hand swelling, redness, and warmth along with stiffness of the hands that lasts 1½ hours each morning. Positive diagnostic studies include a high positive anti-CCP and an elevated ESR. Which of the following is the most appropriate initial treatment option according to the American College of Rheumatology (ACR)?

    A. Ibuprofen
    B. Janus kinase inhibitor
    C. Methotrexate
    D. Occupational therapy
    E. Tumor necrosis factor inhibitor

13. Which of the following laboratory test results is consistent with a diagnosis of fibromyalgia?

    A. Elevated ESR
    B. Positive ANA
    C. Normal CRP
    D. Positive HLA-B27

14. Which of the following diagnoses is commonly associated with polymyalgia rheumatica?

    A. Giant cell arteritis
    B. Polymyositis (PM)
    C. Psoriasis
    D. RA

15. What patient education is most appropriate for patients with rheumatoid arthritis?

    A. Diet has no impact on symptoms.
    B. Exercise during a flare to alleviate symptoms.
    C. Joint damage can be slowed with adequate treatment.
    D. Most patients will need joint surgery within 5 years of diagnosis.
    E. NSAIDs will both provide relief and decrease joint damage.

16. Which clinical manifestation is uncommon in patients with systemic lupus erythematosus (SLE)?

    A. Erosive arthritis
    B. Butterfly rash
    C. Oral mucosal ulceration
    D. Pericarditis

17. Which of the following is the primary treatment of choice for patients diagnosed with polymyalgia rheumatica?

    A. IV pain management
    B. Oral anti-inflammatory medications
    C. Oral glucocorticoids
    D. Topical corticosteroids

18. Which of the following populations is NOT predominantly affected by SLE?

    A. Women
    B. Children
    C. African Americans
    D. Hispanics

19. What are the goals of therapy with the treatment of polymyositis?

    A. Abnormal lab markers return to lower than normal limits
    B. Muscle strength improves/returns
    C. Avoidance of hyperglycemia, reflux, gastric ulcer/bleeding, and infection
    D. Improved sleep-wake cycle

20. Which statement is correct regarding the ANA test?

    A. The ANA test is considered the best marker for disease activity in lupus.
    B. The ANA test is positive in 100% of SLE patients.
    C. Positive ANA test is one of the 11 ACR criteria to be met to determine a diagnosis of SLE.
    D. Renal biopsy is needed for all patients with positive ANA test.

21. Which of the following is a common manifestation of polymyalgia rheumatica?

    A. Small multiple linear pruritic vesicles on top of erythema on right upper extremity
    B. Erythematous and/or violaceous rash on bilateral upper eyelids sometimes with eyelid edema
    C. Pruritic ring-shaped rash, erythematous, scaly and velvety on side of leg
    D. Scaly maculopapular rash sweeping outward across trunk like a tree, with larger oval-shaped macular spot on chest abdomen or back

22. Of the following, which is NOT generally affected by reactive arthritis?

    A. Men
    B. Patients 20–40 years old
    C. African Americans
    D. Caucasians

23. Most patients with reactive arthritis can expect which of the following?

    A. To reach a normal life span
    B. To maintain a near-normal lifestyle
    C. To develop cardiac manifestations, including aortic regurgitation and pericarditis
    D. Both A and B

24. Which new potential treatment regime is being investigated for future use in the treatment of PM?

    A. NSAIDs
    B. Plasmapheresis
    C. Targeting PM-specific autoantibodies
    D. Angiotensin-converting enzyme inhibitors (ACEi)

25. What are the most common autoimmune diseases that present with Sjögren?

    A. Scleroderma and psoriasis
    B. Lupus and rheumatoid arthritis
    C. Multiple sclerosis and Graves disease
    D. Inflammatory bowel disease and celiac disease

26. Which symptom is NOT part of the classic triad of symptoms in reactive arthritis?

    A. Conjunctivitis
    B. Keratoderma blennorrhagicum
    C. Nongonococcal urethritis
    D. Asymmetric oligoarthritis

27. Robin, a 42-year-old Caucasian female, presents to the office with Reynaud phenomenon. She has also noticed that her hands feel stiff, but she attributes that to more computer time at work. What lab test would be appropriate to test for Sjögren?

    A. ANA double-stranded antibody
    B. SPEP/UPEP
    C. Anti-SSA
    D. UACR

28. Lupus nephritis is treated with which of the following?

    A. Combination of calcium and vitamin D
    B. Combination of cyclophosphamide and corticosteroids
    C. Combination of antimalarials and NSAIDs
    D. Cytotoxic agents

29. Patty, a 45-year-old female who recently moved to the area, presents to the office for an introductory physical. She notes that she is having missed menses. PMH is significant for hypothyroidism treated with oral medication and mild hypertension (untreated). She complains about "allergies" that are new to her. Under further questioning, she notes that she has had to start using eye drops. You order an anti-SSA and an anti-SSB and refer her to whom?

    A. Podiatry because she is at risk for increased foot fractures
    B. Allergist for skin testing
    C. Ophthalmology for eye litmus testing
    D. OB/GYN for missed menses

30. Annie is a 58-year-old African Americans female who presents with a well-managed lupus. She has noticed increased complaints of joint pain and wants to know why the increase in symptoms. Upon further questions, she notes that she has had major dental work recently, along with having to strengthen her glasses prescription. What makes you suspicious of Sjögren?

    A. The need for dental work
    B. Annie's age
    C. The underlying lupus diagnosis
    D. All of the above

Section D Pretest: Lower Extremity Disorders

1. Which of the following statements about developmental dysplasia of the hip (DDH) is correct?
   A. Most cases of mild hip instability found on newborn examination will resolve spontaneously and require no intervention.
   B. Untreated DDH can lead to long-term consequences such as avascular necrosis (AVN) of the hip.
   C. Ultrasonography of all infants at birth is recommended as a screening tool for DDH.
   D. Surgery is usually necessary in infants diagnosed with DDH to achieve concentric reduction of the hip and reduce the risk of future OA.

2. Which of the following can identify slipped capital femoral epiphysis (SCFE) on plain films?
   A. Obturator sign
   B. Klein line
   C. Spine line
   D. Straight leg test

3. Which of the following statements should be discussed with the parents of a newborn with DDH?
   A. This disorder cannot be effectively treated.
   B. This disorder does not usually lead to degenerative changes in the joint.
   C. Infants who are treated surgically for DDH should be followed closely by an orthopedist until they have reached physical maturity.
   D. Infants with this disorder often also have visual deficits.

4. Which of the following special tests would be most useful for assessing a patient with meniscal injuries?
   A. Pivot shift
   B. Thessaly
   C. Lachman
   D. Anterior drawer

5. You are performing a newborn examination, and on observation, asymmetric leg creases are noted. You palpate a "clunk" to the left hip when gently performing the Ortolani maneuver. What is your next step in the treatment of this newborn?
   A. Pavlik harness
   B. Ultrasound
   C. Prompt referral to orthopedist
   D. Closed reduction

6. Which of the following clinical manifestations is NOT associated with slipped capital femoral epiphysis (SCFE)?
   A. Obesity
   B. Knee pain
   C. Loss of abduction and internal rotation of the hip
   D. Lower back pain (LBP)

7. Who should be screened for DDH?
   A. Only newborns with obvious risk factors for DDH
   B. Only newborns with physical examination findings suggestive of DDH
   C. Only newborns who are breech at birth
   D. All newborns

8. Aside from the knee examination, what part of the body should be examined in any child with knee pain?
   A. Hips
   B. Ankles
   C. Feet
   D. Shoulders

9. Which one of the following is a risk factor for DDH?
   A. Male sex
   B. Cephalic presenting baby in the third trimester
   C. Tight swaddling
   D. Drug or alcohol exposure during pregnancy

10. Which of the following is NOT a true statement regarding meniscal injuries?
    A. Medial meniscal tears are more common than lateral tears.
    B. Most meniscal injuries affect the red zone, which will not self-heal due to the avascular location.
    C. In the setting of an acute anterior cruciate ligament (ACL) rupture, the lateral meniscus is more likely to be injured.
    D. Meniscal injuries are part of the "unhappy triad": an injury to the ACL, medial collateral ligament (MCL), and meniscus.

11. What is the most appropriate first-line treatment for a patient with a SCFE?
    A. NSAIDs
    B. Closed reduction and hip immobilization
    C. Surgical pinning in situ
    D. Total hip arthroplasty

12. Which of the following are appropriate radiologic views in a suspected right hip fracture?

    A. AP/lateral right proximal femur, AP/lateral right femur, AP pelvis
    B. AP/lateral right proximal femur only
    C. AP/lateral right proximal femur and MRI of the right hip
    D. AP/lateral right and left proximal femur, AP/lateral right femur, AP pelvis

13. A 66-year-old obese patient presents to the clinic with right knee pain for 3 months. He thinks he has a torn meniscus. He reports the knee pain is worse at night and is associated with stiffness to the knee on waking up. What imaging would you want to obtain first in order to diagnose this patient's knee problem?

    A. CT scan
    B. MRI
    C. Arthroscopy
    D. Plain radiography

14. Which of the following is true regarding hip dislocations?

    A. Hip dislocations occur as frequently as hip fractures.
    B. The most common type is an anterior hip dislocation resulting from an MVA.
    C. Patients with total hip arthroplasty are at an increased risk for a hip dislocation.
    D. Plain radiographs are diagnostic and do not require further imaging.

15. Which of the following is not a function of the meniscus?

    A. Stabilizes the AP translation of the tibia relative to the femur
    B. Improves stability and joint congruency
    C. Lubricates articular cartilage
    D. Shock absorbs within the knee

16. A 20-year-old professional tennis player sustains a knee injury after decelerating to chase ball and cutting. She says she felt a "pop" to her knee with sudden onset of pain. On examination, she has a knee effusion and tenderness laterally. She has a positive Thessaly test and a negative Lachman, anterior, and posterior drawer tests. Which of the following choices is the most appropriate diagnostic imaging modality?

    A. Radiography
    B. CT scan
    C. Ultrasound
    D. MRI

17. Which of the following is NOT considered a risk factor leading to avascular necrosis (AVN) of the hip?

    A. Excessive alcohol use
    B. Long-term corticosteroid use
    C. Placement of an intramedullary nail
    D. Total hip arthroplasty

18. A patient presents to the emergency department complaining of knee pain after stopping suddenly from a full sprint and the inability to straighten the leg. What injury do you suspect?

    A. Distal femur fracture
    B. Patellar dislocation
    C. Proximal tibial fracture
    D. Patellar fracture

19. An 82-year-old woman received cannulated screws for a nondisplaced right femoral neck fracture. What is important to tell her and her family?

    A. The risk of a subsequent fracture on the right is low.
    B. There is a risk of AVN of the right femoral head.
    C. She will regain the independence she had before the surgery.
    D. Anticoagulation is not necessary in her age group.

20. Which of the following is considered an intracapsular hip fracture?

    A. Intertrochanteric fracture
    B. Greater trochanter avulsion fracture
    C. Femoral neck fracture
    D. Subtrochanteric fracture

Section E Pretest: Neoplasms

1. Which of the following statements about giant cell tumors of the bone is NOT correct?

   A. Giant cell tumors of the bone are common neoplasms.
   B. Giant cell tumors of the bone typically occur in young adults.
   C. Giant cell tumors of the bone typically occur at the end parts (epiphysis) of long bones.
   D. Giant cell tumors of the bone are aggressive tumors that can destroy the surrounding bone.

2. Which of the following is the most common treatment of metastatic bone disease?

   A. Curative, local field radiation
   B. Palliative, local field radiation
   C. Curative, surgical resection of the tumor
   D. Palliative, surgical resection of the tumor

3. What is the treatment of choice for giant cell tumors?

   A. Anti-inflammatories
   B. Percutaneous ablation
   C. Surgical resection
   D. Radiation therapy

4. A patient was diagnosed with osteoblastoma at lumbar vertebra number 4 (L4) compressing the right nerve root. What is the preferred treatment for osteoblastoma?

   A. Radiation therapy
   B. Chemotherapy
   C. Surgical resection of the tumor
   D. Radioisotope therapy

5. Which imaging test should be performed first in order to characterize a bone tumor?

   A. Biopsy
   B. MRI
   C. Radionuclide scanning
   D. X-rays

6. Which of the following types of cancer does NOT commonly metastasize to skeletal sites?

   A. Lung cancer
   B. Breast cancer
   C. Skin cancer
   D. Prostate cancer

7. A 55-year-old male patient with known lung cancer presenting to the clinic, complaining of new-onset back pain and leg numbness. What is the next most appropriate step?

   A. Complete spine x-rays
   B. CT scans of the spine
   C. Bone scan
   D. Take a thorough medical history and perform physical examination

Section F Pretest: Osteoarthritis

1. In a patient with current knee pain, left knee radiographs reveal moderate tricompartmental OA changes evidenced by joint space narrowing and osteophytes. Examination is consistent with symptomatic left knee OA. Which of the following best describes her diagnosis?

   A. Primary OA
   B. Secondary OA
   C. Inflammatory OA
   D. Infectious OA

2. After extensive trial of physical therapy, NSAIDs, knee bracing, and activity modification, a patient with OA returns requesting additional treatment for persistent moderate pain. Recent left knee MRI confirms moderate tricompartmental OA without evidence of meniscus or ligament injury. Which of the following options would be most appropriate?

   A. Discussing need for sustained opioid analgesia.
   B. Discussing trial of a corticosteroid injection.
   C. Referral for total knee replacement consultation.
   D. Referral for arthroscopic surgery.

3. During your patient's evaluation, she mentions pain and enlargement involving her right index finger distal interphalangeal (DIP) joint location. Radiographs confirm DIP joint space narrowing with bony hypertrophy. Which of the following is the physical examination finding associated with DIP joint enlargement secondary to OA?

   A. Bouchard node
   B. Osler node
   C. Reynaud phenomenon
   D. Heberden node

4. In the Kellgren-Lawrence radiographic grading system, which grade correlates with moderate joint space narrowing?

   A. Grade 1
   B. Grade 2
   C. Grade 3
   D. Grade 4

Section G Pretest: Osteoporosis

1. A 60-year-old Caucasian woman presents to the clinic for health maintenance. Her past medical history is remarkable only for a Colles fracture sustained 6 months ago after a fall while walking her dog. She does not take medications or supplements. She admits to a poor diet and little exercise. On physical examination, her BMI is 22 kg/m². The remainder of her examination is unremarkable. What diagnostic modality should be performed in order to confirm the suspected underlying disease?

   A. Spine and hip radiograph
   B. Dual-energy x-ray absorptiometry (DXA) scan
   C. Serum parathyroid level
   D. Heel ultrasound

2. A 70-year-old man with no significant medical history undergoes a screening DXA scan. His screening labs were unremarkable. The T-score of the hip is −1.2. Which of the following is the most likely diagnosis?

   A. Low bone mass
   B. Osteoporosis
   C. Paget disease of the bone
   D. Rickets

3. A 67-year-old woman with no significant medical history undergoes a screening DXA scan. She is on no medications or supplements. Her screening labs were unremarkable. The T-score of the hip is −2.6. Which of the following is the initial pharmacotherapy of choice?

   A. Calcitonin
   B. Tamoxifen
   C. Alendronate
   D. Teriparatide

4. A 62-year-old postmenopausal woman presents for well-woman examination. She asks about osteoporosis screening. You perform a FRAX calculation, and her 10-year risk for major osteoporotic fracture is 2%. Which of the following would you recommend?

   A. DXA scan
   B. Fall prevention strategies
   C. 24-hour urinary calcium
   D. Begin bisphosphonate therapy

5. Which of the following is a contraindication to oral bisphosphonate therapy?

   A. RA
   B. Parathyroid adenoma
   C. Gastroesophageal reflux disease
   D. Long-term antiepileptic therapy

Section H Pretest: Spinal Disorders

1. What is the gold standard for confirming the diagnosis of lumbar spinal stenosis?

    A. Lumbar spine radiographs
    B. Lumbar spine CT scan
    C. Lumbar spine MRI
    D. Lumbar spine CT with myelogram

2. Which of the following is NOT a treatment option for patients diagnosed with spondylolithesis?

    A. Anti-inflammatory medications
    B. Abdominal core strengthening
    C. Toe-touches
    D. Lumbosacral decompression and fusion

3. A 54-year-old male presents to emergency department with complaints of LBP and numbness to the bilateral legs. He states he was cleaning the gutters and fell off of a ladder. On his way to the emergency department, he urinated himself. An MRI was performed and shows a large herniated disk at the L5-S1 region causing severe spinal stenosis. What is the treatment of choice for this patient?

    A. Epidural steroid injections
    B. Anti-inflammatory medications and an outpatient referral to physical therapy
    C. Lumbosacral discectomy at L5-S1
    D. Lumbosacral discectomy with spinal fusion at L5-S1

4. Bracing is recommended for which of the following patients with scoliosis?

    A. 15-year-old female; Risser 5; Cobb angle 28°
    B. 14-year-old male; Risser 2; Cobb angle 17°
    C. 11-year-old female; Risser 0; Cobb angle 31°
    D. 13-year-old female; Risser 3; Cobb angle 22°

5. Which of the following statements about lumbar spinal stenosis is false?

    A. Patients with lumbar spinal stenosis often find it more comfortable to walk flexed at the hips.
    B. Hyperextension braces are used as adjunct therapy with other means of conservative treatment.
    C. The lumbar spine is the most common area to have spinal stenosis.
    D. Osteophytes or bony spurs on the vertebra may be a cause of spinal stenosis.

6. Where is the most common location for spondylolithesis to occur?

    A. T12-L1

    B. L3-L4
    C. L4-L5
    D. L5-S1

7. Which statement is correct about a patient presenting with lumbar spinal stenosis?

    A. Extension of the lumbar spine alleviates symptoms.
    B. Flexion of the lumbar spine alleviates symptoms.
    C. A positive straight leg raise (SLR) is most often found during physical examination.
    D. Pain is typically unilateral.

8. A 70-year-old woman presents with kyphosis measuring 68°. Neurologic examination is normal, and patient denies back pain. What is the best next step?

    A. Advise the patient to return for follow-up if she develops pain.
    B. Initiate osteoporosis prevention.
    C. Recommend a molded brace.
    D. Refer for surgical correction.

9. A 13-year-old boy presents for a follow-up visit for his adolescent idiopathic scoliosis. Which of the following physical examination findings is least likely to be seen?

    A. Lower extremity weakness
    B. Thoracic rib prominence
    C. Trunk shift
    D. Waist asymmetry

10. Which disease is characterized by a hunchback appearance with a sharp, angulated thoracic hump that worsens with spinal flexion and is associated with back pain?

    A. Postural kyphosis
    B. Adolescent idiopathic scoliosis
    C. Degenerative scoliosis
    D. Scheuermann kyphosis

11. If a patient presents to the office with lower back pain extending to the bilateral legs associated with numbness and tingling, what would be the test of choice for diagnosis?

    A. Lumbosacral CT scan
    B. Lumbosacral MRI
    C. Lateral lumbosacral x-ray
    D. Ultrasound of lumbar spine

12. Which of the following is true regarding lower back pain?

    A. LBP is the #1 reason for doctor visits in the United States.
    B. The most common causes of LBP are lumbosacral strain and vertebral disc herniation.
    C. Most patients with LBP will require surgery to relieve symptoms.
    D. The cause of LBP is easily identified in the majority of patients.

13. Which statement is correct about a patient presenting with spondylolithesis?

    A. Spondyloptosis is a complete disruption between two vertebrae within the spinal column.
    B. Pain is alleviated through continued movement as it keeps the surrounding lumbar muscles in motion.
    C. Surgical treatment should be performed immediately for a grade II slippage.
    D. Spondylolysis, which is usually a precursor to spondylolithesis, is a defect or stress fracture commonly seen in the spinous process of a vertebra.

14. Which of the following is the recommended treatment for a lumbosacral strain?

    A. A 5-day course of oral prednisone
    B. Chiropractic manipulation
    C. NSAIDs, heat, and progressive ambulation
    D. Epidural steroid injection

15. Spondylolysis, which can be a precursor to spondylolithesis, is a defect or stress fracture commonly seen in what vertebra?

    A. L4
    B. L5
    C. S1
    D. L4 and L5

16. A 45-year-old man presents with LBP, burning pain in the left lower extremity, and difficulty ambulating. What finding is expected on physical examination?

    A. A normal neurologic examination
    B. A negative SLR with motor weakness in the left lower extremity
    C. A positive SLR with motor weakness in the left lower extremity
    D. Saddle anesthesia and poor sphincter tone on digital rectal examination

17. What is the recommended initial treatment for a L4-L5 disc herniation?

    A. NSAIDs, heat, and progressive ambulation
    B. Epidural steroid injection at L4-L5
    C. Surgical consult for microdiscectomy
    D. Hydrocodone/acetaminophen, and/or oral methylprednisolone, and rest

18. A 71-year-old male who has a history of a pacemaker fell and slipped this morning in the kitchen. He now complains of LBP extending to the buttock, as well as weakness to the right foot. He is having difficulty walking around his house. What is the test of choice for this patient?

    A. Lumbar CT myelogram
    B. Lumbar MRI without contrast
    C. Lumbar MRI with contrast
    D. Lumbar CT scan with contrast

19. Which of the following is true regarding imaging for LBP?

    A. The majority of patients will require an MRI initially.
    B. It is necessary to obtain plain radiographs in all patients with LBP.
    C. Imaging is necessary since the history and physical examination rarely aid in determining the diagnosis.
    D. Plain radiograph views include AP/lateral of lumbar spine, including lateral view of forward flexion and extension, and oblique views.

Section I Pretest: Upper Extremity Disorders

1. A 24-year-old left hand dominant baseball pitcher complains of a deep left shoulder ache for several months. He denies acute/traumatic injury but has increased his pitching count over this period, and the pain has degraded his performance. His physical examination is significant for pain recreated with range of motion testing and a positive O'Brien test. No numbness or tingling is reported. He would like to

return to his previous level of functionality as soon as possible. Given his age and occupation, which therapeutic intervention would be most appropriate at this time?

A. Orthopedic consultation
B. X-ray
C. Activity modification
D. Narcotic pain relief

2. Which physical examination finding is characteristic of a superior labrum anterior to posterior (SLAP) tear?

A. Neer test
B. Hawkins test
C. Lift off test
D. O'Brien test

3. What is the least invasive first-line treatment for lateral elbow pain?

A. Immobilization of the wrist and/or circumferential compression banding of the forearm
B. Corticosteroid injection
C. Open surgical debridement
D. Arthroscopic debridement

4. What intervention is therapeutic and may aid in diagnosis for SLAP?

A. Narcotic pain relievers
B. System glucocorticoids
C. Corticosteroid injection
D. Hyaluronic acid injection

5. A 35-year-old male contractor presents to the urgent care center complaining of acute elbow pain for the past 3 weeks. He reports an insidious onset of pain localized to the lateral aspect of the joint. The pain is typically aggravated by repetitive forearm twisting using a screwdriver. A physical examination reveals point tenderness pain over the lateral epicondyle, exacerbated by resisted wrist extension. What is the most likely diagnosis?

A. Medial epicondylitis
B. Lateral epicondylitis
C. Fracture of the lateral epicondyle
D. Lateral collateral ligament tear

6. A 55-year-old male machinist presents to the urgent care with a 4-month history of left medial elbow pain. No history of trauma. You assess his condition as an overuse, inflammatory condition with a presumptive diagnosis of medial epicondylitis. Additionally, he reports having numbness (dysesthesias) in the fourth and fifth digits of his left hand for more than a year. What complicating factor would warrant a referral to orthopedics for further evaluation?

A. Posterior interosseous nerve irritation

B. Radial nerve palsy
C. Ulnar neuritis
D. Median nerve compression in the carpal tunnel

7. What is the preferred imaging modality to aid in the diagnosis of a SLAP tear?

A. X-ray
B. MRI
C. MRA
D. CT

8. An 18-year-old female collegiate tennis player presents to your office complaining of medial elbow pain for the past 6 weeks. She denies trauma to the elbow. However, she states that with every forehand shot she is having intense pain over the common extensor muscles of the forearm. A physical examination reveals tenderness over the extensor carpi radialis brevis (ECRB) and condyle of the lateral humerus. Pain was reproduced with resisted middle finger extension (Maudsley test). Plain film radiographs were negative. You prescribe a short course of bracing, activity/sport modification, and nonsteroidal anti-inflammatory medication for the next 2 weeks. Unfortunately, the athlete returns with continued pain despite conservative measures. What is the next treatment option?

A. Corticosteroid injection
B. PRP injections
C. Topical steroid
D. Continued nonsteroidal therapy

9. Which of the following diagnostic assessments is currently considered the diagnostic test of choice for someone in whom you suspect the diagnosis of carpal tunnel syndrome?

A. Nerve conduction study
B. MRI of the wrist
C. Peripheral nerve biopsy
D. Tinel sign

10. A 21-year-old male professional league pitcher presents to your sports medicine clinic with acute medial elbow for the past 3 days. He denies trauma. However, the athlete reports throwing an abnormally high number of pitches in a two game series as a reliever over the weekend. Further history reveals that he was most symptomatic during the cocking phase of his throwing motion. He isolates his pain to the medial aspect of the elbow. An examination of the elbow reproduces pain and laxity of his medial ligaments. What imaging modality would be the best option to rule out a ligamentous injury vs. inflammatory pain?

A. CT scan
B. Positron emission tomography (PET scan)
C. Ultrasound
D. MRI

11. Which peripheral nerve is involved with carpal tunnel syndrome?

    A. Ulnar nerve
    B. Median nerve
    C. Radial nerve
    D. Musculocutaneous nerve

12. Initial treatment for a SLAP tear typically consists of what treatment plan?

    A. Surgery with aggressive physical therapy
    B. Activity modification, NSAIDs/acetaminophen, physical therapy
    C. Activity modification, narcotic pain relief, physical therapy
    D. Sling for 6 months and gradual increase in activity

13. Which of the following clinical stories is most consistent with a diagnosis of median nerve compression of the wrist?

    A. Numbness and tingling into the ulnar side of the hand and fifth digit
    B. Painful paresthesia in the hand waking the patient from sleep in the night
    C. Pain that radiates from the shoulder down into the arm and thumb
    D. Pain and paresthesia radiating from the medial epicondyles into the medial hand

14. A patient with de Quervain tenosynovitis returns to the clinic for follow-up 6 weeks after the birth of her child complaining of continued pain and swelling at the right radial styloid. What is the most appropriate next step in management?

    A. Oral corticosteroid taper
    B. Corticosteroid injection into the first dorsal compartment
    C. MRI of the right wrist
    D. Referral for surgical consult

15. What is the treatment of choice for an individual with carpal tunnel syndrome who has significant motor weakness with thumb abduction and opposition?

    A. Acetaminophen
    B. Wrist splints
    C. Rest and time
    D. Surgical decompression of the nerve

16. Pain reported along the radial styloid process with thumb clenched in a fist and sharp ulnar deviation describes a positive finding of what test?

    A. Tinel sign
    B. Phalen test
    C. Allen test
    D. Finkelstein test

17. Which imaging modality is recommended to confirm the diagnosis of a shoulder dislocation?

    A. MRI
    B. CT
    C. Ultrasound
    D. Plain film

18. In de Quervain tenosynovitis, increased tendon friction due to thickening and swelling of extensor retinaculum is a result of irritation or constriction of which of the following tendon(s)?

    A. Abductor pollicis longus and palmaris longus
    B. Abductor pollicis longus and extensor pollicis brevis
    C. Extensor carpi ulnaris and extensor digitorum
    D. Extensor pollicis longus and extensor pollicis brevis

19. Which of the following is an indication for treating a proximal humerus fracture with open reduction internal fixation (ORIF)?

    A. Failed conservative management
    B. Female gender
    C. Mild bone displacement
    D. Patients age <75

20. Which of the following is consistent with the diagnosis of de Quervain tenosynovitis?

    A. Loss of sensation in affected wrist
    B. Pain located on the ulnar side of wrist
    C. Pain may radiate up the affected forearm
    D. Sudden onset of symptoms

21. What is the most common type of shoulder dislocation?

    A. Superior
    B. Inferior
    C. Anterior
    D. Posterior

22. In which of the following patient populations is there a high incidence of proximal humerus fractures?

    A. Adolescents
    B. Children
    C. Elderly
    D. Middle aged

23. Which of the following is most likely to have a history of de Quervain tenosynovitis?

    A. 30-year-old female golfer
    B. 15-year-old male video gamer
    C. 35-year-old male new father
    D. 75-year-old female gardener

24. Tenderness to palpation at the anatomic snuffbox is indicative of which type of fracture?

    A. Bennett fracture
    B. Distal radius fracture
    C. Distal ulna fracture
    D. Scaphoid fracture

25. Which of the following is considered a potentially useful and conservative treatment option for somebody with carpal tunnel syndrome?

    A. Oral corticosteroids
    B. Rhizotomy
    C. Wearing wrist splints while sleeping
    D. Traction of the cervical spine

26. The fracture displacement in Smith fracture is which of the following?

    A. Ventral
    B. Dorsal
    C. Radial
    D. Ulnar

27. A 27-year-old male has right hand pain after becoming angry and punching a wall. His x-rays show a nondisplaced fifth metacarpal fracture. What is the appropriate treatment?

    A. Ulnar gutter splint with flexion of the metacarpophalangeal (MCP) joints
    B. Ulnar gutter splint with extension of the MCP joints
    C. Volar wrist splint
    D. Splinting the fourth and fifth digits together for immobilization and stability

28. Which nerve is most commonly injured in anterior shoulder dislocations?

    A. Radial
    B. Axillary
    C. Median
    D. Ulnar

29. How will the child's arm with a nursemaid's elbow most often present?

    A. Slight extension at the elbow and supinated forearm
    B. Slight flexion at the elbow and pronated forearm
    C. Slight extension at the elbow and pronated forearm
    D. Slight flexion at the elbow and supinated forearm

30. What is an intra-articular comminuted fracture of the base of the first metacarpal is called?

    A. Galeazzi fracture
    B. Monteggia fracture
    C. Rolando fracture
    D. Bennett fracture

31. Elbow dislocations most commonly occur in what direction?

    A. Posterior
    B. Anterior
    C. Medial
    D. Lateral

32. What is the definition of long head of the biceps (LHB) tendinosis?

    A. Acute inflammation of the tendon sheath
    B. Chronic degenerative changes within the tendon
    C. A complete tear of the LHB tendon
    D. Subluxation of the biceps tendon resulting in pain

33. A 25-year-old male presents with a slowly enlarging mass on the dorsum of his left wrist that has been present for 3 years. He denies any significant symptoms. Physical examination shows a 1 cm nontender, firm, palpable mass that transilluminates. What is the likely diagnosis in this patient?

    A. Lipoma
    B. Ganglion cyst
    C. Colles cyst
    D. Fibroma

34. Which imaging modality is superior in detection of LHB tendinopathy?

    A. Ultrasound
    B. Bone scan
    C. MRI
    D. CT

35. A 20-year-old male presents with a painless, firm mass on the dorsal aspect of his wrist that has been present for 3 weeks. On your examination, the mass transilluminates, and Allen test reveals patent radial and ulnar arteries. What is the most appropriate next step in management?

    A. Referral to an orthopedic oncologist
    B. Surgical excision with wide margins
    C. Observation
    D. Autologous bone marrow aspirate injection

36. Which of the following radiologic evidence would most likely be seen on x-ray in this child with rickets?

    A. Narrowing of the metaphysis
    B. Splicing of the metaphysis
    C. Distinct metaphysis margins
    D. Cupping of the metaphysis

37. Where is the most common anatomic location for a ganglion cyst of the wrist?

    A. Scapholunate joint
    B. Radioscaphoid joint
    C. Scaphotrapezial joint
    D. Radioulnar joint

38. Three weeks after evaluation for LHB tendinopathy, the patient suffers an injury while lifting. Pain is noted in the region of the proximal biceps tendon. Which physical examination finding would indicate a ruptured LHB tendon?

    A. Positive Popeye sign

B. Positive apprehension test

C. Positive speed test

D. Positive Hawkin impingement test

39. What are the most common soft-tissue tumors of the wrist?

A. Lipomas

B. Ganglion cysts

C. Sarcomas

D. Osteomas

40. If a child presented with normal liver and kidney function and elevated serum alkaline phosphatase, which of the following serum lab values would be most indicative of calcipenic rickets?

A. Elevated parathyroid hormone, low inorganic phosphorus, and low calcium levels

B. Normal parathyroid hormone, low inorganic phosphorus, and normal calcium levels

C. Normal parathyroid hormone, low inorganic phosphorus, and low calcium levels

D. Elevated parathyroid hormone, high inorganic phosphorus, and normal calcium levels

41. Which of the following physical examination maneuvers would be most clinically useful in identifying whether your patient's anterior shoulder pain could be due to long head of biceps tendinopathy?

A. Neer impingement sign test

B. Yergason test

C. Drop arm test

D. Apprehension test

42. Which of the following physical examination findings is a common clinical presentation in a child with severe rickets?

A. Flat abdomen

B. Rachitic rosary

C. Microcephaly

D. Lack of dental caries

43. What is the most common anterior chest wall deformity?

A. Pectus excavatum

B. Pectus carinatum

C. Poland syndrome

D. Pigeon chest

44. What type of activities worsen the symptoms associated with thoracic outlet syndrome?

A. Repetitive overhead activities

B. Hyperextension activities of the thoracic spine

C. Sedentary activities

D. Activities that require prolonged standing

45. A 39-year-old male coach was hit on the ride side of his chest with a baseball during practice today. He is complaining of pain to palpation and inspiration. You suspect a rib fracture, but the initial chest x-ray is negative for acute fracture or dislocation. What is your next step?

A. Advise the patient there is no fracture and discharge home.

B. Order an MRI to evaluate for soft-tissue injury.

C. Order a chest CT to further evaluate for rib fracture.

D. Call a code trauma.

46. Which of the following special tests can be used in the diagnosis of thoracic outlet syndrome?

A. McMurray test

B. Phalen test

C. Spurling test

D. Drop arm test

47. Which of the following preventative dosing of vitamin D is the best management for most children to prevent rickets?

A. 100 IU daily

B. 400 IU daily

C. 100 IU weekly

D. 400 IU weekly

48. A 17-year-old female with a history of pectus carinatum presents with right rib pain after being kicked in the ribs during a mixed martial arts practice. You find a single right lateral rib fracture identified on rib films. What is the primary goal of treatment in this patient?

A. Surgical fixation

B. Analgesia

C. Chest wall external splint

D. No treatment

49. Patients with pectus carinatum most often note which of the following as their primary complaint?

A. Severe chest pain

B. Cosmetic concerns

C. Shortness of breath

D. Right upper quadrant abdominal pain

50. A 25-year-old woman with no history of trauma presents with right arm pain. She reports that her right arm is easily fatigable, especially after she swims daily. She denies any history of smoking, hyperlipidemia, or peripheral artery disease. On physical examination, her right upper extremity is pale and cool to the touch, her distal right radial pulse is diminished compared to her left, and she has decreased sensation to her right pinky when she abducts and externally rotates the affected arm. What is the most likely diagnosis?

A. Cervical strain

B. Thoracic outlet syndrome

C. Subclavian steal syndrome

D. Thoracic radiculopathy

51. Which chest wall deformity presents with an increased AP diameter?

    A. Pectus excavatum
    B. Pectus carinatum
    C. Scoliosis
    D. Rib fracture

52. In a patient with thoracic outlet syndrome who presents with acute vascular insufficiency and/or progressive neurologic dysfunction, what is the best treatment modality?

    A. NSAIDs
    B. Botox
    C. Steroids
    D. Surgery

▶ ANSWERS AND EXPLANATIONS TO SECTION A PRETEST

1. **A.** This patient will experience pain first.
2. **A.** Emergent fasciotomy is the definitive treatment for a patient whose clinical findings are consistent with compartment syndrome.

▶ ANSWERS AND EXPLANATIONS TO SECTION B PRETEST

1. **B.** Empiric antibiotics for suspected septic arthritis should be initiated after blood and synovial fluid culture specimens have been obtained. The antimicrobial regimen can be tailored to specific organism(s) once the culture and susceptibility results are known.
2. **C.** The most common organism causing osteomyelitis in adults is *S. aureus*.
3. **D.** Although *S. aureus is* the most common causative organism of septic arthritis, *P. aeruginosa* should be considered in individuals who use IV drugs.
4. **B.** Most cases of septic arthritis arise from hematogenous seeding. Less commonly, joints can become infected through direct inoculation or spread from nearby infected structures.
5. **B.** The recurrence rate of chronic osteomyelitis in adults is 30%.
6. **D.** Atraumatic monoarthritis with joint fluid analysis revealing >50 000 cells/μL, neutrophil predominance, absence of crystals, and Gram-negative bacilli is consistent with septic arthritis and should prompt initiation of empiric cephalosporin.
7. **D.** The definitive diagnosis of septic arthritis is made with synovial fluid culture.

▶ ANSWERS AND EXPLANATIONS TO SECTION C PRETEST

1. **C.** Probenecid is a second-line agent used in the treatment of gout.

2. **D.** The prevalence of AS is ~5% to 6% among people who are HLA-B27 positive. AS is more common among men, and age of onset is typically <40 years.
3. **A.** Chondrocalcinosis is a common finding on knee radiographs of patients with CPPD disease.
4. **B.** Treatment guidelines for AS encourage trialing at least two different NSAIDs, each for at least 2–4 weeks as initial therapy.
5. **B.** Decreased alcohol consumption should be included in this patient's post-treatment education.
6. **C.** Atopic dermatitis is not an extra-articular manifestation of AS. However, psoriasis is.
7. **D.** Polymyalgia rheumatica most commonly affects people aged 60–70 years.
8. **A.** Both fibromyalgia and chronic fatigue syndrome typically present without objective diagnostic findings. The difference is that patients with chronic fatigue syndrome report excessive levels of fatigue. Patients with fibromyalgia often have difficulty sleeping but can still generally function. Depression, morning stiffness, and irritable bowel symptoms including diarrhea are all consistent with a diagnosis of fibromyalgia.
9. **A.** Anti-CCP is both specific and sensitive for RA.
10. **B.** Exercise has been shown to have moderate benefit in patients with fibromyalgia. Corticosteroid injections may be helpful in the treatment of RA, and increasing dietary sodium can improve the symptoms of chronic fatigue syndrome in some patients. Bedrest is counterproductive in patients with fibromyalgia and may increase their symptoms.
11. **A.** The ankle is usually unaffected in polymyalgia rheumatica.
12. **C.** Methotrexate is the most appropriate initial treatment option according to the ACR.
13. **C.** Fibromyalgia is a diagnosis of exclusion and does not have objective laboratory findings. Despite the presence of widespread pain, patients do not have serum indicators of inflammation, such as an elevated ESR or CRP. A positive ANA can be found in SLE and RA. The presence of HLA-B27 is consistent with a diagnosis of spondyloarthropathy, such as AS.
14. **A.** Giant cell arteritis is commonly associated with polymyalgia rheumatica.
15. **C.** Joint damage can be slowed with adequate treatment.
16. **A.** 90% of patients have joint inflammation or early morning stiffness affecting knees, wrists, and hands. Typically, this inflammation does not cause permanent damage (ie, nonerosive arthritis).
17. **C.** Oral glucocorticoid is the primary treatment of choice for patients diagnosed with polymyalgia rheumatica.
18. **B.** Women, African Americans, and Hispanics are more likely to develop SLE.
19. **B.** The most important marker of response to therapy is the improvement muscle weakness.

20. **C.** Positive ANA test is one of the 11 ACR criteria to be met in order to determine a diagnosis of SLE. The other 10 criteria include arthritis, discoid rash, malar rash, photosensitivity, oral ulcers, serositis, hematologic disorders, immunologic disorders, neurologic disorders, or renal disorders.

21. **B.** This is the description of heliotropes or the heliotropic rash that affect bilateral eyelids. Other common cutaneous disease included Gottron sign or papules, or the V or shawl sign.

22. **C.** Reactive arthritis predominantly affects males 20–40 years old, most common in Caucasians.

23. **D.** Most patients with reactive arthritis can expect to reach a normal life span and maintain a near-normal lifestyle. Only 10% of patients will develop cardiac manifestations, including aortic regurgitation and pericarditis.

24. **C.** Future therapies may target specific autoantibodies including the most common associated auto-antibody with PM, Anti-Jo-1.

25. **B.** The most common autoimmune diseases that are correlated with Sjögren are RA and lupus. Between 20% and 50% of patients with RA will present with Sjögren, while 10% to 25% of patients with lupus will develop symptoms of Sjögren.

26. **B.** The classical triad of symptoms in reactive arthritis consists of conjunctivitis, nongonococcal urethritis, and asymmetric oligoarthritis.

27. **C.** While the Anti-SSA is only one of the diagnostic tests needed to confirm a Sjögren diagnosis, it is one of the required objective criteria per international guidelines. An ANA double-stranded antibody is a test for scleroderma, the SPEP/UPEP is a test for multiple myeloma, and the UACR is a screening test for CKD.

28. **B.** Lupus nephritis is treated with a combination of cyclophosphamide and corticosteroids.

29. **C.** If you are worried enough to order lab testing, a referral to ophthalmology is the least aggressive and in this age group, with a past medical history of hypertension, ophthalmology should be offered. There is no increase in fracture rate with Sjögren, nor do you want to start allergy testing until you have ruled out Sjögren. A missed menses in a perimenopausal patient is common.

30. **D.** Annie is at increased risk for secondary Sjögren. Often, patients will have nonspecific symptoms and, only with suspicious questioning, can a differential include Sjögren. Annie has multiple risk factors (age, gender, and autoimmune disease). She has had to go to the dentist and ophthalmologist recently. She is presenting with increased joint pain while having been well controlled for years. Patients do not describe exactly what is listed in the reference books. This is the patient where one needs to be suspicious.

▶ ANSWERS AND EXPLANATIONS TO SECTION D PRETEST

1. **A.** Some hip instability is very common in newborn infants. In fact, most cases of mild hip instability found on newborn examination will resolve spontaneously after birth with normal function without intervention. AVN of the hip is a risk of splinting and surgical intervention, a complication that may arise in treated patients. Ultrasonography is recommended as a screening tool for infants with examination findings or questionable examination findings of DDH, or with identified risk factors for DDH. Although surgery may be recommended by an orthopedic surgeon for the treatment of DDH, this is not usually necessary if DDH is diagnosed early.

2. **B.** The Klein line can identify SCFE on plain films.

3. **C.** DDH can be successfully treated in most cases. Infants with DDH, treated or untreated, have a higher incidence of premature degenerative joint disease in adulthood, but the incidence is lowest in those who receive early treatment. It is important for infants who are treated surgically for DDH to follow up closely with an orthopedist for monitoring of the joint to ensure it develops normally with growth until physical maturity. This disorder is not associated with visual loss.

4. **B.** The Thessaly test is a special clinical test used to diagnose meniscal injuries.

5. **C.** Although the diagnosis of DDH after birth is not an emergency, prompt referral (within a few weeks) to an orthopedist experienced in the diagnosis and treatment of DDH is indicated if the hip is dislocated or dislocatable at any age.

6. **D.** LBP is not associated with SCFE.

7. **D.** Although there remain differing screening recommendations among expert groups within the United States and internationally, the American Academy of Pediatrics recommends screening all newborns for DDH by physical examination at birth and targeted ultrasound screening for infants with multiple risk factors.

8. **A.** The hips should be examined in any child with knee pain.

9. **C.** DDH is more common among infants who are female, in breech position in the third trimester (≥34 weeks' gestation), have a positive family history of DDH, and who have a history of tight lower extremity swaddling. However, some infants diagnosed with DDH have no risk factors.

10. **B.** There are three zones of the menisci. The red zone, which is the vascular region and the outermost third of the meniscus. The red-white zone, which is the junction where the vascular region meets the avascular region and is the middle third of the meniscus. And the white zone, which is the avascular region or

the innermost third of the meniscus. Most meniscal injuries affect the white zone, which will not self-heal due to the avascular location.

11. **C.** Surgical pinning in situ is the most appropriate first-line treatment for a patient with an SCFE.

12. **D.** Radiographic views that should be obtained for complete evaluation of a hip fracture include AP and lateral of affected proximal femur. Additional radiographs (AP and lateral) to include the entire femur are vital to assess for any prosthetic implants that could interfere with surgical intervention or additional fractures. Other images should include AP pelvis (to evaluate for potential pelvic fracture) and AP/lateral of contralateral hip for anatomic comparison. An MRI or CT is indicated if clinical suspicion remains after inconclusive plain radiographs are obtained.

13. **D.** Radiographic examination of the knee would be the first choice of imaging given his age, history, and the suspicion of arthritis as a differential. He very well may also have a degenerative meniscal tear; however, standard radiography should first be used to exclude other sources of knee pain such as OA.

14. **C.** Patients who have undergone total hip arthroplasty are at an increased risk for a hip dislocation. Movements such as hip flexion >90° or adduction of the hip such as crossing one's legs can result in a hip dislocation. Hip dislocations are not nearly as common as hip fractures. A posterior hip dislocation can occur from an MVA. Suspected native hip dislocations require CT imaging to assess additional fractures.

15. **A.** The ACL is the primary restraint to anterior tibial translation, preventing the tibia from sliding anterior to the femur.

16. **D.** MRI is the most sensitive diagnostic imaging test for assessing meniscal injuries. The MRI results can determine the location and severity of the meniscal injury, as well as guide surgical intervention.

17. **D.** Each of the other choices are risk factors for AVN, whereas total hip arthroplasty is the definitive treatment of the disease.

18. **D.** Patellar fracture: A quick stop from a full sprint causes forceful contraction of the quadriceps. If the force of this contraction exceeds the strength of the patella, an avulsions fracture may result, which, in turn, may disrupt the extensor mechanism of the knee. This requires surgical intervention.

19. **B.** Surgical repair of a nondisplaced femoral neck fracture with cannulated screws may result in AVN of the right femoral head due to disruption of the vascular supply to the femoral head. A prior hip fracture is a risk factor for subsequent hip fractures. Nearly half of all patients who sustain a hip fracture do not regain their preoperative independence. Unless contraindicated, all patients, regardless of age, who sustain hip fractures and have surgery will

receive anticoagulants such as low-molecular-weight heparin.

20. **C.** Intracapsular hip fractures include femoral neck fractures and femoral head fractures. Extracapsular fractures include intertrochanteric, subtrochanteric, and greater trochanter avulsion fractures.

▶ ANSWERS AND EXPLANATIONS TO SECTION E PRETEST

1. **A.** Giant cell tumors of the bone are rare neoplasms, typically occurring in young adults at the end parts (epiphysis) of long bones (most often close to the knee). They are aggressive tumors that can destroy the surrounding bone.

2. **B.** In most patients with MBD, treatment is palliative. The most common treatment for MBD patients is local field radiation as it brings maximum pain relief. It may, however, take several months to reach full effect. It results in 60% complete pain relief and >80% partial pain relief.

3. **C.** Surgery is the treatment of choice if the giant cell tumor is determined to be resectable.

4. **C.** Treatment for osteoblastoma involves surgical resection of the tumor without damaging the surrounding structures. Radiation therapy and chemotherapy are not recommended.

5. **D.** X-rays should be the first imaging test performed in order to characterize bone tumors.

6. **C.** The cancer types that most commonly metastasize to the bone include breast, lung, thyroid, kidney, colon, and prostate.

7. **D.** Thorough present and past medical history, family history, and relevant risk factors such as smoking are extremely important. During physical examination, check tenderness around the bones, range of motion of adjacent joints, and perform full neurovascular examination.

▶ ANSWERS AND EXPLANATIONS TO SECTION F PRETEST

1. **A.** Primary OA refers to articular cartilage deterioration without a known cause.

2. **B.** Trial of an intra-articular corticosteroid injection is the most appropriate treatment choice listed. Your patient has not met criteria for arthroscopic or knee replacement surgery. Sustained opioid analgesia is not recommended for knee OA. The best choice of those listed would be discussing trial of a corticosteroid injection.

3. **D.** A Heberden node is bony enlargement of the DIP joint occurring as a result of OA.

4. **C.** Moderate joint space narrowing is described as grade 3 OA in the Kellgren-Lawrence radiographic grading system.

▶ ANSWERS AND EXPLANATIONS TO SECTION G PRETEST

1. **B.** DXA scan is indicated because of multiple risk factors including personal history of a fracture. Heel ultrasound correlates well with DXA of the heel, but not with other areas of the body. She has no reason to suspect secondary causes of osteoporosis, and radiographs are not indicated for assessment of fracture risk.
2. **A.** A T-score of −1 to −2.5 is diagnostic of low bone mass (previously referred to as osteopenia).
3. **C.** This patient has osteoporosis since the T-score is < −2.5. Alendronate is a bisphosphonate, which is the first-line therapy. The selective estrogen receptor modulator (SERM), raloxifene if used more often than tamoxifen; however, SERMs are not considered first-line because bisphosphonates have proven to have better antiresorptive efficacy. The other choices are not considered first line.
4. **B.** This patient is under 65 years of age with a low 10-year risk for major osteoporotic fracture. She benefits from prevention strategies. If she was high risk, she would benefit from a DXA scan, and if trying to exclude secondary causes, a 24-hour urinary calcium could be obtained. She does not meet the indications for pharmacologic therapy at this time.
5. **C.** RA, parathyroid adenoma, and long-term antiepileptic therapy are risk factors for osteoporosis. Oral bisphosphonates cause esophageal irritation and should be avoided in patients with gastroesophageal reflux disease.

▶ ANSWERS AND EXPLANATIONS TO SECTION H PRETEST

1. **C.** Lumbar spine MRI is the gold standard for confirming the diagnosis of lumbar spinal stenosis.
2. **C.** Toe-touches is not a treatment option for patients diagnosed with spondylolithesis.
3. **D.** Lumbosacral discectomy with spinal fusion at L5-S1 is the treatment of choice for this patient.
4. **C.** Bracing is recommended for curves 20° to 40° in patients with a Risser stage of 0, 1, or 2. Curves <20° should be closely monitored, and surgery is an option for curves >40°.
5. **B.** Hyperextension braces are used as adjunct therapy with other means of conservative treatment is not true about lumbar spinal stenosis.
6. **C.** L4-L5 is the most common location for spondylolithesis to occur.
7. **B.** Flexion of the lumbar spine alleviates symptoms in a patient presenting with lumbar spinal stenosis.
8. **B.** A 70-year-old woman is at risk of developing osteoporosis, which can cause kyphosis to progress. Therefore, osteoporosis prevention is recommended.

Physical therapy would also be a reasonable choice. Molded bracing is not currently recommended in skeletally mature patients. Surgery is typically reserved for curves above 80°, or those associated with pain despite conservative therapy.

9. **A.** Thoracic rib prominence, trunk shift, and waist asymmetry are all classic signs of scoliosis. Lower extremity weakness and other neuromotor deficits are unlikely to occur with adolescent idiopathic scoliosis. However, they may be present in scoliosis caused by neuromuscular disease.
10. **D.** Kyphosis is often described as a "hunchback" appearance. Scheuermann deformity becomes more prominent on forward bend test and is often associated with pain, unlike scoliosis or postural kyphosis.
11. **B.** Lumbosacral MRI would be the test of choice for diagnosis in a patient presents to the office with LBP extending to the bilateral legs associated with numbness and tingling.
12. **B.** The most common causes of LBP are low back strain and vertebral disc herniation. The exact cause of symptoms is found in only 12% to 15% of patients. LBP is the second most common reason for health care visits. Most symptoms of LBP can be adequately treated with conservative measures.
13. **A.** Spondyloptosis is a complete disruption between two vertebrae within the spinal column.
14. **C.** Low back strains and sprains should be treated with short-term rest (2 days), ice or heat, NSAIDs, progressive ambulation, and weight loss if indicated.
15. **B.** Spondylolysis, which can be a precursor to spondylolithesis, is a defect or stress fracture commonly seen in L5.
16. **C.** Patients with a lumbar herniated disc will typically have a positive SLR test and decrease motor strength in the lower extremity, specifically in the region that correlates with the affected nerve root. It is rare that a patient would have a normal neurologic examination, especially with his complaints and symptoms. Cauda equina syndrome is not suspected in this patient since he does not complain of urinary or bowel symptoms such as incontinence or retention.
17. **D.** Vertebral disc herniations require an adequate narcotic dose due to the burning nature of the pain. Steroids are often effective. With appropriate medical treatment and rest, >75% of patients will experience relief. Epidural steroid injections are not indicated for herniated discs, and a microdiscectomy is indicated only if conservative measures fail.
18. **A.** Lumbar CT myelogram is the test of choice for this patient.
19. **D.** Most patients do not require imaging of the lumbosacral spine for new-onset LBP. If the patient has no red flag symptoms such as fall or significant injury, fever, weight loss, urinary or bowel complaints, motor or sensory loss in the lower extremities, or

any contributing medical history, no imaging is warranted at this time. If LBP does not resolve with conservative measures, plain radiographs should be obtained before any further imaging, such as MRI or CT. Plain radiograph views include AP/lateral of lumbar spine, lateral view of forward flexion and extension, and oblique views.

▶ ANSWERS AND EXPLANATIONS TO SECTION I PRETEST

1. **A.** Orthopedic consultation would be most appropriate at this time.
2. **D.** O'Brien test is characteristic of a SLAP tear.
3. **A.** Immobilization of the wrist and/or circumferential compression banding of the forearm is correct. Conservative and immediate measures that would promote healing provide eventual pain relief and strengthen the surrounding muscles of the forearm. Answer B is a good option for chronic or recalcitrant (recurrent) epicondylitis. Surgical intervention whether it is a closed or an open procedure is the last option for treatment. Arthroscopic debridement is typically reserved for lateral epicondylitis.
4. **C.** Corticosteroid injection is therapeutic and may aid in diagnosis of a SLAP tear.
5. **B.** Lateral epicondylitis is the most likely diagnosis. Medial epicondylitis occurs on the medial aspect of the elbow at the insertion of the common flexor/pronator muscle group. A fracture or ligamentous injury would be suspected if there was a history of trauma. The onset of symptoms is gradual in this scenario lowering the suspicion of fracture and/or soft-tissue injury.
6. **C.** Ulnar neuritis is correct. The primary nerve associated medial elbow complaints is the ulnar nerve. The ulnar nerve typically affects the fourth and fifth digits of the hand. Further evaluation by an orthopedic specialist would be necessary to address the chronic nature of the likely compressive neuropathy. PIN symptoms are generally associated with lateral epicondylitis. This is often inadvertently caused by prolonged compressive banding. Injuries of the radial nerve are typically associated with trauma (distal third humeral fractures). The median nerve is typically associated with compression within the carpal tunnel of the wrist (carpal tunnel syndrome).
7. **C.** MRA is the preferred imaging modality to aid in the diagnosis of a SLAP tear.
8. **A.** Corticosteroid injection is the most conservative next line treatment option in this scenario. PRP injections are typically a last conservative treatment option before surgical considerations. Topical steroids may be effective over an extended period of time. However, injectable steroids have a more immediate pain-relieving effect. Continuing NSAIDs is not wrong as an adjunctive therapy to other interventions.

9. **A.** Electrodiagnostic studies, specifically a nerve conduction study, are considered the diagnostic study of choice for carpal tunnel syndrome. The study evaluates the neuronal conduction speed through the median nerve as it passes under the transverse carpal ligament.
10. **D.** MRI is the most appropriate imaging modality for soft-tissue anatomy. CT scan is typically reserved for complex bony pathology. PET imaging is a modality used primarily in oncology to detect cancers utilizing radioactive isotopes. Ultrasound is an effective portable tool for immediate or clinical evaluation of soft-tissue structures. However, the sensitivity and efficacy of this modality is user dependent.
11. **B.** Carpal tunnel syndrome is due to compression of the median nerve at the wrist.
12. **B.** Activity modification, NSAIDs/acetaminophen, physical therapy.
13. **B.** Painful nocturnal paresthesia in the hands is a common, classic presentation of carpal tunnel syndrome.
14. **B.** Corticosteroid injection into the first dorsal compartment would be the most appropriate next step in management for this patient. Oral corticosteroids are not indicated in de Quervain tenosynovitis. Surgical treatment is for patients with refractory disease and would be considered if the patient fails to improve with corticosteroid injection therapy. MRI is not indicated unless considering alternate diagnosis. Additionally, in appropriate patients, NSAIDs may be used in conjunction with corticosteroid injection.
15. **D.** If someone who has carpal tunnel syndrome also has motor deficits secondary to nerve compression at the wrist, surgical referral should not be delayed.
16. **D.** Pain with ulnar deviation is a positive finding in Finkelstein test. Tinel sign and Phalen test are used to assess irritation of the median nerve. Allen test is used to assess arterial blood supply of the hand.
17. **D.** Plain film is recommended to confirm the diagnosis of a shoulder dislocation.
18. **B.** In de Quervain tenosynovitis, increased tendon friction due to thickening, and swelling of extensor retinaculum is a result of irritation or constriction of the abductor pollicis longus and extensor pollicis brevis.
19. **A.** Failed conservative management is an indication for treating a proximal humerus fracture with ORIF.
20. **C.** Patients with de Quervain tenosynovitis often complain of pain that radiates up the affected forearm. Pain is typically of gradual onset, located on the radial aspect of the wrist, and patients do not have neurologic symptoms.
21. **C.** The most common type of shoulder dislocation is anterior.
22. **C.** The elderly experience a high incidence of proximal humerus fracture.

23. **A.** A 30-year-old female golfer would have a history consistent with de Quervain tenosynovitis. It most commonly affects women between the ages of 30–50 years. Additionally, activities that require repetitive twisting of the wrist are known to cause to lead to the disease process.

24. **D.** Tenderness to palpation at the anatomic snuffbox is indicative of scaphoid fracture.

25. **C.** Because the natural position while sleeping is to move into a fetal position, which commonly involves flexion of the wrists, repeated compression of the median nerve can happen while sleeping in individuals with carpal tunnel syndrome (essentially Phalen maneuver while sleeping). Wearing wrist splints while sleeping helps prevent this repetitive nerve compression.

26. **A.** The fracture displacement in Smith fracture is ventral.

27. **A.** Ulnar gutter splint with flexion of the MCP joints is the appropriate treatment.

28. **B.** The axillary nerve is most commonly injured in anterior shoulder dislocations.

29. **B.** The child's arm with a nursemaid's elbow will most often present light flexion at the elbow and pronated forearm.

30. **C.** An intra-articular comminuted fracture of the base of the first metacarpal is called a Rolando fracture.

31. **A.** Elbow dislocations are most commonly posterior.

32. **B.** LHB tendinosis refers to degenerative changes in the LHB tendon.

33. **B.** The likely diagnosis in this patient is a ganglion cyst.

34. **C.** MRI is the best imaging modality for evaluation of LHB tendon pathology. MRI arthrogram is superior in detection of common LHB tendinopathy–associated pathologies.

35. **C.** Observation is the most appropriate next step in management.

36. **D.** Classic characteristics seen on imaging of the long bones are widening, fraying, cupping, and splaying of the metaphysis.

37. **A.** The most common anatomic location for a ganglion cyst of the wrist is the scapholunate joint.

38. **A.** Positive Popeye sign indicates distal retraction of the biceps brachii resulting from LHB tendon rupture.

39. **B.** Ganglion cysts are the most common soft-tissue tumors of the wrist.

40. **A.** Calcipenic rickets may be suspected when there is normal liver and kidney function, elevated serum alkaline phosphatase activity, parathyroid hormone, and low inorganic phosphorus and calcium levels. Phosphopenic rickets may be suspected when there is normal liver and kidney function, elevated serum alkaline phosphatase activity, normal parathyroid hormone and calcium, and low inorganic phosphorus levels.

41. **B.** Pain elicited with palpation over the LHB tendon with the patient's elbow flexed to 90° while resisting supination of the patient's forearm indicates positive Yergason test. Yergason test and speed test are clinically useful in the evaluation of LHB tendinopathy. Answers A, C, and D are useful to evaluate for other shoulder pathologies.

42. **B.** Rows of beadlike prominences of the costochondral rib joints, termed *rachitic rosary*, are frequently seen on physical examination (rachitic rosary) as well as on x-ray.

43. **A.** Pectus excavatum is the most common anterior chest wall deformity affecting about 1 in 400 patients.

44. **A.** Repetitive overhead activities worsen the symptoms associated with thoracic outlet syndrome.

45. **C.** Chest CT remains the most sensitive for identifying rib fractures over a PA and lateral chest x-ray.

46. **C.** The Spurling test can be used in the diagnosis of thoracic outlet syndrome.

47. **B.** Most children need about 400 IU (or 600 IU for older children) of daily vitamin D to prevent rickets.

48. **B.** Though this patient has a history of pectus carinatum, the goals of treatment remain analgesia and respiratory care. There is no indication for surgical fixation of the rib or chest wall deformity, and external splints are no longer recommended for rib fractures.

49. **B.** Cosmetic concerns are the most common complaint of patients with pectus carinatum, though respiratory symptoms may be present.

50. **B.** Thoracic outlet syndrome is the most likely diagnosis.

51. **B.** Pectus carinatum typically presents with an increased AP diameter. Pectus excavatum presents with sternal depression. Scoliosis and rib fractures are not usually associated with a change or increase in AP diameter.

52. **D.** Surgery is the best treatment modality.

CHAPTER

225

Compartment Syndrome

Shane Ryan Apperley, MSc, PGCert, PA-R
Jon Slaven, MMS, PA-C

▶ GENERAL FEATURES

- Compartment syndrome is a limb-threatening (irreversible muscle and nerve damage) and occasionally life-threatening condition where osteofascial compartment pressure rises to a level that decreases perfusion.
- The anterior compartment of the leg is the location most commonly affected; however, it can occur anywhere in the body that skeletal muscle is surrounded by fascia, including the forearm, hand, foot, thigh, buttock, shoulder, and paraspinous muscles.
- Most common cause is trauma, specifically secondary to a fracture (69% of cases). Other etiologies include burns, extravasation of intravenous infusion, arterial injury, and tight casts/dressings or external wrappings.
- There is also a chronic compartment syndrome (CCS; also known as exertional compartment syndrome), most often associated with athletic exertion.

▶ CLINICAL ASSESSMENT

- Maintain a high index of suspicion among patients at risk for acute compartment syndrome
- Pain out of proportion to the clinical situation is usually the first symptom of compartment syndrome.
  - Patients will typically require stronger and/or more frequent doses of analgesics but with little to no effect.
  - Pain may be absent in cases of nerve damage and impossible to assess in patients who are sedated.
  - Pain may be difficult to assess in polytrauma patients and in young children who are unable to verbalize.
- On physical examination, pain with passive stretch is the most sensitive finding before the onset of ischemia.
- Other abnormalities may include paresthesia and hypoesthesia (indicative of nerve ischemia in the affected compartment), palpable swelling, absent peripheral pulses (late finding; amputation usually inevitable in this case), and pallor and paralysis (late finding; full recovery is rare).

▶ DIAGNOSIS

- In a patient with intact mental status, diagnosis is based primarily on physical examination.
- If indicated (polytrauma patients, patients who are not alert/unreliable, or patients with inconclusive physical examination findings), compartment pressures can be measured (typically within 5 cm of the fracture site) using a handheld manometer; a difference between the patient's diastolic blood pressure and the compartment pressure of 30 mm Hg or less is indicative of an elevated compartment pressure.
- Plain radiographs of the extremity may be obtained to rule out fracture if suspected but not yet confirmed.

▶ TREATMENT

- Positive clinical findings should always prompt emergent removal of any cast followed by operative intervention in the form of fasciotomy of all involved compartments.
- Postoperative care includes initial dressing of the wound followed by delayed primary closure or skin grafting at 3–7 days following decompression to prevent reoccurrence.
- Nonoperative management is indicated if the difference between the patient's diastolic blood pressure and the compartment pressure is >30 mm Hg. The patient may be placed under close observation or receive hyperbaric oxygen therapy.

Osteomyelitis

Shane Ryan Apperley, MSc, PGCert, PA-R

▶ GENERAL FEATURES

- Osteomyelitis is infection of bone characterized by progressive inflammatory destruction and apposition of new bone. The exact incidence is unknown.
- The most common locations for osteomyelitis include the spine and ribs (dialysis patients), the medial and lateral clavicle (IV drug users), and the feet and decubitus ulcers (diabetes).
- Additional risk factors for osteomyelitis include recent trauma or surgery, poor vascular supply, peripheral neuropathy, and being immunocompromised.
- Key differentials for osteomyelitis include benign tumor, malignant tumor, and a healing fracture.
- The causative organism varies by age of the patient. In adults, *Streptococcus aureus* is most common. Occasionally, *Enterobacter* or *Streptococcus* species are at fault. The mechanism of spread can be hematogenous, contagious spread, or via direct inoculation.
- The recurrence rate of chronic osteomyelitis in adults is 30%. Patients with major nutritional or systemic disorders have a poor prognosis.

▶ CLINICAL ASSESSMENT

- Patients typically report pain and fever (more common in acute osteomyelitis).
- On history, the patient should be asked about the duration of their symptoms, in addition to any prior treatments or risk factors for osteomyelitis.
- On physical examination, the patient may be septic (fever, tachycardic, or hypotensive). On inspection, erythema and edema are commonly seen. Patients may also be tender to palpation, have a draining sinus tract, and/or have a limp/pain inhibition with weight bearing.
- The joints above and below the area of concern should be examined. An assessment of local and/or systemic vascular insufficiency should also be performed.

▶ DIAGNOSIS

- Osteomyelitis can be classified as acute (within 2 weeks), subacute (within 1 to several months), or chronic (after several months). The Cierny-Mader classification (a clinical classification system based on anatomic, clinical, and radiologic features) is also used.
- Despite variable sensitivity and specificity, orthogonal plain radiographs of the affected extremity should be performed in all cases. Note that, for acute osteomyelitis, (i) bone loss must be 50% before evident on plain films and (ii) imaging findings lag behind by 2 weeks.
- CT (eg, to assist in diagnosis and surgical planning), MRI (eg, to diagnose early osteomyelitis), and nuclear medicine (eg, if MRI is not an option) imaging may also be indicated.
- Laboratory studies may include leukocyte count (elevated in one-third of patients with acute osteomyelitis), erythrocyte sedimentation rate (ESR; elevated in 90% of acute and chronic cases), C-reactive protein (CRP; most sensitive test with elevation in 97% of cases), and blood cultures (often negative but used to guide therapy for hematogenous osteomyelitis). Histology and microbiology may also be indicated, including bone culture, which is the gold standard for guiding antibiotic therapy.

▶ TREATMENT

- Treatment is often a combination of culture-directed antibiotics and surgical irrigation and debridement of nonviable tissue.
- Success in treatment is dependent on several factors, including those relating to the patient (eg, nutritional status), the severity of the injury, and the location of the infection.
- Nonoperative treatment options also include hyperbaric oxygen therapy, typically used as an adjunct in refractory osteomyelitis.

- Operative treatment options also include amputation, typically reserved for patients with chronic infection with pervasive wound or bone damage that is unable to be salvaged.

- Complications of osteomyelitis include persistence or extension of infection, sepsis, and malignant transformation (Marjolin ulcer), which has a 1% incidence in chronic osteomyelitis patients.

CHAPTER 227

Septic Arthritis

Janelle Bludorn, MS, PA-C

A 68-year-old woman with diabetes and osteoarthritis status post remote right total knee replacement seeks emergency department care for a 2-day history of atraumatic pain and swelling of her right knee with associated fever. On physical examination, her right knee is warm to the touch with a moderate effusion, and she cannot flex or extend her knee actively or passively due to pain. Which diagnostic study can definitively establish this patient's most likely diagnosis?

▶ GENERAL FEATURES

- Septic arthritis is monoarthritis characterized by intra-articular infection, which may progress to joint destruction.
- Most common pathogen in both native and prosthetic joints is *Streptococcus aureus*, including methicillin-resistant *S. aureus*.
  - Consider *Pseudomonas* in individuals who are immunocompromised or who use intravenous drugs.
  - Consider *Neisseria gonorrhoeae* in sexually active individuals.
  - Polymicrobial infections are rare.
- Although septic arthritis may arise from direct inoculation (eg, intra-articular injection, trauma) or extension of infection from nearby tissues (eg, osteomyelitis), most cases result from hematogenous seeding.
- Large joints are more commonly affected than small joints; the knee accounts for more than half of all cases, followed by wrist, ankle, and hip.
- Individuals with advanced age, underlying arthropathies, joint prosthesis or surgery, intravenous drug use, or immunosuppressed states may be at increased risk.

▶ CLINICAL ASSESSMENT

- Patients present with acute monoarticular arthritis characterized by symptoms of joint pain, swelling, warmth, and decreased mobility, often accompanied by fever.
- Classic physical examination findings include fever and limited active and passive range of motion of the affected joint due to pain and effusion. Examination may also reveal joint warmth, tenderness, erythema, and edema.

▶ DIAGNOSIS

- Definitive diagnosis of septic arthritis requires synovial fluid culture.
  - Synovial fluid arthrocentesis should be performed.
    - Analysis should include cell count with differential, Gram stain, crystal analysis, and culture. If *N. gonorrhoeae* is suspected, nucleic acid amplification testing (NAAT) may be added.
  - Synovial fluid with leukocyte count >50000–150000 cells/μL with neutrophil predominance, positive Gram stain, and positive culture support diagnosis.
- Other diagnostics may be necessary to assess for concurrent complications.
  - Two sets of blood cultures should be obtained before initiation of antibiotic therapy to rule out bacteremia.
  - Joint imaging with radiographs, computed tomography (CT), or magnetic resonance imaging (MRI) provides a baseline assessment of joint condition and may reveal concurrent arthropathy or effusion.

▶ TREATMENT

- The two cornerstones of septic arthritis treatment are joint drainage and antimicrobial therapy.
  - Joint drainage via needle aspiration, arthroscopy, or arthrotomy based on joint affected, infection duration, and suspicion for foreign body.
- Septic arthritis of a prosthetic joint may require prosthesis resection and replacement to obtain source control.

- Initiate empiric antibiotics after blood and synovial fluid culture specimens have been obtained and then tailor antimicrobial regimen to specific organism(s) once the culture and susceptibility results.
  - If synovial fluid Gram stain reveals Gram-positive cocci, start empiric parenteral vancomycin.
  - If synovial fluid Gram stain reveals Gram-negative bacilli, start empiric parenteral cephalosporin.
- Depending upon causative organism and concurrent conditions (eg, bacteremia, endocarditis, osteomyelitis), parenteral antimicrobial therapy may last 2–8 weeks before transitioning to an oral antibiotic regimen.

Case Conclusion

This woman's clinical presentation should raise a high level of suspicion for septic arthritis based on her risk factors of age, immunosuppressed state, and prosthetic joint; her history of acute monoarthritis; and her objective findings of fever, effusion, and painful range of motion. In the emergency department, synovial fluid was collected via bedside arthrocentesis and revealed a leukocyte count of 100 000 cells/µL and Gram-positive cocci. Orthopedic surgery was consulted, and she underwent resection and replacement of the right knee prosthesis. Empiric intravenous vancomycin was initiated while awaiting final culture results.

SECTION C

Inflammatory and Autoimmune Disorders

CHAPTER 228

Gout and Pseudogout

Patricia Higgins, DO

▶ GENERAL FEATURES

- Gout:
  - Metabolic disease in which elevated uric acid levels lead to precipitation of monosodium urate crystals in joint space
  - Result from an increase in the body pool of urate with hyperuricemia, due to either overproduction of uric acid (10% of cases) or decreased renal clearance (90% of cases)
  - Episodic acute and chronic arthritis caused by the deposition of monosodium urate crystals in the joint
  - Most commonly seen in the first metatarsophalangeal joint
  - Most common inflammatory arthropathy, affecting >8 million Americans
    - Elderly males, postmenopausal females, and Black persons are at the highest risk for the development of gout.
    - Patients with a history of hypertension and an elevated body mass index (≥30 kg/m² at age 21 years) are at a risk of developing gout.
  - Patients can develop chronic pain and connective tissue tophi.

- Calcium pyrophosphate dihydrate (CPPD) disease, or pseudogout:
  - Occurs due to the deposition of CPPD crystals in joints.
  - Increased production of inorganic pyrophosphate and decreased levels of pyrophosphatases in the cartilage; crystals form as pyrophosphate combines with calcium.
  - Most commonly seen in patients aged >65 years, with 30% to 50% of cases in persons aged >85 years.
  - Most patients have preexisting joint damage from other conditions (osteoarthritis [OA], rheumatoid arthritis).
  - Knee is the most commonly affected joint.
  - Acute attacks may be precipitated by trauma, surgery, or a rapid decrease in serum calcium.
  - CPPD disease is typically accompanied by a low-grade fever.

▶ CLINICAL ASSESSMENT

- Differential diagnosis of acute monoarticular arthritis includes:
  - CPPD deposition disease (pseudogout), infection, and trauma

- Monoarticular OA and neoplasms
- Psoriatic arthritis: in 60% to 70% of patients, psoriasis precedes joint disease.
- History:
  - Patient presents with sudden development of a warm, red, and tender joint.
  - Precipitating event such as dietary excess, excessive ethanol intake, trauma, surgery, or serious medical illness may be included in the history.
  - Use of diuretics is also a risk factor for the development of gout.
- Physical examination:
  - Patients present with marked swelling and redness in a joint, which develops rapidly.
  - Symptom onset is often at night.
  - The metatarsal joint of the first toe is most often involved.
  - Tarsal joints, ankles, and knees are commonly affected as well.
- CPPD disease:
  - Differential diagnosis includes gout, rheumatoid arthritis, and OA with CPPD (pseudo-OA).
  - In the acute setting, patients present with acute synovitis superimposed on chronically involved joints.
  - Some patients will develop symmetric synovitis (similar to rheumatoid arthritis).
- History and physical examination:
  - Presentation is similar to gout (thus the name pseudogout) with a swollen, red, tender joint; knee is typically involved.
  - Acute attacks may be precipitated by trauma.
  - In up to 50% of cases, a low-grade fever is present.
  - Untreated attacks can last a few days to as long as 4 weeks.

▶ DIAGNOSIS

- Gout (American College of Rheumatology):
  - Rapid development of monoarticular arthritis, characterized by marked swelling and redness
  - Presence of characteristic urate crystals* in joint fluid, or
  - Presence of a tophus, having urate crystals, or
  - Presence of six or more of the following:
    - Asymmetric selling within a joint on radiography
    - Attack of monoarticular arthritis
    - Culture of joint fluid negative for microorganisms (aspirated during acute attack)
    - Development of maximal inflammation within 1 day
    - Hyperuricemia (serum uric acid level of ≥6.8 mg/dL)
    - Joint redness
    - >1 attack of acute arthritis

- Pain or redness in the first metatarsophalangeal joint
- Subcortical cyst without erosions on radiography
- Suspected tophus
- Unilateral attack involving the first metatarsophalangeal joint
- Unilateral attack involving a tarsal joint
- Having a normal serum uric acid level does NOT exclude a diagnosis of gout.
- CPPD disease:
  - Radiographs: punctate and/or linear radiopaque deposits in menisci, cartilage (chondrocalcinosis)
  - Some patient exhibit intervertebral disk and ligament calcification, and spinal stenosis.
  - The definitive diagnosis is made by noting the presence of rhomboid or rod-like crystals in synovial fluid or articular tissue.
  - Under polarized light microscopy, the crystals show positive birefringence.

▶ TREATMENT

- Gout:
  - Reduction of uric acid levels is key in avoiding flares. Patients should limit:
    - alcoholic beverages (especially beer), meat (especially red meat, wild game meat, and organ meat), seafood (especially shellfish and some large saltwater fish), fruit juice, beverages sweetened with high fructose corn syrup, and dairy products.
  - Patients should be instructed to consume more liquids (water).
  - Acute attacks may be treated with NSAIDs, corticosteroids, or colchicine, for best resolution of symptoms; therapy should start within 24 hours of symptom onset.
    - Colchicine does not affect serum urate levels and is usually not as effective if given 72–96 hours into a flare.
    - Colchicine can be used as low-dose prophylaxis (0.6 mg once or twice daily), for up to 6 months, in patients with normal renal and hepatic function during the initiation of antihyperuricemic therapy.
    - Indocin has been the historical NSAID of choice but any NSAID can be used.
    - Rebound flares are common after discontinuation of corticosteroid therapy; after resolution of symptoms, continue steroids in tapering dose over 10–14 days.
    - Allopurinol (urate lowering therapy) can be started during an acute flare IF used with NSAID and colchicine.

*Monosodium urate crystals: negative birefringence under polarized light microscopy

- Serum urate-lowering therapy is recommended for the following patients:
  - Patients with at least two flares per year (one flare per year in patients with chronic kidney disease stage 2 or greater)
  - Patients with tophi
  - Patients with a history of nephrolithiasis
  - Patients with serum uric acid level >9.0 mg/dL.
  - Target serum uric acid levels during therapy: 5–6 mg/dL
  - Allopurinol especially useful in patients who are "stone formers" or who have renal disease; typical starting dose is 100 mg/day.
  - Febuxostat is another option.
  - Probenecid (second-line agent) works by increasing urinary excretion of uric acid; the most common adverse effect is the development of nephrolithiasis.
  - Pegloticase: IV uricase that metabolizes uric acid to allantoin; third-line agent for refractory gout
- Patient education:
  - Avoid diuretics.
- The angiotensin receptor blocker losartan increases the urinary excretion of uric acid.
- Encourage consumption of vegetables and low-fat/nonfat dairy products.
- Limit intake of purine-rich foods, alcoholic beverages (especially beer), and beverages sweetened with high fructose corn syrup.
- Limit coffee consumption to <6 cups per day.
- Control body weight.
- Increase liquid intake to 2 L of water per day (if other comorbidities allow).
- CPPD disease:
  - Joint aspiration, NSAIDs, and intra-articular steroid injections can reduce symptoms to <10 days.
  - In patients with severe polyarticular attacks, a short course of corticosteroids is recommended.
  - For recurrent attacks, patients can be placed on low-dose daily colchicine.
  - Once they develop, there is no effective way of removing CPPD deposits from cartilage and synovium.
  - Anakinra, an interleukin-1 receptor antagonist for daily injection, has been shown effective in otherwise unresponsive cases.

CHAPTER 229

Ankylosing Spondylitis

Chelsey Hoffmann, RD, PA-C

A 32-year old-female presents as an outpatient with a 6-month history of low back pain. The pain started without preceding injury or event. No red flag symptoms are present (loss of bowel or bladder function, saddle anesthesia, weakness, etc). The pain is improved with exercise and NSAIDs. The pain is worse at night. She has a family history of HLAB27 (+). What would be your first choice for diagnostic workup?

nonradiographic ankylosing spondylitis (nr-axSpA). Those with AS will exhibit radiographic abnormalities consistent with sacroiliitis, whereas those with nr-axSpA will have absent or minimal findings on plain radiography. In patients with nr-axSpA, the diagnosis may be supported by sacroiliac (SI) joint inflammation as visualized on MRI or other clinical findings.

▶ GENERAL FEATURES

- Ankylosing spondylitis (AS) is a chronic inflammatory arthropathy affecting the spine and typically presents as chronic back pain in patients aged <45 years.
- Patients with the *HLA-B27* gene are at significantly increased risk of developing AS, though most people who have HLA-B27 do **not** have ankylosing spondylitis.
- Axial spondyloarthritis is subcategorized into (1) AS (also referred to as radiographic axSpA) or (2)

▶ CLINICAL ASSESSMENT

- Almost all patients with AS will report back pain and typically exhibit at least four of the following: age <40 years, insidious onset, improvement with exercise, no improvement with rest, and nocturnal pain.
- The progressive spinal fusion (ie, radiographic "bamboo spine") seen in AS may lead to impairment of spinal mobility and chest expansion. Bamboo spine is typically a late finding of AS and is associated with postural abnormalities such as hyperkyphosis.

- Patients may report alternating or unilateral buttock pain, which may indicate SI joint involvement.
- Hip pain is also frequently reported and is associated with higher degrees of disability and worse prognosis.
- Peripheral arthritis is frequently seen in patients with AS and may include the following joints: ankles, hips, knees, shoulders, and sternoclavicular joint.
- Enthesitis (inflammation of the enthesis, which is the region near the attachment of tendons and ligaments to bones) is a classic feature of AS. Enthesitis may manifest as pain, stiffness, or tenderness with or without edema of the affected area.
- Dactylitis (sausage digits) is characterized by diffuse swelling of toes or fingers.
- Extra-articular manifestations may include: anterior uveitis, inflammatory bowel disease, pulmonary disease, cardiovascular disease, and psoriasis.

▶ DIAGNOSIS

- Laboratory findings are nonspecific, and normal laboratory findings do not rule out nr-axSpA. However, an elevated acute-phase response may be present, including elevated CRP and ESR.
- Plain films of the pelvis (including SI oblique views) and lumbar spine (anteroposterior and lateral views) are beneficial. The radiographic changes of the SI joint are typically graded, as described by the modified New York criteria:
  - Grade 0: Normal
  - Grade 1: Suspicious (but not definite) changes
  - Grade 2: Minimal abnormality—small localized areas of erosion or sclerosis without alteration in the joint width
  - Grade 3: Unequivocal abnormality—moderate or advanced sacroiliitis with one or more of the following: erosions, sclerosis, joint-space widening, narrowing, or partial ankyloses
  - Grade 4: Total ankylosis of joint
- If the suspicion for AS remains high despite negative plain films of the pelvis, consider ordering a pelvic MRI to evaluate for bone marrow edema.

▶ TREATMENT

- Treatment goals include optimization of short- and long-term health-related quality of life through the relief of symptoms, maintenance of function, prevention of complications of spinal disease, and minimization of extraspinal and extra-articular manifestations and comorbidities.
- First-line treatment consists of patient education on the nature of their disease, NSAIDs, PT, OT, and smoking cessation. Smoking is believed to have an adverse effect on AS. Patients should also be screened for depression and should receive psychosocial support.
- Second-line treatment consists of referral to a rheumatologist or other specialist for consideration of corticosteroid injections into affected joints, nonbiologic or biologic medications, or joint replacement for severe pain or damage.
- Referral may be necessary to other specialty areas, such as dermatology, gastroenterology, or ophthalmology, depending upon the presence or absence of other clinical features.
- Prognosis:
  - AS is a chronic disease, which can range from mild to severe in terms of quality-of-life impact. Those with mild disease restricted to a small area of involvement may be able to maintain functional and employment capacity, whereas those with more severe disease may have significant spinal pain and disability.
  - It is felt the availability of biologic medications has improved the prognosis for AS patients as studies have shown reduction in radiographic progression of disease in those patients using biologics.

Case Conclusion

Plain radiographs of the SI joints are sufficient when suspicion is high for diagnosis of AS. If suspicion of this diagnosis remains high given history and physical examination findings, but the plain radiographs are negative, consideration could be given to ordering advanced imaging in the form of MRI of the pelvis, which may show bony edema.

Fibromyalgia

Antoinette Polito, MHS, PA-C

A 42-year-old woman presents to the clinic as a new patient. She has a history of "feeling like my whole body is aching" for the past 3 years. She also describes long-standing difficulty sleeping and near-daily headaches. She adds that she feels "more and more sad and frustrated" about her condition. She has had numerous physical examinations with multiple providers and a lot of blood tests that per her report "show nothing." Your initial physical examination today confirms no objective signs. What pharmacologic treatments are efficacious in patients like this one?

▶ GENERAL FEATURES

- Fibromyalgia (FM) is a syndrome of widespread musculoskeletal pain with multiple points that are tender on palpation.
- The etiology is unknown etiology as is the pathophysiologic mechanism.
- Patients generally appear well and present without objective findings.
- FM was initially presumed to be psychosomatic in nature; now, it is considered a disorder of pain regulation.
- FM shares many features with chronic fatigue syndrome.
- Most common in adults, particularly women, ages 20–55.
- Prevalence is estimated to be 0.2% to 5% in the general population and much higher in some population groups, including patients on hemodialysis and those with autoimmune disorders. Prevalence among women is 8- to 9-fold that of men and prevalence in all groups increases with age.
- The course itself is nonprogressive.

▶ CLINICAL ASSESSMENT

- Typically, patients present with chronic aching pain and stiffness; this usually involves the whole body, but is worst in the neck, shoulders, low back, and hips.
- Fatigue, sleep disorder, headache, morning stiffness, paresthesias, irritable bowel symptoms, and mood and/or cognitive problems (including psychosis) are common.
- Even minor exertion aggravates pain and increases fatigue.
- Objective signs of inflammation are absent, and laboratory studies are normal.
- Physical examination is most often unremarkable, except for "trigger points" of pain produced by palpation of areas such as the trapezius, the medial fat pad of the knee, and the lateral epicondyle of the elbow.

▶ DIAGNOSIS

- FM is a diagnosis of exclusion.
- Differential diagnosis includes rheumatoid arthritis, SLE, hypothyroidism, polymyositis, and polymyalgia rheumatica.
- The diagnosis of FM should be carefully considered in a patient over age 50 and never explains fever, weight loss, or any other objective signs.
- The American College of Rheumatology defines diagnostic criteria for FM as generalized pain for at least 3 months with 11/18 tender points during physical examination.

▶ TREATMENT

- A multidisciplinary approach is most effective.
- Patient education is essential; patients are often reassured to have a diagnosis.
- Cognitive-behavioral therapy with an emphasis on mindfulness training is often helpful.
- Monotherapy can be trialed with medications that have shown modest efficacy: amitriptyline, fluoxetine, duloxetine, milnacipran, chlorpromazine, cyclobenzaprine, pregabalin, or gabapentin. However, <50% of the patients experience a sustained improvement on medications.
- NSAIDs, opioids, and corticosteroids are ineffective.
- Exercise programs are also beneficial.
- Patients whose disease does not respond to initial therapy should be referred for specialty consultation, which may include a rheumatologist, physiatrist, psychiatrist, psychologist, sleep specialist, or pain management specialist.

Case Conclusion

Most patients with FM are relatively young and have had chronic pain without diagnosis for a lengthy period of time. Reassurance, education, referral for behavioral interventions, and a trial of medication will go a long way to effectively treating this disorder. Monotherapy with amitriptyline specifically has been shown to be moderately effective in patients with FM.

Rheumatoid Arthritis

Jennifer Harrington, PA-C, MHS

▶ GENERAL FEATURES

- Rheumatoid arthritis (RA) is a chronic, systemic, inflammatory, peripheral arthritis.
- 1% of the US population suffers from RA.
- RA is 3 times more common in females than in males, most commonly diagnosed between the ages of 40 years and common in patients who suffer from other autoimmune diseases.

▶ CLINICAL ASSESSMENT

- Symmetric peripheral joints are most commonly affected.
- Morning stiffness usually lasts >1 hour.
- The joints may feel better with movement and worse with rest, this is called "gelling."
- Patients often present with constitutional symptoms, including fever, fatigue, or malaise.
- Physical examination of the affected joints may reveal erythema, swelling, and warmth.
- Joint deformities are common in patients with late disease and include ulnar deviation, boutonniere deformity, swan neck deformity, hammer toe, and rheumatoid nodules.

▶ DIAGNOSIS

- Laboratory tests should be ordered if patient has the following findings:
  - >2 swollen joints
  - Tender joints in hands/feet
  - Symptoms >6 weeks
  - Symmetrical pattern of joint involvement
  - Absence of alternative dx
- The following studies should be ordered:
  - Anti-CCP antibodies (anti-cyclic citrullinated peptide): this is both sensitive and specific for RA and is considered the best diagnostic test.
  - Rheumatoid factor: this is often negative initially and is not specific for RA, but is included in European Alliance for Associations of Rheumatology (EULAR) diagnostic criteria and is useful for monitoring patient progress.

- ESR and CRP: these tests are not specific for RA, but they indicate systemic inflammation and are also included in EULAR diagnostic criteria.
- CBC: concomitant anemia is common in RA patients, and thus, CBC should be evaluated; however, it is not part of the EULAR diagnostic criteria.
- A DEXA scan should be ordered once RA is confirmed due to the frequency of early osteoporosis in these patients.
- A score of 6 points or greater in the American College of Rheumatology (ACR)/EULAR criteria is diagnostic of RA:
  - 2–10 large joints involved: 1 point
  - 1–3 small joints involved: 2 points
  - 4–10 small joints involved: 3 points
  - >10 joints involved (including at least 1 small joint): 5 points
  - RF or anti-CCP low positive: 2 points
  - RF or anti-CCP high positive: 3 points
  - Elevated ESR or CRP: 1 point
  - Symptoms that have lasted >6 weeks: 1 point

▶ TREATMENT

- Early treatment with disease-modifying antirheumatic drugs (DMARDs) is mainstay of RA treatment.
- First-line treatment for RA is the DMARD methotrexate, followed by Janus kinase inhibitors and lastly biologic agents such as TNF-α inhibitors.
- Combination therapy with both a DMARD and biologic agent may be necessary in severe RA refractory to monotherapy.
- NSAIDs and corticosteroids can be used as adjunct therapy for symptomatic relief; however, they do not prevent further joint damage.
- Studies have shown that patients may benefit from an anti-inflammatory diet.
- Patients benefit from regular exercise unless they are currently having a flare up of symptoms; at these times, rest should be recommended.

Polymyalgia Rheumatica

Sarah Garvick, MS, MPAS, PA-C

A 72-year-old woman comes to the clinic with stiffness in her shoulders, hips, and neck that occurs for at least 2 hours after she wakes up in the morning. She reports these symptoms started abruptly 2 weeks ago. She denies new activities or medications. Lab results show estimated sedimentation rate (ESR) to be 62 mm/hr and C-reactive protein (CRP) to be 20 mg/L. Which diagnostic studies are indicated for this patient?

▶ GENERAL FEATURES

- Polymyalgia rheumatica (PMR) an inflammatory condition that is best defined by stiffness and pain, specifically in the neck, shoulders, and hips.
- Generally occurs in adults older than age 50, peak occurrence between the ages of 70 and 80 years. Women are affected more than men.
- Exact cause is unknown; giant cell arteritis (GCA) is frequently associated with PMR.
- Differential diagnoses for PMR include: rheumatoid arthritis, osteoarthritis, fibromyalgia, multiple myeloma, and polymyositis.

▶ CLINICAL ASSESSMENT

- Hallmark symptom is morning stiffness and/or pain in the shoulders, neck, and hips.
- Stiffness lasts >30 minutes after awakening and usually involves at least two of the three listed areas.
- Classic finding is the inability to actively abduct the shoulders past 90°.
- Clinical synovitis can occur at the knees, wrists, and metacarpophalangeal joints, but is usually mild. Typically, the feet and ankles will be spared.
- Other, nonspecific, systemic symptoms can include malaise, fatigue, depression, anorexia, weight loss, and low-grade fever.

- The onset of symptoms is often abrupt, but without inciting incident.
- In all patients, GCA must be ruled out at the time of diagnosis. Symptoms of GCA include scalp and temporal artery tenderness as well as jaw claudication.

▶ DIAGNOSIS

- ESR is often markedly elevated at >50 mm/hr (normal: <20 mm/hr).
- The CRP will always be elevated to some degree. A normal CRP (<5 mg/L) can exclude the diagnosis of PMR.
- A complete blood count (CBC) may show a normocytic anemia; however, this is not diagnostic.
- Imaging (ultrasound or magnetic resonance imaging [MRI]) of the affected joints is not necessary for diagnosis, but may confirm synovitis.

▶ TREATMENT

- The mainstay of treatment is low-dose oral glucocorticoids.
- Oral prednisone at a dose of 10–20 mg/day usually controls symptoms quickly.
- The patient should be reassessed every 2–4 weeks.
- A steroid taper can occur once symptoms resolve fully, which, for most patients, is within 1 month.
- If symptoms reoccur, glucocorticoid therapy should be reinstated, possibly at a higher dose.
- Patients should be educated that treatment may continue for up to 2 years.

Case Conclusion

The best diagnostic study for this patient are serum acute-phase reactants, which include CRP and ESR.

A 28-year-old Hispanic woman who is 12 weeks' pregnant came to the clinic today complaining of a macular rash on both of her cheeks, an oral ulcer, and early morning stiffness affecting her knees. She wonders if this is related to her pregnancy. What is the most likely trigger for the disease flare-up?

GENERAL FEATURES

- Systemic lupus erythematosus (SLE) is an autoimmune disorder that affects multiple organs, including the brain, kidneys, and skin.
- Has been associated with certain genetic components, hormonal abnormalities, and exposure to various medications
- Predominantly affects adults aged 20–40 years, with <15% of cases occurring in children
- Older adults diagnosed with SLE, such as postmenopausal women, usually have a milder form.
- Females, African Americans, and Hispanics are more likely to develop SLE, in contrast to Caucasians who have a higher incidence and severity of drug-induced lupus erythematosus (DILE).
- A flare-up of the disease may be triggered by stress, excessive work, sunlight, pregnancy, infection, trauma, surgery, or abrupt discontinuation of medications.

CLINICAL ASSESSMENT

- Clinical presentation includes nonspecific symptoms, such as fever, weight loss, extreme fatigue, and lymphadenopathy.
- Common skin manifestations include a butterfly rash, with sun-induced macules or papules on the face, or a generalized body rash.
- 90% of patients have joint inflammation or early morning stiffness, affecting the knees, wrists, and hands. Typically, this inflammation does not cause permanent damage.
- Other common clinical manifestations are mucosal ulceration (usually oral), reversible alopecia, pleurisy or pericarditis, accelerated atherosclerosis, and high risk for acute myocardial infarction.
- Renal complications such as glomerulonephritis and microvascular thrombosis as well as neuropsychiatric complications such as seizures, psychosis, neuropathies, stroke, and depression are also common.

- Gastrointestinal and ophthalmic manifestations are less common but can be severe and include pancreatitis, hepatitis, and keratoconjunctivitis sicca.
- Thrombocytopenia and hemolytic anemia are frequent early features in pediatric SLE.
- Symptoms in DILE are usually milder, with arthralgia often being the only symptom.

DIAGNOSIS

- Diagnosis is based on classification criteria established by the American College of Rheumatology (ACR).
- Diagnosis of SLE requires that at least 4 of the 11 ACR criteria are met.
- The 11 ACR criteria are broken into the following systems: cutaneous, musculoskeletal, cardiopulmonary, renal, neurologic, and laboratory.
- ACR criteria for the diagnosis of SLE:
  - Antinuclear antibodies
  - Arthritis
  - Discoid rash
  - Hematologic disorder
  - Immunologic disorder
  - Malar rash
  - Neurologic disorder
  - Oral ulcers
  - Photosensitivity
  - Renal disorder
  - Serositis
- In 95% of SLE patients or more, the antinuclear antibodies (ANAs) test is positive.
- The anti-dsDNA antibody test is considered the best marker for disease activity.
- In 95% of DILE patients, the antihistone antibodies test is positive.
- Patients who develop renal complications should undergo a renal biopsy in order to classify the severity and determine treatment.

TREATMENT

- All patients with SLE should practice proper sun protection and have adequate intake of calcium and vitamin D.
- Pharmacologic treatment for SLE patients is highly individualized and depends on disease severity, organ involvement, and symptoms.
- Antimalarial and NSAIDs are useful in the treatment of mild symptoms.

- Oral corticosteroids and cytotoxic agents are used in more severe cases.
- Lupus nephritis is treated with a combination of cyclophosphamide and corticosteroids.
- Better and earlier identification of SLE and more effective treatments have significantly improved survival rates.

Case Conclusion

In this patient, pregnancy is the likely trigger for her flare-up, which can also be triggered by stress, excessive work, sunlight, infection, trauma, surgery, or abrupt discontinuation of medications.

CHAPTER 234

Polymyositis

James A. Gerding, MS, PA-C

A 51-year-old female with right knee osteoarthritis presents to your outpatient clinic with weakness over the past 8 months. She complains of weakness during her initial evaluation after recently moving to the area. She has not had blood work performed or seen a PCP in 10 years and without her regular health maintenance for her age group. She describes bilateral arm weakness with folding laundry or putting away dishes that she used to be able to perform without problem, and difficulty climbing stairs. She also notes a red area on the front of her upper chest as if she was sunburned but does not recall prolonged or intense sun exposure. What is important to evaluate before or concomitantly with the workup of polymyositis (PM) as part of the differential diagnosis?

▶ GENERAL FEATURES

- PM and dermatomyositis (DM) encompass the group idiopathic inflammatory myopathies (IIMs).
- PM is a condition of both proximal symmetric muscle weakness and inflammation of muscles, with a female-to-male predominance of about 2:1. At times, characteristic dermatologic findings are apparent, which includes DM in the diagnosis.
- Associated with genetic, environmental, and geographic predisposition as evidence by immune response activation after specific environmental exposures in genetically susceptible people

▶ CLINICAL ASSESSMENT

- Usually presents with chronic bilateral symmetric proximal muscle weakness. Not caused by fatigue or other causes of immobility like joint disease, shortness of breath, or back pain

- Other signs/symptoms of the disease include: dysphagia, hot/cold intolerance, skin eruptions, photosensitivity, and morning stiffness.
- Common skin findings include: *Heliotrope* rash or erythematous/purple eruption on bilateral upper eyelids with or without edema, Gottron papules or erythematous or purple papule (at times scaled) on dorsal metacarpophalangeal and interphalangeal joints of hand bilaterally, Gottron sign or erythematous or purple patches or macules on extensor surfaces of skin, and Shawl/V sign or hyperpigmented/hypopigmented area of a sun-exposed site, including the upper back (Shawl) or upper anterior chest (V).
- Differential diagnosis includes thyroid disease, drug-induced myopathy, malignancy, muscular dystrophy, or other rheumatologic diseases such as lupus, Sjögren, rheumatoid, or scleroderma.

▶ DIAGNOSIS

- Lab abnormalities include elevation of the following:
  - Creatine kinase (CK), myoglobin, and inflammatory markers such as lactate dehydrogenase (LDH), erythrocyte sedimentation rate (ESR), and C-reactive protein (CRP)
- Workup should include: complete blood count, metabolic panel, liver function tests, and thyroid-stimulating hormone (TSH). Other rheumatologic conditions should be tested for ANA, anti-Ro/SSA, anti-La/SSB, anti-Smith, anti–double-stranded DNA, rheumatoid factor, and serum complement levels.
- Chest x-ray may be useful if there are pulmonary complaints or findings on examination. Usually normal in PM.
- If dermatologic findings present, a skin biopsy by a dermatologist may be useful.

- EMG is very important in determining neuropathic vs. myopathic causes of weakness, findings may show muscle irritability with a myopathic pattern. Muscle biopsy may be performed during EMG.
- Muscle biopsy would confirm diagnosis if it shows necrosis, degeneration, and inflammation.

▶ **TREATMENT**

- Treatment goals are the improvement of muscle strength, the preservation of muscle function, and the avoidance of extramuscular complications or drug complications.
- If DM present, treatment of skin eruptions is also a goal.
- Glucocorticoid therapy is the mainstay of initial therapy. Prednisone at 1 mg/kg/day (max 80 mg) is the most common dosing with tapering over 1 year thereafter pending symptom control. Repeat muscle strength testing should be target of therapy and should direct steroid tapering. Other options include immunomodulators such as azathioprine or methotrexate.
- Hydroxychloroquine can be effective in controlling skin manifestations.

- Adjuncts to pharmacotherapy should include exercise or physical therapy regimes depending on the patient's functional status.
- Future therapy options may target specific autoantibodies such as HLA subgroups or anti-Jo antibodies (the most common auto-antibody) to help direct treatment regimes.
- Referral to PM specialist like a rheumatologist would be reasonable for further testing such as EMG, muscle biopsy, and initiation of therapy after initial workup, including physical examination and lab testing.

Case Conclusion

As part of the workup of PM in this patient who has previous knee arthritis, which could be the etiology of her ambulatory weakness/dysfunction, do thyroid function testing, screening mammography and colonoscopy, knee physical examination and x-ray, and dermatologic examination to evaluate for other rashes.

CHAPTER
235

Reactive Arthritis

Nata Parnes, MD

A 28-year-old man came to the clinic today complaining that for the last week, he has pain in the right knee, swelling and redness, burning pain during urination, and pain and irritation in the left eye. He wonders if this is related to *Shigella* gastrointestinal infection, which he had 3 weeks ago. What will synovial fluid cultures obtained by arthrocentesis from the right knee of this patient probably reveal?

▶ **GENERAL FEATURES**

- Reactive arthritis formerly known as Reiter syndrome is a form of inflammatory arthritis.
- Reactive arthritis develops in response to infection in other parts of the body (cross-reactivity).
- The most common triggers are intestinal infections (*Shigella, Salmonella, Ureaplasma, Yersinia,* or *Campylobacter*) and sexually transmitted infections

(*Chlamydia trachomatis*). It can, however, also appear following group A streptococcal infections.
- By the time the patient presents with symptoms (4-35 days from onset), often the "trigger" infection has been cured or is in remission.
- Reactive arthritis is an RF-seronegative, HLA-B27–linked arthritis.
- Reactive arthritis predominantly affects males 20–40 years old and is more common in Caucasians.
- Patients with HIV are at higher risk of developing reactive arthritis.

▶ **CLINICAL ASSESSMENT**

- Symptoms generally appear 4–35 days (typically 1-3 weeks) from the onset of the episode of the inciting disease (a known infection).
- The clinical mnemonic is "Can't see, can't pee, can't climb a tree," expressing the fact that commonly the eyes, the urine system, and the arms and legs are affected.

- The classic triad consists of conjunctivitis, nongonococcal urethritis, and asymmetric oligoarthritis.
- The classic presentation of the syndrome starts with urinary symptoms such as dysuria (pain during urination) and frequency, which may be accompanied by prostatitis in men or cervicitis, salpingitis, and vulvovaginitis in women.
- Common musculoskeletal manifestations are large joints monoarthritis, asymmetrical inflammatory arthritis of interphalangeal joints, enthesitis (heel pain), Achilles tendinitis, plantar fasciitis, or dactylitis (diffuse swelling of a solitary finger or toe also known as "sausage digit").
- Ocular involvement includes eye redness, pain and irritation, or blurred vision due to conjunctivitis or uveitis.
- Possible mucocutaneous lesions include small hard nodules on the soles of the feet or the palms of the hands called keratoderma blennorrhagicum, recurrent aphthous stomatitis, geographic tongue, and migratory stomatitis.
- 10% of patients, especially those with a prolonged course of the disease, develop cardiac manifestations, including aortic regurgitation and pericarditis.
- Some patients have severe gastrointestinal problems similar to those of Crohn disease.

▶ DIAGNOSIS

- There are no definitive criteria to diagnose the existence of reactive arthritis.
- The American College of Rheumatology (ACR) has published sensitivity and specificity guidelines for typical reactive arthritis, which are based on the presentation of the classic triad: arthritis of >1 month, urethritis/cervicitis, and conjunctivitis.
- In the absence of the classic triad, the presence of keratoderma blennorrhagica is diagnostic of reactive arthritis.
- Synovial fluid cultures obtained by arthrocentesis tend to be negative, suggesting that reactive arthritis is caused by an autoimmune cross-reactivity response to bacterial antigens.
- The urethra, cervix, and throat may be swabbed in an attempt to obtain cultures of the causative organisms. Cultures should also be done on urine and stool samples.
- In 75% of reactive arthritis patients, the genetic marker HLA-B27 is positive.
- C-reactive protein and erythrocyte sedimentation rate are nonspecific tests that can be done to corroborate the diagnosis of the syndrome.

▶ TREATMENT

- The main goal of treatment is to identify and eradicate the underlying infectious source, if still present, with the appropriate antibiotics.
- Nonspecific urethritis may be treated with a short course of tetracycline or NSAIDs.
- Local corticosteroids are useful in the case of iritis.
- In severe cases of reactive arthritis, oral corticosteroids sulfasalazine and immunosuppressants are used.
- Reactive arthritis may be self-limiting, frequently recurring, chronic, or progressive.
- Most patients have severe symptoms lasting from a few weeks to 6 months.
- Repeated outbreaks over many years are common, often eventually resulting in disabling arthritis, heart disease, amyloid deposits, ankylosing spondylitis, immunoglobulin A nephropathy, or aortitis.
- Most patients with reactive arthritis can expect to reach a normal life span and maintain a near-normal lifestyle.

Case Conclusion

This patient has the classic symptoms of reactive arthritis. Synovial fluid cultures obtained by arthrocentesis from the right knee of this patient will probably be negative, suggesting that reactive arthritis is caused by an autoimmune cross-reactivity response to bacterial antigens.

CHAPTER
236

Sjögren Syndrome

Kim Zuber, PA-C, MS
Jane Davis, DNP

▶ GENERAL FEATURES

- Sjögren affects up to 3% of the population.
- Sjögren is often diagnosed as a second autoimmune disorder in a patient with a previous diagnosis of an autoimmune disease, most commonly with rheumatoid arthritis (20%-50%) or lupus (10%-25%).
- Sjögren shows a preference for female gender, 9 of 10 patients are female; a first-degree relative with Sjögren is a risk factor.

- Average age for presentation is 40–60; many females are perimenopausal.
- Sjögren can cause small vessel changes, which lead to skin changes.
- Most common symptoms are dry mouth and/or dry eyes.
- Patients often go multiple years and to multiple medical practitioners before diagnosis is made.

▶ DIAGNOSIS

- Symptoms:
  - Ocular symptoms (at least one): symptoms of dry eyes × 3 m, foreign-body sensation in eye, use of artificial tears >3 times per day
  - Oral symptoms (at least one): symptoms of dry mouth × 3 m, recurrent or persistent swollen salivary glands, need for liquid to swallow dry foods
- Signs:
  - Ocular signs (at least one): abnormal Schirmer test (dry eye test) or positive dye staining of eye surface
  - Histopathology: lip biopsy showing focal lymphocytic sialoadenitis

- Oral signs (at least one): decreased salivary flow, abnormal parotid radiology, abnormal salivary radiology
- Autoantibodies (at least one): anti-SSA (Ro) or anti-SSB (La) or both
- Diagnosis of primary Sjögren requires four of six criteria and must include positive histopathology or autoantibodies.
- Diagnosis of secondary Sjögren requires well-defined connective tissue disease plus one symptom and two objective criteria.

▶ TREATMENT

- There is no cure.
- Treatment is often directed to managing symptoms: eye drops, sugar-free gum, or candies.
- Many patients report decreasing gluten in the diet leads to fewer symptoms, especially joint pain.
- NSAIDs are used for joint pain.
- Dental care with follow-up is vital as decreased saliva leads to caries and loss of teeth.
- Patients should stop the use of antihistamines as these are drying.

SECTION D — Lower Extremity Disorders

CHAPTER 237

Developmental Dysplasia of the Hip

Maureen Heneghan, PA-C, MSHS, MS

A 1-day-old female, born at 39 weeks' gestation by cesarean section for breech presentation, is in the nursery after delivery without complications. On examination of the hips, a "clunk" is palpated on the left hip when the hip is abducted and gentle anterior pressure is placed over the greater trochanter of the proximal femur (Ortolani maneuver). There are no other physical abnormalities.

▶ GENERAL FEATURES

- Abnormal development of hip joint around time of birth or during childhood, including:
  - Dislocated hip: femoral head is out of the acetabulum.

- Dislocatable hip: femoral head pops in and out of the acetabulum.
- Subluxatable hip: femoral head is within the acetabulum, but loose.
- Dysplastic hip: femoral head or acetabulum or both are abnormal.
- Incidence: 1–2 in 1000
- Pathogenesis: multifactorial
- Risk factors: female, breech at ≥34 weeks' gestation, family history (parents or siblings), oligohydramnios, tight swaddling
- Associated with conditions related to decreased fetal movement: torticollis, plagiocephaly, musculoskeletal

anomalies (eg, metatarsus adductus, clubfoot, congenital knee dislocation), firstborn, birth weight >4 kg, multiple gestation pregnancy
- Developmental dysplasia of the hip (DDH) is a treatable disease presenting early in life, but, if neglected, can lead to complications:
  - Untreated or persistence into adolescence or adulthood can result in abnormal gait, functional disability, pain, and early osteoarthritis.
  - Some studies estimate 50% of adults aged <50 years who require hip replacement due to osteoarthritis were found to have underlying hip dysplasia as the etiology.
  - Prognosis depends on severity, age of diagnosis and treatment, and if a concentrically reduced hip joint was obtained.
- This review is limited to typical DDH subtype; hip dysplasia and instability can be associated with teratogenic or neuromuscular subtypes (eg, Ehlers-Danlos syndrome, Down syndrome, arthrogryposis, spina bifida, cerebral palsy).

▶ CLINICAL ASSESSMENT

- Symptoms vary with age and severity:
  - Assess risk factors; typically, DDH is asymptomatic in newborns/infants.
  - Can be present in both hips; more frequently affects left
- Physical examination is the most important component of screening for DDH.
  - Infants <3 months:
    - Asymmetric leg creases, femur length discrepancy
    - Ortolani maneuver: with patient supine and knees flexed, gentle abduction of the hips with anterior pressure over the greater trochanter to feel if there is a palpable clunk as the head of the femur reduces back into the acetabulum. The test will be positive in identifying a dislocated hip that is reducible.
    - Barlow maneuver: with patient supine and knees flexed, gentle adduction of the hips with posterior-directed pressure at the knees to feel if the head of the femur dislocates posteriorly from the acetabulum. Positive test will identify unstable hip that can be passively dislocated. The safety of this maneuver has been questioned. The maneuver should be performed gently; if done frequently or forcefully, it could potentially create instability.
    - Galeazzi/Allis sign: with patient supine and knees flexed, test is positive for unilateral DDH in the leg with the lower knee. The test will not be useful in bilateral DDH.
  - Age 3–12 months:
    - Asymmetric leg creases, femur length discrepancy, limited hip abduction in 90° flexion

- Klisic test: if imaginary line between anterosuperior iliac spine and ipsilateral greater trochanter passes below umbilicus, test is positive.
- Walking age child:
  - Excessive lordosis, prominent greater trochanter, limp
  - Trendelenburg sign/gait/lurch: during ambulation, pelvis drops on side of unsupported leg due to weak muscles on supported leg.

▶ DIAGNOSIS

- Current guidelines on screening techniques to diagnose DDH among expert groups are not uniform as there remains little evidence-based literature to support practices.
  - Most groups (American Academy of Pediatrics, American Academy of Orthopaedic Surgeons, Pediatric Orthopaedic Society of North America, and Canadian DDH Task Force) recommend all newborns be screened for DDH by physical examination at birth and subsequent well visits until 9 months and/or until child is walking.
- The American Academy of Pediatrics, with guidance from the American Academy of Orthopaedic Surgeons, recommends the following DDH surveillance practices:
  - Encourage hip healthy swaddling allowing freedom of hip motion and avoiding forced hip extension and adduction.
  - Consider imaging study in infant with normal physical examination but risk factors of third-trimester breech, family history of DDH, history of improper swaddling, history of abnormal hip examination.
- Ultrasonography is the primary imaging technique for newborns and infants aged <4–6 months with questionable or abnormal examination findings, or with identified risk factors.
- Radiography is generally for diagnosing infants aged >4–6 months.

▶ TREATMENT

- Goal is to obtain and maintain concentric reduction of the hip to enable development of the femoral head and acetabulum and reduce risk of early osteoarthritis.
- If newborn examination is inconclusive, infant should be re-examined at next well visit in 2–4 weeks. If examination remains equivocal at 2–4 weeks:
  - Referral to orthopedist
  - Majority (estimated up to 90%) of neonates with mild hip instability on examination resolve spontaneously after birth with normal function without intervention.
- Infants diagnosed <6 months with hip dislocation or persistently dislocatable or subluxatable hips, or infants <6 months who have acetabular dysplasia without dislocation that persists beyond 6 weeks:

- Referral to orthopedist
  - Abduction splint/brace (Pavlik harness) for 1–2 months; initially full time, and once hip position improves, part-time treatment may be recommended.
  - Closed reduction under anesthesia, spica cast
  - If diagnosed <6 months of age, treatment with Pavlik harness is thought to be successful in about 85% of dislocated hips.
- Infants diagnosed >6 months:
  - Referral to orthopedist if hip is dislocated or dislocatable
    - Reduction under anesthesia (closed or open), spica cast

> **Case Conclusion**
>
> The infant was referred to an orthopedist, and an ultrasound of bilateral hips revealed DDH of the left hip with a diminished alpha angle of ~40° (normal >60°) and 20% coverage of the unossified capital femoral epiphysis by the acetabulum. A Pavlik harness was applied to the infant for 24 hours/day, full time, for 2 months. As the hip position was found to improve on subsequent serial ultrasounds every 2 weeks, the infant was transitioned to nighttime wear of the harness for 1 month following discontinuation of the harness. Ultrasound of the left hip out of the harness at 3 months revealed resolution of DDH.

CHAPTER 238

Slipped Capital Femoral Epiphysis

Lorraine Sanassi, PA-C, DHSc

▶ GENERAL FEATURES

- Slipped capital femoral epiphysis (SCFE) is a pediatric and adolescent hip disorder characterized by displacement of the femoral head on the femoral neck, hindering hip function (Figure 238.1).
- Males are twice as likely as females to develop SCFE, and it is often seen between the ages of 10 and 16 years (boys aged 10-16; girls aged 12-14).
- Occurs at a time when the growth plate of the proximal femur is thickening rapidly under the influence of growth hormone in the absence of the high levels of sex hormones that are responsible for closing and stabilizing the growth plate (prepubertal or early puberty stages)
- The direction of slippage of the femoral head off the femoral neck is always posterior, inferior, and often medial and within the confines of the acetabulum.
- Chronicity:
  - Acute SCFE involves sudden displacement of the femoral head, usually after normal activity.
    - Prodromal symptoms (hip or knee pain, limp, decreased range of motion) for <3 weeks
  - Chronic SCFE is the most common form where the femoral head slips slowly over several months:
    - Prodromal symptoms for >3 weeks
    - Acute on chronic is characterized by 3+ weeks of symptoms with acute exacerbation or change.
- 20% of cases are bilateral, but not necessarily simultaneous, and the left hip is more commonly affected than the right.

- The typical patient is overweight or obese reporting hip pain, medial thigh pain, and/or knee pain.

▶ CLINICAL ASSESSMENT

- General points:
  - If a child or adolescent reports knee pain, the hip must always be examined because knee pain may be referred pain from the hip via the obturator nerve.
  - Obesity should increase the index of suspicion for SCFE because it places more shear forces around the proximal growth plate.
  - Determining the patient's ability to bear weight will identify a stable vs. an unstable SCFE.
    - "Stable" SCFEs allow the patient to ambulate with or without crutches.
    - "Unstable" SCFEs do not allow the patient to ambulate at all; these cases carry a higher rate of complication, particularly of avascular necrosis (AVN).
- In patients with chronic SCFE, there is:
  - A painful limp for several months before complete slippage
  - Referred aching pain in the thigh or knee of the affected leg
  - Loss of abduction and internal rotation of the affected hip
  - Compensatory external rotation of the hip when it is flexed (keeps the posteriorly displaced femoral head in acetabulum)

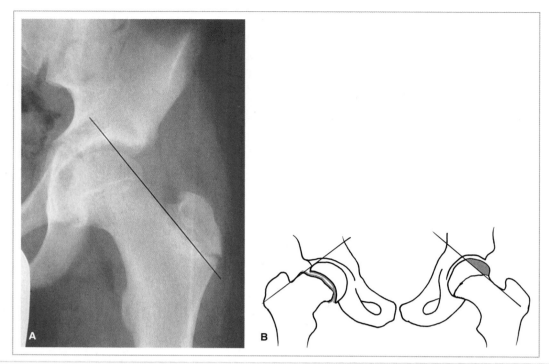

FIGURE 238.1 Slipped capital femoral epiphysis (SCFE): Klein line. A, Normal Klein line, anteroposterior hip. B, Note the abnormal Klein line associated with SCFE, showing no intersection with the femoral epiphysis (left).

- In patients with acute SCFE, there is:
  - A sudden onset of severe hip pain with limping or complete inability to bear weight on affected leg, after little or no trauma
  - Painful, guarded, restricted range of motion of the hip
  - High rate of avascular necrosis in unstable forms

DIAGNOSIS

- Standard anteroposterior (AP) and frog-leg lateral radiographs best identify posterior displacement of femoral head.
  - AP radiograph: the Klein line is drawn straight up the superior aspect of the femoral neck, which should intersect the epiphysis. Lack of intersection suggests an SCFE.
  - Frog-leg radiograph: a straight line through the center of the femoral neck proximally should be at the center of the epiphysis. A line anterior in the epiphysis suggests an SCFE.
- Establishing severity of slippage is important in determining treatment and prognosis. Severity is determined by the percentage femoral head displacement off the femoral neck:
  - Grade I: slippage <33%
  - Grade II: slippage between 33% and 50%
  - Grade III: slippage >50%
- Bone scanning, MRI, and CT scanning are not routinely performed, but may be helpful to confirm the diagnosis of SCFE or more accurately measure the degree of displacement and epiphyseal perfusion.

TREATMENT

- SCFE is usually a progressive disease that requires prompt surgical treatment. Urgency of surgical decisions are based on (1) whether the SCFE is acute, chronic, or acute on chronic; (2) stable vs. unstable; and (3) grade of slippage.
- Because most cases are chronic in nature, it is impossible to manually reduce the femoral head back into its normal anatomic position.
- First-line treatment involves surgical realignment of the femoral head with the femoral neck with insertion of one or two pins across the growth plate (pinning in situ) to prevent further slippage, enhance physeal closure, and reduce morbidity.
- Acute slips may be manually reduced with gentle pressure before fixation; however, caution must be exercised to prevent AVN of the femoral head.
- Prognosis:
  - Following surgery, pain rapidly resolves, and remodeling of the already distorted proximal femur during the remainder of puberty may be favorable enough to improve hip range of motion.
  - With high-grade SCFEs, postsurgical remodeling may not be sufficient with pubertal growth, leaving the patient with a chronic painful limp that requires

repair by proximal femoral osteotomy to reposition the femoral head to improve functional range of motion.

- Evidence suggests that if surgical intervention occurs within 24 hours of SCFE onset, significantly fewer complications occur. If surgical intervention

occurs between 24 and 48 hours, however, the AVN rate dramatically increases.

- Following surgery, the patient is given crutches with protected weight bearing for 6–8 weeks. Physical therapy may be helpful, and most children can then return to full activity once they are pain free with full strength.

CHAPTER
239

Meniscal Injury

Maureen Heneghan, PA-C, MSHS, MS

A 19-year-old male presents to the orthopedic clinic with acute left knee pain. The patient reports twisting his left knee during a basketball game yesterday as he planted his left leg coming down from a block. The patient has associated left knee locking and clicking with squatting. On examination, there is a mild left knee effusion, medial joint line tenderness on palpation, and a positive McMurray test. Laxity was not present, and the rest of the examination was unremarkable.

▶ GENERAL FEATURES

- The menisci are two crescent-shaped fibrocartilage pads (medial and lateral), located within the knee joint between the femoral condyles and tibial plateaus.
- Menisci protect articular cartilage of femur and tibia, acting as shock absorbers, enhancing joint stability and lubrication, and distributing load across the knee joint.
  - Meniscal injury is a significant risk factor for degenerative changes in the tibiofemoral compartment of the knee joint.
- The most common meniscus injury is a meniscal tear.
  - Acute: seen in young patients with history of torsional and axial loading of the knee or sudden acceleration/deceleration coupled with a directional change (cutting maneuver) of the knee; or from a contact injury with varus, valgus, or hyperextension force on the knee during sports
  - Degenerative: seen in older patients as a result of a deterioration process as menisci are less compliant with increasing age; more common in males, obesity increases risk, may be work related
- Less common meniscus injuries:
  - Meniscal cysts: collection of synovial fluid in (parameniscal) or around (perimeniscal) the meniscus, typically associated with meniscal tears

- Discoid meniscus: congenital disorder in which the meniscus (lateral or medial) is thicker than normal and often appears oval rather than crescent in shape and increases risk of meniscal injury
- Meniscal injuries are classified by location, position, and shape:
  - Location:
    - Medial, lateral, or both: most common location of a meniscal tear is medial due to the decreased mobility; the lateral meniscus is more likely to be injured with an acute anterior cruciate ligament (ACL) rupture.
    - Red zone (vascular, outer-third), red-white zone (junction where the vascular meets the avascular region, middle-third), white zone (avascular, inner-third); most meniscal injuries affect the white zone, which will not self-heal due to the avascular location.
  - Position: anterior, middle, posterior-third, root
  - Shape: vertical/longitudinal, bucket handle, oblique/flap/parrot beak, radial, horizontal, complex, root
- Associated conditions:
  - >30% of meniscal injuries are associated with an ACL injury.
  - Meniscal injuries are part of the "unhappy triad": an injury to the ACL, medial collateral ligament, and meniscus

▶ CLINICAL ASSESSMENT

- Symptoms: localized pain to the medial or lateral aspect of the knee, swelling, locking, clicking, catching, pain with ascending or descending stairs, weakness or a sense of buckling or giving away of the knee
- Physical examination: joint line tenderness is the most sensitive physical examination finding, effusion, crepitus, limited range of motion of knee

- Special tests:
  - Accuracy of tests is dependent on skill of the examiner and the severity and location of the injury.
  - Apley compression: with patient prone, knee flexed to 90°, the tibia is internally and externally rotated while placing compression force to the knee joint. The test is positive if the rotation plus compression results in pain or decreased rotation compared to normal knee.
  - Thessaly test: with patient standing on affected leg with the affected knee flexed at 5°, the patient rotates the femur on the tibia internally and externally. This is repeated again with injured knee flexed to 20°. The test is positive if the rotation with flexion results in pain, locking, or catching.
  - McMurray test: with patient supine, the examiner rotates the tibia internally and externally while extending the knee from complete flexion. The test is positive if the rotation plus extension results in pain, locking, or clicking.

▶ DIAGNOSIS

- Diagnosis of meniscal injuries is made by a combination of a comprehensive history, physical examination, and diagnostic imaging.
- Radiographs: plain film to rule out other problems; will not show meniscal injury
- MRI: most sensitive diagnostic imaging test, but has high false-positive rate
  - Information can determine location and severity of injury, as well as guide surgical intervention.

▶ TREATMENT

- Conservative nonoperative treatment vs. surgical management of meniscal injuries is determined by many factors, including characteristics of tear, ability of meniscus to heal, symptoms of patient, and patient lifestyle.

- Nonoperative:
  - First-line treatment for degenerative tears and some acute tears
    - Reduce pain and maintain full motion of knee: rest, ice, compression, elevation, oral nonsteroidal anti-inflammatory pain medications, activity modification
    - Physical therapy, rehabilitation, and muscle strengthening
    - Degenerative meniscal injuries often improve over time with treatment of arthritis.
  - Aspiration and steroid injection for isolated meniscal cysts in young patients
- Operative:
  - For meniscal injuries associated with locking, or if pain persists despite conservative therapy, treatment is to refer to orthopedist for surgical intervention.
    - Preservation of meniscal function is the most important goal of surgery.
    - Left untreated, meniscal injuries can limit activities of daily living, exercise, and sports play and potentially lead to long-term knee problems, such as cartilage wear and arthritis.
  - Knee arthroscopy for meniscal repair vs. partial meniscectomy will depend on tear characteristics.
  - Meniscal transplantation:
    - Consider procedure in young patients with minimal viable meniscal tissue in the knee who are at high risk for developing progression of arthritis.

Case Conclusion

The patient underwent MRI revealing a "double posterior cruciate ligament (PCL) sign," indicating a bucket handle tear of the left medial meniscus. ACL and PCL were intact. Treatment with a month long course of rest, ice, compression, elevation, oral nonsteroidal anti-inflammatory pain medications, activity modification, and physical therapy did not improve the patient's symptoms of pain and locking. Surgical management of left knee arthroscopy, medial meniscal repair, was performed in order to preserve the meniscal biomechanics and protect the knee from further cartilage injury. The patient completed postoperative physical therapy and was able to return to basketball after 16 weeks.

Osgood-Schlatter Disease

Amber Whitmore, PA-C

▶ GENERAL FEATURES

- Osgood-Schlatter disease (OSD) is an overuse injury caused by tension on the patellar tendon where it inserts on the anterior tibial tubercle.
- Chronic tensile stress within the growth plate leads to irritation and inflammation.
- Inflammation results from small injuries to the growth plate with repetitive use before closure of the epiphysis, causing traction injury and microavulsions of the tubercle.
- OSD is most frequently seen in adolescents involved in sports that include activity-related running, jumping, and repetitive bending of the knee.
- OSD occurs most often during puberty when children are likely to go through times of rapid growth; typically in boys ages 13–15 and girls ages 11–13.
- More commonly seen in boys; note that the incidence in girls is growing as their participation in sports increases.
- 20% of children who participate in sports are affected by OSD.
- OSD is self-limited and will resolve with skeletal maturity.

▶ CLINICAL ASSESSMENT

- History:
  - Pain below the kneecap at the bony prominence of the upper shin
  - Aggravated by physical activity, relieved by rest
  - Knee pain worsens with activities such as running and jumping.
  - Participation in the following sports: soccer, football, basketball, ballet, figure skating, or gymnastics
- Physical examination:
  - Local swelling or a prominent bump over the anterior shin, below the kneecap, where the patellar tendon attaches to the tibia
  - Erythema and tenderness to palpation may be noted over the knee.
  - Range of motion, gait, and reflexes should be normal.

▶ DIAGNOSIS

- Patient's age, a comprehensive history, and knee examination are the key to diagnosing OSD.
- Imaging:
  - Radiographs may illustrate OSD but are not confirmatory for the diagnosis.
  - Lateral radiographs can show prominence of the tibial tuberosity with anterior ossicles separating from the proximal tibia.

▶ TREATMENT

- Conservative treatment is recommended for OSD symptoms until the tibial growth plate fuses.
- Patient and family education should include explaining the cause of OSD and reassurance that symptoms will subside with time.
- Lifestyle modifications:
  - Decrease physical activity and limit movements that aggravate the pain.
  - Limit activity based only on symptoms (complete removal from sports has not shown to help).
  - Ice the affected knee for 20 minutes every 2–4 hours and after activity.
  - Wear a knee pad or patellar tendon strap during activity for support.
  - Cross-train with low-impact sports such as cycling or swimming.
- Medication:
  - Over-the-counter medications including acetaminophen and ibuprofen can be used for pain and inflammation.
  - Nonsteroidal anti-inflammatory drugs will help with symptoms but will not shorten the course of OSD.
- Therapy:
  - Physical therapy can help stretch the quadriceps and hamstrings.
  - Strengthening the quadriceps can help stabilize the knee joint.
- Procedures:
  - Casting or bracing to support the knee for 6–8 weeks while it heals may be used in rare cases when symptoms are not alleviated by conservative treatment.
  - Surgical treatment is not recommended and should be avoided around open growth plates.
  - Corticosteroid injections should not be used.
- Complications and prognosis:
  - Bursitis may develop over the aggravated patellar tendon.
  - Symptoms are uncommon after the growth plate closes.
  - Local swelling or chronic pain may persist in rare cases.
- An asymptomatic bony lump (tibial tubercle) may remain on the shin.

Avascular Necrosis

Dawn Colomb-Lippa, PA-C, MHS

▶ GENERAL FEATURES

- Avascular necrosis (AVN) is also known as osteonecrosis; this occurs when there is ischemia and eventually necrosis of a bony region due to comprised vascular supply.
- Necrosis progresses to collapse of the bone which can lead to mechanical failure of the joint.
- The most common regions for AVN are the femoral head, knees, and talus.
- AVN accounts for 5% to 18% of totally hip arthroplasties performed in the United States annually.
  - Cause may be traumatic or atraumatic with major risk factors being: anterior hip dislocation, intramedullary nail placement, fracture of the femoral neck, coagulopathy, and the long-term use of corticosteroids
  - Children with slipped capital femoral epiphysis (SCFE) will be at risk for AVN even after surgical treatment of the disorder.
- AVN of the talus is most frequently associated with talar fracture, which may be occult.
- The incidence of AVN is higher in men than in women and occurs most frequently between the ages of 40 and 65 years.

▶ CLINICAL ASSESSMENT

- History:
  - Patient may have a history of past or present long-term corticosteroid use, prior hip dislocation or fracture, sickle cell disease, or other coagulopathy.
  - Providers should also question the use of alcohol because chronic heavy use may lead to AVN.
  - Hip AVN: patients present with progressively worsening hip pain, which radiates to the groin or buttock region usually without significant trauma history.
  - Talar AVN: patients present with history (generally remote) of ankle trauma, which may include sprain or fracture.
  - Pain in AVN is worse with weight-bearing activities initially but tends to progress eventually to pain at rest.

- Physical examination:
  - Initial examination may be normal.
  - Once the patient is symptomatic, there may be limitation in active range of motion.
    - In hip: loss of internal rotation
    - In ankle: loss or plantar or dorsiflexion
  - Crepitus may be present.
  - Limp may be observed, especially at late stages.

▶ DIAGNOSIS

- The combined use of x-ray, MRI, and physical examination findings can help determine the patient's classification stage.
- Hip: x-rays including anteroposterior (AP) pelvis and frog-leg view of the hip
- Ankle: x-rays including AP and lateral views
  - Findings consistent with AVN include: subchondral fracture (crescent sign), subchondral cysts, flattened femoral head or talar dome, full collapse
- Once signs of AVN are noted on plain films, full collapse will generally occur within 2 years.
- MRI is the most sensitive and specific means of diagnosing AVN of any joint.

▶ TREATMENT

- Precollapse:
  - Medical treatment: judicious use of NSAIDs for discomfort, bisphosphonate use may delay full collapse.
  - Use of ambulatory devices (crutches or walker) to take pressure off the limb during episodes of increased pain may help symptomatically.
  - Surgical procedures: core decompression with the use of bone morphogenic proteins or bone graft
- Postcollapse:
  - Total hip or knee arthroplasty or partial/total ankle arthroplasty are the only definitive treatments of AVN following collapse and mechanical failure of the joint.

Ankle and Foot Fractures

Thomas Gocke, DMSc, ATC, PA-C, DFAAPA

> A 45-year-old female with right foot pain, circumferential swelling, plantar ecchymosis, and difficulty walking tells you that she was out for a trail run, tripped on a tree root, twisted her ankle, and jammed her foot into the ground. She has no allergies and no significant PMHx.

▶ GENERAL FEATURES

- Ankle fracture:
  - Occurs more often in males vs. females
  - Inversion and ankle/foot rotation most common injury mechanism
  - Fracture involving medial and lateral malleolus considered unstable
  - There should always be a concern for interosseous ligament and syndesmosis injuries.
- Metatarsal shaft fractures:
  - Most metatarsal fractures are nondisplaced to minimally displaced and involve the shaft.
  - Injuries result from axial loads, twisting, falls, or repetitive stress.
  - Great toe metatarsal fractures may present an issue with ambulation, weight bearing, and balance.
  - Stress fractures are insidious and cause dorsal foot pain that progresses over >3–4 weeks.
  - Tarsometatarsal injuries result from axial loads, twisting, and falls on plantarflexed foot.
  - 20% tarsometatarsal injuries missed on initial examination.
  - Injury to the tarsometatarsal region is called a Lisfranc injury.
  - No fracture/dislocation = sprain to tarsometatarsal joint
- Lesser toe fractures:
  - Common foot fx, usually closed, and nondisplaced to minimally displaced
  - Injury mechanism; axial load (jammed toe), hyperflexion/hyperextension

▶ CLINICAL ASSESSMENT

- History and physical examination:
  - Ankle fracture:
    - Deformity, swelling, ecchymosis, pain, and inability to bear weight are common.
    - Medial and/or lateral tenderness to palpation corresponding to fracture site over malleoli should alert to fracture.
    - Tenderness to palpation on the proximal fibula should alert to possible interosseous ligament injury (Maisonneuve).
  - Metatarsal fractures:
    - Acute fractures present with focal pain, pain with weight bearing, swelling, and dorsal ecchymosis over site of injury.
    - Stress fx; gradual onset, repetitive activity, weight-bearing pain improves at rest, progressively gets worse over many weeks.
  - Tarsometatarsal joint injury:
    - Fracture presents with pain, swelling, plantar ecchymosis, and inability to weight bear.
    - Point tenderness at metatarsal bases and cuneiforms are usually seen with fractures of these bones.
    - Check pulses, color of extremity, sensory status, and disproportional pain as signs of compartment syndrome.
  - Lesser toe fracture/dislocations:
    - Pain, swelling, ecchymosis, and painful weight bearing are common.
    - Occasionally, toe deformity is noted.

▶ DIAGNOSIS

- Plain x-ray:
  - Ankle fractures: plain x-ray
    - Anteroposterior (AP), lateral, and Mortise
    - Gravity stress view helps with joint instability assessment.
      - Widening ankle mortise (>4 mm) equates to ankle instability.
      - Talus displaced from under the tibial plafond.
    - Widening of the talocrural angle indicates unstable ankle fracture.
      - Normal talocrural angle ~80°
  - Foot injuries plain radiographs:
    - Standing AP, oblique, and lateral
      - AP and oblique show alignment of tarsometatarsal joints, metatarsal shaft, and toe.
      - <3 mm displacement, <10° dorsoplantar angulation acceptable position second to fifth metatarsal shaft fracture

▶ TREATMENT

- Ankle fractures generally require surgery.
  - Initial management, splint/fracture boot, non–weight bearing, elevation, and follow-up in 1 week with orthopedics

- Metatarsal shaft fractures closed, nonangulated, and no joint involvement:
  - Treat conservatively in a rigid sole post-op shoe or fracture boot and crutches. Partial weight bearing as tolerated for 6–8 weeks.
- Fifth metatarsal avulsion and meta-diaphyseal (Jones/Dancer) fracture:
  - Fracture boot immobilization and limited weight bearing 6–8 weeks
- Toe Fx angulated >20° or joint dislocations:
  - Closed reduction, buddy-taping of affected toes (4–6 weeks), post-op shoe
- Factors affecting bone healing:
  - Osteoporosis
  - Tobacco use
  - Diabetes

- Malnutrition
- Compliance
- DVT risks: 30% to 50% risk DVT with lower extremity fx
- Sedentary lifestyle
- Cancer

Case Conclusion

X-rays revealed that the patient suffered a right ankle fracture and an injury to the tarsometatarsal joint. The patient was placed in a well-padded posterior ankle splint, given crutches for non–weight-bearing activity, fracture care instructions, and medication for analgesia. She was schedule to see the orthopedic provider in 5 days.

CHAPTER 243

Hip Fractures and Dislocations

Paige Cendroski, MPAS, PA-C

▶ GENERAL FEATURES

- One of the most common fractures in adults aged 60 years and older; mainly the result of a simple, ground-level fall
- Stress fractures, from overuse and/or osteoporosis, can also occur in the hip/proximal femur.
- Categorized by location of fracture: intracapsular (femoral head or neck) and extracapsular (intertrochanteric and subtrochanteric)
- Risk factors include: osteoporosis, advanced age, female sex, white ethnicity, tobacco and alcohol use, low socioeconomic status, prior hip fracture, and reduced physical activity.
- Identification and treatment will help reduce morbidity and mortality.
- Hip dislocations are relatively uncommon compared to fractures.
  - Native hip dislocations are the result high-velocity trauma.
    - Posterior dislocation far more common than anterior.
- Prosthetic hip dislocations are far more common than native hip dislocations.

▶ CLINICAL ASSESSMENT

- Common symptoms include inability to ambulate after a fall, pain with weight bearing, and/or groin and upper thigh pain.

- A thorough history should be obtained: important factors include other medical comorbidities, history of fractures and/or orthopedic surgeries, hematologic status including bleeding or coagulation disorders, use of anticoagulants or antiplatelets, tobacco and alcohol use, and ambulatory status.
- Physical examination typically reveals a shortened lower extremity on injured side.
- Early ecchymosis is common.
- Tenderness is often noted in the groin rather than lateral aspect of hip.
- Pain generally limits assessment of range of motion (ROM).
- Thorough neurovascular examination of the lower extremities should be performed and documented before surgical intervention.
- Hip dislocations, especially of the native hips, will present with more severe pain after a traumatic injury. Inability to ambulate is common. Often, patients will complain of numbness in the lower extremity due to neurovascular compromise. ROM can rarely be performed nor is it encouraged.

▶ DIAGNOSIS

- Always be suspicious of hip fractures in elderly patients after a fall.
- Anteroposterior (AP) and lateral plain radiographs of the femur are typically diagnostic.
- Radiographs should include the entire femur to assess for additional injuries.

- Other images should include AP pelvis (to evaluate for potential pelvic fracture) and AP/lateral of contralateral hip for anatomic comparison.
- CT or MRI may be required if clinical suspicion of hip fracture remains with no evidence on plain radiographs.
- For suspected hip dislocations, addition radiographs should include internal and external oblique films. A CT of the affected hip is required for suspected traumatic hip dislocations.

▶ TREATMENT

- Surgical intervention within 24 hours is standard of treatment for almost all patients with a hip fracture, regardless of ambulatory status.
  - Goal of surgery includes adequate fracture reduction and stable fixation.
  - Location of hip fractures determines the type of surgical intervention: femoral neck fractures are commonly treated with hemiarthroplasty or cannulated screws.
- Treatment of a native or prosthetic hip dislocation can include a closed reduction with sedation, or it may require surgical intervention.
- Postoperative treatment includes early ambulation with partial weight bearing and advancing weight bearing with physical therapy guidance.
- Deep venous thrombosis prophylaxis is essential: anticoagulation with low-molecular-weight heparin is often utilized, beginning preoperatively and continuing postoperatively.
- Pain control is essential and should always be appropriate for the patient.
- Prognosis:
  - Mortality rate in the elderly status post hip fracture remains near 25% within the first year.
  - Surgical repair of intertrochanteric fractures has a good prognosis; fractures involving the femoral neck have a higher risk of avascular necrosis (AVN).
  - Potential sequelae of hip fractures include pneumonia, deep venous thrombosis and pulmonary embolism, pressure ulcers, and depression.
  - Postoperative complications include surgical site infection including septic joint, periprosthetic fracture, AVN of femoral head, hip dislocation, and nonunion or malunion of fracture.
  - Nearly half of all patients who sustain a hip fracture do not regain their preoperative independence.

CHAPTER
244

Knee Fractures and Dislocations

Nicole Bartoszewski, MPAS, PA-C
Nata Parnes, MD

A 28-year-old male presents to the emergency department after a motorcycle accident, complaining of severe right knee pain and altered distal sensation. He reports feeling his knee "pop out of place then back in." Physical examination reveals hemarthrosis and gross instability of the knee. The popliteal and distal pulses are weak, and sensation in the peroneal nerve distribution is decreased. What is the most dangerous potential complication following a tibiofemoral dislocation?

▶ GENERAL FEATURES

- The knee is highly susceptible to injury, given its anatomic complexity.
- Basic knee anatomy:
  - Bony structures: distal femur, proximal tibia, and patella
  - Soft-tissue structures: medial and lateral meniscus, medial and lateral collateral ligaments, anterior and posterior cruciate ligaments, patellar tendon, and bursas

- Dislocations are classified by location and direction. They may reduce spontaneously before presentation.
- Fractures are classified by location, direction, alignment, comminution, intra-articular vs. extra-articular, and open vs. closed.

▶ CLINICAL ASSESSMENT

- Dislocations:
  - History:
    - Patellar dislocations:
      - Common in young female athletes
      - Lateral dislocations are most common.
      - Typically occur when the foot is planted and a twisting force is applied to the flexed knee in valgus.
      - Patient will report a sudden "buckling" sensation and popping sound followed by severe pain.

- Tibiofemoral dislocations:
  - Infrequent, but a true surgical emergency given the possible associated popliteal artery injury.
  - Anterior dislocations are the more common ones.
  - Result from high energy trauma
  - May be associated with compartment syndrome, injuries to the popliteal artery, peroneal nerve, or stabilizing ligaments
- Physical examination:
  - Clinical findings include deformity, hemarthrosis, ecchymosis, tenderness, swelling, and possible neurovascular deficit.
  - Patellar dislocations:
    - Knee is held in slight flexion, and the patella can be visualized/palpated over the lateral aspect.
    - In patients whose patella reduces spontaneously, the apprehension test is positive.
  - Tibiofemoral dislocations:
    - A gross deformity should be noted, unless it has reduced spontaneously.
- Fractures:
  - History:
    - Complaints of knee pain at the fracture site, as well as pain with weight bearing and decreased/painful range of motion (ROM)
    - Patellar fractures:
      - Most commonly the result of direct trauma or avulsion due to forceful contraction of the quadriceps
    - Distal femur fractures:
      - Most commonly the result of high energy trauma in young males and low energy trauma in elderly osteopenic females
      - Complications: compartment syndrome, fat embolism, adult respiratory distress syndrome, and hemorrhage
    - Tibial fractures:
      - Most common are long bone fractures, with lateral tibial plateau fractures more common than medial ones.
      - Mechanism of injury includes: direct trauma, hyperextension injuries of the knee, and twisting injuries or low energy falls in osteoporotic individuals.
      - May be associated with compartment syndrome, neurovascular injuries, or injuries to stabilizing ligaments
  - Physical examination:
    - Gross deformity and bony tenderness at the fracture site
    - Associated findings: swelling, joint effusion, hemarthrosis, palpable defect, crepitus, decreased ROM, and inability to bear weight
    - Evaluate for open fracture.
    - Thorough neurovascular examination, distal to the injury

- Evaluate the joints above and below the fracture. If the injury is secondary to high energy trauma, look for life-threatening injuries.
- If a patellar fracture is suspected, evaluate the extensor mechanism of the knee.

▶ DIAGNOSIS

- Diagnosis of patellar dislocation can be made clinically.
- Knee radiographs are used to confirm diagnosis of fractures and dislocations. In high energy trauma, pelvis, hip, femur, and ankle radiographs should also be obtained.
- Computed tomography (CT) scan is used when radiographs are inconclusive.
- CT with angiography of the lower extremity may be used to evaluate suspected vascular injury.

▶ TREATMENT

- Dislocations:
  - Reduce urgently after analgesia and sedation have been administered.
  - Repeat neurovascular examination.
  - Immobilize the joint with a long leg splint.
  - Obtain postreduction radiographs to confirm the reduction and evaluate for associated fractures.
  - Outpatient follow up with orthopedics.
  - Patients who have sustained a tibiofemoral dislocation should be admitted for continued vascular monitoring. If any sign of vascular compromise is noted, consult a vascular surgeon urgently.
- Fractures
  - An orthopedic surgeon should be consulted emergently for open fractures, fractures associated with compartment syndrome and neurovascular compromise, as well as for unstable, displaced fractures.
  - Open fractures should be treated with antibiotics, tetanus prophylaxis, irrigation, and debridement, followed by fixation by an orthopedic surgeon.
  - Nondisplaced or minimally displaced, stable fractures can be immobilized in a long leg splint, with recommendations of rest, ice, elevation, analgesics, and no weight bearing. Follow up with orthopedics as an outpatient after 2–3 days.

Case Conclusion

The patient discussed has suffered a tibiofemoral dislocation that spontaneously reduced before arrival. The most dangerous potential complication following a tibiofemoral dislocation is injury to the popliteal artery. The popliteal artery is tethered across the popliteal space, making it susceptible to injury during a knee dislocation. An unidentified popliteal artery injury might result in an above-the-knee amputation after just 8 hours of ischemia.

A 20-year-old athlete presents with a complaint of right knee instability following her soccer game 3 days ago. She recalls that another player slid into the side of her leg, knocking her down after which she was able to weight bear and continue play. Since then, she has noticed that her knee has been swollen, painful, and "gives out" as she walks. Physical examination reveals edema of the medial knee with palpable tenderness in the same region. You suspect a possible medial collateral ligament (MCL) sprain. What finding on physical examination would support this diagnosis?

▶ GENERAL FEATURES

- The knee is a modified hinge joint stabilized by several important ligaments.
- The collateral ligaments are the main stabilizers in the lateral and medial planes.
- An injury to these ligaments generally occurs following a direct contact injury to the knee.
- An MCL injury is more common than a lateral collateral ligament (LCL) injury and usually occurs with a direct blow to the lateral knee (valgus direction).
- Injuries to these structures are sprains and can be classified by grade:
  - Grade 1: ligament sustains traction injury, microtears, but stability is still intact.
  - Grade 2: ligament sustains traction injury, tears, and loses some stability.
  - Grade 3: ligament sustains traction injury, ruptures, and completely loses stability.

▶ CLINICAL ASSESSMENT

- On history, patients:
  - Usually describe a valgus (lateral) or varus (medially) force injury to the knee, commonly during game play
  - May have heard or felt a "pop" in region of injured collateral ligament
  - Often report swelling and pain at joint line
  - Often complain of knee "giving out" with weight bearing

- Findings on physical examination may include:
  - Joint effusion
  - Palpable discomfort at joint line
  - Discomfort and/or instability on valgus stress test suggest medial collateral injury.
  - Discomfort and/or instability on varus stress test suggest lateral collateral injury.
  - Proximal fibular tenderness suggests possible avulsion fracture.

▶ DIAGNOSIS

- Anteroposterior (AP) and lateral x-rays should be ordered when there is any bony tenderness.
- Noncontrast MRI of the knee can confirm the diagnosis.

▶ TREATMENT

- Most MCL and LCL injures can be treated conservatively including:
  - Rest, ice, NSAIDs as needed for swelling and pain
  - Physical therapy to decrease swelling and improve strength and function of knee
  - Hinged bracing with medial and lateral support with gradual return to weight bearing as tolerated
- In cases when conservative treatment has failed or when there is a grade 3 sprain, arthroscopic repair of the ligament may be undertaken using an allograft or autograft.
- Prognosis:
  - The majority of MCL and LCL sprains heal within 2 months and without permanent disability.

Case Conclusion

To support a diagnosis of MCL sprain in your patient above, you perform the laxity of valgus stress test. Stretching the knee in the valgus plane places the MCL under stress and will reveal either pain and/or laxity in MCL injury.

Anterior Cruciate Ligament Injury

Robert O'Brien, MHS, PA-C
Joseph Janosky, MS, PT, ATC

A 15-year-old female presents with her parents to the emergency department complaining of acute onset of right knee pain after a noncontact soccer injury at practice yesterday afternoon. She reports that she quickly cut to avoid an opponent, felt a pop, and immediate difficulty with ambulation. Her parents report that over the course of the evening, there was increased swelling, pain, and limited range of motion. Her parents note that she has been unable to bear full weight on her right leg and experienced an episode of instability while walking down the stairs.

GENERAL FEATURES

- The anterior cruciate ligament (ACL) is the most commonly injured knee ligament.
  - 100 000–200 000 ruptures per year in the United States.
- The pathophysiology of ACL injuries includes both contact and noncontact injuries.
  - Contact injuries often occur from a direct blow to the lateral knee or injuries causing hyperextension to the knee, frequent in rugby, lacrosse, and football.
  - Noncontact injuries occur during sudden deceleration and changes in direction or when an athlete pivots/lands while rotating and laterally bending, frequent in soccer, skiing, and basketball.
- Female athletes are the largest at-risk population for ACL injuries and are 3–8 times more likely to sustain an ACL tear compared to male athletes participating in the same sport or activity.
- Lateral meniscal involvement is frequent with acute ACL tears, medial meniscus involvement is associated with chronic ACL tears.

CLINICAL ASSESSMENT

- Medical history should include inquiring about timing of the injury, mechanism, joint swelling, overall functional ability with ambulation and stairs, recurrent instability, or mechanical symptoms.
- Physical examination findings often include a moderate effusion, limited range of motion, positive Lachman, and anterior drawer sign. If patients are not acutely in pain, it is possible to elicit a positive pivot shift. It is important to perform these special maneuvers on both the affected and unaffected legs to assess for baseline joint laxity.
- Lachman examination is the most sensitive examination: grade 1 = 3–5 mm translation, grade 2 =

5–10 mm translation, grade 3 ≥10 mm translation, A = firm end point, B = no end point.

DIAGNOSIS

- The use of diagnostic imaging is important to assess for concomitant injuries, such as other ligament or meniscal injuries.
- MRI is the primary modality for diagnosis of ACL ruptures.
  - Ultrasound can be used to assist in visualization, assessing effusion, or concurrent collateral ligament injuries.
  - X-rays can be useful to assess for avulsion (Segond) fractures of the proximal lateral tibia, which is pathognomonic for ACL tears.
- MRI findings can include proximal, midsubstance, or distal ACL tears, a buckled posterior cruciate ligament (PCL) (secondary sign of ACL insufficiency), bony contusions of the tibia and femur due to the mechanism of injury, and potential concomitant injuries.
- Patients with 2+ effusions in the outpatient clinic, consideration of arthrocentesis can assist with diagnosis and provide symptomatic relief. Bloody effusions are consistent with ligamentous injuries.

TREATMENT

- Acute management of ACL injuries includes management of swelling with rest, ice, compression, judicious use of NSAIDs, and elevation.
  - Crutches can be advantageous for patients suffering from recurrent instability.
  - Early initiation of physical therapy can help with improving range of motion and controlling edema.
- Nonoperative intervention is reserved for low demand patients with decreased laxity.
  - Associated with increased meniscal and chondral damage
- Surgical intervention is recommended for high-demand sports or occupations or individuals who experience knee instability.
  - Reconstruction is the current gold standard. Graft selection includes autograft for younger patients, including bone-patellar tendon-bone, hamstring, and quadriceps, and allograft for older patients.
  - Promising ongoing research is re-examining the use of ACL repair in carefully selected patients.

- Complications
  - Development of post-traumatic osteoarthritis on radiographs
    - 5% at 2 years, 10% at 5 years, 50% at 10 years
  - Risk of reinjury
    - ACL graft rupture 1.8% to 10.4% within 10 years
    - Contralateral ACL injury 8.2% to 16.0% within 5 years
  - Arthrofibrosis: Stiffness or loss of motion may occur even following surgical repair.

Case Conclusion

The case depicts the initial presentation of an ACL injury, including instability, swelling, and limited range of motion. She was promptly referred to an orthopedic specialist of further evaluation and consideration of surgical intervention. An MRI was ordered, which demonstrated a midsubstance ACL tear. She underwent an ACL reconstruction using autograft hamstrings the following week, followed by several months of physical therapy.

CHAPTER 247

Patellar Tendonitis

Sarah Garvick, MS, MPAS, PA-C

▶ GENERAL FEATURES

- The patellar tendon originates on the inferior pole of the patella and inserts at the tibial tuberosity.
- Patellar tendonitis is an overuse syndrome of the patellar tendon.
- Typically, there is no inciting incident or injury, although patients are usually physically active.
- Weakness and/or tightness of the quadriceps muscles or lower extremity muscle imbalance may contribute to the knee pain.
- Inflammation generally localizes at the midportion of the tendon and toward the insertion point.
- Athletes such as avid runners or walkers or those who participate in explosive jumping activities are most commonly affected.
- Colloquially, patellar tendonitis is referred to as "jumper's knee."

▶ CLINICAL ASSESSMENT

- Patients present with anterior knee pain that has been present for several weeks.
- Typically, there is a history of frequent or new physical activity that involves knee flexion or impact.
- Physical examination findings include:
  - Discomfort in the area of the patella tendon with deep squatting as well as resisted knee extension
  - Tenderness to palpation along the patellar tendon
  - Mild edema around the patellar tendon is possible.
  - Younger patients may go on to develop a painful bump at the insertion of the tendon known as Osgood-Schlatter apophysitis.

- Osgood-Schlatter disease (OSD) is inflammation of the patellar ligament at the tibial tuberosity where the growth plate has not completely closed.
  - Most commonly affects children experiencing growth spurts who also participate in running or jump sports, although pain can continue into adulthood.

▶ DIAGNOSIS

- Patellar tendonitis is a clinical diagnosis; therefore, no imaging is needed to confirm.
- Bedside ultrasound can confirm the diagnosis if performed by a trained clinician.
- Plain film radiographs may be ordered to rule out bony pathology such as arthritis but are not necessary to confirm patellar tendonitis.
- Magnetic resonance imaging (MRI) should be limited to concern for soft-tissue pathology, such as meniscal or ligament tears.

▶ TREATMENT

- Treatment is conservative and limited.
- First steps should include cessation of aggravating activities.
  - Use of ice on the affected area as well as nonsteroidal anti-inflammatory drugs (NSAIDs) for pain relief.
  - Referral to physical therapy should be considered.
  - Patellar tendon strap use can relieve pressure during physical activities.

Ankle Sprain

Shane Ryan Apperley, MSc, PGCert, PA-R
Jon Slaven, MMS, PA-C

▶ GENERAL FEATURES

- Ankle injuries are common, with approximately half of all ankle sprains occurring outside athletic activity.
- This joint is a complex hinged synovial joint formed by the talus, tibia, and fibula (connected by interosseous membrane).
- Ligaments support both medially and laterally.
- ~85% of ankle sprains are inversion sprains (foot falls inward) of the lateral ligaments, mostly commonly the anterior talofibular ligament (ATFL).
- Classified as either grade 1 (mild), grade 2 (moderate), or grade 3 (severe) based on the amount of damage sustained

▶ CLINICAL ASSESSMENT

- Patients typically report pain and swelling (that may present immediately upon injury) in the affected ankle.
- May describe feeling a "pop" at the time of injury
- Most common risk factor is history of at least one previous ankle sprain.
- On physical examination:
  - Ecchymosis and swelling may present around the ankle.
  - Tenderness to palpation over the affected area.
  - Passive and active range of motion (ROM) of the ankle may be decreased.
  - Positive squeeze test and/or external rotation test are suggestive of a syndesmosis injury.

▶ DIAGNOSIS

- Radiographs may be ordered in order to help rule out ankle fracture, which presents similarly.

- Ottawa Ankle Rules should be used to determine need for radiographic imaging. A patient with traumatic ankle pain qualifies for ankle radiographs if they have any of the following:
  - Point tenderness at the posterior edge (of distal 6 cm) or tip of the lateral malleolus
  - Point tenderness at the posterior edge (of distal 6 cm) or tip of the medial malleolus
  - Inability to weight-bear four steps immediately after the injury and in the emergency department
- If indicated, x-rays must include anteroposterior (AP), mortise, and lateral views.

▶ TREATMENT

- The goal of treatment in all ankle sprains is prevention of chronic pain and instability.
- Patients will benefit from RICE therapy (Rest, Ice, Compression, Elevation) as well as from taking nonsteroidal anti-inflammatory drugs (NSAIDs), unless otherwise contraindicated. Physical therapy, including early ROM and proprioception, agility, and endurance training, is also beneficial.
- Patients with a grade 1 ankle sprain can weight-bear as tolerated (WBAT) without the use of a walking aid. Grade 2 (cast-boot) and grade 3 (short leg cast) ankle sprains should be immobilized for at least 2–3 weeks so as to protect the ankle and allow for the healing process to begin. Complete healing can take 3–6 months, and up to 33% of patients still experience some pain in the ankle 1-year postinjury.

CHAPTER
249

Benign Bone Neoplasms

Nata Parnes, MD

An 18-year-old male presents to the clinic complaining of pain in the bony part of his right shin. He further reported that this is an aching pain that is not activity related. It tends to escalate at night to severe pain, and he usually achieves relief with NSAIDs. What should you consider?

▶ GENERAL FEATURES

- Benign bone neoplasms include: osteochondroma, giant cell tumor, and osteoid osteoma.
- Osteochondroma:
  - Most common benign bone tumor and can develop as a single tumor (osteocartilaginous exostosis) or multiple tumors (multiple osteochondromatosis). Malignancy rate is low (<1%).
  - Is a bone and cartilaginous outgrowth of the long bone growth plates?
  - Once a child reaches skeletal maturity, the osteochondroma typically stops growing.
- A giant cell tumor of bone is a rare neoplasm typically occurring in young adults at the ends (epiphyses) of long bones (most often close to the knee).
  - An aggressive tumor that can destroy the surrounding bone
  - Malignancy only occurs in about 2% of cases. However, if malignant degeneration does occur, it is likely to metastasize to the lungs.
- An osteoid osteoma tends to be <1.5 cm in size.
  - It may occur at any age and in any bone in the body, but is most common in males 4–25 years old, and located in the leg or vertebra.

▶ CLINICAL ASSESSMENT

- Osteochondromas are typically asymptomatic:

- Usually discovered only accidentally when an x-ray is done for unrelated reason
- May present as a painless bump near the joints
- Pain may be felt during activity when it is located under a tendon, or there may be neurovascular symptoms if it presses on a nerve or vessel.
- Symptoms of a malignant transformation of osteochondroma constitute pain, swelling, and mass enlargement.
- Giant cell tumors usually cause activity-related pain, restriction of joint motion, and possible swelling.
  - May also present with pathologic fractures at the tumor site or nerve pain with weight bearing
- Osteoid osteoma causes a dull, aching pain that is not activity related and escalates at night to severe pain, but usually can be relieved with NSAIDs.
  - May also cause focal swelling, changes in bone growth, bowing deformity, and muscle atrophy

▶ DIAGNOSIS

- X-rays comprise the first tests performed to characterize bone tumors and may show the following:
  - Osteochondromas may have a stalk (pedunculated osteochondromas) or a broad base (sessiled osteochondromas).
  - Giant cell tumors are lytic, nonsclerotic, and sharply defined bone lesions that grow to the articular surface of the involved bone. Characteristic "soap-bubble" appearance may also be present. When the suspected diagnosis is that of giant cell tumors, a chest x-ray or computed tomography (CT) should be performed to assess for tumor metastases.
  - Osteoid osteomas typically show a round lucency, containing a dense sclerotic central *nidus* (usually <1.5 cm) surrounded by sclerotic bone.

- **CT scans** assist in further characterizing and localizing the bone tumor and are especially helpful in osteoid osteoma.
- **Magnetic resonance imaging (MRI)** is the most accurate method for detecting bone masses in symptomatic cases and depicting the precise morphology of a tumor. MRI can also be used to look for cartilage on the surface of osteochondroma tumors and to depict any vascular complications caused by the tumor. A cartilage cap thicker than 2 cm is a sign of malignant transformation.
- **Radionuclide scanning** shows intense uptake of osteoid osteoma. A handheld detector is used during surgery for localization of the lesion, as well as for confirmation that the entire lesion has been removed.
- **Biopsy.** In biopsies, evidence of multinucleated giant cells is used to diagnose giant cell tumors. A biopsy can also assist in checking for malignant transformations of osteochondroma.

▶ TREATMENT

- Treatments for solitary osteochondroma constitute careful observation over time and regular monitoring of changes in the tumor with the help of x-rays.

- Tumor should be surgically removed: if the lesion is causing pain with activity, if the lesion compress nerve or vessel, or if there is evidence of malignant transformation.
- Surgery is the treatment of choice in cases where a giant cell tumor is determined to be resectable.
  - Patients with tumors that are not amenable to surgery are treated with radiation therapy.
- Osteoid osteoma is treated symptomatically with anti-inflammatories.
  - If this therapy fails or the location of the tumor could lead to growth disturbances, scoliosis, or osteoarthritis, surgical or percutaneous ablation may be considered.

Case Conclusion

This patient's presentation raises suspicion mostly for an osteoid osteoma, which causes a dull, aching pain that is not activity related. It escalates at night to severe pain and may be relieved with NSAIDs. It may also cause focal swelling, changes in bone growth, bowing deformity, and muscle atrophy.

CHAPTER
250

Osteoblastoma and Metastatic Disease Affecting the Bone

Nata Parnes, MD

▶ GENERAL FEATURES

- Cancer of the bone can be classified as primary or metastatic from another region.
- >1.2 million new cancer cases are diagnosed each year, 50% of them may metastasize to the bone and turn into metastatic bone disease (MBD).
  - Most common cancer types that metastasize to the bone include: breast, lung, thyroid, kidney, colon, and prostate cancers.
  - Cancer commonly metastasizes to the spine, pelvis, ribs, skull, upper arm, and long bones of the leg.
- Osteoblastoma is a rare, benign, slow-growing primary bone tumor, affecting mostly males between the ages of 10 and 30 years.
  - Most commonly develops in the spine, leg, hands, and feet

▶ CLINICAL ASSESSMENT

- Most common symptom of MBD is bone pain. It can also cause pathologic fractures and anemia.
- The most common symptoms of osteoblastoma are mild pain and swelling. It typically takes about 2 years of symptoms before diagnosis.
- Osteoblastoma in the spine can cause back pain, muscle spasms, advancing scoliosis, leg numbness, and weakness in the leg or leg pain.
- Thorough current and past medical history, family history, and relevant risk factors, such as smoking, are extremely important.
- Physical examination may reveal tenderness around the bones and pain with or limitation of range of motion of adjacent joints.
- A full neurovascular examination of the area should be performed.

DIAGNOSIS

- X-rays are the first imaging tests performed to characterize bone tumors:
  - Osteolytic bone destruction is characteristic to MBD originating in the lung, thyroid, kidney, or colon.
  - Osteoblastic abnormal new bone formation is characteristic to MBD originating in the prostate, bladder, or stomach.
  - Breast cancer often behaves in a mixed osteolytic and osteoblastic manner.
  - Osteoblastoma lesions are predominantly lytic, with a rim of reactive sclerosis, typically >1.5–2 cm in size although smaller lesions may occur.
- Other imaging tests:
  - Bone scan in MBD is helpful in determining if other bones are also involved.
  - Computed tomography (CT) scans and magnetic resonance imaging (MRI) help further define the tumor, especially when the spine or pelvis are involved.
- Biopsy is often necessary to confirm the diagnosis of MBD including the specific primary tumor type as well as confirming the diagnosis of osteoblastoma.
- Blood tests in suspected MBD should include CBC (anemia, multiple myeloma) and blood chemistry (calcium, alkaline phosphatase).
- Lab tests for patients with suspected specific tumors include urinalysis (blood positive in renal cell carcinoma), thyroid function tests (thyroid tumors), CEA and CA125 (colorectal tumors), prostate-specific antigen (prostate cancer), and serum and urine protein electrophoresis (multiple myeloma).

TREATMENT

- In most patients with MBD, treatment is palliative and is focused on managing pain and bone weakness.
- Treatment for patients with MBD requires a team approach and most commonly includes radiation, medication to control pain, and attempts to prevent further spread of the disease (chemotherapy, endocrine therapy, bisphosphonates) and prevent fractures by surgical methods.
- Several types of radiation therapy are available:
  - The most common is local field radiation.
- Treatment for osteoblastoma involves surgical resection of the tumor without damaging the surrounding structures. Radiation therapy and chemotherapy are not recommended.
- Surgical treatments for osteoblastoma may include: curettage and bone grafting (autograft or allograft), marginal resection of the bone around the tumor, and spinal fusion if support is needed after resection.
- Osteoblastoma recurs in 10% to 20% of patients and can be treated using the same methods.

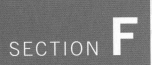

SECTION **F** *Osteoarthritis*

CHAPTER **251**

Osteoarthritis

Lesley Evan Ward, DHSc, MHSc, PA-C

A 64-year-old woman presents with a complaint of gradually worsening 6-month history of medial-sided left knee pain, swelling, and stiffness in the absence of injury. She describes a "grinding sensation" with movement. Her symptoms are constant, moderate (5/10), and aching. Her pain is worse with weight-bearing activity, and she describes difficulty standing from a seated position. Rest usually remits her pain; however, today her pain is constant, and she seeks your consultation and treatment to gain relief. She has no history of drug allergy and has tried acetaminophen without relief. In the absence of contraindication, which medications should be initiated as a first-line treatment?

▶ GENERAL FEATURES

- Osteoarthritis (OA) is the irreversible deterioration of the articular cartilage.
- Primary OA is articular cartilage deterioration without known cause.
- Secondary OA is articular cartilage deterioration resulting from known cause, such as rheumatoid arthritis or previous injury.
- May occur in any joint. Areas commonly affected by OA include the knees, hips, hands, spine, shoulders, elbows, ankles, and feet.
- Risk factors for OA include: older age, obesity, history of joint injuries, family history/genetics, bone deformities/malalignments, exposure to repetitive stresses, and metabolic diseases. Women are more likely to develop OA than men.

▶ CLINICAL ASSESSMENT

- Patients with OA commonly complain of pain in absence of injury, usually worse with overuse and improved with rest.
- Patients may complain of joint "grinding" that usually correlates with crepitus during examination.
- Patients may describe swelling or joint enlargement.
- Assess for malalignment, effusion, erythema, and joint tenderness.
- Common hand-specific OA findings include Heberden (distal interphalangeal [DIP] joint enlargement) and Bouchard nodes (proximal interphalangeal [PIP] joint enlargement). Enlargement and tenderness at the first carpometacarpal (CMC) joint are also common hand-specific findings with first CMC joint (basal joint) OA.

▶ DIAGNOSIS

- Imaging includes three-view radiographs of the affected joint(s).
- Hallmark findings include: joint space narrowing, subchondral sclerosis, and osteophyte formation. MRI is not necessary to diagnose OA, but may be needed in some cases to rule out other potential underlying etiologies.
  - The Kellgren-Lawrence radiographic grading system is widely used to define the severity of OA. The Kellgren-Lawrence system ranges from grade 0 (no radiographic OA changes) to grade 4 (severe OA changes).

- While labs are not necessary to render OA diagnosis, labs may be needed to rule out other potential etiologies, such as rheumatoid arthritis or crystal arthropathy. Synovial fluid analysis may be needed to evaluate for gout, pseudogout, or infection if suspected.

▶ TREATMENT

- Counseling on the importance of low-impact aerobic fitness, self-management programs, and weight loss if indicated.
- Consider orthopedic referral for symptomatic patients who fail conservative measures. If inflammatory arthritis is suspected, rheumatology referral may be needed.
- Physical therapy has been shown to reduce pain and improve strength and mobility.
- Bracing may be beneficial.
- Application of heat, cold, and topical capsaicin may provide symptomatic OA relief.
- Topical or oral NSAIDs should be considered as first-line medications. Acetaminophen can be considered for short-term use in patients unable to take oral NSAIDs. Acetaminophen has been found to be ineffective in the treatment of OA when used for longer durations.
- Intra-articular cortisone injections may be recommended for moderate-to-severe pain.
- Certain patients with knee OA may need arthroscopic treatment in specific cases where loose bodies, concomitant meniscus tears, osteophytes, and mechanical locking symptoms are present.
- Referral for total joint replacement or arthrodesis procedures may be necessary in cases where severity of OA, pain, functional limitations, and failure to respond to conservative interventions indicate need.
- Although opioid treatment for OA is generally not recommended, in certain cases, limited opioid treatment may be considered.

Case Conclusion

NSAIDs are the first-line pharmacologic treatment recommendation for symptomatic OA. Tramadol and duloxetine may be used for symptomatic OA; however, they are not first-line recommendations because of their respective risk profiles.

CHAPTER

252

Osteoporosis

Holly Ann West, MPAS, DHEd, PA-C
Russell Snyder, MD

A 60-year-old Caucasian woman presents to the clinic for health maintenance. Her past medical history is remarkable only for a Colles fracture sustained 6 months ago after a fall while dog walking. She does not take medications or supplements. She admits to a poor diet and little exercise. What should you consider?

▶ GENERAL FEATURES

- Characterized by reduced bone mass with deterioration of structure, resulting in bone fragility and increased risk for fractures
- There is a greater prevalence in women.
- Primary osteoporosis is due to the normal human aging process; secondary results from clinical disorders or the treatment of clinical disorders.
  - A combination of aging and decreased estrogen levels accelerates bone loss. Peak bone mass is reached in the late 20s and early 30s; bone loss is accelerated in the first 5 years of menopause.
- Major osteoporotic fractures include the hip, spine, humerus, or forearm (ie, Colles fracture).

▶ CLINICAL ASSESSMENT

- Evaluate patient for major risk factors including: age, gender, race (white and Asian), low BMI, personal history of adult fragility fracture, family history, medications (eg, glucocorticoids), medical conditions, lifestyle factors (eg, nutrition, smoking, alcohol, decreased physical activity), genetic factors (eg, osteogenesis imperfecta), and estrogen deficiency.
- Screen patients:
  - Without risk factors, women ≥ 65 and men ≥ 70
  - With multiple risk factors (regardless of age)

- With a Fracture Risk Assessment Tool (FRAX) score of ≥9.3% for major osteoporotic fracture
- Most patients are asymptomatic, but fractures may result in pain. Fractured vertebrae may result in kyphosis (dowager hump), tenderness over vertebral bodies, or height loss.

▶ DIAGNOSIS

- Assess bone mineral density (BMD) of the spine and hip with dual-energy x-ray absorptiometry (DXA or DEXA): the gold standard. DXA results are reported as a T-score, which is the number of standard deviations above or below the mean average bone density value for young adult.
  - Normal: ≥−1.0
  - Low bone mass (previously referred to as osteopenia): <−1 to >−2.5
  - Osteoporosis: ≤−2.5
- Obtain labs if concerned about secondary causes (eg, CBC, CMP, 24-hour urinary calcium, 25-hydroxyvitamin D, and TSH).

▶ TREATMENT

- Prevention and lifestyle measures include calcium and vitamin D supplementation, low-impact aerobic activity, weight-bearing and muscle-strengthening exercises, smoking cessation, fall prevention, and, if possible, avoidance of medications that promote bone loss (eg, glucocorticoids).
- Pharmacologic management indicated with hip or vertebral fractures, T-score of ≤−2.5 at the femoral neck or spine (after exclusion of other causes), and/or a T-score between −1 and −2.5 in a high-risk postmenopausal woman.

- Antiresorptives reduce resorption through the inhibition of osteoclastic activity.
  - Bisphosphonates generally considered first-line therapy for menopause-associated bone loss. Oral forms have side effects (esophageal and gastric irritation); rare but serious side effects include osteonecrosis of the jaw and atypical femur fractures, especially with chronic therapy >5 years.
  - Denosumab is an alternative initial treatment option for those intolerant or unresponsive to other therapies and those with renal dysfunction.
  - Selective estrogen receptor modulators (SERMs) exhibit estrogen receptor agonist activity in the bone and reduce spinal fracture risk; however, bisphosphonates have better antiresorptive efficacy.
  - Hormone therapy (HT) is no longer recommended as treatment for osteoporosis but is beneficial in women on HT for menopausal symptoms.

- Calcitonin has a moderate analgesic effect; however, it is only prescribed in certain situations such as pain control in known vertebral compression fractures related to osteoporosis.
- Anabolic agents include exogenous parathyroid hormone and a newer therapy, romosozumab.

> **Case Conclusion**
>
> This patient has many risk factors for osteoporosis (age, race, low body weight, lack of supplementation, poor diet, inadequate physical activity, and a personal history of an adult fragility fracture). Falls from standing are typically atraumatic or cause a sprain/strain vs. a fracture. However, with osteoporosis, this is a common initial presentation.

SECTION H   *Spinal Disorders*

CHAPTER 253   Spinal Stenosis

Alicia Andaloro, PA-C, MS

> A 52-year-old male presents to the office with complaints of lower back pain. He states he was playing football with his son when he first noticed the onset of symptoms. Throughout the night, he then began having right leg numbness. He states that he went to the kitchen to get ice for his back and had a difficult time walking; however, when he bent over, there was some relief.

▶ GENERAL FEATURES

- Spinal stenosis is defined as the narrowing of the spinal canal, lateral recesses, or intervertebral foramina, which may cause bone and/or soft tissue to compress nerve roots.
  - The lumbar spine is the most common site.
  - Sometimes referred to as "pseudoclaudication" or "neurogenic claudication"
- Spinal stenosis may be congenital or acquired. The causes include enlarged osteophytes, degenerative arthritis, hypertrophied ligament flavum, and disc herniations.
- Epidemiology:
  - Patients typically are aged 50 years or older.
  - Males and females are equally affected.

▶ CLINICAL ASSESSMENT

- History:
  - Low back pain
  - Buttock pain
  - Thigh pain that may extend down the entire leg
  - Numbness and/or tingling
  - In severe cases, bladder or bowel incontinence
  - Symptoms tend to progress and typically worsen with increasing time and age.
- Pain characteristics:
  - Aching, burning, cramping, dull fatigue, sharp pain
  - Typically bilateral
  - Worsens with walking, prolonged standing, and lumbar extension

- The classic characteristic is improvement with lumbar flexion.
- Physical examination findings:
  - Examination of the back and lower extremities is often unremarkable early in the disease process.
  - Reduced lumbosacral range of motion, extremity weakness, or foot drop
  - A positive straight leg raise and diminished deep tendon reflexes can be present, but are rare.
  - Patients typically have a positive "stoop" test—when asked to walk briskly, patients assume a stooped position to alleviate pain as they continue walking.

DIAGNOSIS

- The presence of classic symptoms aid in making a diagnosis.
- A lumbosacral MRI with or without contrast is the gold standard—narrowing of the spinal cord will be seen.
  - If there are contraindications to MRI or persistence of symptoms in the absence of MRI findings, a CT myelogram can be used.
- Radiographs may be used to explain the cause of spinal stenosis. Plain x-rays as well as flexion and extension views are common.
- An EMG can help determine nerve root damage to the lower extremities.

TREATMENT

- Conservative treatment:
  - Lifestyle modifications including weight loss, tobacco cessation, and alterations to activities
  - Physical therapy with flexion-based exercises
  - Pain management
    - Oral medications including nonsteroidal anti-inflammatory drugs, opioids, or neuropathic pain medications
    - Epidural corticosteroid or facet joint injections
  - Conservative options should be attempted first unless the patient has neurologic deficits or incontinence, which would prompt emergent surgery.
- Surgical intervention:
  - Lumbar laminectomy
  - Discectomy or foraminotomy
  - Spinal fusion is required for patients needing an extensive foraminotomy or for those who have adjacent-level degeneration after a previous spinal fusion.

Case Conclusion

The patient is a classic example of lumbar spinal stenosis due to his symptoms of lower back pain and right leg numbness. The difficulty he has when walking as well as relief with lumbar flexion would warrant an MRI for this patient.

CHAPTER

254

Scoliosis and Kyphosis

Kristina Stanson, MMS, PA-C

A 12-year-old female presents with concerns of waist asymmetry first noticed by her parents last month during a trip to the beach. She has recently undergone a rapid growth spurt, with a 2-in increase in height over the past 8 months. Physical examination reveals a right thoracic rib hump measuring 8° via scoliometer. What is needed to confirm the suspected diagnosis?

GENERAL FEATURES

- Scoliosis is a lateral curvature of the spine with a Cobb angle >10°.
  - Incidence is similar among males and females, though females are at higher risk of curve progression.
  - Most common type is adolescent idiopathic scoliosis, which typically presents during the adolescent growth spurt.
  - Right thoracic curves (named for the location of the apical vertebral body) are most common. Left thoracic curves may indicate neural axis abnormalities.
- Kyphosis is an exaggerated convex curvature of the thoracic spine measuring >45°.
  - Scheuermann kyphosis is idiopathic osteochondrosis of the thoracic spine, resulting in a wedged appearance of the vertebrae. It typically presents during adolescence, is more common in males, and is often associated with pain.

CLINICAL ASSESSMENT

- In scoliosis, physical examination may reveal lateral curvature of the spine, thoracic and/or lumbar humps, shoulder level and iliac crest level asymmetry, waist asymmetry, and trunk shift.

- Angle of trunk rotation (ATR) is measured with a scoliometer via the Adam forward bend test. Readings <5° are considered within the normal range.
- In kyphosis, physical examination will reveal rounded shoulders or a humpback appearance.
  - Structural kyphosis will become more prominent in spinal flexion, whereas postural kyphosis will diminish.
  - A sharp, angulated curve on forward bend test is indicative of Scheuermann kyphosis.
- Gait and neuromotor function in both conditions are typically normal unless there is an underlying neurologic condition or spinal stenosis.
- Café-au-lait spots and midline skin defects such as hairy patches, dimples, or nevi should alert the provider to investigate other neurologic disorders as the cause of scoliosis such as neurofibramatosis.

▶ DIAGNOSIS

- Anteroposterior (AP) standing full-spine radiograph is recommended for patients with an ATR >5°.
- Cobb angle is measured by drawing lines extending from the superior endplate of the most tilted upper vertebra and the inferior endplate of the most tilted lower vertebra within a curve. Cobb angle >10° is diagnosed as scoliosis.
- A lateral full-spine radiograph is used to identify kyphosis. Anterior wedging of at least three consecutive vertebrae is diagnosed as Scheuermann kyphosis.
- Age of menarche, along with evaluation of skeletal age based on radiographs of the iliac crests (Risser stage), is used to estimate risk of curve progression and guide treatment decisions.
- Magnetic resonance imaging (MRI) is indicated if there is concern for spinal stenosis or other intraspinal abnormalities.

▶ TREATMENT

- Pain associated with spinal deformities can be treated with conservative therapy including anti-inflammatories, application of ice or heat, a flexible lumbar support orthosis, and physical therapy.
- Treatment options for scoliosis include:
  - Skeletally immature patients:
    - Curves 10° to 15°: monitor every 6–12 months with scoliometer checks, followed by an x-ray if any change is noted.
    - Curves >15°: monitor with repeat x-rays every 3 months.
    - Curves 20° to 40°: consider a molded thoracolumbar brace if Risser stage 0, 1, or 2. Braces are worn for 16–23 hours per day until skeletal maturity.
    - Curves >40°: consider surgical intervention.
  - Surgery can be considered for adults with scoliosis >40°, documented curve progression, or decreased quality of life despite conservative therapy.
- Treatment for kyphosis includes:
  - Curves 45° to 60°: physical therapy to improve posture
  - Curves 60° to 80°: bracing is an option for skeletally immature patients.
  - Curves >80°, or unresponsive to conservative therapy: consider surgical intervention.
- Posterior spine instrumentation with fusion is the preferred surgical technique to correct scoliosis and kyphosis.
- Skeletally mature patients should undergo regular monitoring. Osteoporosis prevention and management is key to preventing degenerative buckling of the spinal deformity.
- If left untreated, scoliosis and kyphosis can progress and potentially cause pain, spinal stenosis, cardiopulmonary compromise, and decreased self-esteem due to cosmetic deformity.

Case Conclusion

The diagnosis of scoliosis is confirmed if a full-spine radiograph shows a Cobb angle >10°.

CHAPTER 255

Spondylolithesis

Alicia Andaloro, PA-C, MS

An 18-year-old female presents with her boyfriend to the office complaining of increased lower back pain over the last 2 weeks. She states that she can feel the pain extend into her buttock and down the back of her bilateral thighs. She is a gymnast and is having a very difficult time completing her routines, as the pain increases the more she moves around. She admits that at rest, her pain improves.

GENERAL FEATURES

- Spondylolithesis is a condition of instability in the spinal column, which causes one vertebral body to shift forward in relation to another vertebral body.
- The most common level of occurrence is the L4-L5 vertebra in the lumbar spine.
- Categorized as either congenital, traumatic, degenerative, or pathologic in nature.
  - Common traumatic causes include gymnastics, football, weightlifting, and track and field.
- Commonly, spondylolysis is a precursor to spondylolithesis and occurs when there is a defect or stress fracture in the pars interarticularis of the vertebral arch.
- Males and females are equally affected.

CLINICAL ASSESSMENT

- Classic presentation:
  - Persistent lower back pain or tenderness (most common), worse with hyperextension
  - Lower back stiffness
  - Stiffness in the buttock muscles or hamstrings
  - Posterior thigh pain
  - Numbness and tingling in the legs
  - Pain worsens with activity, improves with rest.
- Physical examination findings:
  - Areas of complaint should be examined for tenderness to palpation.
  - Patients will often present with decreased lumbosacral range of motion, positive straight leg raise, and lower extremity weakness.
  - Patients often walk in short strides with their knees slightly bent.

DIAGNOSIS

- Lateral x-rays should be obtained to evaluate for vertebra slip.
  - Grading system:
    - The diagnosis of spondylolithesis is graded based on the degree of vertebra slip.

- Grade I: <25% slip
- Grade II: 25% to 49% slip
- Grade III: 50% to 74% slip
- Grade IV: 75% to 99% slip
- Grade V: The vertebra has fallen off the vertebra below it. This is the most severe and known as spondyloptosis.
- Lateral x-rays may also reveal stress fractures related to spondylolysis.
- A CT scan or MRI may also be used. These are used when the patient has symptoms of numbness and tingling and will provide more information regarding a fracture, potential disc herniations, or nerve root damage.

TREATMENT

- Conservative treatment:
  - Rest and avoidance of activities, including lifting, bending, and repetitive motions
  - Physical therapy including exercises to increase lumbar range of motion, as well as abdominal core strengthening
  - Hyperextension braces
  - Anti-inflammatory medications
  - Epidural steroid injections
- Surgical intervention:
  - Surgery is indicated for those who have severe or high-grade slippage, vertebral slippage that is progressively worsening, or symptoms that have not improved after conservative treatment.
  - A lumbar spinal fusion with or without decompression of the nerve roots should be performed.

Case Conclusion

The patient was diagnosed with spondylolithesis due to her complaints of increasing pain that has persisted over the last 2 weeks. The classic sign was increased pain with activity and relief with rest. This patient should have lateral x-rays to determine the grade of vertebra slippage.

CHAPTER
256

Low Back Strain and Sprain, Vertebral Disc Herniation, Vertebral Fracture, and Cauda Equina Syndrome

Paige Cendroski, MPAS, PA-C

GENERAL FEATURES

- Low back pain (LBP) accounts for a significant number of outpatient visits, hospital admissions, and emergency department visits; LBP is the second most common reason for visiting a health care provider in the United States.

- It is estimated that 80% of the US population will experience back pain during adulthood; 1% of the US population is chronically disabled due to back problems.
- LBP has various etiologies: depending on the etiology, management ranges from conservative treatment to emergent surgical intervention.
- The most common causes of LBP are low back strain and vertebral disc herniation. The exact cause of symptoms is found in only 12% to 15% of patients.
- Low back strain or sprain can be caused by improper lifting and coupled motions, such as forward and lateral flexion. Age range is widespread.
- Vertebral disc herniations can be the result of improper lifting or twisting but can also occur without the patient's awareness of an inciting injury. Anatomically, the nucleus pulposus herniates into neuroforamina compressing the nerve roots. Typical age for lumbar herniations is 25–55 years.
- Vertebral body fractures can range from pathologic weakening of the bone (elderly) or traumatic injuries. Most osteoporotic compression fractures are located from T12 to L2. Traumatic vertebral fractures can occur following a motor vehicle accident, fall, or jump.
- Cauda equina syndrome is the result of compression of several lumbosacral nerve roots. The cause of this compression can be due to disc herniation, spinal tumors, spinal stenosis, and infections. Cauda equina syndrome can present acutely or have a more chronic presentation.

▶ CLINICAL ASSESSMENT

- Obtaining a detailed history will guide the physical examination and diagnostics. Note location, severity, radiation (SLR). It is important to note any medication usage such as OTC medications to history of narcotic use. Daily activities and history of injury can aid in narrowing differential diagnoses.
- A thorough physical examination for LBP includes gait assessment, inspection/palpation of spine and musculature, ROM of spine and hips, muscle strength and sensation of lower extremities, straight-leg raise (SLR) test, reflexes, and rectal examination if indicated.
- LBP with no referred pain is usually mechanical in nature, such as a strain or sprain. Examination may reveal decreased ROM secondary to pain and tenderness along affected ligaments.
- Leg and buttock pain are usually indicative of nerve root irritation from a herniated disc. Patients will typically complain of burning pain that often radiates into the lower extremities (LEs). Weakness or sensation changes in the lower extremities are common. Location of pain, loss of sensation, and decreased strength in specific areas of the LEs correlate with the level of

nerve root affected. The positive SLR test, which will elicit the radicular pain, supports the diagnosis.
- An elderly patient with a vertebral compression fracture in the lumbar region will commonly present with back pain and may only have decreased ROM of the spine secondary to pain. Patient may have tenderness to palpation at the level of the fracture.
- Progressive motor or sensory loss in the LEs, urinary complaints such as retention or incontinence, or fecal incontinence are highly suggestive of cauda equina syndrome. On examination, saddle anesthesia can be present. A rectal examination can reveal poor anal sphincter tone; and significant decreased muscle strength suggests cauda equina syndrome.

▶ DIAGNOSIS

- A thorough history with abnormal physical examination findings will yield a high suspicion for each of the various lumbar spine pathologies mentioned.
- Red flag symptoms such as fall or significant injury, fever, weight loss, urinary or bowel complaints, motor or sensory loss in the LEs, or any contributing medical history will prompt immediate imaging.
- No imaging is indicated for the clinical suspicion of a lumbar muscle strain or sprain. Plain radiographs are indicated for persistent LBP after 1–2 months of conservative treatment.
- In general, plain radiographs of the lumbar spine should be obtained before further imaging such as MRI, CT, or CT myelogram. Plain radiograph views include anteroposterior (AP) and lateral of lumbar spine with forward flexion and extension.
- A high level of suspicion of a vertebral disc herniation will warrant an MRI with contrast to view the level of herniation and morphology of the disc herniation.
- Plain radiographs of the spine are sufficient for the diagnosis of vertebral fractures. A CT scan is indicated if there is any suspicion of spinal canal involvement.
- For suspected cauda equina syndrome, a CT myelogram or MRI will determine the cause of the syndrome.

▶ TREATMENT

- Low back strains and sprains should be treated with short-term rest (2 days), ice or heat, NSAIDs, progressive ambulation, and weight loss if indicated.
- Mild-to-moderate pain can be treated with acetaminophen or NSAIDs.
- Severe pain can be treated with tramadol, hydrocodone, or oxycodone for no >2 weeks.
- Most disc herniations (75%-80%) are treated successfully with conservative therapies: appropriate dose of narcotic, ice, and rest. Steroids are frequently prescribed with good results. Surgery is indicated in

patients with persistent radicular pain, even with adequate conservative therapies.

- Patients with progressive neurologic deficits, specifically motor function, will require surgery such as a microdiscectomy.
- Treatment of vertebral compression fractures depends on the severity of the symptoms and degree of compression. Conservative measures include oral pain medication, thoracic or lumbar bracing, and physical therapy; patients who have significant pain and/or neurological symptoms may require vertebroplasty (kyphoplasty) or spinal fusion.
- Surgical intervention is indicated in acute cauda equina syndrome.

SECTION **I**

Upper Extremity Disorders

CHAPTER

257

Superior Labrum Anterior to Posterior Tears

Daniel Perez, MPAS

❱ GENERAL FEATURES

- A superior labrum anterior to posterior (SLAP) tear is a disruption to the superior labrum anterior to posterior.
- The labrum is the cartilaginous glove that helps provide stability to the shoulder joint.
- Labral tears can occur secondary to acute injury or chronic overuse.
- The incidence of SLAP tears is unknown, but those who undergo arthroscopy have seen a 6% to 26% incidence.
- SLAP tears are classified into four types using the Snyder Classification System:
  - Type I: labrum fraying with an intact biceps tendon
  - Type II: fraying with damage to the biceps tendon
  - Type III: a tear with no damage to the biceps tendon
  - Type IV: superior labrum tear with tearing to the biceps tendon
- The type of tear can be associated with a patient's condition/activity:
  - Type I: osteoarthritis, rotator cuff arthropathy, age
  - Type II: overhead activities/sports
  - Types III and IV: high-demand occupations, such as baseball pitchers, mechanics
- Shoulder dislocations, repetitive overhead activities such as weightlifting or throwing, fall on an outstretched hand, and lifting heavy objects can predispose to injury.

❱ CLINICAL ASSESSMENT

- Patients may present with acute injury or a week's-to-month's history of chronic shoulder pain.
- Pain may be described as deep and difficult to pinpoint with one finger.
- Patients may report instability of the joint, weakness, and a popping or clicking sensation.
- Pain with overhead and/or lifting activities and limited range of motion secondary to pain may also be reported. However, these symptoms are also consistent with rotator cuff injuries.
- Atrophy of the rotator cuff muscles leading to weakness with abduction and flexion may also be present in older populations.
- Range of motion testing can elicit pain.
- The following special types may help identify a SLAP tear:
  - O'Brien test:
    - Tests for potential labral or acromioclavicular lesions
      - Patient flexes the upper extremity to 90° at the shoulder, arm adducted 10° to 15° and pronate so the thumb faces the floor. Apply downward pressure. Supinate the arm so the hand is in the thumbs up position and apply downward pressure. If more pain is reported with the thumb down and downward pressure is applied, it is considered a positive test.

- Up to 90% positive predictive value
- Sulcus sign:
  - Tests glenohumeral instability of the shoulder
    - Patient is standing or sitting with upper extremities relaxed at their sides. Grasp the elbow and apply downward pressure while observing for a sulcus deformity at the shoulder. Presence of this deformity is considered a positive test.

▶ DIAGNOSIS

- Magnetic resonance arthrogram (MRA) is preferred vs. magnetic resonance imaging (MRI)
- Plain radiographs typically provide no diagnostic assistance but can be useful to rule out other shoulder injuries, such as fractures, osteoarthritis, osteolysis of the clavicle, or dislocations.

▶ TREATMENT

- Treatment should be individualized based on age, activity level, and patient goals.
- Initially, patients begin anti-inflammatories or acetaminophen, activity modification, and physical therapy.

- The glenohumeral approach for a corticosteroid injection may provide temporary pain relief and aid with diagnosis.
- If symptoms do not improve with conservative therapy, orthopedic consultation is appropriate.
- Athletes may require more expedient evaluation by an orthopedist.
- Surgical intervention yields a 6- to 12-month recovery.
  - Surgery involves arthroscopic removal of damaged tissue and anchoring of the labrum to the bone. Sometimes, a biceps tendon release may alleviate symptoms. The surgeon will decide the best method for treatment.

▶ PROGNOSIS

- Most patients recover well with physical therapy. Goals are directed at improving pain-free range of motion and strengthening surrounding muscles.
- Some may continue to experience pain after therapy and have to employ activity modification with aggravating activities.
- Surgical intervention is considered when nonoperative treatment fails to reduce pain sufficiently and/or fails to improve functionality.

CHAPTER 258

Common Overuse Injuries of the Elbow

Steven Kelham, DHSc, PA-C, DFAAPA
Pamela V. Chi, MMSc, PA-C

▶ GENERAL FEATURES

- Lateral epicondylitis (LE):
  - Commonly known as "tennis elbow"
  - An overuse syndrome involving the lateral elbow and extensor tendons of the forearm
  - A usual course could last up to 12–18 months.
  - Epidemiology:
    - Extensor carpi radialis brevis (ECRB) most commonly affected
      - Prime dorsiflexor of the hand and wrist
    - ~1% to 3% of the population
    - 80% to 90% of inflammatory elbow pain
    - Male > female; third and fourth decades of life
  - Etiology:
    - Repetitive motions involving supination and extension of the wrist against resistance
      - Occurs with tennis, use of keyboards, manual work, instruments, and hand shaking

- Degeneration of the ECRB common insertion is often implicated.
  - Degeneration of the hyaline cartilage along with vascular proliferation
- Medial epicondylitis (ME):
  - Commonly known as "golfer's elbow"
  - An acute or chronic condition involving the tendon insertion of the flexor carpi radialis (FCR) and pronator teres (PT).
  - Often associated with ulnar neuritis (cubital tunnel syndrome).
  - Epidemiology:
    - <1% of the population
      - 10% to 20% of inflammatory elbow complaints
    - Male = female; most common in the fourth decade of life
  - Etiology:
    - Repetitive motions involving pronation and wrist flexion with valgus stress

- Occurs with golf, tennis, overhead throwing, occupations involving forceful grip, labor with loads that are >44 lbs, and exposure to vibrations at the elbow
- Common flexor tendon (CFT) degeneration
  - Composed of four forearm flexor muscles and pronator teres
    - Degeneration of pronator teres tendon is most often implicated.
  - The tendon attaches to the medial epicondyle of the humerus and the ulnar collateral ligament (UCL).

▶ CLINICAL ASSESSMENT

- LE:
  - History:
    - Insidious onset of pain over the lateral aspect of the elbow joint with radiation to the upper and lower arm
  - Physical examination:
    - Typically, there is no abnormality on inspection.
    - Range of motion (ROM) is unaffected.
    - Pain will be increased when the wrist is extended with the elbow extended and pronated.
    - Resisted supination such as in gripped hand shaking can also increase pain.
    - Maudsley test: pain in the region of the lateral epicondyle during resisted extension of the middle finger
- ME:
  - History:
    - Insidious onset of pain at the medial aspect of the elbow joint with radiation into the forearm
    - Exacerbated in the cocking phase or early acceleration phase of throwing athletes
    - May include trauma to the elbow, leading to avulsion of the CFT
    - Paresthesias in the ulnar nerve distribution of the hand
  - Physical examination:
    - Tenderness near the medial epicondyle with soft-tissue swelling
    - ROM is preserved.

- Resisted pronation and wrist flexion can exacerbate pain.
- Neurovascular examination:
  - Tenderness over the ulnar nerve in the cubital tunnel
  - Tinel sign; tingling or "pins-and-needles" sensation with taping or percussion of the nerve
  - Decrease two-point discrimination
  - Intrinsic muscle atrophy of the hand

▶ DIAGNOSIS

- Clinical diagnosis is with a proper history and focused examination.
- Basic and advanced imaging may be necessary to assess for trauma, intra-articular pathology, and recalcitrant pain.
  - Plain film radiography
  - Ultrasound
  - Magnetic resonance imaging (MRI)

▶ TREATMENT

- Treatment goals:
  - Manage pain
  - Return to normal function
  - Prevent reoccurrence
- Nonoperative:
  - Rest or minimizing exacerbating activities
  - Ice
  - Counterforce bracing
  - NSAIDs
  - Physiotherapy
  - Corticosteroid injections (LE is more responsive to this therapy than ME)
- Operative:
  - Operative treatment may be indicated if epicondylitis is recalcitrant after 12–18 months of conservative treatment. The nature of the problem also dictates the treatment response.
    - Generally, an arthroscopic/endoscopic procedure is preferred for recalcitrant lateral symptoms.
    - Open procedures are preferred for medial symptoms, given the close proximity to the ulnar nerve.

Carpal Tunnel Syndrome

Tyler D. Sommer, MPAS, PA-C

A 54-year-old female who works at a local convenience store states that she has been experiencing numbness and tingling in her hands intermittently for several months, but this has become progressively worse over the last month. She states that the thumb and index finger are especially involved, and she is frequently woken at night due to pain in the hands.

▶ GENERAL FEATURES

- Carpal tunnel syndrome is considered the most common mononeuropathy, occurring due to compression of the median nerve at the wrist.
- There is 14% lifetime prevalence; it is 3 times more common in women and has a bimodal age of diagnosis at the early 50s and 75–85 years.
- It is commonly associated with repetitive movement or vibrations, frequently occupational, but can occur sporadically as well.
- Carpal tunnel syndrome is also a common finding in pregnant individuals, and it often resolves quickly once the patient is no longer pregnant.

▶ CLINICAL ASSESSMENT

- Median nerve compression occurs due to increased pressure within the carpal tunnel, deep to the transverse carpal ligament at the wrist.
- Tenosynovitis of the flexor tendons of the fingers is the most common cause, whereas others include mass lesions (such as synovial cysts), infection, and fractures of the wrist.
- The classic presentation involves paresthesia, often times painful, within the distribution of the median nerve (the thumb, index finger, middle finger, and radial half of the ring finger, as well as the radial half of the palm).
- More severe cases include motor weakness in the hand, noticeable as weakness with thumb abduction and thumb opposition.
- Severe cases can present with continual numbness and/or atrophy of the musculature of the thenar prominence.
- Being woken from sleep due to painful paresthesia in the hand is highly characteristic of the diagnosis.

▶ DIAGNOSIS

- Tinel sign at the wrist may be positive over the transverse carpal ligament, although the sensitivity and specificity are not high.
- Phalen sign may be more useful and is positive when the patient's symptoms are reproduced while they are holding their hands in wrist flexion for a time.
- Electrodiagnostic studies (nerve conduction studies) are the diagnostic tests of choice and will also assist with grading the severity of disease.
- Ultrasound for evaluation of the diameter of the median nerve at the wrist is becoming increasingly available and useful for diagnosis.
- Rarely, an MRI of the wrist may be necessary for evaluation of a mass lesion, although this is commonly ordered by surgeons if necessary.

▶ TREATMENT

- Conservative measures focus on reducing, eliminating, or modifying activities that seem to exacerbate the patient's symptoms.
- Wearing neutral-position wrist splints, especially while sleeping, can be very helpful.
- Some providers may attempt a local corticosteroid injection into the carpal tunnel, although the literature is mixed on the benefit of this therapy, and it should only be performed by an experienced expert.
- If the patient fails multiple weeks of conservative treatment, and the symptoms are still significant and bothersome, surgical referral is warranted.
- A significant motor deficit or electrodiagnostic results that reveals severe disease are also indications for surgical intervention; surgical referral should not be delayed if motor weakness is present on examination.
- Open and endoscopic decompressive operations are available, depending on the surgeon's preference.

Case Conclusion

With her reports of paresthesia in the distribution of the median nerve, as well as being woken from sleep due to pain in the hands, it is highly likely that the patient has carpal tunnel syndrome. Phalen sign and a neurologic assessment of the hand should be performed, and electrodiagnostic studies would confirm the diagnosis. If motor weakness is present, early surgical referral is warranted.

de Quervain Tenosynovitis

Lindsey Caruthers, MS, PA-C

> A 28-year-old woman who is 34 weeks pregnant presents to the clinic with gradual onset of right radial wrist pain. She states she is having pain in her right wrist with gripping and lifting objects. On examination, she has mild edema and pain with palpation at the right radial styloid.

▶ GENERAL FEATURES

- de Quervain tenosynovitis occurs on the dorsal side of the wrist near the base of the thumb.
- Increased tendon friction due to thickening and swelling of extensor retinaculum is a result of irritation or constriction of the abductor pollicis longus and the extensor pollicis brevis tendons.
- Pain is typically reported around the base of the thumb, most commonly in the dominant wrist.
- Women are more commonly affected than men.
- Typically occurs in patients aged 30–50 years
- The usual cause is repetitive twisting of the wrist.
- Risk factors:
  - Overuse, such as from golf or racquet sports
  - Post-traumatic
  - May occur in pregnancy or postpartum in mothers who lift or hold child with thumb outstretched

▶ CLINICAL ASSESSMENT

- Symptoms are typically of gradual onset and located on the radial side of the wrist.
- Swelling may be present.
- Pain may radiate up to the forearm.
- Pain is made worse by gripping or by raising objects with wrist in neutral position.
- On examination, the patient may complain of pain with palpation of the radial styloid and with resisted radial deviation.
- The neurovascular examination is typically normal.

▶ DIAGNOSIS

- Diagnosis is made primarily through physical examination findings.
- Special tests:
  - Finkelstein test: ask the patient to make a fist with fingers closed over the thumb, then ask the patient to deviate the wrist toward the little finger. Pain with ulnar deviation is a positive finding.
- Radiographs:
  - Anteroposterior/lateral views of the wrist are usually not indicated; however, they can be helpful to rule out basilar thumb arthritis or carpal arthritis.

- Differential diagnosis
- Basilar thumb osteoarthritis (thumb carpometacarpal joint osteoarthritis):
  - Pain is at the base of thumb and made worse by pinching activity.
  - Common in patients over age 50 years
  - Positive grind test: pain and crepitus with passive rotation and axial loading of the joint
  - Radiographs demonstrate loss of joint space between first metacarpal bone and trapezium; may additionally demonstrate bone sclerosis, bone cysts, and osteophytes.
- Carpal tunnel syndrome:
  - Common disorder of the upper extremity and may be associated with pregnancy
  - Pain and paresthesia of the palmar aspect of the thumb, index, and long fingers and radial aspect of the ring finger
  - May be associated with thenar atrophy and weakened pinch
  - Positive Phalen test or Tinel sign
- Scaphoid fracture:
  - Associated with acute trauma
  - Snuffbox tenderness and pain with resisted pronation
  - Radiographs or MRI can help identify fracture.

▶ TREATMENT

- Supportive measures:
  - Rest
  - Ice
  - Activity modification
  - Thumb spica splint for immobilization
- Medication:
  - Nonsteroidal anti-inflammatory drugs (NSAIDs) are typically considered first-line medications for pain.
  - Glucocorticoid injections into the first dorsal compartment are typically very effective and may be considered for refractory pain or when NSAIDs are contraindicated.
- Refer patients for orthopedic consultation for surgical release of first dorsal compartment if symptoms are severe and conservative treatment for 6 months or more has not improved the condition.

Case Conclusion

The patient's history and physical examination, including positive Finkelstein test, is consistent with de Quervain tenosynovitis. At this time, a thumb spica splint and activity modification would be the most appropriate initial treatment. Although typically first-line treatment, NSAIDs are contraindicated in pregnancy.

▶ GENERAL FEATURES

- While it is most commonly referred to as trigger finger, this condition is also known as "stenosing flexor tenosynovitis."
- It is a result of a mechanical impingement of the tendon at the level of the A1 pulley causing pain and locking of the digit.
- The ring finger, long finger, and thumb are the most commonly affected digits.
- Trigger finger has a bimodal age distribution, being predominantly diagnosed in children younger than 8 years and adults aged 40–60 years.
- In adults, it is associated with repetitive movement seen in occupations such as farmers, industrial workers, and musicians.
- It can also be associated with medical conditions, including diabetes mellitus, rheumatoid arthritis, hypothyroidism, gout, and connective tissue disorders.
- In pediatric patients, it is attributed to a developmental condition where the diameter of the flexor pollicis longus tendon is too large for the sheath resulting in tendon entrapment.

▶ CLINICAL ASSESSMENT

- Patients will complain of a catching, popping, or locking sensation, with range of motion of the finger noted at the metacarpophalangeal joint.
- They may note pain with flexion or extension of the finger and stiffness that increases after periods of inactivity.
- Physical examination may reveal a tender nodule, usually over the metacarpophalangeal joint on the palmar surface of the hand.
- An audible snap may be heard with extension of the digit.
- In severe cases, the finger may be locked in flexed position at the interphalangeal joints.

▶ DIAGNOSIS

- Diagnosis is made clinically based on presenting symptoms and physical examination.
- There are no lab tests required for diagnosis.
- If there is a concern regarding an associated, undiagnosed condition, such as diabetes mellitus or rheumatoid arthritis, screening tests for those diseases may be considered.
- Radiographs are not indicated and are performed only if alternative pathology such as fracture, loose bodies, or osteoarthritis is suspected.

▶ TREATMENT

- Rest and avoidance of repetitive motion may improve mild symptoms.
- Patients may use over-the-counter acetaminophen or nonsteroidal anti-inflammatory drugs (NSAIDs) for pain control.
- Corticosteroid injections into the tendon sheath are a mainstay of treatment.
- A 6- to 10-week trial of splinting the digit at night time may be attempted and includes a custom-made hand-based splint that holds the metacarpophalangeal joint at 10° to 15° of flexion, leaving the interphalangeal joints free.
- If conservative treatment is unsuccessful, a surgical procedure called "tenolysis" or "trigger finger release" may be performed.
- Surgical options include open or percutaneous release of the A1 sheath.
- The chief indications for surgical release are failure of splinting and/or injection treatment, locked trigger finger that cannot be reduced or a trigger thumb in infants.
- Research does not support the recommendation of exercise or passive stretching for conservative treatment.

CHAPTER 262

Proximal Humerus Fractures

Shane Ryan Apperley, MSc, PGCert, PA-R
Jon Slaven, MMS, PA-C

▌ GENERAL FEATURES

- Fractures of the proximal humerus are extremely common, typically affecting elderly patients with osteoporosis secondary to a low-energy fall.
- Nonmechanical causes of a fall (ie, cardiac or neurological conditions) should be excluded as should abuse.
- Obese (vs. healthy weight) women are also at significantly higher risk of proximal humerus fracture, especially when postmenopausal.

▌ CLINICAL ASSESSMENT

- Ask if patients are on anticoagulation, are smokers, or if they have a history of osteoporosis.
- Examine for signs of open fracture, skin tenting, or impending necrosis.
- The joints above (shoulder) and below (elbow and wrist) the site of injury should be examined for concomitant injury.
- A complete neurologic examination of the affected extremity should be completed. Particular attention should be paid to the axillary nerve for function and sensation of the lateral deltoid.

▌ DIAGNOSIS

- X-rays should include a three-view shoulder series including a true anteroposterior (AP) view of the glenohumeral joint, a scapular-Y view, and an axillary view.
- The indications for a computed tomography (CT) scan are unclear, but typically reserved for intra-articular involvement, comminuted fracture patterns, and operative planning.

▌ TREATMENT

- Goals of treatment include maximizing function of the shoulder while minimizing the chance of treatment failure.
- Most can be treated conservatively with sling immobilization followed by progressive range of motion (ROM) and physical therapy
- For proximal humeral fractures with moderate-to-severe displacement, open reduction and internal fixation (ORIF) surgery can be performed, if safe to do so. Outcomes are dependent on the preinjury functional status of the patient.

CHAPTER 263

Fractures of the Forearm, Wrist, and Hand

Debra Herrmann, DHSc, MPH, PA-C

▌ GENERAL FEATURES

- Fractures to the forearm, wrist, or hand are common and usually the result of a fall onto an outstretched hand (FOOSH) or a direct blow to the bone.
- The most common fractures of the forearm, wrist, and hand from proximal to distal are:
  - Radial head fracture
  - Nightstick fracture (isolated fracture of the ulna)
  - Monteggia fracture (proximal ulna shaft fracture with radial head dislocation)
  - Galeazzi fracture (distal radius shaft fracture with dislocation of the ulna-radial joint)
  - Colles fracture (distal radius fracture with dorsal displacement of fractured fragments) (Figure 263.1)
  - Smith fracture of the wrist (distal radius fracture with ventral displacement fractured fragments) (Figure 263.2)
  - Scaphoid fracture
  - Boxer fracture (fifth metacarpal fracture)
  - Bennett fracture (intra-articular fracture at the base of the first metacarpal)
  - Rolando fracture (comminuted intra-articular of the base of the first metacarpal)

▌ CLINICAL ASSESSMENT

- Most patients with forearm, wrist, or hand fractures present with a history of injury (eg, FOOSH) with immediate pain, with or without swelling, and with or

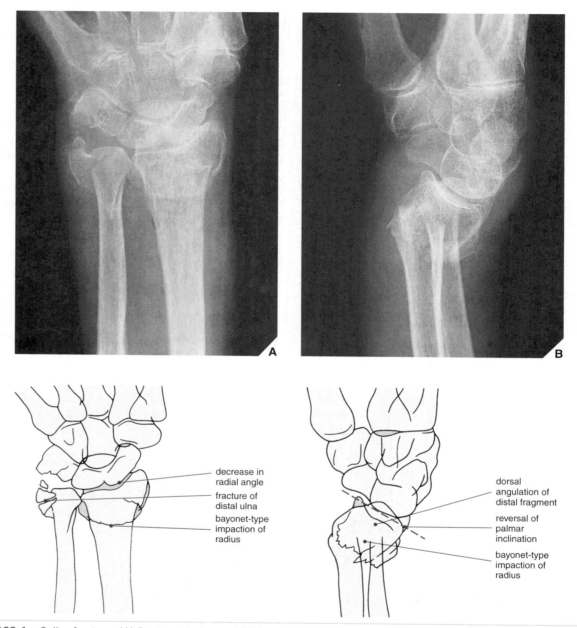

FIGURE 263.1   Colles fracture. (A) Posteroanterior and (B) lateral radiographs of the distal forearm demonstrating the features of Colles fracture. On the posteroanterior projection, a decrease in the radial angle and an associated fracture of the distal ulna are evident. The lateral view reveals the dorsal angulation of the distal radius as well as a reversal of the palmar inclination. On both views, the radius is foreshortened secondary to bayonet-type displacement. The fracture line does not extend to the joint (Frykman type II).

without deformity depending upon the severity of the injury.
- Clinicians must conduct a thorough examination of the arm to include the joint above and below the painful area. Neurovascular status distal to the injury must be assessed as many of the above fractures have associated nerve injury.
- Patients with a radial head fracture have pain along the lateral aspect of the elbow with limited range of motion, particularly pronation and supination.

- A Colles fracture has the classic *dinner-fork* appearance from the dorsal displacement of the fracture fragments.
- A Smith fracture has a *garden-spade* appearance and is often referred to as a reverse Colles fracture because the deformity is ventral rather than dorsal.
- Tenderness in the anatomic snuff box is pathognomonic for scaphoid fracture.
- Boxer fractures are typically the result of someone punching a hard object (eg, a wall).

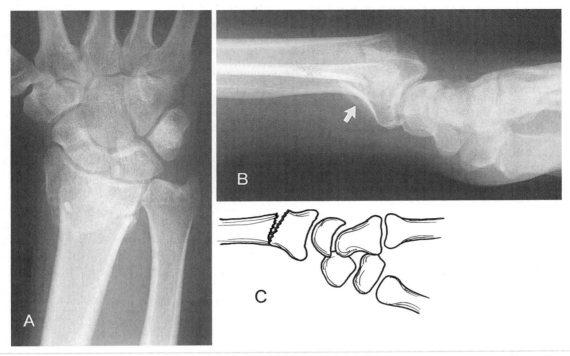

FIGURE 263.2   Smith fracture. A, Posteroanterior wrist. Note the transverse fracture line through the distal radius, with an associated linear density at the fracture site. B, Lateral wrist. Observe the clearly identified fracture line through the distal radius, with impaction at the fracture on the anterior surface (arrow). Associated anterior angulation of the distal fragment has altered the articular plane in this same direction. C, Diagram. The combination of a distal radius fracture with anterior angulation of the articular surface characterizes this fracture deformity.

▶ DIAGNOSIS

- Radiographs: anteroposterior (AP) and lateral views of the injured/painful areas will help confirm the diagnosis of a fracture. Oblique views may be indicated for further fracture definition.
- The radiographs of an occult radial head fracture may show a posterior fat pad as the only abnormality.
- Any patients with snuffbox tenderness (tenderness to palpation of the anatomic snuffbox) are treated for a scaphoid fracture even if the radiographs show no visible fracture of the scaphoid bone. Avascular necrosis of the thumb is a complication of untreated scaphoid fractures.

▶ TREATMENT

- Radial head fracture: long arm splint/cast and sling. Complex fractures often require open reduction and internal fixation (ORIF).

- Nightstick fracture: nondisplaced fractures get a functional brace. Displaced fractures require ORIF.
- Monteggia fracture: ORIF
- Galeazzi fracture: long arm splint/cast. Unstable fractures require ORIF.
- Colles fracture: sugar tong splint/cast
- Smith fracture: reduction (either closed or open) and splint/cast
- Scaphoid fracture: thumb spica splint/cast
- Boxer fracture: ulnar gutter splint/cast with flexion of metacarpal joints
- Bennett fracture: ORIF
- Rolando fracture: ORIF

Dislocations of the Shoulder and Elbow

Debra Herrmann, DHSc, MPH, PA-C

▶ GENERAL FEATURES

- Elbow dislocations:
  - Most common dislocated joint in children
  - Most commonly dislocates posteriorly and is typically caused by a fallen onto an outstretched hand
  - A nursemaid's elbow (also called radial head subluxation) is a common pediatric injury in children aged 1–4 years. This injury is rare past the age of 5 years.
    - Results when sudden longitudinal traction is applied to the patient's hand while the elbow is extended and the forearm is pronated
    - Injury mechanisms include pulling a child up by the hands, swinging a child by holding the hands/wrist, jerking an arm when pulling a child along, or when the child tries to break a fall by reaching an arm out for protection.
- Shoulder dislocations:
  - Account for roughly half of all major joint dislocations and occur from contact sports in the young and from falls in the elderly
  - Most dislocations are anterior, while a small percentage are posterior and inferior.
  - The mechanism of injury:
    - Anterior: blow to the abducted, externally rotated, and extended arm or, less commonly, a blow to the posterior humerus or a fallen onto an outstretched hand
    - Posterior: a blow to the anterior portion of the shoulder, axial loading of an adducted and internally rotated arm, or violent muscle contractions following seizure/electric shock
    - Inferior: axial loading with the arm fully abducted or forceful hyperabduction of the arm

▶ CLINICAL ASSESSMENT

- Elbow:
  - Patient or family describe a mechanism of injury consistent with an elbow dislocation.
  - Patients with elbow dislocations may present with pain, swelling, and deformity of the affected elbow.
  - During the physical examination, it is essential to assess for evidence of open injuries, compartment syndrome, neurovascular status below the injury, and a thorough examination of the shoulder and wrist.
  - For nursemaid's elbow, the child will not want to use the affected limb due to pain.

- Often, the child holds the affected arm in a straight position down by their side or with slight flexion of the elbow with the forearm pronated.
  - On physical examination, the injury will not be evident because there is no associated deformity or swelling.
  - The child may point to the lateral aspect of the elbow when asked where he/she feels pain, and there may be palpable tenderness in this area.
  - The range of motion in the affected elbow is typically normal (if the patient is willing to cooperate), with pain upon supination attempts.
- Shoulder:
  - Patients describe a mechanism of injury consistent with a shoulder dislocation and resist all movements of the shoulder.
  - In all shoulder dislocations, there is a loss of rounded appearance of the shoulder.
  - The way the patient holds their affected arm is dependent upon the type of dislocation:
    - Anterior: affected arm is held in an abducted and externally rotated position.
    - Posterior: affected arm is held in an adducted and internally rotated position.
    - Inferior: affected arm is held above the head and cannot be adducted.
  - During the physical examination, clinicians should assess for other commonly associated injuries with shoulder dislocation, such as axillary nerve damage, rotation cuff tear, labral tear, compression chondral injury of the humerus (Hill-Sachs lesion), and fracture of the anterior/inferior glenoid (Bankart lesion).

▶ DIAGNOSIS

- Elbow:
  - Anteroposterior (AP), lateral, and oblique views of the affected elbow should be obtained.
  - CT scan is recommended for elbow dislocations that seem complicated or highly suspicious for concomitant fracture.
  - The diagnosis for nursemaid's elbow is typically made clinically after obtaining a history with a mechanism of injury consistent with nursemaid's elbow.
    - Radiographs are not necessary and are usually normal. Most clinicians will only order x-rays when they are also concerned about a fracture or an elbow dislocation.

- Ultrasound can confirm the diagnosis of nursemaid's elbow if necessary, but many clinicians will attempt the reduction procedures described below before doing an ultrasound.
- Shoulder: radiographs—AP, lateral, and/or scapular Y-views

▶ TREATMENT

- Elbow:
  - Elbow dislocations are treated nonoperatively with closed reduction techniques and, when necessary, operatively with open reduction techniques.
  - Elbow dislocations must be splinted after reduction, whereas a nursemaid's elbow does not require splinting after closed reduction.
  - Treatment for nursemaid's elbow is a closed reduction of the annular ligament subluxation using a supination technique or hyperpronation technique.
    - Supination technique: apply pressure over the radial head while supinating and flexing the affected elbow.
    - Hyperpronation technique: hyperpronation of the forearm while holding the elbow is slightly flexed.
      - If the reduction technique chosen is successful, the examiner may hear or feel a palpable click, and the child will start using the arm again without pain.
    - Open reduction is rarely required for nursemaid's elbow, as most subluxations can be reduced using the procedures described above.
- Shoulder:
  - Reduction:
    - Anterior dislocation reduction:
      - There are many reduction techniques for anterior dislocations. There is no clear evidence supporting one reduction technique over the other, so the method used is based on clinician preference. Closed reduction techniques may be aided by procedural sedation or intra-articular local anesthesia depending upon the patient condition. Most suggest the following approach:
        - Start with the scapular manipulation technique: while the patient is prone or seated with the affected arm in slight traction and in forward flexion at 90°, stabilize the superior aspect of the scapula while adducting the inferior tip.
      - If scapular manipulation does not work, next try the external rotation technique with or without the Milch technique.
        - External rotation technique: with the patient supine, the affected arm is slowly adducted with elbow flexed to 90° as slow external rotation is applied. Stop when resistance is met and continue when patient is relaxed again.
        - Milch technique: affected arm is positioned overhead. The clinician applies gentle longitudinal traction and external rotation. Stop when resistance is met and continue when patient is relaxed again.
      - When external rotation with or without the Milch technique is unsuccessful, next try the traction countertraction or Stimson technique.
        - Traction countertraction: an assistant applies countertraction with a folded sheet around the chest while the clinician applies traction along the abducted arm.
        - Stimson technique: the patient is prone with the affected arm hanging down. Weight is suspended form the wrist with increasing increments.
  - Posterior dislocation reduction:
    - The severity and duration of the dislocation are factors in determining if a closed or open reduction technique should be used. Often, closed reduction of a posterior shoulder dislocation will require general anesthesia and, therefore, done in the operating room.
    - Reduction involves axial traction on the adducted arm with elbow flexion while applying direct pressure to the posterior aspect of the dislocated humeral head directing it anteriorly.
  - After successful reduction of both an anterior and posterior shoulder dislocation, the arm is immobilized in a neutral position.
  - Postreductions films
  - Immobilization (eg, sling or sling and swath)
  - Physical therapy

Biceps Tendinopathy

Lesley Evan Ward, DHSc, MHSc, PA-C

A 46-year-old man presents with a 6-month history of right (dominant) side anterior shoulder pain. He reports involvement in repetitive lifting at symptom onset. His pain is intermittent, severe, and sharp, worse with lifting, overhead reach, and forceful supination of the forearm. He denies any history of trauma or cosmetic deformity. Which initial treatment options should be initiated if the physical examination findings are consistent with long head biceps (LHB) tendinopathy?

▶ GENERAL FEATURES

- Tendinopathy includes tendonitis and tendinosis.
  - Tendinosis refers to degenerative changes in a tendon.
- The long head of biceps (LHB) brachii tendon origin is located at the supraglenoid tubercle and the superior labrum, and the tendon extends through the bicipital groove inserting distally along with the short head biceps tendon to the radial tuberosity.
- LHB tendinopathy commonly occurs with other shoulder conditions, including rotator cuff impingement syndrome, bursitis, rotator cuff tears, and superior labrum anterior to posterior (SLAP) labral tears. Isolated LHB tendinopathy is seen more commonly in young athletes who are involved in overhead sports.

▶ CLINICAL ASSESSMENT

- Patients usually report pain anteriorly in the region of the bicipital groove, sometimes radiating to the biceps muscle belly.
- Pain is exacerbated by activities that involve shoulder flexion, elbow flexion, and forearm supination.
- Patients may describe history of pain onset after or during repetitive lifting, including overhead lifting, overhead athletic involvement, or biceps exercises.
- In patients who describe painful "clicking" around the bicipital groove, LHB tendon subluxation resulting from underlying subscapularis pathology should be considered.

▶ DIAGNOSIS

- Point tenderness with palpation over the LHB tendon within the bicipital groove is often seen.
- Muscular retraction when biceps brachii is contracted ("Popeye sign") indicates LHB tendon rupture.

- Yergason test: while palpating the LHB tendon, the patient supinates the forearm against resistance with the elbow flexed at 90°. Presence of pain indicates a positive Yergason test, reflecting possible LHB tendon pathology.
- Speed test: with the patient's arm forward flexed to 90°, elbow extended, and forearm supinated, the examiner resists forward flexion. Presence of pain in the bicipital groove indicates a positive Speed test, reflecting possible LHB tendon pathology.
- Examine for painful click along the bicipital groove while patient fully abducts and externally rotates arm. Tenderness or painful click indicates medial LHB tendon instability.
- Relief of pain following corticosteroid injections in the region of bicipital groove suggests LHB tendinopathy.
- Three-view plain film radiographs should be obtained to evaluate for bony abnormalities, osteophytes, or degenerative changes. MRI may be utilized to evaluate the severity of LHB tendon pathology. MRI arthrogram is superior to standard MRI in detection of shoulder pathologies associated with LHB tendinopathy.

▶ TREATMENT

- Initial conservative treatment is recommended, including rest, nonsteroidal anti-inflammatory drugs (NSAIDs), activity modification, and physical therapy.
- If initial conservative management fails, orthopedic referral should be initiated.
- Corticosteroid injection in the region of LHB tendon sheath may help.
- If conservative management fails, then surgical LHB debridement, LHB tenotomy (cutting the proximal LHB tendon), or simultaneous LHB tenotomy and tenodesis (repositioning and anchoring the LHB tendon to the humerus) may be considered.

Case Conclusion

Based on the patient's presentation, initial conservative management considerations for LHB tendinopathy include rest, NSAID if appropriate, activity modification, and physical therapy.

Ganglion Cyst

Lorraine Sanassi, PA-C, DHSc

GENERAL FEATURES

- A ganglion cyst is a noncancerous mucin-filled synovial cyst caused by either trauma, mucoid degeneration (collagen), or synovial herniation.
  - Can be unilobulated, but most are often multilobulated
- Most commonly these are soft-tissue tumors of the hand and wrist, especially on the dorsal aspect of the wrists arising from the scapholunate joint
  - Can also arise from the radioscaphoid or scaphotrapezial joint volarly
  - When located at the distal interphalangeal (DIP) joints, they are termed *mucous cysts* (seen in elderly patients).
- Usually asymptomatic but may cause issues with cosmesis
  - Ganglion cysts arising from the radioscaphoid or scaphotrapezial joint can cause paresthesias, pain, joint instability, weakness, and limitation of motion.
- Occur 3 times as often in women as they do in men
- Predominantly seen in young adults and are rare in children

CLINICAL ASSESSMENT

- Firm and well-circumscribed mass, often fixed to deep tissue, but not to overlying skin, that transilluminates
- With volar wrist ganglions:
  - Assess vasculature by performing the Allen test to ensure radial and ulnar artery flow.
  - Compression of the median nerve cutaneous branches may elicit a sensory or motor nerve palsy.

DIAGNOSIS

- Diagnosis is usually clinical.

- Imaging is not routinely done; however, magnetic resonance imaging, ultrasonography, or x-rays may prove useful in obtaining confirmation of clinical diagnostic findings and ruling out other etiologies.
  - Of note, ultrasound is useful for differentiating a cyst from a vascular aneurysm, especially if aspiration is being considered.

TREATMENT

- Most do not require treatment.
- Surgical intervention is indicated if the patient for cosmetic reasons or if ganglion becomes symptomatic and impairs function.
- Observation is the first line of treatment.
  - In early stages, the cyst can be manually compressed until it bursts and fluid is absorbed.
- Aspiration is the second line of treatment in adults with dorsal ganglions; aspiration typically avoided on the volar aspect of wrist due to risk of injury to the radial artery.
- Open excision (treatment of choice) or arthroscopic excision is required if there is significant pain, limitation of movement, and nerve palsies.
  - Brief splinting of 3–7 days is recommended. Wrist motion within 3–5 days after the procedure can prevent stiffness.
  - Recurrence after surgical excision is most common with volar ganglion cysts.
- Prognosis:
  - Regardless of the method of treatment, recurrence is possible for unknown reasons.
  - Postoperatively, there is statistically significant increases in wrist extension and grip strength.
  - Although some patients reported wrist stiffness after the surgery, motion is usually fully restored by 6 months.

Paget Disease of the Bone

Michelle Kavin, PA-C

GENERAL FEATURES

- Also known as osteitis deformans, Paget disease of the bone is a chronic skeletal disorder characterized by unregulated bone turnover, causing bone enlargement, deformity, and fragility.
- Men and women over 40 years of age are most frequently affected.

- It can affect a single bone (monostotic) or multiple bones (polyostotic).
- It usually affects the femur, spine, skull, sternum, or pelvis.
- Etiology is undetermined but may be associated with genetic factors or viral infection.
- There are three phases of the disease process:
  - The lytic phase where normal bone is resorbed by osteoclasts and bone turnover is increased
  - The mixed phase (lytic and blastic activity) where there is a rapid increase in bone formation by osteoblasts
  - The sclerotic phase, which results in disorganized bone formation and weaker bones

▶ CLINICAL ASSESSMENT

- Most patients are asymptomatic.
- The most commonly reported symptom is local bone pain that is continuous and present at rest.
- When Paget disease affects the skull, patients may complain of headaches or hearing loss.
- Physical examination may reveal bone deformities, such as bowed tibias, an enlarged skull, pelvic alterations, or kyphosis.
- Patients may develop pathologic fractures from the weakened bones.

▶ DIAGNOSIS

- Diagnosis is usually made by an incidental finding on plain radiographs showing sclerotic and lytic areas of the affected bone.

- A bone scan is more sensitive and can detect up to 50% more lesions than can be observed on plain radiographs.
- Laboratory evaluation may reveal an elevated total serum alkaline phosphatase activity, which is a reflection of increased bone formation.
- Bone biopsy is utilized if malignant transformation is suspected.

▶ TREATMENT

- Bisphosphonates are used to achieve remission in Paget disease.
- Surgery is sometimes needed for correction of bone deformities.
- Treatment efficacy is monitored by looking for reduction in serum alkaline phosphatase levels. Alkaline phosphatase is monitored every 3 months for the first 6 months of therapy and then every 6 months thereafter.
- Repeat bone scans and radiographs are not indicated unless the patient reports worsening symptoms.
- Although rare, malignant transformation to an osteosarcoma is possible.
- Other complications may include pathologic fractures, neurologic complications from nerve compression by enlarging bone, high cardiac output, hypercalcemia from excessive breakdown of bone, hyperparathyroidism, osteoarthritis from misshapen bones, and renal calculi.

CHAPTER
268

Rickets

Andrea Rhodes, OTR, MPA, PA-C

A 3-year-old Hispanic male is brought in to see you by his parents for failure to thrive and unusual gait. His weight and height are less than the third percentile for his age. Prenatal history reveals an unremarkable delivery and prenatal course. He was breastfed until 18 months of age. His current diet is primarily vegan. He takes no nutritional supplements. He has bowing of the legs, waddling gait, protruding abdomen, and dental caries. What is the most likely possible risk for vitamin D–deficient rickets?

▶ GENERAL FEATURES

- Rickets refers to alterations at the growth plate before closure due to the insufficient mineralization of bone that leads to the softening and weakening of bones.

- Classified by either the deficiency of vitamin D, calcium, or phosphate
- Two major groups of rickets classification are calcipenic and phosphopenic.
- Calcipenic rickets is the most common cause of rickets worldwide and refers to the deficiency of vitamin D and/or calcium in the diet.
  - Causes of calcipenic rickets include inadequate vitamin D diet intake, renal disease, or vitamin D resistance caused by a genetic defect in vitamin D metabolism or action.
- Phosphopenic rickets may be due to a renal tubular disorder (Fanconi syndrome) or other inherited or acquired defects.
- Risk factors for vitamin D–deficient rickets include infants who are breastfed without vitamin D

supplementation, inadequate sun exposure, dark skin pigmentation, and vegan diets due to the avoidance of dairy products.

▶ CLINICAL ASSESSMENT

- Both calcipenic and phosphopenic rickets display skeletal findings at the wrist and knee where bone growth is rapid, and calcium and phosphorus are needed.
- Classic characteristics seen on imaging of long bones are widening, fraying, cupping, and splaying of the metaphysis.
- Rows of beadlike prominences of the costochondral rib joints, termed *rachitic rosary*, can commonly be visualized on physical examination and seen on x-ray.
- Protruding abdomen and forehead may also be seen as well as curving of the long bones.
- Weight bearing may lead to deformities, such as knock knees and bowlegs.
- Generalized gait disturbances and developmental delay may also be present.

▶ DIAGNOSIS

- The general diagnosis of rickets in a child can be determined by typical clinical or radiographic findings and high levels of alkaline phosphatase.
- In patients with characteristic bone abnormalities, serum alkaline phosphatase (ALP) confirms the diagnosis of rickets and assists in excluding differentials such as hypophosphatasia and Blount disease.

- Measuring serum parathyroid hormone, inorganic phosphorus, and calcium are helpful with further differentiating between calcipenic and phosphopenic rickets.
- Calcipenic rickets may be suspected when there is normal liver and kidney function, elevated serum alkaline phosphatase activity, parathyroid hormone, and low inorganic phosphorus and calcium levels.
- Phosphopenic rickets may be suspected when there is normal liver and kidney function, elevated serum alkaline phosphatase activity, normal parathyroid hormone and calcium, and low inorganic phosphorus levels.

▶ TREATMENT

- Discovering the cause of rickets in your patient helps to guide treatment.
- Nutritional rickets treatment includes daily replacement doses of vitamin D2 (ergocalciferol) or vitamin D3 (cholecalciferol), and treatment is reduced when there is radiographic evidence of healing.
- An alternative protocol, stoss therapy, may be useful when there are compliance issues, and it involves a single dose of high-dose vitamin D.
- Most children need about 400 IU (or 600 IU for older children) of daily vitamin D to prevent rickets.

Case Conclusion

His vegan diet is a possible risk factor for vitamin D–deficient rickets due to the avoidance of dairy products.

CHAPTER
269

Chest and Rib Deformities and Fractures

Janelle Bludorn, MS, PA-C

A 13-year-old male with a history of pectus excavatum presents to the emergency department complaining of worsening chest pain after exercise. He reports trying to exercise more over the last month for soccer tryouts but has been unable to do so secondary to chest pain and shortness of breath. No prior diagnostic imaging is available for review. Why is the patient's past medical history of pectus excavatum important to the diagnostic workup of the chest pain and shortness of breath?

▶ GENERAL FEATURES

- Pectus excavatum is a depression of the sternum, often referred to as "funnel chest."
  - Most common anterior chest wall deformity
  - Higher incidence in males and individuals with connective tissue disorders
  - About one-third of cases noted during infancy; adolescent growth spurts may cause worsened deformity.

- Pectus carinatum is a protrusion of the sternum, often referred to as "pigeon chest."
  - Fairly uncommon chest wall deformity
  - Males and individuals with connective tissue disorders are more commonly affected.
  - 90% of pectus carinatum cases are diagnosed in adolescence when the deformity worsens after a growth spurt.
- Rib fractures often follow blunt trauma to the thorax but may also be atraumatic as in the case of pathologic fractures (eg, metastatic disease) or stress fractures (eg, chronic cough, athletes).
  - Fractures may be displaced or nondisplaced and may cause damage to intrathoracic structures such as the lungs.
  - Flail chest occurs when at least three consecutive ribs are fractured and results in an unstable floating segment that moves paradoxically to the rest of the chest wall.

▶ CLINICAL ASSESSMENT

- Pectus excavatum:
  - History: intolerance to exercise, chest pain, dyspnea, cosmetic concern
  - Physical examination: qualitative (visual assessment) and quantitative (measurement with calipers) assessment of sternal depression. Tachypnea, tachycardia, and systolic murmurs may occur based on the severity of deformity.
- Pectus carinatum:
  - History: cosmetic concerns are most common, but dyspnea on exertion or other respiratory symptoms may be noted.
  - Physical examination: increased anteroposterior diameter due to sternal protrusion. The area of protrusion may be tender to palpation.
- Rib fractures:
  - History: usually localized, reproducible, or pleuritic chest wall pain either suddenly with preceding blunt trauma or gradually with risk factors for atraumatic fractures such as cancer or athletic activities
  - Physical examination: point tenderness with or without crepitus and ecchymosis. Decreased breath sounds may be present in the setting of concurrent pneumothorax or pulmonary contusion.

▶ DIAGNOSIS

- Pectus excavatum is a clinical diagnosis, but diagnostics can assess defect severity, impact on thoracic structures, and need for surgical intervention.
  - Computed tomography (CT) can be used to calculate the pectus severity index (PSI), a ratio of lateral thoracic diameter and distance between the sternum and the spine. PSI of ≤ 2.5 is normal.

- Pulmonary function testing (PFT) is indicated, but is often normal.
- Electrocardiogram and echocardiography may reveal right axis deviation and right ventricular obstruction, respectively, and based on disease severity.
- Pectus carinatum is a clinical diagnosis; diagnostics can be useful in intervention planning.
  - Plain radiographs of the chest can assess deformity severity.
  - CT can be used to calculate the PSI. For pectus carinatum, a lower number is indicative of more severe deformity.
- Most rib fractures and associated lung injuries can be diagnosed on posteroanterior and lateral plain films of the chest; dedicated rib series radiographs and chest CT are more sensitive and can be obtained if clinical suspicion is high but initial plain films are unrevealing.

▶ TREATMENT

- Surgical intervention timing and approach for pectus excavatum is controversial, but is considered in the presence of at least two of the following: PSI >3.25, deformity causing cardiac abnormalities, abnormal PFTs, or prior repair failure.
  - Surgical interventions are often performed in late childhood to adolescence. Minimally invasive and open procedures are both available.
- Pectus carinatum treatment is mostly cosmetic.
  - Bracing can be used for mild-to-moderate disease, whereas surgical interventions are indicated for more severe deformities.
- Pain control and respiratory care (ie, incentive spirometry) for rib fractures is key to minimize complications, such as pneumonia and atelectasis due to splinting. NSAIDs, opiates, transdermal lidocaine, and nerve blocks are analgesia options.
  - Most rib fractures take about 6 weeks to heal.
  - Patients with fewer than three isolated rib fractures without findings suggestive of associated intrathoracic injury can usually be managed outpatient.
  - Patients with flail chest or fractures resulting chest wall deformity should be considered for surgical fixation.

Case Conclusion

Shortness of breath and chest pain with exercise in an adolescent patient with a history of pectus excavatum may indicate underlying cardiopulmonary structural disease. Diagnostics including a CT scan of the chest, electrocardiogram, and echocardiogram may determine disease severity, impact on other structures, and the need for possible surgical intervention.

Thoracic Outlet Syndrome

Lorraine Sanassi, PA-C, DHSc

▶ GENERAL FEATURES

- Thoracic outlet syndrome (TOS) refers to a variety of signs and symptoms related to compression of the brachial plexus and the subclavian vessels, as they exit the clinical thoracic outlet by local structures in the area just above the first rib and behind the clavicle.
- Most often seen in patients who engage in repetitive motions of extreme shoulder abduction and external rotation (swimmers, water polo, baseball, tennis players)

▶ CLINICAL ASSESSMENT

- Initial presentation is dependent on whether the compression is vascular, neurogenic, or nonspecific.
  - Pure vascular TOS is rare.
    - More common in younger patients who are athletes
    - Venous obstruction: upper extremity swelling, venous distention, or diffuse arm or hand pain
    - Arterial obstruction: be color changes of their affected upper extremity, claudication, or diffuse arm or hand pain (including the forearm)
      - Initially symptoms are mild due to collateral flow, causing patients to seek medical evaluation after ischemic changes occur (ulceration, gangrene, absent pulses).
  - Pure neurogenic TOS is also rare.
    - Compression of the brachial plexus
    - Presents with painless atrophy of the intrinsic muscles of the hand, leading to difficulty grasping (such as a racket or ball)
    - Sensory loss or paresthesias are common.
    - Radicular pain in the affected upper extremity may be seen.
  - A combination of neurovascular symptoms is the most common presentation.
  - Nonspecific type:
    - Unexplained pain in the arm, scapular region, and cervical region
- Physical examination:
  - General assessment:
    - Posture (poor posture can be damaging for the scapular and neck muscles)
    - Symmetry of both arms (muscle bulk may be decreased in affected extremity, sensation and strength may be diminished)
    - Active and passive range of motion of the neck and shoulder

- Vascular TOS:
  - Arterial obstruction: pallor, a weak or absent pulse, and coolness of the upper extremity; decreased blood pressure >20 mm Hg in the affected arm
  - Venous obstruction: edema and cyanosis of the upper extremity; distended veins in the shoulder or chest
- Neurogenic TOS:
  - Gilliatt-Sumner hand: atrophy of the abductor pollicis brevis with lesser involvement of the interossei and hypothenar muscles; decreased sensation along the ulnar nerve distribution
- Nonspecific type:
  - Nonfocal; diffuse upper extremity pain with guarding
- Special tests:
  - Spurling test: patient's head is placed in extension and lateral flexion, axial compression applied by the examiner to the patient's head in an effort to recreate radicular pain
  - Adson maneuver: loss of the radial pulse in the affected arm by rotating head to the ipsilateral side with extended neck following deep inspiration
  - Wright test: loss of the radial pulse in the affected arm by progressively hyperabducting and externally rotating the patient's affected arm while assessing the ipsilateral radial pulse
  - Roos stress test: patient positioning both shoulders in abduction and external rotation of 90° with elbow flexion at 90°. The patient then opens and closes hands over a period of 3 minutes. Reproduction of symptoms or a sensation of heaviness or fatigue is considered a positive test result.

▶ DIAGNOSIS

- Diagnosis is usually made clinically with the assistance of special maneuvers.
- With unclear history or physical examination findings consider:
- Laboratory:
  - To exclude systemic disease and inflammation: blood glucose level, complete blood cell (CBC) count, erythrocyte sedimentation rate (ESR), basic metabolic panel, thyrotropin level, and rheumatologic workup, if indicated
- Imaging:
  - Radiography: cervical spine, upper thoracic spine, chest, shoulder, and clavicle radiographs

- Computed tomography (CT) scanning and magnetic resonance imaging (MRI)
- Magnetic resonance angiography (MRA) for suspected arterial vascular TOS
- Venography and duplex scanning or suspected venous vascular TOS
- Electrodiagnostic studies for suspected neurogenic TOS

▶ TREATMENT

- Surgery: indicated for acute vascular insufficiency and progressive neurologic dysfunction. Anticoagulants are also used to treat acute arterial or venous occlusion.
- Nonoperative treatment: rest, nonsteroidal anti-inflammatory drugs (NSAIDs), cervicoscapular strengthening exercises, transcutaneous nerve stimulation, and biofeedback. Interscalene injection of anesthetic agents, steroids, or botulinum toxin type A (BTX-A) have also been useful.
- Physiotherapy for pain control and range of motion improvement
- Avoidance of repetitive motions, stressful lifting, and overhead work
- Prognosis:
  - Symptoms recur in 15% to 20% of patients.
  - Nerve injury is the most serious postoperative complication after thoracic outlet decompression.
  - Symptoms resolve with conservative therapy in ~90% of individuals.
  - Most patients are able to return to their previous lifestyle without difficulty.
  - Return to sports following treatment varies per person is highly dependent on the type of TOS, the presence of contributing factors, the treatment plan, the response to treatment, and the sport played.

Section A Pretest: Closed Head Injury

1. Which of the following is a component of the definition of post-concussion syndrome (PCS)?
   A. Inability to recall the events before the concussion
   B. Having signs or symptoms of neurologic deficit immediately after a traumatic force to the head
   C. Having a least one symptoms of concussion for at least 4 weeks after injury
   D. Inability to balance with eyes closed 2 weeks after an injury

2. What pathology often accompanies acute intracranial hemorrhage?
   A. Decreased intracranial pressure (ICP)
   B. Elevated ICP
   C. Hydrocephalus
   D. Ischemic stroke due to thrombosis

3. Which of the following medicine may be used to treat headache pain in the first 48 hours of concussion?
   A. Ibuprofen
   B. Naproxen
   C. Amitriptyline
   D. Acetaminophen
   E. Amantadine

4. Which of the following is classified as traumatic intracranial hemorrhage?
   A. Berry aneurysm rupture
   B. Epidural hemorrhage
   C. Scalp laceration
   D. Traumatic brain injury (TBI)

5. A 17-year-old female soccer player jumps to head a ball and makes head-to-head contact with an opponent. She falls to the ground, stands and tries to run but stumbles. She is removed from the game and evaluated with a series of questions and examination maneuvers. She notes headache and some dizziness. She insists on returning to the game. Which of the following does NOT increase the likelihood that she has a concussion?
   A. Headache
   B. Dizziness
   C. Ability to return to play
   D. Stumbling with trying to run

6. What adjunct therapy is associated with better outcomes in intracranial hemorrhage?
   A. Hyperthermic therapy
   B. Hyperventilation
   C. Hypothermic therapy
   D. Seizure prophylaxis

7. Which of the following is the most important aspect of treatment for an initial concussion?
   A. Initiate a week-long rest period
   B. Supply the patient with a medication to help treat their symptoms
   C. Ice packs to the head and neck to decrease cerebral blood flow
   D. Removal from their activity to avoid additional head trauma

Section B Pretest: Demyelinating Disorders

1. A 26-year-old male presents with fatigue and progressive bilateral lower extremity weakness over the last week following several days of nausea, vomiting, and diarrhea. Physical examination reveals decrease in deep tendon reflexes. Which of the following is the most likely diagnosis?
   A. Multiple sclerosis (MS)
   B. Myasthenia gravis

C. Guillain-Barré syndrome (GBS)
D. Huntington disease

2. Which is the most predictive factor of the progression of MS disease and subsequent disability?
   A. Patient age at presentation
   B. Patient gender
   C. Number of lesions on initial brain MRI
   D. Patient nutritional status

3. Which of the following is considered first-line treatment for patients with Guillain-Barré syndrome?
   A. High-dose corticosteroids
   B. Hemodialysis
   C. Plasma exchange
   D. Continuous positive airway pressure

4. Which of the following represents the most sensitive diagnostic test for most cases of MS?
   A. Inflammatory markers
   B. CT of the brain
   C. Lumbar puncture (LP) with CSF analysis
   D. T2-weighted MRI of the brain

5. Which of the following is correct regarding GBS?
   A. Vaccines have not been associated with developing GBS.
   B. Pain treatment with opioids is an important component of GBS management.
   C. Autonomic nervous system is not affected by GBS.
   D. Albuminocytologic dissociation supports the diagnosis.

6. Which factor is linked to an increased incidence of MS?
   A. Age <35 years
   B. Vitamin D deficiency
   C. Living in tropical regions
   D. Male gender

7. Which factor is associated with an increase incidence of GBS?
   A. *Campylobacter jejuni*
   B. Poliomyelitis
   C. Diphtheria
   D. *Borrelia burgdorferi*

8. Which symptom pattern is distinctive for the most common classification type of MS?
   A. Relapsing-remitting course progressing to steady decline
   B. Worsening neurologic function without relapse
   C. Periods of stable disability with intermittent exacerbations
   D. A single isolated episode of varying neurologic symptoms

9. Which of the following represents the most sensitive diagnostic test for most cases of GBS?
   A. LP and CSF analysis
   B. Serum inflammatory markers
   C. Gadolinium contrast MRI of the brain
   D. Serum blood culture

10. Which of the following is considered first-line treatment for acute exacerbations of MS symptoms?
    A. Methotrexate
    B. High-dose corticosteroids
    C. Vitamin D supplementation
    D. NSAIDs

11. A diagnosis of MS should be considered in a healthy 28-year-old female who presents with which of the following conditions?
    A. Amaurosis fugax
    B. Bilateral cataracts
    C. Retinal detachment
    D. Optic neuritis

Section C Pretest: Infectious Disorders

1. What pathogen is most commonly responsible for meningitis?
   A. Enterovirus
   B. *Haemophilus influenzae*
   C. *Streptococcus pneumoniae*
   D. West Nile virus

2. What pathogen is most commonly responsible for encephalitis?
   A. Coxsackievirus A
   B. Enterovirus
   C. Herpes simplex virus (HSV)
   D. Varicella zoster virus

3. What physical examination finding would necessitate a CT be performed before LP?
   A. Brudzinski positive
   B. Hypotension
   C. Kernig positive
   D. Papilledema

4. What CSF findings are expected in a patient with encephalitis?
   A. Lymphocyte-predominant pleocytosis, elevated glucose, normal protein
   B. Lymphocyte-predominant pleocytosis, normal glucose, elevated protein

C. Neutrophil-dominant pleocytosis, elevated glucose, normal protein

D. Neutrophil-dominant pleocytosis, normal glucose, elevated protein

5. Following a close exposure, what is the most appropriate chemoprophylaxis for family members living with a patient diagnosed with bacterial meningitis?
   A. Ampicillin
   B. Cefotaxime
   C. Ciprofloxacin
   D. Rifampin

Section D Pretest: Movement Disorders

1. A 33-year-old woman presents with strange dance-like movements of her hands that she has noticed over the past year. She also reports some mild changes in memory and increasing irritability during this time period. Her father died in his early 50s from a motor vehicle accident and experienced similar symptoms. What is the most likely diagnosis in this patient?
   A. Amyotrophic lateral sclerosis
   B. Tourette syndrome (TS)
   C. Huntington disease
   D. Myasthenia gravis

2. Which age group is typically affected by tics?
   A. 0-15
   B. 15-20
   C. 40-60
   D. 60-80

3. A patient is being evaluated for chorea and dementia. The patient's father had similar symptoms and died at age 55. Which test is most appropriate to confirm a diagnosis of Huntington disease?
   A. PET scan
   B. MRI
   C. CT
   D. Genetic testing

4. Which of the following is the first-line pharmacologic treatment for essential tremor?
   A. Levodopa
   B. Botulinum toxin injections
   C. Propanolol
   D. Alcohol

5. A patient with Huntington disease currently on no medications presents with worsening chorea. Which of the following medications may help treat this disease manifestation?
   A. Pyridostigmine
   B. Sertraline
   C. Tetrabenazine
   D. Prednisone

6. What would be the first-line medication to treat the bradykinesia, rigidity, and tremor in a patient with Parkinson disease (PD)?
   A. Trospium
   B. Midodrine
   C. Carbidopa/levodopa
   D. Amantadine

7. What is the mode of inheritance for Huntington disease?
   A. Autosomal recessive
   B. Autosomal dominant
   C. X-linked recessive
   D. X-linked dominant

8. A patient with PD presents to the clinic with lightheadedness when going from sitting to standing. Blood pressure is 130/80 when seated and drops to 100/70 with standing. Her medications include carbidopa/levodopa, lisinopril, and atorvastatin. Your next step would be:
   A. Start midodrine
   B. Discontinue lisinopril
   C. Increase carbidopa/levodopa
   D. Stop atorvastatin

9. A 10-year-old girl presents with fever, chorea, and migratory joint pain. Past medical history is negative other than an untreated sore throat 4 weeks ago. An antistreptolysin O (ASO) titer was positive. What is the most likely diagnosis?
   A. Acute rheumatic fever
   B. Huntington disease
   C. Cerebral palsy
   D. Thyrotoxicosis

10. Which of the following is correct regarding essential tremor?
    A. Present with movement
    B. Present at rest
    C. Commonly unilateral
    D. Associated with gait disturbances

11. Which of the following is the most common comorbidity of patient with Tourette Syndrome?
    A. Obsessive-compulsive disorder (OCD)
    B. Conduct disorder
    C. Attention deficit hyperactivity disorder (ADHD)
    D. Oppositional defiant disorder

12. A 67-year-old woman presents to your primary care office complaining of worsening tremor in her hands. She reports an associated shaking in her voice, which is worse at the end of the day. Her mother had a similar tremor, eventually leading to an inability to write legibly, and the patient is concerned it could be the same thing. On physical examination, you notice a tremor that is localized to her hands and only present when she tried to complete a task. It is not present at rest. Which of the following is the most likely diagnosis?
    A. Essential tremor
    B. Parkinson's Disease
    C. Alcohol withdrawal
    D. Anxiety

13. Which of the following is a defining diagnostic clue for TS from other hyperkinetic movement disorders?
    A. Ability to temporarily voluntarily suppress movement or vocalization
    B. Repetitive, stereotyped movement or vocalization
    C. Lack of awareness of urge to perform movement or vocalization
    D. Varying severity and periods of waxing and waning

14. Which of the following ages is a common time for the presentation of essential tremor?
    A. Before age 18
    B. People in their 30s
    C. Between 45 and 55 years
    D. After age 70

15. What is the first-line treatment in patients with TS and tics that cause psychological, social, physical, or other functional problems?
    A. Counseling and Supportive Care Only
    B. Guanfacine
    C. Clonidine
    D. Habit Reversal Training

Section E Pretest: Neurocognitive Disorders

1. A 72-year-old woman comes to your office for her annual physical. Her daughter reports that her mom had been doing fine until a few weeks ago when her mom's memory ability to remember new information abruptly worsened. Her speech is unchanged, and she has no motor deficits. Which is the most likely cause of her new dementia?
    A. Alzheimer disease
    B. Dementia with Lewy bodies
    C. Frontotemporal dementia
    D. Vascular Dementia

2. Which of the following is the most likely cause of delirium in an elderly patient?
    A. Myocardial infarction
    B. Urinary tract infection
    C. Stroke
    D. Diabetic ketoacidosis

3. A diagnosis of dementia cannot be made until which of the following have been ruled out?
    A. Presence of *APOE4* gene
    B. Depression
    C. Hyperthyroidism
    D. Vitamin B6 deficiency

4. Why should a clinician order a comprehensive metabolic profile in a patient with delirium?
    A. To evaluate possible diabetic ketoacidosis
    B. To identify an underlying metabolic derangement
    C. Hyperkalemia is common in patients with delirium
    D. To assess for vitamin deficiencies

5. Which of the following medications is indicated in moderate-to-severe Alzheimer disease?
    A. Antidepressants such as trazodone
    B. Antipsychotics such as quetiapine
    C. Cholinesterase inhibitors such as donepezil
    D. NMDA receptor antagonists such as memantine

6. What is the prevalence of delirium in the intensive care unit?
    A. 10%
    B. 25%
    C. 50%
    D. 100%

7. Which of the following is a dementia mimic?
    A. Huntington disease
    B. Normal pressure hydrocephalus
    C. PD dementia
    D. Vascular dementia

8. Which of the following medications is potentially useful to treat agitation in acute delirium?
   A. Fluoxetine
   B. Lorazepam
   C. Zolpidem
   D. Haloperidol

9. Which of the following is the most common presentation of Alzheimer disease?
   A. A patient comes to the office and reports he got lost while driving home from work.

   B. A patient comes to the office complaining of memory loss.
   C. A patient is brought to the office by her husband who reports her memory loss.
   D. A patient is brought to the office by her husband who reports her speech has changed.

Section F Pretest: Peripheral Nerve Disorders

1. A 35-year-old administrative assistant presents with paresthesias in the first three digits and radial aspect of the fourth digit in her right hand that awaken her from sleep. On examination, mild atrophy of the thenar muscles in the right hand is noted. What is the most likely diagnosis?
   A. Cubital tunnel syndrome
   B. Carpal tunnel syndrome
   C. Radial mononeuropathy
   D. de Quervain tenosynovitis

2. A 52-year-old man presents with low back pain (LBP), radiating pain from his left thigh to beyond his knee, sensation decreased in the medial left calf, 3/5 strength in knee extension and ankle dorsiflexion, and patellar reflex is 1+. What nerve root is likely affected?
   A. L2
   B. L3
   C. L4
   D. L5

3. Which of the following is true regarding myelopathy?
   A. Spinal nerve roots are compromised in myelopathy.
   B. Most patients can be managed with conservative therapies.
   C. A common presenting symptom includes pain in one extremity.
   D. Patients will often present with gait disturbances and numbness and clumsiness of the hands.

4. An MRI reveals a C6-7 disc herniation compromising the C7 nerve root on the right. What are the correlating symptoms and examination findings for a C7 radiculopathy?
   A. Bilateral shoulder pain with normal muscle strength and no changes in sensation

   B. Right shoulder and arm pain, tingling sensations in lateral forearm; 3/5 strength right wrist extension, and 1+ biceps and brachioradialis reflex
   C. Right shoulder and arm pain, tingling sensations in right middle finger; 3/5 strength right triceps and wrist flexion and 1+ triceps reflex
   D. Right shoulder and arm pain; decreased sensation lateral arm; 2/5 strength in right deltoid and biceps and 1+ biceps reflex

5. Which of the following patients with peripheral neuropathy would most likely warrant referral to a neurologist?
   A. A patient with an asymmetric, non–length-dependent neuropathy
   B. A patient with sensory-predominant symptoms
   C. A patient with a length-dependent, symmetric symptoms
   D. A patient with a slow and gradual onset of symptoms over the past 6 months

6. What is the recommended initial management for suspected cervical radiculopathy symptoms <1-month duration and no history of trauma?
   A. MRI of C-spine with contrast to confirm diagnosis
   B. CT scan of C-spine to rule out fracture
   C. Prompt referral to spine surgeon for surgical intervention
   D. NSAIDs and physical therapy for traction modalities

7. A 47-year-old woman with a 15-year history of type 2 diabetes presents with new complaints of burning pain in the toes that has ascended into her feet over the past several months. She has experienced difficulty falling asleep as the presence of her bedsheets aggravates the

pain. Physical examination reveals absent Achilles reflexes and decreased sensation to light-touch in the bilateral feet. In addition to controlling her diabetes, what medication class would be most appropriate to address this patient's symptoms?
A. Tricyclic antidepressant (TCA)
B. Selective serotonin reuptake inhibitor
C. Steroids
D. Opiates

8. A 25-year-old male presents to the emergency department (ED) with ascending limb weakness and numbness that have progressed over the past 7 days. Initially, the problem was confined to the lower extremities, but now his upper extremities are also affected and today he has developed shortness of breath. His past medical history is significant for a diarrheal illness 1 month ago. Examination reveals diaphoresis, inability to fully close his eyes, diffuse and bilateral weakness and sensory loss in the proximal and distal upper and lower extremities, and globally absent reflexes. Given the most likely diagnosis, what is the most appropriate treatment?
A. Discharge the patient on oral steroids.
B. Administer thrombolytics.
C. Admit the patient and administer intravenous immunoglobulin.
D. Prescribe gabapentin and discharge the patient with a physical therapy consult.

9. Which of the following is true regarding cervical radiculopathy?
A. The most common etiology of radiculopathy in younger patients is spondylosis.
B. The C6 and C7 nerve roots are most commonly affected.
C. Common presenting symptoms include pain in the upper and lower extremities.
D. Most patients will require surgical intervention for cervical radiculopathy.

10. Which of the following signs on physical examination may point to a central rather than peripheral cause of sensory loss?
A. Decreased reflexes
B. Atrophy
C. Weakness
D. Increased tone

Section G Pretest: Primary Headaches

1. Which of the following is the most common type of primary headache?
A. Tension
B. Cluster
C. Migraine
D. Acephalic migraine

2. Which of the following is the first-line pharmacologic treatment for migraine headaches?
A. Triptans
B. Aspirin
C. NSAIDs
D. 100% oxygen

3. Which of the following is true regarding cluster headaches?
A. They are bilateral.
B. They are induced by bright lights.
C. They may be increased during times of stress.
D. There is no effective treatment.

4. A 27-year-old man who presents to your primary care office is complaining of worsening headaches over the last week that are so severe that they limit his activities of daily living. He reports that he has had headaches for several years and assumed that they were migraines. They occur daily for several days to weeks and then resolve. They tend to occur when he is under stress. Nothing seems to alleviate the pain, although resting helps. The headaches are localized to his right eye and temple and are associated with eye watering and rhinorrhea. He denies change in vision or cognition. Which of the following is the most likely diagnosis?
A. Migraine
B. Tension-type headache
C. Cluster headache
D. Acephalic migraine

5. Which of the following is true regarding migraines?
A. They are caused by vascular constriction.
B. Those with aura are at increased risk for cardiovascular disease.
C. They have the same pathophysiology as cluster headaches.
D. They are differentiated from tension headaches by level of severity and disability to the patient.

Section H Pretest: Seizure Disorders

1. A 30-year-old female with no past medical history presents to the ED with history of "whole body shaking." She then passed out. She is currently unconscious, but vital signs are stable. Blood sugar is 450. Which of the following is the most likely diagnosis for her neurologic condition?
   A. Epilepsy
   B. Seizure
   C. Conversion disorder
   D. Munchausen by proxy
   E. Aura

2. A patient presents with new-onset seizure-like activity. Which of the following would NOT be a part of the normal workup?
   A. Toxicology screen/drug panel
   B. CBC/BMP
   C. UA/urine hcg
   D. CT of the head
   E. Electromyelogram (EMG)

3. What is the most common etiology for seizures?
   A. Fever
   B. Trauma
   C. Tumor
   D. Idiopathic
   E. Hyperglycemia

4. A patient with known epilepsy seizes continuously for 30 minutes and is turning blue. You administer oxygen and immediately give a benzodiazepine. Why is the most important reason to administer this in this circumstance?
   A. You need them to calm down for intubation.

   B. They are having a panic attack and you want to stop it.
   C. This is status epilepticus and a neurologic emergency.
   D. Stopping delirium tremens is of utmost importance.
   E. That is not the correct medication to give.

5. A 35-year-old patient with no PMH except for known epilepsy seizes and goes flaccid on his left side. Family from out of country has flown in for the weekend and has not seen him seize before. They ask what this is called with him going flaccid. You state that most likely this is which of the following?
   A. Idiopathic
   B. Ischemic stroke
   C. Todd paralysis
   D. Hemiplegic migraine
   E. MS exacerbation

6. A 3-year-old baby presents to the ED with a seizure per family. He has an acute otitis media and a fever of 104.2 °F. The family wants him admitted for further workup. You advise the family with which of the following?
   A. You are correct. We will admit him.
   B. We need further workup before making a definitive disposition.
   C. There is no need. This is just a febrile seizure with a known etiology.
   D. We need to keep monitoring him in the ED because the cause is idiopathic.
   E. After giving an IM dose of antiseizure medications, we will discharge him home.

Section I Pretest: Vascular Disorders

1. A 58-year-old female presents with sudden-onset, focal neurologic deficits of right upper extremity weakness and facial droop. Which of the following is the most appropriate initial diagnostic study?
   A. MRI
   B. CT
   C. Electroencephalography (EEG)
   D. LP

2. Which medication is used as treatment for complex regional pain syndrome?
   A. Gabapentin
   B. Cyclobenzaprine
   C. Sertraline
   D. Acetaminophen

3. Which of the following is a risk factor for subarachnoid hemorrhage (SAH)?
   A. Type 1 diabetes mellitus
   B. Collagen vascular diseases
   C. Hypothyroidism
   D. Cluster headaches

4. About how many Americans suffer a cerebrovascular accident (CVA) each year?
   A. 700 000
   B. 1.8 million
   C. 200 000
   D. 50 000

5. The description the patient gives of the headache associated with SAH is which of the following?
   A. A headache that is like being stabbed in the right eye with an icepick
   B. A headache that is on the right side of the head and is associated with visual changes
   C. A headache over the whole head that is associated with photophobia and nausea
   D. A headache that arose slowly and is like a hatband fitted around the head.

6. What are the most common brain tumors in adults?
   A. Meningiomas
   B. Glial tumors
   C. Brain metastases
   D. Schwannomas

7. What is the definitive treatment for SAH?
   A. Neurosurgery to clip or coil the aneurysm
   B. Nimodipine to stop vasospasm
   C. Seizure prophylaxis to prevent hypoxemia
   D. Watchful waiting with the patient in a neurocritical care unit

8. Which of the following terms describes pain to nonpainful stimuli?
   A. Allodynia
   B. Dystonia
   C. Hyperalgesia
   D. Causalgia

9. Which statement is correct with regards to central nervous system tumors in children?
   A. More common in African Americans
   B. More common in females
   C. More common in Asian/Pacific Islanders
   D. The least common solid tumor

10. Which of the following is considered an important reversible cause of transient ischemic attacks (TIAs) and CVAs that should be addressed adequately if found?
    A. Inflammatory bowel disease
    B. Carotid artery stenosis
    C. Atrial fibrillation
    D. Two of the above
    E. None of the above

11. Which of the following are the most common brain tumor in children?
    A. Astrocytic tumors
    B. Ependymal tumors
    C. Meningiomas
    D. Medulloblastomas

12. A 57-year-old female presents with pain in her right arm for 1 week. The patient denies any trauma to this extremity; however, she does admit to a carpal tunnel release surgery 2 months before the start of her pain. She denies any neck or back pain. She describes the pain as deep, burning, and throbbing. She also reports her arm is extremely sensitive to touch and appears more swollen than her left arm. Physical examination reveals a slightly cyanotic, mottled right arm with generalized pain of the entire extremity. Pulses are intact (2+) and ROM is limited. Neurologic examination is normal. Radiographs obtained of the right arm and hand are normal. What is the most likely diagnosis?
    A. Cervical radiculopathy
    B. Peripheral vascular disease
    C. Carpal tunnel syndrome
    D. Complex regional pain syndrome

13. Which of the following errors lead to missed diagnosis of SAH?
    A. Neuroradiologists call too many findings SAH in error.
    B. Provider believes that an LP is indicated in all potential SAH cases.
    C. Provider believes that patient does not look unwell enough to have SAH.
    D. Provider believes that the headache is too severe to be an SAH.

14. Increased hair growth of the affected limb found in a patient with complex regional pain syndrome is an example of what type of change?
    A. Vasomotor
    B. Sudomotor
    C. Motor
    D. Trophic

15. The most common cause(s) of a CN IV palsy is/are?
    A. Head trauma
    B. Intracranial hemorrhage
    C. Congenital CN IV palsy
    D. Both A and C

16. Which of the following patients is more likely to develop complex regional pain syndrome?
    A. 10-year-old boy who fractured his clavicle
    B. 62-year-old female with a Colles fracture
    C. 37-year-old male who sprained his ankle playing basketball
    D. 25-year-old male after a recent anterior cruciate ligament repair

17. In a patient experiencing an ischemic CVA for 1 hour who has no contraindications, which of the following is the treatment of choice?
    A. Bed rest
    B. Heparin and Coumadin
    C. Aspirin 325 mg PO
    D. IV tissue plasminogen activator (tPA)

18. A 35-year-old obese female presents to the ED complaining of new-onset binocular horizontal diplopia, a headache that is worse when she is lying flat, and blurred vision. MRI shows signs of increased pressure in the brain, and LP has an opening pressure of 40 cm H_2O. Based on the suspected diagnosis, what CN is most likely responsible for her diplopia?
    A. Abducens nerve
    B. Oculomotor nerve
    C. Trochlear nerve
    D. Trigeminal nerve

19. Which of the following most accurately describes one of the main differences between a cerebral vascular accident (CVA) and a transient ischemic attack (TIA)?
    A. CVAs do not cause any permanent neurologic injury.
    B. TIAs always reveal abnormalities on a CT scan of the head.
    C. Symptoms of a TIA last <24 hours.
    D. CVAs are always preceded by TIAs.

20. A 40-year-old female with a history of a pituitary adenoma presents to the ED with a severe headache "worst headache of her life" and altered consciousness. On examination, you note ophthalmoplegia and facial hypoesthesia, the lesion localizes to the cavernous sinus, and there is a concern for pituitary apoplexy. What is the initial imaging modality recommended?
    A. MRI of the brain with and without contrast
    B. CT of the head without contrast
    C. CTA of the head and neck with and without contrast
    D. Catheter angiogram

21. Which one of the CNs that is responsible for controlling eye movements is the most commonly injured?
    A. Oculomotor nerve
    B. Trochlear nerve
    C. Abducens nerve
    D. Optic nerve

22. A 55-year-old female with a recent history of a fall resulting in head trauma presents to your clinic complaining of vertical binocular diplopia that is resolved when she closes either eye. You suspect that she has a traumatic right fourth nerve palsy. On examination,

what field of gaze would you expect her diplopia would be worse?
    A. Left gaze and right head tilt
    B. Right gaze and left head tilt
    C. Right gaze
    D. Her diplopia will be equal in all fields of gaze.

▶ ANSWERS AND EXPLANATIONS TO SECTION A PRETEST

1. **C.** PCS is generally defined as having at least one symptom for at least 4 weeks after a head injury. Answer A is incorrect as this is the definition of retrograde amnesia. Answer B is incorrect as this is the definition of a concussion. Answer D is incorrect as most often 4 weeks is used as the cutoff for PCs.

2. **B.** Increased ICP due to hemorrhage and swelling often accompanies traumatic intracranial hemorrhage. Hydrocephalus may occur later in the course of the recovery but is not an acute finding. Ischemic stroke is unrelated to intracranial hemorrhage.

3. **D.** Acetaminophen should be recommended over NSAIDs for acute headache in the first 48 hours due to the theoretical increased risk of bleeding caused by NSAIDs. Answers A and B are incorrect as they are NSAIDs. Answer C is incorrect as TCAs are considered in the treatment of HA for PCS, not in the acute phase. Answer E is incorrect as amantadine may be considered for cognitive deficits in PCS. It does not have a role in treatment of acute headache.

4. **B.** Although TBI often accompanies intracranial hemorrhage, patients can suffer TBI without having a bleed. Berry aneurysm rupture is considered a hemorrhagic stroke.

5. **C.** Although some athletes may be able to return to play, this is not related to the diagnosis of concussion. Answers A and B are incorrect because those are symptoms that may be present with a concussion. Answer D is incorrect because motor instability after a head injury is a sign that a concussion may be present. Seeing this should increase the index of suspicion for this injury.

6. **D.** Seizure prophylaxis with an antiepileptic drug is the only listed strategy that has improved outcomes in patients with traumatic intracranial hemorrhage. Decreased CO_2 (hypocarbia) was thought to help prevent cerebral edema for a period of time and so patients were previously hyperventilated; however, this has been shown of no benefit and can cause cerebral vasoconstriction.

7. **D.** The most important first step in the management of concussion is removal from the activity to help decrease the risk of subsequent injury. Answer A is incorrect because a full week of mental and physical rest may not be needed. Answer B is incorrect because although a medicine may be needed for symptoms,

after removing them from play, a history and physical examination should be performed. Answer C is incorrect as there is currently no evidence to support cold packs in the initial treatment of concussion.

▶ ANSWERS AND EXPLANATIONS TO SECTION B PRETEST

1. **C.** GBS is the most likely diagnosis.
2. **C.** Number of lesions on initial brain MRI is the most predictive factor of the progression of MS disease and subsequent disability.
3. **C.** Plasma exchange is considered first-line treatment for patients with GBS.
4. **D.** T2-weighted MRI of the brain represents the most sensitive diagnostic test for most cases of MS.
5. **D.** Albuminocytologic dissociation supports the diagnosis of GBS.
6. **B.** Vitamin D deficiency is linked to an increased incidence of MS.
7. **A.** *C. jejuni* is associated with an increase incidence of GBS.
8. **C.** Periods of stable disability with intermittent exacerbations are distinctive for the most common classification type of MS.
9. **A.** LP and CSF analysis is the most sensitive diagnostic test for most cases of GBS.
10. **B.** High-dose corticosteroids are considered first-line treatment for acute exacerbations of MS symptoms.
11. **D.** A diagnosis of MS should be considered in a healthy 28-year-old female who presents with optic neuritis.

▶ ANSWERS AND EXPLANATIONS TO SECTION C PRETEST

1. **A.** Enterovirus is most commonly responsible for meningitis.
2. **C.** HSV is most commonly responsible for encephalitis.
3. **D.** Papilledema would necessitate a CT be performed before LP.
4. **B.** Lymphocyte-predominant pleocytosis, normal glucose, and elevated protein are expected in a patient with encephalitis.
5. **C.** Ciprofloxacin is the most appropriate chemoprophylaxis for family members living with a patient diagnosed with bacterial meningitis.

▶ ANSWERS AND EXPLANATIONS TO SECTION D PRETEST

1. **C.** This patient most likely has Huntington disease, an inherited movement disorder associated with a triad of motor, behavioral, and cognitive dysfunction. Patients with myasthenia gravis, amyotrophic lateral sclerosis, or TS typically do not display chorea.
2. **A.** Symptoms in TS are first noticed between the ages of 2 and 15 years, but typically occur by age 11. Severity of the tics peaks between the ages of 10 and 12 years, followed by improvement during adolescent years and adulthood.
3. **D.** Genetic testing is the most appropriate way to confirm the diagnosis in patients with a family history of Huntington disease. Neuroimaging may help support the diagnosis or rule out other differentials but is no longer used for confirmatory purposes.
4. **C.** Propanolol is the first-line pharmacologic treatment for essential tremor.
5. **C.** Tetrabenazine and other dopamine depleting or blocking medications can help treat chorea in patients with Huntington disease. Sertraline and other selective serotonin reuptake inhibitors may be indicated to treat depression, but not chorea, in Huntington disease.
6. **C.** Carbidopa/levodopa is used to treat bradykinesia, rigidity, and tremor. Trospium is used for urinary incontinence in PD, midodrine is second line for treating orthostatic hypotension if medication adjustment is not successful, and amantadine treats dyskinesias from levodopa.
7. **B.** Huntington disease is transmitted in an autosomal dominant manner.
8. **B.** Discontinue Lisinopril. The first step in treating orthostatic hypotension in a Parkinson patient is to decrease or discontinue antihypertensives.
9. **A.** This patient most likely has acute rheumatic fever. Sydenham chorea is an important potential etiology of chorea and should be considered in children with evidence of prior group A streptococcal (GAS) infection. The patient also has migratory joint pain and fever, which can support a diagnosis of acute rheumatic fever.
10. **A.** Essential tremor is present with movement.
11. **C.** The most common comorbidities in TS include ADHD (occurring in ~60%) and OCD (occurring in ~27%).
12. **A.** Essential tremor is this patient's most likely diagnosis.
13. **A.** The ability to temporarily voluntarily suppress tics and premonitory symptoms that precede tics are hallmark features that differentiate TS from other hyperkinetic movement disorders. Although tics in TS are repetitive, stereotyped, and can vary in severity with periods of waxing and waning, these are not defining features from other hyperkinetic disorders. Patients are often aware of the urge to perform movements or vocalizations as they experience premonitory symptoms.
14. **D.** A common time for the presentation of essential tremor is after age 70.
15. **D.** Habit Reversal Training (with Comprehensive Behavioral Intervention for Tics) is indicated in patients with TS and tics that cause psychological, social,

physical, or other functional problems. Guanfacine and clonidine are the only two Food and Drug Administration (FDA)–approved pharmacologic agents for TS and ADHD. Counseling and supportive care is only indicated for patients with mild cases of TS with completely nondisabling tics.

▶ ANSWERS AND EXPLANATIONS TO SECTION E PRETEST

1. **D.** Vascular dementia is the most likely cause of her new dementia.
2. **B.** Urinary tract infection is the most likely cause of delirium in an elderly patient.
3. **B.** A diagnosis of dementia cannot be made until depression has been ruled out.
4. **B.** A clinician should order a comprehensive metabolic profile in a patient with delirium to identify an underlying metabolic derangement.
5. **D.** NMDA receptor antagonists such as memantine are indicated in moderate-to-severe Alzheimer disease.
6. **C.** The prevalence of delirium in the intensive care unit is 50%.
7. **B.** Normal pressure hydrocephalus is a dementia mimic.
8. **D.** Haloperidol is potentially useful to treat agitation in acute delirium.
9. **C.** The most common presentation of Alzheimer disease is a patient brought to the office by her husband who reports her memory loss.

▶ ANSWERS AND EXPLANATIONS TO SECTION F PRETEST

1. **B.** This patient presents with neuropathic symptoms that match the distribution of the medial nerve and are consistent with carpal tunnel syndrome. The patterns of motor and sensory dysfunction in cubital tunnel syndrome and radial mononeuropathy do not match this presentation.
2. **C.** L4 radiculopathy will present with pain in the anterior thigh and anterior tibial region; sensation changes in the medial calf and foot; and decreased strength in knee extension and ankle dorsiflexion. The patellar reflex is hyporeflexic in an L4 radiculopathy.
3. **D.** Patients with myelopathy often present with the complaint of difficulty ambulating and numbness in the hands. More than one extremity is affected in most cases of myelopathy. The spinal cord is compressed in myelopathy, and a prompt referral to a spine surgeon is necessary to prevent progressive neurologic deterioration.
4. **C.** C7 radiculopathy will present with pain in the neck, shoulder, and middle finger; sensation changes in the palm, index and middle fingers; and decreased

strength in wrist flexion, finger extension, and triceps. The triceps reflex is hyporeflexic in a C7 radiculopathy.
5. **A.** Referral to neurology and electrodiagnostic studies are vital in patients with acute or subacute neuropathies, rapidly progressive symptoms, motor or autonomic predominant neuropathies, asymmetric or non–length-dependent neuropathies, hereditary neuropathies, and severe or disabling neuropathies.
6. **D.** Most cervical radiculopathies are self-limited and can be treated with conservative measures. Medications include NSAIDs, acetaminophen, or an appropriate dose narcotic if patient has moderate-to-severe pain. Imaging is not indicated for symptoms <2 months and no history of injury. Referral to a spine surgeon is warranted in the presence of trauma or if symptoms persist >2 months with adequate conservative treatment.
7. **A.** This patient most likely has distal symmetric polyneuropathy secondary to diabetes. First-line medications for neuropathic pain include the anticonvulsants gabapentin and pregabalin, TCAs, and serotonin norepinephrine reuptake inhibitors. In this case, a TCA would be a reasonable, given the comorbid insomnia.
8. **C.** This presentation is consistent with a diagnosis of GBS. The patient presents with symmetric, ascending weakness, sensory loss, areflexia, and concern for involvement of the CNs and respiratory muscles. The appropriate treatment would be admission, intravenous immunoglobulin or plasma exchange, and monitoring the patients for respiratory failure, dysautonomia, and cardiac arrhythmias.
9. **B.** The C6 and C7 nerve roots are most commonly affected in cervical radiculopathies. Herniated discs are the most common cause of cervical radiculopathies in younger patients. Common presented symptoms include pain in one arm with or without sensation changes. Most cases are managed with conservative therapies and are self-limited.
10. **D.** Signs such as hyperreflexia or increased tone may be evidence of a central rather peripheral cause of sensory or motor abnormalities. Weakness and sensory complaints may be caused by central or peripheral nervous system dysfunction, so weakness alone cannot differentiate between a central or peripheral cause.

▶ ANSWERS AND EXPLANATIONS TO SECTION G PRETEST

1. **A.** Tension is the most common type of primary headache.
2. **C.** NSAIDs are the first-line pharmacologic treatment for migraine headaches.
3. **C.** Cluster headaches may be increased during times of stress.
4. **C.** Cluster headache is the most likely diagnosis.

5. **B.** Those with aura are at increased risk for cardio-vascular disease.

ANSWERS AND EXPLANATIONS TO SECTION H PRETEST

1. **B.** Seizure is the most likely diagnosis for her neurologic condition. While seizures and/or epilepsy can be considered in the differential diagnosis, the likely diagnosis here is new-onset diabetes.
2. **E.** If any ancillary testing would be done, it should be an EMG.
3. **D.** Most seizures (>50%) are idiopathic.
4. **C.** This is status epilepticus and a neurologic emergency. If they are seizing with a known seizure disorder, the likely cause is not a panic attack. Although a benzodiazepine can stop a panic attack, it is also an indication in patients with status epilepticus to stop those as well. That is most likely what this is.
5. **C.** Todd paralysis is the name for this phenomenon. It usually resolves on its own spontaneously but is a postictal finding in some patients with seizures, often confused as a stroke.
6. **C.** A febrile seizure is the likely cause here. Although these can recur, the likelihood is that patients who have these may never have them again, though do carry a risk for seizures later in adult life if you suffer these as a child.

ANSWERS AND EXPLANATIONS TO SECTION I PRETEST

1. **B.** Anytime CVA is suspected as a possible diagnosis, a CT scan of the head without contrast should be ordered immediately and ideally performed within 25 minutes of arrival.
2. **A.** Gabapentin is used as treatment for complex regional pain syndrome.
3. **B.** Collagen vascular disease is a risk factor for SAH.
4. **A.** Each year in the United States, 700 000 individuals suffer CVA. Roughly 500 000 of these are experiencing their first CVA, whereas 200 000 are experiencing a subsequent attack.
5. **C.** A patient with SAH describes the headache as over the whole head and associated with photophobia and nausea.
6. **C.** The most common brain tumors in adults are brain metastases.
7. **A.** The definitive treatment for SAH is neurosurgery to clip or coil the aneurysm.
8. **A.** Allodynia describes pain to nonpainful stimuli.
9. **C.** Tumors in children are more common in those of Caucasian and of Asian/Pacific Island ethnicity.
10. **D.** Atrial fibrillation and carotid artery stenosis are both fairly common causes of embolic stroke. If discovered in diagnostic valuation of someone who has experienced a CVA or TIA, these should be adequately treated to prevent another event.
11. **A.** The most common brain tumors in children are astrocytic tumors.
12. **D.** Complex regional pain syndrome is the most likely diagnosis.
13. **C.** When a provider believes that a patient does not look unwell enough to have SAH, this leads to misdiagnosis.
14. **D.** Increased hair growth of the affected limb found in a patient with complex regional pain syndrome is an example of trophic change.
15. **D.** Head trauma and congenital CN IV palsy are the most common causes.
16. **B.** A 62-year-old female with a Colles fracture is more likely to develop complex regional pain syndrome.
17. **D.** If there are no contraindications to administration of IV tPA, this is the treatment of choice for a person experiencing an ischemic CVA of <3 hours (4.5 hours in some circumstances). Contraindications are common, however, and the next best treatment would be aspirin.
18. **A.** The abducens nerve is most likely responsible for her diplopia (most common cause of a CN VI palsy is from increased ICP caused by a mass, edema, or hemorrhage or is microvascular).
19. **C.** TIAs produce symptoms that last <24 hours. If symptoms and neurologic injury last >24 hours, it is a CVA and results in permanent neurologic injury. CVAs are not always preceded by TIAs, although TIAs should be considered a warning that a CVA could occur soon.
20. **B.** CT of the head without contrast is the initial imaging modality recommended.
21. **C.** The abducens nerve is the most commonly injured CN.
22. **A.** Left gaze and right head tilt would be worse (sensorimotor examination will be notable for a hypertropia in the affected eye that is worse in the contralateral gaze and in the ipsilateral head tilt).

CHAPTER 271

Concussion and Post-Concussion Syndrome

Christopher Miles, MD

A 17-year-old female soccer player jumps to head a ball and makes head-to-head contact with an opponent. She falls to the ground, stands and tries to run but stumbles. She is removed from the game and evaluated with a series of questions and examination maneuvers. She notes headache and some dizziness. She insists on returning to the game.

▶ GENERAL FEATURES

- Concussions occur from a direct blow to the head, a rotational force of the head, or force to another area of the body that causes head acceleration/deceleration.
- Cause an alteration of the function of the neurons (not structure), leading to deficit in one or more neurologic faculties. These deficits generally resolve spontaneously.
- Loss of consciousness may occur, but is not required to diagnose a concussion.
- ~90% of sport-related concussions (SRCs) are resolved by 14 days.
- Post-concussion syndrome (PCS) is defined as at least one symptom from concussion present for at least 4 weeks.
- Concussion and PCS are considered neuropsychiatric conditions.

▶ CLINICAL ASSESSMENT

- Suspect concussion in anyone who has sustained a blow to the head or a force to the body, causing rapid head position change with symptoms or sign of neurologic deficit.
- Patients may note or providers may identify concussive symptoms from the following domains:
  - Physical: headache, dizziness, head pressure, photophobia, phonophobia, ear ringing, blurred or double vision, fatigue, nausea/vomiting, or not feeling "right"
  - Cognitive: amnesia, difficulty remembering, confusion, disorientation, feeling in a fog, feeling slowed down, inability to focus or concentrate, or feeling stunned

  - Emotional: sadness, anxiety, nervousness, irritability, emotional lability, anger, crying
    - Signs may include stumbling or poor balance, poor testing on memory or concentration, slurred speech, dazed appearance or staring, eye tracking difficulties, nystagmus, pupillary changes, loss of consciousness, or just not acting normally.
- Sport Concussion Assessment Tool (SCAT5), Balance Error Scoring System (BESS), and Vestibulo-Occular Motor Screening (VOMS) yield the most comprehensive assessment for concussion.

▶ DIAGNOSIS

- Any deficits in the domains above after a contact or force should lead to the diagnosis of concussion.
- Imaging is not necessary for the diagnosis of concussion, but should be considered to rule out more severe injury with:
  - Loss of consciousness, vomiting, worsening of symptoms from baseline, high-velocity trauma, Glasgow Coma Scale <15, palpable skull fracture, or significant focal neurologic deficit
- PCS is diagnosed when symptoms last >4 weeks.
- Rule out other causes of prolonged symptoms such as cervicogenic headaches (cervical spine pathology), visual disturbances, inner ear dysfunction, mood- or stress-related changes, vestibular dysfunction, or a new headache syndrome.

▶ TREATMENT

- Most important step is removal of patient from sport or other risky activity at diagnosis (or suspected injury). Data show continuing to participate on same day after injury prolongs symptoms.
- Once diagnosed, mental and physical rest for at least 48 hours should be initiated.

- Light aerobic activity with no risk of head injury after a minimum of 48 hours, if no worsening of symptoms, may be therapeutic.
- NSAIDs should be avoided in the first 48 hours. Acetaminophen can be used as needed in the first 48 hours for pain.
- Rest is important. There is no need to wake an athlete to check on symptoms.
- Once symptoms have resolved, a slow Return to Learn (RTL) and a Return to Play (RTP) should be initiated. These should incrementally reintroduce mental and physical activity in a staged sequence.
- Academic accommodations may be needed for students to RTL.
- Medications may be used to address the specific symptoms.
  - Headache may be treated with TCAs or topiramate.
  - Cognitive symptoms may be treated with amantadine.
  - Attention deficit may need stimulant medications.
- Treatment is often multidisciplinary with physical therapy, vestibular therapy, psychological therapy, and close follow-up.

Case Conclusion

Our case highlights a few key elements. Female athletes are at a higher risk of concussion than their male counterparts. This patient has both symptoms (headache and dizziness) and signs of a concussion (motor instability). Often times, despite symptoms, athletes will request or demand to return to the game. Our task is to keep any athlete with a suspected concussion out of play to minimize the risks associated with an additional head trauma.

CHAPTER 272

Traumatic Intracranial Hemorrhage

Ian Smith, MMS, PA-C, APA-C

An 86-year-old woman who fell at the nursing home presents to the emergency department with altered level of consciousness. Staff who witnessed the fall say she tripped on her walker and on the way down she hit her forehead, landing on her left side. She has a small skin tear above her left eyebrow and is confused with a Glasgow Coma score (GCS) of 13. What should be included in the differential diagnosis list as you evaluate this patient?

▶ GENERAL FEATURES

- Traumatic intracranial hemorrhage encompasses a variety of head bleeds, including intraventricular, intraparenchymal, subarachnoid, subdural, and epidural hemorrhage.
- The most common cause is falls, followed by motor vehicle collisions.
- Risk factors include men as they generally engage in more risky behavior patterns and geriatric patients as their balance and gait change.

▶ CLINICAL ASSESSMENT

- Most common presenting symptom is altered level of consciousness. Patients may also describe headache, amnesia, loss of consciousness, dizziness, blurred or double vision, nausea, and/or vomiting.
- Providers should have a high index of suspicion when patient reports a loss of consciousness, amnesia, or has altered level of consciousness on evaluation in the setting of trauma, including ground-level falls.
- Complete neurologic examination, including mental status assessment and GCS, should be performed.
- Often accompanied by traumatic brain injury and/or diffuse axonal injury, which have significantly worse outcomes.

▶ DIAGNOSIS

- Noncontrasted head CT is the mainstay of the diagnosis.
- Hyperattenuating fluid within the affected area is often the accompanying radiologic finding noted on CT evaluation of the head.
- Basic laboratory evaluation, such as a complete blood count, metabolic panel, and coagulation studies, should be obtained in preparation for urgent neurosurgical intervention.

▶ TREATMENT

- Immediate consultation with the neurosurgical service is vital.
- Treatment is centered on maintaining support for injured brain tissue.
  - Maintenance of normal blood pressure, temperature, oxygenation, coagulation profiles, as well as intracranial pressure (ICP) is vital to ensure further damage is prevented.
- In patients with decreased GCS, an ICP monitor may be required.
- Elevated ICP is treated in a step-wise manner with upright patient positioning, hypertonic saline, hyperosmolar therapy, sedatives, and chemical paralysis.

- Intervention with craniotomy or hemicraniectomy may be required if pharmacologic management is unsuccessful at preventing increased ICP.
- In addition to quality neurocritical care, adjunct therapy in traumatic intracranial hemorrhage, which has been shown to improve outcomes, includes resumption of statin therapy, seizure prophylaxis, and β-blocker therapy.

Case Conclusion

Patients with decreased GCS in a traumatic mechanism should always be considered for possible intracranial hemorrhage.

SECTION B   *Demyelinating Disorders*

CHAPTER 273   Guillain-Barré Syndrome

Catherine Shull, PA-C, MPAS

▶ GENERAL FEATURES

- Guillain-Barré syndrome (GBS) is an immune-mediated progressive paralytic, polyneuropathy involving peripheral nervous system.
- Commonly triggered by acute respiratory or gastrointestinal infections, causing nerve demyelination and axonal injury
- Causative triggers can include infections such as *Campylobacter jejuni* (about 30% cases), Epstein-Barr, *Mycoplasma pneumoniae*, *Haemophilus influenzae*, HIV, cytomegalovirus, and Zika virus.
- Occurs more often in patients with Hodgkin disease, lymphoma, systemic lupus erythematosus, after surgery/trauma, or bone marrow transplantation. Certain vaccines have triggered GBS to include H1N1 influenza and other influenza A immunizations.
- GBS subtypes: acute inflammatory demyelinating polyneuropathy (AIDP; most common), acute motor axonal neuropathy (AMAN; second most common), acute motor-sensory axonal neuropathy (AMSAN; rare), and Miller Fisher syndrome (MFS; rare)
- Affects any age (rare in <2 years old) with annual incidence of 1 or 2 of 100 000
- GBS progresses in three stages: (1) initial phase with symptom evolution lasting a few days up to 6 weeks, (2) plateau phase lasting weeks to months, and (3) recovery phase with remyelination, which can last weeks to months but, in severe cases, can last up to 2 years or more and without complete improvement.

▶ CLINICAL ASSESSMENT

- Common prodromal infection symptoms may present with fever, nasal congestion with rhinorrhea, sore throat, cough, and diarrhea.
- Majority of patients report severe and deep aching pain in the back and legs that is worse with movement. Pediatric patients may have pain before weakness.
- Ascending symmetrical weakness in lower extremities can progress and involve the upper extremities and respiratory muscles.
- Moderate-to-severe pain in muscles and joints can be seen in acute phase.
- Sensory and possible cranial nerve involvement may develop.
- Autonomic problems can accompany the presentation with orthostatic hypotension, urinary retention, and syncope.
- Physical examination signs depend upon the GBS subtype but can include flaccid muscular weakness, decreased or absent deep tendon reflexes (AMAN with hyperreflexia), decrease in light-touch sensation, cranial nerve deficits, arrhythmias, hypotension, or hypertension.

▶ DIAGNOSIS

- History and physical examination are extremely valuable in making the GBS diagnosis. Brighton criteria involving history, clinical presentation, and diagnostic testing are used to assure diagnosis and exclude mimics.

- Lumbar puncture (LP) with cerebrospinal fluid (CSF) may show increased protein by week 3 without lymphocytosis (albuminocytologic dissociation). Can also test for antibodies in CSF.
- Neuroimaging with gadolinium contrast MRI of the spine can identify nerve root enhancement, supporting diagnosis of GBS.
- Nerve conduction studies are abnormal after 2 weeks into clinical progression of GBS with specifics dependent upon subtype.

▶ TREATMENT

- Early diagnosis is critical. Hospital admission for supportive care is necessary. Mechanical ventilation may be required for respiratory failure.

- Primary treatment is immune modulation therapy involving intravenous immunoglobulin (IVIG) or plasma exchange (PLEX). Neuropathic pain treatment is important to include.
- The multidisciplinary medical team should involve specialists in neurology, pulmonology, physical therapy, occupational and speech therapy, psychology, and rehabilitation medicine.
- Clinical improvement most commonly seen in the first year. Patients <40 years have better outcomes, usually resulting in a complete recovery.

CHAPTER
274

Multiple Sclerosis

Catherine Shull, PA-C, MPAS

▶ GENERAL FEATURES

- Chronic and incurable autoimmune inflammatory disorder characterized by central nervous system (CNS) demyelination
- Unknown exact cause—possible genetic, immune mediated, and environmental influences (factors, elements)
- Classic histopathologic sign is white matter plaque formed after CNS myelin and axon destruction.
- Classification types include (1) relapsing-remitting (R-R), affecting about 85% of multiple sclerosis (MS) patients having periods of stable neurologic disability with intermittent acute exacerbation; (2) primary progressive (PP) characterized by worsening neurologic functioning without relapse; (3) secondary progressive (SP) having initial R-R progression then changing to a steady neurologic decline; and (4) clinically isolated syndrome (CIS) is a first episode of focal or multifocal neurologic decline presentation not specifically meeting all MS diagnostic criteria but having increased risk for later flares that can lead to diagnosis of MS.
- Mean age of diagnosis is 30 years old.
- R-R affects women 3:1 over men. Primary progressive affects both genders equally.
- First-degree relative risk increase is about 3%, with specific allele DRB1*1501 in HLA being primary cause. Higher incidence of MS is associated with history of cigarette smoking, vitamin D deficiency, obesity, and Epstein-Barr infection.
- Should be considered in any patient under age 50 years who has neurologic symptoms lasting for several days to weeks that spontaneously resolve

▶ CLINICAL ASSESSMENT

- Medical disorders that present similarly to MS include thyroid dysfunction, vitamin B12 deficiency, HIV infection, Lyme disease, and vasculitis. Avoid misdiagnosis with appropriate evaluation.
- Clinical presentation and course variable, but symptoms occur in specific episodes lasting >24 hours, most commonly 8 weeks, and separated by at least a month or more.
- Symptoms are determined by lesion location: most common presentations are fatigue, unilateral optic neuritis with blurred vision and eye movement pain, diplopia, vertigo, trigeminal neuralgia, facial sensation loss and motor disturbances, gait ataxia with poor balance, intentional or postural tremors, hemiparesis or sensory changes, Uhthoff phenomenon with increase in body heat worsening symptoms, Lhermitte syndrome with electrical radiation of pain down spine with cervical flexion, bladder urgency or retention, constipation, erectile dysfunction, depression, and cognitive impairment.
- Physical examination may reveal abnormalities in mental status, cranial nerves, deep tendon and plantar reflexes, sensation, motor, and cerebellar function.
- Common findings include impaired visual acuity and color vision, Marcus Gunn pupil, asymmetrical pupillary response to light, limited extraocular movements, nystagmus, dysarthria, hyperreflexia, extensor plantar response, ascending paresthesias, decrease in proprioception and vibration sense, intentional tremor, spastic muscle tone, and ataxia.

DIAGNOSIS

- Gadolinium-enhancing T2 MRI of the brain and spinal cord are the most sensitive imaging tests to diagnose R-R MS.
- Cerebrospinal fluid (CSF) may show oligoclonal banding presence (two or more).
- Other lab tests can assist in ruling out other diagnoses: CBC with differential, complete metabolic panel, vitamin B12, methylmalonic acid, ESR, CRP (inflammatory markers), TSH, ANA, HIV, RPR, and CSF analysis.
- Neurologist specializing in MS should be involved in the diagnosis of this condition.

TREATMENT

- Goals to decrease symptom severity and duration during flares and restrict disability progression for improvement in quality of life
- The number of lesions noted in the initial T2 MRI of the brain upon MS diagnosis is the most reliable predictor of disability over time. CNS oligoclonal banding presence indicates higher risk for symptomatic flares.

- Expedited and accurate diagnosis is important with early referral to neurology for initiation of disease-modifying therapy (DMT).
  - Decreases disease progression
  - Reduces relapse frequency
  - Targets inflammatory mechanism of MS but does not repair demyelination
- Relapse episode treatment involves a short course of oral or IV high-dose corticosteroids and symptom-specific treatment.
- Nonpharmacologic treatment includes occupational and physical therapy, neuropsychology, clinical psychology, speech therapy, nutrition, nursing, and social services.
- Exercise with progressive resistance training, aerobics, balance training, and stretching increase mobility and reduce fatigue.
- Cognitive-behavioral therapy and mindfulness training also improve stress, anxiety, and depression associated with MS diagnosis.
- Factors that affect mortality include diagnosis age, MS classification type, delay in starting DMTs, and the degree of disease complications.

SECTION C Infectious Disorders

CHAPTER 275 Meningitis and Encephalitis

Stephen Noe, DMS, MPAS

A 22-year-old man is brought into the emergency department for a 12-hour history of fever, chills, rhinorrhea, and headache. He recently began feeling stiffness in his neck and became concerned. Physical examination reveals an ill-appearing male who has a documented fever of 39 °C (102.2 °F). His mental status is intact, and he can flex the neck fully but with complaints of increased pain when doing so. Kernig and Brudzinski signs are negative. CSF findings reveal a neutrophil-predominant pleocytosis, elevated protein, and low glucose. In addition to dexamethasone, what is the most appropriate antimicrobial therapy?

GENERAL FEATURES

- Meningitis:
  - Inflammatory condition of the meningitis, specifically of the pia and arachnoid
  - Most common etiology in US adults hospitalized for meningitis is enterovirus (50.9%), followed by unknown etiology (18.7%), bacterial (13.9%), herpes simplex virus (HSV; 8.3%), noninfectious (3.5%), fungal (2.7%), arboviruses (1.1%), and other viruses (0.8%).

- Providers cannot reliably differentiate viral meningitis from bacterial meningitis clinically, diagnostic testing is necessary to differentiate.
- Encephalitis:
  - Neurologic emergency, which can lead to severe morbidity and mortality
  - Pathophysiology of encephalopathy is similar to viral/aseptic meningitis, where the brain is inflamed most commonly related to a viral infection; however, other etiologies include autoimmune, bacterial, and fungal infections.
  - HSV 1 is the most common viral etiology of encephalitis.
  - Though symptoms generally begin with an influenza-like presentation with fever, headache, and myalgias, patients often present much sicker appearing than aseptic meningitis and require emergent care related to mental status changes, personality changes, and seizures.

CLINICAL ASSESSMENT

- Fever, headache, neck stiffness (nuchal rigidity), and altered mental status are classic symptoms of meningitis, and a combination of two of these occurs in 95% of adults presenting with bacterial meningitis.
- Fever, seizures, or other focal neurologic deficits attributed to brain parenchyma are the classic symptoms of encephalitis, with encephalopathy symptoms of altered mental status is required.
- Patient history for both meningitis and encephalitis should focus on the patient's presenting symptoms, including fever, headache, photophobia, vomiting, the presence of seizures, the presence of neurologic symptoms, mental status changes, and/or personality changes.
- Additional history should focus on immunization status, ill community exposures, travel history, contact with animals, fresh water, mosquito, or tick bites.
- Physical examination for both meningitis and encephalitis includes a full neurologic evaluation.
  - Testing should include all cranial nerves, motor and sensory systems, and the reflexes.
  - Brudzinski sign:
    - Patient in the supine position
    - Examiner passively raises the patient's head while preventing the patient from rising.
    - Flexion of the patient's hips and knees after passive flexion of the neck is a positive Brudzinski sign.
  - Kernig sign:
    - Patient in the supine position with hips and knees in flexion
    - Examiner attempts to passively extend the patient's knee with a flexed hip.
    - In a positive sign, pain prevents full extension of knee due to inflammation of sciatic nerve.

- Must also include a general examination, with emphasis on the ears, sinuses, cardiac, and respiratory systems
- Patients with bacterial meningitis are generally more ill appearing.

DIAGNOSIS

- Mainstay of diagnosis for both meningitis and encephalitis remains the lumbar puncture (LP) with CSF analysis.
- LP must be preceded by neuroimaging (computerized tomography) to rule out herniation syndrome minimally in the following situations:
  - Focal neurologic deficits
  - Evidence of increased intracranial pressure (eg, papilledema)
  - History of CNS disease
  - Hypertension with bradycardia
  - Immunosuppression
  - Seizures
- CSF findings in aseptic/viral meningitis and encephalitis may include a slight lymphocytic pleocytosis, normal glucose, and normal to slightly elevated protein, although they may be normal.
- CSF polymerase chain reaction (PCR) testing for enterovirus, West Nile virus, HSV, and varicella zoster, when positive, may be used to halt unnecessary antibiotic use or in the setting of encephalitis.
  - Cerebrospinal fluid PCR for HSV has a sensitivity and specificity of over 95% for HSV encephalitis.
- Bacterial meningitis typically reveals a neutrophil pleocytosis, low glucose, and elevated protein.
- CSF culture is the gold standard testing for bacterial meningitis and has high yield, whereas viral PCR testing has had mixed results for viral meningitis.
- Repeat CSF testing is not necessary unless the patient is not improving 48 hours following initiation of antibiotic therapy.
- Serum diagnostic studies may include serum C-reactive protein and procalcitonin.
  - C-reactive protein has a high negative predictive value but a much lower positive predictive value.
  - Procalcitonin is sensitive (96%) and specific (89%-98%) for bacterial causes of meningitis.

TREATMENT

- Cardiovascular and hemodynamic support is initial mainstay of therapy for both meningitis and encephalitis.
- Initiate broad-spectrum empiric antibiotics after blood cultures are drawn and the LP is performed.
  - Antibiotics should not be delayed if there is any lag time in performing the LP.
  - Acyclovir is a time-critical life-saving treatment for HSV encephalitis and should be commenced before LP if this is delayed for any reason.

- Neonatal meningitis is typically caused by *Streptococcus agalactiae* (group B *Streptococcus*; GBS) and *Escherichia coli*.
- For all other ages, the majority of meningitis cases are caused by *Streptococcus pneumoniae* (pneumococcus) and *Neisseria meningitidis* (meningococcus).
- Antibiotic selection and duration of use is age-based set against the most common pathogen:
  - Infants younger than 1 month:
    - Ampicillin plus cefotaxime
  - Toddlers 1–23 months of age:
    - Vancomycin plus ceftriaxone
  - Children to adults aged 2–50 years:
    - Vancomycin plus ceftriaxone
  - Adults over 50:
    - Vancomycin plus ceftriaxone plus ampicillin
- Dexamethasone should be given before or at the time of initial antibiotics while awaiting the final culture results in all patients older than 6 weeks with suspected bacterial meningitis.
- Seizure control is commonly needed in the acute phase of encephalitis.
- Prognosis/health maintenance:
  - Neurologic sequelae following meningitis are rare in children, but may include developmental delays that may be permanent, failure to reach developmental milestones, lowered IQ/decreased academic performance, hearing loss (reversible) to deafness, seizures, and mortality.
  - Neurologic sequelae may include focal neurologic deficits, seizure disorder, cardiorespiratory failure, and mortality.
  - Many patients with encephalitis will have residual physical and neuropsychological issues and require a multidisciplinary approach to ongoing care.
  - Vaccines have decreased the incidence of meningitis include *Haemophilus influenzae* type B, *S. pneumoniae*, and *N. meningitidis*.
  - Chemoprophylaxis following close exposures is indicated and includes the use of rifampin, ceftriaxone, and ciprofloxacin, though rifampin resistance has been documented.

Case Conclusion

In this patient with CSF finding of neutrophil-predominant pleocytosis, elevated protein, and low glucose, ceftriaxone plus vancomycin is warranted in addition to dexamethasone.

SECTION D
Movement Disorders

CHAPTER 276
Huntington Disease

Carrie Smith Nold, MPA, PA-C

A 33-year-old woman presents with strange dance-like movements of her hands that she has noticed over the past year. She also reports some mild changes in memory and increasing irritability during this time period. Her father died in his early 50s from a motor vehicle accident and experienced similar symptoms.

▶ GENERAL FEATURES

- Huntington disease is a hereditary movement disorder inherited in an autosomal dominant pattern.
  - Expanding trinucleotide repeat disorder caused by an increase in the number of nucleotide (CAG) repeats in the coding sequence of the huntingtin gene on chromosome 4, which causes central nervous system damage.
  - A larger number of repeats correlates with earlier disease manifestation.
- Onset is typically between the ages of 25 and 45 years; fewer than 10% of cases are a juvenile type with onset at or before age 20 years.
- Huntington disease can occur in all ethnic groups but has a higher prevalence in Europe, North America, and Australia than Asia.

CLINICAL ASSESSMENT

- Consists of a triad of abnormal cognitive, behavioral, and motor features; symptoms typically start gradually and progress slowly over the course of the disease
- Most patients develop dementia but may have milder cognitive changes earlier in the course of the disease.
- Patients may experience irritability, depression, anxiety, obsessive-compulsive disorder, suicidal ideation, and psychosis.
- Motor symptoms include irregular and involuntary muscle jerks and body movements (chorea) and impairment of voluntary movement.
  - Patients may display motor impersistence, such as the inability to sustain tongue protrusion or keep their eyes closed.
  - Patients may attempt to incorporate the chorea into purposeful action (parakinesia).
  - Later in the course of the disease, patients may have a reduction in chorea with increasing parkinsonian features.
- In contrast to the adult type, the juvenile variant consists of bradykinesia and rigidity and may be accompanied by seizures.
- Patients may also experience gait disturbances, oculomotor dysfunction, dysarthria, and weight loss; patients can develop type 2 diabetes and other neuroendocrine abnormalities.

DIAGNOSIS

- A diagnosis of Huntington disease is strongly suspected in a patient with chorea and a family history of Huntington disease. Occasionally, there is no known family history.
- Genetic testing is the most definitive way to confirm a suspected clinical diagnosis.
  - Genetic testing also can be used in asymptomatic patients with a positive family history.
  - Genetic testing should be done with proper genetic counseling.
- Neuroimaging can help support the diagnosis and rule out alternative diagnoses.
  - CT or MRI may demonstrate cerebral atrophy or atrophy of the caudate nucleus.
  - Positron emission tomography (PET) may demonstrate reductions in striatal metabolic rate.
- Laboratory and other diagnostic studies can help exclude other medical disorders associated with chorea, including drug toxicity, Sydenham chorea, thyrotoxicosis, electrolyte disorder, and systemic lupus erythematosus.

TREATMENT

- Huntington disease has no cure. Current treatment is symptomatic, but investigations into disease-modifying and genetic treatments are ongoing.
- Chorea may be treated with dopamine-blocking or depleting agents such as tetrabenazine, deutetrabenazine, and typical and atypical antipsychotics, but treatment may cause adverse reactions, including worsening of other aspects of the disease.
  - Tetrabenazine and deutetrabenazine can cause secondary parkinsonism and depression.
  - Antipsychotics can also treat psychosis and behavioral disturbances but have the potential to cause tardive dyskinesia, neuroleptic malignant syndrome, confusion, postural hypotension, weight gain, and drowsiness.
- Patients require monitoring for mania and suicidal ideation and may require treatment of anxiety and depression.
- No medication has shown to be clearly effective to treat the dementia associated with Huntington disease.
- All patients should be referred to a neurologist; management should involve an interprofessional team.
- Depending on the disease presentation, patients may benefit from physical, occupation, or speech therapy.
- Prognosis:
  - Huntington disease is usually fatal within 15–20 years after onset.
  - Successive generations may have an expansion of trinucleotide repeats, resulting in an earlier and more severe phenotype (also known as "anticipation"); this is worse in paternal inheritance.

Case Conclusion

The patient presents with a classic example of Huntington disease, displaying the triad of cognitive, behavioral, and motor features. Additionally, the patient has an onset of symptoms in the typical range of most adults, and there is concern for a family history with her father having experienced similar symptoms. Genetic testing confirmed the diagnosis.

Parkinson Disease

Sonya Peters, PA-C

A 72-year-old male presents to the clinic with concerns of a tremor that has been present in his left hand for the past year. He recently developed a mild tremor in his right hand as well. The tremor is present when doing a task like brushing his teeth. However, it seems to be more severe when he is just resting his arms. He also describes difficulty walking and feeling unstable or off balance. His son notes that there is always a pause before his father starts to walk. Once he starts walking, he leans forward and takes small steps. The physical examination reveals a slow shuffling gait, a resting "pill-rolling" tremor (left hand worse than the right hand), and cogwheel rigidity is present on the left upper extremity. It is also noted that his voice is soft and monotone, and his speech is slow.

▶ GENERAL FEATURES

- Parkinson disease is the most common cause of parkinsonism, a syndrome manifested by rest tremor, rigidity, bradykinesia, and postural instability.
- It is a motor system disorder.
- The cause is still unknown, but the mechanism of the disorder involves degenerative loss of dopaminergic neurons in the brain.
- Typically occurs in patients aged 60 years or older, with a mean age at diagnosis of 70.5 years
- Presentation is usually asymmetric.

▶ CLINICAL ASSESSMENT

- Four cardinal features of Parkinson disease:
  - Bradykinesia
  - Rigidity (cogwheel or lead pipe rigidity), resistance to passive range of motion
  - Resting tremor
  - Postural and gait instability
- Related symptoms may include:
  - Loss of smell
  - Hypomimia (masked facial expression)
  - Writing changes: it may be harder to write and writing may appear smaller.
  - REM sleep behavior disorder
  - Insomnia
  - Depression/anxiety
  - Visual hallucinations

- Speech impairment, including palilalia (involuntary repetition of a phrase or word), hypophonia (soft speech), and hypokinetic dysarthria (slowed speech, monotony of pitch and loudness, imprecise enunciation of consonants)
- Orthostatic hypotension
- Problems with bladder control and erectile dysfunction
- Constipation
- Dysphagia (may develop with more advanced disease)
- Cognitive impairment (typically minor until late disease)

▶ DIAGNOSIS

- Diagnosis is made on clinical findings and requires the presence of two of the following four cardinal features:
  - Bradykinesia
  - Rigidity (cogwheel or lead pipe rigidity), resistance to passive range of motion
  - Resting tremor
  - Postural and gait instability
- Presentation is typically asymmetric, and there is a clear and dramatic benefit from dopaminergic therapy.
- Neuroimaging is usually nondiagnostic in the evaluation of suspected Parkinson disease, but an MRI of the brain may be performed to exclude structural abnormalities that could mimic Parkinson disease.

▶ TREATMENT

- Treat according to symptoms of the disease:
  - Bradykinesia, rigidity, and tremor:
    - Carbidopa/levodopa
    - To extend the benefit of levodopa between doses:
      - Dopamine agonists (pramipexole, ropinirole, rotigotine)
      - Monoamine oxidase type B inhibitors (selegiline, rasagiline, safinamide)
      - Catechol-O-methyltransferase inhibitors
    - To decrease levodopa-induced dyskinesias:
      - Amantadine
    - Deep brain stimulation if motor symptoms insufficiently managed with medication therapy
  - Physical therapy can help treat gait instability, constipation, dysphagia, and speech impairment.
  - Insomnia:
    - Melatonin

- Orthostatic hypotension:
  - Decrease or discontinue drugs that lower blood pressure
  - Treatment with midodrine or fludrocortisone may become necessary if medication adjustment is not therapeutic.
- Erectile dysfunction:
  - Phosphodiesterase inhibitors
- Urinary Incontinence:
  - Trospium

Case Conclusion

This is a classic example of Parkinson disease. The patient was over 60 years old and presented with initial tremor being unilateral and later involving the other limb. He had a resting tremor ("pill rolling"), bradykinesia (slow "shuffling gait"), cogwheel rigidity, hypophonia (soft speech), and hypokinetic dysarthria (slowed speech, monotony). The patient also mentioned gait instability. He has all four of the cardinal features of Parkinson disease (bradykinesia, rigidity, resting tremor, and gait instability).

CHAPTER 278
Myasthenia Gravis

Tamara S. Ritsema, PhD, MPH, PA-C/R

▶ GENERAL FEATURES

- Myasthenia gravis (MG) is caused by an autoimmune attack on the acetylcholine receptor (AChR), causing failure of signal transmission from nerve to muscle at the level of the neuromuscular junction (NMJ).
- MG is a disease of young women and older men. Infants born to women who have MG may also have transient myasthenia of the newborn. The prevalence of MG is thought to be 20–40 per 100 000 people.
- While the progressive fatiguability of muscles is nearly pathognomonic for MG, other diseases to consider include amyotrophic lateral sclerosis, multiple sclerosis, Lambert-Eaton myasthenic syndrome, statin-induced myopathy, and generalized fatigue.

▶ CLINICAL ASSESSMENT

- Patients typically complain of increasing difficulty in performing repetitive activities such as climbing stairs or chewing.
- Muscle fatiguability generally waxes and wanes.
- >50% of MG patients report some ocular symptoms, most commonly ptosis and diplopia. About 15% of people with MG solely have symptoms in the facial musculature.
- Physical examination is very helpful. Examine the patient to assess for typical patterns of weakness associated with stroke or radiculopathies. Patients with MG often are not diagnosed quickly because they either do not have weakness on examination at rest or their weakness seems to not conform to a known pathophysiologic pattern.
- It is crucial to attempt to fatigue muscles in the examination of the patient. You can ask the patient to lift a heavy textbook or purse repetitively. When the patient reaches a point of fatigue, then conduct traditional manual muscle testing to formally assess for weakness.
- Another approach to provoking fatigue is to ask the patient to hold arms out parallel to the floor and look up to the ceiling. Record how long they can maintain eye position and arm position. As treatment begins to take hold, this time should lengthen.

▶ DIAGNOSIS

- A positive test for the acetylcholine receptor antibody (AChR-Ab) is confirmatory for MG. While 90% of MG patients will have positive AChR-A tests, some patients develop other types of antibodies, such as muscle-specific receptor tyrosine kinase (MUSK) antibodies that also prevent neural transmission to the muscle.
- A quick screening test for MG can be performed for patients with ptosis in almost any clinical setting. Applying an icepack to the eyelid for 2 minutes. Reassess ptosis immediately after removing the icepack. If ptosis is improved, it is likely the cause of the ptosis is MG.
- Electrophysiologic studies can confirm MG, especially in cases in which serology is negative but symptoms are highly suggestive. The most commonly used test is repetitive nerve stimulation, which is about 80 sensitive. Much less commonly used, but much more sensitive, are single-fiber electromyography tests.

▶ TREATMENT

- Treatments are aimed at increasing the amount of acetylcholine in the NMJ, suppressing the autoimmune attack against the NMJ, or modulating the immune response by surgically removing the thymus.
- Pyridostigmine is typically the initial therapy for most patients with MG. This medication leaves more acetylcholine

in the NMJ, improving the ability of the muscle to perform repetitive movements. Most patients tolerate this medication well, although GI side effects are common.

- Treatment with pyridostigmine is often combined with immunosuppressive medications such as prednisone, azathioprine, and myocophenolate for long-term prevention of worsening symptoms.

- Many medications used for other illnesses can abruptly worsen MG. Commonly used medications that should be avoided in MG included benzodiazepines, sedatives, opiates, fluoroquinolones, and aminoglycosides. Anesthesia with neuromuscular blocking agents can be associated with prolonged ventilator time and slow recovery of muscle strength after the procedure.

CHAPTER 279

Essential Tremor

Adrian Banning, DHSc, MMS, PA-C

▶ GENERAL FEATURES

- Essential tremor (also known as intentional tremor or benign essential tremor) is a movement disorder that presents most often as a bilateral tremor but may present unilaterally.
- Most common movement disorder
- Affects ~5% of the US population
- Family history of resting tremor common
- Often presents in those over 70 years old, but can present in childhood
- 5–10 Hz tremor present with posture or with intentional movement in hands.
- Can affect head movements and voice
- Must be differentiated from Parkinson disease, does not present with other Parkinson disease symptoms:
  - Parkinson disease is characterized by a resting tremor.
  - Slower tremor than essential tremor at 4–6 Hz
  - Parkinson commonly unilateral
  - Parkinson may be associated with pill-rolling movements, muscular rigidity, and changes in gate.
- Can progress enough as to interfere with activities of daily living

- Patients may report that their tremor is worse at the end of the day.
- May improve after alcohol consumption

▶ CLINICAL ASSESSMENT

- Tremor with intentional movement evident
- Neurologic examination inspecting for other focal neurologic deficits warranted

▶ DIAGNOSIS

- Diagnosis is clinical.
- Imaging is unnecessary.

▶ TREATMENT

- Mild symptoms may not require treatment.
- Symptoms severe enough to interfere with activity of daily living can be treated with 20–120 mg of propranolol daily or primidone, 12.5–150 mg TID.
- Botulinum toxin may be used for voice or limb tremor.
- Surgical therapies that target the thalamus ventrointermediate nucleus (VIN) may be beneficial in severe cases.

CHAPTER 280

Tourette Syndrome

Paul Gonzales, MPAS

An 11-year-old cis-gendered girl presents to the clinic with her parents who are concerned about her repetitive outbursts, which she appears to be aware of. In addition, she tends to repetitively blink and shrug her shoulders, but is able to suppress this if she focuses. She is not making friends at school, and teachers are starting to label her as a "troublemaker" in class. What diagnostic workup would be indicated for this patient to confirm the most likely diagnosis?

▶ GENERAL FEATURES

- Tourette syndrome (TS) is a complex movement and neurobehavioral disorder occurring in children that results from disturbances in the cortico-striatal-thalamic-cortical (mesolimbic) circuit, which leads to disinhibition of the motor and limbic system.
- TS is characterized by multiple motor, and phonic tics believed to be caused by social, environmental, and genetic factors.

- Tics are abrupt, short-lived, occasional movements (motor tics) or vocalizations (phonic tics) that are often preceded by irresistible urges or sensations to perform a tic, followed by feelings of relief after performing the tic.
- The ability to temporarily voluntarily suppress tics and premonitory symptoms that precede tics are hallmark features that differentiate TS from other hyperkinetic movement disorders.
- TS affects cis-gendered males more often than cis-gendered females by ~4:1. Studies have solely been conducted in cis-gendered individuals.

▶ CLINICAL ASSESSMENT

- The stereotypical presenting complaint of TS is with motor tics (80% of patients) or phonic tics (20%), although generally it becomes a combination of the two.
- Simple motor tics include facial grimacing, eye blinking, and shoulder shrugging. Complex motor tics include more coordinated movements, such as kicking, jumping, body gyrations, bizarre gait, copropraxia, and echopraxia.
- Phonic tics include barking, moaning, throat clearing, hollering, and grunting. Complex phonic tics can include coprolalia (in 40% of cases), echolalia, and palilalia.
- Symptoms are first noticed between the ages of 2 and 15 years, but typically occur by age 11. Severity of the tics peak between the ages of 10–12 years, followed by improvement during adolescent years and adulthood.
- Aggravating factors may include stress, anxiety, anger, excitement, fatigue, or illness.
- Tics may evolve over time with varying severity and periods of waxing and waning.
- The most common comorbidities in TS include attention deficit hyperactivity disorder (ADHD; occurring in ~60%) and obsessive-compulsive disorder (OCD; occurring in ~27%).
- Approximately one-third of tics resolve completely, one-third improve, and one-third remain without improvement.
- The neurologic examination is often normal with the exception of tics.

▶ DIAGNOSIS

- TS is purely a clinical diagnosis requiring multiple motor and at least one phonic tic (present for some part during illness, not necessarily concurrent) with onset before age 21 (*DSM-5* criteria require onset before age 18).

- Tics must occur many times per day, nearly every day, or intermittently for at least 12 months.
- Anatomic location, frequency, number, type, complexity, or severity of tics must change over time.
- These involuntary movements and noises cannot be better explained by another medical condition.
- History and direct observation or video recording is key to a solid diagnosis. A diagnosis generally does not require any diagnostic testing.
- Although not required for diagnosis, neuroimaging such as CT or MRI of the head is unremarkable in patients with TS.
- Electroencephalogram (EEG) can be utilized to rule out the possibility of seizure, if suspected.

▶ TREATMENT

- Mild TS and nondisabling tics require only counseling and supportive care.
- Habit Reversal Training (with Comprehensive Behavioral Intervention for Tics) is indicated in patients with TS and tics that causes psychological, social, physical, or other functional problems.
- If Habit Reversal Training is not an option or tics are debilitating, treatment with tetrabenazine is recommended. Alternatively, fluphenazine or risperidone can be used.
- For patients with comorbid conditions such as TS and ADHD or OCD, behavioral interventions are preferred to medication. If medication is needed, treatment options should be selected that treat both tics and the comorbid condition.
- Guanfacine and clonidine are the only two FDA-approved pharmacologic agents for TS and ADHD.
- Cognitive-behavioral therapy (CBT) is first-line therapy for TS and OCD, but for more severe cases of OCD, CBT and selective serotonin reuptake inhibitors (SSRIs) are indicated.

Case Conclusion

This is a classic presentation of a patient with TS. Onset of tics (both phonic and motor) is between the ages of 2 and 15 years. The tics are repetitive, she is aware of them, and she is able to suppress them momentarily at will; the tics are also affecting her daily life. No diagnostic testing is indicated for a patient with TS as the diagnosis is a clinical one.

CHAPTER
281

Delirium

Tamara S. Ritsema, PhD, MPH, PA-C/R

▶ GENERAL FEATURES

- Delirium is a syndrome characterized by acute changes in cognition and level of consciousness. Delirium is most common in elderly patients with an infection or other acute serious illnesses, such as myocardial infarction, stroke, diabetic ketoacidosis, or alcohol/drug withdrawal.
- People with delirium have a higher mortality rate than other patients with similar underlying medical conditions that are not delirious.
- Patients with preexisting dementia, Parkinson disease, advanced hepatic or renal disease and those with a history of substance abuse are more likely to become delirious.
- Delirium is exceedingly common in hospitalized patients, and particularly in patients in intensive care environments. In several studies, the prevalence of delirium in ICUs was found to be >50%.

▶ CLINICAL ASSESSMENT

- Patients are often brought to medical attention by a family member who reports that the patient is newly disoriented or confused over the past 1–3 days. Families often report that the patient's confusion waxes and wanes.
- Patients with delirium are often difficult to interview. They may not be able to remember the questions they are asked, or report reliable answers. They are often agitated by the process of conducting a history and physical examination. Several validated assessments, including the Confusion Assessment Method, can be used to assess patients with delirium.
- Physical examination of the patient should seek to determine the underlying cause of the delirium. Examine ears, mouth, throat, neck, lungs, heart, abdomen, and vasculature. Conduct a full body skin examination looking for evidence of substance abuse, bedsores, or cellulitis.

▶ DIAGNOSIS

- While nearly any type of infection or serious medical illness can cause delirium, infections of the urinary tract and lungs are the most common etiologies.
  - Urinalysis (with culture) and chest x-ray should always be obtained, along with a comprehensive metabolic panel and a complete blood count.
- Further testing should be guided by the patient's history and physical examination. Clinicians may consider requesting an EKG, head CT, troponin, throat culture, lipase, blood and urine screens for toxins, and obtaining CSF if meningitis or subarachnoid hemorrhage is on the differential diagnosis. EEG is not commonly obtained unless the clinician suspects subclinical seizures or a metabolic encephalopathy with a characteristic EEG pattern.

▶ TREATMENT

- The most effective treatment for delirium is to treat the underlying cause of the delirium (infection, stroke, metabolic abnormality, myocardial infarction, etc).
- Patients with delirium are at high risk for other sequelae while delirious.
  - Ensure patient is receiving adequate nutrition and hydration.
  - Institute standard nursing measures to prevent skin breakdown, aspiration, contractures, and other consequences of longer term hospitalization.
- Manage agitation by providing gentle re-orientation, verbal reassurance, and touch. If family members are not available, the presence of a professional sitter can help avoid the need for pharmacologic intervention.
- The use of antipsychotics should be limited to patients with severe delirium. Use of sedatives is not supported by the best evidence. Haloperidol, although not formally FDA approved for use in delirium, is viewed as the safest of the antipsychotics in this patient population.

Dementia

Tamara S. Ritsema, PhD, MPH, PA-C/R

GENERAL FEATURES

- The cognitive losses that we group together as "dementia" are caused by several neurodegenerative conditions, including Alzheimer disease (AD), vasculopathies, dementia with Lewy bodies, Parkinson disease dementia, and frontotemporal dementia.
- Many other pathologies such as Huntington disease, alcoholism, and multiple system atrophy can also cause dementia. Some dementia patients have more than one cause for their illness.
- Other diseases, such as depression or normal pressure hydrocephalus, can mimic dementia. Certain medications, such as anticholinergics and antihistamines, also cause dementia symptoms. However, unlike dementias, once these diseases are properly treated or medications discontinued, the cognitive losses resolve.

CLINICAL ASSESSMENT

- Patients typically do not complain of memory loss. They are brought in by a family member who reports that the patient forgets new information while typically retaining memories of events in the past.
- Families of patients with vascular dementia will report that the patient's cognitive function remains relatively stable over time, with abrupt worsening at specific times. Families of patients with AD will report a slow, inexorable decline overall with "better" and "worse" days along the way.
- Families will also report that the patient has difficulty with executive function and carrying out daily tasks, is losing verbal fluency, or is displaying behavioral changes such as social withdrawal, anxiety, or aggressiveness.
- Patients typically deny or downplay memory loss when queried. They may insinuate that their family is "making it up" or is "out to get me."
- Physical examination is typically unrevealing, but the PA should evaluate closely to detect signs of stroke or of other systemic diseases that could be causing these symptoms.

DIAGNOSIS

- Bedside cognitive assessment with a test such as the Mini Mental State Examination will reveal that patients cannot easily form new memories and may have difficulty with attention, language, or multistep processes. All patients should be also screened for depression.
- Patients should be screened for hypothyroidism and vitamin B12 deficiency. Patients with risk factors should be screened for HIV and neurosyphilis.
- MRI is useful for ruling out other potential causes of dementia, such as occult stroke, brain tumor, subdural hematoma, or normal pressure hydrocephalus.
- Genetic testing for APOE4 or other mutations is not recommended.
- Most patients in whom a primary dementia is suspected should undergo formal neuropsychological testing to identify specific deficits and to establish a baseline against which future progression can be measured.
- *DSM-5* criteria for dementia are:
  - Evidence from the history and clinical assessment that indicates a significant cognitive impairment in at least one of the following cognitive domains: learning and memory, language, executive function, complex attention, perceptual motor function, social cognition
  - The impairment must represent a significant decline from a previous level of functioning.
  - The cognitive deficits must interfere with independence in everyday activities.
  - The disturbances must not be caused be delirium or be better accounted for by another medical disorder.

TREATMENT

- Treatments for dementias caused by AD have limited effectiveness. Treatment for other causes of dementia should be aimed at controlling the underlying pathology, which will slow the progression of the dementia.
- Two classes of drugs have been approved for the treatment of AD: cholinesterase inhibitors and NMDA receptor antagonists. Cholinesterase inhibitors may be used in early dementia. NMDA receptor antagonists are indicated for patients with moderate-to-severe AD and may be used in combination with cholinesterase inhibitors.
- When dementia patients have worsening behaviors, thoroughly investigate for nondementia causes, such as urinary tract infection, worsening arthritis, pneumonia, and constipation.
- Sedatives and antipsychotics have limited usefulness in treating behavioral manifestations of dementia. Their benefits are often outweighed by the adverse effects caused by these medications.

CHAPTER

283

Radiculopathy

Paige Cendroski, MPAS, PA-C
Jon Levy, MD

▶ GENERAL FEATURES

- Radiculopathy is defined as a condition in which compressed spinal nerve roots results in neurologic symptoms, such as pain, weakness, numbness, and tingling in the extremities.
- Presentation varies depending on the location of the affected nerve root: the distribution of symptoms correlates with the affected nerve root.
- Lumbosacral radiculopathy is most followed by cervical and then thoracic radiculopathies.
- Etiologies of radiculopathy include degenerative changes (spondylosis), disc herniation, infection, tumors, trauma, and vascular conditions.
- Cervical radiculopathy is often caused by disc herniation in the younger population and spondylosis with increased age. The C6 and C7 nerve roots are the most commonly affected.
- Differential diagnoses of cervical radiculopathy include shoulder pathology (rotator cuff or labral injury), cervical spine strain, brachial plexus pathology, and other peripheral neuropathies.
- Lumbar radiculopathy is often caused by disc herniation, spinal stenosis, and spondylolisthesis. The L5 nerve root is the most commonly affected nerve root in the lumbosacral spine.
- Myelopathy (cord compression) is often mistaken for radiculopathy. Multiple extremities can be affected in myelopathy; radiculopathy commonly involves one extremity.
  - Gait disturbances and paresthesia of hands are common complaints; patients rarely complain of pain; bowel and/or bladder dysfunction can occur.

▶ CLINICAL ASSESSMENT

- A detailed history will guide the physical examination and diagnostics.

- Note location of symptoms, radiation in a dermatomal pattern, duration, and recurrence. Radiculopathy is primarily unilateral. Note weakness in the myotomes and sensation changes in the dermatomal patterns.
- Radiculopathy can present with extremity pain with or without sensory and motor dysfunction.
- Risk factors for radiculopathies include manual labor such as heavy lifting, obesity, smoking, and poor posture.
- The presence of any "red flag" symptoms should heighten the suspicion of a more urgent diagnosis: fever, weight loss, bowel or bladder dysfunction, saddle anesthesia, rapid neurologic deterioration, history of malignancy, or other significant medical comorbidities.
- Physical examination should include inspection and palpation of spine, ROM of spine, neurologic examination, reflexes, and gait assessment. See chart for specific nerve root radiculopathies.
- A rectal examination is indicated to assess sphincter tone if the patient complains of bowel or bladder changes or saddle anesthesia.
- Special examinations include the Spurling or distraction tests for cervical radiculopathy and the straight leg test for lumbar radiculopathy.
- Myelopathy findings can include abnormal gait, hyperreflexia, positive Babinski or Hoffman reflex, or clonus.

▶ DIAGNOSIS

- Primary imaging consists of plain radiographs: anteroposterior (AP), lateral, and oblique views of cervical or lumbar spine. These images can reveal disc space or foraminal narrowing, osteophytes, or spondylolisthesis. Flexion and extension views can reveal instability.
- Radiographs should be obtained in the setting of trauma or if a patient continues to have neck or back pain >1 month with conservative treatment.

- MRI is the imaging modality of choice and can support the diagnosis of radiculopathy: Benefits of an MRI include no radiation exposure, and it provides good visualization of soft tissues and neural structures.
- A CT scan should be obtained in suspected fractures.
- EMGs can be obtained to help differentiate nerve root involvement from other neurologic conditions.

▶ TREATMENT

- Conservative treatment includes oral analgesics, either NSAIDs or an appropriate dose narcotic. A short course of oral corticosteroids can also be prescribed.
- Physical therapies, including cervical traction and avoidance provocative activities, may be helpful. Immobilization with a soft cervical collar may provide relief for cervical radiculopathy.
- Referral to an orthopedic or neurosurgical spine surgeon is indicated in any spine trauma or when symptoms persist after conservative treatment.

- Surgery is indicated for persistent symptoms exceeding 2 months with conservative measures, motor deficits, or increasing pain.
- When indicated, surgical laminectomies and discectomies provide successful outcomes.
- Prompt referral to a surgeon is indicated for suspected myelopathy, as surgery is often warranted.
- Prognosis:
  - Most (>80%) of radiculopathies are self-limited and can be managed with nonsurgical modalities.
  - Most patients with lumbar radiculopathy secondary to a herniated disc will be successfully treated with conservative therapies.
  - Up to one-third of patients with cervical radiculopathy and one-fourth of those with lumbar radiculopathy will experience a recurrence after initial improvement.
  - Patients with myelopathy will exhibit gradual neurologic deterioration and have a risk of catastrophic injury if not identified and treated.

Common Cervical and Lumbosacral Radiculopathies				
Nerve Root	Pain Distribution	Sensory Disturbance	Motor Weakness	Reflex Affected
C5	Neck, shoulder, scapula	Lateral arm	Deltoid and biceps	Biceps and brachioradialis reflex
C6	Neck, shoulder, scapula, lateral arm	Lateral forearm	Wrist extension and biceps	Biceps and brachioradialis reflex
C7	Neck, shoulder, middle finger	Palm, index and middle finger	Wrist flexors Finger extension Triceps	Triceps reflex
L2	Anterior upper thigh	Anterior upper thigh	Hip flexion	–
L3	Anterior thigh and knee	Anterior thigh	Hip flexion, knee extension	–
L4	Anterior thigh, anterior tibial area	Medial calf and foot	Ankle dorsiflexion and knee extension	Patella reflex
L5	Dorsum foot	Lateral leg, Dorsal surface of foot	Great toe dorsiflexion Ankle dorsiflexion	–
S1	Lateral foot	Lateral foot	Ankle plantarflexion and eversion	Achilles

CHAPTER 284

Peripheral Neuropathy

Carrie Smith Nold, MPA, PA-C

A 47-year-old woman with a 15-year history of type 2 diabetes presents with new complaints of burning pain in the toes that has ascended into her feet over the past several months. She has experienced difficulty falling asleep as the presence of her bedsheets aggravates the pain. Physical examination reveals absent Achilles reflexes and decreased sensation to light-touch in the bilateral feet.

▶ GENERAL FEATURES

- Peripheral neuropathy (PN) has a prevalence of 2% to 8%, which increases with age and the diagnosis of diabetes.
- Classified by the pattern of distribution:
  - Distal symmetric polyneuropathy (DSPN) is most common and presents with symptoms in a diffuse, length-dependent pattern.

- Typically presents with sensory complaints in a stocking-glove pattern with weakness later
- Diabetes is the most common cause.
- Mononeuropathies present with neuropathic symptoms in the distribution of one nerve. Carpal tunnel syndrome is the most common mononeuropathy.
- Mononeuropathy multiplex presents with neuropathic symptoms in the distribution of multiple, noncontiguous nerves.
  - Acute or subacute pain is a common presenting symptom. Symptoms are frequently asymmetric and non–length dependent.
  - Mononeuropathy multiplex may require urgent evaluation as it can be associated with underlying conditions such as vasculitis.
- Causes of PN are diverse and include:
  - Hereditary causes such as Charcot-Marie-Tooth
  - Immune-mediated causes such as Guillain-Barré syndrome
  - Toxin and drug-induced cases such as heavy-metal exposure, alcohol abuse, or chemotherapeutic agents
  - Vitamin-related abnormalities such B12 deficiency
  - Systemic diseases such as diabetes, infections, vasculitis, connective tissue disease, paraneoplastic syndromes, paraproteinemias, and thyroid, liver, or renal disease
    - Diabetes is the most common cause of PN in the developed world.
    - Diabetes can be associated with multiple patterns of PN, although DSPN is the most common.

CLINICAL ASSESSMENT

- Patients should be asked about family history of neuropathy, current medical conditions, past medical history, possible toxin exposure, and medication use.
- Establishing the onset and progression is important:
  - The onset for chronic neuropathies is >12 weeks.
  - The onset for acute neuropathies is <4 weeks, and the onset for subacute neuropathies is 4–12 weeks.
- Symptoms may include sensory complaints such as burning pain or numbness; motor complaints such as weakness; or autonomic complaints such as dizziness, syncope, erectile dysfunction, or sweating and circulatory abnormalities.
- Signs may include difficulties with pain, light-touch, temperature, vibratory, or proprioception testing; weakness and muscle atrophy; decreased or absent deep tendon reflexes, or gait abnormalities and a positive Romberg sign.
- Physical examination should include a thorough neurological examination, including mental status, cranial nerves, reflexes, various sensory modalities, and a motor examination.
- Patients may show evidence of autonomic dysfunction or of an undiagnosed systemic disease, which may be responsible for the PN.
- Signs such as hyperreflexia or increased tone may be evidence of a central rather peripheral cause of sensory or motor dysfunction.

DIAGNOSIS

- Patients with diabetes should be screened at visits for signs or symptoms of PN.
- Electrodiagnostic studies can confirm the presence of PN and establish the pattern of distribution, underlying pathophysiology, and type of nerve fibers affected.
- Focused laboratory studies may include:
  - Blood glucose, serum B12 with metabolites, and serum protein immunofixation electrophoresis
  - Other commonly ordered studies include a complete blood count, comprehensive metabolic panel, erythrocyte sedimentation rate, thyroid testing, and urinalysis.
- Additional laboratory studies or diagnostic testing should be based on the patient presentation and differential diagnosis.
  - Cerebrospinal fluid analysis is typically low yield outside suspected infectious, neoplastic, or demyelinating PN.
  - Genetic testing may be indicated in suspected hereditary neuropathies.
  - Autonomic testing and nerve and skin biopsies are not done routinely but may be useful.
- Patients with acute or subacute neuropathies, motor or autonomic predominant neuropathies, hereditary neuropathies, or asymmetric neuropathies should be referred to a neurologist.
- Patients with mild, sensory-predominant DSPN may not require immediate referral.
- Urgent evaluation and treatment are warranted for patients with acute and rapidly progressive neuropathies, which may indicate a serious underlying cause such as Guillain-Barré syndrome or vasculitis.

TREATMENT

- When possible, the underlying cause should be addressed and treated.
- Patients may still be left with symptoms.
- Symptomatic control includes addressing neuropathic pain, gait instability, and foot care.
  - First-line medications for neuropathic pain include gabapentin and pregabalin, tricyclic antidepressants, and serotonin norepinephrine reuptake inhibitors.
  - Physical and occupational therapy can help address gait issues and the need for adaptive equipment.
- 25% of the time no underlying etiology is discovered. Patients can be treated symptomatically in the absence of progression or other red flags.

Case Conclusion

This patient displays classic signs and symptoms of DSPN, including burning pain, difficulties with light-touch, and absent deep tendon reflexes that occur in a length-dependent pattern. Electrodiagnostic studies could confirm the diagnosis.

CHAPTER
285

Primary Headaches: Tension Headache, Migraine Headache, and Cluster Headache

Adrian Banning, DHSc, MMS, PA-C

▶ GENERAL FEATURES

- Cluster headaches are rare, estimated to present in only 0.1% of the population.
  - More common in males
  - Present as a combination of severe unilateral trigeminal area pain, ipsilateral autonomic symptoms, and general restlessness
  - Thought to be result of abnormal activity in the hypothalamus, trigeminovascular system, and autonomic nervous system
  - Pain can be so severe as to induce suicidality.
- Tension headaches or tension-type headaches (TTH) are the most common type of primary headache.
  - Present as "band-like" or squeezing sensation from brow to occipital region
  - Usually bilateral
  - Result of neck tension, poor body mechanics, and stress
- Migraine headaches are the second most common type of primary headache.
- There are several forms, but only about 20% to 25% of people have characteristic migraine aura of visual disturbances that accompany a "classic migraine."
  - Groups of headache attacks over 4 hours to 3 days.
  - Thought to be caused by multifactorial pathophysiology
  - Can be provoked or worsened by stimulation from the environment. Migraine symptoms may be preceded with a prodromal phase where the patient may feel fatigue or perceive lights or sounds differently.
  - Patients who experience migraine with aura are at in increased risk for cerebrovascular and cardiovascular disease.
  - More common in females than in males, family history of migraines is common.

▶ CLINICAL ASSESSMENT

- Cluster headaches: typically present with excruciating unilateral pain, ipsilateral eye lacrimation, and ipsilateral rhinorrhea
- TTHs: headache with mild neck tension may be noted, but no other physical examination findings are associated with TTHs.
- Migraine:
  - Diagnostic criteria are that they have at least two of the following features:
    - Moderate to severe in intensity
    - Throbbing and unilateral
    - Worse with movement
    - Accompanied by at least nausea, vomiting
    - Sensitivity to sound or light. They are not simply severe tension headaches, but are a neurologic disorder thought to be caused by multifactorial pathophysiology.
- Can also present with aura, but without pain, a condition known as acephalic migraine. In those cases, vertigo may be a predominant feature.
- Neurologic examination should be unremarkable. If focal neurological deficits are present, this indicates a need for further workup.

▶ DIAGNOSIS

- History is the most important diagnostic component.
- Imaging is not needed in the diagnosis of primary headache in the absence of focal neurologic deficits.

▶ TREATMENT

- Cluster headaches can be aborted with subcutaneous sumatriptan, nasal inhalation zolmitriptan, 100% nasal canula oxygen, or 4% to 10% lidocaine sprayed into the ipsilateral nostril.

- Prophylactic medications for cluster headaches include verapamil and lithium. An ECG before and after administration or dosage increase of verapamil is warranted. Lithium can alter thyroid function, and TSH levels should be checked regularly.
- TTHs can be treated with aspirin, acetaminophen, or NSAIDs along with relaxation techniques. Triptans are not indicated in the treatment of TTHs.
- First-line treatment for migraines is avoidance of triggers and nonpharmacologic methods like stress reduction.
  - First-line pharmacologic treatment is NSAIDs, followed by ergotamine or dihydroergotamine and triptans.

- Prophylactic treatment should be considered in patients who have four or more migraines per month. Avoidance of known triggers is the primary nonpharmacotherapeutic consideration. Side effects of the medication used for migraine prophylaxis may be considerable and need to be considered before prophylaxis is initiated. Pharmacologic prophylaxis includes β-blockers like propranolol or metoprolol; antidepressants including venlafaxine, nortriptyline, and amitriptyline; and anticonvulsants such as valproate and topiramate. Regular injections of onabotulinum toxin A is also used as migraine prophylaxis.

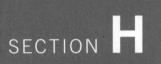

SECTION H

Seizure Disorders

CHAPTER 286

Focal and Generalized Seizures and Status Epilepticus

Rob Estridge, BA, BS, MPAS, PA-C

▶ GENERAL FEATURES

- Seizures are an electrical disturbance in the brain that manifest themselves clinically as focal or generalized pending the origination of the abnormal neuronal discharge. Focal seizures arise from one part of the brain and symptoms can be isolated, whereas generalized seizures are holocephalic and result in loss of consciousness.
- Epilepsy is a clinical condition characterized by two or more recurrent seizures unprovoked by systemic or acute neurologic insults.
- >50% of seizures are idiopathic, but known causes include trauma and congenital defects.
- Majority of seizures arise from the temporal lobe.
- Seizures are defined as focal or partial if they arise from one part of brain, as opposed to generalized if they come from the whole brain.
- Herpes simplex encephalitis is a leading cause of refractory temporal lobe seizures that can be difficult to control with a mortality rate of >70% without antivirals and high still with treatment.

- Status epilepticus is a neurologic emergency defined by a seizure >30 minutes or a series of epileptic seizures during which function is not regained between the events in a 30-minute period.
- Sudden unexpected death in epilepsy (SUDEP) is a rare phenomenon but is well known where patients who seize become hypoxic and can die as a consequence; mostly young and mostly at night.
- Mortality for patients with epilepsy is 2–3 times higher than that for patients without and usually due to underlying disease and that from status epilepticus is higher.

▶ CLINICAL ASSESSMENT

- History is the most significant portion of the workup, especially in looking for genetic abnormalities, history of head injury, history of febrile seizures, and family history of seizures.
- Fever can elicit unprovoked febrile seizures, especially in children which is usually benign and does not warrant workup.

- Physical examination is typically normal for these patients, except when seizing and in which case you would see abnormalities pending the origination of the seizure cerebrally.
- Diagnostic tests may include complete blood count, electrolytes, urinalysis, pregnancy test if female, toxicology screen, and CT/MRI and consideration of lumbar puncture if no previous history.
- Definitive diagnosis of a seizure is visualization of a seizure-like episode while on (ideally video) EEG.
- A postictal state is common after a seizure and can present as confusion, agitation, or even Todd paralysis where you may find profound motor weakness, mimicking a stroke.

▶ TREATMENT

- Goal of treatment is complete cessation of seizures, though this is not always possible.

- Treatment strategy involves minimizing amount of medication and side effects.
- Monotherapy is ideal but may not be achievable.
- Recommended medications for focal epilepsy are: lamotrigine, oxcarbazepine, and, if failure, consider carbamazepine, gabapentin, or topiramate.
- Recommended medications for generalized epilepsy are valproate, lamotrigine, or slightly less superior is topiramate.
  - Treatment for status epilepticus consists of airway management, circulatory support, and serial doses of benzodiazepines to halt seizures.
  - Refractory cases require a load or bolus of AEDs and may require intubation and sedation.
- Surgical intervention may be considered in cases such as stereoelectroencephalography (SEEG), vagal nerve stimulator placement, temporal lobectomy, lesionectomy, or even hemispherectomy.

SECTION I   *Vascular Disorders*

CHAPTER
287

Cerebral Vascular Accident and Transient Ischemic Attack

Tyler D. Sommer, MPAS, PA-C

A 73-year-old male is brought to the ED via EMS after his daughter found him at home confused and with a facial droop. His symptoms began about 35 minutes ago. What do you do?

▶ GENERAL FEATURES

- Cerebrovascular disease is characterized by stenosis or rupture of cerebral vasculature.
  - Risk factors include increasing age, hypertension, and those risk factors associated with atherosclerosis.
- Transient ischemic attacks (TIAs) are characterized by focal ischemia causing neurologic deficit that lasts for <24 hours, commonly <1–2 hours.
  - If the neurologic deficit lasts for >24 hours, it is a cerebrovascular accident (CVA), commonly known as a stroke, and results in permanent neurologic injury.

- CVA is the third leading cause of death in the United States; ~700 000 Americans are affected by CVA each year, with several of these being subsequent attacks.
- About 80% to 85% of CVAs are ischemic in nature, resulting from either thrombotic or embolic blockage of blood flow to a portion of the brain.
- About 15% to 20% of CVAs are hemorrhagic in nature, resulting from rupture of a diseased artery, often times in the presence of uncontrolled hypertension; this hemorrhage causes an intraparenchymal hematoma with surrounding edema.

▶ CLINICAL ASSESSMENT

- TIA and CVA can present with identical signs and symptoms; the main difference between the two is in the duration of time as discussed above.

- Onset of symptoms is usually quite abrupt, and the symptoms depending on where in the brain the stroke is occurring.
- Because the symptoms depend on the location of the lesion, symptoms can often indicate where the stroke is based on cerebral arterial distribution.
- Depending on the location of the lesion, strokes can result in unilateral hemiparesis, facial droop, dysarthria, aphasia, memory loss, confusion, sensory disturbances, cranial nerve palsy, gait disturbances, vertigo, vision loss, and so on.
- Symptoms are generally contralateral to the affected hemisphere, such as the contralateral arm, face, or leg.

DIAGNOSIS

- If a stroke is suspected based on clinical presentation, a CT of the head without contrast should be performed immediately, ideally within 25 minutes of arrival.
- The CT scan is used to exclude hemorrhagic stroke, but findings may be normal during the initial 6–24 hours of an ischemic stroke.
- Intraparenchymal hematoma due to hemorrhagic CVA is quickly visible on a CT and requires much different treatment than an ischemic stroke.
- Diffusion-weighted MRI or perfusion CT scans can be performed after the initial noncontrast CT to define the distribution and extent of an ischemic infarction.
- Other diagnostic tests that should be considered immediately include coagulation studies, electrocardiogram, serum glucose, and general metabolic labs.
- In stable patients receiving treatment, other studies may include echocardiogram, Holter monitor, carotid ultrasound, and tests for hypercoagulable conditions.

TREATMENT

- Patients with ischemic strokes should be considered for treatment with IV tissue plasminogen activator (tPA), ideally within 3 hours and generally not >4.5 hours after the onset of symptoms.
- Patients with ischemic strokes who are not the candidates for tPA should receive aspirin immediately.
- Treatment for hemorrhagic stroke is largely supportive and sometimes involves surgery; neurosurgery should be consulted immediately if hemorrhage is found.
- Attempts to lower blood pressure during an acute stroke are often not advised, especially in ischemic CVA.
- If important reversible causes of TIA and CVA are identified with diagnostic studies, such as carotid artery stenosis or atrial fibrillation, these should be adequately addressed.
- TIAs leave no permanent damage but indicate that the patient is at high risk for CVA and should be treated medically as such.
- Around 25% of individuals who recover from a first CVA will experience another CVA within the next 5 years, highlighting the importance of secondary prevention.

Case Conclusion

Because the patient is presenting with an acute neurologic deficit consistent with a CVA, a CT of the head without contrast is immediately indicated. Treatment depends on whether it is an ischemic stroke or a hemorrhagic stroke.

CHAPTER
288

Subarachnoid Hemorrhage and Cerebral Aneurysm

Tamara S. Ritsema, PhD, MPH, PA-C/R

GENERAL FEATURES

- Subarachnoid hemorrhage (SAH) is a rupture of a blood vessel or cerebral aneurysm into the subarachnoid space where cerebrospinal fluid (CSF) usually flows. Rapid flow of blood into the subarachnoid space quickly raises intracranial pressure and causes abrupt onset of a severe headache.
- People with hypertension, smoking history, a family history of SAH, moderate to heavy alcohol use, and postmenopausal women are at higher risk for SAH.

- While the most common cause of SAH is rupture of aneurysm, patients may also have SAH due to trauma, ruptured arteriovenous malformations, or congenital collagen vascular disorders.

CLINICAL ASSESSMENT

- The stereotypical presenting complaint of SAH is an abrupt onset of the worst headache of a patient's life (aka "thunderclap" headache). The headache tends to be nonfocal in distribution, not unilateral like migraine or cluster headaches.

- SAH should be on the differential diagnosis in all patients with an unusually severe headache. Missed diagnosis in early SAH is a substantial cause of patient morbidity and of provider medicolegal liability.
- Common associated symptoms include neck stiffness, nausea/vomiting, and photophobia. Associated seizures are very poor prognostic factor.
- Misdiagnosis of SAH is common. One of the most common errors is to assume that because a patient is awake, is not vomiting, and does not have focal neurologic deficits that they are not "sick enough" to have SAH. Providers may fail to consider an SAH in their differential diagnosis, not obtain a history specific enough to SAH, and fail to order a CT or may not understand the potential limitations of CT in assessment of SAH.

▶ DIAGNOSIS

- All patients in whom an SAH is suspected should undergo immediate CT scan of the head without contrast.
- In the majority of cases, if the CT is negative in a patient in whom SAH is suspected, a lumbar puncture should be obtained to examine CSF for the presence of red blood cells.

- Recent evidence suggests that reliable patients whose pain clearly started within the last 6 hours may be safely discharged based on a negative head CT performed on a high-resolution CT scanner with an experienced neuroradiologist reading the scan.
- Draw basic lab tests such as a complete blood count, a metabolic panel, and coagulation studies in case the patient needs urgent neurosurgery.

▶ TREATMENT

- Patients with SAH require expert neurosurgical care. Patients should be treated in or transferred to a hospital with a high-volume neurosurgical service and neurologic critical care facilities. Patients cared for at such facilities have better long-term outcomes.
- Treatment is generally aimed at stopping the bleeding and lowering the elevated intracranial pressure. Many patients require surgery to clip or to place a coil in the aneurysm to stop the current bleed and prevent future bleeds.
- Important adjunct treatments include seizure prophylaxis; prevention of vasospasm with nimodipine; appropriate intravenous hydration; and continuous neurologic, neurovascular, and cardiologic monitoring for hypoxia, hypoglycemia, and worsening neurologic deficits.

CHAPTER 289

Neoplasms of the Central Nervous System

Maryellen Blevins, MPAS, PA-C
Nata Parnes, MD

A 1-year-old girl of Asian ethnicity who presents to the emergency department with her mother stating that the child has been irritable, crying, and having periodic nausea and vomiting, but no fever or diarrhea. The mother notes that the child is not acting like her usual self and the symptoms have worsened over the last few weeks. The urine analysis and an ear, throat, and abdominal examination are normal. What is the appropriate imaging study?

▶ GENERAL FEATURES

- Adults:
  - Incidence or primary central nervous system (CNS) tumors occur at a rate of 30 per 100 000 persons.
  - Higher mortality in males

- Between 85% and 95% of all primary CNS tumors are brain tumors.
- Meningiomas and glial tumors constitute two-thirds of all primary brain tumors.
- Schwannomas, meningiomas, and ependymomas constitute over three-fourths of primary spinal tumors.
- Brain metastases are the most common brain tumors in adults, with lung cancer being the most common primary source.
- Children:
  - Incidence is 5.95 cases per 100 000.
  - Most common solid tumor in children
  - 60% of tumors are malignant, and malignant CNS tumors make up 15% to 20% of all childhood malignant tumors.

- More common in boys
- They are the leading cause of death from cancer.
- The most common brain tumors are astrocytic tumors.
- The most common malignant tumors are medulloblastomas.
- 40% to 60% of spinal tumors are ependymal tumors.
- Overall:
  - Tumors are classified using the WHO (TNM) system while in children the *International Classification of Childhood Cancer (ICCC)* can be used.
  - Tumors are more common in people of Caucasian ethnicity (in children, they are equally common in those of Asian/Pacific Island ethnicity).
  - Risk factors are not usually known unless there is presence of genetic risk factors or exposure to ionizing radiation.
  - Survival depends on age and type of tumor.

▶ CLINICAL ASSESSMENT

- Location, size of tumor, increase in intracranial pressure (ICP), and compression of surrounding structures affect symptom presentation.
- Symptoms of brain tumors include tension-like headaches (which may present as irritability in infants), seizures, visual changes, nausea/vomiting, changes in personality, mental capacity, and concentration.
- Symptoms of spinal tumors include changes in bowel habits, trouble urinating, weakness/numbness in arms/legs, and gait disturbances.
- In infants, macrocephaly may be present due to increase in ICP and unfused cranial sutures.

▶ DIAGNOSIS

- CT: R/O hemorrhages, calcifications, skull lesions
- MRI: soft-tissue evaluation including R/O abscesses, arteriovenous (AV) malformations, and infarctions

- Biopsy: performed by open surgery or stereotactic surgery (needle biopsy)—no glucocorticosteriods before biopsy

▶ TREATMENT

- Consult neurology.
- Surgery:
  - Complete or near-complete removal of tumor (used for diagnosis and also to decrease ICP since total elimination is rare)
- Radiation:
  - Dependent on tumor type
  - Conformal radiation therapy targets size and shape of the tumor
  - Intensity-modulated radiation therapy
  - Stereotactic radiosurgery
  - Conventional external beam—usually used in children
- Chemotherapy:
  - High dose or combination of systemic therapy
  - Intrathecal chemotherapy
  - Intratumoral chemotherapy
- Active surveillance:
  - Monitor tumor growth by imaging.
- Supportive therapy:
  - Symptom relief
  - Palliative care for tumors with poor prognosis
  - Pediatric survivors often experience neurologic, cognitive, endocrine, and psychological complications, which need long-term care.
  - >70% of children with brain tumors live for <5 years after diagnosis.
- Targeted therapy:
  - Monoclonal antibody therapy

> **Case Conclusion**
>
> The most appropriate imaging of the brain is head CT, which can reveal brain/skull lesions, hemorrhages, and calcifications.

CHAPTER 290

Complex Regional Pain Syndrome

Lauren Trillo, PA-C

▶ GENERAL FEATURES

- Characterized by spontaneous and evoked regional pain that is disproportionate in severity to any known cause
- Most commonly affects the distal extremities, upper greater than lower, and peaks in incidence at 50–70 years. Women are more likely than men to develop complex regional pain syndrome (CRPS).
- Prominent autonomic and inflammatory changes in the region of pain distinguish CRPS from other chronic pain conditions.

- There are two subtypes of CRPS:
  - Type I (formerly known as reflex sympathetic dystrophy) refers to patients without evidence of a peripheral nerve injury. This represents about 90% of clinical presentations.
  - Type II (formerly known as "causalgia") refers to cases of known peripheral nerve injury.
- Many patients improve spontaneously after a year, with some progressing to chronic CRPS.

▶ **CLINICAL ASSESSMENT**

- Onset of symptoms typically occurs within 4–6 weeks of an inciting event.
- Most common trigger is fractures. Other triggers include sprains, contusions, crush injuries, and surgery. Up to 10% of cases occur without a clear precipitating factor.
- Main symptoms include:
  - Pain: the most prominent and debilitating symptom. Often described as a deep, burning, stinging, or tearing sensation
  - Sensory changes: extreme hyperalgesia and allodynia (pain to nonpainful stimuli) commonly in a stocking/glove distribution
  - Motor impairments: functional motor impairment related to pain, with some developing central motor symptoms (tremor, myoclonus, dystonic postures, and impaired initiation of movement)
  - Autonomic symptoms: change in skin temperature, skin color, sweating, and/or edema
  - Trophic changes: increased hair growth, increased or decreased nail growth, contraction and fibrosis of joints and fascia, and/or skin atrophy.

▶ **DIAGNOSIS**

- The diagnosis is based solely on clinical signs and symptoms; however, objective medical tests may be needed to exclude other treatable conditions.
- International Association for the Study of Pain diagnostic criteria:
  - Continuing pain disproportionate to an inciting event
  - Must include at least one symptom in three of the four categories:
    - Sensory: hyperesthesia and/or allodynia
    - Vasomotor: temperature asymmetry and/or skin color changes and/or skin color asymmetry
    - Sudomotor/edema: edema and/or sweating and/or sweating asymmetry

- Motor/trophic: decreased range of motion and/or motor dysfunction (weakness, tremor, dystonic posture) and/or trophic changes (hair, nail, skin)
- Must display at least one sign at the time of evaluation in two or more categories:
  - Sensory: hyperalgesia (to pinprick) and/or allodynia
  - Vasomotor: evidence of temperature asymmetry and/or skin color changes and/or asymmetry
  - Sudomotor/edema: edema and/or sweating changes and/or sweating asymmetry
  - Motor/trophic: decreased range of motion and/or motor dysfunction (weakness, tremor, dystonia) and/or trophic changes (hair, skin, nails)
- No other diagnosis better explains the signs and symptoms.

▶ **TREATMENT**

- Immediate treatment is important and is best achieved through a comprehensive, interdisciplinary treatment regimen.
- Physical and occupational therapy are first-line treatments.
- Pharmacologic therapy includes topical lidocaine cream/patches, topical capsaicin cream, nonsteroidal anti-inflammatory drugs (NSAIDs), bisphosphonates, tricyclic antidepressants, gabapentin/pregabalin, carbamazepine, and opioids. Corticosteroids may be considered if inflammation is present.
- Behavioral therapy is helpful in reducing pain-related fear, pain intensity, and disability.
- Patients who are unresponsive to conservative treatment or have progressive symptoms should be referred to a pain management specialist.
  - Interventional procedure options include sympathetic ganglion nerve blocks, intravenous regional sympathetic blocks, spinal cord stimulation, and surgical sympathectomy.

CHAPTER
291

Cranial Nerve Palsy

Jeanette Elfering, MHS, PA-C

A 60-year-old male with a past medical history of prostate cancer currently in remission and hypertension presents to the emergency department with new-onset binocular diplopia and ptosis of the right eyelid that started 1 month ago and has progressively worsened. On examination, you note complete ophthalmoplegia of the right eye with ptosis and anisocoria that is greater in the dark than in the light. Neurologic examination is also remarkable for decreased sensation in the V1 and V2 distribution of the trigeminal nerve.

▶ **GENERAL FEATURES**

- 12 cranial nerves (CNs): some function solely as sensory neurons or motor neurons; a few have dual functions of both sensory and motor neurons.
  - Olfactory nerve (CN I, sensory): sense of smell
  - Optic nerve (CN II, sensory): visual acuity
  - Oculomotor nerve (CN III, motor): eye movements; pupillary constriction and accommodation, muscle of upper eyelid

- Trochlear nerve (CN IV, motor): eye movements (intorsion and downgaze)
- Trigeminal nerve (CN V, both sensory and motor): somatic sensation from the face, mouth, cornea; muscles of mastication
- Abducens nerve (CN VI, motor): eye movements (abduction)
- Facial nerve (CN VII, both sensory and motor): controls the muscles of facial expression; taste from anterior tongue; lacrimal and salivary glands
- Vestibulocochlear nerve (CN VIII, sensory): hearing; sense of balance
- Glossopharyngeal nerve (CN IX, both sensory and motor): sensation from posterior tongue and pharynx; taste from posterior tongue; carotid baroreceptors and chemoreceptors; salivary gland
- Vagus nerve (CN X, both sensory and motor): autonomic functions of the gut; cardiac inhibition; sensation from larynx and pharynx; muscles of vocal cords; swallowing
- Spinal accessory nerve (CN XI, motor): shoulder and neck muscles
- Hypoglossal nerve (CN XII, motor): movements of the tongue
- Etiologies for any CN palsy are very broad and can include vascular (microvascular or vascular malformations), infectious, inflammatory, autoimmune, neoplastic, compressive, traumatic, congenital, idiopathic, or iatrogenic causes.
- CN III etiologies: most common cause of a pupil-sparing CN III palsy is microvascular injury or disease; most common cause of a pupil involving CN III palsy is related to compression of the third nerve by either an intracranial aneurysm or a pituitary tumor.
- CN IV etiologies: most common cause of a CN IV palsy is trauma or decompensation of a congenital fourth nerve palsy.
- CN VI etiologies: most commonly injured ocular CN; most common cause of a CN VI palsy is from increased intracranial pressure caused by a mass, edema, or hemorrhage or is microvascular.
- Isolated CN III, IV, or VI palsy in a patient aged >50 years and with atherosclerotic risk factors is most likely caused by a microvascular injury or disease; rarely, a microvascular palsy can be arteritic in nature (related to a vasculitis).
- Risk factors for CN III, IV, and VI nerve palsies include microvascular conditions (hypertension, diabetes, hypercholesterolemia, arteriosclerosis, and smoking), inflammatory conditions, intracranial mass, intracranial hemorrhage, meningitis, encephalitis, cavernous sinus thrombosis, or neurosurgical intervention.

▶ CLINICAL ASSESSMENT

- A full CN and neurological examination should always be performed. Visual acuity should also be assessed in each eye separately.

- Dilated fundus examination can be normal, may show papilledema (in cases of increased intracranial pressure), or an infiltrative lesion (in cases of malignancy or autoimmune conditions).
- Symptoms can include vertical or horizontal binocular diplopia (diplopia resolves with either eye closed), ptosis, ocular pain, decreased vision, or headache.
- If a subarachnoid bleed is the suspected cause of the palsy, the patient could present with leptomeningeal irritation.
- CN palsies caused by increased intracranial pressure, the patient might also complain of a headache that is worse in the supine position, pulsatile tinnitus, or transient vision obscurations.
- CN III palsy:
  - Determine if it is a complete (ptosis, restriction in elevation, depression, extorsion, and adduction) or partial CN III palsy and if it is pupil involving (patient will have anisocoria worse in the light, then dark) or pupil sparing. If the pupil is involved, then you must consider a compressive etiology related to an aneurysm or pituitary tumor.
  - Sudden onset of a painful CN III palsy with associated meningeal signs is suggestive of a subarachnoid hemorrhage from aneurysmal rupture or pituitary apoplexy.
  - Pupil sparing is more likely associated with an ischemic process.
  - Typically, the patient will present with their eye stuck in the abducted position.
- CN IV palsy:
  - Patient will have difficulty looking down toward the nose, resulting in vertical diplopia. Sensorimotor examination will be notable for a hypertropia in the affected eye that is worse in the contralateral gaze and in the ipsilateral head tilt.
- CN VI palsy:
  - The affected eye will be stuck in the adduction position (toward the nose), causing an esotropic appearance. Diplopia will be worse in the direction of the palsied muscle and gets better in the contralateral gaze.
- Lesions involving multiple CNs often produce unilateral or bilateral ophthalmoplegia. Associated symptoms and signs will help you to localize where the lesion resides.
- A lesion causing a CN III, IV, or VI palsy can be localized to either the nucleus, fascicle, subarachnoid space, cavernous sinus (consists of CN III, CN IV, CN VI, V1, V2, and the internal carotid artery), or orbital apex (can result in CN II, CN III, CN IV, CN VI, and CN V1 palsies and/or pupil involvement).

▶ DIAGNOSIS

- CN examination and patient symptoms will help you determine which CN are affected.
- Neuroimaging to rule out compressive, hemorrhage, or inflammatory pathology

- In an acute setting, a computed tomography (CT) of the brain with and without contrast is the preferred imaging modality. Magnetic resonance imaging (MRI) of the brain and orbits with and without contrast should also be obtained once an intracranial hemorrhage is ruled out. A magnetic resonance angiogram (MRA) or CT angiogram (CTA) is also needed to assess for aneurysmal etiology.
- Laboratory tests include: hemoglobin A1C, comprehensive metabolic panel (CMP), lipid profile, complete blood count (CBC), erythrocyte sedimentation rate (ESR), C-reactive protein (CRP), rapid plasma reagin (RPR), Lyme titer, antinuclear antibody (ANA) test, and rheumatoid factor (RF). Laboratory workup should be tailored to the most likely etiology.
- Lumbar puncture should be considered if MRI and laboratory work is negative or if you suspect that the CN palsy is caused by increased intracranial pressure.

▶ TREATMENT

- Depends on underlying etiology:
  - Vascular: control risk factors to prevent future complications or reoccurrence. Consider starting antiplatelet therapy.
  - Compressive: surgical resection, radiation, or chemotherapy
  - Inflammatory/autoimmune: corticosteroids and/or immunosuppression
  - Neoplastic: treat underlying cancer
  - Infectious: antimicrobials, antifungals, or antivirals depending on the suspected pathogen
- If the patient is diplopic, occlude either eye or use prisms to help alleviate their diplopia.
- If CN palsy is due to microvascular ischemia, it should resolve within 3–6 months; if it does not, then additional workup is required.

Case Conclusion

The case patient is a classic example of multiple CN palsies. CN III, IV, and VI were affected resulting in complete ophthalmoplegia with ptosis and anisocoria in the right eye, and CN V (V1 and V2 distributions) were affected resulting in decreased sensation on the right side of the face, localizing the lesion to the cavernous sinus. MRI of the brain and orbits showed an enhancing lesion most suggestive of metastatic prostate cancer. He was started on chemotherapy and managed by his oncology team.

CHAPTER 292

Cerebral Palsy

Lauren Wiley, PA-C

▶ GENERAL FEATURES

- Cerebral palsy (CP) refers to a heterogeneous group of conditions involving permanent, nonprogressive, motor dysfunction that affects muscle tone, posture, and movement.
- These conditions are because of abnormalities of the developing fetal or infantile brain.
- The disorder is not progressive but may change over time as the central nervous system matures.
  - The overall prevalence of CP is ~2 per 1000 live births.

▶ CLINICAL ASSESSMENT

- Symptoms of the condition are motor abnormalities, altered sensation/perception, intellectual disabilities, communication and behavior difficulties, dystonia, seizure disorders, and musculoskeletal complications.
  - Early signs/risks of developing CP include history of prematurity, low birth weight, multiple gestation, infection, and known brain dysmorphology.

- CP is characterized by abnormalities of motor activity, tone, and posture.
- Different subtypes: spastic CP (with multiple subtypes), dyskinetic CP, and ataxic CP:
  - Spastic diplegia: 13% to 25% of cases: lower limbs are more affected than upper limbs.
  - Spastic hemiplegia: 21% to 40% of cases: one side of the body is affected; the arm is typically more affected than the leg.
  - Spastic quadriplegia: 20% to 43% of cases: all limbs affected.
  - Dyskinetic subtype: 12% to 14% of cases: characterized by involuntary movement. Contractures are not common, variable degree of dysarthria and intellectual disability.
  - Ataxic subtype: 4% to 13% of case: ataxic movements, widespread disorder of movement function
    - In severely affected individuals, an attempted voluntary movement may evoke a primitive reflex, co-contraction of agonist and antagonist muscles, and mass movements.

DIAGNOSIS

- The diagnosis is usually made at the age of 12–24 months.
  - There is no single test to rule in or out CP, so if suspected, a detailed developmental assessment should be performed and hearing and vision should be evaluated. Motor milestones should be evaluated regularly.
  - The most common motor delays in child with CP are:
    - Not sitting by 8 months
    - Not walking by 18 months
    - Early asymmetry of hand function before 1 year of age
  - In child without CP, most motor reflexes related to posture disappear between 3 and 6 months. In CP, these reflexes disappear later.
  - A sign of CP may be seen when an infant is held in vertical suspension, the appropriate response is for the infant to assume the sitting position. Persistent extension of the legs may suggest CP.
  - Neurobehavioral signs suspicious for CP are excessive docility or irritability. A history of poor feeding may be present.
    - The Gross Motor Function Classification System (GMFCS) is used to categorize functional motor impairment in CP.
      - The subtype and GMFCS allow providers to assess a global impression of the child's condition severity.
    - The GMFCS is also useful for tracking responses to interventions.

TREATMENT

- Treatment is focused on maximizing the child's functional status. The mainstay of treatment is supportive care.
- PT/OT is a vital part of CP management.
- Braces/orthotics/standers/mobility devices help many children to provide proper alignments, promote function and delay, or prevent joint contractures.
- Dystonia first-line management is benzodiazepines, and second line is levodopa. Deep brain stimulation can be used in patients with severe dystonia.
- Tone management is usually managed with pharmacologic and surgical intervention.
  - The first line for spasticity is baclofen or benzodiazepines. Second line is Botox injections for localized treatment.
  - Surgery can be done to release and lengthen muscle tendons but is reserved for severe cases.
- Associated conditions include intellectual disability, neurodevelopmental disorders, epilepsy, vision problems, speech and hearing impairment, feeding difficulties, growth failure, GI disorders, sialorrhea, pulmonary disease, orthopedic disorders, osteopenia, chronic pain, and sleep disorders.

PART XII

Psychiatry and Behavioral Health Pretest

Section A Pretest: Abuse

1. You are working in the emergency department and are seeing a 32-year-old female patient who complains of vaginal spotting. Her last menstrual period (LMP) was 1 week ago, her cycle length is typically regular, and she takes no oral birth control or hormones and does not believe she is pregnant. She is sexually active with her boyfriend, and they typically use condoms. She denies vaginal itching, burning, or rashes. She endorses vaginal pain as well as the bleeding, which she describes as more than spotting but less than a steady flow. She denies clotted blood. She is extremely reluctant to do a pelvic examination, but after a period of shared decision-making, you are able to help her understand the procedure and agree to a pelvic examination. Upon examination, she has multiple abrasions to the posterior fourchette and labia, all of which are tender to touch and two that are oozing blood. Upon further questioning, she admits that an acquaintance raped her at a party last night. What of the following should comprise your response?
   A. Immediately call the police yourself—this is a crime and must be reported.
   B. Insist that the patient call the police, explaining to her that you know that she should report this as a crime.
   C. Discuss with her reporting options, forensic examination for evidence collection.
   D. Discuss reporting options, forensic examination, PEP for HIV protection, and STI treatment options and, using shared decision-making, help her make a set of decisions that work for her.

2. Your next patient in the urgent care is a 25-year-old female, 14 weeks' pregnant, gravida 2, para 1, who is complaining of abdominal pain. She denies nausea and vomiting, but she also endorses some cramping and vaginal spotting. Upon examination, she is tender along the left flank and also in the suprapubic area. There is some faint bruising along the left flank, and she also has some bruising around her left eye. You question her about domestic violence and safety in the home, and she admits that her husband "got pretty angry with her" but that things are better now, and she denies feeling unsafe in her home. In addition to ensuring her home safety and safety planning, what other question should you ask her?
   A. Whether or not she wants to leave her husband
   B. If her husband used his hands, arms, or anything else to choke or strangle her (nonfatal strangulation) as part of this or any other abusive episode
   C. If there are other children or weapons in the house
   D. Both B and C
   E. All of the above

Section B Pretest: Anxiety Disorders

1. If a patient fails an SSRI for first-line treatment of generalized anxiety disorder (GAD), the next drug of choice would be which of the following?
   A. Benzodiazepine
   B. Antipsychotic
   C. Anticonvulsant
   D. A different SSRI

2. The Generalized Anxiety Disorder 7-item scale (GAD-7) is used to assess the severity of anxiety in an anxious patient.
   A. True
   B. False

3. First-line treatment for specific phobia is lorazepam or alprazolam.
   A. True
   B. False

Section C Pretest: Autism Spectrum Disorder

1. Autism-specific screening is recommended by the American Academy of Pediatrics at which of the following ages?
   A. 6 and 12 months
   B. 9 and 18 months
   C. 15 and 36 months
   D. 18 and 24 months

2. Which of the following are risk factors for autism spectrum disorder (ASD)?
   A. Older sibling with ASD
   B. Young parental age
   C. Limited or no breastfeeding
   D. Late or no prenatal care

3. In order to meet the *DSM-5* diagnostic criteria for ASD, children must demonstrate which of the following?
   A. Deficits in social communication
   B. Stereotypical hand movements
   C. Picky eating habits
   D. Intellectual disability

4. The evaluation of a child with suspected ASD should include which of the following labs or diagnostic tests?
   A. Lead level
   B. CBC
   C. Urinalysis
   D. MRI

Section D Pretest: Bipolar Disorder

1. Which of the following diagnostic criteria is consistent with *DSM-5* diagnosis for bipolar disorder?
   A. Bipolar I is characterized by at least one episode of mania of at least 1-week duration and associated with hospitalization, functional impairment, and possible depressive and hypomanic episodes.
   B. Bipolar I is characterized by a history of major depressive and hypomanic episodes, but no mania.
   C. Bipolar I is characterized by periods of depression and hypomanic symptoms for at least 2 years in adults that do not meet diagnostic criteria for major depressive or hypomanic episodes.
   D. Bipolar I is characterized by significant change in weight or appetite, insomnia, psychomotor agitation, fatigue, indecisiveness, and recurrent thoughts of death or suicide.

2. A 32-year-old patient suffers from a chronic mood disturbance with long periods of depressed mood, fatigue, and occasional periods of irritability. He does not remember a symptom-free period that lasted more than a few weeks. He denies alcohol, prescription medication, and illicit drug use. The symptoms have not resulted in any social or functional impairments in his life or led to hospitalization. What is the most likely diagnosis?
   A. Bipolar disorder type 1
   B. Cyclothymic disorder
   C. Dissociative disorder
   D. Major depression

3. A 50-year-old patient is experiencing acute mania with significant psychotic features and has recently started lithium and risperidone. What is the best short-term adjunctive medication to reduce agitation and cause sedation in this patient?
   A. Clonazepam
   B. Clonidine
   C. Gabapentin
   D. Paroxetine

Section E Pretest: Conduct Disorder

1. Which statement is true regarding conduct disorder?
   A. Conduct disorder is prevalent in the general population (>25%).
   B. It is not feasible to try to obtain information from the child.
   C. Patients exhibit a lack of remorse, empathy, and have poor academic performance.
   D. Respect for authority figures.
   E. Treatment leads to a good prognosis.

2. When using pharmacologic treatment of conduct disorder, which statement is true?
   A. No pharmacologic treatment is used.
   B. Patients are compliant on medications.
   C. Pharmacologic treatment is given only when the patient is inpatient.
   D. Treat the comorbidities.
   E. Use off-label medications.

Section F Pretest: Depressive Disorders

1. Which of the following is NOT a criterion of major depressive disorder (MDD)?
   A. Feelings of worthlessness
   B. Weight loss of 20 lb while dieting
   C. Recurrent thoughts of death
   D. Inability to make decisions

2. Which antidepressant should NOT be used in a patient with a history of seizures?
   A. Fluoxetine
   B. Duloxetine
   C. Mirtazapine
   D. Bupropion

3. Which of the following is NOT considered high risk for suicide completion?
   A. Adolescent female
   B. Past suicide attempt
   C. Family history of suicide
   D. Older male

4. Which of the following statements is true?
   A. Phototherapy has been proven effective for all types of MDD.
   B. Antidepressants should never be continued indefinitely.
   C. All patients should begin with cognitive-behavioral therapy (CBT) before medication.
   D. Children may present with a primarily irritable mood instead of depressed mood.

Section G Pretest: Feeding and Eating Disorders

1. You are suspicious that your patient has an eating disorder. She denies binging, purging, or withholding food, but admits to exercising 6-8 hours daily. Which of the following is NOT *DSM-5* diagnostic criteria for diagnosing anorexia nervosa (AN)?
   A. Distorted body image
   B. Intense fear of gaining weight
   C. Amenorrhea
   D. Significantly low body weight

2. An 18-year-old female presents to your office for an annual sports physical. She has not menstruated in 6 months. Her BMI is 16. Physical examination finds eroded dentition and calluses on the back of her hands. She reports eating mostly vegetables as she is concerned about excess body fat. What is her likely diagnosis?
   A. Bulimia nervosa
   B. Anorexia nervosa
   C. Binge eating disorder
   D. Avoidant/restrictive food intake disorder

3. A patient presents for follow-up of anorexia nervosa. She has been seeing a multiple disciplinary group to help her manage; however, she has not gained weight as expected. She has not resumed menstruation either. She is a freshman in college and is struggling to maintain a 4.0. She feels the need for perfectionism. What medication might you consider in this patient?
   A. Olanzapine
   B. Lorazepam
   C. Sertraline
   D. Bupropion

4. A 16-year-old patient presents to primary care for occasional heartburn and a puffy cheek. Review of systems and history of present illness note several episodes of a puffy cheek over the past 6 weeks, increased exercise, and three dental caries treated by a dentist over the past 6 weeks. The heartburn is not associated with any other GI symptoms and resolves with antacid. Vital signs, BMI, and physical examination are within normal limits. Serum biochemistries reveal hypokalemia and a metabolic alkalosis,

but no other abnormalities. What is the most likely diagnosis?
   A. Anorexia nervosa
   B. Bulimia nervosa
   C. Suppurative parotitis
   D. Viral parotitis

5. A young female comes in for evaluation wearing multiple layers of clothing despite it being a hot summer day. You note her BMI is 17. How should you further evaluate this patient?
   A. Consider screening her for an eating disorder using the SCOFF questionnaire.
   B. Consider asking the patient to void and then wear a medical gown before re-taking her vitals.
   C. Ask her about her diet and exercise routine.
   D. All of the above.

6. A 24-year-old patient presents to a university student health clinic for a sports-related clearance examination. She denies any significant past medical or surgical history, but notes she struggles to maintain a consistent body weight. Temperature is 98.7 °F, blood pressure (BP) is 110/68 mm Hg, pulse is 65 beats per minute, respirations are 12/min, and BMI is 19.5. On examination, dental enamel erosions and calluses on the knuckles of both hands are noted. Which of the following results are most likely to be found on laboratory testing today?
   A. Increased chloride, potassium, and bicarbonate
   B. Increased chloride, decreased potassium, decreased bicarbonate
   C. Decreased chloride and potassium, increased bicarbonate
   D. Decreased chloride, potassium, and bicarbonate

Section H Pretest: Attention Deficit Hyperactivity Disorder

1. Which of the following disorders is most likely in a young boy who struggles to remain focused and complete daily tasks both at home and at school?
   A. Attention deficit hyperactivity disorder
   B. Autism
   C. Conduct disorder
   D. Learning disability

2. Which of the following symptoms best describe behaviors seen in patients with attention deficit hyperactivity disorder?
   A. Impulsive and inattentive
   B. Focused and reliable
   C. Dependent and organized
   D. Compliant and timely

3. Which of the following should be used initially to diagnose the patient with attention deficit hyperactivity disorder?
   A. Comprehensive history
   B. Physical examination
   C. Laboratory testing
   D. Neuroimaging

4. Which of the following drug classes is best utilized to treat attention deficit hyperactivity disorder?
   A. Psychostimulants
   B. Antidepressants
   C. Antipsychotics
   D. Mood stabilizers

Section I Pretest: Obsessive-Compulsive Disorder

1. Which of the following medications should NOT be considered as a first choice for a patient with obsessive-compulsive disorder?
   A. Fluoxetine
   B. Citalopram
   C. Escitalopram
   D. Venlafaxine

2. Which of the following disorders is frequently associated with obsessive-compulsive disorder?
   A. Personality disorders
   B. Mood disorders
   C. Schizophrenia
   D. Post-traumatic stress disorder (PTSD)

3. Which of the following would be an example of a compulsion?
   A. Thinking of hurting the neighbor
   B. Worried if the oven was left one
   C. Washing hands 4 times before leaving the bathroom
   D. The belief that sex is evil

4. Which of the following forms of psychotherapy shows the most efficacy in the treatment of obsessive-compulsive disorder?
   A. CBT with an emphasis on exposure with a response prevention
   B. Behavioral therapy
   C. Classic Freudian psychoanalysis
   D. Exposure therapy

5. Which of the following would be an example of an obsession?
   A. Washing hands 4 times before leaving the bathroom
   B. Checking to make sure the oven is turned off multiple times before leaving the house
   C. Muttering "abracadabra" 13 times before turning the car on
   D. Fear that while driving you ran over a pedestrian

Section J Pretest: Personality Disorders

1. What type of personality disorder has an extreme lack of self-confidence, needs reassurance, become clingy, and allows others to run their life?
   A. Dependent
   B. Narcissistic
   C. Paranoid
   D. Antisocial
   E. Avoidant

2. What is considered a cluster A personality disorder?
   A. Avoidant
   B. Dependent
   C. Histrionic
   D. Obsessive
   E. Schizoid

3. While attending the Emmy Awards, an actor has an angry outburst when he is not selected for the award. He mentions to others that he is a far better actor than the winner and that they cannot measure his skills by any award. The actor feels he was not selected for the Emmy because of jealousy by those on the committee. What is the treatment for this disorder?
   A. Antipsychotic medications
   B. Inpatient treatment
   C. Patient cooperation
   D. Psychotherapy
   E. Therapist confrontation of patient

4. An impeccably dressed 32-year-old male presents for workup after a routine physical examination revealed elevated BP. He demands that he should be seen by the head of cardiology since no mere minion could be capable of handling his case. He states that his general well-being has never been better, he is able to accomplish 10 times as much as any of his colleagues, and that over the past week, he is not even needed to sleep. When asked about illicit drug use, he becomes irate, threatening that he knows important people and can cause trouble if his integrity continues to be impugned. Laboratory tests are unremarkable. What pharmacotherapeutic adjunct would be most appropriate in his treatment?
A. Alprazolam
B. Atenolol
C. Clomipramine
D. Clonidine
E. Valproate

Section K Pretest: Schizophrenia Spectrum and Psychotic Disorders

1. When a patient presents with hallucinations in the clinic, what history question(s) is/are most important to rule out potential causes?
   A. When did the symptoms start?
   B. Do you use illicit or legal drugs?
   C. Have any family members had similar symptoms?
   D. Can you explain the symptoms you are having?
   E. All of the above

2. What is an example of a nonbizarre delusion?
   A. A working 30-year-old male with the belief that he can fly if he "just flaps his hands just right"
   B. A 65-year-old who believes that all should bow down to him because he is the god of the world's chrome
   C. A 22-year-old who believes that the vice president is from Venus
   D. A 50-year-old female believes her husband of 30 years is unfaithful with her best friend despite both denying the claims, stating "I just know it"

3. You have just confirmed that your 25-year-old male patient has schizophrenia. He initially presented with auditory hallucinations, and the frequency of symptoms is increasing. What is the best option for proceeding with treatment?
   A. Recommend starting olanzapine (Zyprexa), therapy, with patient and family education
   B. Recommend starting haloperidol (Haldol), therapy, and continue with only family support groups
   C. No medications are needed at this time, patient education and therapy only with follow-up in a few days
   D. Recommend oral fluoxetine (Prozac) daily, family therapy, and education that this condition likely will not improve

Section L Pretest: Somatic and Dissociative Disorders

1. A 23-year-old female presents to your office with multiple complaints. This is her third visit in 6 months. Today, she is complaining of recurrent headaches, intermittent low back pain, and epigastric pain for 1 month that have sometimes prevented her from going to work. At prior visits over the past year, you have ordered labs and studies for diarrhea, vomiting, and excessive menstrual bleeding but found no medical or substance-induced cause for these symptoms. Which of the following is the most appropriate treatment for this patient?
   A. Schedule her with one provider 4 times a year for hour-long office visits
   B. Do not work up any more symptoms

C. Dismiss her from the practice for malingering

D. Schedule her with a single medical provider

2. Which of the following is a symptom of functional neurologic symptom disorder?
   A. Constipation
   B. Paralysis
   C. Tinnitus
   D. Ageusia

3. A 33-year-old female patient presents to your office requesting an MRI because she is convinced that she has brain cancer. This is her third visit in 6 months with this request. Prior to this, she was sure that she had ovarian cancer. Which of the following is the most likely diagnosis?
   A. Somatic symptom disorder
   B. Illness anxiety disorder

C. Factitious disorder

D. Functional neurologic symptom disorder

4. What is a possible risk if and/or when a patient diagnosed with dissociative amnesia recovers a memory?
   A. Suicide attempt
   B. Seizure disorder
   C. Fugue state
   D. Temporal lobe impairment

5. Which of the following is a risk factor for dissociative identity disorder?
   A. Male gender
   B. History of childhood trauma
   C. High socioeconomic level
   D. Autism spectrum disorder

Section M Pretest: Substance Use and Addictive Disorders

1. Which of the following describes tolerance of a substance?
   A. Consumption amounts that increase the likelihood of health consequences
   B. Needing to increase the amount of a substance to achieve the same desired effect
   C. Body's response to the abrupt cessation of a drug
   D. Spending excessive time getting/using/recovering from the drug use

2. Which of the following medications is indicated for the treatment of opioid withdrawal?
   A. Varenicline
   B. Bupropion
   C. Naltrexone
   D. Buprenorphine

3. A 52-year-old-male comes to the office with his wife for a routine office visit. You have been this patient's provider for many years and have noticed the patient is not as friendly or outcoming as he used to be and avoids looking at you directly. On physical examination, you notice fine tremors in his hands. He also

reports he was recently let go from his job for absenteeism. The patient's wife admits she is concerned about her husband's alcohol consumption. What is your next step?
   A. Administer a screening tool such as AUDIT or CAGE questionnaires.
   B. Order labs.
   C. Admit the patient for further workup.
   D. Refer for counseling.

4. Alcohol withdrawal commonly requires the use of what class of drugs?
   A. Benzodiazepines
   B. Antidepressants
   C. Narcotics
   D. Stimulants

5. Withdrawal from which substance does NOT generally require medication?
   A. Alcohol
   B. Cocaine
   C. Marijuana
   D. Opioids

Section N: Trauma- and Stress-Related Disorders

1. An 8-year-old boy has been fighting at school since moving to a new city 3 months ago. His mother reports he is anxious and nervous about going to school and has asked to stay home. Prior to moving, he loved school. Based on the above, which of the following is the most likely diagnosis?
   A. Oppositional defiant disorder
   B. Generalized anxiety disorder
   C. Adjustment disorder
   D. Conduct disorder

2. How is narcolepsy diagnosed?
   A. Polysomnography
   B. Multiple sleep latency test
   C. Sleep diary
   D. Hypocretin level

3. A 20-year-old female presents to clinic with complaints of trouble sleeping, poor concentration, and increased irritability. She reports no longer being able to drive since witnessing a fatal car accident 2 weeks ago and she avoids the area where the accident happened. She admits to often replaying the accident in her head and says it feels like the accident is happening again. She has nightmares about the wreck and finds it difficult to laugh. Which of the following diagnoses is correct?
   A. Post-traumatic stress disorder
   B. Acute stress disorder
   C. Generalized anxiety disorder
   D. Adjustment disorder with anxiety

4. A 22-year-old female presents to the OB/GYN for her annual checkup. She takes folic acid, propranolol for performance anxiety, sumatriptan, fluoxetine, and has an intrauterine device. Which medication puts the patient at highest risk of suicidal ideation?
   A. Propranolol
   B. Sumatriptan
   C. IUD
   D. Fluoxetine

5. A 35-year-old patient presents to clinic complaining of daytime sleepiness. Which of the following symptoms is most closely correlated with narcolepsy?
   A. Daytime sleepiness
   B. Sleep paralysis
   C. Hallucinations
   D. Cataplexy

6. A 45-year-old male presents to your primary care office for a routine follow-up visit for hypertension and type 2 diabetes. During the visit, he discusses the difficulties of coping with the recent death of his wife, stating that he feels alone and sometimes feels that life would be better if he were not alive. You state: "I know this must be a difficult time for you and I am so sorry you have been having these thoughts." Which of the following is the best initial response to the patient?
   A. "Do you feel like ending your life?"
   B. "Have you attempted suicide recently or in the past? Do you have a plan?"
   C. "When did you first notice having thoughts that 'life would be better if you weren't alive,' and how often do you have these thoughts?"
   D. "Do you have a gun or other weapon available?"
   E. "Do you think you would benefit from antidepressants?"

7. A 24-year-old presents to the clinic complaining of "sleep attacks." This has been occurring for the past 4 months. He fell asleep driving once and had a minor accident. He works as a waiter and often works double shifts. He is going to school at night (online). He estimates he gets 2-3 hours of sleep at night and takes a 1-hour nap between school and work. What will help determine the diagnosis?
   A. Clinical diagnosis
   B. Actigraphy
   C. Sleep Medicine referral
   D. Polysomnography

8. A 30-year-old male veteran presents to your office for increased frequency of insomnia. He states he keeps having nightmares about his times overseas and does not feel as though he can cope with these memories anymore. You suspect he may have suicidal thoughts and ask, "Have you ever thought about killing yourself?" to which he replies he has. Which of the following is the next best question to ask?
   A. "What stops you from killing yourself?"
   B. Ask patient about frequency, duration, intensity of suicidal ideations.
   C. Seek out the patient's family members and ask if they can confirm the patient's report.
   D. "Do you have a plan in place?"

9. Which of the following is considered first-line treatment of nightmares in post-traumatic stress disorder?
   A. Melatonin
   B. Hydroxyzine
   C. Trazodone
   D. Prazosin

10. A 19-year-old is diagnosed with narcolepsy type 1. What medication may be used to treat the associated cataplexy symptoms?
    A. Modafinil
    B. Methylphenidate
    C. Venlafaxine
    D. Zolpidem

11. A 34-year-old nurse reports to clinic complaining of feeling like she is going crazy. She started working the night shift 4 months ago and feels like her life has not been right since then. She is often sleepy at work and is afraid she is going to make an error. During her off time, she tries to spend the day engaged in activities with her children. She is always tired but cannot sleep, she is often moody, causing stress with her family. She has gained weight, and today her BP was elevated. What is the first-line treatment?
    A. Melatonin
    B. Cognitive behavioral therapy
    C. Sertraline
    D. Modafinil

12. A 14-year-old male presents to your primary care office at the request of his mother due to "dramatic mood changes." On further examination without the parent present, you find scars along his forearms bilaterally. He states he has been feeling more stressed and depressed recently. He expresses fear that there is a gun accessible in the house. Which is the next best step in the management for this patient?
    A. Call back in patient's mother and discuss your concerns with both patient and mother.
    B. Admit patient to hospital for further care and observation.
    C. Same-day appointment with behavioral health provider/psychiatrist/emergency department for further evaluation.
    D. Express concerns to child's mother only and admit to hospital.
    E. Trial patient on an SSRI and follow-up in several days.

13. Which of the following statements is true about post-traumatic stress disorder?
    A. PTSD can only be diagnosed in children and adults older than 6 years.
    B. Having a strong support group is a protective factor against PTSD.
    C. PTSD symptoms must be met within 6 months of the traumatic event.
    D. A patient rarely has another comorbid diagnosis with PTSD.

14. A 30-year-old female presents with symptoms of depression. After further investigation, she admits to occasional suicidal ideation and thoughts of death, but no clear plan has been established. After further questioning, she admits a previous suicide attempt using alcohol and acetaminophen ~5 years ago. Which level of risk would you diagnose this patient as?
    A. Low
    B. Moderate
    C. High
    D. Severe

15. A 70-year-old man presents to your office for feelings of depression. He admits to suicidal ideation, specifies a plan for killing himself, and has meticulously gone through and rehearsed his plan using his handgun. Upon questioning, he states that he has good relationships with his children and has some friends at the local coffee shop. Which of the following is the most appropriate treatment for this patient?
    A. Inpatient hospitalization; if the patient refuses hospitalization, consider involuntary commitment if state permits.
    B. Call the therapist and send the patient there immediately.
    C. Create a safety plan with the patient and admit them to the hospital.
    D. Encourage the patient to contact family members, consider initiation of antidepressant, collaborate with other health care providers.

▶ ANSWERS AND EXPLANATIONS TO SECTION A PRETEST

1. **D.** Survivors of sexual assault frequently feel disenfranchised and powerless. One of the most helpful things that you can do for a survivor is to help them regain their own personal power, especially in control over their physical being. The initial response to disclosure carries a strong tendency to direct the course of the survivor's recovery long term, including predicting the severity, length, and likelihood of developing PTSD, anxiety disorders, and depression. Option D is the best choice because it highlights shared decision-making, nonjudgmental option presentation. It is also the best choice because it mentions a thorough explanation of the survivor's prophylactic options, including an informed discussion about PEP.

2. **D.** Nonfatal strangulation in the context of domestic violence relationships raises the homicidality risk of future violent episodes exponentially. Asking about and screening for nonfatal strangulation episodes during any interview about domestic violence is a crucial part of identifying potentially fatal interactions. Weapons in the home (particularly handguns, whether loaded or unloaded) also carries an almost 200% increase in fatality risk in future

domestic violence incidents. Asking about handguns and other safety measures in the home is also crucial to identify high-risk domestic violence relationships. Asking about children in the home is also essential, for several reasons. Having a child in the home who is not the biological child of the abuser also raises the homicide risk. It is well-documented that children who witness or experience domestic violence (an example of an adverse childhood event, or ACE) are more likely to have long-term physical and mental health sequelae. Therefore, it is important to ensure that children are safe and experience as little domestic violence or other ACEs as possible. Answer A is not an acceptable choice because the psychology of "staying or going" in domestic violence relationships is often very complicated and difficult to elucidate, especially when otherwise stressed.

▶ ANSWERS AND EXPLANATIONS TO SECTION B PRETEST

1. **D.** If a patient fails treatment with one SSRI, it is reasonable to try a different drug from the same class or an SNRI.
2. **B.** The GAD-7 is a tool used to screen for anxiety, whereas the Hospital Anxiety Depression Scale can be used to assess the severity of a patient's anxiety.
3. **B.** Treatment for specific phobia should start with CBT with exposure therapy. Benzodiazepines can be used if CBT is ineffective.

▶ ANSWERS AND EXPLANATIONS TO SECTION C PRETEST

1. **D.** Autism-specific screening is recommended by the American Academy of Pediatrics at 18 and 24 months.
2. **A.** An older sibling with ASD is a risk factor for ASD.
3. **A.** Children must demonstrate deficits in social communication to meet the *DSM-5* diagnostic criteria for ASD.
4. **A.** The evaluation of a child with suspected ASD should include lead level.

▶ ANSWERS AND EXPLANATIONS TO SECTION D PRETEST

1. **A.** Bipolar I is characterized by at least one episode of mania of at least 1-week duration and associated with hospitalization, functional impairment, and possible depressive and hypomanic episodes.
2. **B.** Cyclothymic disorder is defined by periods of hypomanic symptoms and periods of depressive symptoms (lasting at least 2 years in adults or 1 year in children/adolescents) that do not meet diagnostic requirements for a hypomanic and depressive episode.

Bipolar disorder type 1 involves at least one manic episode of at least 1 week duration and associated with hospitalization, functional impairment (eg, social, occupational), or psychotic features.

3. **A.** The use of lithium plus an antipsychotic or valproate plus an antipsychotic is appropriate as a first-line pharmacologic approach for a patient with bipolar disorder with a severe manic or mixed episode. Severely ill or agitated patients may also require short-term adjunctive treatment with a benzodiazepine, such as clonazepam. Antidepressants, such as paroxetine, should be tapered or discontinued, if possible, during an acute manic episode.

▶ ANSWERS AND EXPLANATIONS TO SECTION E PRETEST

1. **C.** Patients who are diagnosed with conduct disorder present with no remorse for crimes they have committed, they have no empathy or regard for anyone and tend to have a poor academic performance due to either learning disabilities or lack of caring about their schoolwork.
2. **D.** There is not a specific medication to treat conduct disorder. It is necessary to treat the comorbid conditions. Some off-label medications may be used by the mental health community. Patients are usually not compliant with treatment.

▶ ANSWERS AND EXPLANATIONS TO SECTION F PRETEST

1. **B.** Weight loss of 20 lb while dieting is not a criterion of MDD.
2. **D.** Bupropion should not be used in a patient with a history of seizures.
3. **A.** An adolescent female is not considered high risk for suicide completion.
4. **D.** Children may present with a primarily irritable mood instead of depressed mood.

▶ ANSWERS AND EXPLANATIONS TO SECTION G PRETEST

1. **C.** Amenorrhea is not the *DSM-5* diagnostic criteria for diagnosing AN.
2. **B.** AN is her likely diagnosis.
3. **A.** Consider olanzapine in this patient.
4. **B.** This patient presenting with electrolyte disturbance (eg, hypokalemia and metabolic alkalosis), oral health issues, normal BMI, and likely parotid gland enlargement is suspicious for bulimia nervosa. In anorexia, the BMI is usually decreased. In suppurative parotitis, an ill patient and significant physical examination findings (eg, fever, erythema, tenderness, or purulence) would be expected. In viral parotitis,

swollen, tender parotid gland(s) with low-grade fever would be typical.

5. **D.** Further evaluate this patient by screening her for an eating disorder using the SCOFF questionnaire, asking the patient to void and then wear a medical gown before re-taking her vitals, and asking her about her diet and exercise routine.

6. **C.** The patient likely has bulimia nervosa with purging as evidenced by her dental enamel erosions. Patients who self-induce vomiting can develop hypochloremic, hypokalemic metabolic alkalosis as purging results in loss of hydrogen and chloride ions.

▶ ANSWERS AND EXPLANATIONS TO SECTION H PRETEST

1. **A.** ADHD is a neurobehavioral disorder that predominately affects boys between the ages of 4 and 18 years. It is characteristic of symptoms that affect daily living in two or more settings (in this case, home and school).

2. **A.** The classic presentation of ADHD is an impulsive and inattentive individual.

3. **A.** A comprehensive history allows the practitioner to diagnose ADHD. To date, there are no physical examinations, labs, or imaging results for definitive diagnosis.

4. **A.** Psychostimulants (methylphenidate, dextroamphetamine) are the most effective drugs to treat ADHD. They work by increasing levels of norepinephrine in the brain, which increases the ability to focus. Patients with ADHD may have other comorbidities that will benefit from antidepressants, antipsychotics, and/or mood stabilizers.

▶ ANSWERS AND EXPLANATIONS TO SECTION I PRETEST

1. **D.** Venlafaxine should not be considered as a first choice for a patient with OCD.

2. **B.** Mood disorders are frequently associated with OCD.

3. **C.** Washing hands 4 times before leaving the bathroom is a compulsion.

4. **A.** CBT with an emphasis on exposure with a response prevention shows the most efficacy in the treatment of OCD.

5. **D.** Fear that while driving you ran over a pedestrian is an example of an obsession.

▶ ANSWERS AND EXPLANATIONS TO SECTION J PRETEST

1. **A.** Dependent personalities need reassurance and depend on others to make decisions for them. They become clingy with those close to them.

2. **E.** Cluster A consists of schizoid, schizotypal, and paranoid personality disorders.

3. **D.** Treating a narcissistic personality disorder is difficult. If the patient does not eventually cooperate, there is less a chance for success. Narcissistic personality disorders do well in a program that has family, group, and individual therapy sessions. Medications are not helpful in these patients unless there are comorbid conditions, such as depression. Those with comorbidities and newly diagnosed sometimes do respond in an inpatient residential facility because of intense focus on a daily basis.

4. **E.** Medication use for narcissistic personality disorder is generally adjunctive, used to target comorbid features such as hypomania seen in this case. Drugs with abuse potential and those with high risk in overdose should be avoided.

▶ ANSWERS AND EXPLANATIONS TO SECTION K PRETEST

1. **E.** When a patient presents with hallucinations in the clinic, ask all of those questions.

2. **D.** A 50-year-old female believes her husband of 30 years is unfaithful with her best friend despite both denying the claims, stating "I just know it" is an example of a nonbizarre delusion.

3. **A.** Recommend starting olanzapine (Zyprexa), therapy, with patient and family education for this patient.

▶ ANSWERS AND EXPLANATIONS TO SECTION L PRETEST

1. **D.** Schedule her with a single medical provider.

2. **B.** Paralysis is a symptom of a functional neurologic symptom disorder.

3. **B.** Illness anxiety disorder is the most likely diagnosis.

4. **A.** Suicide attempt is a possible risk if and/or when a patient diagnosed with dissociative amnesia recovers a memory.

5. **B.** History of childhood trauma is a risk factor for dissociative identity disorder.

▶ ANSWERS AND EXPLANATIONS TO SECTION M PRETEST

1. **B.** Needing to increase the amount of a substance to achieve the same desired effect describes tolerance of substance.

2. **D.** Buprenorphine is indicated for the treatment of opioid withdrawal.

3. **A.** Administer a screening tool such as AUDIT or CAGE questionnaires.

4. **A.** Alcohol withdrawal commonly requires the use of benzodiazepines.

5. **C.** Withdrawal from marijuana generally does not require medication.

▶ ANSWERS AND EXPLANATIONS TO SECTION N PRETEST

1. **C.** Adjustment disorder is the most likely diagnosis.
2. **B.** Narcolepsy is diagnosed with MSLT.
3. **B.** Acute stress disorder is the correct diagnosis.
4. **D.** Fluoxetine puts the patient at highest risk of suicidal ideation.
5. **D.** Cataplexy is most closely correlated with narcolepsy.
6. **C.** "When did you first notice having thoughts that 'life would be better if you weren't alive,' and how often do you have these thoughts?"
7. **A.** This is a clinical diagnosis.
8. **B.** Ask patient about frequency, duration, intensity of suicidal ideations.
9. **D.** Prazosin is considered first-line treatment of nightmares in PTSD.
10. **C.** Venlafaxine may be used to treat the associated cataplexy symptoms.
11. **B.** CBT is the first-line treatment.
12. **C.** Same-day appointment with behavioral health provider/psychiatrist/emergency department for further evaluation is the next best step in management for this patient.
13. **B.** Having a strong support group is a protective factor against PTSD.
14. **B.** This patient is moderate risk.
15. **A.** Inpatient hospitalization; if the patient refuses hospitalization, consider involuntary commitment if state permits.

CHAPTER
293

Child Abuse, Elder Abuse, Domestic Violence, and Sexual Abuse

Katherine Thompson, MCHS

▶ GENERAL FEATURES

- *Interpersonal violence* is an umbrella term that includes domestic violence, sexual assault, child abuse, elder abuse, and human trafficking.
- Domestic violence, also called intimate partner violence, is defined by the presence of behaviors of power and control within a relationship.
- Sexual assault includes rape, unwanted sexual touching, sexual harassment, and attempted rape.
- Elder abuse includes neglect, physical abuse, sexual abuse, financial abuse, and verbal abuse of those generally over the age of 65 years.
- Child abuse includes sexual abuse, physical abuse, neglect, verbal abuse, mental abuse, exploitation, and other subcategories against those under the age of 18 years.
- One in three women and one in eight men will experience sexual assault in their lifetime. One in four women and one in eight men will experience violence within a relationship. More than 80% of victims of sexual assault will know their perpetrator.

▶ CLINICAL ASSESSMENT

- Diagnosis of interpersonal violence is typically made through any combination of patient disclosure, routine screening, clinical judgment and patient interviewing, reporting from concerned relatives or friends, or law enforcement involvement.
- Differential for domestic violence may include accidental injury, although injury patterns tend to differ between accidental injury and inflicted harm.
- Differential for child abuse may include nonintentional abusive behaviors, particularly neglect.
- Differential for child sexual abuse varies broadly, but can include nonspecific findings, from hymenal notches (that may masquerade as loss of hymenal tissue in young girls) to nonspecific vaginal erythema or bleeding that may be unrelated to sexual abuse.

- Physical examination, lab studies, and imaging for domestic violence are specific to the injury patterns or areas of concern, but should always include a verbal assessment for nonfatal strangulation and traumatic brain injury.
- Physical examination, lab studies, and imaging for child abuse typically focus on the type of abuse and areas of concern; may include an x-ray skeletal survey, which often identifies untreated or previously healed fractures.
- Other modalities for assessment include forensic interviewing techniques used to encourage children to discuss difficult topics without prompting, coaching, or other techniques that could affect the suspected veracity of the confession.

▶ DIAGNOSIS

- Criterion for diagnosis for all forms of interpersonal violence is based on a wide continuum of considerations, including age and mental status of the victim, suspected type of abuse or violence, and status of disclosure (or lack thereof).

▶ TREATMENT

- Criterion for treatment of domestic violence is based on evaluation of physical condition, including evaluation for nonfatal strangulation. Similar to a trauma assessment, diagnosis and treatment is based on injuries present and the mechanisms of injury.
- Criterion for treatment of child abuse is grounded by informed discussion with parents, a high degree of suspicion, activation of the child protective services, and diagnosis and treatment of existing physical injuries depending on the mechanisms of injury.
- Criterion for treatment of elder abuse should be highly sensitive for neglect and nonphysical abuse, multiple types of longitudinal abuse, and consider mental health conditions that may create barriers around reporting or recalling incidents of abuse.

- Criterion for treatment of sexual assault should include counseling on prophylactic treatment for STIs, monitoring for hepatitis, HIV (if PEP is not selected) and syphilis, and treatment for any injuries.
- Prophylactic recommendations for STIs/pregnancy postsexual assault:
  - Chlamydia, gonorrhea, trichomonas: 250 mg IM ceftriaxone, 1 g oral azithromycin, and 2 g oral metronidazole (in a single dose)
  - HIV: discussion with patient about likelihood of contracting HIV from various unsafe sexual practices, possibility of side effects, and necessary medications
  - Hepatitis B: at least two immunizations must be given postexposure prophylaxis (PEP). If previously immunized, a single booster should be considered.
  - Pregnancy: emergency contraception is given using Plan B or a similar medication; an IUD can be considered as an alternative within 72 hours.
- Complications:
  - Acute and chronic complications from interpersonal violence can include: acute stress reactions, anxiety, STIs, infections or complications from injuries, insomnia, PTSD, depression, chronic pain syndromes, fibromyalgia, heart disease, IBS, dyspareunia, chronic pelvic pain, and even death.

SECTION **B** *Anxiety Disorders*

CHAPTER
294

Generalized Anxiety Disorder, Phobias, and Panic Disorder

Amy M. Klingler, MS, PA-C, DFAAPA

A 32-year-old female presents to clinic with concerns of uncontrollable worry, irritability, poor sleep, and poor appetite for the past 6 months. She reports that as a result of her symptoms, she quit her job and prefers to stay at home to avoid situations where she must talk to other people. What should you consider?

GENERAL FEATURES

- Generalized anxiety disorder (GAD) is characterized by persistent, excessive, uncontrollable worry that causes distress. It interferes with the patient's ability to function normally.
- If the anxiety is situational or related to a specific object, it is referred to as a *phobia*, whereas episodic anxiety is a panic disorder.
- Patients often seek medical care for panic attacks because they are difficult to distinguish from other medical emergencies.
- Patients with anxiety disorders commonly report physical complaints related to a heightened state of arousal, including insomnia, fatigue, headaches, and pain of the neck, shoulders, or back.

CLINICAL ASSESSMENT

- A comprehensive history should include past medical history noting illnesses, medications, and adverse drug reactions; personal and family psychiatric history; and social history, including stressful life events, caffeine, nicotine, alcohol and illicit drug use, and abuse and neglect.
- Tests can be ordered to rule out a physical cause for symptoms when indicated by history and physical examination, including complete blood count, comprehensive metabolic panel, thyroid-stimulating hormone, electrocardiogram, and urine or blood toxicology.
- The Generalized Anxiety Disorder 7-item scale (GAD-7) can be used to screen for symptoms of anxiety, whereas the Hospital Anxiety Depression Scale can be used to assess the severity of GAD.

DIAGNOSIS

- The *Diagnostic and Statistical Manual of Mental Disorders* (Fifth Edition; *DSM-5*) criteria are used to identify GAD, phobias, and panic disorders.
- GAD requires the presence of:

- Persistent feelings of worry and anxiety present on most days for at least 6 months
- Difficulty controlling the worry
- Anxiety and worry associated with three or more of the following symptoms (only one item is required in children), with at least some of the symptoms present for more days than not for the past 6 months:
  - Restlessness or feeling keyed up or on edge
  - Being easily fatigued
  - Difficulty concentrating or mind going blank
  - Irritability
  - Muscle tension
  - Sleep disturbance
- Anxiety, worry, or physical symptoms cause clinically significant distress or impairment in social, occupational, or other important areas of functioning.
- The disturbance is not attributable to the physiologic effects of a substance (medication or drug of abuse) or other medical condition.
- Panic attacks are episodes of sudden, intense fear without a specific trigger that cause significant physical symptoms, such as palpitations, shaking, shortness of breath, diaphoresis, and/or a sense of impending doom.
- A diagnosis of panic disorder requires presence of recurrent, unexpected panic attacks, and 1 month of either worry about future attacks or a change in behavior due to the attacks.
- Panic disorder can occur with or without agoraphobia, fear, and avoidance of situations that can cause panic. Agoraphobia is classified as a separate anxiety disorder.
- Specific phobia involves anxiety about a specific object or situation. The object or situation almost always provokes immediate anxiety. It is actively avoided or endured with intense anxiety, which is out of proportion to the actual danger. The anxiety related to a phobia is persistent, typically lasting for 6 months or more, and the anxiety or avoidance causes significant distress.

▶ TREATMENT

- Anxiety disorders can be treated with medication or cognitive-behavioral therapy (CBT) or a combination of both. Specific phobias are usually treated with CBT with exposure therapy.
- Selective serotonin reuptake inhibitors (SSRIs), selective norepinephrine reuptake inhibitors (SNRIs), and buspirone are effective anxiety treatments. A short course of benzodiazepines can abort panic attacks and treat specific phobias, if CBT is ineffective.
- Patients usually achieve full clinical effect of SSRIs and SNRIs after 4-6 weeks. Partial response to medication can be treated with dose titration. If no response at a therapeutic dose, the initial drug should be tapered off and another agent prescribed from the same or a different class of medications.
- Options for second-line treatment include benzodiazepines, tricyclic antidepressants, gabapentin or pregabalin, and some anticonvulsants.
- Duration of treatment for anxiety disorders should be at least 12 months. Patients who stop sooner than 12 months are more prone to relapse.

Case Conclusion

The patient is exhibiting symptoms of GAD and agoraphobia because she is avoiding situations that may cause her anxiety. She did not describe panic attacks or major depressive disorder.

SECTION C

Autism Spectrum Disorder

CHAPTER 295

Autism Spectrum Disorder

Kristy Luciano, PA-C

▶ GENERAL FEATURES

- Autism spectrum disorder (ASD) covers a range of neurodevelopmental disorders characterized by early-onset impairments in social communication and interaction.
- Restricted and repetitive behavior patterns, interests, or activities are common.
- The term *autism spectrum disorder* covers a broad range of severity, including individuals who need some assistance to patients who need substantial support.

- According to the CDC, 1 in 54 children have been identified with autism.
  - ASD is nearly 5 times more common in boys (1 in 42) than in girls (1 in 189).
  - The exact cause of ASD is unknown; etiology appears to be multifactorial and includes genetic and environmental factors.
  - A relationship between thimerosal containing vaccines and autism has been robustly disproven.
- The median age of diagnosis is after age 4 years, although many parents may have concerns about their child's development by age 15 or 18 months.
- A delay in diagnosis is significant as prognosis is best with aggressive early intervention.

▶ CLINICAL ASSESSMENT

ASD should be considered in children who are evaluated for developmental concerns or behavioral, social, or emotional problems.

- History:
  - Identify risk factors such as:
    - Older sibling diagnosed with ASD
    - Genetic conditions such as fragile X syndrome
    - Child born to older parents
  - Ask parents if they have concerns about their child's language, hearing, or behavior.
  - Patients with ASD may demonstrate selective hearing (eg, a child may respond to noise in the environment, but not a parent calling his or her name).
  - Inquire about nonverbal communication such as abnormalities in eye contact.
  - Ask about relationships with or interest in peers.
  - Children diagnosed with ASD may be inflexible or have fixated interests, which can lead to behavior problems at home or difficulty relating to or engaging with peers.
  - Identify children with stereotyped motor movements such as hand flapping or stereotyped speech such as repetitive vocalizations.
- Developmental surveillance and screening:
  - Developmental surveillance should occur at every well-child visit.
  - The American Academy of Pediatrics recommends administering standardized developmental screening tests at 9, 18, and 30 months.
  - Recommended screening tools include:
    - Ages and Stages Questionnaires (ASQ)
    - Parents' Evaluation of Developmental Status (PEDS)
  - Autism-specific screening is recommended by the American Academy of Pediatrics at ages 18 and 24 months.
    - Modified Checklist for Autism in Toddlers, Revised, With Follow-Up (M-CHAT-RF)

- A positive screening test should be followed by a thorough diagnostic evaluation.

▶ DIAGNOSIS

- Based on comprehensive assessment of patient via structured interviews, observation, behavioral and cognitive assessments, and medical examination
  - Ideally, children with suspected ASD undergo evaluation by a team of child specialists with experience in the diagnosis of ASD.
  - Feedback from teachers and caregivers is useful.
- All children with suspected ASD should have an audiology evaluation and lead screening.
- *DSM-5* diagnostic criteria include:
  - Symptoms should be present from early childhood and in different contexts or settings.
  - Two principal categories of symptoms:
    - Deficits in social communication and social interaction
    - Restrictive and repetitive behavior patterns
- A reliable diagnosis can often be made by age 2 years.
- If the patient has an intellectual disability or the clinician has concerns about a specific genetic or neurologic disorder, consider referral to a developmental pediatrician, geneticist, or child neurologist.

▶ TREATMENT

- There is no cure for ASD.
- Goals of therapy include improving quality of life and functional independence. Treatment plans should include goals focusing on family support.
- At the first sign of developmental delay, a child should be referred for early intervention evaluation and services.
  - If the child's age ≥3 years, refer to the local school district.
- Treatment consists of intensive therapies that should be started as soon as possible.
  - This often includes speech and occupational therapy as well as social skills training.
  - Parent training and education may decrease behavioral issues in children.
- Interventions such as behavioral strategies are used to address communication, social skills, behavioral issues, and academic problems.
- Medication may be used to support behavior management (eg, challenging behaviors such as irritability) or treat comorbid psychiatric diagnoses.
  - Aripiprazole and risperidone are the only FDA-approved medication for irritability in children with ASD.

CHAPTER
296

Bipolar Disorder

Reamer L. Bushardt, PharmD, PA-C, DFAAPA
Teri L. Capshaw, MBA

A 57-year-old patient presents to a primary care provider with complaints of anxiousness and irritability for the past 2 months. The patient recently relocated for work and endorses poor sleep for the past several weeks. He has hyperlipidemia and a long history of depression and anxiety with two prior psychiatric admissions (in his 20s and 30s) for depression. He underwent electroconvulsive therapy during the first admission and reports prior treatment with various antidepressants, lithium, and carbamazepine. His current medications are lithium carbonate (30-day supply filled 75 days ago), sertraline, and pravastatin (30-day supply filled 25 days ago for both). What is the best next step to evaluate and manage his symptoms?

▶ GENERAL FEATURES

- *DSM-5* defines bipolar disorder as a group of brain disorders that cause fluctuation in an individual's mood, energy, and ability to function.
  - Three basic types of bipolar disorders: bipolar I disorder, bipolar II disorder, and cyclothymic disorder (cyclothymia):
    - For bipolar symptoms that do not match basic types, the term *unspecified bipolar and related disorders* is used.
  - Bipolar I disorder is defined by manic episodes that last at least 7 days, or by manic symptoms that are so severe that the person needs immediate hospital care.
    - Depressive episodes usually occur as well, and episodes of depression with mixed features are also possible.
  - Bipolar II disorder is defined by a pattern of depressive episodes and hypomanic episodes, but not the type of manic episodes seen in bipolar I disorder.
  - Cyclothymic disorder is defined by periods of hypomanic symptoms and periods of depressive symptoms (lasting at least 2 years in adults or 1 year in children/adolescents) that do not meet diagnostic requirements for a hypomanic and depressive episode.

- Estimated prevalence of bipolar disorder in US adults is 2.8%, and average onset is at 25 years of age.
- Bipolar I rates are similar among males and females; bipolar II is more common in women.
- Multifactorial interactions among genetic and environmental factors (eg, chronic stressors, physical or sexual abuse) likely contribute to the pathogenesis.
  - Appears highly heritable and shares inheritance patterns with schizophrenia and major depressive disorder
- Comorbid psychiatric disorders and/or substance use disorders often occur.
- Bipolar disorder is associated with increased risk of suicidality and premature death.

▶ CLINICAL ASSESSMENT

- Diagnosis is based on history, mental status examination, and exclusion of other causes of symptoms.
  - Consider bipolar disorder in individuals presenting with depression or symptoms of mania.
  - Screening tools (eg, Mood Disorder Questionnaire) can help identify bipolar disorder in the general population.

▶ DIAGNOSIS

- Diagnosis based on criteria within the *DSM-5*:
  - Bipolar 1:
    - At least one manic episode of at least 1-week duration and associated with hospitalization, functional impairment (eg, social, occupational), or psychotic features
    - May have prior depressive episode, and hypomanic episodes may also occur
    - May have labile mood between episodes that does not meet diagnostic criteria for depression, hypomania, or mania
    - Additional clinical features may be seen (eg, anxious distress, mixed features, rapid cycling,

melancholic features, atypical features, mood-congruent or incongruent psychotic features, catatonia, seasonal pattern, or peripartum onset)
- Bipolar II:
  - History of major depressive and hypomanic episodes, but no mania
  - Additional clinical features may be seen (eg, anxious distress, mixed features, rapid cycling, melancholic features, atypical features, mood-congruent or incongruent psychotic features, catatonia, seasonal pattern, or peripartum onset)
- Cyclothymia:
  - Periods of depression and hypomanic symptoms for at least 2 years in adults (or 1 year in children/adolescents) that do not meet diagnostic criteria for major depressive or hypomanic episodes
  - No period without symptoms lasting > 2 months
  - May occur with anxious distress and may resemble bipolar I or II with rapid cycling due to frequent mood changes

▶ TREATMENT

- Multidisciplinary approach to management is used because of chronic, relapsing, and remitting nature of bipolar disorder.
  - Drug therapy is a mainstay of treatment for bipolar I and II.
  - Psychoeducation supports patients in detecting/managing early symptoms as well as with stress management and healthy lifestyle interventions.
  - Various psychosocial interventions have shown benefits (eg, symptom management in acute depressive episodes, improved treatment adherence, relapse prevention, and improved quality of life).
    - In person with depressive symptoms, commonly use cognitive-behavioral therapy (CBT), interpersonal and social rhythm therapy (IPSRT), or family-focused therapy (FFT)
    - For maintenance and relapse prevention, may use CBT, IPSRT, FFT, peer support, or cognitive/functional remediation therapy
- Drug therapy depends on clinical presentation and symptoms.
  - For acute mania or hypomania:
    - Mood stabilizer (eg, lithium, divalproex) or second-generation antipsychotic (eg, quetiapine, ziprasidone, olanzapine, aripiprazole)

- Consider discontinuing antidepressant until patient's mood is stabilized due to potential for rapid cycling and exacerbation of mania/hypomania.
- For acute agitation with mania or depression:
  - Antipsychotic or benzodiazepine (oral)
    - Consider intramuscular options if rapid management indicated.
- For bipolar depression:
  - Mood stabilizer or second-generation antipsychotic
  - Consider adjunctive antidepressant only if monotherapy mood stabilizer is not sufficient to manage symptoms and in combination with an adequate mood stabilizer.
- For maintenance therapy:
  - Consider same medication used for acute symptoms or switch to another mood stabilizer (eg, lithium, divalproex, quetiapine, lamotrigine).
- Inpatient treatment considered with acute mania, and with risk of harm to self or others
- Electroconvulsive therapy (ECT) may be used in treatment of refractory cases, rapid care is needed, or other scenarios (eg, psychotic symptoms, catatonia, severe suicidality, food refusal leading to nutritional compromise, prior history of favorable response to ECT).
- Regularly evaluate patients with bipolar disorder for:
  - depressive, manic, and hypomanic symptoms
  - suicide risk
  - sleep symptoms/hygiene
  - comorbidities, including substance use disorder(s)
  - adherence to treatment
  - general health
  - drug safety (including laboratory monitoring specific to prescribed medications)

Case Conclusion

Based on history and clinical presentation, the patient likely has bipolar disorder (eg, probably bipolar II if no manic episodes have occurred) with his symptoms the result of stress from a major life event, poor sleep, and medication issues (eg, nonadherence to lithium, use of an antidepressant without adequate mood stabilizer therapy). Screening for substance use, suicidality, and verifying the diagnosis using a questionnaire or *DSM-5* criteria is appropriate, and prior medical records may be helpful. Temporary discontinuation of antidepressant, use of a mood stabilizer, stress reduction, and patient education would be considered.

CHAPTER 297

Conduct Disorder

Michelle Heinan, EdD, PA-C
Lauren Anderson, MMS, PA-C

A 13-year-old male presents to your clinic due to aggressive behavior. His parents have not been able to control him. In past year, he has been intimidating and picking fights at school. He pulled a knife on a boy during his last fight. He has been caught shoplifting multiple times and has been staying out all night at least 6 times in the last month. He also set fire to a neighbor's pool deck.

▶ GENERAL FEATURES

- Conduct disorder is a repetitive and persistent pattern of aggressive and/or defiant behavior in which age-appropriate expectations are not followed.
- The disruptive behavior may occur at home, school, or in public.
- It is thought to be caused by neurobiologic factors such as reduced noradrenergic function and right temporal lobe and gray matter volumes, psychological factors such as lower IQ, and social factors such as low socioeconomic status, lack of parental involvement in childbearing, and harsh discipline.
- Prevalence is around 1% in school-aged children but significantly increases into adolescence with a male-to-female ratio of 2:1.
- Symptoms after onset are highly variable and differ with age.

▶ CLINICAL ASSESSMENT

- Disruptive behaviors will fall into four major categories: aggression toward people and/or animals, destruction of property; deceitfulness or theft, and serious violations of rules that persist and worsen.
- There are several associated features that are predictive of impairment, including problems with anger management, understanding social cues, family and peer relationships, aggression, low self-esteem, substance abuse, learning, or underachievement.

- Patients will minimize problems.
- Parents will report that they have been unable to control their child's behavior.

▶ DIAGNOSIS

- Diagnosis depends on differentiating between regular experimentation and risk-taking behavior from behaviors that seriously cause harm and are antisocial.
- Medical history and neuropsychological assessment should be included.
- Interview parents, child, teachers, law enforcement (if indicated), and caregivers. The child should be observed as they interact with family.
- Comorbidities include ADHD, depression, substance misuse, anxiety, bipolar disorder, learning disabilities, PTSD, and developmental disorders.
- Differential diagnoses should include new onset of psychotic disorders, mood disorders, and substance abuse. A urine drug screen may be considered.
- Psychological tests are completed by mental health professionals to make the diagnosis.
- *DSM-5* criteria: pattern of persistent and relative behavior that violates age-appropriate norms and rights of others. Must meet 3 of 15 criteria in the last 12 months and at least 1 of the criteria within the last 6 months.
- Aggression to people and animals: bullies and intimidates people, initiates fights, uses weapons on others to cause physical harm, confronts and steals from others, and cruelty to animals and people to inflict physical harm
- Destruction of property: arson, vandalism
- Deceitfulness and theft: theft; shoplifting, cons others out of things or favors
- Serious violation of rules: before age 13 years, stays out at night or stays out all night (at least twice), or runs away from home for a period of time or truancy

TREATMENT

- Long-term treatment may include placement at a residential facility to provide structure.
- Anger management, behavioral therapy, family therapy, and psychotherapy
- Parent training is provided to learn to set limits, set up a routine, provide clear direction, have consequences for poor behavior, and reward positive behaviors.
- Special education is needed if learning disability identified.
- Multisystemic therapy for the family and child to improve child behavior, family dynamics, and functioning at school
- Pharmaceuticals are used only in treating comorbidities, such as ADHD, depression, and impulse problems.

- Relapse rates are high.
- Prognosis depends on how early intervention was started, comorbidities, age at the time behaviors appeared, and parental criminal activity.

Case Conclusion

This child meets criteria for conduct disorder based on engaging in at least 3 of the 15 *DSM-5* criteria and 1 in the last 6 months. The criteria met are (1) intimidating, (2) initiating fights, (3) using a knife, (4) staying out all night, (5) shoplifting, and (6) setting fire to a neighbor's pool deck.

SECTION **F**   *Depressive Disorders*

CHAPTER **298**

Major Depressive Disorders and Bereavement Disorders

Victoria Specian, MSCP, PA-C

GENERAL FEATURES

- Major depressive disorder (MDD) has a multifactorial etiology: genetic, biochemical, psychodynamic, and socioenvironmental.
- Grief is a normal reaction to a significant loss, such as bereavement, natural disaster, or serious medical illness, and can share many symptoms of MDD.
- Predominant feelings of emptiness and loss tend to come in waves and lessen over days to weeks.
- Bereaved individuals may develop MDD if symptoms are severe and persist beyond acute grieving.

CLINICAL ASSESSMENT

- Diagnosis is made via clinical interview based on *DSM-5* criteria.
- Rule out a previous manic or hypomanic episode because bipolar disorder commonly presents initially as depression.
- Persistent depressive disorder (dysthymia) should be ruled out in patients complaining of depressed feelings for a 2-year period (or 1 year in children).
- Basic lab work can rule out other diagnoses.

DIAGNOSIS

- *DSM-5* criteria:
  - Diagnosis includes one of the following two symptoms: (1) depressed mood or (2) loss of interest or pleasure, along with five (or more) of the following SIG E CAPS mnemonic for a 2-week period:
    - Sleep (insomnia or hypersomnia)
    - Interest (loss of interest/pleasure in activities)
    - Guilt (feelings of worthlessness or inappropriate guilt)
    - Energy decreased or fatigue
    - Concentration decreased
    - Appetite decreased or increased
    - Psychomotor agitation or retardation
    - Suicidal ideation
  - Symptoms must cause significant distress or impairment in social, occupational, or other important areas and cannot be attributed to substance use or another condition.

TREATMENT

- For severe MDD, the combination of SSRIs and cognitive-behavioral therapy (CBT) has proven most effective.
- Antidepressants take anywhere from 4 to 6 weeks to reach full effectiveness.
- If remission is not obtained with an adequate dose and trial, then it is recommended to:
    - switch classes of antidepressant
    - add another antidepressant, such as bupropion or mirtazapine
    - add one of the three FDA-approved atypical antipsychotics: quetiapine XR, aripiprazole, or brexpiprazole
- TCAs and MAOIs, though effective in treating depression, are no longer the first-line treatments because of side effects and possible drug/food interactions.
- Electroconvulsive therapy (ECT), vagus nerve stimulation (VNS), transcranial magnetic stimulation (TMS), and esketamine are reserved for treatment-resistant MDD and are not available in all areas.

SECTION G *Feeding and Eating Disorders*

CHAPTER 299 Anorexia Nervosa

Sara Hoyle, MSPA

GENERAL FEATURES

- Psychological disorder characterized by a significantly low body weight, distorted body image, and an intense fear of gaining weight
- The average age of onset is 17.5 years.
- Lifetime prevalence of 0.9% in women and 0.3% in men.
- Mortality rate is 5% to 10%, one of the highest of all psychiatric conditions.
- Anorexia nervosa (AN) has a low probability of recovery (50%) and a high probability of comorbid psychiatric conditions.
- AN and malnutrition can impact most organ systems.
    - Refeeding syndrome is a potentially fatal complication that can occur as a result of fluid and electrolyte shifts during aggressive nutritional rehabilitation.

CLINICAL ASSESSMENT

- Diagnosed clinically in patients with low body weight associated with severe dietary restriction or weight loss behaviors and that excludes other causes for weight loss
- Several screening tools are available, such as SCOFF, Eating Disorder Screen for Primary Care (ESP), and Eating Attitudes Test (EAT).

- Patients often present with symptoms such as:
    - Hypotension
    - Weakness or fatigue
    - Palpitations
    - Amenorrhea or infertility
    - Constipation

DIAGNOSIS

- Diagnosis by *DSM-5* requires all of the following:
    - Restricted energy intake relative to requirements, leading to a significantly low body weight
    - Intense fear of weight gain
    - Distorted body image
    - Further classified it into two types: binging/purging or restricting, with severity based on BMI
- Laboratory testing and imaging is individualized and may vary based on a patient's symptoms. Examples include:
    - For all patients, consider doing UA, CBC, and CMP.
    - If amenorrheic, consider FSH, LH, PRL, TSH, and hCG.
    - To assess bone health, consider vitamin D level and DEXA scan.
    - If severe AN or history of palpitations, consider an EKG.

TREATMENT

- Outpatient therapy preferred, but inpatient treatment considered if patient is unstable or is at high risk for medical complications.
- Treatment requires multidisciplinary management, including a dietitian, counselor, and primary care provider to coordinate and manage other health issues that arise, such as constipation.
  - Nutritional rehabilitation (refeeding) works toward restoring weight and normal eating patterns.
    - Refeeding syndrome is rare, but potentially fatal. Severely malnourished patients need close monitoring to avoid refeeding syndrome.
  - Psychotherapy with a counselor or psychiatrist may focus on cognitive-behavioral therapy (CBT) to help overcome reluctance to increase calories and challenge distorted beliefs about themselves and food.
  - Pharmacologic management is limited.
    - Olanzapine can be used in patients who do not gain weight following nutritional rehabilitation plus psychotherapy.
    - Antidepressants are not first line and should be used with caution. Tricyclic antidepressants should be avoided due to risks of cardiotoxicity in malnourished patients, and bupropion is contraindicated due to higher incidence of seizures.
- Numerous general medical complications may affect multiple organ systems as a result of weight loss and malnutrition. Treatment for complications includes nutritional replenishment. Many complications resolve with weight gain.
- Be aware of and address potential behaviors that interfere with treatment. For example, a patient may attempt to manipulate a provider's assessment of their weight by wearing multiple layers of clothing or hiding weights in their clothes, so a standard policy could be weighing all patients in a gown and standing on the scale backward where the patient cannot see their weight.

CHAPTER
300

Bulimia Nervosa

Reamer L. Bushardt, PharmD, PA-C, DFAAPA

A 28-year-old woman presents to her gynecology practice for an annual visit, with no complaints. Her BMI is 25 kg/m². On examination, the provider notes signs of poor oral health and bilaterally enlarged parotid glands. Upon further interview about her health behaviors and exploration of risk factors, the patient reports she binge eats on pasta and bread a couple of times per week and feels anxious most days. What would be the most appropriate next step to assess the patient for an eating disorder?

GENERAL FEATURES

- Bulimia nervosa (BN) is a serious, potentially life-threatening eating disorder characterized by recurring episodes of excessive eating ("binging" or binge eating) and compensatory behaviors to avoid weight gain.
- Prevalence is 2% to 3% for women and 0.5% for men.
  - Most common in young women
- Binging behavior is associated with a perceived loss of control.
- Examples of compensatory behaviors to prevent weight gain are self-induced vomiting, misuse of laxatives, fasting or excessive exercise, and diuretic use.
  - These can result in serious medical complications, such as electrolyte disturbances, GI tract injury, oral health problems, and premature death.

- BN is frequently associated with comorbid psychiatric illness (eg, mood and anxiety disorders) and other psychological signs and symptoms (eg, social withdrawal, self-harm behaviors, low self-esteem).
  - Comorbid mental illness as well as history of suicidal or self-harm ideation increase risk of death in patients with eating disorders.

CLINICAL ASSESSMENT

- Diagnosis is primarily based on history.
  - Interview-based assessment tools (eg, Eating Disorders Assessment for *DSM-5*, EDA-5) exist.
  - Additional input gathered from physical examination, laboratory testing (eg, basic metabolic panel), psychological evaluation, and other diagnostic studies (eg, ECG) to assess for medical complications and associated conditions
- Potential medical complications of BN:
  - Local adverse effects of vomiting:
    - Persistent gastric acid reflux leading to dysphagia and dyspepsia, hematemesis, perimolysis, oral mucositis, and cheilitis
  - Acid-base and electrolyte abnormalities:
    - Metabolic alkalosis and hypokalemia are the most common abnormalities.

- Effects of excessive laxative use (eg, hypokalemia or local GI effects such as rectal prolapse, diarrhea, hemorrhoids, hematochezia, cathartic colon syndrome)
- Sialadenitis (parotid gland enlargement)

▶ DIAGNOSIS

- According to *DSM-5*, BN is present if these criteria are met:
  - Recurrent episodes of binge eating, as characterized by:
    - Eating, within any 2-hour period, an amount of food that is definitively larger than what most individuals would eat in a similar period of time under similar circumstances
    - A feeling that one cannot stop eating or control what or how much one is eating
  - Recurrent inappropriate compensatory behaviors in order to prevent weight gain
  - The binge eating and inappropriate compensatory behaviors occur, on average, at least once a week for 3 months.
  - Self-evaluation is unjustifiability influenced by body shape and weight.
  - The disturbance does not occur exclusively during episodes of anorexia nervosa.
- Severity is described as:
  - Mild: an average of one to three episodes of inappropriate compensatory behaviors per week
  - Moderate: an average of four to seven episodes of inappropriate compensatory behaviors per week
  - Severe: an average of 8-13 episodes of inappropriate compensatory behaviors per week

- Extreme: an average of 14 or more episodes of inappropriate compensatory behaviors per week

▶ TREATMENT

- A multidimensional approach is used, with cognitive-behavioral therapy (CBT) as a first-line treatment.
- Interpersonal therapy is a second-line, evidence-based treatment for adults with BN.
- Family-based treatment or CBT is preferred in adolescents.
- Limited evidence exists on role of pharmacotherapy in BN.
  - Considered adjunctive to psychotherapy (eg, fluoxetine that is FDA approved for treatment of BN and can decrease binge eating and vomiting).
  - Pharmacotherapy can be used to treat comorbid psychiatric condition(s).
- Assess nutritional intake for all patients (regardless of weight/BMI).
- Medical complications may require targeted treatment but often improve or resolve as underlying BN is managed.

Case Conclusion

The diagnosis of an eating disorder is primarily based on patient history; thus, the provider should gather additional historical information and assess within *DSM-5* criteria. A guided-interview tool for eating disorders could be used to structure the history-taking. In addition, the patient reports anxiety symptoms, and this should be explored in the context of the *DSM-5* or with a screening tool for common anxiety and mood disorders.

SECTION **H**   *Attention Deficit Hyperactivity Disorder*

CHAPTER
301

Attention Deficit Hyperactivity Disorder

Ashley Fort, MPAS

▶ GENERAL FEATURES

- Attention deficit hyperactivity disorder (ADHD) is one of the most common neurobehavioral disorder of childhood, affecting 2% to 9.5% of school-aged children and adolescents.

- ADHD predominantly affects boys.
- The etiology of the disease is correlated with genetics and environmental factors (eg, prematurity, low birth weight, intrauterine growth restriction, history of brain injury and certain genetic syndromes, prenatal

tobacco exposure, socioeconomic disadvantage, and environmental exposure to lead).
- Diagnosis is established between the ages of 4 and 18.
- Patients with ADHD experience academic and/or behavioral problems that cause significant impairment.
- Symptoms of ADHD can include inattention, hyperactivity, or impulsivity.

▶ CLINICAL ASSESSMENT

- Evaluation for ADHD should determine if a behavior meets the diagnostic criteria and can rule out other conditions that mimic ADHD or cause similar symptoms.
- A thorough history and clinical interview provides a comprehensive analysis of the patient's past medical, family, and social history along with any other factors that may affect the patient's functioning.
- Behavior rating scales completed by parents, teachers, and/or caregivers will assess the number and magnitude of symptoms. Examples of these rating scales include:
  - Behavior Assessment System for Children (BASC-3)
  - National Institute for Children's Health Quality (NICHQ) Vanderbilt Assessment Scale
  - Conner's Comprehensive Behavior Rating Scale (CBRS)
  - Swanson, Nolan, and Pelham-IV Questionnaire (SNAP-IV)
  - Conners-Wells' Adolescent Self-Report Scale
- Neurologic imaging and blood tests are indicated if there is strong evidence for neurologic pathology or other conditions.
- Comorbid conditions are common and may include learning or language disorders, neurodevelopmental disorders, psychological and behavioral conditions, autism spectrum disorder, sleep disorder, depression or anxiety, and oppositional defiant or conduct disorder, so testing for these is important, based on the patient's presentation.

▶ DIAGNOSIS

- The diagnosis of ADHD is made when a patient's behavior meets the *DSM-5* criteria:
  - Behavior that is developmentally inappropriate
  - Symptoms are present before age 12.
  - Symptoms are present for 6 months or more.
  - Symptoms are present in two or more settings.
  - Symptoms clearly interfere with function at home, school, work, or peer settings.
  - Symptoms are not explained by another medical disorder.
- Based on symptomology, the diagnosis of ADHD can be further classified into three subtypes:
  - Primarily inattentive

- Primarily hyperactive-impulsive
- Combined type

▶ TREATMENT

- Current research suggests the most effective management is a combination of medication and behavioral treatment.
- Psychostimulants have proven useful for children with moderate-to-severe ADHD. The most commonly prescribed psychostimulants are methylphenidate and amphetamine.
- Behavioral therapy may improve behaviors that cause impairment. This involves clear communication between parents and teachers about expectations and strategies for improvement in the classroom. Students benefit from academic interventions, such as task modifications, reinforcement for on-task behaviors, organizational skills training, and homework strategies.
- Patient education, particularly for parents, is key for optimal treatment and understanding the condition, accepting and complying with treatment plan, and communicating progress.
- Adults dealing with ADHD are also most successful with the use of psychostimulants and behavioral therapy. Behavioral therapy can involve cognitive therapy, dialectical therapy, or life coaching. When combined with proper education, these interventions can assist in identifying where ADHD symptoms are causing the most challenges and allow for transformation of these negative patterns.
- Complications:
  - Children with ADHD often experience problems associated with poor school performance and have increased rates of dropping out of school.
  - Social impairments cause some to have low self-esteem and lead to substance abuse.
  - Impulsive behavior can lead to increased rates of accidents and teen pregnancies/STIs.
  - Comorbid disorders, such as anxiety, depression, and conduct disorder, often exist.
- Prognosis:
  - Hyperactive and impulsive symptoms tend to decrease with age.
  - 50% to 70% of patients continue to have significant inattentiveness, restlessness, and impulsivity into adulthood.
  - Owing to negative stigma and misunderstanding of ADHD and its appropriate use of stimulants, there is a high tendency for treatment and follow-up noncompliance. This leads to many individuals experiencing a poor quality of life secondary to financial, legal, and social problems.

CHAPTER

302

Obsessive-Compulsive Disorder

Paul "PJ" Koltnow, MS, MSPAS, PA-C

▶ GENERAL FEATURES

- Obsessive-compulsive disorder (OCD) causes persons to experience repetitive intrusive thoughts, images, or urges, which are known as obsessions. These persons then engage in repetitive behaviors, either mental or physical, that they feel they "must" perform to help alleviate the anxiety caused by the obsession.
- Aggression, sex, and religion are common obsessional themes.
- These mitigating behaviors (compulsions) can take the form of repetition (eg, washing hands, putting things in specific orders or checking) or mental activities (eg, praying, counting, repeating words).
- Obsessions become recurring and persistent and are not pleasurable or voluntary, rather they are intrusive and unwanted. The person will then engage in compulsions in an attempt to counteract or avoid the anxiety and distress.
- These obsessions and/or compulsions cause significant impairment in daily functioning.

▶ CLINICAL ASSESSMENT

- Onset usually occurs in the mid-20s, though can be seen in childhood.
- 76% of patients have a lifetime history of an anxiety disorder and 63% have a lifetime history of a mood disorder, which is often major depressive disorder.
- Females are slightly more affected than males. The lifetime prevalence in the general population is around 2% to 3%.
- Most people with OCD realize their obsessions are irrational.
- It is important to rule out other physiologic effects, such as medication side effects, drug abuse, or another medical condition.

- There are certain themes that are common and include:
  - Cleaning: fears of contamination
  - Symmetry: insisting items are symmetrical, repeating, in a specific order
  - Taboo thoughts: sexual or religious obsessions
  - Harm: thoughts or images about harming self or others, checking compulsions

▶ DIAGNOSIS

- If OCD is suspected, an evaluation of impact on daily functioning is performed via diagnostic interview.
  - Yale-Brown Obsessive Compulsive Scale (Y-BCOS) or Children's (CY-BCOS) Scale
- Providers should obtain a baseline assessment followed by routine reassessment to determine treatment effectiveness.
- There are no lab or imaging tests to identify OCD.
- Diagnostic criteria are defined by the *DSM-5*. The following is an abridged version.
  - Presence of obsessions or compulsions or both:
    - Obsessions as defined by:
      - Recurrent and persistent thoughts, urges, or images that are unwanted and cause significant distress, or impairment in social, occupational, or other important areas of functioning
    - The individual attempts to reduce these thoughts, urges, or images, with some other thought or action known as compulsions.
    - Compulsions may involve mental tasks, such as counting or praying, or they may involve physical rituals, such as repeated handwashing or checking the state of an object.
  - Rule out substance abuse, medical disorders, or another mental condition.

TREATMENT

- Adults:
  - Treatment involves using a form of cognitive-behavioral therapy (CBT) called "exposure with response prevention" as well as pharmacotherapy.
  - Two classes of serotonergic antidepressants are strongly supported by randomized trials for OCD.
    - Consider a selective serotonin reuptake inhibitor (SSRI) antidepressant (eg, fluoxetine, fluvoxamine, sertraline, paroxetine, or sertraline).
    - If not responding to SSRI, consider clomipramine, a tricyclic antidepressant.
- Children:
  - CBT is the psychotherapy of choice for children.
  - SSRIs are the first-line choice for pediatric OCD.
    - Either fluoxetine, fluvoxamine, or sertraline has been shown to be safe and effective in children.

SECTION **J**   *Personality Disorders*

CHAPTER
303

Personality Disorders

Michelle Heinan, EdD, PA-C
Mary Beth Babos, PharmD, BCPS

During history-taking at a wellness examination, a 32-year-old reports anxiety over career indecision. She states she is not good enough for most jobs that her family and friends suggest, despite their reassurance and assistance. She fears she cannot answer interview questions without help. What treatment is appropriate for this patient?

GENERAL FEATURES

- Impairments in personality functioning and pathologic personality traits.
- Persistent and uncompromising in social and personal situations
- Distress in functional, social, and occupational areas
- Develops in adolescence into early adulthood
- The *DMS-5* defines 10 personality disorders in three clusters:
  - Cluster A: "odd, eccentric" includes schizoid, schizotypal, paranoid
  - Cluster B: "dramatic, erratic" includes histrionic, borderline, narcissistic, antisocial
  - Cluster C: "anxious, fearful" includes obsessive compulsive, dependent, avoidant

- Four features are common to all:
  - Distorted thinking
  - Problematic emotional responses
  - Altered impulse control
  - Interpersonal difficulties
- Prevalence in the United States:
  - Cluster A, 4%
  - Cluster B, 2%
  - Cluster C, 4.2%
- Associated with decreased quality of life, poor health, and premature death
- Etiology is complex, involving genetic and environmental factors.
- Risk factors:
  - Family history:
    - Personality disorders
    - Psychiatric conditions
    - Substance use disorders
  - Early adverse childhood experience
- Traits:
  - Anger, attention-seeking, blame-placing, emotional lability, lacking insight, inflexibility, difficulty with social cues, feeling exploited, and intolerance of boredom

▶ CLINICAL ASSESSMENT

- Review personality traits related to relationships, behavior, impulsivity, emotional expression, reality, and self-identity.
- Interview patient's associates to assess changes.
- Check for comorbidities or substance use when symptoms emerge during adulthood.

▶ DIAGNOSIS

- Based on symptoms described and objective observations during assessment
- Diagnostic criteria established in the *DSM-5:*
  - Not a situational response
  - Deviation from behavior expected norms in at least two areas (ie, cognition, affectivity, interpersonal functioning, impulsivity)
  - Traits are maladaptive, inflexible, cause distress, have persisting pattern.
- More than one disorder may co-occur.
  - Tendency for disorders within the same cluster to co-occur
  - May co-occur with other psychiatric diagnoses
  - *DMS-5* attempts to reduce overlap using dimensional vs. categorical approach.
- Cluster A personality disorders:
  - Paranoid: mistrustful, paranoid, suspicious that others aim to hurt or humiliate them
  - Schizoid: detached from relationships, limited in emotional expression, often loners
  - Schizotypal: superstitious, discomfort in social situations, no close relationships, feelings of "sixth sense"
- Cluster B personality disorders:
  - Antisocial: "psychopaths," aggressive, irresponsible, remorseless, with disregard for others. Often involved in criminal activity. Diagnosis cannot be made until 18 years of age.
  - Borderline: mood fluctuations, impulsivity, unstable relationships, and poor self-image
  - Histrionic: shallow, dramatic, attention-seeking, emotional, demanding, and impulsive
  - Narcissistic: self-centered, superiority act covers delicate self-esteem, prioritizes power and success, requires extensive attention, and lacks empathy
- Cluster C personality disorders:
  - Avoidant: feels inadequate, fears being judged or embarrassed, reclusive due to avoidance of social contact
  - Dependent: helpless, indecisive, forms relationships for constant reassurance through ingratiating behavior, abandonment fears lead to clingy behavior
  - Obsessive compulsive: inflexible due to need for perfection and order; fear of mistakes or preoccupation with detail leads to difficulty in task completion

▶ TREATMENT

- Psychotherapy is the first-line treatment.
- Exercise, journaling, and stress management are often helpful.
- Isolation and substance use should be avoided.
- Pharmacotherapy is adjunctive, targets symptoms, and may have a greater role with active comorbid disorders.
  - Medications are used primarily in acute situations and withdrawn with crisis resolution.
  - Examples of drugs used with target signs/symptoms:
    - Antipsychotics: low dose for anger control, hallucinations, and paranoia
    - Mood stabilizers: for anger, anxiety, impulse control, and depressed mood
    - Antidepressants: small effect for anxiety and anger
    - Omega-3 fatty acids: moderate evidence to reduce recurrent self-harm
- Tolerability and adverse effect profile should factor in medication selection.
- Most patients will improve over time with psychotherapy; thus, attempts at medication taper are recommended.

Case Conclusion

In this case, the presentation is suspicious for a Cluster C personality disorder and further diagnostic screening is warranted. Psychotherapy would be a first-line treatment if the diagnosis is established.

CHAPTER

304

Schizophrenia Spectrum and Psychotic Disorders

Marie Pittman, DMSc, MPAS, PA-C, RDH

▶ GENERAL FEATURES

- Schizophrenia is a chronic psychiatric disorder characterized by a combination of positive symptoms, such as hallucinations, delusions, and negative symptoms such as social withdrawal, affective flattening, or lack of motivation, associated with broad impairment in cognitive function.
- Age of onset for schizophrenia and other psychotic disorders is the early 20s in men and late 20s in women.
- Exact etiology is unknown; thought to be linked to dopamine overstimulation.
- Schizophrenia prevents adequate self-sustained living (work, social, family life, etc) owing to chronic or recurrent psychosis for 6 months or longer. Psychosis is associated with positive and negative symptoms:
  - Positive symptoms (symptoms present that should not be):
    - Hallucinations: sensory input that is not there (auditory, visual, olfactory, somatic, gustatory). Auditory hallucinations are the most common.
    - Delusions: fixed false beliefs, can be bizarre or nonbizarre
    - Disorganized speech
    - Disorganized behavior
    - Catatonic behavior
  - Negative symptoms (symptoms that should be present but are not):
    - Flat affect
    - Impairments in cognition
    - Attention deficits
    - Loss of executive function
    - Alogia
    - Apathy
    - Anhedonia
    - Social withdrawal
- Mood and anxiety symptoms appear more commonly than in the general population.

- Patients can show neurologic disturbances and metabolic disturbances.
- Those with predominantly negative symptoms are the least likely to respond to treatment.
- Suicide rates are higher in persons with schizophrenia.
- Other schizophrenia spectrum disorders:
  - Brief psychotic disorder: sudden onset of one or more positive psychotic symptoms and resolution within the month. Typically linked to a marked stressor.
  - Schizophreniform disorder: all criteria of schizophrenia met, but the disease state is from 1 to 6 months in duration.
  - Schizoaffective disorder: schizophrenia with manic episodes or significant depression. Usually, psychosis presents at a different time than the mood episodes.
  - Psychotic mood disorders: psychotic episodes are associated with mood episodes.
  - Substance-induced psychotic disorder: psychotic symptoms are in association with substances or withdrawal of those substances. Resolves once the patient is sober. Common drugs include hallucinogens, dopamine agonists, psychostimulants, alcohol, and sympathomimetics, among others.
  - Psychosis due to a medical condition: the medical condition causes psychosis. Ensure that you have ruled out other medical conditions before a diagnosis of schizophrenia. Examples include, but are not limited to, brain neoplasm, HIV/AIDS, CVA, dementia, Parkinson disease, and seizure disorder.
  - Delusional disorder: delusions present without meeting criteria for schizophrenia. Patients can typically function normally. There are several types: grandiose, erotomanic, jealous, persecutory, somatic, or mixed.

- Schizotypal personality disorder: a personality type that does not meet the delusions or hallucinations needed to be classified as schizophrenia. There is a long life pattern of odd and/or eccentric behaviors and beliefs.
- Schizoid personality disorder: little interest in social relationships or intimacy. These patients typically do not have psychosis but do show negative symptoms as found in schizophrenia. May precede schizophrenia or delusional disorder.
- Pervasive developmental disorders: delayed development of social and communication skills, can present with psychosis or negative symptoms.

CLINICAL ASSESSMENT

- History of present illness and overall history from the patient and family/friends is crucial.
- May take multiple visits to rule out different causes, especially with a poor history (common)
- Use tests to rule out other causes of psychosis:
  - Do urine toxicology screenings, bloodwork, or breath tests to rule out substance use.
  - Testing to rule out medical conditions (ie, CVA or TBI, Wilson disease, porphyria, syphilis, dementia, etc).
- Baseline labs and information needed:
  - Baseline BMI, waist circumference, heart rate, BP, and signs of extrapyramidal syndrome (EPS) and tardive dyskinesia (TD) should be measured before initiation of pharmacotherapy.
  - Baseline labs are needed before starting antipsychotic medications. These include CBC, thyroid function tests, lipid profile, and CMP (particularly paying attention to electrolytes, fasting glucose, liver function, and renal function). EKGs should also be obtained in those with prior cardiac issues and/or those put on medications that can cause QT prolongation. Monitor labs throughout treatment.

DIAGNOSIS

- Schizophrenia diagnosis is typically one of exclusion.
- *DSM-5* criteria:
  - Two or more of the following symptoms are present for 6 months with at least 1 month of active symptoms:
    - Delusions
    - Hallucinations
    - Disorganized speech (eg, frequent derailment or incoherence)
    - Grossly disorganized or catatonic behavior
    - Negative symptoms (ie, affective flattening, alogia, or avolition)
  - The clinical diagnosis is made based on these characteristic signs and symptoms, time course, adverse impact on functional capacity, and idiopathic nature.
- The diagnosis should rule out all other issues (ie, medical, substances, no major depressive, manic, or mixed episodes have occurred with psychosis symptoms).

TREATMENT

- Negative symptoms are difficult to treat.
- Antipsychotics are used to reduce symptoms and promote return-to-normal daily functioning. Multiple forms of intake are available depending on needs. Doses should be titrated to therapeutic as quickly as tolerated.
  - First-generation "typical" antipsychotics are older antipsychotics (ie, chlorpromazine [Thorazine], haloperidol [Haldol], and many more).
  - Second-generation "atypical" antipsychotics are newer and have fewer EPS symptoms (clozapine [Clozaril], risperidone [Risperdal], quetiapine [Seroquel], ziprasidone [Geodon], olanzapine [Zyprexa], and many more).
- Side effects of first-generation antipsychotics are more common. EPS is less often seen with second-generation antipsychotics. Continual maintenance is necessary. Examples of side effects and treatments include:
  - EPS: involuntary movements; can be painful. Decrease dosing of medications or change medications. Benztropine (Cogentin) is used to treat and prevent EPS.
  - TD: permanent involuntary movement of the face, arms, and/or trunk. Educate patients before starting medications for acceptance of risks. Discontinue immediately if suspected TD.
  - Hyperprolactinemia: if concerned, check blood prolactin levels. Discontinue or decrease the dosing of the medication. Females and males can have growth of breast tissue and galactorrhea. Decreased libido and amenorrhea are also possible.
  - Watch for xerostomia, constipation, difficulty urinating, hypotension, ejaculatory failure, and sedation and adjust treatment accordingly.
- Therapy is imperative, although antipsychotics are the mainstay. Noncompliance is very common with these disorders.

CHAPTER

305

Somatic and Dissociative Disorders

Ann McDonough-Madden, MHS, PA-C

▶ GENERAL FEATURES

- According to the *DSM-5*, somatoform disorders include somatic symptom disorder (SSD), illness anxiety disorder (IAD), functional neurologic symptom disorder (FNSD), and factitious disorder. Dissociative disorders include dissociative amnesia, depersonalization/derealization disorder, and dissociative identity disorder (DID).
- Somatoform disorders are physical manifestations of psychological stress, with SSD being the most prevalent. All disorders, except for factitious disorder, are most likely to be seen in the primary care setting.
- Dissociative disorders, characterized by a disruption in the normal integration of consciousness, memory, identity are rare and thought to be a reaction to extreme trauma in a patient's life. Associated with risk of suicide.

▶ CLINICAL ASSESSMENT

- SSD: >6-month history of somatic complaints with a variety of symptoms, such as pain and fatigue marked by excessive thoughts, feelings, or behaviors related to the somatic symptoms. Patient may report being sickly all their life and have a history of consulting many health care providers.
- IAD: a variant of SSD and new to the *DSM-5*. Greater than 6-month preoccupation with having or acquiring a serious illness. May have somatic complaints but they are mild compared to the preoccupation with being seriously ill. Formerly known as hypochondriasis.
- FNSD: dramatic presentation involving sensory and motor complaints of the neurologic system. Common complaints are paralysis, numbness, mutism, and blindness. Associated with dissociative symptoms such as derealization and depersonalization.

- Factitious disorder: purposeful and deceptive misrepresentation of physical or psychological signs or symptoms. Primary gain for patient is attention rather than an external reward, such as worker's compensation or avoiding legal issues.
- DID: the presence of two or more distinct identity states. Formerly known as multiple personality disorder. Risk factors include history of interpersonal physical and sexual abuse.
- Dissociative amnesia: characterized by the inability to recall important autobiographical information. Patients often have a history of trauma, child abuse, and victimization.
- Depersonalization/derealization disorder: recurrent or sustained feelings of feeling alien to oneself. Can be depersonalization where the patient describes feeling physically or emotionally numb. Derealization is the feeling that the patient is not connected to the outside world.

▶ TREATMENT

- Somatoform disorders: regularly scheduled medical office visits with the same provider for SSD and IAD along with referral for psychotherapy. Treat coexisting anxiety and depression if present.
- FNSD: initiate treatment at once, including behavioral or insight-focused therapy. Patients with FNSD often recover spontaneously.
- Dissociative disorders: trauma-focused therapy for DID; supportive psychotherapy (trauma-informed care, cognitive-behavioral therapy, and dialectical-behavioral therapy) with pharmacologic intervention if there is coexisting anxiety and depression for dissociative amnesia and derealization/depersonalization disorder.

Substance Use and Addictive Disorders

CHAPTER

306

Substance Use and Addictive Disorders

Paula Miksa, DMS, PA-C

▶ GENERAL FEATURES

- *DSM-5* combines *DSM-IV* of substance abuse and substance dependence into a single disorder (substance use disorder or SUD, measured on a continuum of mild to severe).
  - Separate use disorders exist for specific substances (eg, alcohol, opioid, stimulant).
  - Mild SUD requires the presence of two to three symptoms, moderate requires four to five, and severe requires six or more symptoms.
  - An important characteristic is an underlying change in brain circuits that may persist beyond detoxification, particularly in individuals with severe disorders.
- According to the American Society of Addiction Medicine, addiction is a treatable, chronic medical disease involving complex interactions among brain circuits, genetics, the environment, and an individual's life experiences.
  - In addiction, patients use substances or engage in behaviors that become compulsive and often continue despite harmful effects.
- Tolerance occurs when people need to increase the amount of a substance to achieve the same desired effect. The "desired effect" might be the desire to avoid withdrawal symptoms, or the desire to get high.
- Withdrawal is the body's response to the abrupt cessation of a drug once the body has developed a tolerance to it. The resulting cluster of (very unpleasant and sometimes fatal) symptoms is specific to each drug.
- Risky use of alcohol or other drugs are consumption amounts that increase the likelihood of health consequences (eg, injury, interpersonal problems, medical consequences).

▶ CLINICAL ASSESSMENT

- *DSM-5* recognizes multiple SUDs:
  - Alcohol, cannabis, hallucinogens, inhalants, opioids, sedatives, hypnotics or anxiolytics, stimulants, and tobacco

▶ DIAGNOSIS

- SBIRT (Screening, Brief Intervention, and Referral to Treatment) is a comprehensive, integrated, public health approach to delivery of early intervention and treatment services for persons with SUDs.
- Diagnosis is based on a pathologic set of behaviors related to the use of that substance. These behaviors fall into four main categories: impaired control, social impairment, risky use, and pharmacologic indicators (tolerance and withdrawal).
- Risk factors can be assessed in an office setting through screening tools. Most guidelines and organizations identify AUDIT (Alcohol Use Disorders Identification Test) as a validated and useful tool. CAGE (cut-annoyed-guilty-eye) questionnaire is primarily able to identify alcohol dependence or abuse—it does not have questions about quantity or frequency of drinking; however, it can be modified to fit any substance by simply replacing alcohol with the substance in question. A third tool is T-ACE (tolerance, annoyed, cut down, eye-opener).
  - AUDIT consists of 10 items with score ranging from 0 to 40.
  - When a patient answers "yes" to two or more questions on the CAGE questionnaire, the sensitivity is 60% to 90% and the specificity 40% to 60% for SUDs.

▶ TREATMENT

- The best approach to treating patients with SUDs involves a combination of counseling and social support. Medications are approved to treat some SUDs, but not all. Brief psychological or behavioral interventions are first-line treatment.
- Brief interventions by a primary care clinician consist of one to four brief (5-15 minutes) encounters with motivational interviewing, nonjudgmental feedback, recommendations for behavior change, goal setting, and making plans for follow-up.
- Patients with moderate-to-severe SUD may additionally benefit from participation in mutual support groups, 12-step programs, and may require referral to a specialist for treatment that may involve longer term counseling and medication management.
- Nonpharmacologic modalities also include education, coping skills, relaxation therapy, family therapy, various types of psychotherapy (individual and group therapy), health and nutritional counseling, lifestyle changes, and aftercare programs.
- Some forms of dependence require intensive detoxification, rehabilitation, and/or ongoing medication.
- Withdrawal symptoms may occur during discontinuation of a substance, especially if the use was prolonged or heavy.

- Approved medications should be used in conjunction with psychosocial interventions. Pharmacologic therapy includes:
  - Alcohol withdrawal: the use of benzodiazepines, such as diazepam (Valium) or chlordiazepoxide (Librium), as well as thiamine, folic acid, and multivitamin administration.
  - Opioid withdrawal: naloxone fully reverses all effects of opioids. Symptoms of opioid withdrawal can be rendered more tolerable by administration of α-2 adrenergic agonists, benzodiazepines, antiemetics, and antidiarrheals. Buprenorphine (Suboxone) can both induce and treat opioid withdrawal, depending on the timing of its administration. Naltrexone can block the effects of exogenously administered opioids. Used once a patient is opioid free for at least 7-10 days.
  - Tobacco withdrawal: nicotine and tobacco cravings can be treated with nicotine transdermal patches, nasal spray, gum, lozenges, inhaler, and antidepressants, such as bupropion (Zyban) or varenicline (Chantix).
  - Marijuana, phencyclidine (PCP), and hallucinogen withdrawal: usually do not require medication; however, anxiolytics can be used.
  - CNS depressants such as sedatives, benzodiazepines, or hypnotics: treatment requires gradually tapering the medication. Pentobarbital can be used if patients are experiencing severe symptoms.

SECTION **N**   *Trauma- and Stress-Related Disorders*

CHAPTER **307**   # Post-traumatic Stress Disorder and Adjustment Disorder

Victoria Specian, MSCP, PA-C

▶ GENERAL FEATURES

- Post-traumatic stress disorder (PTSD) is characterized by the triad of re-experiencing the event, avoidance of stimuli associated with the trauma, and increased arousal symptoms.
- A majority of Americans have experienced at least one potentially traumatic event in their lifetime.
- The risk of a trauma resulting in PTSD is dependent on several factors, including gender (female), history of previous trauma, and family history of anxiety disorders.

- The course of PTSD is variable, with half of all cases resolving within 3 months.
- PTSD not resolved within the 3 months often becomes chronic, with significant impact on occupational, physical, and interpersonal functioning.

▶ CLINICAL ASSESSMENT

- Diagnosis is made via clinical interview based on *DSM-5* criteria.

- PTSD can occur any time along the life span, with the onset of symptoms most often within 3 months following the trauma.
- Acute stress disorder (ASD) should be considered in symptoms that have lasted between 3 days and 1 month, because symptoms must be present for at least 1 month to be considered PTSD.
- Symptoms must cause distress or impairment in social, occupational, or other area of functioning.

▶ DIAGNOSIS

- *DSM-5* criteria:
  - Exposure to an actual or threatened death, serious injury, or sexual violence in one (or more) of the following ways:
    - Directly experiencing the traumatic event
    - Personally witnessing the event as it occurred to others
    - Learning of a traumatic event to a close family member or friend
    - Experiencing repeated exposure to aversive details of the traumatic event
  - Presence of one or more intrusive symptoms associated with the traumatic event:
    - Recurrent, involuntary, and intrusive memories
    - Recurrent distressing dreams related to the trauma
    - Flashbacks in which the individual feels or acts as if the trauma is reoccurring
    - Intense or prolonged distress at exposure to cues that resemble an aspect of the trauma
    - Physiologic reactions to cues that resemble an aspect of the trauma
  - Persistent avoidance of stimuli associated with the traumatic event in at least one of the following:
    - Avoidance of memories, thoughts, and feelings of the trauma
    - Avoidance of external reminders (people, places, or things) of the trauma

- Negative changes in cognitions or mood associated with the traumatic event in at least two of the following:
  - Inability to remember aspects of the trauma
  - Persistent, exaggerated negative beliefs about oneself and others
  - Persistent, distorted cognitions regarding the cause or consequence of the trauma
  - Persistent negative emotional state
  - Diminished interest or participation in significant activities
  - Feeling detached from others
  - Inability to experience positive emotions
- Alterations in arousal and reactivity associated with the traumatic event, as evidenced by two or more of the following:
  - Irritable behavior and angry outbursts
  - Self-destructive or reckless behavior
  - Hypervigilance
  - Exaggerated startle response
  - Difficultly concentrating
  - Sleep disturbances

▶ TREATMENT

- Psychological therapy, antidepressants, and symptom-directed pharmacotherapy are mainstays of treatment.
- SSRIs remain the gold standard for psychopharmacologic treatment of PTSD.
- TCAs, MAOIs, and atypical antipsychotics are other options, but their side-effect profiles should be considered.
- Comorbid psychiatric conditions need to be concurrently managed.
- To address anxiety symptoms associated with PTSD, buspirone, β-blockers, benzodiazepines, and α-2 agonists are all popular choices.
- Benzodiazepines are generally considered for short-term use only in ASD because of the concern for tolerance and dependence.
- Trauma-focused cognitive-behavioral therapy and EMDR (eye movement desensitization and reprocessing) are effective.

CHAPTER 308

Sleep-Wake Disorders

Teresa Bigler, DHEd, PA-C

▶ GENERAL FEATURES

- There are more than 60 types of sleep disorders in seven major sleep categories.
- The most common include inadequate sleep syndrome, circadian sleep-wake rhythm disorders (including shift-work disorder, jet lag, etc), and narcolepsy type 1 or type 2.

- Common symptoms of sleep-wake disorders include excessive daytime sleepiness (EDS), with or without insomnia, to the extent that it interferes with the person's ability to perform their specified duties (work, school, home responsibilities, etc).
- Differential diagnoses for EDS are extensive and include sleep disorders (obstructive sleep apnea [OSA]

or central sleep apnea [CSA], periodic limb movement disorder, parasomnias), medical and psychiatric disorders (nocturia, chronic pain, depression, anxiety), medications and drug use, or environmental stimuli that lead to fragmented sleep.

- Insomnia is described as a recurrent difficulty falling and staying asleep despite adequate opportunity.
  - Most adults will report at least a few episodes of insomnia.
  - Short-term insomnia is usually related to a specific stressor.
  - Chronic insomnia occurs at least 3 times per week for at least 3 months.
- Narcolepsy is a sleep disorder with EDS. It often occurs in conjunction with cataplexy and other symptoms, such as disturbed sleep at night, sleep paralysis, and hypnagogic and hypnopompic hallucinations.
  - Narcolepsy type 1:
    - Characterized by recurrent irresistible attacks of daytime sleepiness and low or absent cerebrospinal fluid (CSF) hypocretin-1 levels, with or without cataplexy
    - Sleepiness usually occurs in monotonous situations not requiring active participation.
    - Usually begins in the teenage years or early 20s
    - Possible etiologies include genetic factors, autoimmune processes, and unidentified environmental factors.
  - Narcolepsy type 2:
    - Characterized by recurrent irresistible attacks of daytime sleepiness without cataplexy
    - It may be caused by neurologic disorders, including tumors, multiple sclerosis, myotonic dystrophy, Prader-Willi syndrome, Parkinson disease, or head trauma.
- Patients with narcolepsy are at an increased risk of depression and anxiety; it is unclear if this is a manifestation of the disorder or a result of the disease.
- Narcolepsy patients are at an increased risk for car accidents and may have problems with employment due to medications, required naps, and sleep attacks. They may have additional psychosocial strain.

▶ CLINICAL ASSESSMENT

- A thorough history, with emphasis on daily routine and sleep habits (bedtime, wake time, how long to fall asleep, naps [intentional or sleep attacks], number of hours allotted vs. actual sleep, number of awakenings, feeling refreshed after sleep, current or remote shift work), should be performed.
- Reviewing the patient's medications, including times of dosing, is essential.
- Screening tools for daytime sleepiness, such as the Epworth Sleepiness Scale, can be used to determine a subjective measurement of the patient's daytime sleepiness and to monitor treatment success.

- Physical examination is typically normal. Physical examination should focus on other common causes of EDS, including OSA and CSA, and other neurologic conditions.
- Specific evaluation for narcolepsy includes questions about cataplexy, hypnagogic hallucinations, and sleep paralysis.

▶ DIAGNOSIS

- Most sleep-wake disorders are diagnosed clinically. The patient can complete a sleep diary over a 2-week period to assist with detection of sleep patterns. Actigraphy may provide additional information, but is not required for the diagnosis.
- Symptoms of daytime impairment are present in insomnia; insomnia should be considered when symptoms cannot be better explained by another sleep disorder.
  - Depression and anxiety are common comorbidities in patients with insomnia.
  - Medical conditions, medications, drugs, and other sleep disorders may contribute to or be exacerbated by insomnia.
- Patients with suspected narcolepsy should be referred to a sleep medicine center. Diagnosis is made using an overnight polysomnogram (PSG) that must show 6 hours of unfragmented sleep (to exclude other primary sleep disorders) followed by a daytime multiple sleep latency test (MSLT, also known as a nap test) to objectively measure how long it takes a patient to fall asleep and achieve REM sleep during 4-5 naps space throughout the day.

▶ TREATMENT

- The treatment for sleep-wake disorders is to align the timing of the sleep cycle with the desired sleep-wake cycle for the patient.
- Cognitive-behavioral therapy (CBT) is the cornerstone of treatment, starting with sleep hygiene and a strict sleep-wake schedule, with adequate time allotted for sleep (7-8 hours for adults). The use of supplemental melatonin is controversial.
- Treatment of concurrent sleep disorders should be emphasized (eg, OSA).
- Treatment goals for insomnia include improving sleep quality and improving daytime symptoms.
  - The short-term goal is to reduce the stress of not sleeping. Nonbenzodiazepine benzodiazepine receptor agonists (BZRAs) may be used for up to 2 weeks.
  - Cognitive-behavioral therapy for insomnia (CBT-i) is the most effective treatment for chronic insomnia, but it may not be easily available.
  - Over-the-counter sleep aids are usually not effective in this setting. Choice of medication may include BZRAs, doxepin, or ramelteon. Drug choice should be based on patient characteristics.

- Treatment for narcolepsy includes:
  - Scheduled naps, stimulants (caffeine, modafinil, amphetamines), and treatment of cataplexy with norepinephrine or serotonin reuptake inhibitors
  - When prescribing stimulants, a patient contract may be required to limit misuse or diversion of drugs.
  - A strict sleep schedule and medication schedule must be maintained to achieve remission of symptoms.

- Once symptoms are controlled, patients should be followed by sleep medicine at least annually.
- Common complications of sleep-wake disorders include daytime sleepiness and impairment that can lead to significant problems with neurocognitive functioning and lead to motor vehicle accidents, loss of jobs, stress on relationships, physical and mental health, and so on.

CHAPTER 309

Suicide and Intentional Overdose

Chris Gillette, PhD
Lindsey Mitchell, MS, MPAS, PA-C
Stephanie Daniel, PhD

▶ GENERAL FEATURES

- Characterized by a potentially self-injurious behavior with at least some intent to die
- Those at highest risk include patients with depression and other mental health disorders, substance abuse, easy access to firearms, being male, being a veteran of the armed forces, and being an adolescent *or* elderly
- Prescription and OTC medications may cause or be associated with suicide ideation and suicide attempts.
- Youth: nonopioid pain relievers, antidepressants used most often and are less lethal than drugs used by adults
  - Adults: alcohol, benzodiazepines, cocaine, and opioids used most often

▶ CLINICAL ASSESSMENT

- History:
  - Threatening to hurt/kill oneself:
    - Elderly: making statements such as, "I don't want to be a burden"
    - Talking or writing about killing/hurting oneself
  - Insomnia
  - Purposelessness/hopelessness
  - Dramatic mood changes
  - Previous suicide attempt
  - Major physical illnesses
  - Central nervous system disorders
  - Mental illnesses, including:
    - Mood disorders
    - Schizophrenia
    - Anxiety disorders, including PTSD
    - Substance use disorder
    - Personality disorders or attention deficit hyperactivity disorder, conduct disorder (antisocial behavior, aggression)

- Anhedonia (inability to feel pleasure)
- Family history of suicide or exposure to suicide
- Chaotic family history
- Lack of social support/isolation
- Local cluster of suicide
- Physical examination:
  - Ask clear questions to patients you suspect may be feeling suicidal about thoughts/feelings regarding suicide.
  - Ask questions from the Columbia-Suicide Severity Rating Scale (C-SSRS).
  - Prior suicide attempt is strongest predictor of future suicidal behavior. Ask if patient has attempted suicide in the past, even if no recent suicidal thinking.
  - If patient is having suicidal thoughts, ask about frequency, duration, and intensity.
  - After discussing frequency, duration, and intensity, inquire about planning.
  - After discussing planning, determine intent to carry out the plan and whether patient believes plan is to be lethal or injurious.
  - Look for any disagreement between what you see (objective findings) and what the patients tells you about their suicidal state (subjective findings).
  - When possible, and always with adolescents, seek to confirm patient's reports with information from family member, spouse, and close friend.
    - People are more likely to tell a family member than a health care provider about suicidal thoughts.

▶ DIAGNOSIS

- Clinicians should make diagnosis on basis of all available information and use own judgment.

- If a patient has suicidal ideation or any past attempt(s) within past 2 months:
  - Low risk:
    - Patient has thoughts of death only; no plan or behavior.
  - Moderate risk:
    - Patient has suicidal ideation, but limited suicidal intent and no clear plan, may have had previous attempt.
  - High risk:
    - Patient has suicide plan *and* has prepared or rehearsed behavior.

▶ TREATMENT

- For all levels of risk:
  - Record risk assessment, rationale, treatment plan; continue to monitor via repeat interviews, follow-up contacts, and collaborate with other providers.
  - If patient has therapist, call them in presence of patient.
- Low risk:
  - Encourage social support involving family members, close friends, and community resources including therapy services.
- Moderate risk:
  - Create a safety plan.
  - Consider:
    - Pharmacologic treatment with psychiatric consultation
    - Alcohol/drug assessment/referral
    - Individual/family therapy referral to evidence-based treatment
  - Encourage social support.
- High risk:
  - If patient has:
    - Good social support, intact judgment
      - Take action to prevent the plan.
      - Collaboratively develop a safety plan.
      - Consider
        - Pharmacologic treatment with psychiatric consultation
        - Alcohol/drug assessment/referral
        - Individual/family therapy referral to evidence-based treatment
        - Encourage social support involving family members, close friends, and community resources
  - If patient has/is:
    - Severe psychiatric symptoms/acute precipitating event, access to lethal means, poor social support, impaired judgment, unable to collaborate in developing safety plan, or unsafe environment
      - Hospitalize or call 911 or local police if no hospital available.
        - If patient refuses hospitalization, consider involuntary commitment if state permits.

Section A Pretest: Disorders of the Pulmonary Circulation

1. Which of the following patients should be referred to an expert pulmonary hypertension (PH) center?

   A. Patient with delayed diagnosis of HIV with elevated pulmonary pressures and functional tricuspid regurgitation
   B. Patient with exacerbation of left-sided heart failure with hypervolemia
   C. Patient with COPD and mild elevation of pulmonary pressures
   D. Patient with an acute pulmonary embolism (PE) following an international flight

2. A 45-year-old previously healthy man presents with shortness of breath, and the diagnosis of a small PE is confirmed. He lives with his wife, who is a nurse, and his adult daughter, who is a physician assistant. What treatment, if any, should be initiated?

   A. Admission to the hospital to start a 2-week course of intravenous heparin.
   B. Admission to the hospital for heparin bridge therapy for 5 days while starting oral rivaroxaban.
   C. Outpatient treatment with oral apixaban.
   D. Treat the patient with an initial dose of low-molecular-weight heparin (LMWH), followed by a daily VKA (warfarin).
   E. Discharge this patient to outpatient treatment with oral edoxaban.

3. A 35-year-old woman presents to the emergency department complaining of shortness of breath and feeling that something is not right. She thinks she may have "passed out." She has a history of ovarian cancer in remission. Her initial workup includes a positive D-dimer of 1200 ng/mL. Her computed tomographic pulmonary angiography (CTPA) was positive for a PE. Which medication is the initial treatment of choice?

   A. Intravenous heparin followed by rivaroxaban
   B. Intravenous heparin and warfarin (a VKA)
   C. Oral edoxaban only
   D. LMWH

4. During a routine office visit, a 46-year-old woman with SLE notes that she has had worsening fatigue and shortness of breath for the past few weeks. If you are suspecting she may have pulmonary HTN, which would be the most appropriate initial study to obtain?

   A. Right heart catheterization
   B. Vasoreactivity study
   C. Transthoracic echocardiogram
   D. Chest CT

5. A 72-year-old female presents to the office with complaints of unilateral leg swelling and shortness of breath after a recent lengthy automobile trip. Her past medical history is unremarkable. Her vital signs include a BP of 136/86, a heart rate of 82, respiratory rate 20, and oxygen saturation of 89% on room air. Physiologically, what has most likely has caused her diagnosis?

   A. Venous stasis
   B. Endothelial injury
   C. Hypercoaguability
   D. Volume overload

6. A patient with confirmed pulmonary arterial hypertension (PAH) who is asymptomatic at rest but who develops shortness of breath with normal daily activities would fall into which WHO functional class?

   A. WHO class I
   B. WHO class II
   C. WHO class III
   D. WHO class IV

7. Which of the following medications is most appropriate to manage nonreactive PAH?

   A. Nifedipine
   B. Phenylephrine
   C. Warfarin
   D. Epoprostenol

8. A 68-year-old man presents to the emergency department via EMS after being found down at home. He is breathing on his own. Vital signs reveal a temperature of 35 °C, heart rate of 120 and regular, respiratory rate of 24, and BP of 84/44. He has a past medical history of prostate cancer, HTN, and hyperlipidemia. Repeat vital signs reveal a BP of 60/40. You decide to start vasopressors. His D-dimer is 1340 ng/mL. Which classification of PE are you suspecting in this patient?

   A. Submassive
   B. Massive
   C. Subsegmental
   D. Saddle
   E. Nonmassive

Section B Pretest: Obstructive Pulmonary Disease

1. Goals for the treatment of COPD include which of the following?

    A. Increase exercise tolerance
    B. Reduce disease progression
    C. Prevent exacerbations
    D. Improved symptoms
    E. All of the above

2. What is considered a positive sweat chloride test?

    A. ≥60 mmol/L
    B. ≤60 mmol/L
    C. ≥30 mmol/L
    D. ≥45 mmol/L

3. Which of the following is required to confirm a diagnosis of COPD?

    A. CT scan of the chest
    B. Spirometry
    C. Chest x-ray
    D. Peak flow meter

4. In what inheritance pattern does cystic fibrosis (CF) occur?

    A. Autosomal dominant
    B. Autosomal recessive
    C. X-linked dominant
    D. X-linked recessive

5. Initial treatment for a patient diagnosed with COPD is based on which of the following?

    A. ABCD assessment tool
    B. Exacerbation history
    C. Assessment of airflow limitation
    D. Assessment of symptoms
    E. All of the above

6. Which of the following classes of medication for asthma is a quick reliever or rescue medication?

    A. An inhaled long-acting β2-agonist
    B. An inhaled corticosteroid
    C. An inhaled long-acting muscarinic agent
    D. An inhaled short-acting β2-agonist (SABA)

7. Appropriate treatments for a patient with COPD include:

    A. Inhaled medication
    B. Pulmonary rehabilitation
    C. Oxygen therapy
    D. Nutritional support
    E. All of the above

8. What is a characteristic finding on a chest x-ray in a patient with severe CF?

    A. Diffuse pulmonary infiltrates
    B. Tram-track opacities
    C. Cardiomegaly
    D. Normal chest x-ray

9. The most important risk factor for COPD is which of the following?

    A. Industrial pollutants
    B. Genetic predisposition
    C. Tobacco use
    D. Obesity

10. CF-related diabetes is managed with which of the following?

    A. Metformin
    B. Diet and exercise
    C. Insulin
    D. GLP-1 inhibitor

11. An indicator of very poorly controlled asthma would be the need to use an inhaled SABA when?

    A. Before physical education class each day
    B. One to two nights per month
    C. More than once a day
    D. <2 days per week

Section C Pretest: Other Pulmonary Disorders

1. Which of the following is a risk factor for obstructive sleep apnea (OSA)?

   A. Hypertension
   B. Diabetes
   C. Obesity
   D. Stroke

2. What is the recommended tidal volume in patients with ARDS who are mechanically ventilated?

   A. 6 mL/kg ideal body weight
   B. 6 mL/kg actual body weight
   C. 10 mL/kg ideal body weight
   D. 10 mL/kg actual body weight

3. A 56-year-old man presents to the clinic complaining of daytime somnolence. He states even though he sleeps all of the time, he still is tired and he sleeps better in his chair. He has a history of diabetes with neuropathy and takes gabapentin 3 times a day. His A1C was 10.5. His BMI is 52. In addition to lifestyle modifications, what treatment option may best address these symptoms?

   A. Advise him his symptoms are most like due to his medical conditions and medications
   B. Refer him to sleep medicine for evaluation of OSA
   C. Refer him to physical therapy for physical deconditioning
   D. Refer to endocrinology for diabetes management

4. Which of the following is a direct cause of lung injury that is associated with ARDS?

   A. Acute pancreatitis
   B. Blood product transfusion
   C. Sepsis
   D. Pneumonia

5. A 50-year-old female presents to clinic for HTN follow-up. She is on three medications, but her BP is high in clinic today. She has OSA and was prescribed PAP therapy, but does not like using her machine. How do you manage this patient?

   A. Increase dose of current medication
   B. Educate her on the importance of PAP use for BP control
   C. Add another medication
   D. Refer her for a PSG

6. Which of the following is part of the case definition of ARDS?

   A. Onset greater than 10 days after injury
   B. Direct or indirect pulmonary injury
   C. Unilateral opacity on chest x-ray
   D. Respiratory failure in the setting of left atrial HTN

7. A 25-year-old man presents to clinic complaining of daytime sleepiness. What physical examination finding would lead you to suspect OSA?

   A. Neck circumference 18 in
   B. BMI 29
   C. Pedal edema
   D. Tonsils 1+

8. A 58-year-old man with influenza pneumonia and diffuse, bilateral opacities on chest x-ray has worsening FiO_2 requirements. He is currently intubated with a tidal volume of 6 mL/kg ideal body weight, and his FiO_2 is 75%. Arterial blood gas on those settings is as follows: 7.30/36/60/18. In addition to his respiratory failure, he has acute renal failure, elevated transaminitis, and is hypotensive, requiring vasopressor support. Echocardiogram demonstrates normal cardiac function. Classification of the severity of the patient's ARDS as mild, moderate, or severe is dependent on which of the following?

   A. Presence of noncardiogenic pulmonary edema
   B. Number of opacities on chest x-ray
   C. PaO_2/FiO_2 ratio
   D. Presence of multisystem organ failure

9. Which of the following patients is at risk for central sleep apnea (CSA)?

   A. 65-year-old with HTN and diabetes
   B. 58-year-old with coronary artery disease
   C. 64-year-old with heart failure
   D. 38-year-old with BMI >40

10. Which of the following physical examination findings is associated with respiratory distress syndrome (RDS) in the newborn?

    A. Bounding peripheral pulses
    B. Diminished lung sounds
    C. Elevated core temperature
    D. Pulmonary flow murmur

11. Which stage of ARDS is typically seen after the first week and tends to last 2-3 weeks?
    A. Fibroproliferative stage
    B. Fibrotic stage
    C. Exudative stage
    D. Transudative stage

12. Which of the following best explains the increasing incidence of RDS in the newborn with decreasing gestational age?
    A. Expression of pulmonary surfactant in lung tissue after 20 weeks' gestation
    B. Expression of sodium channels on epithelial cells after 20 weeks' gestation
    C. Inactivation of pulmonary surfactant by protein leak into airspaces
    D. Inactivation of pulmonary surfactant by intrapulmonary shunting of blood

13. Antenatal corticosteroids are most efficacious in reducing morbidity and mortality associated with RDS in the newborn when administered during which of the following time periods?
    A. 18-22 weeks' gestation
    B. 23-34 weeks' gestation
    C. After 34 weeks' gestation
    D. Before 18 weeks' gestation

14. Of the following, which is the most common presenting symptom of aspiration?
    A. Altered mental status
    B. Cough
    C. Pink, frothy sputum
    D. Wheezing

15. Which of the following best explains how exogenous surfactant improves the clinical course of RDS in the newborn?
    A. Enhances lung tissue maturation
    B. Increases pulmonary fluid absorption
    C. Prevents cytokine-mediated inflammatory response
    D. Reduces alveolar surface tension

16. Which of the following statements about obesity hypoventilation syndrome (OHS) is true?
    A. It is more common in men.
    B. It is also known as Pickwickian syndrome.
    C. Blood gasses reveal retention of carbon monoxide and depletion of oxygen.
    D. It is irreversible.

17. A patient with newly diagnosed OHS presents to discuss his treatment options with the sleep specialist. Which of the following is indicated?
    A. PAP titration study
    B. Initiation of a high-protein diet
    C. Pulmonary rehabilitation program
    D. Initiate inhaled steroids

Section D Pretest: Pleural Disease

1. What diagnostic criteria is used to help distinguish exudative vs transudative effusions?
   A. Hounsfield units on the CT scan
   B. Light's criteria
   C. Paracentesis
   D. Pleural fluid cytology

2. A chest radiograph with decreased lung markings at the peripheral lung fields is indicative of?
   A. Hemothorax
   B. Pleural effusion
   C. Pneumonia
   D. Pneumothorax

3. A transudative pleural effusion is most likely related to what etiology?
   A. Heart failure
   B. Pneumonia
   C. PE
   D. Tuberculosis (TB)

4. Treatment of a hemothorax often involves which of the following?
   A. Pleurodesis
   B. Thoracentesis
   C. Tube thoracostomy
   D. Watchful waiting with oxygen therapy

Section E Pretest: Pulmonary Neoplasms

1. Which of the following is a common site of malignancy metastases?

   A. Skin
   B. Lung
   C. Small bowel
   D. Stomach

2. Lung cancer screening criteria recommend targeting at-risk individuals aged 55-80 years with a 20 pack-year history and smoking cessation within what period of time?

   A. Within the past 15 years
   B. Within the past 18 years
   C. Within the past 20 years
   D. Within the past 25 years

3. What is the most common cause of lung cancer?

   A. Smoking
   B. Radiation
   C. Environmental exposures
   D. Pulmonary fibrosis

4. What stage is a tumor that is confined to the lung, but cancer has spread to lymph nodes outside the lung but within the chest cavity?

   A. I
   B. II
   C. III
   D. IV

5. What is the most common cancer-related death worldwide?

   A. Breast
   B. Lung
   C. Colon
   D. Liver

Section F Pretest: Respiratory Infections

1. Which of the following medications is considered in effective antibiotic option when treating a patient infected with *Bordetella pertussis*?
   A. Penicillin
   B. Clarithromycin
   C. Ciprofloxacin
   D. Vancomycin

2. Which of the following, if present, is an indication for hospitalization in a patient with acute bronchiolitis?
   A. Office pulse oximetry of 96% on room air
   B. Patient age being older than 7 months
   C. A chest x-ray showing patchy atelectasis
   D. RDS with poor urination and oral intake

3. Which of the following is true regarding preventive measures of *B. pertussis*?
   A. There is no vaccination effective for *B. pertussis*.

   B. Vaccination with acellular pertussis is only safe after the age of 10 years.
   C. Immunity is acquired by adulthood, so booster immunizations are not advised after 18 years of age.
   D. All pregnant women should receive a dose of Tdap during each pregnancy.

4. Patients who are more at risk for severe complications of RSV include all of the following, except which of the following?
   A. Prematurity at birth
   B. History of congenital birth defects
   C. A patient who is age <2 months
   D. A patient who is age >2 months

5. An 18-month-old female presents to the emergency department with RDS. The patient has had an upper respiratory infection for 2-3 days when she awoke

from sleep with inspiratory stridor and a "barky cough." Which of the following is helpful in differentiating this as croup rather than bronchiolitis?
A. High-grade fevers
B. The child's age of 18 months
C. Improvement of symptoms with aerosolized racemic epinephrine
D. Expiratory stridor

6. A 6-month-old patient presents to your clinic with a fever, cough, decreased appetite, and wheezing. Which of the following statements would most likely be true about their initial symptoms?
A. 48 hours earlier this patient likely would have had nasal discharge.
B. 36 hours earlier this patient most likely would have had vomiting.
C. 36 hours earlier this patient most likely would have had diarrhea.
D. 48 hours earlier this patient likely would have stopped eating and drinking.

7. In a patient with suspected pertussis is suspected, which stage of the illness is characterized by periodic attacks of violent coughing, often times with an inspiratory whoop sound, and sometimes posttussive emesis?
A. Paroxysmal stage
B. Catarrhal stage
C. Convalescent stage
D. Mediocre stage

8. All of the following are examples of lower respiratory infections that can occur in RSV, except which of the following?
A. Bronchiolitis
B. Pneumonia
C. Acute respiratory failure
D. Rhinorrhea

9. Which of the following laboratory findings is common in children who are having a *B. pertussis* infection?
A. CBC reveals neutropenia.
B. CBC reveals lymphocytosis.
C. CBC reveals thrombocytopenia.
D. CBC always reveals a normal WBC count.

10. An 8-month-old presents with rhinorrhea, sneezing, and cough for the past 3 days. His mom states that his cough became worse this morning. The patient shows RDS with nasal flaring. You note the use of accessory muscles for respiration and audible wheezing without crackles can be heard on auscultation. Which of the following questions should you ask to help guide your treatment plan?
A. Is he allergic to aspirin?
B. Has he been eating and drinking normally?
C. Does anyone in the house smoke?
D. Have you noticed any rashes?

11. Which of the following is NOT considered an indication for hospitalization in an infant diagnosed with bronchiolitis?
A. Temperature >100.5 °F
B. Age <3 months
C. SpO$_2$ <95% on room air
D. Respiratory rate >70 breaths per minute

12. A 67-year-old male presents with chief complaint of a nonproductive cough, congestion, and rhinitis. This has been ongoing for the past 4 days. Though suspecting acute bronchitis, which of the following signs would suggest further diagnostic workup?
A. Temperature of 100.2 °F
B. Rhonchi that clear with cough
C. Dullness to percussion of right lateral lung field
D. Heart rate of 98 beats per minute

13. Which of the following pathogens is the most common cause of pneumonia?
A. *Pneumocystis jirovecii*
B. *Mycoplasma pneumonia*
C. Pseudomonas aeruginosa
D. *Streptococcus pneumoniae*

14. A 40-year-old male, heavy smoker, presents to your office with a low-grade fever and sudden onset of dry cough for the past 6 days. You diagnose him with acute bronchitis. What is the most appropriate management at this time?
A. Oral corticosteroid 5-day tapered dose pack
B. Doxycycline 100 mg PO BID for 10 days
C. Give the patient an albuterol inhaler
D. Increased fluids and acetaminophen

15. Which of the following risk factors increases a patient's risk of developing fungal pneumonia?
A. Age of 65 years or older
B. Current smoker
C. Occupation as a farm worker
D. Infection with viral URI

16. Which of the following is considered the confirmatory diagnostic study for suspected pertussis?
A. Elevated WBC count
B. Paroxysmal coughing attacks
C. Isolation of *B. pertussis* on specialized culture media after nasal pharyngeal swab
D. Chest x-ray revealing a reticular pattern and basilar lung infiltrates

17. A 72-year-old female with a history of COPD comes to your outpatient clinic complaining of cough, tactile fever, and increased work of breathing. The patient's vital signs are all within normal limits. Chest radiograph shows a left lower lobar pneumonia. You elect to treat the patient outpatient with oral antibiotics. Which of the following treatments would be most appropriate?
A. Doxycycline
B. Amoxicillin plus doxycycline

C. Levofloxacin

D. TMP/SMX

18. Which of the following represents the most common pathogen for acute bronchitis?

A. *S. pneumoniae*

B. *Pseudomonas*

C. *Mycoplasma*

D. Respiratory viruses

19. Which of the following is true regarding diagnosing pneumonia?

A. Diagnosis is definitively confirmed by physical exam.

B. Any opacity on chest x-ray is definitive for diagnosis of pneumonia.

C. Diagnosis requires sputum aspirate and culture.

D. History, physical exam, and chest x-ray are typically sufficient workup for ambulatory care.

Section G Pretest: Restrictive and Fibrotic Pulmonary Diseases

1. Which of the following symptoms is commonly seen in patients with idiopathic pulmonary fibrosis?

A. Productive cough

B. Progressive decrease in exercise tolerance

C. Chest pain

D. Lower extremity edema

2. Which of the following best explains the etiology of sarcoidosis?

A. Autoimmune

B. Idiopathic

C. Inflammatory

D. Vascular

3. You have a follow-up with a patient with a cough and confirmed TB-positive diagnosis. Upon chest radiograph, you notice an "eggshell" appearance of widespread opacities. Which diagnosis of pneumoconiosis is the most likely?

A. Silicosis

B. Asbestosis

C. Talcosis

D. Coal workers

4. A chest x-ray demonstrating pulmonary sarcoidosis with bilateral upper lobe parenchymal involvement without hilar adenopathy is classified as which stage?

A. Stage I

B. Stage II

C. Stage III

D. Stage IV

5. What is the average survival of patients diagnosed with pulmonary fibrosis?

A. 2-5 years

B. 8-10 years

C. 15 years

D. 1 year

6. A healthy patient presents for routine examination and is incidentally found to have hilar lymphadenopathy. Biopsy confirms sarcoidosis. Of the following, which is the most appropriate treatment plan?

A. Inhaled beclomethasone

B. Oral prednisone

C. Oral methotrexate

D. Surveillance

7. Which of the following pathology results is most consistent with a diagnosis of sarcoidosis?

A. Fibrosis

B. Necrotizing granuloma

C. Noncaseating granuloma

D. Microangiopathy

8. When explaining the treatment to a patient with the diagnosis of pneumoconiosis, which of the following is true?

A. Supportive care for symptoms and further prevention is the standard.

B. Lung transplantation is a first-line treatment option.

C. Prevention of pneumoconiosis will not be beneficial to the patient or their family.

D. Oral albuterol and steroids are mainstream treatment.

9. When diagnosing pneumoconiosis, what is a key component?

A. Immediate symptoms following exposure

B. Documented exposure

C. Response to albuterol treatment

D. Co-diagnosis with cancer

10. Your patient of 25 years presented a few weeks ago with dyspnea and prior asbestos exposure. After an extensive workup, you confirm that the patient has

malignant mesothelioma. Which is true about this condition?

A. CT will show honeycombing and reticular opacities.

B. Pleural plaques on CXR and ferruginous bodies on tissue biopsy are present.

C. Radiology shows perilymphatic marginated nodules with hilar node enlargement.

D. No abnormalities are typically seen on CT or CXR with this condition.

▶ **ANSWERS AND EXPLANATIONS TO SECTION A PRETEST**

1. **A.** Patient with delayed diagnosis of HIV with elevated pulmonary pressures and functional tricuspid regurgitation.

2. **C.** In patients with low-risk PE, and whose home circumstances are adequate, outpatient treatment is reasonable. Option A is incorrect. Intravenous heparin is used as a bridge to oral agents such as dabigatran, edoxaban, and VKA treatment, however, not for 2 weeks. Option B is incorrect as this patient could be started on oral rivaroxaban without the need for bridge treatment with heparin. Option D is incorrect as LMWH is only recommended for the initial treatment of cancer-related thrombus and not as a bridge to an oral agent. Option E is incorrect as oral edoxaban requires pretreatment with parenteral anticoagulation.

3. **D.** The recommended treatment of cancer-related thrombus is with LMWH for 3 months. Option A is incorrect because rivaroxaban can be used as a solo treatment without the need to pre-treat with intravenous heparin. Option B is incorrect as there are better options to be used, according to the ACC. Option C is incorrect because oral edoxaban requires pretreatment with parenteral anticoagulation.

4. **C.** Transthoracic echocardiogram is the most appropriate initial study to obtain.

5. **A.** This patient's risk factor of limited mobility can lead to venous stasis.

6. **B.** A patient with confirmed PAH who is asymptomatic at rest but who develops shortness of breath with normal daily activities is WHO class II.

7. **D.** Epoprostenol is most appropriate to manage nonreactive PAH.

8. **B.** A massive PE refers to the hemodynamic compromise and not necessarily the size of the thrombus. Option A is incorrect, as submassive PE does not cause systemic hypotension. Option C is incorrect, as subsegmental PE is peripheral and does not include the more proximal pulmonary arteries. Option D is incorrect as a saddle PE may be present; however, they are still either massive, submassive, or nonmassive, depending on the severity of hemodynamic

compromise. Option E is incorrect as this patient has systemic hypotension requiring vasopressors.

▶ **ANSWERS AND EXPLANATIONS TO SECTION B PRETEST**

1. **E.** All of the above answers are goals in the treatment of COPD.

2. **A.** A positive sweat chloride test is ≥ 60 mmol/L.

3. **B.** Spirometry is required to confirm the diagnosis of COPD.

4. **B.** CF occurs in an autosomal recessive pattern.

5. **E.** All of the above are required to properly treat a patient with COPD.

6. **D.** An inhaled SABA is a quick reliever or rescue medication for asthma.

7. **E.** All of the above are appropriate treatments for a patient with COPD.

8. **B.** Tram-track opacities is a characteristic finding on a chest x-ray in a patient with severe CF.

9. **C.** Tobacco has been found to be the most important risk factor for developing COPD.

10. **C.** CF-related diabetes is managed with insulin.

11. **C.** Needing to use an inhaled SABA more than once a day is an indicator of very poorly controlled asthma.

▶ **ANSWERS AND EXPLANATIONS TO SECTION C PRETEST**

1. **C.** Obesity is a risk factor for OSA.

2. **A.** The recommended tidal volume in patients with ARDS who are receiving mechanical ventilatory support is 6 mL/kg ideal body weight. This minimizes the risk of barotrauma.

3. **B.** Refer him to sleep medicine for evaluation of OSA.

4. **D.** Pneumonia results in direct injury to the lung. Lung injury in the setting of sepsis alone (excluding pneumonia as the underlying cause) would result in indirect injury.

5. **B.** Educate her on the importance of PAP use for BP control.

6. **B.** The diagnostic criteria for ARDS are direct or indirect pulmonary injury, bilateral opacities on chest x-ray, acute onset (within 1 week of injury), and absence of left atrial HTN.

7. **A.** A neck circumference 18 in would lead you to suspect OSA.

8. **C.** Severity of ARDS is defined by the $PaO_2:FiO_2$ ratio: mild $PaO_2:FiO_2$ >200 and ≤ 300, moderate $PaO_2:FiO_2$ >100 and ≤ 200, and severe $PaO_2:FiO_2$ ≤ 100.

9. **C.** A 64-year-old with heart failure is at risk for CSA.

10. **B.** Diminished lung sounds is associated with RDS in the newborn.

11. **A.** The clinical course seen in ARDS can be divided into three stages. The initial stage is the early

exudative stage, seen for the first 7-10 days. This is followed by the fibroproliferative stage and, finally, the fibrotic stage. Not every patient experiences all three stages.

12. **A.** Expression of pulmonary surfactant in lung tissue after 20 weeks' gestation best explains the increasing incidence of RDS in the newborn with decreasing gestational age.

13. **B.** Antenatal corticosteroids are most efficacious in reducing morbidity and mortality associated with RDS in the newborn when administered at 23-34 weeks' gestation.

14. **B.** Cough is the most common presenting symptom of aspiration.

15. **D.** Exogenous surfactant improves the clinical course of RDS in the newborn by reducing alveolar surface tension.

16. **B.** Pickwickian syndrome. There is no known gender prevalence in OHS. Blood gasses reveal retention of carbon dioxide, not monoxide. OHS is reversible with weight loss.

17. **A.** PAP titration is the appropriate treatment for OHS. Other correct treatment options include supervised weight loss programs and consultation to endocrinology.

▶ ANSWERS AND EXPLANATIONS TO SECTION D PRETEST

1. **B.** While Hounsfield units and pleural fluid cytology can help analyze the density and content of the pleural fluid, Light's criteria identify pleural fluid as exudative vs. transudative in nature.

2. **D.** An upright chest radiograph will demonstrate fluid at the bases, often obscuring the costophrenic angle or blunting the diaphragm in hemothorax and pleural effusion. Pneumonia is often demonstrated by hazy opacity within the lung parenchyma.

3. **A.** In the United States, the most often associated cause of pleural effusion is heart failure. Although PE may be associated with a transudative process, most often, it is identified as an exudative process along with the other two infectious etiologies.

4. **C.** Watchful waiting is inappropriate with even a small hemothorax as complications such as empyema are likely. Pleurodesis and thoracentesis are more appropriate in pleural effusion. Hemothorax requires a chest tube placed for evacuation blood within the pleural space.

▶ ANSWERS AND EXPLANATIONS TO SECTION E PRETEST

1. **B.** Common sites of metastasis include lung, lymph nodes, brain, bone, liver, and adrenal glands.

2. **A.** US Preventive Services Task Force recommends those aged 55-80 years who have a 20 pack-year smoking history and currently smoke or have quit within the past 15 years to have a low-dose CT scan.

3. **A.** Smoking is the leading cause of and the largest risk factor for lung cancer. In addition, secondhand smoke exposure has caused many lung cancer deaths.

4. **D.** Stage IV is confined to the lung, but cancer has spread to lymph nodes outside the lung but only inside the chest cavity.

5. **B.** Lung cancer is the most common cause of cancer deaths in both men and women.

▶ ANSWERS AND EXPLANATIONS TO SECTION F PRETEST

1. **B.** Recommended treatment options for individuals with suspected or confirmed pertussis, as well as any of their close contacts over the past 3 weeks, include erythromycin, clarithromycin, azithromycin, and trimethoprim-sulfamethoxazole.

2. **D.** RDS with poor urination and oral intake is an indication for hospitalization in a patient with acute bronchiolitis.

3. **D.** Women who are pregnant should also receive a dose of Tdap during in each pregnancy, regardless of their prior vaccinations and optimally between 27- and 36-weeks' gestation.

4. **D.** A patient who is age >2 months is not at risk for severe complications of RSV.

5. **D.** Croup is an upper respiratory illness with inflammation in the larynx causing inspiratory stridor and a harsh, barky cough. Bronchiolitis is a lower respiratory illness with inflammation in the bronchioles causing expiratory wheezing and a wet cough. Treatment for both can begin at home with humidified air. Both conditions affect patients in this age group and are associated with low-grade fevers and are often preceded by upper respiratory symptoms. Racemic epinephrine would improve symptoms of both croup and bronchiolitis.

6. **A.** This patient likely would have had nasal discharge 48 hours earlier.

7. **A.** The paroxysmal stage is characterized by a classic whooping cough that occurs in paroxysmal attacks, manifest by a "whoop" sound during inspiration. Post-tussive vomiting is common during this stage.

8. **D.** Rhinorrhea does not occur in RSV.

9. **B.** An elevated WBC count is a common finding in pertussis, often times as high as 15-20 000 cells/μL and is characteristically lymphocytosis.

10. **B.** To help guide your treatment plan, ask, "Has he been eating and drinking normally?"

11. **A.** Temperature >100.5 °F is not considered an indication for hospitalization in an infant diagnosed with bronchiolitis.

12. **C.** Dullness to percussion of right lateral lung field would suggest further diagnostic workup.
13. **D.** Regardless of the underlying comorbidities or age, *S. pneumoniae* remains the most common cause of pneumonia.
14. **D.** The most appropriate management is increased fluids and acetaminophen.
15. **C.** Patients who have exposure to soil and animal excreta or are immunosuppressed are at increased risk of developing fungal pneumonia.
16. **C.** The diagnosis of pertussis is established and confirmed by isolation of *B. pertussis* on specialized culture media. PCR assay is also becoming increasingly available and is also confirmatory.
17. **C.** Levofloxacin would be most appropriate.
18. **D.** Viruses account for 85–95% of acute bronchitis cases.
19. **D.** The diagnosis of pneumonia is typically made due to the combination of history and physical examination suggestive of pneumonia with a chest x-ray significant for pulmonary infiltrate.

▶ ANSWERS AND EXPLANATIONS TO SECTION G PRETEST

1. **B.** Progressive decrease in exercise tolerance is commonly seen in patients with idiopathic pulmonary fibrosis.
2. **B.** The etiology of sarcoidosis is idiopathic.
3. **A.** Silicosis is most likely.
4. **C.** A chest x-ray demonstrating pulmonary sarcoidosis with bilateral upper lobe parenchymal involvement without hilar adenopathy is classified as stage III.
5. **A.** The average survival rate of patients diagnosed with pulmonary fibrosis is 2-5 years.
6. **D.** Surveillance is the most appropriate treatment plan.
7. **C.** Noncaseating granuloma is most consistent with a diagnosis of sarcoidosis.
8. **A.** Supportive care for symptoms and further prevention is the standard.
9. **B.** When diagnosing pneumoconiosis, documented exposure is a key component.
10. **B.** Pleural plaques on CXR and ferruginous bodies on tissue biopsy are noted.

SECTION **A** *Disorders of the Pulmonary Circulation*

CHAPTER
310

Pulmonary Embolism

Douglas D. Long, DMSc, PA-C

▶ GENERAL FEATURES

- Pulmonary embolism (PE) refers to a blood clot traveling to, or originating within, the pulmonary vasculature. Pulmonary emboli may cause symptoms ranging from mild discomfort to hemodynamic collapse.
- Clot formation typically requires one or more of Virchow triad: endothelial damage, venous stasis, and hypercoagulability.
- Risk factors include surgery, pregnancy, trauma, cancer, prolonged travel or immobility, obesity, increased age, smoking, exogenous estrogen use, hospitalization, and hypercoaguable disorders or states, such as cancer or thrombophilia. A history of proximal deep venous thrombosis (DVT) is present in up to 50% of patients.
- Incidence increases with age: after 45 years, the lifetime risk of developing venous thromboembolism (VTE) is 8%.
- ~70% of patients with symptomatic PE also present with a DVT.

▶ CLINICAL ASSESSMENT

- The classic presentation of an acute PE may include dyspnea, pleuritic chest pain, and cough. Syncope, dizziness, and hemoptysis are less common presenting symptoms.
- Physical examination may be notable for tachypnea, accentuated second heart sound, tachycardia, and signs of poor peripheral and/or end-organ perfusion.
- Massive PE results in shock or persistent hypotension (ie, a systolic blood pressure <90 mm Hg, need for vasopressors, or a decrease in the systolic blood pressure by ≥40 mm Hg from baseline for 15 minutes or longer despite resuscitation).

▶ DIAGNOSIS

- Laboratory tests and diagnostic imaging should be used in concert with clinical pretest probability and clinical decision tools.

- D-Dimer laboratory testing may be useful in intermediate-risk patients. An elevated D-dimer in these patients should trigger additional imaging studies.
- Computed tomographic pulmonary angiography (CTPA) is the preferred imaging modality for diagnosis of PE.
- Ventilation-perfusion (VQ) scan maybe utilized if CT is not available or the patient is allergic to contrast dye.
- Echocardiogram may be normal or may show signs of RV dysfunction and/or dilation. McConnell sign, akinesia of the mid free wall with increased motion at the apex, is a distinct finding specific to PE.
- EKG may show sinus tachycardia, T wave inversions in the precordial and/or inferior leads (RV strain pattern), or the classic "$S_IQ_{III}T_{III}$" pattern with a deep S wave in lead I, Q-wave in lead III, and T wave inversion in lead III.

▶ TREATMENT

- Patients with massive PE should be treated with immediate systemic thrombolysis.
- Options for the treatment of submassive PE (those with signs of RV strain or dysfunction) should be individualized to the patient; options include catheter-directed thrombolysis, surgical thrombectomy, or anticoagulation alone.
- Anticoagulation therapy is the mainstay of treatment for most patients and may be adequate for patients with low-risk PE. Options include warfarin, DOACs, and low-molecular-weight heparin.
- Patients who are at low risk for complications with adequate home support may have treatment as an outpatient.
- Some low-risk patients with a subsegmental PE and no evidence of DVT may be appropriate for surveillance only.

Pulmonary Hypertension

Brendan Riordan, MPAS, PA-C

▶ GENERAL FEATURES

- Pulmonary hypertension (PH) is a broad term referring to elevated blood pressures in the pulmonary vasculature.
- Defined as a mean arterial pulmonary pressure (mPAP) >20 mm Hg at rest as measured by right heart catheterization
- Further defined by the World Health Organization (WHO) categories based on etiology:
  - Group 1: pulmonary arterial hypertension (PAH)
  - Group 2: PH caused by left-sided heart disease
  - Group 3: PH caused by hypoxemia or chronic lung disease
  - Group 4: PH caused by chronic thromboembolic disease (CTEPH)
  - Group 5: PH caused by diseases with unspecified or multifactorial mechanisms (eg, sickle cell disease, sarcoidosis)
- Multiple subclassifications exist, most notably within group 1: idiopathic, heritable, drug/toxin induced, connective tissue disorders, HIV, portal hypertension (HTN), congenital, schistosomiasis

▶ CLINICAL PRESENTATION

- Symptoms are often absent or attributable to other conditions (ie, other existing cardiopulmonary disease).
- Symptoms may include dyspnea on exertion and exercise intolerance; these may worsen if right ventricular (RV) failure occurs.
- Physical examination findings are often absent (a prominent P2 heart sound may initially be auscultated).
- Additional symptoms and physical examination findings will be related to concomitant disease state (especially groups 2-5) or development of RV failure (eg, widely split S2, murmur of tricuspid regurgitation, increased jugular vein distention [JVD])
- Initial recommended study is a transthoracic echocardiogram (TTE) to estimate pulmonary pressures and assess for tricuspid regurgitation and/or RV dysfunction, and assess for LV dysfunction as a contributing etiology.

▶ DIAGNOSIS

- Additional diagnostic workup should focus on assessment for lung disease, venous/pulmonary artery thromboembolism, or other possible contributing diagnoses.
- Gold standard for diagnosis is a right heart catheterization with direct measurement of pulmonary artery pressures, confirming the diagnosis.
- Patients with PAH are organized into a risk category (low, intermediate, high) based on history and diagnostics including 6-minute walking distance (6MWD), cardiopulmonary exercise testing, natriuretic peptide (BNP) levels, and invasive hemodynamics.

▶ TREATMENT

- Patients with PAH or severe PH should be referred to an expert center for further diagnostics and management.
- Management of patients with PH groups 2-5 is generally supportive and directed toward treatment of their underlying disease.
  - Some patients may benefit from diuresis and/or supplemental oxygen therapy for symptom relief.
  - Patients with CTEPH may be considered for surgical thrombectomy and systemic anticoagulation.
- Treatment options depend on whether or not the HTN responds to calcium channel blockers (vasoreactive). Treatment options for nonreactive PAH include endothelin receptor antagonists, phosphodiesterase-5 inhibitors, guanylate cyclase stimulators, and prostacyclin analogues/receptor agonists; pharmacologic support may involve single agents or combinations (determined by risk and functional class); these patients are best managed by PAH expert centers owing to their complexity.
- Patients who remain symptomatic despite optimal pharmacologic therapies may be considered for a surgical atrial septostomy (creation of passage between right and left atria to unload right side and improve left-sided cardiac output) and/or lung transplantation.

CHAPTER

312

Chronic Obstructive Pulmonary Disease

Bethany Dunn, PA-C, DC

▶ GENERAL FEATURES

- Chronic obstructive pulmonary disease (COPD) is a condition of chronic inflammatory response in the airways and lungs characterized by progressive airflow limitation and accompanied by respiratory symptoms (dyspnea, cough, and/or sputum production).
- Also referred to as emphysema or chronic bronchitis
- COPD is a leading cause of morbidity and mortality worldwide
- Most common risk factor for COPD is smoking of tobacco products.
- COPD often coexists with other comorbidities that may have a significant impact on the disease course.

▶ CLINICAL ASSESSMENT

History often includes exposure to risk factors (tobacco smoke, occupational exposure, indoor air pollution, passive exposure to cigarette smoke, socioeconomic status).

- Symptoms of COPD include dyspnea, chronic cough, sputum production, and intermittent dyspnea.
- Symptoms of COPD exacerbation include acute worsening of dyspnea and/or cough; change in the volume, color, or consistency of sputum; fever if inciting event is infection.
- Exacerbations and/or hospitalizations are often recurring and frequent.
- Examination may be notable for cyanosis, clubbing, barrel chest, the use of accessory muscles, pursed-lip breathing diminished breath sounds, and rhonchi/wheezing.

▶ DIAGNOSIS

- Diagnosis is confirmed through spirometry/pulmonary function testing, which detects the presence and severity of airflow limitation.

- The presence of a post-bronchodilator FEV_1/FVC <0.70 confirms the presence of persistent airflow limitation. GOLD Classification Grade is determined by FEV_1.
- Chest x-ray is not usually useful to establish a diagnosis of COPD but may be notable for hyperinflation, flattened diaphragms, bullous disease, and increased bronchovascular markings.
- Computed tomography of the chest is not routinely recommended, except for COPD patients who meet the criteria for lung cancer risk assessment or who are being evaluated for lung transplantation.

▶ TREATMENT

Acute exacerbation:

- Short-acting β-2 agonists with or without anticholinergics
- Corticosteroids (oral or IV) for 5-14 days
- Antibiotics in severe exacerbations or if there is evidence of infection
- Supplemental oxygen and bilevel noninvasive positive pressure ventilation as needed
- Severe respiratory compromise may require ICU admission and mechanical ventilation.

Chronic disease:

- Reduce exposure to risk factors; smoking cessation
- Nonpharmacologic therapies including physical activity, pulmonary rehabilitation (3 times per week for 8 weeks), nutritional support (heart healthy diet), and oxygen therapy. Vaccines (influenza and pneumovax) should be discussed and encouraged.
- Initial pharmacotherapy should be based on the refined GOLD ABCD assessment tool and GOLD pharmacologic treatment algorithms using an escalation/de-escalation approach. Pharmacologic therapies include short-acting bronchodilators, long-acting muscarinic

receptor agonists (LAMA), long-acting β-2 agonists (LABA), inhaled corticosteroids, combination inhaled medications, roflumilast, and long-term daily antibiotic therapy.

- Pulse oximetry should be utilized to evaluate a patient's arterial oxygen saturation and need for supplemental oxygen therapy. Initiate oxygen if Sao_2 is at or below 88% or if Pao_2 is at or below 55 mm Hg.

CHAPTER 313

Cystic Fibrosis

Katelyn Adler, MSPAS, PA-C

▶ GENERAL FEATURES

- Cystic fibrosis (CF) is a multisystem, autosomal recessive disorder caused by a mutation in the cystic fibrosis transmembrane conductance regulator (*CFTR*) gene, responsible for encoding chloride channels.
- Chloride channel dysfunction leads to thick secretions in the respiratory, gastrointestinal, endocrine, and reproductive systems.
- Affects ~30 000 people in the United States and 80 000 people worldwide, most commonly Caucasians (1:3000 live births)
- Leads to a shortened life span in patients, usually due to severe respiratory disease. Median age of death is ~30 years.

▶ CLINICAL ASSESSMENT

- Respiratory:
  - Productive cough, shortness of breath, decreased exercise tolerance, and hemoptysis
  - Frequent lung infections due to bacterial colonization, most commonly with *Staphylococcus aureus*, *Haemophilus influenzae*, and *Pseudomonas aeruginosa*
  - Physical examination findings include sinus tenderness, purulent nasal discharge, nasal polyps, crackles on lung examination, increased anteroposterior chest diameter, and digital clubbing.
- Gastrointestinal:
  - Meconium ileus at birth and distal intestinal obstructive syndrome (DIOS) in older patients
  - Pancreatic insufficiency, presenting as steatorrhea, weight loss, poor growth, and vitamin deficiency
  - Biliary cirrhosis and gallstones
- Endocrine:
  - CF-related diabetes develops in ~30% of adults requiring treatment with insulin.
- Reproductive:
  - Male infertility due to the absence of the vas deferens

▶ DIAGNOSIS

- ~65% of new diagnoses occur in asymptomatic newborns due to newborn screening (NBS). A positive NBS does not confirm the diagnosis of CF but requires further investigation with sweat chloride testing and/or genetic testing.
- A positive sweat chloride result (≥60 mmol/L) is considered diagnostic and should be followed by genetic testing.
- A *CFTR* gene analysis may result in >1800 identified mutations, with the most common being a deletion of bases coding for phenylalanine at the 508th position (F508del). Approximately 85% of patients have at least one copy of the F508del mutation.
- Other modalities to monitor disease include chest x-ray, revealing bronchiectasis, and pulmonary function tests, revealing a mixed obstructive and restrictive pattern.

▶ TREATMENT

- Patients are typically managed at multidisciplinary clinics, including visits with pulmonology, nutrition, genetics, psychology, and physical therapy.
- Pulmonary therapies may consist of airway clearance, inhaled medications, antibiotics, and CFTR modulators. These therapies are taken daily and sometimes even multiple times daily.
  - Airway clearance is recommended in all patients with CF. Typically, inhaled bronchodilators and inhaled mucolytics, like hypertonic saline, are used first, followed by postural drainage or vest therapy.
  - Inhaled antibiotics, aztreonam and tobramycin, are used daily in those colonized with *P. aeruginosa*. During exacerbations, patients are treated with oral or IV antibiotics based on sputum cultures.
  - CFTR modulators (Kalydeco, Symdeko, Trikafta) correct the defective CFTR protein, allowing the transport of chloride to the cell surface, decreasing the viscosity of secretions.
- Extrapulmonary disease may require treatment with pancreatic enzyme supplementation, laxatives, and insulin.
- Early referral to a transplant center for lung transplantation is encouraged in those with severe disease.

Asthma

Alan Brokenicky, MPAS, PA-C

GENERAL FEATURES

- Heterogeneous disease usually characterized by chronic airway inflammation/hyperresponsiveness producing symptoms reversible airflow limitations
- Common disease affecting ~8% to 10% of the population
- Slightly more common in male children (younger than 14 years) and in female adults
- Genetic predisposition
- Prevalence, hospitalizations, and fatal asthma have all increased in the United States over the past 20 years.
- Risk factors:
  - Hospitalization rates have been highest among Black/African American patients and children, and death rates are consistently highest among Black/African American patients aged 15-24 years.
  - Predisposing factors include:
    - Personal or family history of atopy
    - Obesity
  - Asthma triggers include inhaled allergens or irritants:
    - Smoke
    - Chemical fumes
    - Air pollution
    - House dust mites (often found in pillows, mattresses, upholstered furniture, carpets, and drapes)
    - Cockroaches
    - Cat dander
    - Seasonal pollens
  - Other precipitants of asthma include exercise, upper respiratory tract infections, rhinosinusitis, postnasal drip, aspiration, gastroesophageal reflux, weather/atmospheric changes, and stress.

CLINICAL ASSESSMENT

- Asthma is characterized by episodic wheezing, shortness of breath, chest tightness, and cough. Excess sputum production is common.
  - "Wheezing" does not have a standard meaning for patients and may be used by those without a medical background to describe a variety of sounds, including upper airway noises emanating from the nose or throat.
  - Cough may be dry or productive of clear mucoid or pal-yellow sputum.
  - The frequency of symptoms is variable. May range from infrequent, brief episodes to nearly continuous symptoms.
  - Asthma symptoms are frequently worse at night; circadian variations in bronchomotor tone and bronchial reactivity reach their nadir between 3 AM and 4 AM, increasing symptoms of bronchoconstriction.

- Physical examination findings:
  - Auscultation:
    - Asthmatic wheezing usually involves diffuse sounds of different pitches, starting and stopping at various points in the respiratory cycle and varying in tone and duration over time.
  - Signs of severe airflow obstruction:
    - Tachypnea, tachycardia, prolonged expiratory phase of respiration (decreased I:E ratio), and a seated position with use of extended arms to support the upper chest (tripoding).
    - Airflow may be too limited to produce wheezing, and the only diagnostic clue on auscultation may be globally reduced breath sounds with prolonged expiration.
    - Use of the accessory muscles of breathing (eg, sternocleidomastoid) during inspiration and a pulsus paradoxus (>12 mm Hg fall in systolic blood pressure during inspiration) are usually found only during severe episodes.
  - Other findings:
    - Nasal mucosal swelling, increased secretions, and polyps are often seen in patients with allergic asthma.
    - Eczema, atopic dermatitis, or other allergic skin disorders may also be present.

DIAGNOSIS

- Pulmonary function testing:
  - Tests of airflow limitation are critical tools in the diagnosis of asthma.
    - Airflow obstruction is indicated by a reduced FEV_1/FVC ratio.
    - Significant reversibility of airflow obstruction is defined by an increase in 12% or more and 200 mL in FEV_1 or FVC 10-15 minutes after inhaling a short-acting bronchodilator.
  - Bronchial provocation testing with inhaled histamine or methacholine may be useful when asthma is suspected but spirometry is nondiagnostic.
  - Peak expiratory flow (PEF) measured during a brief, forceful exhalation, using a simple and inexpensive device; limited diagnostic value.
- Laboratory findings:
  - No blood tests are available that can determine the presence or absence of asthma or gauge its severity.
  - Arterial blood gas measurements may be normal during a mild asthma exacerbation or may reveal hypercapnia, hypoxia, and respiratory alkalosis.
- Imaging:
  - Chest radiograph is typically normal in patients with asthma but may be useful in ruling out alternative diagnoses.

▶ TREATMENT

- Acute exacerbations:
  - Administer supplemental oxygen to maintain SpO_2 >93%.
  - Administer inhaled short-acting β-2 agonist (SABA), such as albuterol; consider continuous nebulized treatment for severe exacerbations.
  - Administer ipratropium to patients with moderate-to-severe exacerbations.
  - Administer systemic steroids to speed resolution and prevent relapse of symptoms.
  - IV magnesium sulfate administration may reduce hospital admissions in adults with acute asthma.
  - Reserve antibiotic administration for those patients with signs/symptoms of bacterial infection.
  - Intubation and mechanical ventilation for patients with impending respiratory failure.
- Long-term management:
  - Prescribe a SABA to all patients for acute symptom control along with an inhaled corticosteroid (ICS).
- The Global Initiative for Asthma (GINA) recommends a stepwise approach to the management of asthma in adults and children older than 12 years based on disease severity:
  - Step 1: Preferred reliever: as-needed ICS and rapid-onset long-acting β agonist (LABA) such as formoterol. Preferred controller: as-needed low-dose ICS/ LABA.
  - Step 2: Preferred reliever: as-needed low-dose ICS/ LABA. Preferred controller: daily low-dose ICS plus as-needed SABA or as-needed low-dose ICS/LABA.
  - Step 3: Preferred reliever: as-needed low-dose ICS/ LABA for patients prescribed with maintenance and reliever therapy. Preferred controller: low-dose ICS/ LABA (used as needed with SABA reliever) or ICS/ LABA (as both controller and reliever).
  - Step 4: Preferred reliever: as-needed low-dose ICS/ LABA for patients prescribed with maintenance and reliever therapy. Preferred controller: low-dose ICS/ LABA (as both reliever and controller) or medium-dose ICS/LABA (used with as-needed SABA).
  - Step 5: Preferred reliever: as-needed low-dose ICS/ LABA for patients prescribed with maintenance and reliever therapy. Preferred controller: high-dose ICS/ LABA; refer for phenotypic assessment and add-on treatments.
- Alternative treatments include mast cell stabilizers, antileukotrienes, or methylxanthines.
- Patient education, risk factor/trigger avoidance, allergy testing, specialist referral, and frequent follow-up are important elements of care.

SECTION **C** *Other Pulmonary Disorders*

CHAPTER **315**

Sleep Apnea

Teresa Bigler, DHEd, PA-C

▶ GENERAL FEATURES

- Sleep apnea is a sleep-related breathing disorder that is classified as obstructive (OSA), central (CSA), or mixed (central and obstructive).
- OSA, the most common sleep-related breathing disorder, is characterized by the collapse of the upper airway during sleep, leading to apneas (complete blockage of airway) and/or hypopneas (partial blockage of the airway), resulting in arousals from sleep.
- OSA risk factors: obesity (BMI > 35), craniofacial and upper airways abnormalities (crowded airway), neck size (>17 in in men, >16 in in women), male gender, and older age
- CSA is characterized by repetitive cessation of airflow and ventilation during sleep caused by decreased or absent central respiratory drive.
- CSA is often the result of other medical conditions, such as heart failure, central nervous system pathology, or medications (especially opioids).

- Associated medical conditions: heart disease (hypertension, atrial fibrillation, heart failure, myocardial infarction), type 2 diabetes, gastroesophageal reflux disease, transient ischemic attacks, and stroke

CLINICAL PRESENTATION

- Daytime sleepiness is one of the most common presenting symptoms.
- Other symptoms include frequent nocturnal arousals; sleep interrupted by snoring, choking, or gasping; teeth grinding; frequent nocturia; waking up unrefreshed; and morning headaches. The severity of symptoms does not correlate with the severity of sleep apnea.
- OSA: on physical examination, the patient may have a large neck. Inspection of the facial structures includes evaluation of the relative size and shape of the mandibular and maxillary structures, oropharyngeal airway may reveal a high arched palate, large tongue with scalloping, elongated or edematous uvula, enlarged tonsils, evidence of crossbite, or bruxism. The Mallampati classification for airway narrowing is used to stratify risk of OSA. Nasal passages may reveal nasal polyps, septal deviation, or limited airflow with nasal collapse during inspiration.
- Pediatric patients with OSA present with symptoms of sleep deprivation, including irritability, hyperactivity, behavioral problems, and poor school performance.

DIAGNOSIS

- STOPBANG and Epworth Sleepiness Scale are useful OSA screening tools.
- Patients with suspected sleep apnea should be referred to a sleep medicine clinic.
- A polysomnography (PSG) is the gold standard test to diagnose sleep apnea and distinguish between OSA, CSA or mixed apneas.
- Sleep apnea is classified as mild, moderate, or severe.
- In pediatric patients, an apnea-hypopnea index >1/ hour with symptoms or hypoventilation is considered diagnostic for OSA.

- A "split-night" study can be used to establish the diagnosis and perform a positive airway pressure (PAP) titration to determine the optimal treatment pressures. The airway pressure prevents the collapse of the airway.

TREATMENT

- Patients with mild OSA with daytime symptoms may benefit from conservative therapy (positional therapy, weight loss, oral appliances) or PAP therapy.
- Treatment for moderate-to-severe OSA is PAP therapy. Common options include CPAP (continuous) and BiPAP (bilevel), determined during the PAP titration portion of the PSG. Pressures may be fixed or automatically adjusting (auto-CPAP or auto-BiPAP). If a patient has CSA or mixed apneas, a BIPAP with a spontaneous timed breathing feature (BiPAP-ST) is the treatment of choice.
- Surgical referral may be indicated for anatomic problems. Patients with craniofacial abnormalities should be evaluated by oral maxillary facial surgery (OMFS), and patients with nasal obstruction should have their airway evaluated by ENT.
- For pediatric patients, first-line therapy is surgical. Refer to ENT for adenotonsillectomy; if symptoms remain or patient is not a good surgical candidate, PAP therapy can be initiated.
- Complications:
  - Untreated, patients with moderate-to-severe sleep apnea have a higher all-cause mortality rate; specifically, there is a higher risk of cardiovascular events and ischemic strokes.
  - Many comorbid conditions are exacerbated by untreated sleep apnea, including hypertension, arrhythmias, heart failure, metabolic syndrome, diabetes, depression, and any condition that can be exacerbated by sleep deprivation, such as migraine headaches and seizures.

Acute Respiratory Distress Syndrome

Katie Hanlon, MMS, PA-C

A 70-year-old woman with a history of tobacco use presents with a fever, shortness of breath, and productive cough with nonbloody sputum for 1 week. On examination, her heart rate is 112 beats per minute and regular, she is tachypneic with SpO_2 80% on room air, improving to 92% on 6 L nasal cannula (NC). Her blood pressure is 98/55 mm Hg. Chest x-ray demonstrates diffuse bilateral infiltrates, and she is admitted with pneumonia and sepsis. The patient has persistent hypoxemia and worsening respiratory status despite broad-spectrum antibiotics and supplemental oxygen. Her BNP is normal, and a transthoracic echocardiogram demonstrates normal cardiac function. How should the patient's deteriorating respiratory status be managed?

GENERAL FEATURES

- Acute respiratory distress syndrome (ARDS) is acute lung injury due to proliferation of inflammatory mediators characterized by hypoxemia and bilateral radiographic infiltrates in the absence of cardiogenic pulmonary edema.
- Multiple etiologies are a result of either direct or indirect pulmonary insult:
  - Direct lung injury: pneumonia, aspiration, inhalation injury
  - Indirect lung injury: sepsis, severe trauma, shock, blood product transfusion, acute pancreatitis:
    - Sepsis is the most common cause of ARDS.
- Associated with high mortality (27%-45% depending on severity)

CLINICAL ASSESSMENT

- Acute onset: within 1 week of clinical insult or new respiratory symptoms
- Typically manifests as dyspnea, tachypnea, and hypoxemia, with evolution to respiratory failure
- Common symptoms include dyspnea, cough (productive or nonproductive), and pleuritic chest pain.
- History may point to less typical etiologies of ARDS, such as prior blood product transfusion, trauma to chest, burns, or inhalation injury.
- Physical examination findings depend on underlying etiology but may include:
  - Tachypnea, tachycardia, diffuse crackles, accessory muscle use during respiration

  - Altered mental status, cyanosis, diaphoresis
- Clinical course is often characterized by progressive hypoxemia with increasing supplemental oxygen requirements and/or mechanical ventilator support.
  - Severe hypoxemia may persist, and the patient may become ventilator dependent with radiographic progression of airspace disease to a reticular pattern.
  - Complications may include barotrauma due to positive pressure mechanical ventilation and nosocomial infections.

DIAGNOSIS

- Clinical diagnostic criteria:
  - Respiratory symptoms of acute onset ($\leq$7 days)
  - Hypoxemia with severity determined by PaO_2/FiO_2 ratio based on arterial blood gas analysis:
    - Mild: PaO_2/FiO_2 ratio 200-300
    - Moderate: PaO_2/FiO_2 ratio 100-200
    - Severe: PaO_2/FiO_2 ratio <100
  - Bilateral pulmonary infiltrates on chest x-ray or CT scan
  - Absence of left atrial hypertension
- Exclusion of acute cardiogenic pulmonary edema: BNP with or without transthoracic echocardiogram
- Classically described as three pathologic stages:
  - Early exudative stage: first 7-0 days; nonspecific lung injury with acute and chronic inflammation and edema
  - Fibroproliferative stage: after 7-10 days; typically lasts 2-3 weeks
    - Resolution of pulmonary edema
    - Characterized by proliferation of alveolar cells
  - Fibrotic stage: development of fibrosis and remodeling of normal lung architecture

TREATMENT

- Supportive management of hypoxemia: administration of supplemental oxygen. Select patients may be the candidates for high-flow NC; however, the many patients with ARDS require intubation and mechanical ventilation.
- Mechanical ventilation with low tidal volume strategy (6 mL/kg ideal body weight):

- Maintain SpO_2 88% to 95% or PaO_2 goal of 55-80 mm Hg to minimize oxygen toxicity
- Plateau pressure of ≤30 cm H_2O to minimize barotrauma
- Conservative fluid management; avoid volume overload
- Severe disease may benefit from neuromuscular blockade and prone positioning.
- Treat underlying etiology

Case Conclusion

This case illustrates ARDS as a result of the most common form of ARDS—sepsis. The patient is septic due to pneumonia, which means she has had both direct and indirect injuries to her lungs. Her presentation meets the clinical criteria for ARDS diagnosis, and she should be intubated and provided supportive management of both sepsis and respiratory failure.

CHAPTER 317
Respiratory Distress Syndrome in the Newborn

Stephanie Hull, EdS, MMS, PA-C

▶ GENERAL FEATURES

- Respiratory distress syndrome (RDS) in the newborn, formerly hyaline membrane disease, is the most common cause of respiratory distress in the preterm infant.
- A deficiency of pulmonary surfactant production in the immature lung and inactivation of pulmonary surfactant by protein leak into airspaces results in poor lung compliance and atelectasis from alveolar collapse.
- Atelectasis leads to injury of the respiratory epithelium and alveolar capillary endothelium, which can trigger a cytokine-mediated inflammatory response.
- Pulmonary edema results from inflammation, reduced pulmonary fluid absorption (sodium channels expressed on epithelial cells increases with gestational age in parallel with the surge in pulmonary surfactant production), and low urine output.
- Hypoxemia results from the ventilation/perfusion mismatch with intrapulmonary right-to-left shunting of blood past large regions of poorly ventilated lung and extrapulmonary shunting across the foramen ovale and patent ductus arteriosus.
- Highest incidence in infants born at <30 weeks' gestation as pulmonary surfactant is not expressed in the lung until around 20 weeks' gestation.

▶ CLINICAL ASSESSMENT

- Signs of respiratory distress—including tachypnea, hypoxia, nasal flaring, expiratory grunting, and intercostal, subxiphoid, and subcostal retractions—develop minutes to hours after birth.
- Lung sounds are often decreased on pulmonary auscultation despite increased work of breathing.

- Pallor, cyanosis, diminished peripheral pulses, peripheral edema, and low urine output are often noted.

▶ DIAGNOSIS

- The classic chest radiograph findings are low lung volume and diffuse reticulogranular ground-glass appearance with air bronchograms.
- Hypoxemia is noted on arterial blood gas. The $PaCO_2$ may be normal or slightly elevated initially but increases as RDS worsens.

▶ TREATMENT

- Prevention of preterm delivery allows time for lung maturity and pulmonary surfactant production.
- Antenatal corticosteroid administration enhances lung maturation and release of pulmonary surfactant. All pregnant women at 23-34 weeks' gestation at increased risk of preterm delivery within the next 7 days should receive corticosteroids. The efficacy of antenatal corticosteroids at 34-37 weeks' gestation is uncertain.
- Oxygenation and ventilation supported with supplemental and positive airway pressure through noninvasive measures or intubation and mechanical ventilation.
- Exogenous surfactant therapy, most often administered via endotracheal tube, is most effective when given within the first 30-60 minutes of life.
- Uncomplicated RDS not treated with exogenous surfactant typically resolves by 1 week of age, marked by spontaneous diuresis followed by improvement in lung function. Administration of exogenous surfactant dramatically improves lung function and shortens the clinical course.

CHAPTER 318

Aspiration, Foreign-Body Aspiration, Aspiration Pneumonitis, and Aspiration Pneumonia

Gayle Bodner, MMS, PA-C
Kristin Lindaman, MMS, PA-C

▶ GENERAL FEATURES

- Foreign-body (FB) aspiration is a serious, potentially life-threatening condition and one of the leading causes of accidental death in children.
  - Can be acute or undetected and tolerated for longer periods of time
  - Larger FBs have increased risk of acute asphyxiation.
  - Food, coins, and small parts from toys are common aspirates in children.
  - Often occurs in children younger than 4 years
  - Slightly greater prevalence in boys and in children with neurologic disorders. Contributing factors in this population include immature swallowing coordination, smaller airway diameters, less developed dentition, easy distractibility, or oral exploration by putting things in their mouth.
- Risk factors for aspiration in adults include anesthesia, intoxication, loss of consciousness, gastroesophageal reflux disease, vomiting, swallowing dysfunction secondary to chronic neurologic disease, age-related degeneration in glottal function and gag reflex, as well as gastrointestinal and respiratory devices and procedures, including emergent endotracheal intubation.
  - Bone fragments, seeds, teeth, and metallic FBs are common aspirates in this population.
  - Aspiration of oropharyngeal secretions and gastric contents are more likely to be associated with aspiration pneumonitis and aspiration pneumonia (PNA).
- Aspiration pneumonitis: chemical injury due to inhalation of acidic gastric contents. Increasing acidity, food particulate, and volume of aspirated gastric content all lead to greater severity of pneumonitis.
- Aspiration pneumonia: the inhalation of oropharyngeal or upper gastrointestinal infectious contents into the lower respiratory tract causing an infection. Risk factors include those noted above as well as dementia, prolonged supine position, poor dentition, esophageal disorders, malnutrition, and tube feeding. Can lead to increased length of hospital stay, morbidity, and mortality.

▶ CLINICAL ASSESSMENT

- History may include witnessed aspiration event, though many aspiration events are unwitnessed and high clinical suspicion is necessary.

- Children tend to present acutely with choking and cough. May be accompanied by wheezing, stridor, and indicators of increased work of breathing, such as grunting and retractions.
- Larger or prolonged obstruction may include signs of severe respiratory distress including altered mental status and cyanosis, which is a medical emergency.
- Children with lower airway FBs may have subtle symptoms and present with respiratory complaints.
- Aspiration in adults can have a range of presentations from acute events to asymptomatic (particularly in elderly patients) or subtle chronic symptoms such as cough or recurrent pneumonias. Unilateral wheezing or decreased breath sounds may not always be present.
- In children, FB aspiration can present equally in right and left bronchial trees; in older children and adults, FB aspiration occurs more frequently in the right bronchial tree because of its vertical orientation.
- Common presenting symptoms of aspiration pneumonitis include cough and dyspnea. Depending on severity, patients may also present with increased work of breathing, hypoxia, low-grade fever, and pink/frothy sputum production. Typically, symptoms are self-limited and resolve within 24-48 hours.
- Aspiration pneumonia may have presentation comparable to aspiration pneumonitis; however, sputum is generally purulent, and fever may be higher.

▶ DIAGNOSIS

- Radiographic imaging is indicated in stable patients with suspected aspiration or FB obstruction.
- When the upper airway obstruction is suspected, posteroanterior (PA) and lateral soft-tissue x-ray views of the neck should be obtained. If obstruction is suspected below the larynx, PA and lateral chest x-ray should be obtained and may show a radiopaque FB, unilateral hyperinflation, atelectasis, and/or mediastinal shift.
- FBs are often radiolucent, and x-rays may be negative; CT is indicated for adults with high clinical suspicion. For children, bronchoscopy may be pursued if there is high clinical suspicion. Confirmation of the diagnosis is done via laryngoscopy by direct visualization of objects above the vocal cords or, if below, via bronchoscopy.
- In patients with aspiration pneumonitis, chest x-ray findings may be normal within the first 24 hours. In

mild cases, chest x-ray may show infiltrate in dependent lung fields; in severe cases, diffuse bilateral infiltrates may be seen.

- Chest x-ray in patients with aspiration pneumonia may reveal infiltrates in the dependent lung segments.

▶ TREATMENT

- When obstruction is associated with acute asphyxiation, basic life support maneuvers, oxygenation, and secure airway management, including advanced airways, may be needed. If these interventions are unsuccessful, emergent tracheotomy or cricothyrotomy may be required.
- In stable, nonasphyxiating FB aspiration, diagnostic and therapeutic rigid bronchoscopy under sedation or general anesthesia is recommended.
- For aspiration pneumonitis, utilize supportive measures such as suction of aspirated material and airway secretions and management of hypoxemia (supplemental oxygen and continuous positive airway pressure [CPAP] or mechanical ventilation, in severe cases).

- Bronchoscopy may be indicated for removal of liquid contents. Corticosteroids and prophylactic antibiotics are not recommended for pneumonitis.
- According to the Infectious Disease Society of America (IDSA) guidelines, aspiration pneumonia treatment mirrors community-acquired PNA guidelines and can be summarized as follows:
  - Outpatient:
    - For patients without comorbidities, monotherapy with amoxicillin, doxycycline, or a macrolide are acceptable options.
    - For patients with comorbidities, combination therapy with a β-lactam and macrolide or monotherapy with a respiratory fluoroquinolone is recommended.
  - Inpatient:
    - Antibiotic therapy recommendations depend on the severity and risk for MRSA and *Pseudomonas aeruginosa*.
    - Empiric coverage for anaerobic bacteria is no longer routinely recommended.
- Important adjunct management of aspiration includes assessment of swallow function and aspiration risk mitigation.

CHAPTER 319

Obesity Hypoventilation Syndrome

Ilana Borukhov, MSPAS, PA-C

▶ GENERAL FEATURES

- Obesity hypoventilation syndrome (OHS) is a metabolic, hormonal, cardiovascular, and respiratory complication of obesity caused by a failure to compensate for excessive weight on the respiratory system.
- Historically known as Pickwickian syndrome
- Results from a combination of pathologic processes including sleep disorder breathing (from mild-to-severe OSA), progressive retention of serum bicarbonate, a diminished respiratory drive, structural and functional respiratory impairment, reduced lung volumes, reduction of airway diameter, and airway smooth muscle structure and function.
- Leptin resistance plays an important role in the decreased ventilatory drive (diminished response to elevated CO_2).
- The main characteristics of OHS are:
  - Obesity (BMI >30 kg/m^2)
  - Daytime alveolar hypoventilation (wake P_{CO_2} > 45 mm Hg)
  - Sleep disordered breathing
  - Absence of other conditions such as primary pulmonary disease, skeletal restrictions, neuromuscular weakness, hypothyroidism, pleural pathology

- Associated with:
  - Reduced quality of life
  - Pulmonary HTN
  - Right heart failure
  - Insulin resistance
- The prevalence of OHS in the US adult population is ~0.3% but may be underestimated because of insufficient screening, misdiagnosis, or lack of confirmatory testing. Prevalence in specific groups is:
  - BMI 30–35: 8%–12%
  - BMI > 40: 18%–31%
  - BMI > 50: 50%

▶ CLINICAL ASSESSMENT

- Daytime symptoms: hypersomnolence, fatigue, morning headaches, impaired concentration and memory, depression, shortness of breath
- Nocturnal symptoms: poor sleep quality, frequent nocturnal awakenings, observed apneas, from mild to loud snoring, choking and gasping during sleep
- Physical examination findings:
  - General: elevated BMI, increased abdominal girth, neck circumference >16″ (female) and >17″ (male)

- Decreased O_2 saturation by pulse oximetry
- Skin: cyanosis or flushing (due to compensatory erythrocytosis)
- ENT: crowded upper airway, Mallampatti III or IV, macroglossia, micrognathia, retrognathia, high-arched palate, tonsillar hypertrophy, wide-neck circumference
- Increased right heart/venous pressures resulting in jugular venous distension, hepatomegaly, bilateral pedal edema
- Psych: anxiety, delirium (due to severe hypercapnia)

▶ **DIAGNOSIS**

- Nocturnal polysomnography with continuous CO_2 monitoring is the diagnostic gold standard and will show a sustained elevation of CO_2 >55 mm Hg or an increase of 10 mm Hg or more in CO_2 levels during sleep compared to wake.
- Laboratory tests:
  - BMP may show an elevated serum bicarbonate (>27 mEq/L).
  - CBC may show polycythemia, elevated RBC, and/or elevated hematocrit.
  - Thyroid function testing may reveal severe hypothyroidism as underlying cause.
  - Arterial blood gas may show hypercapnia ($Paco_2$ > 45 mm Hg) and/or hypoxemia (Pao_2 < 70 mm Hg).
- Pulmonary function tests (PFTs):
  - May show restrictive ventilatory defect, reduced expiratory reserve volume, and functional residual capacity
  - Normal PFTs do not exclude the diagnosis.

- Chest x-ray and CT chest may show:
  - Elevated hemi-diaphragms
  - Cardiomegaly, right ventricular hypertrophy
- Transthoracic echocardiogram may show signs of cor pulmonale: right ventricular hypertrophy, right atrial enlargement, and elevated pulmonary artery pressures.

▶ **TREATMENT**

Treatment is aimed at prevention and controlling any disease manifestations that are detected during workup.

- Health lifestyle modifications: weight loss through diet and exercise
- Endocrine, bariatric surgery, and dietitian consultations should be offered.
  - Weight loss can reverse OHS.
- Treatment of thyroid and cardiovascular disorders if present
- Treatment with continuous positive airway pressure (CPAP) or bilevel positive airway pressure (BiPAP) device
- Supplemented oxygen may be necessary in addition to PAP therapy.
- Tracheostomy in severe cases
- Reassess sleep disorder breathing after 3 months of continuous therapy.
- Complications:
  - Left untreated, complications may develop:
    - Depression, irritability, increased risk for motor vehicle or heavy machinery accidents, hypertension, right heart failure (cor pulmonale), secondary erythrocytosis, pulmonary hypertension, respiratory failure, increased mortality.

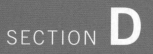

SECTION **D**

Pleural Disease

CHAPTER **320**

Pleural Effusion, Pneumothorax, and Hemothorax

Ian Smith, MMS, PA-C, APA-C

▶ **GENERAL FEATURES**

- Pleural effusions:
  - Occur when excess fluid collects in the potential space between the visceral and parietal pleura
  - There are a variety of causes for effusions; however, the most common cause of pleural effusion in the United States is heart failure.

- Pleural effusions can be classified as transudative or exudative in nature, based on the protein content of the fluid.
- Pneumothorax:
  - Occurs when air accumulates in the pleural space. Pneumothoraxes can occur spontaneously or secondary to traumatic injuries.

- Accumulation of fluid, blood, or air within the pleural space can be asymptomatic, but more often causes some element of collapse of the surrounding lung parenchyma.
- Hemothorax occurs when blood collects in the pleural cavity and is most often traumatic in nature.

CLINICAL ASSESSMENT

- Pleural effusion:
  - Patients will often complain of shortness of breath, cough, or chest pain and may exhibit hypoxia, tachypnea, or tachycardia.
  - On examination of the affected side of the chest, breath sounds may be diminished, decreased, or absent tactile fremitus, and percussion of the chest may demonstrate dullness in the patient with a pleural effusion.
  - The patient should be examined further for any possible etiology of the pleural effusion.
- Pneumothorax:
  - Classically, spontaneous pneumothorax occurs in the tall, thin man in his 20s with a smoking history.
  - On examination of a patient with a pneumothorax, the affected side will have absent or diminished breath sounds and tympany on percussion.
- Hemothorax is often secondary to traumatic injuries such as rib fractures.

DIAGNOSIS

- Chest radiograph is the most common first-line diagnostic evaluation of a patient with pleural pathology; the chest radiograph should be done upright, as fluid or blood may layer out across the pleura in the supine patient.
  - Pneumothorax demonstrates a lack of lung markings at the peripheral lung field or the mediastinum with or without associated lung collapse.
- Increasingly, bedside ultrasound is a rapid, effective, and highly sensitive evaluation tool for chest pathology.
  - Hemothorax and pleural effusion will be indistinguishable on ultrasound.
  - Pneumothorax will present as absent pleural sliding on ultrasound.

- A CT scan of the chest is the most sensitive evaluation for pleural effusion, hemothorax, or pneumothorax.
  - CT will further quantify density and amount of fluid present.
  - Pneumothorax seen on CT scan, but not on chest x-ray, is classically known as an occult pneumothorax.
- Tension pneumothorax is a clinical diagnosis seen with signs of decompensation, hypoxia, hypotension, tachycardia, tracheal deviation (away from the affected side), and absent breath sounds (on the affected side). Immediate intervention with chest decompression is necessary to prevent further decompensation and death.
- Lab testing of a patient with pleural effusion involves analysis of the pleural fluid after thoracentesis, including protein and LDH, cytology, and sometimes culture if empyema is suspected.
- Light's criteria help identify an exudative effusion by comparing pleural fluid protein and LDH content to serum levels.

TREATMENT

- Patient support is the basis of treatment, ensuring airway and ventilatory maintenance is continued during evaluation and treatment.
- Pleural effusion:
  - Transudative effusions are often effectively treated via the underlying etiology, such as diuresis in heart failure.
  - Thoracentesis is required for diagnosis and treatment in all pleural effusions, except known cases of heart failure or cirrhosis with previously diagnosed pleural transudative effusion.
- Pneumothorax:
  - Evacuation of the traumatic pneumothorax or hemothorax is generally accomplished with tube thoracostomy.
  - Occult pneumothorax may be treated with watchful waiting and oxygen therapy.
  - In tension pneumothoraxes, rapid identification and finger thoracostomy or needle decompression is required before further patient decompensation.
- In the case of recurrent pleural effusion or pneumothorax, pleurodesis may be considered to ensure obliteration of the pleural space and help prevent recurrence.

CHAPTER
321
Pulmonary Nodules
Melissa Ricker, PA-C

▶ GENERAL FEATURES

- A solitary pulmonary nodule (SPN) is a common incidentally identified radiologic abnormality described as a solid, subsolid, or ground-glass mass that is <30 mm in diameter and surrounded by pulmonary parenchyma.
- Patients at high risk of a malignant etiology include those with a history of cigarette smoking, emphysema, pulmonary fibrosis, known malignancy, family history of malignancy, hazardous fume or asbestos exposures, and African American race.
- Small size (<20 mm), smooth contour, well-defined margins and the presence of calcifications are suggestive of, but not diagnostic for, benign pathologies.
- Larger size (>20 mm), lobulated contour, and irregular margins are highly suspicious of, but not diagnostic for, malignant pathologies. Note there is considerable overlap in the internal characteristics of benign and malignant pathologies.
- The most common causes of SPN include benign cysts, benign tumors, current infection, scarring from remote infections, autoimmune disease, congenital malformation, and lung or other cancer.
- SPNs >30 mm are commonly referred to a lung masses.

▶ DIAGNOSIS

- With nearly all SPNs incidentally found on chest imaging, patients typically do not present with a specific complaint or classic physical examination finding.
- There is no individual laboratory test that yields a definitive diagnosis.
- A low-radiation technique chest CT is the preferred imaging modality for standardized follow-up.
- Solid nodule(s):
  - Low-risk patients with a solid nodule <6 mm have a low likelihood of malignancy, and CT follow-up is not recommended.
  - High-risk patients with a solid nodule >8 mm should have a repeat CT or positron emission tomography (PET) scan in 3 months.
  - High-risk patients with a solid mass >30 mm have a high likelihood of malignancy and should be referred for surgical resection.
  - High- or low-risk patients with a solid nodule size between 6 and 8 mm should have a repeat CT in 6-12 months.
  - High- or low-risk patients with multiple solid nodules: imaging is optional for nodules <6 mm in size; nodules >6 mm should have repeat CT in 3-6 months.
- Subsolid nodule(s):
  - Ground-glass and subsolid nodules <6 mm have a low likelihood of malignancy, and CT follow-up is not recommended.
  - Ground-glass and subsolid nodules >6 mm should have a CT repeated in 6 months to confirm presence. If confirmed, should be referred for surgical resection.
  - Multiple ground-glass and subsolid nodules should have a CT repeated in 3-6 months.
- If the SPN remains stable after the above-recommended follow-up, the risk/benefit of serial imaging should be discussed. If growth or altered morphology is observed, refer for biopsy.
- Decisions regarding choice of diagnostic procedure depend on the SPN size and location, availability of the procedure, and regional expertise.
  - For peripherally located SPNs, transthoracic needle biopsy vs. surgical resection is preferred.
  - For centrally located SPNs, endobronchial biopsy is preferred.
- If SPN sampling is nondiagnostic or suspicious for malignancy, a diagnostic wedge resection by video-assisted thoracic surgery (VATS) is the preferred diagnostic procedure.

TREATMENT

- The Fleischner Society is an international and multi-disciplinary society that maintains the guidelines for management of SPNs. Most recently updated in 2017, these guidelines have standardized follow-up examination and noninvasive treatment of diseases of the chest but do not apply to those younger than 35 years, immunocompromised patients, or those with existing malignancy.
- Definite treatment of the SPN is based on histological diagnostic findings, recommendations from a multidisciplinary team, surgical candidacy, and patient preference.

CHAPTER 322

Lung Cancer

Brittany Strelow, MS, PA-C

GENERAL FEATURES

- Malignancy originating in the airways or pulmonary parenchyma
- The most common cause of cancer deaths in both men and women.
- Classified primarily as either:
  - Small cell lung cancer (SCLC):
    - Known for metastatic spread and aggressive rate of growth
    - Limited-stage SCLC, 5-year survival is 15% to 25%.
    - Extensive-stage SCLC is <1%.
  - Non–small cell lung cancer (NSCLC):
    - Accounts for 85% of all lung cancers
  - Other cell types:
    - Lung neuroendocrine (carcinoid) tumors
- Risk factors:
  - Smoking:
    - Dose dependent
    - Risk persists for years after quitting
    - Includes secondhand exposure
  - Radiation exposure
  - Environmental toxins:
    - Radon
    - Asbestos
    - Metals
      - Arsenic, chromium, and nickel
    - Ionizing radiation
    - Polycyclic aromatic hydrocarbons
  - Pulmonary fibrosis
  - Genetic factors
- Screening:
  - US Preventive Services Task Force recommends those aged 55-80 years who have a 30 pack-year smoking history and currently smoke or have quit within the past 15 years to have a low-dose screening CT scan.

CLINICAL ASSESSMENT

- Majority of patients have advanced disease at clinical presentation.

- Symptoms:
  - Dyspnea
  - Persistent cough
  - Hemoptysis
  - Chest pain
  - Hoarseness
  - Pleural involvement
  - Postobstructive pneumonia
  - Superior vena cava syndrome
  - Pancoast syndrome
  - Bone pain
  - Headache
  - Malaise
  - Seizures
  - Fatigue
  - Anorexia
  - Weight loss
  - Paraneoplastic syndromes:
    - Hypercalcemia
    - SIADH secretion
    - Cushing syndrome
- Evaluation:
  - Includes lactate dehydrogenase (LDH), CBC, comprehensive metabolic panel, to assess for evidence of extrapulmonary involvement
  - Imaging:
    - Chest radiography: findings may include solitary pulmonary nodule, hilar mass, nonresolving infiltrate/consolidation, mediastinal lymph node involvement, pleural effusions.
    - Contrast-enhanced CT of the chest and abdomen/pelvis: may show primary lung lesions and/or metastatic lesions.
    - PET to evaluate for distant metastasis
    - MRI to evaluate for brain metastasis
- Biopsy to confirm diagnosis via:
  - Bronchoscopy
  - Endobronchial ultrasound (EBUS)
  - CT guidance
  - Medical thoracoscopy

- Video-assisted thoracoscopic surgery (VATS)
- General staging (also staged by TNM8 system)
  - Stage I:
    - The tumor is confined to the lung with no lymph node involvement.
  - Stage II:
    - The tumor is confined to the lung but has spread to lymph nodes in the lung.
  - Stage III:
    - The tumor is confined to the lung; cancer has spread to lymph nodes outside the lung but remains within the chest cavity.
  - Stage IV:
    - Cancer has spread outside the chest wall.
  - Common sites of metastasis:
    - Contralateral lung
    - Lymph nodes
    - Brain
    - Bone
    - Liver
    - Adrenal glands

▶ TREATMENT

- SCLC:
  - Very responsive to chemotherapy and radiotherapy but has a high rate of relapse
  - Limited-stage disease (stages I-III):
    - Considered surgical intervention/resection for solitary nodules without regional lymph node involvement
    - Chemotherapy with concurrent radiation therapy
  - Extensive-stage disease (stage IV):
    - Chemotherapy is first line
    - Often, disease is too extensive to be encompassed in a safe, tolerable radiation field.
- NSCLC:
  - Treatment depends on the stage and the patient's general health.
  - STAGE I:
    - Surgical resection
  - STAGE II:
    - Surgical resection
  - STAGE III:
    - Concurrent chemotherapy and radiation therapy. On occasion, surgery is also considered.
  - STAGE IV:
    - Palliative chemotherapy accompanied by palliative radiation therapy for symptomatic sites (eg, painful bone metastasis, spinal cord compression, superior vena cava syndrome, postobstructive pneumonia) and brain metastases
    - Patients may choose to forego these therapies and pursue hospice care.

SECTION **F**

Respiratory Infections

CHAPTER

323

Pertussis

Tyler D. Sommer, MPAS, PA-C

▶ GENERAL FEATURES

- Pertussis is an acute infection of the bronchial tree caused by the Gram-negative rod *Bordetella pertussis*, a highly contagious pathogen transmitted by respiratory droplets.
- Commonly known as "whooping cough"
- Most commonly affects children under the age of 5 years, most significantly affects those under 2 years or age, and can occur in any season.

- Mortality is highest in infants under the age of 1 year, while adults and older children generally experience a milder illness.
- Pertussis is a vaccine-preventable illness; those at highest risk are unvaccinated and immunocompromised children.

▶ CLINICAL ASSESSMENT

- The incubation period is typically 6-14 days. The illness can last 6-8 weeks and is broken down into three distinct stages:

- Catarrhal stage: initial 1-2 weeks, characterized by low-grade fevers, nasal congestion, sneezing, and a mild cough. Most contagious phase.
- Paroxysmal stage: the fever subsides, and the characteristic whooping cough begins in paroxysmal attacks, characterized by a "whoop" sound during inspiration. Post-tussive vomiting is common.
- Convalescent stage: begins about 4 weeks after the initial onset. Coughing attacks become less frequent, slowly fading over 2-4 weeks. Patients are no longer contagious during this stage.

▶ DIAGNOSIS

- Diagnostic testing options include:
  - Polymerase chain reaction (PCR) assay of nasopharyngeal swab
  - B. pertussis on specialized culture media (Bordet-Gengou agar) of nasopharyngeal swab
  - Serology of blood, saliva, or throat swab
- White blood cell count is usually significantly elevated, commonly in the range of 15-20 000/μL, with predominant lymphocytosis.

▶ TREATMENT

- Antibiotic treatment should be prescribed for all suspected or confirmed cases of pertussis and is most effective when prescribed during the catarrhal stage.
  - Drug of choice is erythromycin.
  - Effective alternatives include azithromycin, clarithromycin, and trimethoprim-sulfamethoxazole.
- Antibiotic therapy may shorten contagious duration and decrease the severity of the paroxysmal stage.
- Individuals who are known to have been in close contact with an active case of pertussis within 3 weeks of the onset of the cough should also be treated antibiotics.
- Pertussis vaccination is advised for all infants and is combined with the diphtheria and tetanus toxoid vaccinations (DTaP).
- Adolescents between 11 and 18 years of age who have completed the DTaP vaccination series prior should receive a single dose of Tdap for booster immunization. Adults of all ages should receive a single dose of Tdap at some point as well.
- Women who are pregnant should also receive a dose of Tdap during in each pregnancy, regardless of their prior vaccinations and optimally between 27- and 36-weeks' gestation.
- Lasting immunity is not generally conferred by vaccination or survival of the disease

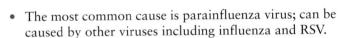

CHAPTER 324

Croup

Sonya Peters, PA-C

A 2-year-old boy presents with 1 day of a runny nose and a barking cough that wakes him from sleep. His parents have observed labored breathing today. Vital signs include temperature 100 °F, heart rate (HR) 110 beats per minute, blood pressure 90/60, RR 30, and oxygen saturation 98% on room air. Physical examination reveals inspiratory stridor at rest with mild intercostal retractions. Lung auscultation is clear without wheezing, rales, or rhonchi. What is the best treatment plan for this patient?

▶ GENERAL FEATURES

- Upper airway respiratory condition that leads to swelling of the larynx and trachea
- Most common in children 6-36 months of age but can be seen in children as young as 3 months. It is uncommon in children >6 years old.
- More common in boys

- The most common cause is parainfluenza virus; can be caused by other viruses including influenza and RSV.
- Most cases occur in the fall or early winter.

▶ CLINICAL ASSESSMENT

- Typical signs and symptoms of croup include:
  - Barking cough
  - Labored breathing
  - Hoarseness
  - Inspiratory stridor
  - Low-grade fever
- Signs of more severe croup include:
  - Stridor at rest
  - Intercostal or suprasternal retractions
  - Cyanosis
- Signs and symptoms are typically worse at night and last 3-5 days.

▶ DIAGNOSIS

- Typically, a clinical diagnosis is based on characteristic symptoms.
- Lateral neck radiography may show characteristic narrowing of the trachea (steeple sign).
- Imaging and laboratory tests are typically not required for diagnosis.

▶ TREATMENT

- Mild croup may be treated at home with the following modalities:
  - Hydration
  - Humidified or cooled air
  - Antipyretics (if needed)
- Moderate-to-severe croup is treated in the emergency department (ED) setting with the following modalities:
  - Supplemental oxygen
  - Comforting the child/limiting agitation, which can worsen symptoms
  - Nebulized (racemic) epinephrine
  - Steroids (dexamethasone or prednisolone)
- Patients should be observed for treatment response before discharge home.
- Patients with persistent respiratory compromise or repeated visits should be hospitalized.

Case Conclusion

After evaluating the patient, administer oral dexamethasone and observe for resolution of retractions. The boy is saturating 98% on room air. In this circumstance, humidified air may be therapeutic but was not an option. Two liters of oxygen on nasal cannula is unlikely to be beneficial and may cause oxygen toxicity, given his already normal oxygen saturation. The boy had stridor at rest and had suprasternal retractions. These symptoms put him in the moderate-to-severe croup category, and the boy should be kept in the ED until he is more stable. Croup is a clinical diagnosis based on characteristic symptoms of the infection; it is not necessary to get a chest x-ray to diagnose croup. Dexamethasone is a common medication administered with croup to improve symptoms.

CHAPTER 325

Respiratory Syncytial Virus

Paul "PJ" Koltnow, MS, MSPAS, PA-C

▶ GENERAL FEATURES

- Respiratory syncytial virus (RSV) is one of the most common respiratory infections in infants and children.
- It follows a seasonal pattern and, in the northern hemisphere, it is most active in the fall and early spring, with a peak occurrence in January or February.
- RSV can cause severe lower respiratory infections and accounts for >70% of bronchiolitis and 40% of pneumonia in young children.
- Children who were born premature, very young infants, those with a history of congenital heart disease, and those who are immunocompromised are at higher risk for complications.
- Reinfection is common.
- May be associated with the development of asthma later in life

▶ CLINICAL ASSESSMENT

- May present as a lower respiratory tract infection, including bronchiolitis (most common in infants), bronchospasm, pneumonia, or acute respiratory failure
- Early infections may present with upper respiratory symptoms, such as nasal congestion or rhinorrhea; later infections may include fever (50%), poor feeding, coughing, or wheezing.
- Physical examination may be notable for increased respiratory rate, wheezing, or crackles. Nasal flaring, chest retractions, and tachypnea are concerning for respiratory distress.
- Clinical signs of dehydration or hypovolemia may be present.

▶ DIAGNOSIS

- Diagnosis is typically made clinically.
- Chest x-ray is mainly used to rule out other potential causes of symptoms. Findings may include hyperinflation and patchy atelectasis, but these are nonspecific.

▶ TREATMENT

- Usually self-limited
- Monitor respiratory status and fluid status.
- Reasons for hospitalization include pulse oximetry of <90% on room air; respiratory rate of >70 breaths a minute; toxic appearance, poor feeding, or dehydration.
- If hospitalized, supportive care may include supplemental oxygen support, fluids for hydration, and nutrition support.

Acute Bronchitis

Alan Brokenicky, MPAS, PA-C

▶ GENERAL FEATURES

- Acute bronchitis is a lower respiratory tract infection involving the large airways (bronchi), without evidence of pneumonia, occurring in the absence of chronic obstructive pulmonary disease.
- Acute bronchitis is among the most common adult outpatient diagnoses, with ~100 million ambulatory care visits in the United States each year.
- Highest incidence is in the fall and winter.
- Most common causes:
  - Viruses: influenza A and B, parainfluenza, coronavirus types 1-3, rhinoviruses, respiratory syncytial virus (RSV), human metapneumovirus.
  - Bacterial causes are uncommon (<10%) and include *Bordetella pertussis*, *Mycoplasma*, and *Chlamydia*.
  - Noninfectious: asthma, pollution, smoking tobacco, or cannabis

▶ CLINICAL ASSESSMENT

- Symptoms are typically self-limited, resolving within 1-3 weeks and characterized by acute onset of persistent cough. May also involve:
  - Sputum production
  - Wheezing
  - Low-grade fever
- Physical examination may be notable for:
  - Low-grade fever

- Wheezing or rhonchi on lung auscultation that improves with coughing

▶ DIAGNOSIS

- The diagnosis clinical based on history and physical examination.
- Testing is generally reserved for:
  - Cases in which pneumonia is suspected
  - Clinical diagnosis is uncertain, or when results would change management
- Chest x-ray may be useful to exclude pneumonia in patients with a high clinical suspicion or abnormal vital signs.
- Laboratory tests are typically not indicated.

▶ TREATMENT

For most patients with acute bronchitis, symptoms are self-limited and resolve in 1-3 weeks.

- Antibiotics are not recommended for uncomplicated bronchitis.
- Reassurance and symptom control are the cornerstones of care, including antitussives, expectorants, and decongestants.
- Bronchodilators such as β-2 agonists may reduce cough in adult patients with airflow obstruction.

Acute Bronchiolitis

Alan Brokenicky, MPAS, PA-C

▶ GENERAL FEATURES

- Bronchiolitis is an infectious clinical condition characterized by upper respiratory symptoms (eg, rhinorrhea) followed by lower respiratory inflammation, resulting in wheezing and increasing respiratory effort in children under the age of 2 years.
- The most common lower respiratory tract infection in infants and children ≤2 years of age and is the leading cause for hospitalization in children <1 year of age.

- Cases primarily occur in the fall and winter.
- Most often caused by respiratory syncytial virus (RSV) and transmitted by direct contact with contaminated secretions.
- Increases risk for dehydration as blocked nasal passages inhibit feeding while increased work of breathing and a higher metabolic rate contribute to increased insensible losses
- Risk factors for severe disease:
  - Prematurity (gestational age ≤36 weeks)
  - Low birth weight

- Age <12 weeks
- Chronic pulmonary disease, particularly bronchopulmonary dysplasia (also known as chronic lung disease)
- Anatomic defects of the airways
- Hemodynamically significant congenital heart disease
- Immunodeficiency
- Neurologic disease
- Tobacco smoke exposure

▶ CLINICAL ASSESSMENT

- History:
  - The usual course of RSV bronchiolitis is 1-3 days of fever, rhinorrhea, and cough, followed by wheezing, tachypnea, and respiratory distress.
  - Additional associated symptoms include irritability, cyanosis, and poor feeding.
  - Symptoms typically last 7-21 days and are often the worst in the first week of the illness.
- Physical examination:
  - Often reveals tachypnea with a shallow, rapid respiratory pattern
  - Lung auscultation may reveal diffuse wheezing and/or crackles.
  - Nasal flaring, use of accessory muscles, fever, cyanosis, retractions, and a prolongation of the expiratory phase may be present, depending on the severity of illness.
  - May include signs of dehydration/hypovolemia including dry mucous membranes, tachycardia, lethargy, delayed capillary refill, inadequate urine output, and a sunken fontanelle

▶ DIAGNOSIS

- Bronchiolitis is diagnosed clinically.
- Diagnostic testing may help rule out secondary or co-morbid bacterial infection, complications, or other conditions in the differential diagnosis, particularly in children who have preexisting cardiopulmonary disease.
- Laboratory findings:
  - Laboratory tests are not routinely indicated.
  - Rapid viral diagnosis can be made by identification of viral antigens in nasopharyngeal secretions.
- Radiology:
  - Chest radiographs should only be obtained if there is a high suspicion of alternative or additional diagnoses such as bacterial pneumonia.
  - Radiologic findings are generally nonspecific and may include air trapping, consolidation, and collapse.

▶ TREATMENT

- Patients can typically be managed as outpatients with close observation for disease progression.
- Infants and young children with severe disease usually require hospitalization for observation and treatment.

Treatment consists of supportive care including hydration, supplemental oxygen, suctioning of secretions, and close monitoring.

- High-flow nasal cannula, CPAP, and endotracheal intubation may be indicated in severe disease.
- The antiviral ribavirin should be considered only in selected infants and young children with severe illness or at high risk for serious RSV disease.

CHAPTER
328

Pneumonia

Joy Moverley, DHSc, MPH, PA-C

▶ GENERAL FEATURES

- Lower respiratory tract infection caused by a variety of pathogens and differentiated by setting of infection (community-acquired pneumonia [CAP], nosocomial or hospital-acquired pneumonia [HAP], and ventilator-acquired pneumonia [VAP])
- Leading cause of morbidity and mortality worldwide
- Risk factors include:
  - Older age
  - Chronic comorbidities including diabetes mellitus, asthma, and chronic obstructive pulmonary disease
  - Dental/periodontal disease
  - Smoking
  - Alcohol overuse
  - Opioid use
  - Liver, heart, and kidney disease
- Most common community-acquired pathogens: *Streptococcus pneumoniae* and respiratory viruses
  - Pathogens are only identified in one-third of CAP diagnoses.
- Bacterial pneumonia:
  - Other typical bacterial pathogens include:
    - *Haemophilus influenzae*
    - *Moraxella catarrhalis*
    - *Staphylococcus aureus*
    - Group A streptococci

- Atypical (not visualized by Gram stain or traditional culture techniques) pathogens include:
  - *Legionella* spp
  - *Mycoplasma pneumoniae*
  - *Chlamydia pneumoniae*
  - Microbes involved in aspiration pneumonia may include microaerophilic bacteria and anaerobic bacteria.
- Viral pneumonia :
  - Most common pathogens:
    - Influenza A and B viruses
    - Respiratory syncytial virus (RSV)
    - Coronavirus
- Fungal pneumonia:
  - Specific risk factors: immunosuppression, workers with exposure to animal excreta in endemic areas (often farm workers)
  - Most common pathogens:
    - Opportunistic fungi:
      - *Pneumocystis jirovecii*
      - *Aspergillus*
    - Endemic fungi (if appropriate for regional area):
      - Histoplasmosis
      - Coccidioidomycosis
      - Blastomycosis
      - Cryptococcosis
- HIV-related pneumonia:
  - Opportunistic pathogens including *Pneumocystis jirovecii* pneumonia (PJP), fungal pathogens, parasites, and less common viral pathogens such as cytomegalovirus (CMV) should be considered, especially in patients with a CD4 count <200 cells/μL.
  - Pneumocystis pneumonia (caused by *P. jirovecii* or PJP) is the most common AIDS-defining opportunistic infection in the United States.
  - Typical sources of bacterial and viral infection remain common in patients with HIV.
  - HIV-associated tuberculosis (TB) is most common among those who use intravenous (IV) drugs.

▶ CLINICAL ASSESSMENT

- History:
  - Cough (with or without sputum production)
  - Dyspnea
  - Pleuritic chest pain
  - Fever
  - Chills
  - Fatigue
  - Malaise
  - Anorexia
- Physical examination:
  - Fever, tachycardia, tachypnea
  - Labored breathing
  - Adventitious lung sounds: crackles/rales, rhonchi
  - Tactile fremitus, egophony, dullness to percussion
  - Lymphadenopathy
  - Rashes

▶ DIAGNOSIS

- Chest x-ray may be significant for infiltrate.
  - CT scan may be ordered if immunocompromised patient with high risk for pneumonia and negative chest x-ray.
  - The American Thoracic Society/Infectious Disease Society of America do not recommend obtaining a follow-up chest radiograph in patients whose symptoms have resolved in the first 5-7 days.
- Patients only requiring outpatient treatment do not typically need further diagnostics.
- Specific considerations:
  - Bacterial
    - CBC may show leukocytosis and neutrophilia.
    - Most often present with lobar consolidation on radiograph.
    - Urinary antigen testing for *S. pneumonia* is available, but not universally recommended.
    - Legionella testing should be ordered if suspected.
  - Viral:
    - If seasonally appropriate, test for respiratory viruses via viral culture or rapid antigen test (influenza, adenovirus, parainfluenza, RSV, human metapneumovirus, epidemic coronaviruses)
    - For immunocompromised patients, consider quantitative PCR for CMV.
  - Fungal:
    - CBC may show eosinophilia, neutropenia, or leukopenia.
    - Consider PCR-based assays or non–culture-based tools (galactomannan [GM] or β-D-glucan [BD]) in high-risk patients or suspected cases.
    - Urine culture for Cryptococcus or Blastomycosis
  - HIV related:
    - CD4 count should be ordered to correlate risk of opportunistic infection.
      - Sinusitis and bronchitis can occur at any CD4 count.
      - Bacterial pneumonia and TB can occur when the CD4 count is above 500 cells/μL.
      - Disseminated fungal disease, PJP, and CMV typically only occur when CD4 count is below 200 cells/μL.
    - Radiographic findings for PJP are nonspecific, including "ground-glass" appearance with bilateral airspace infiltrates. PCR testing for PJP is available.
    - Patients with TB and HIV often have atypical radiographic appearance, about 30% having upper lobe cavitation or opacification. Tuberculin skin test cannot reliably rule out active or latent TB infection in patients with CD4 count <300 cells/μL.

▶ TREATMENT

- Treatment is generally started empirically before the causative pathogen is identified.

- Patients with normal vital signs and no comorbidities usually present with mild severity and can be treated in an outpatient setting.
- CURB-65 and Pneumonia Severity Index (PSI) scores can be used to help determine need for hospital admission. High-risk features include advanced age, altered mental status, tachypnea and other abnormal vital signs, hypotension, severe laboratory derangements, and hypoxia.
- Bacterial:
  - Outpatient therapy of CAP:
    - Low-risk patients should be given monotherapy with amoxicillin, doxycycline, or a macrolide (in areas where pneumococcal resistance is known to be low).
    - In higher risk patients (comorbidities, immune compromise, recent antibiotic use), treatment options include:
      - Monotherapy with a respiratory fluoroquinolone OR
      - Combination therapy of a β-lactam (amoxicillin/clavulanate OR a cephalosporin) PLUS coverage of atypical organisms (a macrolide OR doxycycline)
  - Inpatient therapy of CAP:
    - First-line options include a respiratory fluoroquinolone OR a combination of β-lactam (such as ceftriaxone) PLUS a macrolide (such as azithromycin).
  - Inpatient therapy of HAP and VAP
    - Broad-spectrum antibiotics covering Gram-negative bacteria including *Pseudomonas*
      - Piperacillin-tazobactam
      - Cefepime
      - Carbapenems (such as meropenem)

- PLUS
- Add one of the following for patients at risk for MRSA:
  - IV vancomycin
  - IV linezolid
- Viral:
  - Most viral pathogens are treated with supportive care and monitoring of symptoms.
  - For patients with confirmed influenza, start antiviral treatment as soon as possible with a neuraminidase inhibitor such as oseltamivir.
  - For confirmed CMV infection, start appropriate antiviral treat (ganciclovir or foscarnet).
- Fungal:
  - Amphotericin B at doses appropriate for the known pathogen is typically first-line therapy.
  - Consultation with infectious disease specialists is recommended.
- HIV related:
  - Patients with HIV who present with typical features of pneumonia plus consolidation on x-ray should be treated for the most common CAP pathogens.
  - Fluoroquinolones can delay the diagnosis for TB. Initially, TB can respond to fluoroquinolone antibiotics. If high risk for TB, obtain appropriate testing before administering treatment.
  - Immunocompromised patients are more likely to experience significant complications, such as empyema, bacteremia, and endocarditis.
  - Consider HIV in any patient who fails to respond to treatment.
- For all patients, to prevent CAP, recommend smoking cessation, universal influenza vaccination, and pneumococcal vaccination for at-risk patients.

SECTION **G**	*Restrictive and Fibrotic Pulmonary Diseases*
CHAPTER **329**	**Idiopathic Pulmonary Fibrosis** Katelyn Adler, MSPAS, PA-C

▶ GENERAL FEATURES

- Idiopathic pulmonary fibrosis (IPF) is a progressive fibrotic interstitial pneumonia with no known specific cause.

- Risk factors include:
  - Cigarette smoking
  - Environmental exposures
  - GERD
  - Sleep apnea

- Most commonly affects men aged 50-75 years
- Poor prognosis with typical survival from the time of diagnosis of 2-5 years

▶ CLINICAL ASSESSMENT

- Symptoms typically include nonproductive cough and gradual-onset dyspnea on exertion with decreased exercise tolerance.
- May include acute exacerbations with rapid worsening of symptoms associated with fever
- Patients may report a history of exposure to metal or wood dust.
- Physical examination may reveal clubbing of digits and fine bibasilar crackles on lung auscultation.

▶ DIAGNOSIS

- Chest x-ray may reveal bilateral opacities with a reticular pattern typical of interstitial processes.

- CT of the chest may reveal ground-glass opacities and diffuse reticular opacities (honeycombing).
- Pulmonary function tests demonstrate a restrictive pattern, decreased total lung volume and residual volume, and a normal to increased FEV_1/FVC ratio.
- Echocardiography may reveal pulmonary hypertension.
- Bronchoalveolar lavage, transbronchial biopsy, and surgical biopsy are reserved for cases in which the diagnosis cannot be determined by imaging.

▶ TREATMENT

- Currently, no treatment improves survival in patients with IPF.
- Encourage smoking cessation
- Oxygen therapy for patients with hypoxemia at rest or with exercise
- Early referral for lung transplantation evaluation

CHAPTER 330

Pulmonary Sarcoidosis

Caroline Sisson, MMS

▶ GENERAL FEATURES

- Sarcoidosis is an inflammatory disease characterized by the formation of immune granulomas with multiple manifestations, including pulmonary, dermatologic, cardiac, optic, hepatic, renal, and musculoskeletal.
- Pulmonary involvement is the most common manifestation.
- Occurs more commonly in women and in Black patients
- Often presents in the third or fourth decade of life
- Clinical course is variable, including asymptomatic disease, sustained remission with treatment, or chronic disease.

▶ CLINICAL ASSESSMENT

- Presentation may include:
  - Cough, dyspnea, and chest pain
  - Constitutional symptoms (fever, malaise, and weight loss)
  - New skin lesions, changes in vision, polyarthritis
  - Renal or hepatic impairment
  - Heart palpitations, exercise intolerance, dizziness, or syncope may signal cardiac involvement.

- Pulmonary examination is often unrevealing. Wheezing may be present and is associated with airway obstruction from traction bronchiectasis related to fibrotic changes.
- Clubbing of finger and/or toenails may be present in patients with fibrotic disease.
- A 6-minute walk may demonstrate significant oxygen desaturation.
- Physical examination may also be notable for lymphadenopathy.
- Dermatologic manifestations include erythema nodosum, which carries a more favorable prognosis. Ocular involvement may include uveitis or involvement of the lacrimal glands, conjunctiva, and other extraocular structures.
- Hepatomegaly may be present in patients with hepatic involvement.

▶ DIAGNOSIS

- Chest x-ray classically features bilateral hilar lymphadenopathy. May also be notable for nodules, reticular opacities, masses, consolidation, or fibrosis.
- CT scan of the chest may show mediastinal/hilar lymphadenopathy, nodules, masses, or consolidation,

ground-glass opacities (including the "reverse halo sign"), fibrosis, and mosaic attenuation with air trapping.
- Radiographic involvement in pulmonary disease is grouped in stages:
  - Stage I: hilar adenopathy alone
  - Stage II: hilar adenopathy with parenchymal involvement, upper lobe predominant
  - Stage III: parenchymal involvement with minimal or no hilar adenopathy
  - Stage IV: advanced fibrotic changes
- Spirometry may be unrevealing or demonstrate restriction.
- Diagnosis is confirmed by biopsy demonstrating non-caseating granulomas. Common biopsy sites are skin lesions or lymph nodes. Endobronchial ultrasound (EBUS) is recommended for hilar node biopsy.
- ACE levels are often elevated, but this finding is neither specific nor sensitive.
- Additional workup should screen for extrapulmonary disease including ophthalmologic examination, CBC, EKG, serum calcium, serum creatinine, and alkaline phosphatase.

- If pulmonary hypertension is suspected, transthoracic echocardiogram can be performed as screening with right heart catheterization for confirmation. If cardiac involvement is suspected, cardiac MRI is recommended.

▶ TREATMENT

- Oriented toward a goal of remission of symptoms or preventing organ or life-threatening disease
- Patients without symptoms or evidence of organ-threatening disease should be routinely monitored for progression.
- Systemic corticosteroids are the mainstay of treatment and may be used long-term balancing the risk of adverse effects and relapse of symptoms. In some cases of single organ, isolated symptoms, such as skin lesions or cough, topical steroids can be used.
- Other immunosuppressant medications like methotrexate or azathioprine can be used in those intolerant of steroid therapy or with refractory disease.

CHAPTER 331

Pneumoconiosis

Marie Pittman, DMSc, MPAS, PA-C, RDH

▶ GENERAL FEATURES

- Pneumoconiosis is group of fibrotic occupational pulmonary diseases characterized by lung damage caused by the inhalation of dust particles and inorganic substances.
- Acutely, can result in transient hypersensitivity pneumonitis. With chronic irritation, the damage becomes permanent.
- Pneumoconiosis is subdivided into four categories based on lesion findings:
  - Fibrogenic (ie, silica, coal, talc, asbestos)
  - Benign or inert (ie, iron, tin barium)
  - Granulomatous (ie, beryllium)
  - Giant cell associated with hard metal inhalation (ie, cobalt)
- Pneumoconiosis conditions are differentiated by the cause of the disease. They include:
  - Silicosis: associated with inhalation of silica (ie, quartz, sandstone, granite). Most widespread pneumoconiosis is in the United States. At-risk occupations include mining, quarrying, drilling, and sandblasting. Increases risk for tuberculosis (TB).

- Asbestosis: occurs from naturally occurring fibrous magnesium silicate usually found in insulation material. Commonly manifests as pleural disease. Findings include ferruginous bodies within the lung parenchyma. Asbestos increases the risk for bronchogenic carcinoma. Exposure may occur from mining/milling, construction and insulation work, or indirect exposure through airborne particles in the home or workplace. Malignant mesothelioma is also strongly linked to asbestos exposure.
  - Coal worker's pneumoconiosis: occurs due to the deposition of coal dust particles (including silica) in the lungs; coal miners are at the highest risk.
  - Berylliosis: also known as chronic beryllium disease (CBD). Clinically resembles sarcoidosis. At-risk populations include those living near beryllium manufacturing plants and/or working in dental, computer, nuclear, and aerospace industries.
  - Talcosis: exposure to crystalline hydrous magnesium silicate in occupations such as ceramics, paper, plastics, rubber, paint, and cosmetics

- Vineyard sprayer's lung disease: occupational exposure to "Bordeaux mixture" that contains calcium hydroxide
- Hard metal pneumoconiosis: exposure to dust produced from substances such as cobalt. At-risk occupations include jewelers.
- Silo-filler's lung: a non–dust-related occupational disease. The disease is seen in those inhaling silo gas, which is linked to NO_2 inhalation.
- Byssinosis: resultant from long-term inhalation of dust related to farming. Most commonly associated with raw cotton, flax, hemp, and, possibly, sisal. Typically presents as acute or subacute disease.
- Bagassosis: occurs in workers with inhaled fibrous material from sugarcane processing
- Smoking increases risk for severe lung disease.

▶ CLINICAL ASSESSMENT

- History may contain clues to occupational or other exposure.
- The severity of pneumoconiosis spans from asymptomatic disease with incidental findings to symptomatic and life-limiting disease.
- Patients typically present with progressive dyspnea.
- Examination may be notable for inspiratory crackles, cyanosis, and/or clubbing of fingers.

▶ DIAGNOSIS

- The patient must show four criteria to diagnose pneumoconiosis:
  - Documented exposure
  - Defined latent period
  - Recognized features of the disease
  - Exclusion of other more common diseases
- Diagnosis typically made with history, physical examination, and imaging.
- Typical findings in common pneumoconioses:
  - Coal worker's pneumoconiosis: coal macules form, mostly in the upper lung fields. Lungs take on the color of the coal. As fibrosis progresses, CXR findings change from initial millimeter sized nodules to large fibrotic lesions.
  - Silicosis: small round opacities/nodules throughout the lungs, "eggshell" calcifications
  - Asbestosis: linear streaking at lung bases and in the pleural lining. Pleural plaques are common. Evidence of malignant mesothelioma is strongly associated with asbestos exposure.
- Pulmonary function tests will typically show decreased diffusing capacity for carbon monoxide (DLCO) and, in later disease, a restrictive and/or obstructive lung disease pattern.
- Biopsy can be used to confirm diagnosis.
  - Asbestosis will show ferruginous bodies on histopathology.

▶ TREATMENT

- Prevention is key: education for workers, masks and other forms of occupational protective equipment
- Avoid additional exposure to prevent further damage.
- Treatment is mostly supportive as disease process is irreversible.
  - Steroids show mixed benefit.
  - Bronchodilators may with obstruction/airflow limitation.
  - Keep vaccinations up to date.
  - Supplemental oxygen if needed.
- Lung transplantation is an option for some patients.

Section A Pretest: Breast Disorders

1. A 60-year-old Caucasian female is diagnosed with left breast mastitis. You treat her with antibiotics, and though her condition has not worsened, it has not improved. What type of carcinoma should you be concerned about?

   A. Invasive ductal carcinoma (IDC)
   B. Inflammatory breast cancer
   C. Ductal carcinoma in situ (DCIS)
   D. Lobular carcinoma in situ (LCIS)

2. Which of the following is the first-line treatment for fibrocystic breast changes?

   A. Cooper's ligament support
   B. Diclofenac topical anti-inflammatory gel
   C. Excision of the tissue
   D. Needle aspiration of cystic fluid

3. A 27-year-old female, G1P1, 3 weeks postpartum, has been diagnosed with left breast mastitis. Which antibiotic should NOT be prescribed for this patient, based on her history?

   A. Flucloxacillin
   B. Amoxicillin-clavulanate
   C. Trimethoprim-sulfamethoxazole
   D. Erythromycin

4. A 47-year-old female is diagnosed with HER-2–positive, estrogen receptor–negative breast cancer. Which of the following should be done at baseline and sequentially?

   A. Pelvic ultrasound (U/S)
   B. Dual-energy x-ray absorptiometry (DEXA) scan
   C. Echocardiography
   D. Pelvic MRI

5. You are seeing a new patient today in the office whom you have diagnosed with left breast mastitis, and she is currently breastfeeding her 3-week-old infant. What lab should be drawn on this patient to aid in diagnosis?

   A. No labs are needed
   B. CBC
   C. BMP
   D. CRP

6. Which of the following immunohistologic subtypes of breast occurs more often in premenopausal African American women?

   A. Estrogen receptor positive, HER-2 negative
   B. Estrogen receptor positive, HER-2 positive
   C. Estrogen receptor negative, HER-2 positive
   D. Estrogen receptor negative, HER-2 negative

7. A patient breastfeeding her 3-week-old infant was just diagnosed with a left breast abscess as confirmed by ultrasonography. Breast aspiration of this abscess was performed, and she is now taking antibiotics as prescribed. What other information is important to review with this patient?

   A. Immediately stop breastfeeding and begin formula feeds via a bottle.
   B. Immediately stop breastfeeding but continue to pump and dump breast milk.
   C. Continue to breastfeed but only via the unaffected breast.
   D. Continue to breastfeed, as usual, if tolerable.

8. Which of the following breast masses are not under hormonal influences?

   A. Breast cyst
   B. Fat necrosis
   C. Fibroadenoma
   D. Galactocele

9. A 52-year-old female presents with a chief complaint of a right breast mass she felt while taking a shower 2 months ago. She states it is not painful and was hoping it would go away with her next menses. Her past medical history (PMH) is noncontributory, and her family history (FH) is significant for one maternal aunt with postmenopausal breast cancer. Upon physical examination, there is a 2-cm mobile, firm mass along the upper outer quadrant of the right breast. There is no nipple discharge, inversion, or induration. No axillary lymphadenopathy is palpated. A diagnostic mammogram is ordered, and the results indicate a spiculated mass; the breast U/S reveals posterior acoustic shadowing with irregular borders of the mass. Which of the following is the most likely diagnosis?

   A. DCIS
   B. LCIS
   C. Infiltrating ductal carcinoma
   D. Fibroadenoma

10. Which of the following is the most common presentation of a fibroadenoma?

A. Painful solitary, unilateral mass noted in the upper outer breast quadrant

B. Painless diffuse, rope-like tissue found unilaterally near the areola

C. Painless well-defined, mobile mass noted in the upper outer breast quadrant

D. Painful bilateral, breast mass most commonly found in the upper outer breast quadrant

Section B Pretest: Gynecologic Disorders

1. A 28-year-old woman presents to the office complaining that her menstrual cycle is late. She has not had a menstrual period for 3 months and is concerned she may be pregnant, although she takes oral contraceptives, and a urine pregnancy test was negative. Her cycle is usually every 30 days and has been so since she was 14. She states that she started a new job 6 months ago and has been working 14- to 16-hour days. Her appetite is normal, but she gets 6 hours of sleep each night. She denies any fatigue, weight gain, hot flashes, insomnia, and polydipsia. She takes no medications other than the oral contraceptives. What other factor might be contributing to her late menstrual cycle?

A. Stress

B. Inadequate caloric intake

C. Menopause

D. Hypothyroidism

2. A 28-year-old G0 presents with a chief complaint of abnormal bleeding. Upon further questioning, she states the bleeding occurs primarily after intercourse. On physical examination, the physician assistant (PA) visualizes a friable pedunculated lesion protruding from the cervical os. Which of the following is the most likely diagnosis?

A. Uterine fibroid

B. Cervical cancer

C. Endocervical polyp

D. Cervical condyloma

3. Which of the following is the first step in the clinical management of amenorrhea?

A. Order an abdominal MRI

B. Order serum β-hCG

C. Order a progesterone challenge test

D. Order serum estradiol and progesterone testing

4. A 23-year-old, sexually active G0 female patient presents to your office for a routine well visit. Which of the following recommendations do you make based on US Preventive Services Task Force (USPSTF) recommendations for cervical cancer screening?

A. Pap smear is not indicated in her age group.

B. Pap smear is indicated only if she is sexually active.

C. Pap smear with HPV co-testing is indicated every 3 years.

D. Pap smear alone is indicated every 3 years until she turns 30.

5. Which of the following is the most common cause of secondary amenorrhea?

A. Asherman syndrome

B. Primary hypothyroidism

C. Pregnancy

D. Opioid use

6. A 32-year-old G1P1 female with a history of cigarette smoking is diagnosed with early-stage squamous cell carcinoma of the cervix. Which of the following is true regarding her diagnosis?

A. Tobacco use is a risk factor for cervical squamous cell carcinoma.

B. She will not be able to have more children because an oophorectomy is required.

C. Her cancer could have been prevented if she had used condoms consistently.

D. She will not be able to have more children after surgical conization or radical trachelectomy.

7. A 49-year-old G4P4 presents with heavy menstrual bleeding on and off for several years. She states she had used combination oral contraception until she was 45 years and then stopped it due to concerns

about breast cancer. She states the bleeding seems to be getting worse with each menstrual cycle and now is having some dyspareunia. Her last Pap test was 1 year ago and normal. Upon physical examination, the uterus is found to be enlarged at ~12 weeks, and a urine pregnancy test is negative. Which of the following is the next best step in evaluating this patient?

A. Perform an endometrial biopsy.
B. Perform a Pap test.
C. Order a pelvic MRI.
D. Order a pelvic U/S.

8. A 40-year-old G3P2A1 female reports vaginal spotting after sex for the past 3 months. She has no history of sexually transmitted infections (STIs) and is in a monogamous relationship. She does not use contraception. Her last cervical Pap smear was normal ~1 year ago. On speculum examination, you observe a small, friable cervical lesion at the three o'clock position. What is the most appropriate next step?

A. Obtain a cervical Pap smear and HPV testing
B. Obtain a cervical Pap smear, HPV testing, and cervical cultures for gonorrhea and chlamydia
C. Obtain a biopsy of the cervical lesion
D. Follow the American Society for Colposcopy and Cervical Pathology (ASCCP) guidelines for cervical cancer screening and defer her Pap smear at this time

9. Which of the following is a common female cause of infertility?

A. Abnormal spermatogenesis
B. Varicocele
C. Sperm transport disorder
D. Endometriosis

10. Your patient's screening Pap smear reveals a low-grade squamous intraepithelial lesion (LSIL). High-risk HPV co-testing returns positive. You ask the patient to return to the office for a cervical colposcopy. When counseling your patient about her Pap smear results, which of the following do you tell her?

A. LSIL on Pap smear is a normal finding, and colposcopy is being recommended just for precautions.
B. LSIL on Pap smear usually correlates with mild dysplasia (CIN1) on histology.
C. LSIL on Pap smear usually correlates with moderate (CIN2) or severe (CIN3) dysplasia on histology.
D. LSIL on Pap smear is a concerning finding with high likelihood of progression to cervical squamous cell carcinoma.

11. Which of the following is the most common cause of primary amenorrhea?

A. Turner syndrome
B. Testicular feminization
C. Kallman syndrome
D. Pituitary tumor

12. You are seeing a 60-year-old patient who has a history of squamous cell carcinoma of the cervix at age 38. She has a surgical history of radical hysterectomy with bilateral salpingectomy and upper vaginectomy. She reports painful intercourse that has worsened since she experienced menopause. She denies vaginal bleeding or discharge. Her last examination and vaginal Pap smear were normal 1 year ago. Which of the following is the best next step?

A. Recommend that she return to her oncologist as soon as possible for an examination
B. Advise her that sexual dysfunction is common after cervical cancer, and she should use vaginal lubricants
C. Perform a pelvic examination and vaginal Pap smear
D. Discuss that this cannot be related to her cancer, because cervical cancer treatment has no long-term side effects

13. What is the most likely cause of ovarian torsion?

A. Low-dose estrogen-containing pills
B. Ectopic pregnancy
C. Uterine mass
D. Ovarian mass

14. A 46-year-old G3P3 presents with a chief complaint of heavy menstrual bleeding for about 6 months. She states she is also having occasional hot flushes. Her FH is significant for a maternal aunt with colon cancer and maternal grandmother with uterine cancer. Which of the following should be ruled out?

A. Hereditary breast and ovarian cancer (HBOC)
B. Lynch syndrome
C. Li-Fraumeni syndrome
D. Multiple endocrine neoplasia

15. Which is NOT a risk factor for vaginal prolapse?

A. Nulliparity
B. Obesity
C. Chronic cough
D. Maternal history of prolapse

16. A 16-year-old Caucasian G0 is brought to the office by her mother with complaints of heavy menstrual bleeding since menarche at age 14. The patient states she bleeds about every 28 days, but the bleeding lasts

up to 10 days, and she has to use tampons and pads or she will bleed through her clothes. She denies any history of pelvic or abdominal trauma. A urine pregnancy test is negative, and a CBC is pending. Which of the following tests would be most appropriate in the initial workup of this patient?

A. Hemoglobin electrophoresis
B. vWF antigen
C. D-Dimer
D. Liver enzymes

17. Which of these requires urgent management?

A. Prolapse that can be reduced but falls back down
B. Keratinization of the prolapsed vaginal epithelium
C. Stress urinary incontinence that the patient believes is due to the prolapse
D. Inability to reduce the prolapse into the vagina, causing pain

18. A 52-year-old G2P2 presents with heavy menstrual bleeding. She states her menses are now lasting 7-10 days but are still occurring monthly. PMH is significant for estrogen receptor–positive breast cancer for which she takes tamoxifen. Which of the following is the next best step in managing this patient?

A. Perform an endometrial biopsy.
B. Order an MRI.
C. Prescribe tranexamic acid.
D. Insert a progestin-secreting intrauterine device (IUD).

19. A 66-year-old postmenopausal female presents with two episodes of vaginal bleeding after exercising at her gym. Which of the following is the most appropriate recommendation?

A. She should avoid strenuous exercise for 2 weeks and the bleeding will resolve.
B. She should be evaluated for endometrial cancer with an MRI of the pelvis.
C. The bleeding is likely due to vaginal atrophy, and she should be prescribed vaginal estrogen cream.
D. She should be evaluated for endometrial cancer with endometrial sampling.

20. What is the term for cervical motion tenderness associated with pelvic inflammatory disease (PID)?

A. "Caviar sign"
B. "Chandelier sign"
C. "Coffee sign"
D. "Cradle sign"

21. You are counseling a 52-year-old patient who was diagnosed with endometrioid-type endometrial cancer after a dilation and curettage was performed for irregular menstrual bleeding. She is a good surgical candidate and has no significant comorbidities. You tell her that all of the following will be removed during surgery, except which of the following?

A. Cervix and uterus
B. Ovaries and fallopian tubes
C. Lower vagina and vulva
D. Pelvic and para-aortic lymph nodes

22. Which of the following is a risk factor for PID?

A. IUD insertion 5 months ago
B. Age 40 years
C. Prior history of PID
D. Monogamy

23. You are seeing a patient for her gynecologic well visit. She recently heard about a family friend who was diagnosed with uterine cancer, and after learning that it is the most common gynecologic cancer, she is now afraid that she might also be at risk. You review the risk factors and protective factors with her. Which of the following is a protective factor for uterine cancer?

A. Use of a levonorgestrel-containing IUD
B. Nulliparity
C. Endometrial hyperplasia
D. Lynch syndrome mutations

24. Which of the following is the best treatment for a premenopausal woman with ovarian torsion without an ovarian mass?

A. Detorsion and conservation
B. Salpingo-oophorectomy
C. Observation
D. Unilateral tubal ligation

25. Which of the following is a possible treatment modality for uterine cancer?

A. Surgery
B. Pelvic radiation therapy
C. Chemotherapy
D. All of the above

26. Which of the following histologic types of uterine cancer is relatively uncommon and is associated with a poor prognosis?

A. Uterine sarcoma
B. Squamous carcinoma
C. Endometrioid adenocarcinoma
D. Epithelial tumors

27. A 62-year-old postmenopausal presents to the ED with right-sided pelvic pain. A transvaginal (TVUS) and transabdominal U/S was performed. There was decreased color flow on the transabdominal Doppler when evaluating the right ovary. A 5-cm solid mass was noted on the ovary. What would be the next step in management?

A. Detorsion and conservation
B. Salpingo-oophorectomy
C. Observation
D. Unilateral tubal ligation

28. For a female patient younger than 35 years, infertility is the failure to conceive after how many months?

    A. 9
    B. 12
    C. 15
    D. 18

29. Which of the following is accurate advice for a patient that states she forgot to take her combined hormonal contraception (CHC) pill for 2 days?

    A. Avoid sexual intercourse for 2 weeks.
    B. Start a new pill pack.
    C. Take two pills today, two pills tomorrow, and continue with the remaining pills at the usual time and use a condom for the next week.
    D. Take all the missed pills immediately and continue taking the remaining pills at the usual time.

30. What is the most common presenting symptom of PID?

    A. Yellow, serous vaginal discharge
    B. Milky, white vaginal discharge
    C. Unilateral upper abdominal pain
    D. Bilateral lower abdominal pain

31. Which of the following organisms are mostly common associated with the development of pelvic inflammatory disease?

    A. *Chlamydia trachomatis, Neisseria gonorrheae, Gardnerella vaginalis*
    B. *Clostridium difficile, Acinetobacter baumannii, Pseudomonas aeruginosa*
    C. *Salmonella typhi, Mycobacterium tuberculosis, Candida auris*
    D. *Klebsiella pneumoniae, Clostridium sordelli, Corynebacterium bovis*

32. Beyond prevention of unplanned pregnancy, what other benefits may some contraception provide?

    A. Reduce symptoms of endometriosis
    B. Treatment of vasomotor symptoms in menopausal women
    C. Weight loss in overweight women
    D. Reduces stress incontinence

33. Which diagnostic test is highly sensitive and specific for pelvic inflammatory disease?

    A. nucleic acid amplification test (NAAT)
    B. hCG
    C. Pelvic U/S
    D. No single diagnostic test is highly sensitive and specific for PID

34. Which of the following medications could reduce the efficacy of combined hormonal contraception?

    A. Citalopram
    B. Lamotrigine
    C. Metformin
    D. Prednisone

35. Which of the following is a diagnostic test for the male partner in an initial infertility workup?

    A. Hysterosalpingogram
    B. Antral follicle count
    C. Anti-Müllerian hormone
    D. Semen analysis

36. Which of the following is NOT associated with irritant dermatitis?

    A. Scented soaps or gels
    B. Wet incontinence pads
    C. Routine bathing rather than showering
    D. Cleaning the genital area with hot water

37. Which of the following medications is commonly prescribed by primary care physicians to induce ovulation?

    A. Medroxyprogesterone
    B. Danazol
    C. Letrozole
    D. Drospirenone

38. Which of the following is NOT true of lichen sclerosis?

    A. It is contagious.
    B. It is a chronic, noncurable condition.
    C. It is treated with topical superpotent steroid ointment.
    D. It may lead to scarring of the vaginal introitus and vulvar cancer.

39. Which of the following is a component of fertility education and guidance?

    A. Increased use of lubricants
    B. Healthy diet and exercise
    C. Ejaculation multiple times daily
    D. Coitus daily for 7 days postovulation

40. A 17-year-old female, G0, presents to the clinic with bilateral pelvic pain and abnormal vaginal discharge for the past 2 weeks. Her last menstrual period (LMP) was 1 week ago, and her pregnancy test is negative. The patient states that she has exchanged sex for drugs with at least four partners in the past 6 months. She has noticed symptoms for the past 2-3 weeks. What is the most likely diagnosis?

    A. Pregnancy
    B. Chlamydia cervicitis
    C. Urinary tract infection
    D. Cervical cancer

41. Which of the following women should be offered a cervicitis test of cure 4 weeks after treatment?

    A. Women who have symptoms that persist after treatment
    B. All women under the age of 25 whose symptoms resolve after treatment
    C. Pregnant women
    D. Both A and C

42. A 24-year-old female, G2P1, presents to the office stating that she has been having postcoital bleeding for the past 2 months. Her LMP was normal 2 weeks ago. She states that she has a new sexual partner who she has been with for 3 months. She uses oral contraceptives and denies missing or mistaking them. What test would most likely confirm your diagnosis?

    A. Cervical swab for gonorrhea and chlamydia
    B. Pregnancy test
    C. Blood test for syphilis and HIV
    D. All of the above

43. Which of the following is a cystocele?

    A. Prolapse of the apical vagina
    B. Prolapse of the bladder against the anterior vaginal wall
    C. Prolapse of the uterus into the vaginal cavity
    D. Prolapse of the small intestines against the posterior vaginal wall

44. A 21-year-old female presents to the ED with a 1-week history of low-grade fever (99 °F), bilateral pelvic pain, and a yellow vaginal discharge. On her gynecologic examination, you note a copious amount of cervical mucopurulent discharge and cervical motion tenderness. You order cervical swabs and diagnose her with pelvic inflammatory disease. The patient states that she has had multiple sexual partners in the past 3 months and diagnosis and treatment of chlamydia 6 months ago. What will your treatment plan consist of?

    A. Presume that the patient has both gonorrhea and chlamydia due to her high-risk sexual behavior and treat her for both infections as they commonly coexist.
    B. Treat this patient for chlamydia only because it is the most common cause of PID.
    C. Send the patient home and do not treat the patient with any medications until the cultures are received because you do not want to treat her unnecessarily.
    D. Admit the patient to the hospital and observe her symptoms.

45. Your 32-year-old female patient is considering trying to conceive in the next year and PMDD, but lifestyle interventions are not helping her mood. What option would you consider next?

    A. Fluoxetine
    B. Olanzapine
    C. Lithium
    D. Amitriptyline

Section C Pretest: Obstetrics

1. A 23-year-old woman presents with lower abdominal pain since the morning. She reports spotting but attributes this to the onset of her period. She describes the pain as worse than her usual menstrual cramps. Vital signs are stable. Which of the following is the initial step in her evaluation?

    A. Abdominal ultrasonography
    B. Pelvic examination
    C. Pregnancy test
    D. TVUS

2. What is the first-line pharmacologic treatment for gestational diabetes (GDM)?

    A. Metformin
    B. Glyburide
    C. NPH
    D. Asparte
    E. Empagliflozin

3. A patient is diagnosed with a tubal ectopic pregnancy. In which of the following circumstances would you offer medical management with methotrexate?

    A. Gestational sac size of 3.0 cm
    B. Patient is breastfeeding her first child
    C. Presence of cardiac activity
    D. Serum β-hCG of 25 000 IU/L

4. When should women deliver if she has diet-controlled GDM?

    A. 36 weeks
    B. 37 weeks
    C. 38 weeks
    D. 39 weeks
    E. 40 weeks

5. A patient who is Rh(D) negative has an ectopic pregnancy. Because of potential for fetomaternal bleeding and the patient's Rh(D) negative status, which of the following might be indicated to prevent RhD alloimmunization?

A. Methotrexate
B. Progesterone
C. Rho(D) immunoglobulin
D. Estrogen

6. Which of the following tests should be avoided in the diagnosis and monitoring of GDM?

A. Plasma fasting glucose
B. 1-hour postprandial glucose
C. 2-hour postprandial glucose
D. Hemoglobin A1c

7. A 23-year-old woman presents with lower abdominal pain since the morning. She reports spotting but attributes this to the onset of her period. She describes the pain as worse than her usual menstrual cramps and just before arrival experienced a syncopal episode. Her blood pressure (BP) is 90/60 mm Hg, pulse is 125/min. Physical examination reveals LLQ tenderness with guarding. TVUS reveals no intrauterine pregnancy and a left adnexal mass with free fluid in the cul-de-sac. Which of the following is indicated now?

A. Methotrexate
B. Expectant management
C. Laparoscopy
D. Await serial β-hCG results

8. How often should a woman with history of GDM be screened for type 2 diabetes after delivery?

A. Recheck for GDM every 1-3 years if the 4- to 12-week postpartum test is normal.
B. Recheck for GDM every 5 years if the 4- to 12-week postpartum test is normal.
C. Recheck every 3 months for the first 5 years after delivery if postpartum test is normal.
D. Recheck every 3 months for the first 1 year after delivery if postpartum test is normal.

9. A 32-year-old female, G0P0, presents with complaints of persistent nausea and vomiting for 1 week and cannot tolerate liquids. She appears dehydrated on examination and is actively vomiting. Her LMP was 6 weeks ago, and she reports vaginal spotting that began today. Her β-hCG is 125 000 mIU/mL. What should you do next?

A. After termination, advise to wait 2 months before attempting to get pregnant again.
B. Evacuate the uterus.
C. Get an U/S.
D. Treat the vomiting with antiemetics and IV fluids and discharge once symptoms resolved.

10. Which of the following is the most common site of ectopic pregnancy?

A. Abdominal wall
B. Fallopian tube
C. Ovary
D. Cervix

11. A 40-year-old female has just finished 6-month surveillance of hCG after a partial molar pregnancy. The hCG has been zero for 4 months. The patient would like to attempt to get pregnant again, but she is worried about increased risks in the future pregnancy. How should you counsel your patient?

A. She should be advised to avoid pregnancy.
B. The pregnancy will have similar complications as the general population.
C. There is a significant increase in risk of a molar pregnancy.
D. There is an increased risk of gestational trophoblastic neoplasia (GTN).

12. Which of the following is the most appropriate intervention in a patient at 36 weeks' gestation who presents with a BP of 162/110 mm Hg?

A. Begin antihypertensive therapy with IV labetalol or hydralazine.
B. Recheck BP in 4 hours.
C. Begin 81 mg of aspirin daily.
D. Institute diet and lifestyle modifications.

13. Which of the following is a risk factor for the development of placenta previa?

A. Singleton pregnancy
B. Decreased maternal age
C. Previous cesarean delivery
D. Female fetus

14. Which of the following best describes when delivery is indicated in a patient with preeclampsia without severe features and BP of <160/110 mm Hg?

A. When the patient reaches 36 weeks 0 days
B. At 37 weeks 0 days unless the patient develops complications
C. When the patient is not adherent with antihypertensive medication
D. If the fetal weight is below the 10th percentile

15. Which of the following physical examination components is contraindicated before obtaining a pelvic U/S in a pregnant patient who presents with vaginal bleeding?

A. Fetal heart tones
B. Fundal height
C. Dilation and effacement
D. Urinalysis

16. Which of the following is a severe feature of preeclampsia?

    A. Urine protein dipstick of 2+
    B. BP > 140/90 mm Hg on two separate occasions
    C. A 24-hour urine protein of 310 mg
    D. Doubling of hepatic transaminases

17. Which of the following is a finding in magnesium toxicity?

    A. Dilated pupils
    B. Tachypnea
    C. Hyporeflexia
    D. Hyperreflexia

18. A patient presents at 34w6d with a BP of 162/112 mm Hg and thrombocytopenia. Which of the following is the best course of action?

    A. Initiate biweekly nonstress tests and oral labetalol.
    B. Administer labetalol, a course of corticosteroids, and plan for delivery.
    C. Begin oral nifedipine and recheck BP in 24-48 hours.
    D. Begin oral labetalol and plan on delivering at 37 weeks' gestation.

19. Separation of the placenta from the uterine wall is associated with the development of which condition?

    A. Acute disseminated intravascular coagulation (DIC)
    B. Placenta previa
    C. Cervical insufficiency
    D. Anemia polycythemia sequence

20. Within a few hours after delivery, where should the fundus of the uterus be located?

    A. In the prepregnancy location in the pelvis
    B. About a finger's breadth below the pregnant uterus measurement
    C. At the level of the umbilicus
    D. Depends on the size of the fetus delivered

21. Which of the following activities is contraindicated for a patient with known placenta previa after 20 weeks' gestation?

    A. Walking 20 minutes per day
    B. Lying on the left side while sleeping
    C. Driving a car
    D. Vaginal intercourse

22. Which of the following symptoms would a patient report during the first trimester of pregnancy?

    A. Excessive fetal movement
    B. Nausea/vomiting
    C. Regular uterine contractions
    D. Increased energy

23. Which of the following is associated with an increased risk of developing placental abruption?

    A. Folic acid supplementation
    B. Motor vehicle accident
    C. Walking 30 minutes per day
    D. Maternal hypotension

24. How is a patient determined to be in labor?

    A. Rupture of membranes with or without regular uterine contractions
    B. Fetal distress with contractions
    C. Regular contractions with vaginal bleeding
    D. Regular uterine contractions and progressive cervical dilation

25. Which of the following physical examination techniques should be used to estimate fetal weight and position before delivery?

    A. McDonald's method
    B. Speculum examination
    C. Bishop score
    D. Leopold's maneuvers

26. Which diagnostic test is confirmatory for multiple gestation?

    A. Quantitative human chorionic gonadotropin (β-hCG)
    B. Alpha fetoprotein (AFP)
    C. Doppler fetal heart tones
    D. Obstetric U/S

27. Routine screening for which of the following is necessary during prenatal care?

    A. Diabetes
    B. Group B *Streptococcus* (GBS)
    C. Blood type and Rh with antibody screen
    D. All of the above

28. Which of the following symptoms is common in a multiple gestation pregnancy?

    A. Decreased severity of morning sickness
    B. Late fetal movement
    C. Weight loss
    D. Increased fatigue

29. A 41-year-old G2P0 spontaneous abortion x one presents for her initial prenatal visit at 11 weeks' gestation. She is found to be Rh negative, and her antibody screen is positive. Which of the following is the best choice for next steps?

    A. Perform an U/S to check for evidence of fetal hydrops.
    B. Refer to maternal-fetal medicine.
    C. Administer anti-D immunoglobulin and recheck at 28 weeks.
    D. Nothing needs to be done at this point.

30. Which of the following is a risk factor for multiple gestation?

    A. Primigravida
    B. Advanced maternal age
    C. Conception without the use of infertility treatments
    D. Low maternal weight

31. Which of the following statements is most true about Rh incompatibility in pregnancy?

    A. Most cases of Rh incompatibility are caused by the presence of D antigens.
    B. Most cases of Rh incompatibility are caused by the presence of D antibodies.
    C. The most common Rh antigen in humans is C.
    D. The most common Rh antigen in humans is E.

32. Which of the following is a component of prenatal anticipatory guidance for multiple gestation?

    A. Less weight gain is recommended than with a singleton pregnancy.
    B. No additional folic acid supplementation is recommended.
    C. Delivery should be scheduled before 40 weeks' gestation.
    D. No additional daily caloric intake is recommended.

33. The process by which the body forms antibodies to Rh (D) is called?

    A. Alloimmunization
    B. Heteroimmunization
    C. Autoimmunization
    D. Contraimmunization

34. Diagnosis of cervical insufficiency is made by which of the following?

    A. Uterine tocodynamometry
    B. pH examination of vaginal secretions
    C. Based on a history of previous preterm delivery
    D. U/S measurements of cervical length and width

35. Which physical examination finding is consistent with multiple gestation?

    A. Decreased maternal heart rate
    B. Uterine size large for gestational age
    C. Lower than expected weight gain
    D. Decreased maternal BP

36. A patient who is Rh negative and antibody screen negative delivers an Rh-positive baby via normal spontaneous vaginal delivery. Which of the following statements describes the next best step?

    A. Administer anti-D immunoglobulin at her 6-week postpartum visit.
    B. Recheck her antibody screen at her 6-week postpartum visit.
    C. Administer anti-D immunoglobulin within 72 hours postpartum.
    D. Check the baby's antibody screen and administer anti-D immunoglobulin if negative.

37. Which of the following is a risk factor for cervical insufficiency?

    A. Uterine contractions
    B. History of mechanical dilation
    C. Use of vaginal progesterone
    D. Vaginal bleeding

38. The most common presentation of cervical insufficiency is which of the following?

    A. Vaginal bleeding
    B. Uterine contractions
    C. Asymptomatic cervical dilation
    D. Rupture of membranes

39. Which of the following is a pathognomonic finding for rupture of membranes?

    A. Nitrazine paper turns blue
    B. Ferning
    C. Positive fetal fibronectin
    D. Cervical dilation

40. Which of the following is NOT a complication of shoulder dystocia?

    A. Clavicular fracture
    B. Hypoxic ischemic encephalopathy
    C. Erb palsy
    D. Klumpke palsy
    E. Nuchal cord

41. Which of the following is an appropriate intervention for a stable patient with confirmed preterm prelabor rupture of membranes at 32w4d?

    A. Administration of magnesium sulfate for neuroprotection
    B. Immediate induction of labor with prostaglandins
    C. Administration of amoxicillin-clavulanic acid for prophylaxis
    D. One course of corticosteroid injections for fetal lung maturity

42. Which of the following is NOT a common risk factor for shoulder dystocia?

    A. Fetal macrosomia
    B. Previous shoulder dystocia
    C. Premature delivery
    D. GDM
    E. Prolonged pregnancy

43. A patient at 30w2d gestation with no known medical allergies who has confirmed rupture of membranes should be given which of the following antibiotics for prophylaxis?
    A. Ciprofloxacin
    B. Ceftriaxone
    C. Ampicillin
    D. Gentamycin

44. Which of the following should be initiated in all patients who present with prelabor rupture of membranes after 24 weeks' gestation?
    A. Screening for GBS and prophylactic treatment when appropriate
    B. Prophylactic treatment of HSV with acyclovir
    C. Magnesium sulfate for fetal neuroprotection
    D. A single course of corticosteroids for fetal lung maturity

▶ ANSWERS AND EXPLANATIONS TO SECTION A PRETEST

1. **B.** Inflammatory breast cancer presents similarly to that of a breast infection, with an acute onset of symptoms such as edema, erythema, and peau d'orange. If you suspect and treat for an infection with no improvement, inflammatory breast cancer should be worked up.

2. **A.** 85% of women with fibrocystic breast changes will improve with a better fitting bra and more support for the breast tissue. Reassurance after benign imaging can sometimes be the only treatment needed for women as well.

3. **C.** Trimethoprim-sulfamethoxazole should not be prescribed for women who are breastfeeding children under the age of 4 weeks. In addition, this is a pregnancy category C medication, where all others listed are pregnancy category B.

4. **C.** HER-2–targeted therapies are associated with left ventricular ejection fraction decline and heart failure. Current guidelines recommend testing at baseline and sequentially. It may be appropriate to assess bone density in a postmenopausal patient, but current guidelines do not recommend a baseline and sequential DEXA for HER-2–positive breast cancer patients. A pelvic U/S and MRI may be appropriate if a pelvic mass was palpated or if the patient was experiencing abnormal uterine bleeding.

5. **A.** There is no routine lab required for mastitis as it is typically a clinical diagnosis.

6. **D.** Estrogen receptor–negative, HER-2–negative, also called triple-negative or basal, breast cancer is more common in premenopausal African American women.

7. **D.** Continue to breastfeed as usual to prevent milk stasis, which can harbor bacteria.

8. **B.** Breast cysts and fibroadenomas are both thought to occur due to fluctuations in estrogen and progesterone hormone levels, whereas galactoceles occur during lactation when there is significant prolactin influence. Fat necrosis is a benign condition that occurs commonly as a result of breast trauma and not hormonal changes.

9. **C.** IDC is the most common invasive breast cancer and typically presents as a palpable breast mass with spiculation and irregular borders on radiographic imaging. DCIS and LCIS do not present as a palpable breast mass, but evidence of DCIS or LCIS can be seen in women with IDC. Fibroadenomas are benign masses that have smooth, round edges on imaging.

10. **C.** Simple fibroadenomas are typically painless, well-defined, solitary lesions that are mobile under the skin. They have been termed "breast mouse" because of the ease with which they move under the skin. The most common location for a fibroadenoma, like fibrocystic breast changes, is the upper outer breast quadrant.

▶ ANSWERS AND EXPLANATIONS TO SECTION B PRETEST

1. **A.** Functional hypothalamic GnRH deficiency can be caused by emotional stress among other causes. This patient states that her appetite is normal, and she does not have symptoms of hypothyroidism, such as weight gain and fatigue. She does not have symptoms of menopause.

2. **C.** Endocervical polyps are benign growths that typically appear as pedunculated lesions arising from the endocervical canal and protruding through the cervical os. They are easily removed via cervical polypectomy. Uterine fibroids will rarely protrude through the cervical os. Cervical cancer can present with postcoital bleeding but will typically not present as a solitary pedunculated lesion protruding from the os. Cervical condyloma will appear as raised, cauliflower-like flesh-colored lesions and is often only visualized via colposcopy.

3. **B.** All women with amenorrhea should have serum hCG measured.

4. **D.** USPSTF Guidelines for Cervical Cancer Screening include cervical cytology alone every 3 years in women between the ages of 21 and 29 years. HPV co-testing may be added starting at age 30.

5. **C.** Pregnancy is the most common cause of secondary amenorrhea.

6. **A.** Tobacco use is a risk factor for squamous cell carcinoma of the cervix. Additional risk factors include

early sexual activity, multiple sexual partners, and the HPV virus. Condoms are ~70% effective at preventing HPV transmission. Oophorectomy is recommended for women with adenocarcinoma, as the ovaries are a site of possible metastatic disease in cervical adenocarcinoma only. Women who undergo fertility-sparing treatment for early-stage cervical cancer have an increased risk of pregnancy complications, including preterm birth. However, surgical conization and radical trachelectomy are options for fertility preservation in patients with cervical cancer.

7. **D.** Order a pelvic U/S. An endometrial biopsy is indicated to rule out endometrial hyperplasia or malignancy, but it is advised to obtain an U/S to rule out anatomic pathologies such as leiomyoma, polyps, and adenomyosis first, although an U/S-guided saline infusion followed by biopsy would be appropriate as well. This patient had a normal Pap 1 year ago so does not need another Pap until 3-5 years after her last one, depending on if she had co-testing. An MRI can detect pelvic pathology but is more expensive and is not the preferred initial imaging modality.

8. **C.** Although usually asymptomatic, patients with invasive cervical cancer may present with postcoital bleeding. Women with a visible cervical lesion on speculum examination should undergo biopsy for further evaluation.

9. **D.** Common causes of female infertility include ovulatory disorders, endometriosis, abnormalities of the Fallopian tubes, and uterine adhesions.

10. **B.** Abnormal results of a Papanicolaou test can include ASCUS, LSIL, HSIL, or atypical glandular cells. LSIL usually correlates with mild dysplasia on histology, whereas HSIL usually correlates with moderate or severe dysplasia.

11. **A.** Gonadal dysgenesis, including Turner syndrome, accounts for ~43% of primary amenorrhea cases.

12. **C.** Long-term cervical cancer survivors should have annual pelvic examinations and vaginal cytology to evaluate for disease recurrence. Dyspareunia in this case may be related to vaginal atrophy, vaginal stenosis, and/or vaginal shortening due to her surgical treatment for cervical cancer.

13. **D.** Ovarian mass is the most likely cause of ovarian torsion.

14. **B.** Lynch syndrome (also known as nonpolyposis hereditary colorectal cancer) is associated with various cancers due to genetic mutations. The most common malignancies include colorectal cancer, endometrial cancer, breast cancer, and other GI cancers.

15. **A.** History of pregnancy, obesity, chronic cough, and maternal history of prolapse are all risk factors for vaginal prolapse.

16. **B.** Von Willebrand disease can present in young women as heavy menstrual bleeding. The PMH should include questions about other bleeding episodes such as epistaxis or prolonged bleeding after dental procedures or minor lacerations. The PMH should include questions about other inheritable coagulopathies.

17. **D.** Urgent management is required if the prolapse cannot be reduced.

18. **A.** Perform an endometrial biopsy. Women who take tamoxifen who present with heavy menstrual bleeding should be ruled out for endometrial hyperplasia and cancer as tamoxifen acts as an agonist on the endometrium. Tranexamic acid would be appropriate in the management of a patient with heavy menstrual bleeding once malignancy has been ruled out.

19. **D.** All women who present with postmenopausal bleeding must be evaluated for endometrial cancer. The best way to evaluate postmenopausal bleeding is through tissue diagnosis, either with endometrial biopsy or with dilation and curettage.

20. **B.** Cervical motion tenderness (chandelier sign) and adnexal tenderness on bimanual examination are characteristic findings of PID.

21. **C.** Surgical intervention for endometrial cancer includes total hysterectomy, bilateral salpingo-oophorectomy, and pelvic and para-aortic lymph node dissection. The lower vagina and vulva are not affected. Additional treatment, including vaginal brachytherapy, external beam radiation therapy, or systemic chemotherapy, may be considered based on postoperative disease staging.

22. **C.** Risk factors include multiple sexual partners, age younger than 25 years, prior history of PID, and a sexual partner with an STI.

23. **A.** Factors that reduce risk of uterine cancer include combination oral contraceptives, levonorgestrel IUD, and physical activity. The highest risk factor for uterine cancer is exposure to unopposed estrogen. Families with Lynch syndrome mutations are also at increased risk of uterine cancer.

24. **A.** Detorsion and ovarian conservation is recommended for most premenopausal women. Ovarian cystectomy is preformed if a benign mass is present. Patients with an obviously necrotic ovary or a mass that is suspicious for malignancy require salpingo-oophorectomy. Observation is not indicated as ovarian conservation is less successful when the longer torsion is in place. Unilateral tubal ligation is not medically indicated.

25. **D.** Treatment options for uterine cancer depend on histology and staging and include surgery, vaginal brachytherapy, external beam pelvic radiation, chemotherapy, and endocrine therapy.

26. **A.** The mesenchymal tumors, including sarcomas, are rare and carry a worse prognosis than other types of uterine cancer. Endometrioid adenocarcinoma is the most common histologic type of uterine cancer and has a favorable prognosis.

27. **B.** Because this patient has ovarian torsion with a mass and is postmenopausal, the next step would be to remove the ovary for further pathological evaluation.

28. **B.** Infertility is the failure to conceive after 12 months of unprotected sexual intercourse. In female patients older than 35 years, infertility is the failure to conceive after 6 months of unprotected sexual intercourse.

29. **C.** A patient who misses two consecutive oral contraceptive pills can catch up by taking two pills a day for two days and should use backup birth control for 7 days. Full instructions for late or missed doses can be found at https://www.cdc.gov/reproductivehealth/unintendedpregnancy/pdf/248124_fig_2_3_4_final_tag508.pdf.

30. **D.** The most common presenting symptom of PID is bilateral lower abdominal pain lasting for 1-2 weeks.

31. **A.** The organisms most commonly associated with the development of PID are *C. trachomatis*, *N. gonorrheae*, and *G. vaginalis*.

32. **A.** Contraception can reduce symptoms of endometriosis. Some forms of contraception can result in weight gain, not weight loss. Vasomotor symptoms should be treated with hormone therapy, not oral contraceptives.

33. **D.** PID is generally diagnosed based on clinical presentation without additional diagnostic studies; no single diagnostic test is highly sensitive and specific for PID.

34. **B.** Reduced efficacy of combined hormonal contraception occurs with several anticonvulsants, including lamotrigine; consider an alternate method.

35. **D.** Initial diagnostic studies for the male partner include LH, FSH, total testosterone, and a semen analysis.

36. **C.** The act of bathing itself is not associated with development of irritant dermatitis. Use of scented bath products, such as shower gels or bubble bath, may be. These agents can also dry out the vulvar skin.

37. **C.** If anovulation is identified, letrozole or clomiphene is prescribed to induce ovulation.

38. **A.** The exact cause of lichen sclerosis is unknown. It is thought to be immune mediated and may have a genetic predisposition. It is not contagious between sexual partners.

39. **B.** Encourage lifestyle modifications, healthy diet, and exercise. Vaginal intercourse daily or every other day for 7 days before ovulation is recommended. Male partners should ejaculate no more than once daily to avoid sperm count depletion. Discourage the use of lubricants or intravaginal products.

40. **B.** The patient is at high risk for infectious cervicitis, most likely chlamydia, because of her young age and sexual history. Her symptoms are most likely due to infection. Her menstrual cycle is normal, and her pregnancy test is negative. Cervical cancer is unlikely, given her age and symptoms of bilateral pelvic pain.

Urinary tract infection is less likely due to abnormal vaginal discharge and postcoital bleeding complaints.

41. **C.** Pregnant patients should always have a follow-up test of cure. Patients who have been treated for cervicitis and complain of persistence or recurrence of symptoms should be offered a test of cure. Patients who report complete resolution of symptoms after treatment do not need a test of cure.

42. **B.** A cervical swab is the best method to diagnose this patient with infectious cervicitis based on her symptoms of postcoital bleeding and new sexual partner. A pregnancy test will less likely make the diagnosis because the patient is on oral contraception and reports normal menstrual cycles. Blood tests are not used to diagnose her infectious cervicitis but can be used to diagnose other sexually transmitted infections (STIs).

43. **B.** Cystocele is a prolapse of the bladder against the anterior vaginal wall. Vaginal vault prolapse is a prolapse of the apical vagina. Uterovaginal prolapse is prolapse of the uterus into the vaginal cavity. Enterocele is the prolapse of the small intestines against the posterior vaginal wall.

44. **A.** The patient most likely has pelvic inflammatory disease due to infectious cervicitis caused by chlamydia and/or gonorrhea and her history demonstrates high-risk sexual behavior; therefore, she should presumptively be treated for both based on her symptoms to prevent complications, including tubo-ovarian abscess. The patient may or may not be admitted to the hospital, but treatment should not be delayed.

45. **A.** SSRIs and SNRIs are best utilized for mood-predominant symptoms, and patients who are trying to conceive. Pharmacotherapy can be used if lifestyle interventions are not alleviating symptoms.

▶ ANSWERS AND EXPLANATIONS TO SECTION C PRETEST

1. **C.** Any woman of reproductive age presenting with abdominal pain and vaginal bleeding first needs a pregnancy test. Results provide valuable information for the remainder of the steps such as physical examination and U/S. Pelvic examination and TVUS, although useful in diagnosis, are not the initial step.

2. **C.** NPH is first line for treatment in GDM. Glyburide and metformin are both second line. Other oral medications are not recommended in the treatment of GDM and may lack safety for fetus.

3. **A.** A diameter of >3.5 cm, presence of cardiac activity on TVUS, and initial hCG concentrations of >5000 IU/L have lower success rates. Breastfeeding is an absolute contraindication to methotrexate.

4. **E.** If GDM is controlled with diet and there are no other complications, a woman may deliver at 40 weeks.

5. **C.** After an antepartum event such as an ectopic pregnancy when fetomaternal bleeding has been documented, the Rh(D)-negative patient may be a candidate for Rh(D) immunoglobulin.

6. **D.** A1c should not be used to monitor or diagnose GDM because of the rapid turnover of RBCs and changing hemodynamic needs associated with pregnancy.

7. **C.** This patient is presenting with signs and symptoms of a ruptured ectopic pregnancy with hemodynamic instability. Emergent laparoscopy is indicated. This then excludes the answers of methotrexate and expectant management. Serial hCGs can be done after laparoscopy but are not done emergently.

8. **A.** This screening should occur indefinitely as the risk of developing T2DM is up to 60% in the next 5-10 years.

9. **C.** Get an U/S. This patient is presenting with symptoms of hyperemesis gravidarum and an hCG level significantly higher than expected. You should consider the possibility of gestational trophoblastic disease (GTD). GTD may be confirmed with an U/S. You would not want to evacuate the uterus without an U/S confirming the possibility of GTD. And patients should not attempt to get pregnant for at least 6 months after evacuation.

10. **B.** The most common site of an ectopic is the fallopian tube with 80% in the ampullary segment.

11. **B.** After GTD, the risks for complications in pregnancy are similar to the general population, except for a slight increase in another molar pregnancy. There is no increased risk of malignant GTN in future pregnancies.

12. **A.** The patient has severe hypertension and must be managed expeditiously with IV labetalol or hydralazine. Oral nifedipine can be used if IV access cannot be obtained. Patients with one elevated BP <160/110 mm Hg should have another BP check at least 4 hours apart before a diagnosis can be made. Patients with chronic hypertension should begin aspirin therapy at 12 weeks' gestation.

13. **C.** Risk factors for the development of placenta previa include a previous history of placenta previa, previous C-section delivery, male fetus, and multiple gestation.

14. **B.** Delivery should occur at 37 weeks unless the patient develops complications. Delivery would be indicated sooner if complications develop, such as oligohydramnios, HELLP, placental abruption, and rupture of membranes.

15. **C.** Digital examination of the vagina is contraindicated in any pregnant patient over 20 weeks' gestation presenting with painless vaginal bleeding until ultrasonography rules out placenta previa.

16. **D.** Doubling of hepatic transaminases is a hallmark of preeclampsia with severe features. Other severe features include thrombocytopenia (platelets <100 000 cells/mm^3) and an increase in creatinine concentration to >1.1 mg/dL. BP >140/90 mm Hg is not specific for preeclampsia with severe features.

17. **C.** Loss of deep tendon reflexes indicated magnesium toxicity; hence, patellar reflexes are checked periodically while the patient is receiving magnesium sulfate.

18. **B.** The patient has preeclampsia with severe features as evidenced by the elevated BP and thrombocytopenia. The workup should also assess renal function and measurement of hepatic transaminases. Delivery is considered definitive management, but in a patient with severe features, waiting until 37 weeks would not be correct. The patient with preeclampsia with severe features should be started on an IV antihypertensive such as labetalol, and the patient should be given a course of corticosteroids for fetal lung maturity with plans to deliver the infant.

19. **A.** Acute DIC is associated with significant placental separation.

20. **C.** Within a few hours after delivery, the uterine fundus should be located at the level of the umbilicus.

21. **D.** Patients with placenta previa should avoid orgasm, putting any item into the vagina, and moderate or strenuous exercise after 20 weeks' gestation.

22. **B.** Nausea and vomiting are common during the first trimester of pregnancy, along with fatigue rather than increased energy. Fetal movement is typically felt between 18-20 weeks in the second trimester. Regular uterine contractions occur during labor.

23. **B.** Risk factors for placental abruption include abdominal trauma (motor vehicle accident, domestic abuse), cocaine use, smoking tobacco, and hypertension.

24. **D.** Regular uterine contractions and progressive cervical dilation indicate the onset of labor; this can occur with or without spontaneous rupture of membranes. Fetal distress is not typically observed in normal labor. Regular contractions with vaginal bleeding indicate a complication of pregnancy, not onset of labor.

25. **D.** Leopold's maneuvers are a series of four maneuvers to assess the position of the fetus before delivery.

26. **D.** First-trimester U/S examination confirms the presence of more than one fetus.

27. **D.** Routine prenatal care includes screening for diabetes by week 28, GBS between weeks 34-37 and blood type and Rh with antibody screen are included in the initial prenatal lab examination.

28. **D.** Patients with multiple gestation may report increased severity of morning sickness, early fetal movement, and increased fatigue.

29. **B.** Refer to maternal-fetal medicine. The patient will have serial serum anti-D titers and ultrasonographic imaging to assess for erythroblastosis fetalis and fetal hydrops. Hydrops due to alloimmunization is difficult to diagnose in the first trimester as it can appear to mimic fetal aneuploidies. A patient who is Rh negative with a negative antibody screen should receive anti-D immunoglobulin at 28 weeks.

30. **B.** Maternal age, ethnicity, maternal FH, high maternal BMI, and a history of prior pregnancies are risk factors for nonidentical multiple gestation.

31. **B.** The presence of antibodies to Rh(D) is the most common cause of Rh incompatibility.

32. **C.** Delivery for a multiple gestation pregnancy should be scheduled before 40 weeks' gestation to reduce the incidence of fetal mortality. Specific timing of delivery is dependent on the chorionicity and amnionicity. Additional caloric intake and folic acid supplementation is recommended.

33. **A.** Often, the terms alloimmunization and isoimmunization are used interchangeably when describing Rh incompatibility. The most common ways it is written is maternal alloimmunization and Rh isoimmunization.

34. **D.** U/S measurements demonstrating changes in cervical length and width are used to diagnose cervical insufficiency.

35. **B.** Physical examination may reveal excessive weight gain and uterine size that is large for gestational age.

36. **C.** Administer anti-D immunoglobulin within 72 hours postpartum. Six weeks is too long to wait to provide protection for the mother, and there is no need to recheck the antibody screen postpartum. It is also unnecessary to check the newborn's antibody screen as the Rh is positive.

37. **B.** Risk factors for cervical insufficiency include history of mechanical dilation, cervical procedures, cervical biopsies, anatomic malformations, and connective tissue disorders.

38. **C.** Most women with cervical insufficiency present with asymptomatic cervical dilation.

39. **B.** The presence of ferning under microscopic analysis is diagnostic of amniotic fluid rupture. Nitrazine paper that turns blue can occur in the presence of semen, blood, and some bacteria. Fetal fibronectin has a high false-positive rate. Cervical dilation (and effacement) has nothing to do with rupture of membranes as they are separate events.

40. **E.** A nuchal cord is not a complication of shoulder dystocia, but all other listed complications can occur at variable incidence rates in cases of shoulder dystocia.

41. **D.** A single course of corticosteroid is recommended for fetal lung maturity. Magnesium sulfate is indicated if the patient is <32 weeks and delivery is imminent. Immediate induction is not indicated, and the use of prostaglandins in PPROM is associated with higher risk of chorioamnionitis. Amoxicillin-clavulanic acid is not recommended as it is associated with a higher risk of fetal necrotizing enterocolitis.

42. **C.** Premature delivery is not a risk factor as fetal size is typically smaller, decreasing the chance of fetal shoulder impaction.

43. **C.** The current recommendation is 48 hours of ampicillin plus erythromycin; if the patient has not delivered after 48 hours, an extra 5 days of oral amoxicillin and erythromycin is advised. Ciprofloxacin is contraindicated in pregnancy. Ceftriaxone can be used for bacterial pneumonias, gonorrhea, and PID. Gentamycin is not a first-line antibiotic in pregnancy as it is associated with ototoxicity and nephrotoxicity.

44. **A.** GBS screening and prophylactic treatment is always recommended. The only exception would be if a patient had delivered a prior GBS-positive infant; in that circumstance, the patient is considered to be GBS positive and will be given antibiotics. Prophylactic treatment of HSV is recommended if the patient has a history of genital HSV. Magnesium sulfate is indicated if the gestation is <33 weeks and delivery is imminent. Corticosteroids are recommended when the gestation is <37 weeks.

CHAPTER

332

Mastitis and Breast Abscess

Katlin Bates, MSPAS

▶ GENERAL FEATURES

- Mastitis is an inflammation of breast tissue that can occur with or without microbial infection. A rare complication of mastitis is breast abscess, which is an infection within the breast tissue.
  - Mastitis is common in lactating women, especially prima gravida, due to nipple trauma associated with breastfeeding and/or clogged ducts from milk stasis.
    - If associated with breastfeeding, mastitis will often occur within the first 3 months following delivery.
  - *Staphylococcus aureus* is the most common cause of mastitis and breast abscess, but it can also be caused by methicillin-resistant *S. aureus* (MRSA).
    - Other less common causes include *Streptococcus pyogenes*, *Escherichia coli*, *Bacteroides* species, *Corynebacterium* species, and coagulase-negative staphylococci.
  - Women who develop mastitis should continue to breastfeed, or pump, to empty the breast and aid in resolution of the infection.
  - Women who are not lactating can still develop mastitis; however, they should undergo evaluation to rule out inflammatory breast cancer, which can mimic mastitis.
  - Though chronic types of mastitis exist, they are rare and usually seen in immunocompromised individuals.

▶ CLINICAL ASSESSMENT

- Mastitis is a clinical diagnosis that will present unilaterally.
  - Patient may complain of pain, edema, warmth to the breast, nipple discharge, change in sensation of the nipple, itching, and/or lump.
- During the history, patient may note systemic symptoms such as fever, chills, fatigue, and malaise.
- Clinical examination will elicit one breast that is larger than the other with notable erythema.
  - Affected breast will be tender to palpation.
  - Axillary adenopathy may be appreciated.

- A breast abscess has similar symptoms but will be localized on the breast with an area of induration and fluctuance.

▶ DIAGNOSIS

- A thorough history and clinical breast examination is essential to diagnosis.
- Laboratory tests are not routinely indicated in mastitis and/or breast abscess.
- Breast ultrasound should be considered to rule out breast abscess in women with persistent symptoms.

▶ TREATMENT

- For a patient with mastitis, supportive measures with warm compresses should be encouraged.
  - If breastfeeding, the patient should be encouraged to continue breastfeeding or pumping (to prevent milk stasis). Anti-staphylococcal antibiotics (such as dicloxacillin) should be utilized for a duration of 5-7 days (which can be increased to 10-14 days if needed) to clear infection and prevent an abscess.
    - If risk factors for MRSA are present, consider trimethoprim-sulfamethoxazole (if infant is >1 month old and is low risk for glucose-6-phosphate dehydrogenase deficiency) or clindamycin (which should be used with caution due to the potential for infant gastrointestinal disturbance).
  - Over-the-counter analgesics may be used if needed for pain control.
- Should a breast abscess develop, the patient should be treated with incision and drainage (I&D) in addition to antibiotics.
  - Smoking cessation must be encouraged to decrease the risk of subsequent abscess.
  - If breastfeeding, the patient may continue to breastfeed unless limited by the pain, the incision is within the infant's latch, or the antibiotics the mother is taking are not safe for the child.

Breast Cancer

Elyse Watkins, DHSc, PA-C, DFAAPA

▶ GENERAL FEATURES

- Breast cancer is the most common malignancy diagnosed in women in the United States.
- One in eight women will be diagnosed with a breast malignancy in her lifetime.
- Risk factors for breast cancer: nulliparity, later age at first birth, exogenous estrogen and progestin use, tobacco use, and alcohol use.
- Nonmodifiable risk factors: advancing age, genetic mutations, early menarche and late menopause, family history of breast and/or ovarian cancer (particularly premenopausal), and personal history of radiation therapy to the chest.
- Women with BRCA mutations are at higher risk for developing breast cancer, but <10% of women with breast cancer will have a known mutation.
- Infiltrating ductal carcinoma is the most common histologic subtype of breast cancer.
- Inflammatory breast cancer is the least common but is generally more aggressive than other subtypes.
- Immunohistochemical biomarkers are used to define prognosis and treatment options.
  - The four immunohistochemical biomarkers that comprise breast cancer subtypes are: Luminal A (estrogen receptor positive, progesterone receptor positive, HER-2 negative, Ki-67 low), Luminal B (estrogen receptor positive, progesterone receptor positive, HER-2 positive or negative, Ki-67 high), HER-2 positive (estrogen receptor negative, progesterone receptor negative, HER-2 positive), Basal (estrogen receptor negative, progesterone receptor negative, HER-2 negative; also called triple negative).
- Triple-negative breast cancer is the most aggressive, and prevalence is highest among premenopausal African American women.

▶ CLINICAL ASSESSMENT

- A palpable breast mass is evident in only about 30% of patients with breast cancer.
- Inflammatory breast cancer classically presents with skin dimpling, an orange-peel appearance of the skin, erythema, and induration.
- Inflammatory breast cancer can mimic mastitis and breast abscess; any assumed mastitis that does not respond to antibiotic therapy should be evaluated for inflammatory breast cancer.

- The physical examination of a patient with a breast mass must include palpation of axillary lymph nodes.
- Other physical examination findings may include nipple retraction, sanguineous nipple discharge, anatomic distortion, and skin discoloration.

▶ DIAGNOSIS

- Diagnostic mammography with ultrasound is the initial imaging modality.
- Common imaging findings in patients with invasive breast cancer include spiculation, anatomic distortion, irregular mass shape, and posterior acoustic shadowing.
- Suspicious lesions should undergo ultrasound-guided core-needle biopsy.
- The pathology report will include information on hormone receptivity, human epidermal growth factor receptor 2 (HER-2) overexpression status, and other immunohistologic markers that are used to help stratify risk of recurrence.
- Breast MRI is used to quantify the extent of disease and helps with presurgical planning.
- Genetic counseling is offered to determine whether screening for hereditary breast cancer is appropriate.

▶ TREATMENT

- Treatment depends upon immunohistochemical results, age of patient, extent of disease, evidence of recurrence, and patient expectations.
- Surgical options include lumpectomy or mastectomy with axillary staging of disease.
- Most patients can undergo sentinel lymph node biopsy during lumpectomy or mastectomy; this approach mitigates the development of upper extremity lymphedema.
- Invasive breast cancers are also treated with radiation therapy, usually postoperatively.
- Radiation and chemotherapy before surgery is called neoadjuvant therapy and is used when disease is locally advanced, and the patient is considered at high risk.
- Chemotherapeutic regimens depend upon immunohistochemical results, evidence of recurrence, and staging of disease.
- Estrogen receptor–positive breast cancer patients will receive either a selective estrogen receptor modulator

(SERM) or an aromatase inhibitor, depending on the patient's age and menopausal status. Aromatase inhibitors are drug of choice for postmenopausal breast cancer. SERMs are the standard initial treatment for premenopausal women.

- Patients who take aromatase inhibitors should have their bone density assessed and be given a bisphosphonate to help protect against osteoporosis.
- Patients with HER-2–positive breast cancer receive HER-2–targeted therapies.

- HER-2–targeted therapies can be cardiotoxic and are associated with decreased left ventricular ejection fraction and heart failure; therefore, cardiac function must be monitored.
- Patients with triple-negative breast cancer receive a taxane- or anthracycline-based chemotherapy regimen.
- Targeted therapies are in development for triple-negative metastatic breast cancer.

CHAPTER 334

Benign Breast Masses: Fibroadenoma and Fibrocystic Breast Changes

Tanya Fernandez, MS, PA-C, IBCLC

A 24-year-old woman presents to the office with concern for a painless, lump in her right breast. It was discovered about a month ago and is not enlarging or changing in size or shape and does not have any overlying skin changes. She denies nipple discharge, current or recent pregnancy, and the use of herbal or prescription medications. What is the most appropriate initial evaluation modality?

▌ GENERAL FEATURES

- Fibroadenomas typically occur in women between the ages of 15 and 30 years.
- Pathophysiology of fibroadenomas: excess proliferation of stromal and epithelial tissue in the breast secondary to estrogen and progesterone receptor sensitivity.
- Simple fibroadenomas can be confused with breast neoplasms, breast abscess, galactocele, fat necrosis, lipomas, and breast cysts. In addition, fibroadenomas can be classified as simple, complex, giant, and juvenile, all of which should be differentiated from a phyllodes tumor, if it is found to be changing rapidly.
- Fibrocystic breast changes peak in the mid-40s and continue through perimenopause.
- Elevated estrogen and decreased progesterone levels cause the hyperproliferation of connective tissue and cyst formation found in fibrocystic breast changes.

▌ CLINICAL ASSESSMENT

- Fibroadenomas present as unilateral, painless breast lump.
- On clinical breast examination, a fibroadenoma presents as a solitary mobile, smooth, and discrete mass with a well-defined shape. Multiple masses or bilateral lumps can be found but are only noted in 20% of fibroadenomas.
- Fibrocystic breast changes present with diffuse bilateral breast pain with an irregular and rope-like texture on palpation.
- Fibrocystic breast pain may be cyclical or constant with a corresponding increase in breast tissue size in the upper outer quadrant before menses.

▌ DIAGNOSIS

- Depending on the age of the patient, imaging of a breast mass could include a targeted breast ultrasound (US) or a diagnostic mammogram.
- The American College of Radiology (ACR) recommends that women under the age of 30 undergo diagnostic breast US; however, after the age of 40, women should be directed to undergo diagnostic mammogram, often in combination with US.
- The majority of fibrocystic breast changes can be diagnosed by breast US alone.

- Definitive diagnosis of fibroadenoma is based on the histopathology from a core-needle biopsy or excisional tissue sample.
- Fine-needle aspiration of a breast cyst is reserved for simple cysts (no internal echoes or solid components on U/S) with signs of infection or inflammation or complicated cysts (low-level echogenic debris without solid components on U/S); however, complex cysts (masses with thick walls/septa, cystic and solid components on U/S) are evaluated with core-needle biopsy, given the need to evaluate the solid components.

▶ TREATMENT

- If the biopsy-confirmed fibroadenoma is not causing the patient any symptoms, the lump can be left in place. Many fibroadenomas regress after menopause.

- Complex fibroadenomas may warrant excision, as there is a slightly increased risk of cancer. Shared decision-making is important, as excision is not without risks such as scarring, dimpling, mammographic changes, and damage to the nerve and breast duct system.
- Reassurance and a better fitting bra that improves support of Cooper's ligament improve symptoms of fibrocystic breast changes in 85% of patients. Topical diclofenac can be an adjuvant to bra adjustments.

Case Conclusion

The patient has symptoms of a classic simple fibroadenoma. Given the patient's age of <40 years, the ACR recommends breast US for initial evaluation.

Galactorrhea and Gynecomastia

Tanya Fernandez, MS, PA-C, IBCLC

▶ GENERAL FEATURES

- Galactorrhea:
  - Type of physiologic discharge from the nipple that resembles breast milk but occurs in a patient who is not actually lactating
  - Pathologic breast discharge is characterized by spontaneous, unilateral, discharge that is bloody, serous, or serosanguinous.
  - The most common cause of galactorrhea is hyperprolactinemia secondary to a prolactinoma. Other endocrine disorders, medications, chronic renal failure, chronic subareolar abscess, and some chest wall lesions/trauma should also be considered when investigating the underlying cause of galactorrhea.
  - Both physiologic galactorrhea and gynecomastia occur in times of extreme hormonal changes. Galactorrhea and gynecomastia seen in the neonate are usually transient and resolve without intervention. Galactorrhea can be seen during menarche and menopause for women, whereas gynecomastia can be seen during adolescence and is much more common in the elderly male.
- Gynecomastia:
  - Gynecomastia, or the benign enlargement of breast stroma in males, can be physiologic or pathologic and is related to hormonal influences.

- Gynecomastia occurs when there is either a decrease in androgen effect or an increase in estrogen effect. The increase in estrogen effect often occurs due to an increase in aromatase activity. Underlying causes of gynecomastia to consider when evaluating a patient include hypogonadism, hormone-producing tumors, medications, chronic liver disease, malnutrition, and hyperthyroidism. Gynecomastia mimics most commonly include lipomastia (pseudogynecomastia), subareolar abscess, and, more rarely, breast cancer.

▶ CLINICAL ASSESSMENT

- Galactorrhea:
  - Typically a thin, watery, milk-like discharge from both breasts and originates from multiple breast ducts. Galactorrhea is most common in postpartum females (aged 20-35 years) who have repeated nipple stimulation, whether that be from hand expression, clothing friction, or sexual intimacy.
  - A thorough medication review may also uncover the underlying cause for both galactorrhea and gynecomastia.
    - Medication classes associated with hyperprolactinemia with subsequent galactorrhea include hormonal therapy, psychiatric medications

(antidepressants, antipsychotics, anxiolytics), chronic opioids, and some antihypertensives, such as methyldopa and verapamil.

- Double vision and headaches can be an indicator of a prolactinoma.
- Gynecomastia:
  - Gynecomastia is typically bilateral, although it can be unilateral. Unilateral presentation raises more red flags for the possibility of a pathologic cause.
  - Early gynecomastia, especially in adolescents, can be painful to palpation; however, older adults tend to note less pain than their younger counterparts.
  - Differentiate between gynecomastia and pseudogynecomastia (fat deposition) by palpating for a ridge of glandular tissue that is concentric from the nipple and symmetric between the two sides. Inability to palpate a rubbery or firm mass may indicate pseudogynecomastia.
  - Medications noted to increase aromatase activity and subsequently cause gynecomastia include antihypertensives (diuretics, ACE inhibitors, β-blockers), spironolactone, statins, antidepressants, first-generation antihistamines, NSAIDs, Parkinson meds, proton-pump inhibitors, and some muscle relaxants.
  - In addition to the breast examination, patients with gynecomastia should be evaluated for the most common underlying causes of pathologic gynecomastia, including signs of hyperthyroidism (goiter, lid lag, exophthalmos, tachycardia), liver disease (ascites, hepatosplenomegaly, skin and nail changes, caput medusae), and hypogonadism (small testes).

▶ DIAGNOSIS

- Galactorrhea:
  - Often made based on history and physical examination alone
  - Given the interplay of hormones and prolactin levels, many practitioners will rule out pregnancy with a urine pregnancy test and will evaluate prolactin and thyroid-stimulating hormone (TSH) levels in a patient with galactorrhea.

- If prolactin levels are elevated and indicate the possibility of a prolactinoma, high-resolution CT or MRI is the imaging modality of choice for detecting microadenomas.
- Galactorrhea due to nipple stimulation does not require further evaluation beyond the initial workup indicated above.
- Gynecomastia:
  - Diagnosis is usually made by history and physical examination.
  - Consider serum testosterone level in older men with other findings suggestive of hypogonadism. However, if history and physical examination do not reveal an underlying medication or obvious pathologic cause for the gynecomastia, serum levels of luteinizing hormone (LH), follicle-stimulating hormone (FSH), testosterone, estradiol, and human chorionic gonadotropin (hCG) are recommended to evaluate for underlying cause.
  - If gynecomastia is unilateral and associated with nipple discharge or retraction, skin changes, a firm or fixed mass or any axillary node enlargement, a workup for breast cancer should be initiated with diagnostic imaging.

▶ TREATMENT

- Galactorrhea:
  - Galactorrhea due to nipple stimulation requires reassurance and elimination of the stimulus.
  - Hyperprolactinemia secondary to hormonal therapy or medications should improve with cessation of the causative medication, whereas prolactinomas will require the addition of a dopamine agonist for the treatment of bothersome symptoms.
  - Surgical resection and radiation therapy are reserved for macroadenomas and pituitary stalk masses that continue to increase in size.
- Gynecomastia: physiologic gynecomastia requires no intervention other than reassurance and re-evaluation every 6 months. Treat the underlying cause of pathologic gynecomastia.

CHAPTER

336

Amenorrhea

Renee Andreeff, EdD, PA-C, DFAAPA

▶ GENERAL FEATURES

- Amenorrhea is the absence or abnormal cessation of menstrual cycles in a woman of reproductive age and can be classified as primary or secondary.
- Primary amenorrhea is the absence of menstrual bleeding at age 15 in women who exhibit normal growth and signs of secondary sexual characteristics. Causes can be divided into three main categories:
  - End-organ disorders including chromosomal abnormalities (such as Turner syndrome) that cause gonadal dysgenesis, Müllerian agenesis, and ovarian failure
  - Outflow tract obstruction such as imperforate hymen, transverse vaginal septum, testicular feminization, and vaginal agenesis or atresia
  - Central regulatory disorders including hypothalamic and pituitary disorders. Examples include Kallmann syndrome, brain/pituitary tumors, TBI, and congenital gonadotropin-releasing hormone (GnRH) deficiency
- Secondary amenorrhea is defined as cessation of menstrual cycles for three or more consecutive cycles in women with previously normal menstrual cycles or cessation of menstrual cycles for >6 months in women with previously irregular menstrual cycles.
  - The most common cause of secondary amenorrhea is pregnancy.
  - Other causes can be divided into four main categories:
    - Anatomic abnormalities, including Asherman syndrome (intrauterine adhesions) or cervical os stenosis
    - Ovarian dysfunction such as polycystic ovary syndrome (PCOS) or ovarian failure due to torsion, postsurgical infection, tumor, radiation, chemotherapy, or premature ovarian failure

- Pituitary dysfunction caused by pituitary adenomas, primary hypothyroidism, or medications such as haloperidol, metoclopramide, estrogen, phenothiazine, monoamine oxidase inhibitors, tricyclic antidepressants, and opioids
- Central nervous system or hypothalamic disorders such as sellar masses and functional hypothalamic GnRH deficiency
- Functional hypothalamic GnRH deficiency is characterized by a decrease in hypothalamic GnRH secretion. Causes include eating disorders such as anorexia nervosa, excessive exercise, nutritional deficiencies, severe illness, and emotional stress.

▶ CLINICAL ASSESSMENT

- Evaluation of primary amenorrhea should begin at age 15 in girls who exhibit secondary sexual characteristics and at age 13 in girls who do not exhibit secondary sexual characteristics.
- History should be focused depending on suspicion for primary or secondary amenorrhea.
- Ask patients about contributing family history, history of neonatal crisis, short stature, and hyperandrogenism.
  - Other important past medical history questions may include possibility of pregnancy, history of endometrial scarring, weight changes, recent stress or illness, and use of medications. Screen patients for eating disorders, acne, hirsutism, libido, galactorrhea, headaches, visual field changes, fatigue, polyuria, and polydipsia. Include questions related to estrogen deficiency, such as hot flashes, vaginal dryness, and poor sleep.
- Patients with secondary amenorrhea should be assessed for risk factors for endometrial hyperplasia and/or cancer. These include obesity, age over 40 years,

history of polycystic ovarian syndrome, and previous history of hyperplasia.

- Document body mass index (BMI). Low BMI may indicate disordered eating, stress, or excessive exercise. BMI > 30 is frequently seen in patient with PCOS.
- Physical examination of primary amenorrhea should include Tanner staging, Turner syndrome features, and the presence or absence of the vagina and uterus.
- Physical examination for secondary amenorrhea should include assessment of cranial nerves and visual fields, hyperandrogenism (hirsutism, striae, acne, and hyperseborrhea), dental erosions, galactorrhea, and vaginal anatomic defects along with signs of estrogen deficiency.
- Patients with PCOS may have elevated BMI, whereas women with eating disorders and athletes may have BMI < 20 kg/m^2.

▶ DIAGNOSIS

- Pregnancy testing via serum β-human chorionic gonadotropin should be performed in all women, even if the patient denies sexual activity.
- Laboratory testing may include follicle-stimulating hormone (FSH), luteinizing hormone (LH), thyroid-stimulating hormone (TSH), prolactin, and testosterone levels.

- Pelvic and transvaginal ultrasound or magnetic resonance imaging (MRI) can evaluate anatomic abnormalities of the vagina, cervix, and uterus.
- MRI or computed tomography (CT) of the hypothalamus and pituitary may be used to assess central nervous system tumors.
  - If the uterus is abnormal or absent, FSH and LH are elevated to obtain a karyotype analysis.
    - A progesterone challenge test can assess the presence or absence of sufficient estrogen. If patient does not experience withdrawal bleeding with the progesterone challenge, an estrogen-progesterone challenge test can assess for uterine outflow obstruction or hypergonadotropic hypogonadism.

▶ TREATMENT

- Directed toward underlying pathology and helping a woman to achieve fertility if desired.
- Induction of ovulation can occur for most women with the use of medications (dopamine agonist, clomiphene citrate, insulin-secreting agents, and gonadotropins), except for women with premature ovarian failure.

CHAPTER
337

Cervical Cancer

Johanna D'Addario, PA-C

▶ GENERAL FEATURES

- The highest incidence of cervical cancer is in women between the ages of 40 and 49 years.
- Squamous cell carcinoma (SCC) and adenocarcinoma are the most common types.
- Cervical intraepithelial neoplasia (CIN) and cervical carcinoma are strongly associated with high-risk human papillomavirus (HPV) infection.
  - HPV infection is extremely common, affecting up to 80% of the population.
  - While the majority of HPV infections are transient and resolve within 6-24 months, HPV types 16 and 18 are more likely to progress to CIN and cervical SCC.
  - Condoms are ~70% effective at preventing HPV transmission.

- The HPV vaccine series was originally recommended for females between the ages of 9 and 26 years and for males between the ages of 9 and 21 years, and its FDA approval was expanded to age 45, for certain patients, in 2018.
- Risk factors related to high-risk HPV infection and cervical cancer include:
  - Early onset of sexual activity
  - Multiple sexual partners
  - Low socioeconomic status
  - Immunosuppression
  - Tobacco use (increases risk of cervical SCC)
  - Oral contraceptive pills

▶ CLINICAL ASSESSMENT

- Screening includes cervical cytology (Papanicolaou test) and HPV testing.

- Conventional cytology and liquid-based cytology have similar sensitivity and specificity for diagnosis of high-grade CIN.
- HPV testing is more sensitive than cytology alone in the diagnosis of CIN2 or CIN3.
- Abnormal cervical cytology and/or HPV infection are followed by cervical colposcopy and tissue sampling.
- The US Preventive Services Task Force provides the following screening recommendations:
  - Cervical cytology alone every 3 years in women between the ages of 21 and 29 years.
  - Cervical cytology alone every 3 years, or cervical cytology plus HPV testing every 5 years in women between the ages of 30 and 65 years.
  - No screening for women under 21 or over 65 with history of prior adequate screening.
  - No screening for women who have had a hysterectomy, unless a prior history of CIN2 or higher, in which case screening of the vaginal apex should be continued for 20 years after the last abnormal test result.
- The American Society for Colposcopy and Cervical Pathology (ASCCP) has developed a clinical algorithm for cervical cancer screening and management of abnormal cervical cytology.
- Although usually asymptomatic, patients with invasive cervical cancer may present with abnormal vaginal or postcoital bleeding, bladder symptoms, back pain, or pelvic pain.
- Women with a visible cervical lesion or ulceration on speculum examination should undergo biopsy, regardless of cytology results.

▶ DIAGNOSIS

- Abnormal results of a Papanicolaou test include:
  - Atypical squamous cells of unknown significance (ASCUS)
  - Low-grade squamous intraepithelial lesions (LSILs)
  - High-grade squamous intraepithelial lesions (HSILs)
  - Atypical glandular cells
- LSIL usually correlates with mild dysplasia (CIN1) on histology.
- HSIL usually correlates with moderate (CIN2) or severe (CIN3) dysplasia on histology.

- A high-grade lesion extending beyond the basement membrane of the cervical epithelium is consistent with a diagnosis of cervical cancer.
- Endocervical curettage, colposcopy-directed cervical biopsy, or lesion excision aid in the diagnosis.
- Staging is based on the International Federation of Gynecology and Obstetrics (FIGO) guidelines and includes:
  - Tumor size
  - Depth of invasion
  - Surrounding tissue involvement
  - Distant metastases (common sites include the lung, liver, and bone)
- CT, MRI, and PET imaging can be used to assess disease extension and lymphovascular space invasion.

▶ TREATMENT

- Surgical management:
  - Simple or radical hysterectomy based on disease stage
  - Because cervical adenocarcinoma has risk of ovarian metastasis, oophorectomy is recommended.
- For women with early-stage disease who wish to preserve fertility, conization with negative margins or radical trachelectomy (removal of the cervix) may be possible.
  - Women should be counseled on the risk of pregnancy complications, including preterm birth.
- Adjuvant therapy includes platinum-based chemotherapy and/or radiation therapy with external beam radiation or high-dose intracavity brachytherapy.
- Bevacizumab (Avastin) has been shown to improve survival compared with standard chemotherapy alone.
- Long-term effects of cervical cancer treatment include sexual dysfunction, cystitis, proctitis, ovarian failure, infertility, and chronic pelvic pain.
- Recurrence usually occurs within the first 3 years after treatment.
  - Patients should be followed every 3-6 months for the first 2-5 years after treatment.
  - Long-term cervical cancer survivors should have annual pelvic examinations and vaginal cytology to evaluate for disease recurrence.

Abnormal Uterine Bleeding

Elyse Watkins, DHSc, PA-C, DFAAPA

▶ GENERAL FEATURES

- Heavy menstrual bleeding is bleeding that results in >80 mL of blood loss and/or lasts for >7 days per menstrual cycle.
- Intermenstrual bleeding is bleeding that occurs at irregular intervals and is >80 mL per episode.
- It is difficult to quantify blood loss in milliliters, so asking the patient about the number of pads/tampons used and frequency of changing them is essential. Soaking through a pad/tampon every hour is abnormal.
- Postmenopausal bleeding is caused by endometrial cancer until proven otherwise, although, in most cases, the patient's abnormal uterine bleeding (AUB) will be caused by genital atrophy.

▶ CLINICAL ASSESSMENT

- Evaluate the patient for hemodynamic stability.
- A thorough history, including obstetric history, and physical examination are critical to narrow the differential diagnosis.
- Assess the onset, duration, and timing of the bleeding. Inquire about recent trauma or abdominopelvic surgeries.
- Determine whether the bleeding occurs postcoitally or if the bleeding is accompanied by pelvic or abdominal pain.
- The review of systems should include questions about bruising, fatigue, tachycardia, shortness of breath, bleeding from the nose or gums, pelvic bloating, and early satiety.
- Assess for the presence of hypercoagulable risk factors and a history of a thromboembolic event as some of the treatments for AUB include estrogens, progestins, and tranexamic acid, contraindicated in patients with a history of a thromboembolic event and all should be used with caution in patients with hypercoagulable risk factors.
- Past medical history should include questions about endocrinopathies, coagulopathies, malignancies, and previous episodes of a similar presentation.
- The PALM-COIEN system is useful when assessing the patient with AUB.
  - P: polyp (uterine and endocervical)
  - A: adenomyosis
  - L: leiomyoma
  - M: malignancy (cervical and uterine cancer; endometrial hyperplasia)
  - C: coagulopathy (inherited or acquired)
  - O: ovarian dysfunction (PCOS; perimenopause)
  - E: endometrial (can include pelvic inflammatory disease and endometritis)
  - I: iatrogenic (intrauterine systems; exogenous hormone use; antiplatelet and anticoagulant medications)
  - N: not yet classified
- A patient with a positive pregnancy test who presents with abnormal bleeding in the first trimester has an ectopic pregnancy until proven otherwise.
- Rule out endometrial hyperplasia and endometrial cancer in women with AUB who are taking a selective estrogen receptor modulator such as tamoxifen and in patients with PCOS who are chronically amenorrheic or oligomenorrheic.
- Patients with AUB and who have a family history of colon, endometrial, breast, ovarian, and gastrointestinal cancer should be referred to a genetics counselor to be tested for Lynch syndrome (hereditary nonpolyposis colorectal cancer). Lynch syndrome can cause endometrial cancer.

▶ DIAGNOSIS

- Perform a pregnancy test on all reproductive-aged women.
- Laboratory evaluation of heavy menstrual bleeding also includes a complete blood count. However, in an acute bleeding episode, the hemoglobin and hematocrit might not yet be decreased.
- In episodes of acute heavy bleeding, type and cross, PT, aPTT, and fibrinogen are usually indicated.
- Consider checking for von Willebrand disease with a vWF antigen, particularly in younger patients.
- A pelvic and transvaginal ultrasound can determine anatomic abnormalities, such as leiomyoma and adenomyosis.
- An endometrial thickness measured with ultrasound >4 mm in a postmenopausal woman requires tissue sampling to rule out endometrial hyperplasia and cancer.

▶ TREATMENT

- Treatment depends upon the underlying cause.
- Once malignancy and pregnancy have been ruled out, several pharmacologic therapies can be considered.
- Long-term management with estrogen and progestin can be considered in reproductive-aged women without an underlying malignancy and without risk

factors/contraindications for the use of estrogen and progestin.

- Progestin-secreting intrauterine systems can be used in reproductive-aged women without a malignancy or known contraindications.
- Tranexamic acid is an antifibrinolytic and is an option for women with cyclic heavy menstrual bleeding and acute heavy menstrual bleeding.
  - A contraindication for tranexamic acid includes a history of thromboembolic disease.

- Patients who present with acute heavy menstrual bleeding can receive intravenous conjugated equine estrogen if they do not have contraindications to estrogen use (thromboembolic disease, breast cancer, uterine cancer).
- Other options for treating heavy menstrual bleeding once malignancy has been ruled out include endometrial ablation, uterine artery embolization if leiomyoma is present, and definitive surgical management with hysterectomy.

CHAPTER 339

Endometrial Cancer

Johanna D'Addario, PA-C

GENERAL FEATURES

- The most common gynecologic cancer in the United States
- Histologic types of uterine epithelial tumors include:
  - Endometrioid adenocarcinoma (75%-80% of cases)
  - Serous carcinoma (10%)
  - Clear cell adenocarcinoma (4%)
  - Mucinous adenocarcinoma (1%)
  - Squamous carcinoma (<1%)
- Mesenchymal tumors make up a small minority of uterine cancers:
  - Carcinosarcoma
  - Leiomyosarcoma
  - Adenosarcoma
  - Endometrial stromal sarcoma
- Endometrial hyperplasia secondary to unopposed estrogen stimulation is a precursor to endometrial cancer.
  - Women with an intact uterus who take estrogen therapy require progesterone for uterine protection.
  - Hyperplasia is categorized by architecture (simple/complex) and cytology (typical/atypical).
  - The highest risk of progression to cancer occurs in women with complex atypical hyperplasia.
  - Hysterectomy can prevent progression to cancer in women with atypical hyperplasia.
- Other risk factors for endometrial cancer include obesity, age, family history or genetic predisposition, early menarche, late menopause, nulliparity, tamoxifen use, polycystic ovarian syndrome, and diabetes mellitus.
  - Lynch syndrome caused by a pathogenic variant in one of the mismatch repair genes *MLH1*, *MSH2*, *PMS2*, or *MSH6* is associated with a significantly increased lifetime risk of endometrial cancer along with other types of cancer.

- Cowden syndrome, caused by a variant in the *PTEN* gene, is a less common inherited condition associated with increased risk of endometrial cancer.
  - Research indicates a possible increased risk of serous endometrial cancer in women with a pathogenic variant in the *BRCA1* gene.
- Protective factors include combination oral contraceptives, levonorgestrel IUD, and physical activity.

CLINICAL ASSESSMENT

- All postmenopausal bleeding must be evaluated.
- Patients may be asymptomatic or present with abnormal uterine bleeding or discharge.
- Some women may have atypical glandular cells (AGUS) on screening Pap smear.
- Advanced disease can present with abdominal pain, pelvic pain, or bloating.

DIAGNOSIS

- Diagnosis is made by tissue sampling with endometrial biopsy, dilation and curettage, or on surgical pathology after hysterectomy.
- The International Federation of Gynecology and Obstetrics (FIGO) staging system is determined by:
  - Grade of tumor (histologic differentiation)
  - Depth of myometrial invasion
  - Lymphatic vascular space invasion
- The National Comprehensive Cancer Network (NCCN) recommends universal testing of endometrial cancers for microsatellite instability, which can be indicative of a germline Lynch syndrome mutation.

- Imaging evaluation includes chest radiograph, pelvic MRI, or CT scan of the chest, abdomen, and pelvis.
- PET/CT scan can be used if metastatic disease is suspected.
- Uterine serous and clear cell carcinomas are more likely to spread beyond the uterus, and imaging or CA-125 tumor marker may be helpful to evaluate disease status.

▶ TREATMENT

- The NCCN provides clinical guidelines for the treatment of uterine tumors based on histologic type, grade, and stage.
- Surgical management includes exploratory laparoscopy or laparotomy, total hysterectomy, bilateral salpingo-oophorectomy, pelvic washings, and pelvic and para-aortic lymph node dissection.
- Patients with early (FIGO stage IA) endometrial cancer may require no postoperative intervention and can be observed only.

- Patients with more advanced disease require adjuvant treatment, which may include:
  - Vaginal brachytherapy
  - External beam pelvic radiation therapy
  - Platinum-based chemotherapy
- Post-treatment surveillance:
  - Regular pelvic examinations
  - CA-125 levels (only if initially elevated)
  - Imaging based on symptoms or concern for disease recurrence
- Recurrence is managed with surgery, chemotherapy, radiation, or endocrine therapy.
- Targeted therapies based on molecular and genetic abnormalities in the tumor are a novel approach.
- Prognosis:
  - Endometrioid adenocarcinoma, the most common histologic type, has a good prognosis.
  - Serous carcinoma, clear cell carcinoma, and uterine sarcoma have worse outcomes with lower 5-year survival rates.

CHAPTER 340

Ovarian Torsion

Joy Moverley, DHSc, MPH, PA-C

A 38-year-old cisgender female presents to the ED with sudden and severe right-sided pelvic pain, nausea, and vomiting. The patient's urine hCG was negative. What do you think could be causing this patient's symptoms?

▶ GENERAL FEATURES

- Ovarian torsion is the complete or partial rotation of the ovary on its ligamentous supports, which can impede its blood supply.
- Ovarian torsion initially causes compression of the ovarian vein and lymphatic vessels, impeding venous outflow and lymphatic flow. Owing to the muscular nature of their walls, arteries are less compressible.
- Continued arterial infusion with decreased or absent venous and lymphatic drainage leads to ovarian enlargement, edema, ischemia, and, possibly, ovarian infarction and necrosis.
- Adnexal torsion (the fallopian tube twisting along with the ovary) may occur.

- The utero-ovarian ligament attaches the medial pole of the ovary to the lateral pelvic wall.
- The suspensory ligament of the uterus (infundibulopelvic ligament) attaches the ovary to the lateral pelvic wall and contains the ovarian artery, ovarian vein, ovarian nerve plexus, and lymphatic vessels.
- In ovarian torsion, the ovary typically rotates around both the suspensory ligament of the uterus and the utero-ovarian ligament.
- Risk factors:
  - Pregnancy (about 20% of cases)
  - Ovarian mass such as a benign ovarian cyst or neoplasm. In adult women, a physiologic ovarian cyst or neoplasm >5 cm in diameter is the most common cause of ovarian torsion.
  - Being of reproductive age (median age is 28 years)
- In a woman with acute pelvic pain and an adnexal mass, exclude ectopic pregnancy, a ruptured ovarian cyst, tubo-ovarian abscess, and appendicitis.
- The right ovary is most commonly affected (60% of cases).

▶ CLINICAL ASSESSMENT

- Prompt diagnosis is crucial to preserving ovarian and tubal function but can be challenging because symptoms are relatively nonspecific.
- History:
  - Sudden, unilateral moderate-to-severe pelvic pain
  - Nausea and vomiting
  - Recent diagnosis of adnexal mass
  - Inciting event such as vigorous activity
  - Rare: genital tract bleeding
- Physical examination:
  - Low-grade fever in some patients
  - Elevated heart rate or BP related to severe pelvic pain
  - Pelvic and/or abdominal tenderness frequently is not present.
  - A palpable mass is not always present.
  - Peritoneal signs are suggestive of adnexal necrosis.
- Laboratory evaluation:
  - Pregnancy testing (β-hCG)
  - Torsion risk is increased in pregnancy.
  - Exclude ectopic pregnancy
  - Complete blood cell count
    - Rarely, torsion causes hemorrhage that can result in anemia.
    - Leukocytosis may occur with adnexal necrosis and subsequent infection.
    - Both anemia and leukocytosis are nonspecific but suggestive of severe adnexal damage.

▶ DIAGNOSIS

- Imaging:
  - Pelvic ultrasound
    - Both transvaginal and transabdominal recommended
    - May show an ovary that is rounded and enlarged, with heterogeneous stroma relative to contralateral ovary due to edema and vascular congestion
    - May elicit pain with intravaginal probe during ultrasound on ipsilateral side of mass
    - May show multiple small peripheral follicles, the "string of pearls" similar to polycystic ovarian syndrome but with edema and acute pain
    - May show displaced ovary to the anterior of uterus and free fluid
  - Doppler flow ultrasound can evaluate blood flow to the ovary.
  - MRI is helpful when ultrasound results are equivocal but is not routinely done because of the cost and time required. If done, an MRI typically will show an enlarged, edematous, displaced ovary with coiled vessels if contrast is used.
  - CT is not often used, but an enlarged and edematous ovary may be seen in abdominal workup. Enhancement may be absent with contrast administration.
  - Direct visualization is the definitive diagnosis.

▶ TREATMENT

- Expedient evaluation is the mainstay of treatment to preserve ovarian function.
- Surgery:
  - The combination of the patient's symptoms, signs, and ultrasound findings guides the decision to proceed.
  - Detorsion and ovary conservation is recommended for most premenopausal women.
    - Salpingo-oophorectomy is reasonable for postmenopausal women.
    - Perform ovarian cystectomy to treat benign ovarian mass.
    - If an ovarian mass is suspicious for malignancy, regardless of the age of the patient, a salpingo-oophorectomy and pathology evaluation is required.
- Preventing recurrence:
  - Oral contraceptives may be administered for ovarian cyst suppression.
  - Unilateral or bilateral oophoropexy may be performed, although no long-term studies have evaluated fertility after this procedure.

Case Conclusion

Ovarian torsion should be considered in all sudden pelvic pain patients, especially if a history of an ovarian mass. This patient should undergo a Doppler flow ultrasound to confirm blood flow to the ovary. If torsion is identified, she should promptly undergo detorsion and conservation of her ovary.

Pelvic Inflammatory Disease

Jennifer Johnson, BS, MPAS, DMSc

▶ GENERAL FEATURES

- Pelvic inflammatory disease (PID) is an infection of the female upper genital tract, involving at least one of the following: uterus, fallopian tubes, or ovaries.
- Risk factors include multiple sexual partners, age younger than 25 years, prior history of PID, and a sexual partner with a sexually transmitted infection (STI).
- The majority of PID cases are caused by sexually transmitted pathogens.
- The organisms most commonly associated with the development of PID are *Chlamydia trachomatis*, *Neisseria gonorrhoeae*, and *Gardnerella vaginalis*. Infections may be polymicrobial.
- IUD placement is associated with an increased risk of developing PID, though this risk is limited to the first 3-4 weeks immediately following insertion.

▶ CLINICAL ASSESSMENT

- The most common presenting symptom is bilateral lower abdominal pain lasting for 1-2 weeks.
- Cervical motion tenderness (chandelier sign) and adnexal tenderness on bimanual examination are characteristic findings of PID.
- Fever >101 °F, purulent cervical discharge, cervical friability, and/or nausea may be present.
- Findings that necessitate inpatient treatment include pregnancy, pelvic abscess, severe illness, severe nausea/ vomiting, and infection that is refractory to treatment.

▶ DIAGNOSIS

- Perform urine hCG to rule out an ectopic pregnancy.

- Perform nucleic acid amplification test (NAAT) for *C. trachomatis* and *N. gonorrhoeae*.
- PID is generally diagnosed based on clinical presentation without additional diagnostic studies; no single diagnostic test is highly sensitive and specific for PID.

▶ TREATMENT

- Promptly initiate broad-spectrum antibiotics that cover Gram-negative organisms, anaerobes, *C. trachomatis*, and *N. gonorrhoeae*. CDC STI treatment guidelines are updated regularly and should be consulted for treatment recommendations.
- An intramuscular cephalosporin plus doxycycline is an appropriate regimen in the outpatient setting. Consider the addition of metronidazole for patients with a history of a recent gynecologic procedure.
- Inpatient antimicrobial treatment consists of an intravenous cephalosporin plus oral doxycycline. Intravenous clindamycin plus intravenous gentamicin is an acceptable alternative regimen.
- Severe or refractory cases may require inpatient care or surgical treatment.
- Re-evaluate the patient 72 hours after initiating treatment.
- Patients with IUDs who decline removal require close clinical monitoring.
- Evaluate and treat sexual partners.
- Patients should refrain from sexual activity during treatment.
- Complications of untreated PID include infertility, ectopic pregnancy, and chronic pelvic pain.

Contraception

Gina Brown, MPAS

A 30-year-old female is requesting contraception. Her medical history includes obesity and treatment for chlamydia 2 weeks ago. She has two children who were both "unplanned" because of the difficulty in remembering to take an oral contraceptive pill daily. She also reports using an injectable contraceptive for 5 years in her early 20s. What form of contraception would you recommend to her now?

▶ GENERAL FEATURES

- Contraception is the prevention of unwanted pregnancy and can be either reversible or permanent.
- Permanent forms include a variety of surgical procedures that result in either male or female sterilization.
- Reversible forms can be subdivided into hormonal and nonhormonal. Alternately, they can be subdivided into long-acting, short-acting, and emergency formulas.

- Nonhormonal options include fertility awareness with periodic abstinence or barrier use during ovulation, lactational amenorrhea, barrier methods such as male and female condoms, diaphragm, sponge, and spermicide. The copper-containing intrauterine device (IUD) is also hormone free.
- Hormonal options include combination hormonal contraceptives (CHC) that contain both estrogen and progestin and are available in oral forms, vaginal rings and transdermal patches, or progestin-only contraceptives that are available in oral forms, injections, subdermal implants, and as IUDs.
- Efficacy of methods varies from about 72% to 99.95% within the first year of typical use. Fertility awareness, condoms, sponge, and spermicides are the least effective in preventing pregnancy, whereas implants, IUDs, and sterilization have the highest efficacy.

▶ CLINICAL ASSESSMENT

- Evaluation of the female patient who is requesting contraception includes past medical history, sexual history, history of present health, and personal preferences. The goal of the provider should be to guide the patient toward the most effective method that is appropriate for the individual.
- Contraindications or significant cautions should be considered when starting a patient on contraception with the following health conditions:
  - IUDs should be avoided if uterus has abnormal shape, in cases of unresolved cervical cancer, endometrial cancer, some cases of gestational trophoblastic disease, current PID or cervicitis, recent septic abortion, postpartum sepsis, current pregnancy, or unexplained vaginal bleeding.
  - All hormonal contraceptives should be avoided in patients with current or recent breast cancer. The copper-containing IUD is a safe alternative.
  - Estrogen-containing contraception (CHC) should be avoided for 21-30 days postpartum depending on breastfeeding, as well as in patients with any increased risk of thromboembolism, all patients who have migraines with aura, in diabetic patients with known end-organ damage, in symptomatic gallbladder disease, hypertension, various heart or liver diseases, systemic lupus erythematosus with positive antiphospholipid antibodies, and in smokers who are age 35 years or more.
  - A comprehensive list of diseases and risks of contraception can be found at https://www.cdc.gov/reproductivehealth/contraception/pdf/summary-chart-us-medical-eligibility-criteria_508tagged.pdf.
- Some forms of contraception are FDA approved for treatment of endometriosis, heavy menstrual bleeding, and acne; some include iron or folic acid supplementation.

- Other considerations for patient selection:
  - Efficacy of some methods is decreased in obese women.
  - Efficacy of some methods is decreased when combined with certain medications, including some anticonvulsants and antimicrobials.
  - Progestin component carries various potential androgenic effects.
  - There is an association with hormonal contraception and first-time diagnosis of depression, especially among adolescents.
  - Avoiding hormone-free intervals (such as placebo pills) may improve symptoms of dysmenorrhea or premenstrual syndrome.
  - Compliance and preference of daily, weekly, monthly, or longer protocols. Hormonal IUDs remain effective up to 5 years and the copper IUD is effective for up to 10 years.
  - Sexually transmitted infection (STI) should be resolved before placing IUD.
- Emergency contraception can be taken orally after intercourse to prevent pregnancy. If implantation has already occurred, it is not effective. Over-the-counter forms can be used up to 3 days after intercourse. The copper IUD can be used up to 5 days after intercourse; its mechanism of action depends on if fertilization or implantation has occurred.

▶ TREATMENT

- Discussion and/or provision of contraception should occur at annual health assessments beginning at age 13. Adolescents who use contraception at first intercourse are less likely to have an unplanned pregnancy.
- Education includes clarifying misconceptions; the most common reason for not using contraception when not planning pregnancy is that the patient thought they could not get pregnant.
- Starting contraception may cause temporary side effects that usually resolve. If persistent breakthrough bleeding, consider increasing either estrogen or progestin. If persistent nausea, breast tenderness, or headache, consider decreasing either estrogen or progestin. If persistent low mood, decrease progestin. If persistent increase in appetite, acne, or hirsutism, choose a different progestin with fewer androgenic properties.
- Missed doses generally require 7 days of backup contraception, such as condoms, if 48 hours or more has passed since the last dose or application. Restart the missed contraception immediately.

Case Conclusion

Subdermal implant of etonogestrel would be most appropriate at this time. Owing to the previous failure for daily regimen, a long-acting contraception is preferred. The patch has decreased efficacy with obesity. The implant is preferred as her recent STI needs confirmed resolution.

Infertility

Jennifer Johnson, BS, MPAS, DMSc

GENERAL FEATURES

- Infertility is the failure to conceive after 12 months of unprotected sexual intercourse. In female patients older than 35 years, infertility evaluation is appropriate after 6 months of unprotected sexual intercourse.
- Roughly, 85% of couples trying to conceive will conceive within 12 months.
- Infertility can result from congenital and systemic disorders, as well as acquired diseases.
- Common causes of female infertility include ovulatory disorders, endometriosis, abnormalities of the Fallopian tubes, and uterine adhesions.
- Common causes of male infertility include endocrine disorders, spermatogenesis abnormalities, and sperm transport disorders.
- In 10% to 15% of couples, no identifiable cause for infertility can be determined. The prognosis for these couples is worse than for couples in whom a cause is identified.

CLINICAL ASSESSMENT

- Both the male and female partners should be thoroughly assessed for causes of infertility.
- Obtain a complete history from both partners, including menstrual history, prior illnesses, sexually transmitted infection (STI) history, current medical illnesses, medications, potential toxic exposures, contraceptive history, and sexual practices. It is important to verify that the couple has been trying to conceive via unprotected vaginal intercourse without the use of contraceptives.
- Ascertain if either partner has conceived prior. Determine the number of pregnancies, miscarriages, and live births.
- Perform a thorough physical examination on both partners, including a genitourinary examination. Assess the female partner for breast and cervical/uterine abnormalities and assess the male partner for testicular abnormalities and varicoceles. The physical examination is often unremarkable when evaluating for infertility.
- Infertility can result in significant stress for both partners. Screen for anxiety and depression as part of the infertility assessment.

DIAGNOSIS

- Diagnostic testing is aimed at identifying structural or hormonal abnormalities that may contribute to infertility.
- Initial diagnostic studies for the female partner include thyroid-stimulating hormone, luteinizing hormone (LH, to identify a surge before ovulation), luteal-phase progesterone, day 3 serum follicle-stimulating hormone (FSH) and estradiol, total testosterone, anti-Müllerian hormone, antral follicle count, and hysterosalpingogram. Consider pelvic ultrasound if uterine myomas or ovarian cysts are suspected, and laparoscopy should be considered if endometriosis is suspected.
- Initial diagnostic studies for the male partner include LH, FSH, total testosterone, and a semen analysis. Normal semen analysis makes male factors contributing to infertility less likely.
- Abnormal results for any serum diagnostic tests or the semen analysis warrant referral to a reproductive endocrinologist for additional testing. Karyotyping may be considered for both partners.

TREATMENT

- Counsel patients on lifestyle modifications, healthy diet, and exercise and avoidance of alcohol, tobacco, and illicit drugs when trying to conceive.
- Many patients lack understanding of the physiology of conception. Education should be provided on ovulation and the importance of timed, frequent coitus. Vaginal intercourse daily or every other day for 5-7 days before ovulation is recommended. Male partners should ejaculate no more than once daily to avoid sperm count depletion. Discourage the use of lubricants or intravaginal products.
- If a cause of infertility is identified on examination or through diagnostic testing, focus treatment on correcting or mitigating the cause. If anovulation is identified, prescribe letrozole or clomiphene to induce ovulation.
- Patients who are refractory to initial treatment have multiple causal factors resulting in infertility or in whom no abnormalities are identified after diagnostic testing is complete should be referred to a reproductive endocrinologist. Specialized infertility treatments include advanced medical therapy, intrauterine insemination, in vitro fertilization, and surrogacy.

Vaginal and Vulvar Disorders

Taryn Smith, PA-C

GENERAL FEATURES

- Vulvar itching may be attributed to multiple, and at times coexisting, etiologic factors.
- The differential of a vulvovaginal itch should include candidiasis, lichen sclerosis, irritant dermatitis, and vulvar intraepithelial neoplasia (VIN), vulvar carcinoma, and other causes based on history and physical exam.
- Lichen sclerosis causes chronic itching in the genital region. It should be considered if the patient has a yeast infection that recurs or does not respond to treatment. Vaginal discharge is not typical of this condition.
- Lichen sclerosis is chronic and progressive. Early diagnosis and management can help prevent long-term consequences such as scarring of the vaginal introitus and development of vulvar cancer.
- Irritant dermatitis may be quite common, particularly if scented cleaning products, wet wipes, or direct heat are used in the genital area. Wet incontinence pads may also cause maceration and irritation of the skin.
- The vulvar skin is prone to over drying and irritation when the natural oil layer is removed.

CLINICAL ASSESSMENT

- Chronic itching of the vulva should prompt a careful examination of the external genitalia and surrounding skin. Note the appearance of the clitoral hood and clitoris, labia majora and minora, and the perineum.
- Ask the patient to identify the pruritic areas with her fingers and the aid of a mirror, if needed.
- Biopsy may be indicated, particularly if changes to vulvar hygiene and a course of topical steroid ointment do not lead to resolution of itching.
- VIN and vulvar cancer should be considered if itching or visible lesions do not improve. For this reason, follow-up is recommended if a patient is diagnosed with chronic vulvar pruritis.

DIAGNOSIS

- The classic vulvar appearance of lichen sclerosis is thinned, blanched skin, often in a "figure-of-eight" pattern that includes the bilateral labia and the perineum. Loss of labial and/or clitoral hood architecture is seen in more advanced cases.
- Contact dermatitis often results in an erythematous, excoriated, dry rash.
- Satellite lesions are more consistent with vulvar candidiasis. Topical steroid use may change the appearance from classic features, so lack of these should not rule out the diagnosis.

TREATMENT

- Management and prognosis are, in large part, dependent on the diagnosis.
- The goal of treatment for lichen sclerosis is to prevent progression and identify any precancerous or cancerous lesions promptly. Cure is not possible.
- The mainstay of treatment for lichen sclerosis is patient education on self-care and self-examination and the use of a superpotent steroid ointment. Once the itching is controlled, the steroid ointment should be used twice weekly indefinitely to help prevent progression.
- In cases of lichen sclerosis, an annual examination by a practitioner with expertise in vulvar care is recommended.
- Steroid ointment is preferred to cream because it contains fewer additives and absorbs better.
- Treatment for irritant dermatitis is removal of the offending agent(s) and protecting the skin as it heals. This may be achieved by consistent use of a barrier ointment, such as Vaseline. The patient should be counseled that resolution may take weeks or months to achieve.
- Treatment for vulvar candidiasis is topical or oral antifungal, depending on the extent of tissue involvement and presence of complicating factors such as recurrence and chronic disease states. If diabetic, counsel the patient on the importance of blood sugar control.
- Recurrent or persistent itching despite adherence to treatment should prompt consideration of re-biopsy of any suspicious lesions to check for progression to precancer or cancer.

Cervicitis

Gladys Wilkins, MSPAS, PA-C

▶ GENERAL FEATURES

- Cervicitis is an inflammation of the uterine cervix.
- Most commonly caused by a sexually transmitted infection (STI) but can also be caused by mechanical or chemical irritation, radiation, malignancy, or systemic inflammatory diseases
- Urethritis can occur concomitantly in women with cervicitis.
- *Chlamydia trachomatis* is the most common cause of infectious cervicitis and may coexist with gonococci. Other infectious causes include herpes simplex virus (HSV), trichomoniasis, and *Mycoplasma genitalium.*
- Untreated infection can lead to tubo-ovarian abscess, pelvic inflammatory disease, chronic pelvic pain, infertility, and ectopic pregnancy.
- Complications in pregnancy including spontaneous abortion, premature rupture of membranes, and preterm delivery
- Routine screening for chlamydia, gonorrhea, and trichomonas is recommended in all sexually active women under the age of 25 and for older women with risk factors.

▶ CLINICAL ASSESSMENT

- Perform a complete gynecologic and sexual history including age of menarche, last menstrual period, gravida/para, history of pap smear and pap smear results, history of STI, number of sexual partners in the past 3 months as well as number of new partners, condom use, the use of other methods of contraception, exchange of sex for money or drug, and known exposure to STIs.
- Physical examination should include pelvic examination with inspection of the vulva, vagina, and cervix, noting abnormal appearance of vaginal and cervical secretions (mucopurulent, creamy, yellow, frothy, milky) and the presence of any lesions or ulcerations and bimanual examination.
- Evaluate pH of vaginal/cervical discharge, wet mount of vaginal discharge, and laboratory tests for chlamydia, gonorrhea, trichomonas, and mycoplasma.
- Perform urinalysis to rule out pregnancy and urinary tract infection.

▶ DIAGNOSIS

- Purulent or mucopurulent (yellow) vaginal discharge is characteristic of chlamydia or gonorrhea.
- Punctate cervical hemorrhage (strawberry cervix) is a classic finding in *Trichomonas vaginalis* infection.
- Vesicular lesions can indicate HSV infection.
- Genital malodor may be associated with bacterial vaginosis infection or retained foreign body.
- Erosive cervical lesions are concerning for cancer and should be evaluated with pap smear, colposcopy, biopsy, and/or gynecologic oncology referral.
- The presence of cervical motion tenderness and pelvic or abdominal pain may indicate pelvic inflammatory disease.
- Nucleic acid amplification test (NAAT) is the most reliable for the diagnosis of gonorrhea, chlamydia, and mycoplasma and can be performed on vaginal, endocervical, or urine samples for the evaluation of cervicitis.

▶ TREATMENT

- Antimicrobial agents are used to treat specific infections.
- Both patient and partner should abstain from sexual intercourse for 7 days or until completion of therapy.
- The Centers for Disease Control Guidelines for first-line treatment are as follows:
  - Gonorrhea: ceftriaxone 250 mg intramuscularly with azithromycin 1 g PO (both in a single dose regardless of chlamydia testing results)
  - Chlamydia: azithromycin 1 g PO once or doxycycline 100 mg PO BID for 7 days
  - *M. genitalium*: azithromycin 1 g PO once
  - Trichomoniasis: metronidazole 500 mg BID for 7 days or tinidazole 2 g PO as a single dose
  - HSV (initial infection): valacyclovir 1000 mg PO BID for 7-10 days or acyclovir 400 mg PO TID or 200 mg PO 5 times daily for 7-10 days
- Presumptive treatment is recommended for patients when classic symptoms are present and culture is pending, partner has tested positive for an STI and other situations with clinician discretion.
- Consider treatment for both gonorrhea and chlamydia, in areas where gonorrhea is prevalent or in women with significant risk factors.

- Always test for syphilis and HIV in patients diagnosed with any STI.
- If a patient tests positive for an STI, she should be re-tested 3-4 months after treatment because repeat infections are common. Test for a cure at 3-4 weeks after treatment is not recommended unless the patient is pregnant, symptoms persist, noncompliance with treatment is a concern, or there is concern for reinfection.
- Use caution when treating pregnant patients to assure antimicrobial is not contraindicated.
- Counsel patients regarding STD prevention.

CHAPTER
346

Uterine Prolapse

Taryn Smith, PA-C

▶ GENERAL FEATURES

- Vaginal prolapse is a common complaint among women, particularly those who are postmenopausal, have experienced pregnancy, and are overweight or obese.
- Prolapse may also run in families, be associated with collagen disorders, and is more common in those with a history of increased intra-abdominal pressure (eg, chronic straining due to constipation).
- Vaginal prolapse may represent any combination of the following: cystocele (bladder pushing down the anterior vaginal wall), uterovaginal (uterus telescoping down the vaginal cavity), vaginal vault prolapse (collapse of the apical wall after hysterectomy), rectocele (rectum pushing into posterior vaginal wall), or enterocele (small intestines pushing into the posterior wall).
- Prolapse is generally not painful but may be associated with a sense of pressure in the vagina.

▶ CLINICAL ASSESSMENT

- On pelvic examination, a soft mass is noted either protruding from the vaginal introitus or is found within the vaginal cavity. It is usually reducible with gentle pressure. Isolation of the individual vaginal walls with aid of a single speculum blade may be helpful.
- A patient who believes her bladder is prolapsed may actually have one of the other types of prolapse, or a combination of them.
- If long-standing, the prolapsed vaginal epithelium may appear keratinized or eroded if it has been protruding past the vaginal introitus.
- Vulvovaginal atrophy is a common concurrent examination finding but is not required for the diagnosis.
- Hard stool may be palpable in the rectum through the posterior vaginal wall, particularly if the patient is constipated.

- Urinary incontinence is frequently a concurrent condition but may not be directly related to the prolapse. Reduction of the prolapse can worsen stress urinary incontinence. A cystocele can lead to overflow urinary incontinence.

▶ DIAGNOSIS

- Prolapse is a clinical diagnosis, based on examination. Imaging is usually not required.
- Specialists use a numerical system called the POP-Q to map the degree of laxity of each vaginal wall.
- Describing the prolapse with the aid of a diagram or model can help the patient appreciate the nature of the changes.
- In cases of advanced or highly symptomatic prolapse, a referral to a urogynecologist or general gynecologist may be preferred.

▶ TREATMENT

- Options for the management of prolapse include expectant management, pelvic floor physical therapy, fitting for an intravaginal pessary, or surgical correction.
- The choice of treatment is based on the degree of bother to the patient and if any alarming signs and symptoms are present, such as an inability to empty the bladder.
- Vaginal intercourse is typically safe despite the presence of prolapse.
- A prolapsed bladder can be gently reduced by the patient to facilitate emptying of the bladder.
- A prolapse that can be reduced but falls back down is not an emergency but should be managed for patient comfort.
- A prolapse that cannot be reduced may be a surgical emergency and requires immediate evaluation.

CHAPTER 347

Ovarian Cancer

Kelly Marie Joy, MS, MSPAS, PA-C

A 63-year-old G0P0 female presents to her primary care provider complaining of abdominal bloating and early satiety. The patient reports her last menstrual period (LMP) at 56 years of age. She denies any postmenopausal bleeding. The patient also denies a family medical history of ovarian cancer (OC). Physical examination is positive for a large abdominal mass. The mass is firm, mobile, and extends from the pelvis to slightly above the umbilicus. The serum cancer antigen (CA-125) level is 75 U/mL (0-35 U/mL), and the pelvic ultrasound (U/S) is positive for a 22-cm complex cystic mass on the left ovary. This patient is referred for surgical resection of left ovarian tumor.

Histologic examination of the resected ovarian mass is mostly likely to suggest which diagnoses?

▶ GENERAL FEATURES

- OC is the fifth most common cause of cancer death in women and is the leading cause of mortality from gynecologic malignancy.
- Because the symptoms are vague and because there is no effective screening protocol for early detection, OC is often diagnosed at an advanced stage with a low rate of survival.
- Histologic types of OC:
  - Epithelial
    - Accounts for ~90% of all malignant OC
    - Risk factors include age, hereditary risk, early menarche, late menopause, and nulliparity.
    - Reduced risk is associated with parity, breast-feeding, and oral contraceptive use.
  - Germ cell:
    - Begin in reproductive cells. Usually unilateral and occur more frequently in young women
    - Dysgerminomas, teratomas, and endodermal sinus tumors are included in this category.
  - Sex cord-stromal:
    - Composed of various combinations of granulosa, theca, Sertoli, and Leydig cells
    - Granulosa-stromal cell tumors included in this category demonstrate increased estrogen secretion and can be associated with:
      - Pseudoprecocity in young girls, menstrual irregularities in reproductive-aged women, and postmenopausal bleeding in older women
  - Metastatic carcinomas to the ovary:
    - ~5% of ovarian tumors are metastatic.
    - Most frequently from the female genital tract, breast, or gastrointestinal tract

- Other very rare types
- The majority of cases occur sporadically without familial risk.
- ~10% of OC is associated with a known hereditary genetic mutation.
  - In hereditary syndromes, OC tends to present at a younger age.
  - Hereditary breast ovarian cancer (HBOC) syndrome and hereditary nonpolyposis colorectal cancer (HNPCC) syndrome or Lynch syndrome are the two main hereditary syndromes associated with increased risk for OC.
    - Epithelial ovarian cancer (EOC) is the most common OC type in HBOC and Lynch syndromes.

▶ CLINICAL ASSESSMENT

- The symptoms of OC may include:
  - Pelvic/abdominal pain
  - Pain with intercourse
  - Pelvic/abdominal bloating
  - Early satiety
  - Gastroesophageal reflux
  - Bowel dysfunction
  - Bladder dysfunction
  - Hormone imbalance
  - Abnormal uterine bleeding
- Physical examination findings may include:
  - Pelvic/abdominal mass
  - Pelvic/abdominal pain with palpation
  - Ascites

▶ DIAGNOSIS

- Diagnosis can only be made through the histologic examination of a resected ovarian tumor.
- The following preoperative evaluation results suggest increased malignancy risk in a patient with an adnexal mass:
  - Exclusion of other conditions
  - Pelvic U/S findings:
    - Bilateral tumors
    - Complex cystic masses >8-10 cm in diameter
    - Masses that increase in size or complexity within 2 months of initial imaging
  - CA-125 elevation
- If there is a low risk of malignancy, a period of expectant management may be considered.
- If there is a high risk for malignancy, patients are referred for surgical mass resection.

- Labs:
  - CA-125 is a useful tumor marker.
    - Often used for initial evaluation and for surveillance
    - Does not identify specific types of OC
    - Can be elevated in noncancerous conditions such as endometriosis
    - Normal levels do not rule out cancer.
  - Serum LDH, AFP, and hCG are useful for both diagnosis and postoperative surveillance of germ cell malignancies.
  - Inhibins and anti-Müllerian hormones (AMH) are useful markers for granulosa-stromal cell tumors.
- Additional imaging:
  - Chest x-ray should be considered to rule out metastasis.
  - CT and MRI:
    - May be useful to determine the presence or extent of lymphadenopathy and metastases
  - PET scan:
    - May contribute to the specificity of a CT scan

▶ TREATMENT

- Treatment based on surgical staging
- Surgery:
  - The primary treatment for OC
  - Typically includes total abdominal hysterectomy, BSO, surgical staging, and tumor debulking
- Adjuvant therapy:
  - Includes chemotherapy and radiation

Case Conclusion

Epithelial histotypes including high-grade serous carcinoma are the most common OC type. The average age at the time of diagnosis of serous carcinoma is 61. This patient also reports nulliparity and late menopause, which are the risk factors for serous carcinoma.

CHAPTER 348

Premenstrual Dysphoric Disorder

Brittany Strelow, MS, PA-C

A 32-year-old female G1P1 with no past medical history presents to primary care with a history of mood swings, irritability, and fatigue that have been present for the past year and resolve after menses begins. She also notes that symptoms are significantly distressing and are starting to affect her work and friendships. Patient began menarche at age 11. Last menstrual period (LMP) was 1 week ago. Menstrual cycles are on average 30 days, with 6 days of bleeding. She is also experiencing physical symptoms in addition to fatigue before menstruation. Which symptoms are associated with premenstrual dysphoric disorder (PMDD)?

▶ GENERAL FEATURES

- PMDD is a severe variant of premenstrual syndrome (PMS).
- Physical and behavioral symptoms of PMDD interfere with normal daily activities.
- Symptoms follow a predictable pattern over most menstrual cycles.

▶ CLINICAL ASSESSMENT

- Symptoms begin in the late luteal phase (5 days before the onset of menses).
- Symptoms resolve after menses begin (within 4 days of the onset of menses).
- Symptoms last an average of 6 days per month.
- Symptoms occur during three or more consecutive menstrual cycles
- Physical signs and symptoms may include:
  - Bloating
  - Breast tenderness
  - Fatigue
  - Changes in sleep and eating habits
  - Headaches
  - Hot flashes
- Evaluation:
  - Daily Record of Severity of Problems (DRSP)
    - Kept for at least 2 months to show exacerbations of signs and symptoms before menses and resolution after menses
    - Consists of 17 common PMS symptoms
    - Patients rate each symptom on a six-point scale, ranging from 1 (none at all) to 6 (extreme).

- Patients should be screened for anxiety, depression, and substance abuse.
- Physical examination is usually unremarkable.
- Laboratory testing to exclude other medical conditions may include:
  - CBC (anemia)
  - Thyroid-stimulating hormone (TSH) (hyperthyroidism or hypothyroidism)
  - If menstrual cycles are irregular:
    - Follicle-stimulating hormone (FSH)
    - Prolactin
    - Serum human chorionic gonadotropin (hCG)

▶ DIAGNOSIS

- According to the *Diagnostic and Statistical Manual of Mental Disorders*, Fifth Edition (*DSM-5*), the criteria for PMDD include:
  - Symptoms present in most menstrual cycles in the preceding year.
  - At least five symptoms present the week before the onset of menses.
  - Symptoms *improve* within a few days after the onset of menses.
  - *Minimal* or absent symptoms in the week after menses
  - One (or more) of the following symptoms must be present:
    - Mood swings, feeling suddenly sad or tearful, or increased sensitivity to rejection
    - Irritability or anger or increased interpersonal conflicts
    - Depressed mood, feelings of hopelessness, or self-deprecating thoughts
    - Anxiety, tension, and/or feelings of being keyed up or on edge
  - One (or more) of the following symptoms additionally present, to reach a total of *five* symptoms:
    - Decreased interest in usual activities
    - Subjective difficulty in concentration
    - Lethargy, easy fatigability, or marked lack of energy
    - Marked change in appetite, overeating, or specific food cravings
    - Hypersomnia or insomnia
    - A sense of being overwhelmed or out of control
    - Physical symptoms such as breast tenderness or swelling, joint or muscle pain, a sensation of "bloating," or weight gain
  - Symptoms are associated with clinically significant distress or interference with work, school, usual social activities, or relationships with others.
  - Not an exacerbation of symptoms of another disorder
  - Symptoms are not attributable to the physiologic effects of a substance or another medical condition.

- Differential diagnosis:
  - Mood and/or anxiety disorders
  - Menopause transition
  - Hypothyroidism
  - Hyperthyroidism
  - Substance abuse
- Patients diagnosed with PMDD have a higher risk of suicidality.

▶ TREATMENT

- Lifestyle interventions:
  - Exercise:
    - Moderate activity 3-4 times weekly for >30 minutes
  - Relaxation techniques:
    - Mindfulness, meditation, yoga
  - Healthy nutrition
  - Adequate sleep
- Pharmacologic treatment:
  - Based on severity and type of symptoms
  - Combined therapy may be appropriate
  - Regimens:
    - Continuous
      - Effective for low-level symptoms during non-premenstrual intervals
      - Most effective for severe physical symptoms
      - Convenient and simple
    - Luteal-phase therapy:
      - Started on cycle day 14
      - Discontinued at the onset of menses
      - Less expensive and fewer side effects
      - Higher doses may be needed to treat symptoms.
    - Symptom-onset therapy:
      - Begins at point of symptom onset
      - Discontinued first few days of menses
- Antidepressant:
  - Best for mood-predominant symptoms and patients who do not desire contraception
  - More effective if taken continuously rather than during the luteal phase only
  - Selective serotonin reuptake inhibitors (SSRIs) or serotonin-norepinephrine reuptake inhibitors (SNRIs) effective in PMDD include:
    - Fluoxetine
    - Sertraline
    - Other SSRIs and SNRIs also likely equally effective:
      - Venlafaxine
      - Citalopram
- Oral contraceptive:
  - Best for physical manifestations
  - Patient desires contraception

- Can be used if other indications for hormonal therapy are present:
  - Menorrhagia
  - Acne
  - Irregular cycles
- Continuous or extended combination (estrogen and progesterone) regimens to decrease hormonal fluctuations
  - Suppress ovulation and improve physical and behavioral symptoms

- Special consideration for the progestin drospirenone
  - Pose a slightly increased absolute risk of venous thromboembolism compared to oral contraceptives containing levonorgestrel

Case Conclusion

Physical symptoms such as bloating, breast tenderness, fatigue, changes in sleep and eating habits, and headaches can be experienced by patients with PMDD the week before menstruation.

CHAPTER 349

Dysmenorrhea

Danielle O'Laughlin, PA-C, MS

▶ GENERAL FEATURES

- Dysmenorrhea refers to painful menstrual cramps and is classified as either primary or secondary.
- Primary dysmenorrhea is defined as painful menses without underlying pathology. This generally starts shortly after menarche and is more common in young women.
  - The diagnosis of primary dysmenorrhea can be made by history alone if pain is reported during the first 3 days of the menstrual cycle.
- Secondary dysmenorrhea is defined as painful menses with underlying pathology and typically occurs in women slightly older than with primary dysmenorrhea.
  - The diagnosis of secondary dysmenorrhea often requires pelvic examination and additional workup.
  - Endometriosis is the most common cause of secondary dysmenorrhea.
- Risk factors:
- Age:
  - Teens to early 20s for primary dysmenorrhea; 20s-40s for secondary dysmenorrhea
- Family history of dysmenorrhea/genetics
- Nulliparity
- Onset of menarche before age 12
- Low BMI (<20 kg/m^2) or high BMI (>30 kg/m^2)
- Long-term menstrual cycles
- Heavy menstrual flow
- Smoking
- Mental health issues, such as depression, anxiety, and disrupted social support networks

▶ CLINICAL ASSESSMENT

- History and physical examination:

- History alone can be used to diagnosis primary dysmenorrhea. Pelvic examination is generally not required.
- Secondary dysmenorrhea often requires pelvic examination, which can be normal.

▶ DIAGNOSIS

- The diagnosis of primary dysmenorrhea can be made clinically in adolescents who meet criteria with pain in the first 3 days of the menstrual cycle.
- Sexually active adolescents should be screened for chlamydia and gonorrhea.
- In women with secondary dysmenorrhea, pelvic examination may be normal or may show signs of PID. Transvaginal or transabdominal ultrasound may demonstrate adenomyosis, leiomyoma, or ovarian or bowel endometrioma.

▶ TREATMENT

- Treatment for primary dysmenorrhea can be started immediately. First-line therapy is use of nonsteroidal anti-inflammatory drugs (NSAIDs). Other treatments include cyclooxygenase-2 (COX-2) inhibitors, oral contraceptives, topical heat, and high-frequency transcutaneous electrical nerve stimulation (TENS).
- Treatment for secondary dysmenorrhea depends on the underlying cause. If endometriosis is the cause, treatment is aimed at hormonal suppression, conservative laparoscopic surgical debulking, and occasionally hysterectomy.

Menopause

Holly Ann West, MPAS, DHEd, PA-C

▶ GENERAL FEATURES

- Characteristics of the transitional states of menopause:
  - Early perimenopause = variable time frame marked by inconsistent ovulation
  - Late perimenopause = ovarian estrogen production fluctuates unpredictably and some or all cycles are anovulatory, resulting in menstrual irregularities and menopausal symptoms
  - Menopause = cessation of estrogen production marked by amenorrhea for 12 consecutive months; median age is 51.4
  - Postmenopause = persistent hypoestrogenism
- Premature menopause (formerly referred to as premature ovarian failure but is now termed *primary ovarian insufficiency*) = menopause age <40 years
- Surgical menopause = menopause secondary to bilateral oophorectomy with or without hysterectomy

▶ CLINICAL ASSESSMENT

Manifestations of perimenopause and menopause are due to estrogen deficiency. A complete history to elicit severity and the impact on quality of life is an essential component of the evaluation.

Evaluate for the following:
- Menstrual cycle irregularity secondary to oligo-ovulation and anovulation, which may begin in late reproductive years
- Vasomotor symptoms (ie, hot flashes or hot flushes) occur in 68% to 93% of women and may be first physical manifestation of declining estrogen production.
  - Characterized by sudden sensation of heat with flushing and perspiration, especially in the upper trunk, face, and neck. Some experience chills, palpitations, or tachycardia.
  - Episodes can occur throughout the day but are common at night (referred to as "night sweats").
- Sleep disturbances (eg, insomnia, nighttime and early waking) are often caused by the hot flashes.
- Mood changes such as depression and anxiety; worsened by sleep deprivation
- Genitourinary syndrome of menopause (GSM):
  - Vulvovaginal atrophy occurs when estrogen-dependent tissue in the vagina become atrophied (atrophic vaginitis).
    - Symptoms: vaginal dryness, pruritis, burning, spotting, and dyspareunia
    - Physical examination findings: pale vaginal wall lacking rugae, introital narrowing, decreased moisture, and diminished turgor of the vulvar skin
  - Lower urinary tract symptoms include urgency, frequency, and urge incontinence.
- Skin and hair changes such as decreased skin elasticity, increased facial hair, scalp hair loss, and acne
- Long-term effects of estrogen deficiency:
  - Increased rate of bone loss for the first 5 years of menopause
  - Increased cardiovascular disease risk due to dyslipidemia (increase total cholesterol and LDL; decrease in HDL)
  - Dementia; however, there is no clear evidence that dementia is menopausal related

▶ DIAGNOSIS

- In healthy perimenopausal women who present with irregular menstrual cycles and exhibit menopausal symptoms, perimenopause can be diagnosed.
  - Rule out other causes of abnormal uterine bleeding, including endometrial neoplasia.
- In healthy perimenopausal women who have 12 months of amenorrhea, menopause can be diagnosed.
  - A high serum follicle-stimulating hormone is not required to make a diagnosis of perimenopause or menopause but can be confirmatory.

▶ TREATMENT

- Hot flashes
- Lifestyle modifications (eg, use fans, dress in layers that can be removed, avoid triggers such as caffeine, alcohol, spicy foods)
- Nonhormonal therapies:
  - Serotonin-norepinephrine reuptake inhibitors (SNRIs) such as venlafaxine and selective serotonin reuptake inhibitors (SSRIs) such as paroxetine
  - Gabapentin
  - Clonidine
- Systemic hormonal therapy (HT):
  - Goals are to relieve menopausal symptoms affecting quality of life.
  - Requires an individualized patient approach weighing risk/benefit: suggest lowest effective dose for shortest duration necessary.
  - In women without a uterus: continuous estrogen-only therapy (ET); FDA-approved formulations include oral, transdermal (patch, cream, gel, mist), vaginal ring, or injectable options.

- In women with an intact uterus: estrogen plus progestin therapy (EPT) or estrogen plus a selective estrogen receptor modulator (SERM; bazedoxifene) to prevent endometrial hyperplasia
- Contraindications to ET include undiagnosed abnormal uterine bleeding; known or suspected estrogen-dependent neoplasia, breast cancer, active or previous venous thromboembolic event (pulmonary embolus [PE] or deep vein thrombosis [DVT]), stroke, transient ischemic attack, myocardial infraction, and active liver disease.
- Risks of ET include thromboembolic disease (DVT, PE, thrombotic stroke).

- Risks of EPT include slight increased risk of breast cancer.
- Lower genital tract atrophy:
  - Vaginal moisturizers and lubricants
  - Low-dose vaginal estrogen; FDA-approved formulations include tablets, creams, and ring.
  - Oral SERM (ospemifene)
- General treatment information:
  - HT is no longer indicated solely for the prevention of chronic diseases (coronary heart disease, osteoporosis, cognitive function, dementia), but there is osteoporosis benefit for women on HT.

CHAPTER 351

Vaginitis

Danielle O'Laughlin, PA-C, MS
Dawn Colomb-Lippa, PA-C, MHS

A 28-year-old G0P0 sexually active female on oral contraceptive pills presents to clinic with 1 week of vaginal discharge. She describes intermittent itching and irritation of the vulva and vagina and dysuria. Discharge is described as white, thick, and curdy. The physical examination revels white, thick, and curdy discharge with mild erythema to the vulva and vagina.

GENERAL FEATURES

- Vaginitis, also called vulvovaginitis, is inflammation of the vagina, which can cause discharge, pruritus, and pain.
- Other vaginitis symptoms can include dyspareunia, dysuria, odor and vulvar burning, pruritus, or pain.
- Vaginitis is commonly caused by a fungus (candidiasis), a protozoon (*Trichomonas*) or a disruption of the normal vaginal flora (bacterial vaginosis).
- History and physical examination, including wet mount and pH measurement, can aid in the diagnostic evaluation of vaginitis.
- Risk factors for vaginitis depend on the cause:
  - Candidiasis risk factors include a change in the vaginal pH, use of oral contraceptive pills, pregnancy, diabetes, and recent antibiotic use.
  - Trichomonas risk factors include sexual activity and multiple sexual partners.
  - Bacterial vaginosis risk factors include sexual activity, multiple sexual partners, douching, cigarette smoking, social stressors (homelessness, poverty, safety concerns), and lack of hydrogen peroxide–producing lactobacilli.

CLINICAL ASSESSMENT

- The history and physical examination findings are specific to the cause.
  - Candidiasis presents with increased discharge (white, thick, curdy), dysuria and vulvar/vaginal pruritus, and burning. Vulvar and vaginal erythema is often found.
  - Trichomonas presents with increased discharge (white/gray/yellow or green, frothy), increased odor, dysuria, and pruritus. Vaginal or cervical erythema (strawberry cervix) can be present.
  - Bacterial vaginosis presents with increased discharge (white, thin, homogeneous) and a fishy odor.

DIAGNOSIS

- Diagnosis relies on history and physical examination, which includes assessment of the vaginal secretions by wet mount and measurement of the vaginal pH. Each vaginitis cause has a specific wet mount characteristic and pH range. The normal vaginal pH is 3.8-4.5.
  - Candidiasis:
    - pH <4.5
    - Hyphae or spores present on wet mount
    - Positive *Candida* culture
  - Trichomonas:
    - pH >4.5
    - Motile trichomonads with increased white cells on wet mount
    - Rapid antigen and nucleic acid amplification test (NAAT)

- Bacterial vaginosis:
  - pH >4.5
  - Amsel's criteria (must meet 3/4): pH >4.5, thin watery discharge, >20% clue cells on wet mount, positive whiff test (amine odor after adding 10% potassium hydroxide to discharge)
  - Nugent score: Gram stain scoring system (must score 7-10)

▶ TREATMENT

- Treatment varies based on the cause of vaginitis and medication available.
  - Candidiasis:
    - Intravaginal use of the azoles (butoconazole, clotrimazole, miconazole, tioconazole, or terconazole) at varying doses OR
    - Oral fluconazole once at 150 mg
  - Trichomonas:
    - Oral metronidazole once at 2 g; metronidazole 500 mg twice a day for 7 days; OR tinidazole once at 2 g
  - Bacterial vaginosis:
    - Oral metronidazole 500 mg twice a day for 7 days; tinidazole 2 g for 3 days; tinidazole 1 g

for 5 days; clindamycin 300 mg twice daily for 7 days
  - Intravaginal 0.75% metronidazole gel one 5 g application daily for 5 days; 2% clindamycin cream one 5 g application every night for 7 days; clindamycin ovules 100 mg once at bedtime for 3 days
- Prognosis:
  - With proper treatment of candidiasis, trichomonas, and bacterial vaginosis, the prognosis is good.
  - Patients with bacterial vaginosis have higher risks of other sexually transmitted infections, pelvic inflammatory disease, infertility, cervicitis, endometritis, cystitis, postgynecologic and postpartum infections, preterm delivery, and cervical intraepithelial neoplasia.

Case Conclusion

The classic symptoms of candidiasis include an increased white, thick, and curdy vaginal discharge; dysuria; pruritus; and burning. Physical examination often reveals white, thick, and curdy vaginal discharge with vulvar and vaginal erythema. The diagnosis can be made by the presence of spores and hyphae on wet mount. The vaginal pH is <4.5.

CHAPTER 352

Endometriosis and Leiomyomas

Catherine Nowak, MS, PA-C, DFAAPA

A 26-year-old woman presents to your primary care office for a follow-up visit for chronic pelvic pain. She has been having low pelvic pain associated with her menstrual periods for over 5 years. She states she and her partner have stopped using contraceptive methods and have been trying to conceive for almost a year without success. She reports no abnormal uterine bleeding. What is the most likely cause of her chronic pelvic pain and infertility?

▶ GENERAL FEATURES

- Endometriosis:
  - The presence of endometrial tissue found outside the uterus; most common locations are in the pelvis or on the ovary.
  - Common finding in women who complain of pelvic pain and/or infertility
  - Endometrial implants respond to changes in estrogen and can thicken and bleed like endometrium, causing pain.

- The definitive cause is unknown, but the most widely accepted theory is that of retrograde menstruation where endometrial cells in the menstrual blood implant outside the endometrium. Other theories include vascular and lymphatic dissemination, coeleomic (body cavity) metaplasia, and immune dysfunction that allow proliferation of the endometrial tissues outside the endometrial cavity.
  - Most common in nulliparous women in their 20s and 30s
  - Frequently associated with infertility
  - Risk factors: family history, exposure to diethylstilbestrol (DES) in utero, early menarche, heavy menstrual flow, and shorter menstrual cycles (<27 days)
  - Protective factors: parity, longer duration of lactation, late menarche
- Leiomyomas (uterine fibroids):
  - Benign tumor of the uterus that is classified according to its location. Intramural fibroids are located in the uterine wall; submucosal fibroids are located below the endometrium and may extent into the

uterine cavity; subserosal fibroids originate from the myometrium and may extend out of the uterus. Fibroids may also be found on the cervix or broad ligament. They may be pedunculated.

- Often asymptomatic and found incidentally on imaging
- Risk factors include nulliparity, obesity, early menarche, Black race, age > 40.
- Women with uterine fibroids are at increased risk for endometrial cancer.
- Leiomyomas are estrogen dependent and may enlarge during pregnancy and reduce in size after menopause.
- Most common indication for hysterectomy

▶ CLINICAL ASSESSMENT

- Endometriosis:
  - Triad of dysmenorrhea, dyspareunia, and infertility
  - Dysmenorrhea may start 1-2 days before menses and persist during and for several days after menses.
  - Women may report pain with bowel movements and/or urination.
  - May be asymptomatic and found incidentally during surgery or pelvic imaging
  - Women may present with infertility as adhesions can block fallopian tubes and inflammation associated with endometriosis can interfere with movement of, or damage, egg or sperm.
  - Physical examination findings depend on the size and location of endometrial implants and may include decreased mobility of cervix or uterus, fixed or retroverted uterus, cervical motion tenderness, and adnexal mass.
- Leiomyomas:
  - Women may present with prolonged, heavy menstrual bleeding; pelvic pressure or fullness; infertility or obstetric complications; urinary frequency or incomplete bladder emptying; or constipation.
  - Physical examination can identify an enlarged, irregularly shaped, nontender uterus.

▶ DIAGNOSIS

- Endometriosis:
  - No pathognomonic findings for endometriosis
  - Serum cancer antigen (CA125) may be elevated in women with endometriosis and other benign and cancerous diseases, so it is not recommended as a screening test.
  - Transvaginal ultrasound or MRI may show ovarian cysts or nodules or the rectovaginal septum or bladder.
  - Laparoscopy may be performed for definitive diagnosis by direct visualization.

- Leiomyomas:
  - Transvaginal ultrasound is the initial diagnostic imaging test of choice.
  - Sonohysterography or hysteroscopy may be used to visualize the endometrial cavity.
  - MRI reserved for complicated cases and before surgical intervention.
  - Laboratory tests are generally not indicated unless evaluating for anemia, pregnancy, or ruling out other causes of menorrhagia.

▶ TREATMENT

- Endometriosis:
  - Goals of treatment include pain management, preservation of fertility, prevention of complications related to intrapelvic cysts, and adhesions.
  - Treatment options include:
    - Medical management with NSAIDs, combined hormonal contraceptives (commonly used extended cycle), progestin contraceptives (IUD, implant, injection, pill), gonadotropin-releasing agonists/antagonists, and aromatase inhibitors.
    - Surgical management with conservative surgery to remove endometrial implants or, less common, hysterectomy with bilateral salpingo-oophorectomy
- Leiomyomas:
  - Goals of treatment are to relieve symptoms, decrease uterus size, and increase fertility.
    - Treatment may not be necessary if asymptomatic.
    - Medical therapy may include GnRH analogs, raloxifene, mifepristone, progestin, or danazol.
  - Surgical/procedural therapy:
    - Hysterectomy—definitive procedure
    - Myomectomy: removal of fibroid only, fertility-preserving procedure
    - Uterine artery embolization, radiofrequency ablation
    - Myolysis: laparoscopic surgery that coagulates vessels by electric current that supply blood to the fibroid, causing it to shrink
    - Endometrial ablation: destroys the lining of the uterus resulting in inability to become pregnant

Case Conclusion

Endometriosis is a common cause of infertility because adhesions can obstruct the fallopian tubes and pelvic inflammation can affect fertilization of the egg by sperm. Since the patient is trying to conceive she should be referred for evaluation and consideration of fertility preservation.

CHAPTER 353

Ovarian Cysts and Polycystic Ovary Syndrome

Leocadia Conlon, PhD, MPH, PA-C

A 20-year-old female complains of left lower quadrant dull pain that began 2 days before the start of her menses. Her last menstrual period (LMP) was 7 days ago. Physical examination shows left lower quadrant (LLQ) tenderness with deep palpation, no rebound or guarding, and unremarkable pelvic examination without cervical motion tenderness. Transvaginal ultrasound demonstrates a left ovarian complex cyst, 5.2 cm in diameter, with a thick crenulated vascular wall ("ring of fire"). Urine pregnancy test is negative. What is the next best step in this patient's management?

▶ GENERAL FEATURES

- Ovarian cysts:
  - An ovarian cyst is a sac filled with fluid or other tissue that forms in, or on, an ovary.
  - Ovarian cysts are classified as functional (physiologic) cysts or ovarian cystic neoplasms.
  - Functional ovarian cysts derive mass from accumulation of intrafollicular fluids and are the most common ovarian cyst in prepubertal and reproductive-aged women. Types of functional ovarian cysts include: follicular cysts, corpus luteum cysts, and theca lutein cysts.
    - Follicular cysts occur when a follicle fails to rupture and continues to grow. Most are 2–5 cm in diameter, but may grow as large as 15 cm.
    - Corpus luteum cysts occur when the corpus luteum (formed after ovulation and release of oocyte) fails to involute and continues to grow.
    - Follicular and corpus luteum cysts can be hemorrhagic. Granulosa layer of ovary is avascular at time of ovulation; after ovulation, it becomes vascularized by thin-walled vessels, which erupt easily, giving rise to hemorrhagic cysts.
    - Theca lutein cyst is a luteinized follicular cyst that forms as a result of overstimulation from high human chorionic gonadotropin (hCG) levels. Often seen in multiple gestations or ovarian hyperstimulation (as in fertility treatment). Ovaries can enlarge up to 20-30 cm in diameter.
  - Ovarian cystic neoplasms derive mass from cellular proliferation.
    - Teratoma (dermoid) cysts arise from single germ cell and may contain mature tissue from any of the three germ layers: ectodermal (skin and hair), mesodermal (muscle, urinary), or endodermal (GI, lung) origin.
    - Endometrioma filled with menstrual blood and endometrial tissue. Either from retrograde menstruation or bleeding from endometric implant itself. Form as a result of endometriosis.
    - Serous or mucinous cystadenoma cysts arise from surface epithelial cells and are lined by cells similar to those lining the fallopian tubes.
- Polycystic ovary syndrome (PCOS):
  - Complex endocrine disorder characterized by ovarian dysfunction and hyperandrogenism. Initial discovery of PCOS described women with enlarge ovaries and multiple small follicular cysts. However, multifollicular ovarian morphology is not present in all patients with PCOS, which has led to a shift away from focusing on the presences of multiple cysts.

▶ CLINICAL ASSESSMENT

- Ovarian cysts:
  - Most ovarian cysts are asymptomatic and found incidentally.
  - If symptomatic, may present with dull ache or pelvic fullness. Symptoms of pain are often exacerbated by certain activities, such as exercise. Sharp or severe pain is concerning for complication of ovarian cyst rupture or torsion.
  - Complications of functional ovarian cysts and ovarian cystic neoplasms include hemorrhage, ovarian torsion, and cyst rupture. Teratomas can rarely cause immune-mediated encephalitis.
  - Symptoms of ovarian cysts may mimic tubal pregnancy, pelvic inflammatory disease, and ovarian malignancy.
- PCOS:
  - Presenting signs and symptoms of PCOS are associated with ovarian dysfunction (menstrual irregularities) and/or cutaneous hyperandrogenism (hirsutism and/or moderate-severe acne).
  - Menstrual irregularities most often present with complaints of secondary amenorrhea due to anovulatory cycles. Some patients may also experience oligomenorrhea or dysfunctional uterine bleeding.
  - Hirsutism is the presence of dark coarse hair growth in a male-like pattern (upper lip, chin, sideburns, neck, periumbilical, chest, upper back, around nipple area). Dark hair growth on arms and lower legs is not hirsutism. Use of a validated numerical scale, such as the modified Ferriman-Gallwey scale, to assess hirsutism is recommended.

- Acne associated with clinical hyperandrogenism of PCOS should be suspected when moderate-to-severe acne is resistant to standard acne treatments.
- Clinical presentation of menstrual irregularities and cutaneous hyperandrogenism as potential signs of PCOS are often overlooked in adolescents due to difficulty distinguishing between manifestations of PCOS and normal physiologic changes of puberty.
- PCOS is associated with increased lifelong risk for complications of metabolic and reproductive health to include obesity, insulin resistance, impaired glucose tolerance, type 2 DM, cardiovascular disease, fatty liver disease, infertility, endometrial hyperplasia, and endometrial cancer.
- Complications of PCOS, such as infertility, may be the initial clinical presentation in patients with a delayed diagnosis. PCOS is the most common cause of female infertility in the United States.
- Research has demonstrated negative impact on quality of life and increased prevalence of anxiety and depression in both adolescents and adults with PCOS.

▶ DIAGNOSIS

- Ovarian cysts:
  - Ultrasound is gold standard for diagnosis of ovarian cysts. Transvaginal ultrasound (TVUS) is preferred.
  - MRI is used for inconclusive or definitive results. CT is discouraged for evaluation of ovarian cysts due to poor discrimination of soft-tissue and radiation exposure.
  - Most ovarian cysts and neoplasms are benign; classified according to cell type and histologic appearance as benign, borderline (low malignancy potential), or invasive.
  - Follicular cysts appear smooth, thin walled, and unilocular.
  - Corpus luteum cysts have varied sonographic characteristics: they can appear complex and often demonstrate brightly colored ring because of high vascularity (termed *ring of fire*). Because of their more complex appearance on ultrasound, corpus luteum cysts are referred to as the "great imitator." Ring of fire is also a finding in ectopic pregnancies.
  - Theca lutein cysts are often bilateral, multiple smooth-walled cysts.
  - Teratomas (dermoid cysts) display distinct linear demarcations on sonography where there is fat-fluid or hair. Cysts are unilocular and usually contain one area of localized growth of dermoid material that protrudes into the cyst cavity, referred to as the Rokitansky protuberance.
  - Cystadenomas are thin walled on ultrasound, unilocular or multilocular, and range in size from 5 to 20 cm.

- Endometriomas are noted as complex cysts on ultrasound with old blood contained in the cyst characterized as chocolate-colored fluid. Thus, the classic appearance on ultrasound is referred to as "chocolate cysts."
- Sizes of ovarian cysts can range from a 2-3 mm to 20-30 cm in diameter for some cysts (eg, theca lutein cysts and teratomas).
- PCOS:
  - PCOS is a diagnosis of exclusion. Must rule out other causes of menstrual irregularities and/or hyperandrogenism: pregnancy, thyroid dysfunction, hyperprolactinemia, and nonclassic congenital adrenal hyperplasia.
  - Diagnostic criteria differ for adolescents and adults because of similarities between PCOS symptoms and normal findings in puberty.
  - 2013 Endocrine Society Clinical Practice Guidelines recommend the Rotterdam Criteria for the diagnosis of PCOS in adult women. Rotterdam requires that two of the following three findings are present AND exclusion of other causes: (1) menstrual irregularities, (2) clinical hyperandrogenism (hirsutism or moderate-severe acne) or biochemical (elevated serum testosterone), or (3) multifollicular (polycystic) ovarian morphology on sonography.
  - 2015 Pediatric Endocrine Society Practice Guidelines recommend the following criteria for the diagnosis of PCOS in adolescents: otherwise unexplained (exclusion of other causes) combination of menstrual irregularities that persist 2 years after menarche and evidence of biochemical (elevated testosterone levels) or clinical hyperandrogenism. Clinical hyperandrogenism in this population is defined as moderate-to-severe hirsutism. Acne is not considered evidence of clinical hyperandrogenism to meet diagnostic criteria.
  - Ultrasound evidence of polycystic ovarian morphology (PCOM) is not indicated in adolescents. Ovarian volume is increased in puberty, and follicle size changes with age, with the greatest number of small follicles present during adolescence. The presence of PCOM in an adolescent who does not have hyperandrogenism/irregular menses does not indicate a diagnosis of PCOS.

▶ TREATMENT

- Ovarian cysts:
  - Management recommendations vary based on size, age (premenopausal vs. postmenopausal), and characteristics of cyst (benign vs. indeterminate vs. potentially malignant).
  - Ovarian cysts with malignant qualities require surgical evaluation in all age groups.

- Most functional cysts resolve spontaneously within 6 months of identification. Usually expectant management unless there are complications of cyst rupture or ovarian torsion.
- Management may include serial TVUS, serum CA125, MRI, and/or surgical evaluation.
- For patients who experience multiple recurrence of symptomatic functional ovarian cysts, combined hormonal oral contraception suppresses ovarian activity and protects against ovarian cyst formation. Incidence of functional ovarian cysts increases with progestin-only contraception.
- Endometriomas, repeat TVUS in 6-12 weeks, if persistent, follow with yearly TVUS.
- Teratomas (dermoid cysts), in most cases, require surgical removal. Little evidence to support surveillance of dermoid cysts.
- PCOS:
  - Lifestyle modification is the first-line treatment for all patients with PCOS.
  - Additional treatment should be individualized to optimize symptom relief and reduce risk of long-term complications.
  - Combined oral hormonal contraceptives are recommended for menstrual irregularities and clinical hyperandrogenism (hirsutism and/or moderate-severe acne).

- Metformin helps to improve metabolic/glycemic abnormalities associated with PCOS and can also help with regulation of menses.
- Combined oral hormonal contraceptives and metformin can be used together and are beneficial and safe to use in adolescents with PCOS.
- Screen women with PCOS for diabetes and other metabolic complications, such as obesity and hypertension, throughout their life span.
- Evaluate for mood disorders (anxiety and depression).
- Patients with prolonged history of anovulatory cycles associated with PCOS should be evaluated for endometrial hyperplasia and risk of endometrial cancer.
- Clomiphene is the first-line therapy for PCOS-associated infertility.

Case Conclusion

This patient most likely has a functional ovarian cyst. The most appropriate management is to monitor symptoms and repeat ultrasound in 6-12 weeks to ensure resolution.

SECTION C *Obstetrics*

CHAPTER 354 Ectopic Pregnancy

Holly Ann West, MPAS, DHEd, PA-C

▶ GENERAL FEATURES

- An ectopic pregnancy is a pregnancy implanting anywhere other than the endometrium of the uterine cavity.
  - The most common site is the fallopian tubes, with 80% in the ampullary segment; other sites include ovarian, abdominal, cornual (interstitial), cervical, and cesarean scar.
- A heterotopic pregnancy = an ectopic pregnancy co-occurs with an intrauterine pregnancy (IUP) (more common in women who under in vitro fertilization)
- Ectopic pregnancy remains one of the leading causes of death in the first trimester; rupture of the structure where implantation occurs can result in life-threatening hemorrhage.

- Risk factors:
  - Up to 50% have no known risk factors; however, major risks include previous ectopic pregnancy, acute or recurrent pelvic inflammatory/infectious processes (pelvic inflammatory disease, salpingitis, chlamydia and gonorrhea infections), prior pelvic or fallopian tube surgery, infertility, and women who undergo tubal sterilization and then experience sterilization failure.
  - In women who have assisted reproductive technology, tubal factor infertility and embryo transfer are associated with an increased risk of ectopic pregnancy.
  - Less significant risk factors include advanced age and smoking.
  - Note: In women with an intrauterine device (IUD), an ectopic is less likely because pregnancy is less likely; however, if a pregnancy occurs, there is a higher chance of a tubal pregnancy.

▶ CLINICAL ASSESSMENT

- Any sexually active woman of reproductive age with amenorrhea followed by vaginal bleeding and/or abdominal or pelvic pain should be evaluated for an ectopic pregnancy.
- Initial evaluation of signs of hemodynamic stability and/or acute abdomen is crucial because a ruptured ectopic can be life-threatening
- Abdominal examination to evaluate for acute abdomen signs (severe pain, rebound tenderness, rigidity and guarding)
- Pelvic examination to include a speculum examination (to identify source and volume of bleeding) and bimanual examination (to elicit cervical motion tenderness or palpation of an adnexal mass)

▶ DIAGNOSIS

- Evaluate potential pregnancy using a combination of β-hCG measurements and transvaginal ultrasonography (TVUS). If pregnancy is confirmed, determine whether this is a normal intrauterine or an abnormal pregnancy (eg, ectopic, incomplete or complete abortion).
  - TVUS is used to determine the presence of free fluid in the pelvic cul-de-sac (worrisome for rupture) and the location of pregnancy; a definitive IUP (visualization of a gestational sac with a yolk sac or embryo) eliminates an ectopic, except in cases of heterotopic pregnancy.
    - Visualization depends on gestational age and β-hCG levels.
      - The absence of an IUP on TVUS with a β-hCG above the discriminatory zone of 3500 IU/L is

suspicious of an ectopic pregnancy or a failed pregnancy.
  - Note: The term *Pregnancy of Unknown Location* is used as a transient diagnosis in instances where an ectopic has not been visualized and a failed IUP has not been excluded.
- Initial quantitative β-hCG is obtained to establish the discriminatory zone (the level above which an intrauterine gestational sac should be visualized by TVUS).
- Because a single level cannot diagnose viability or location of a gestation, serial (every 48-72 hours) quantitative β-hCG may be necessary to follow the trend or monitor spontaneous resolution.
  - Early normal pregnancies show a curvilinear rise in hCG until a plateau at 100 000 mIU/mL by 10 weeks of gestation.
  - A failure to rise, a plateau, or a decrease is concerning for a failing pregnancy.
- Other laboratory testing may be indicated (CBC, blood type, and screen for potential transfusion and to determine the need for anti-D immunoglobulin in RhD-negative women; baseline renal and liver function for potential methotrexate administration).

▶ TREATMENT

- Patients can be managed medically, surgically, or expectantly; the decision should be guided by clinical, laboratory, and imaging findings as well as patient-informed choice.
- Medical management with intramuscular methotrexate (MTX):
  - MTX is a folic acid antagonist to stop the growth of the ectopic. Although not an FDA-approved indication, MTX is used for medical management.
  - Candidates for medical management with MTX include:
    - Ectopic <3.5 cm
    - No cardiac activity on TVUS
    - Initial β-hCG <5000 IU/L
    - Patients who are hemodynamically stable, have no contraindications to MTX, and are able to comply with serial β-hCG measurements
  - MTX has numerous contraindications; examples include IUP, ruptured ectopic, immunodeficiency, breastfeeding, and inability of patient to follow-up.
  - Serial β-hCG measurements at 4- and 7-day postinjection
    - If decline by at least 15%, measure weekly until undetectable.
    - If no decline, may need second round of MTX or surgery.
- Surgical management of tubal ectopic:
  - Surgical indications include contraindications or concerns of MTX, failed MTX therapy, signs and

symptoms of impending or ongoing rupture, or if the patient desires a concurrent surgical procedure (eg, sterilization).
- Laparoscopic (preferred) and laparotomy:
  - Linear salpingostomy—removal of pregnancy
  - Segmental resection—removal of affected tubal segment
  - Salpingectomy—removal of entire tube
- Followed with post-therapy serial quantitative β-hCG measurements

- May need MTX postoperatively
- Expectant management:
  - Remains an option only for a small proportion of women in which the risk of tubal rupture is minimal
  - Carries the risk of tubal rupture, hemorrhage, and emergency surgery.

CHAPTER

355

Gestational Trophoblastic Disease

Sara Lolar, MS, PA-C, DFAAPA

▶ GENERAL FEATURES

- Gestational trophoblastic disease (GTD) is defined as the abnormal proliferation of pregnancy-related trophoblastic tissue in the placenta.
- All GTDs have malignant potential.
- 80% to 90% of GTD are noninvasive or localized tumors called hydatiform mole or molar pregnancy.
  - Complete moles do not have any fetal tissue.
  - Partial moles have fetal tissue, but often deformed and nonviable.
- 15% to 20% of GTD is malignant and is referred to as gestational trophoblastic neoplasia (GTN).
  - GTN includes invasive moles, choriocarcinomas, and placental-site trophoblastic tumors.
  - Risk of GTN increased with complete moles (15% to 20%) and is relatively rare following partial moles (<5%).
  - Increased risk with maternal age (≥45) and history of prior molar pregnancy
  - Early detection of GTD has not decreased the overall rate of GTN.

▶ CLINICAL ASSESSMENT

- Vaginal bleeding is the most common symptom (>90%).
  - Bleeding can be variable—light to heavy, sudden to intermittent.
  - Caused by tissue separating from the decidua
- Human chorionic gonadotropin (hCG) is usually higher than expected for gestational age, sometimes elevated >100 000 mIU/mL.
  - Caused by hCG secreted by the growing trophoblastic tissue
- Uterus is often large for gestational age.
  - Caused by growth of tumor or retained blood clots

- Multiple theca lutein cysts can cause enlargement of ovaries.
- Other classic signs such as hyperemesis gravidarum, pregnancy-induced hypertension before 20 weeks of gestational age, and hyperthyroidism are more common in complete moles.
  - These signs are seen less frequently now because of earlier diagnosis with modern ultrasounds and modern laboratory testing of hCG.
- Partial moles present more insidiously, without classic symptoms.
  - Often misdiagnosed and treated as a missed or incomplete abortion and the diagnosis is only discovered on pathology.

▶ DIAGNOSIS

- Suspect GTD in a patient with vaginal bleeding and an hCG higher than expected for gestational age.
- Elevated hCG acts as a tumor marker.
  - Important to obtain a baseline to use for future monitoring
- Ultrasonography is the diagnostic method of choice.
  - Will demonstrate numerous discrete anechoic, cystic spaces with central heterogeneous mass
    - With a partial mole, fetal tissue may be noted. Often, results in delayed diagnosis.
    - The classic "snowstorm pattern" or "Swiss cheese pattern" is uncommon on modern ultrasounds.
- If GTD suspected, check a thyroid panel, CBC for anemia, and liver enzymes, renal function, and chest x-ray for possible metastasis, as clinically indicated.
- Any products of conception should be sent for pathology.

▶ TREATMENT

- Partial and complete moles are treated the same.
- All Rh-negative women should receive Rh immunoglobulin.
- The uterus should be evacuated by suction curettage and sent to pathology to confirm the diagnosis of GTD.
  - Medication-only evacuation not currently recommended.
  - May consider hysterectomy for those at high risk for GTN or those who no longer desire fertility
    - This does not obviate the need for monitoring as below.
  - May consider chemoprophylaxis in high-risk complete molar pregnancies.
- Surveillance of hCG levels for at least 6 months following evacuation.
  - hCG level should be monitored weekly until zero for 3 weeks.
  - Then monthly for 6 months
- All patients should be started on contraception.
  - A new pregnancy during surveillance makes it difficult to interpret hCG levels and will complicate management.
- GTN may be confirmed on pathology, or if persistent positive hCG after 6 months, or if levels plateau or rise during the 6-month surveillance period.
- Patient may pursue another pregnancy after completing the surveillance period.
  - Complications are similar to those of general population, except for a slight increased risk of another molar pregnancy.

CHAPTER 356

Gestational Diabetes

Joy Moverley, DHSc, MPH, PA-C

▶ GENERAL FEATURES

- Gestational diabetes (GDM) is diagnosed in the second or third trimester of pregnancy in a patient not previously known to have diabetes before gestation.
- Risk factors:
  - Race/ethnicity of high risk including Latina, Native American, Asian, Pacific Islander, and Black
  - Over 35 years old
  - Body mass index >26 kg/m^2
  - History of glucose intolerance, polycystic ovarian syndrome, severe obesity, or adverse pregnancy outcomes associated with GDM
  - First-degree relative with known diabetes
  - History of delivering a baby over 9 lb
  - Hypertension
  - Physical inactivity
- During pregnancy, the placenta secretes diabetogenic hormones (eg, growth hormone, corticotrophin-releasing hormone, human placental lactogen, and progesterone), promoting insulin resistance and carbohydrate intolerance. If pancreas cannot compensate for insulin resistance due to functional β-cell deficits, GDM occurs.

▶ CLINICAL ASSESSMENT

- Maternal complications:
  - Preeclampsia
  - Gestational hypertension
  - Cesarean delivery
  - Maternal birth trauma
- Fetal complications:
  - Spontaneous abortion and fetal demise
  - Fetal anomalies
  - Macrosomia and large for gestational age infant
  - Neonatal hypoglycemia
  - Neonatal hyperbilirubinemia
  - Neonatal hypertrophic cardiomyopathy
  - Infant birth trauma

▶ DIAGNOSIS

- Screening recommendations:
  - At first prenatal visit if high risk for undiagnosed diabetes
    - If results are normal and two or more risk factors for GDM are present, screening should be repeated between 24 and 28 weeks.
  - All asymptomatic pregnant women at 24-28 weeks' gestation
- The ADA Standards of Medical Care in Diabetes recommends two strategies for diagnosis. Diagnostic cutoffs differ between two tests. Only one abnormality is needed to make the diagnosis of GDM.
  - "One-step" 75 g oral glucose tolerance test (OGTT) after an 8 hour fast with glucose measurements at 0, 1, and 2 hours

- Diagnostic criteria includes:
  - Fasting plasma glucose of 92 mg/dL
  - 1-hour plasma glucose of 180 mg/dL
  - 2-hour plasma glucose of 153 mg/dL
- "Two-step" nonfasting 50 g glucose load test (GLT) screen measured at 1 hour followed by a fasting 100 g OGTT measured at 0, 1, 2, and 3 hours for those who screened positive with the GLT
  - Diagnostic criteria for GLT (50 g oral glucose):
    - 1-hour plasma glucose >139 mg/dL
  - Diagnostic criteria for the 3-hour GLT includes:
    - Fasting plasma glucose > 95 mg/dL
    - 1-hour plasma glucose > 180 mg/dL
    - 2-hour plasma glucose > 155 mg/dL
    - 3-hour plasma glucose > 140 mg/dL
- A1c levels for GDM are less preferable because of physiologic changes in red blood cell turnover and physiologic dilution anemia. Further, A1c does not provide information on postprandial hyperglycemia, which causes macrosomia.

▶ TREATMENT

- Glycemic control through physical activity and medical nutrition therapy are first line.
  - If after 2 weeks unable to obtain normal glucose levels, consider medication therapy.
- Target glucose levels include:
  - Fasting glucose <95 mg/dL
  - 1-hour postprandial <140 mg/dL
  - 2-hour postprandial <120 mg/dL
- Monitoring glucose daily is recommended, continuous glucose monitors can be helpful for some patients to recognize patterns.
- Medications:
  - Insulin is the medication of choice if further intervention is needed.

- Intermediate-acting insulin (NPH) is most commonly prescribed.
- Glargine and detemir are also safe.
- Insulin does not cross the placenta barrier at measurable level.
- Oral medications occasionally used in GDM include metformin and/or glyburide.
  - Metformin is more likely to cross placental barrier than glyburide but is associated with lower risk of neonatal hypoglycemia and less maternal weight gain than insulin.
- Consideration for delivery:
  - Ultrasound should be performed to determine risk-benefit for a scheduled cesarean delivery if fetal weight estimated to be >4500 g.
  - Women meeting recommended control for GDM may deliver at 40 weeks.
  - Women managed by medications should deliver between 39 0/7 and 39 6/7 weeks.
  - If poorly controlled, GDM may deliver earlier based on risks of stillbirth vs. prematurity between 37 0/7 and 38 6/7 weeks.
- Postpartum recommendations:
  - Medications for diabetes are typically discontinued upon delivery.
  - Monitor glucose levels until 6-week follow-up appointment and retest for diabetes at that time with OGTT.
    - Women with GDM are at high risk of developing T2DM. Recheck for GDM every 1-3 years if the postpartum test is normal.
  - Consider enrolling in Diabetes Prevention Program to delay or prevent the diagnosis of T2DM postpartum.

CHAPTER 357

Hypertensive Disorders in Pregnancy

Elyse Watkins, DHSc, PA-C, DFAAPA

▶ GENERAL FEATURES

- Hypertensive disorders of pregnancy are a leading cause of maternal and perinatal morbidity and mortality.
- Four classifications:
  - Preeclampsia, with or without severe features, or eclampsia
  - Preexisting (chronic) hypertension

- Preeclampsia or eclampsia with superimposed chronic hypertension
- Gestational hypertension, previously called pregnancy-induced hypertension
- Risk factors for gestational hypertension and preeclampsia include primiparity, diabetes, chronic hypertension, advanced maternal age, multiple gestation, obesity, systemic lupus erythematosus,

antiphospholipid syndrome, renal disease, history of preeclampsia or thrombocytopenia, and in vitro fertilization.

- Complications of severe hypertension (systolic BP of 160 mm Hg or greater, diastolic BP of 110 mm Hg or greater) during gestation:
  - Maternal: stroke, acute kidney injury, heart failure, myocardial infarction, hypertensive cardiomyopathy, placental abruption, death
  - Fetal: growth restriction, preterm delivery, congenital heart disease, stillbirth, neonatal death

▶ CLINICAL ASSESSMENT

- Patients may be asymptomatic, or may complain of headaches, visual changes (scotoma, photopsia), upper abdominal or epigastric pain, or swelling in the extremities.
- Auscultate the lungs for evidence of pulmonary edema and assess for peripheral edema.

▶ DIAGNOSIS

- Criteria for preeclampsia without severe features (both must be met):
  - BP >140/90 mm Hg on two occasions 4 hours apart (or 160/110 mm Hg on one occasion)
  - Proteinuria >300 mg over 24 hours or a urine protein/creatinine ratio >0.3 mg/dL
- Criteria for preeclampsia with severe features:
  - BP >140/90 mm Hg on two occasions 4 hours apart (or 160/110 mm Hg on one occasion) AND thrombocytopenia (platelets <100 000 cells/mm^3), increase in creatinine concentration to >1.1 mg/dL, and doubling of hepatic transaminases
  - A quantified proteinuria of >5 g in 24 hours is no longer required.
  - The patient may be negative for proteinuria. A urinary dipstick for proteinuria usually is not sufficient for diagnosis.
  - Pulmonary edema and visual or cerebral changes constitute severe features of preeclampsia.
- Rule out molar pregnancy in a patient who develops preeclampsia before 20 weeks' gestation.
- Eclampsia is defined as new-onset seizures in a patient with preeclampsia and without a known seizure disorder.
- Gestational hypertension:
  - BP of 140/90 mm Hg or greater after 20 weeks' gestation on two separate occasions 4 hours apart without the development of proteinuria or other end-organ dysfunction
  - Gestational hypertension is considered severe when systolic BP is 160 mm Hg or greater and/or diastolic BP is 110 mm Hg or greater.

- Up to 50% of patients with gestational hypertension develop preeclampsia, so monitor patients closely.
- Preeclampsia or eclampsia with superimposed chronic hypertension:
  - Proteinuria and/or other evidence of end-organ manifestations developing after 20 weeks' gestation in a patient with chronic hypertension (BP of 140/90 mm Hg or greater) who did not have proteinuria or end-organ manifestations before 20 weeks' gestation

▶ TREATMENT

- General principles:
  - Women with BP <160/105 mm Hg are generally not treated with antihypertensive therapy but should have twice-weekly BP and urine protein checks.
  - Patients should monitor fetal movements daily.
  - Most clinicians will initiate antihypertensive therapy when diastolic BP is 105 mm Hg or greater.
  - Patients may have nonstress tests and serial ultrasounds to assess fetal health.
  - Women with BP of 160/110 mm Hg or greater should be managed expeditiously with antihypertensive therapies, such as IV labetalol or hydralazine. Oral nifedipine can be used if IV access is not available.
    - Angiotensin-converting enzyme inhibitors and angiotensin-receptor blockers are not recommended for pregnant patients.
  - Lifestyle modifications, such as diet and exercise, limiting caffeine intake, and alcohol cessation, are recommended for all pregnant patients.
  - The American College of Obstetricians and Gynecologists recommends starting low-dose aspirin (81 mg/day) at 12 weeks' gestation to prevent preeclampsia in women with chronic hypertension and who are at high risk for developing preeclampsia.
- Most women will become normotensive within the first week postpartum, but may have elevated BP well through 6 weeks postpartum, so close follow-up is necessary.
- All patients with a hypertensive disorder during pregnancy should have a BP check at 72 hours postpartum and again at 7-10 days because preeclampsia and eclampsia can develop during the postpartum period. Educate patients on signs and symptoms.
- The definitive treatment of preeclampsia and eclampsia is delivery.
- Preexisting (chronic) and gestational hypertension:
  - The oral antihypertensive drugs of choice for outpatient management of hypertension are labetalol, nifedipine, and methyldopa.
  - Ongoing evaluation of gestational hypertension includes weekly or twice-weekly nonstress tests; weekly BP monitoring; weekly urine protein,

platelets, and hepatic transaminases; and ultrasound evaluation every 3 weeks.
- Preeclampsia without severe features:
  - Management algorithms depend on gestational age and the presence or absence of severe features.
  - In patients with BP <160/110 mm Hg and without severe features, delivery is indicated when the patient reaches 37 weeks 0 days.
  - Delivery is indicated earlier if patients develop HELLP syndrome (hemolysis, elevated liver enzymes, low platelets); have abnormal ultrasound findings (fetal weight <5th percentile or oligohydramnios); have persistently low biophysical profiles (6/10 or less); other maternal or fetal abnormalities; or rupture of membranes.
  - Patients with BP >160/110 mm Hg should receive IV labetalol or hydralazine. Oral nifedipine can be used if IV access is not available.
- Preeclampsia with severe features:
  - Pregnant patients at <34 weeks' gestation with severe features should be admitted to labor and delivery for continuous fetal monitoring, maternal BP and urine output monitoring, corticosteroid administration, and laboratory evaluation for renal function and the development of HELLP.
- Consider delivery for patients at 34 weeks 0 days and later following a course of antenatal corticosteroids (if not already done), or immediate delivery if there is evidence of fetal distress, ruptured membranes, oliguria, serum creatinine of 1.5 mg/dL or greater, pulmonary edema, HELLP syndrome, eclampsia, platelets of fewer than 100,000 cells/mm^3, coagulopathy, or placental abruption.
- Magnesium sulfate should be considered to prevent seizure activity.
  - Magnesium toxicity can cause loss of deep tendon reflexes, respiratory depression, and cardiac arrest.
  - Magnesium toxicity can be reversed with the IV administration of calcium gluconate.
  - Magnesium sulfate is also neuroprotective to the fetus.
  - Contraindications for magnesium sulfate include myasthenia gravis and renal impairment.
- Eclampsia:
  - Acute management includes maintaining adequate oxygenation, treating hypertension with IV labetalol or hydralazine, preventing recurrent seizure activity with magnesium sulfate, and evaluating the patient for immediate delivery.

CHAPTER
358

Late Complications: Placenta Previa and Placental Abruption

Jennifer Johnson, BS, MPAS, DMSc

▶ GENERAL FEATURES

- Placenta previa:
  - Obstetric complication resulting from the placenta completely or marginally covering the internal cervical os
  - The classic presentation is bright red, painless vaginal bleeding in the second or third trimester.
  - Risk factors for the development of placenta previa include a previous history of placenta previa, previous C-section delivery, and multiple gestation.
- Placental abruption:
  - Premature detachment of the placenta from the uterine wall, often following recent abdominal trauma
  - It typically occurs in pregnancies over 20 weeks' gestation.
  - It is most common in patients younger than 20 years and older than 35 years. Other risk factors include cocaine use, smoking tobacco, and hypertension.

▶ CLINICAL ASSESSMENT

- Placenta previa:
  - Should be suspected in any pregnant patient over 20 weeks' gestation with painless vaginal bleeding
  - Digital examination of the vagina is contraindicated in any pregnant patient over 20 weeks' gestation presenting with painless vaginal bleeding until ultrasonography rules out placenta previa. Digital pelvic examination in a patient with placenta previa can result in severe, life-threatening hemorrhage. Evaluation with a sterile speculum may be performed before ultrasound.
- Placental abruption:
  - Ultrasound should be performed before pelvic examination to rule out placenta previa.

- Bleeding may be mild to profuse and comes in waves with palpable uterine contractions. Acute disseminated intravascular coagulation (DIC) is associated with significant placental separation.
- Maternal blood pressure and fetal heart rate should be monitored for signs of distress.
- Assessing for Rh status, fetal-maternal transfusion, and bleeding disorders may also be indicated.

▶ DIAGNOSIS

- Placenta previa:
  - Diagnosis is made by visualizing the placenta by ultrasound.
  - Assess the patient for Rh status, fetal-maternal transfusion, and bleeding disorders.
  - Placenta previa may be an incidental ultrasonography finding in an asymptomatic, second-trimester patient.
  - Patients with asymptomatic placenta previa should be monitored via ultrasonography at 28 weeks for migration of the placenta and resolution of the condition.
- Placental abruption: diagnosis is made by ultrasound, which allows visualization of the retroplacental hematoma.

▶ TREATMENT

- Placenta previa:
  - Patients with placenta previa should avoid orgasm, inserting any item into the vagina, and moderate or strenuous exercise after 20 weeks' gestation.
  - Persistent placenta previa in the third trimester is treated with bedrest. Women may be hospitalized in the case of bleeding.
  - Tocolytics may be used to suppress contractions if they accompany bleeding.
  - Corticosteroids should be administered to women with bleeding due to placenta previa between 24 and 34 weeks' gestation to promote lung maturity.
  - Decision regarding cesarean section or vaginal delivery depends on the location of the placenta and maternal and fetal status.
- Placental abruption:
  - Hemodynamic status of mother, gestational age, and severity of abruption will determine treatment options.
  - Patient should be admitted for diagnostic testing and monitoring.
  - C-section delivery may be required for maternal and fetal stabilization.
  - Transfusion may be required.
  - A facility with a neonatal intensive care unit is preferred if the fetus is preterm.

CHAPTER
359

Normal Pregnancy, Prenatal Care, Labor and Delivery, and Postpartum Care

Jennifer Norris, MSPAS, PA-C

▶ GENERAL FEATURES

- Normal pregnancy/prenatal care:
  - A pregnancy lasts 40 weeks from the date of the first day of the last menstrual period (LMP). It is divided into three trimesters.
    - The first trimester is from 1 to 13 weeks' gestation. In the first trimester, patients are usually fatigued, may experience some nausea/vomiting, and may experience slight cramping and even some spotting during implantation. Patients do not yet feel fetal movement in the first trimester.
    - The second trimester is 13.1-26 weeks. Patients in their second trimester usually feel well; they have more energy, less nausea/vomiting; they start to experience fetal movement (as early as 18 weeks for multiparous patients and about 20 weeks for nulliparous patients), and the uterus/fetus begins to grow out of the pelvic cavity.
    - The third trimester is 26.1 weeks to delivery. Patients may begin to experience fatigue as the pregnancy progresses, feel lots of fetal movement, and may experience "practice" contractions (Braxton-Hicks) on and off until they go into labor.
  - Normal labor and delivery:
    - Labor is defined as progressive cervical dilation with continued uterine contractions. Patients may

experience rupture of membranes before delivery. The color and consistency of the fluid should be evaluated and documented.

- Labor is divided into three phases. Phase 1 consists of the latent and active phase and is the phase in which the cervix becomes fully dilated. Phase 2 starts with complete dilation and ends with the delivery of the fetus. Phase 3 starts with the delivery of the fetus and ends with delivery of the placenta.

- Postpartum care:
  - Postpartum care starts with the delivery of the placenta. The immediate postpartum period is the riskiest for the patient. In the first few hours after delivery, the uterus remains large and heavy vaginal bleeding or a postpartum hemorrhage may occur if the uterus does not become firm.
  - The postpartum period lasts ~6 weeks after delivery. Lochia (vaginal bleeding and discharge) should slow and stop completely at the end of the postpartum period.

▶ CLINICAL ASSESSMENT

- Normal pregnancy/prenatal care:
  - The first prenatal visit should include a complete history, including patient's past medical history and family history concentrating on bleeding issues and genetic diseases. A complete physical examination should be conducted, including a speculum examination with Pap, cultures for sexually transmitted diseases and bacterial infections. Labs should include CBC, hCG quantitative, HIV, hepatitis panel, rubella status, syphilis, blood group and Rh (antibody screen), and urine culture. Other labs may be added dependent upon the history obtained, random glucose or hemoglobin A1C, hemoglobinopathy workup/electrophoresis, CMP, anemia workup, and so on.
  - For a normal pregnancy without complications, prenatal visits occur at standard intervals.
    - From the first prenatal visit until 28 weeks, 1 visit per month. From 28 to 36 weeks: 1 visit every 2 weeks
    - After 36 weeks until delivery: 1 visit each week
  - Every prenatal visit should include vital signs, weight of the patient, urine dipstick for specific gravity, ketones, protein and sugars, fundal height measurement, and fetal assessment with Doppler or ultrasound.
  - Patients with a normal weight/BMI should anticipate gaining about 30 lb during the pregnancy.
  - Fundal height is obtained using the McDonald's method with the patient supine and is the measurement from the symphysis pubis to the top of the fundus. At 20 weeks, the fundus should be approximately at the umbilicus and measure 20 cm. With normal fetal growth, every week gestation after 20 weeks should equal the measurement obtained in centimeters.

  - Every nondiabetic patient should be screened for gestational diabetes at 24-28 weeks with either a one- or two-step test.
    - Two-step screen: 1-hour glucose challenge test (50 g oral glucose); if abnormal, a 3-hour glucose test (100 g) should be ordered as confirmation with blood sugar measurements taken fasting, 1, 2, and 3 hours.
    - One-step oral glucose tolerance test: 75 g oral glucose with fasting, 1- and 2-hour blood sugar measurements.
  - Screen patients for group B *Streptococcus* (GBS) with culture at 34-37 weeks' gestation. GBS is a bacteria woman carries in the vagina that poses no risk to them; however, the fetus could become infected if exposed during normal delivery. Patients should be educated to report GBS status when in labor so that they may be treated appropriately to decrease the risk of transmission to the fetus.
  - During routine prenatal care, education should include breastfeeding, circumcision, preterm labor signs, danger signs, and labor signs. Childbirth education and parent education classes can also be encouraged.

- Normal labor and delivery:
  - Continuous fetal monitoring and uterine tocodynamometry should occur during the labor process. A healthy fetus can tolerate the stress of contractions. Fetal distress implies intolerance to contractions and may indicate the need for a cesarean section.
  - Labor progress should be monitored to ensure the patient remains on the labor curve. Labor progress is evaluated by cervical examination, which includes dilation, effacement, and fetal station. Calculation of a Bishop score can be determined from the cervical examination and is a good indicator of the likelihood of vaginal delivery.
  - Leopold's maneuver consists of four steps that are done in a systematic way to confirm fetal position; this should be done with every laboring patient. With the patient supine, palpate starting at the fundus to determine the consistency, shape, and mobility of the fetal part, continue palpating bilaterally moving inferiorly on the uterus to determine the direction of the fetal back. Palpate just above the symphysis pubis to determine the presenting part and lastly apply deep pressure into the pelvic outlet to determine the cephalic prominence.
  - Upon admission, fetal weight should be estimated through palpation. This allows for preparation of delivery complications, including shoulder dystocia or cephalopelvic disproportion.

- Postpartum care:
  - Begins immediately after birth. It ends ~6 weeks after delivery. It can be considered the fourth trimester of pregnancy.
  - Reduction in size of the uterus occurs after delivery. Within a few hours, the uterus should be firm, midline, and at the level of the umbilicus. The uterus should continue to decrease in size until it returns to the prepregnant state. In the postpartum period, the fundus should be palpated for consistency and location to ensure it remains firm and continues to decrease in size.
  - The site of the placental insertion heals by exfoliation. Lochia (discharge and vaginal bleeding) should continue to decrease during the postpartum period as the site heals and the uterus returns to its prepregnant state.
  - Patients should be seen at 6 weeks postpartum to evaluate uterus and breasts and to discuss birth control if not already planned.
  - Breastfeeding during this time helps to contract the uterus after delivery and provides antibodies to the baby.

▶ DIAGNOSIS

- Normal pregnancy/prenatal care:
  - Patients experience amenorrhea and usually take a home pregnancy test. The pregnancy can be confirmed with a qualitative test (urine or blood) and with a quantitative test (blood). The pregnancy should be confirmed to be intrauterine with ultrasound. The date of the LMP along with measurements obtained with ultrasound are used to determine an estimated date of confinement (EDC) or estimated due date (EDD). Patients should be encouraged to seek prenatal care as soon as they have a positive pregnancy test. Early prenatal care has been shown to decrease maternal and fetal morbidity and mortality.
- Normal labor and delivery:
  - Patients experiencing regular uterine contractions should be evaluated for cervical change and for rupture of membranes. During the evaluation for labor, fetal status should also be monitored.
  - Patients in labor should be admitted for delivery.
- Postpartum care:
  - During the 6 weeks after delivery, patients should be monitored for signs of uterine infection. If lochia develops a foul odor, uterus becomes tender, or a fever develops, the patient should be evaluated for endometritis, including drawing a white count and obtaining vaginal cultures.
  - Patients should also monitor for signs of mastitis. Erythema, edema, tenderness, and abnormal nipple discharge are common with mastitis.

▶ TREATMENT

- Normal pregnancy/prenatal care:
  - Patients should be prescribed prenatal vitamins as soon as possible, before conception is best. Folic acid is needed for neural tube development and the neural tube closes before a patient misses her period.
  - Patients may need to take iron supplements if found to be anemic. Pregnant women frequently experience constipation so, if adding iron, a stool softener should also be prescribed.
  - Urine or vaginal infections should be treated when diagnosed in pregnancy, even if asymptomatic. Untreated infections could cause preterm labor and delivery.
  - Consideration of medication for chronic diseases should be reviewed. Every medication a patient is taking needs to be evaluated for safety during pregnancy and may need to be changed or dosed accordingly. Medications for thyroid disease, epilepsy, and hypertension are common medications that need to be changed and/or adjusted during pregnancy.
  - If a patient is diagnosed with HIV, medication should be started as soon as possible to decrease the viral load and to decrease the risk of transmission to the fetus.
  - If a patient has a known history of herpes simplex, they should be placed on suppressive therapy around 34 weeks' gestation.
  - Patients should have Tdap immunizations between weeks 27 and 36 of each pregnancy, regardless of the interval since last Tdap, to help prevent pertussis in infants.
  - Patients should be educated on the importance of compliance with prenatal visits. Patients should understand how to determine fetal kick counts and should know the signs of infection and labor.
- Normal labor and delivery:
  - Patients in labor should be admitted to the hospital for continuous monitoring of the fetus.
  - Patients positive for GBS should have antibiotics administered before delivery.
  - Pain management can be offered via IV, epidural placement, or local anesthesia.
  - Labor progress should be monitored, and with complete dilation, patient should be encouraged to push.
  - In the event of fetal distress or labor progress stalls, cesarean section should be considered.
  - Neonate should be evaluated with Apgar scores at 1 and 5 minutes after birth.
- Postpartum care:
  - If patients are seronegative for rubella, they should be vaccinated postdelivery. Rubella infection is teratogenic to the fetus and vaccination after delivery will offer protection for subsequent pregnancies.

- Location of the fundus of the uterus and lochia should be monitored in the postpartum period. Uterus should remain nontender, and lochia should become absent. If endometritis develops, patients should be given antibiotics after cultures are obtained and most likely readmitted to the hospital.
- Breasts should be full but soft during breastfeeding and milk production. If signs of mastitis develop, antibiotics should be given and patients should continue to breastfeed or pump.

- Birth control options should be discussed and prescribed if patient has not already started a method.
- Medication adjustments should be made during the 6-week postpartum visit. Patients may start back on prepregnancy medications and/or dosing adjustments should be considered. Safety in breastfeeding should be considered with each medication.

CHAPTER
360

Multiple Gestation

Jennifer Johnson, BS, MPAS, DMSc

▶ GENERAL FEATURES

- Multiple gestation is a pregnancy with more than one fetus.
- Maternal age, ethnicity, maternal family history, high maternal BMI, and a history of prior pregnancies are risk factors for nonidentical multiple gestation.
- Twins are the most common form of multiple gestation, occurring in 3.3% of pregnancies; higher order multiples (triplets or more) occur less frequently.
- The use of assisted reproductive technologies significantly increases the likelihood of multiple gestation. In vitro fertilization (IVF) is associated with an increase in both nonidentical and identical twin pregnancies.
- Multiple gestation pregnancies are at increased risk for preterm delivery, preeclampsia, gestational diabetes, abnormal placental function, and delivery complications.

▶ CLINICAL ASSESSMENT

- Multiple gestation is often an incidental finding on early first-trimester ultrasound examination.
- Ultrasound to assess chorionicity (number of placental chorions) and amnionicity (number of amniotic sacs) is important as shared chorion and amnion may place fetuses at higher risk of complications. Optimal timing for this ultrasound is after 7 weeks until early second trimester. Monochorionic fetuses are at risk for twin-twin transfusion syndrome.
- Ultrasound examination for fetal survey is recommended between 18 and 22 weeks.
- Patients with multiple gestation may report increased severity of morning sickness, early fetal movement, and increased fatigue.

- Physical examination may reveal excessive weight gain and uterine size that is large for gestational age.
- It is vital to obtain accurate gestational dates and a thorough history that assesses risk factors for multiple gestation.

▶ DIAGNOSIS

- Quantitative human chorionic gonadotropin (β-hCG) levels will be elevated, though this finding does not exclude a singleton pregnancy.
- Multiple gestation is a cause of elevated α-fetoprotein (AFP) levels.
- Assessment of fetal heart tones via Doppler may reveal multiple heartbeats.
- In the majority of cases, multiple gestation is diagnosed by first-trimester ultrasound examination, which confirms the presence of more than one fetus.

▶ TREATMENT

- Prenatal anticipatory guidance should include expected weight gain and nutritional recommendations for multiple gestation. This includes increased requirements of folic acid, vitamins, minerals, and daily caloric intake. Patients may require medical therapy or intravenous rehydration if morning sickness is severe.
- Weekly antepartum fetal testing starting at 32 weeks including nonstress test (NST), biophysical profile (BPP), evaluation of amniotic fluid levels, and Doppler velocimetry.
- Delivery should be scheduled prior 40 weeks' gestation. Specific timing of delivery is dependent on the chorionicity and amnionicity.

Rh Incompatibility in Pregnancy

Elyse Watkins, DHSc, PA-C, DFAAPA

> A 22 year-old G1P0 presents for her initial prenatal visit. She is found to be O negative, and her antibody screen is negative. When should she receive her first anti-D immunoglobulin injection?

GENERAL FEATURES

- A person's blood type can be A, B, O, or AB.
- The Rhesus factor (Rh) is reported as a positive or negative result.
- The most common Rh in humans is D, but other antigens include C, c, E, e, and G.
- A person who is Rh positive means they have evidence of Rh antigen on the red blood cell surface.
- A person who is Rh negative does not have evidence of the antigen, so exposure to Rh positive blood will result in the development of antibodies. This is referred to as alloimmunization.
- Alloimmunization occurs when there is mixing of Rh-positive blood in a person with Rh negative blood, usually due to a procedure during pregnancy, such as chorionic villus sampling or amniocentesis.
  - An Rh-negative woman who experiences an early pregnancy loss may also be at risk if the pregnancy was Rh positive.
- Alloimmunization will not adversely affect the first pregnancy but rather will negatively affect subsequent pregnancies.
- Rh incompatibility that is untreated can result in erythroblastosis fetalis and fetal hydrops.
- Erythroblastosis fetalis leads to pericardial effusion, heart failure, and ascites.
- Fetal hydrops is diagnosed when two or more of the following is present: polyhydramnios, ascites, pleural effusion, pericardial effusion, increased placental thickness, or increased fetal skin thickness.
- If intrauterine death does not occur, the newborn can develop kernicterus.

CLINICAL ASSESSMENT

- Alloimmunization is asymptomatic for the gravid patient.

DIAGNOSIS

- All pregnant women are screened at the initial obstetric visit. Rh negative women will be tested again at 28 weeks for Rh factor and presence or absence of anti-Rh(D) antibodies.

TREATMENT

- Prevention of alloimmunization is critical through screening all gravid patients.
- Women who are Rh negative and do not have a positive antibody screen receive anti-D immunoglobulin at 28 weeks and within 72 hours postpartum (if the fetus is Rh positive).
- Women who are Rh negative and antibody screen negative should also receive anti-D immunoglobulin if any potential mixing of blood occurs, such as with first-trimester bleeding or an invasive procedure.
- Women who are found to have a positive antibody screen must be referred to a maternal fetal medicine specialist for serial anti-D serum titers and ultrasonographic imaging.
- Increased middle cerebral artery peak systolic velocity is highly indicative of fetal anemia.
- Fetal anemia can be managed with fetal transfusions up until 32 weeks' gestation.
- Delivery should occur by 34 weeks' gestation.

Case Conclusion

Plan to administer anti-D immunoglobulin at 28 weeks' gestation. The patient will have a repeat antibody screen before immunization and as long as it remains negative, she can receive the immunoglobulin. Immunoglobulin would only be given at this visit if she was experiencing a threatened abortion or if she were undergoing an invasive procedure.

Cervical Insufficiency

Jennifer Norris, MSPAS, PA-C

▶ GENERAL FEATURES

- Cervical insufficiency is defined by the American College of Obstetrics and Gynecology (ACOG) as the inability of the cervix to maintain a pregnancy past the second trimester in the absence of uterine contractions.
- Often asymptomatic. Painless dilation and/or cervical shortening occur without regular uterine contractions, vaginal bleeding, or leaking of fluid.
- Inherited risk factors for cervical insufficiency include anatomic malformations and connective tissue disorders.
- Acquired risk factors include a history of cervical procedures, cervical biopsies, and mechanical dilation.
- Patients with a previous preterm delivery without contractions are presumed to have cervical insufficiency and are at highest risk.
- Patients with previous documented or suspected cervical insufficiency should be monitored diligently during subsequent pregnancies.
- Patients with documented cervical insufficiency may be offered a prophylactic cervical cerclage placed in the first trimester.

▶ CLINICAL ASSESSMENT

- Patients are asymptomatic. Patients with vaginal bleeding, leaking of fluid, or regular uterine contractions should be evaluated for other causes.
- Routine prenatal care should include regular cervical examinations throughout the pregnancy and should occur at increased frequency (sometimes with every visit) in patients at high risk for cervical insufficiency. It may be difficult to discern cervical length or a cervical funnel with a manual cervical examination, especially with a closed cervix.
- Speculum examination may reveal visual cervical dilation, exposed or bulging membranes or rupture of membranes.
- Examination of cervical length and dilation should be evaluated with ultrasound. Serial measurements with ultrasound can demonstrate cervical changes early.
- Physical examination otherwise is unremarkable, no contractions are found on uterine tocodynamometry, and fetal status is usually reassuring.

▶ DIAGNOSIS

- Diagnosis is made with cervical visualization via speculum examination or with manual vaginal examination revealing an open, dilated, or shortened cervix before term. All patients should be placed on external fetal monitoring including uterine contraction monitoring to ensure no signs of labor are present and fetal status is reassuring.
- Patients should be screened for signs of infection, including serum blood tests, urine culture, and vaginal cultures.
- Examination with a speculum should include screening for gonorrhea, chlamydia, bacterial vaginosis, trichomoniasis, and yeast.
- Rule out for rupture of membranes using the fern test and pH examination using nitrazine.
- Ultrasound should measure cervical length and width. Placenta placement and amniotic fluid level should be documented.

▶ TREATMENT

- Cervical cerclage may be offered prophylactically for a patient with a history of a previous preterm delivery due to cervical insufficiency. A prophylactic cerclage is placed early in the second trimester.
- Vaginal progesterone or IM hydroxyprogesterone may be offered in addition to a cervical cerclage or may be prescribed as an alternative option for a patient with a history of a previous preterm delivery and/or documented cervical insufficiency.
- Rescue cerclage may be offered later in the second trimester if patient displays no signs of infection and membranes are intact. Placement of a rescue cerclage carries risks of infection, bleeding, and loss of pregnancy.
- Patients diagnosed with cervical insufficiency, with cervical cerclage in situ, or taking progesterone should be counseled on pelvic rest and should avoid sexual intercourse.
- Cervical cerclage remains in place until 36-week gestation or if labor begins and tension is noted on the cerclage.

Premature Rupture of Membranes

Elyse Watkins, DHSc, PA-C, DFAAPA

A 28-year-old G1P0 presents at 30 weeks' gestation with a chief complaint of "I think my water broke." Her pregnancy has been uncomplicated up to this point. What is the next best step in assessing this patient?

▶ GENERAL FEATURES

- Premature rupture of membranes is also called prelabor rupture of membranes (PROM) and refers to spontaneous rupture of the amniotic sac before the onset of uterine contractions.
  - If it occurs ≥37 weeks' gestation, it is called PROM.
  - If it occurs <37 weeks' gestation, it is called preterm prelabor rupture of membranes (PPROM).
- PPROM is the leading cause of prematurity in the United States.
- Gravid patients who experience PROM are at risk for developing chorioamnionitis, placental abruption, and umbilical cord prolapse.
- Fetuses are at risk of significant morbidity and mortality due to the above and the sequelae of prematurity, including respiratory distress and pulmonary hypoplasia.
- Risk factors for PPROM include history of PROM or PPROM, amniotic infections, a shortened cervix, tobacco and/or illicit drug use, polyhydramnios, low socioeconomic status, bleeding in the second and third trimesters, and low body mass index.

▶ CLINICAL ASSESSMENT

- Gravid patients with suspected PROM/PPROM should undergo a sterile speculum examination to check for pooling which is the presence of amniotic fluid in the posterior fornix of the vagina or on the speculum.
- A sterile speculum examination includes the use of sterile gloves and a sterile speculum.
- Patients in whom PROM/PPROM is suspected should not have a nonsterile digital cervical examination.

▶ DIAGNOSIS

- The diagnosis can sometimes be made by visualizing amniotic fluid pooling on the speculum or in the vaginal fornix, or coming from the os.
- A small amount of fluid can be obtained with a sterile swab and placed on a slide.
- Ferning is the pathognomonic finding if amniotic fluid is present.
- Nitrazine paper will turn blue in the presence of amniotic fluid because of its alkaline pH, but blood, semen, and some bacteria can also cause alkaline pH.

- Various rapid noninvasive immunoassays have been developed to help aid in the diagnosis of membrane rupture.
- Fetal fibronectin (FFN) has a high negative predictive value, but positive FFNs are not clinically useful.
- Other tests for amniotic proteins can be used as adjuncts to standard means of diagnosis as they are associated with high false positives.
- Ultrasonographic measurements of amniotic fluid can also be performed.

▶ TREATMENT

- Regardless of gestational age, management includes assessing the mother for infection, bleeding, and onset of labor.
- Treatment largely depends upon gestational age.
  - <24 weeks:
    - There is insufficient evidence to recommend the use of corticosteroids (for fetal lung maturity) or magnesium sulfate (for neuroprotection) before viability (23 weeks).
    - Group B *Streptococcus* prophylaxis and tocolytics are not recommended before viability.
    - Antibiotics can be considered to help prevent chorioamnionitis.
  - For all PPROM/PROM >24 weeks:
    - Perform a vaginorectal swab for group B *Streptococcus* and treat the patient accordingly.
    - A patient with a history of genital herpes simplex should be given prophylactic acyclovir; if active lesions or prodromal symptoms are present, the patient should undergo cesarean delivery.
  - 24w0d-33w6d:
    - Expectant management with careful monitoring of maternal and fetal signs and symptoms is appropriate unless delivery is imminent.
    - A single course of corticosteroids is recommended for fetal lung maturity.
    - The current recommendations are 12 mg of intramuscular betamethasone given 24 hours apart for two doses or 6 mg of intramuscular dexamethasone given every 12 hours for four doses.
    - Prophylactic antibiotics are recommended. A standard regimen is intravenous ampicillin and erythromycin (or azithromycin if erythromycin is unavailable or not tolerated) for 48 hours.
    - If delivery has not occurred, oral antibiotics should be continued and include amoxicillin plus erythromycin for 5 days.

- Amoxicillin-clavulanic acid is not recommended because of the association with fetal necrotizing enterocolitis.
- Neuroprotection with magnesium sulfate is recommended if the patient is <33 weeks and delivery is imminent.
  - 34w0d-36w6d:
    - A single course of corticosteroids is recommended if not previously administered.
  - Term (37 weeks+):
    - Induction of labor with oxytocin is recommended; however, expectant management for up to 14 hours may be offered if the patient is afebrile and there is no evidence of maternal or fetal distress.
    - Induction of labor with prostaglandins can be considered but carries a higher risk of chorioamnionitis.

Case Conclusion

Perform a sterile speculum examination. While the speculum is in place, check for pooling. Never perform a digital examination on a patient with suspected rupture of membranes unless delivery is imminent. Ultrasound can be used if other modalities are inconclusive.

CHAPTER 364

Breech Presentation and Shoulder Dystocia

Alyssa Abebe, PA-C
Madison Lewis, BS

A 31-year-old female patient has been in active labor for 10 hours and is currently in the second stage of labor with confirmed breech presentation. The fetal heart monitor indicates late decelerations with the mother's attempts to push during each contraction. Upon pelvic examination, the physician assistant notices that the fetal trunk has been fully delivered, but that the fetus is not progressing through the birth canal.

▶ GENERAL FEATURES

- Breech presentation:
  - The presenting part of the fetus in breech presentation is the buttocks or feet.
    - Three different types of breech presentation:
      - Frank breech: fetus is flexed at the hips with the feet near the face (pike position).
      - Complete breech: flexion of the hips and knees (tucked position)
      - Incomplete breech: one or both hips are extended or one or both legs are extended.
- Shoulder dystocia:
  - Obstetric emergency.
    - While shoulder dystocia most commonly occurs after delivery of the fetal head, it can also occur in breech deliveries after delivery of the fetal legs and trunk.
    - Risk factors for shoulder dystocia include, but are not limited to, fetal macrosomia, maternal diabetes, operative delivery, a past medical history of shoulder dystocia, and gestational age >42 weeks.
  - Over 50% of shoulder dystocia cases occur independent of risk factors.
  - Brachial plexus injuries, specifically Erb palsy and Klumpke palsy, hypoxic ischemic encephalopathy, and humeral or clavicular fractures can all occur as a result of delivery in the presence of shoulder dystocia.
  - Fundal pressure should be avoided as it can lead to an exacerbation of shoulder impaction, uterine rupture, or fetal injury.

▶ CLINICAL ASSESSMENT

- Breech presentation:
  - Can be evaluated using Leopold's maneuvers on transabdominal examination. A hard, mobile structure will be palpable at the uterine fundus and/or soft mass may be palpable at the pelvic bone.
  - Fetal heart tones may be auscultated higher in the abdomen.
- Shoulder dystocia:
  - Shoulder dystocia involves the mechanical obstruction of one or both shoulders in the pelvis, typically at the level of the maternal pubic symphysis, during vaginal delivery.
  - Anterior shoulder impaction is more common and typically occurs at the maternal pubic symphysis.

- Posterior shoulder impaction usually occurs at the maternal sacral promontory.
- "Turtle sign" is commonly seen in cases of shoulder dystocia and involves the delivery and subsequent perineal retraction of the fetal head.

▶ DIAGNOSIS

- Ultrasound can confirm the diagnosis of breech presentation.
- Shoulder dystocia:
  - The occurrence of physical obstruction during vaginal delivery is associated with:
    - Inability to promote delivery of the fetal shoulders with the use of manual gentle traction of the fetal head in downward motion
    - Head-to-body interval lasting >60 seconds in duration
    - Need for additional delivery maneuvers

▶ TREATMENT

- Breech presentation:
  - Before labor and delivery, external version may be performed to change the position of the fetus.
  - Vaginal delivery of a fetus in breech presentation is complicated; most are delivered via cesarean section.
- Shoulder dystocia:
  - First-line maneuvers:
    - McRoberts maneuver—the maternal hips are placed into a position of hyperflexion so that the thighs are against the abdomen.
    - Suprapubic pressure—using a fist, pressure is applied to the region just above the maternal pubic bone.
  - Second-line maneuvers:
    - Rotational maneuvers to manipulate the fetal shoulders
    - Posterior axillary traction to facilitate delivery of the posterior arm and shoulder
  - Other (heroic) measures:
    - Clavicular fracture—an intentional fracture of the fetal clavicle is performed by pulling it in an outward direction.
    - Zavanelli maneuver—a combination of manipulating the fetal head through rotation, flexion, and elevation back into the uterus, followed by cesarean section.
    - Abdominal rescue—the fetal shoulders are rotated after a low transverse hysterotomy is performed to facilitate vaginal delivery.
    - Symphysiotomy—a last resort method that involves making an incision in the fibrous cartilage of the symphysis pubis

Case Conclusion

This is a classic example of shoulder dystocia with breech presentation because the fetal shoulders were mechanically obstructed during vaginal delivery even after attempted downward traction. Shoulder dystocia is an obstetrical emergency that can also be characterized by mechanical obstruction during delivery in the presence of a head to body interval lasting for longer than 60 seconds or obstruction only relieved by additional, more involved maneuvers. Such maneuvers include, but are not limited to, the McRoberts maneuver, suprapubic pressure, rotational maneuvers, posterior axillary traction, and even clavicular fractures.

CHAPTER 365

Fetal Distress

Elyse Watkins, DHSc, PA-C, DFAAPA

A 33-year-old G2P1 Asian female is undergoing continuous external fetal heart rate (FHR) monitoring during the first stage of labor, and a sinusoidal pattern is noted. Sinusoidal patterns are associated with profound fetal anemia, sepsis, narcotics, and chorioamnionitis. This pattern is a harbinger of poor fetal outcomes. What steps should be taken to assess this abnormal fetal heart rate tracing?

▶ GENERAL FEATURES

- Fetal distress during labor is evidenced by specific changes in the external fetal heart monitor (tocodynamometer, also called cardiotocography [CTG]), internal monitor with a scalp electrode, or through analysis of fetal scalp blood gas analysis and lactate measurements.
- Passage of meconium into the amniotic fluid is also a sign of fetal distress.
- Distress is due to disruptions in fetal oxygenation.
- The fetus receives oxygen from the maternal circulation. Maternal oxygenation occurs along a spectrum, from the cardiopulmonary system to distal blood vessels and continuing to the uterus, placenta, and umbilical cord.

- Disruptions in oxygen distribution can occur at any point along the spectrum.
- The most common cause of fetal distress during labor is uterine hyperstimulation, resulting in tachysystole, or excessive uterine contractions.
  - If tachysystole is present, the uterine stimulant should be reduced or removed.
  - If a patient is in the second stage of labor and actively pushing, allowing her to rest may alleviate distress.
- Other common causes include uncontrolled asthma, pulmonary embolus, respiratory depression, compression of the inferior vena cava, hypotension, hypovolemia, vasculopathy, vasoconstriction, uterine overstimulation, uterine or placental rupture, umbilical cord compression, and umbilical cord prolapse.
- Inadequate oxygenation results in fetal hypoxemia. This leads to hypoxia, metabolic acidosis, and metabolic acidemia (pH < 7), which can result in significant morbidity and mortality of the newborn.

CLINICAL ASSESSMENT

- Noninvasive monitoring of fetal well-being is accomplished with CTG.
- Invasive monitoring of fetal well-being is accomplished with fetal scalp blood gas and lactate analysis.
- Intermittent external fetal heart monitoring typically begins around 32 weeks' gestation when there is an underlying maternal or fetal issue that has been diagnosed. Examples include maternal diabetes, maternal hypertension, and fetal anomalies.
  - Women who are considered advanced maternal age often undergo biweekly testing.
  - Patients undergo at least 20 minutes of external monitoring twice weekly.
- Continuous monitoring occurs during labor. Changes in the FHR can be reassuring or worrisome, depending on the finding (see "Diagnosis" section).
- In low-risk laboring patients, the FHR tracing should be reviewed at least every 30 minutes in the active phase of the first stage of labor and at least every 15 minutes in the second stage of labor.
- High-risk patients should be evaluated at least every 15 minutes in the active phase of the first phase of labor and at least every 5 minutes in the second stage of labor.
- Sustained episodes of fetal tachycardia (FHR >160 beats per minute) or fetal bradycardia (FHR <110 beats per minute) require further investigation.
- Common maternal causes of fetal tachycardia include certain medications or illicit drugs (sympathomimetics, cocaine, and methamphetamines) and hyperthyroidism. Fetal causes include metabolic acidemia and anemia.

- Common maternal causes of fetal bradycardia include certain medications (opioids, magnesium sulfate), hypoglycemia, and hypothermia. Fetal causes include cardiac anomalies and impairment in fetal oxygenation.
- Several other variables are considered when assessing the FHR via external fetal monitoring, including baseline heart rate, variability of heart rate, sinusoidal pattern of regular variability, and decelerations, which can be variable, early, late, and/or prolonged.
- Prolonged decelerations are associated with poor fetal outcomes. They are evidenced by decreases of at least 15 beats per minute in the baseline FHR that lasts for at least 2 minutes. Prolonged decelerations occur when oxygenation is disrupted and, as such, is a worrisome finding. Prolonged decelerations that last ≥5 minutes in the presence of reduced variability and fetal bradycardia require emergent intervention. FHR findings are classified into three categories.
  - Category I: normal baseline FHR; moderate variability; no variable, late, or prolonged decelerations. This is normal and reassuring.
  - Category II: findings that do not fit in category I or III. Close monitoring should still occur.
  - Category III: absent variability and one of the following: recurrent late decelerations, recurrent variable decelerations, sustained bradycardia (for at least 10 minutes), or sinusoidal pattern for at least 20 minutes. This is abnormal and requires further assessment.
- Fetal scalp blood analysis can be used to definitively diagnose hypoxia and acidemia in the setting on non-reassuring external monitoring.
- Fetal health can also be assessed with a biophysical profile (BPP). The BPP encompasses external FHR monitoring plus ultrasound evaluation of fetal breathing, fetal movement, fetal tone, and measurement of amniotic fluid.
- The modified BPP (mBPP) includes external FHR monitoring plus amniotic fluid measurement.

DIAGNOSIS

- The diagnosis of fetal distress is made when there are non-reassuring findings on external or internal fetal monitoring, abnormal fetal scalp blood gas or lactate, meconium in the amniotic fluid, or an abnormal BPP or mBPP.

TREATMENT

- The treatment of fetal distress depends upon the underlying cause and persistence of non-reassuring findings.
- Several steps should be undertaken when any FHR tracing is abnormal.

- A: Assess the oxygenation pathway (maternal to fetal).
- B: Begin noninvasive corrective measures as recommended (see below).
- C: Clear any obstacles that would inhibit rapid delivery.
- D: Delivery.
- Noninvasive corrective measures include applying supplemental oxygen, administering an intravenous fluid bolus, changing maternal position to take pressure off the inferior vena cava and increase venous return to the heart, and reducing or stopping uterine stimulants, such as oxytocin.

- Laboring women who remain supine or semi-recumbent often experience a change in FHR variability.
- When non-reassuring findings persist or hypoxia/acidemia is present, delivery must be expedited.
- When vaginal delivery cannot be accomplished in a rapid manner, cesarean delivery is necessary.

Case Conclusion

When an FHR tracing is abnormal assess maternal to fetal oxygen pathway, begin noninvasive corrective measures, clear obstacles that may inhibit delivery, and prepare for eminent delivery.

CHAPTER 366

Postpartum Hemorrhage

Elyse Watkins, DHSc, PA-C, DFAAPA

A 23-year-old female is brought to the emergency department, having delivered a baby at home with a doula within the past hour. She is pale and unable to answer questions. Her nightgown is blood soaked, and her vital signs include a blood pressure of 94/60 mm Hg with a pulse of 110 beats per minute. What is the next intervention?

▶ GENERAL FEATURES

- Postpartum hemorrhage (PPH) is defined as a blood loss of 1000 mL or more or signs and symptoms of hypovolemia within the first 24 hours after delivery and up until 12 weeks postpartum, regardless of method of delivery.
  - Early or primary PPH occurs within the first 24 hours, whereas secondary PPH occurs after the first 24 hours.
  - The vast majority of PPH occurs within the first 24 hours of delivery.
- PPH is the leading cause of maternal mortality globally.
- The etiology of PPH can be classified by using the 4 Ts mnemonic: tone (uterine atony), trauma (lacerations, rupture, inversion), tissue (retained placental fragments), and thrombin (coagulopathies).
- Uterine atony is the most common cause of PPH.
  - Uterine atony is due to dysfunctional hypocontractility of the myometrium during the immediate puerperium.

- Risk factors for uterine atony include the presence of leiomyomata, multifetal gestations, polyhydramnios, and large for gestational age fetuses, chorioamnionitis, placental abruption, a placenta that implants into the lower uterine segment; and antenatal treatment with magnesium sulfate (used for neuroprotection in preeclampsia with severe features and eclampsia) and nifedipine (used for hypertension in pregnancy).
- Other risk factors for PPH include antepartum hemorrhage, augmented labor, maternal anemia, primiparity, prolonged labor, maternal obesity, fetal macrosomia, inherited or acquired coagulopathies (such as HELLP syndrome, von Willebrand disease, and disseminated intravascular coagulopathy [DIC]).

▶ CLINICAL ASSESSMENT

- The initial assessment must address hemodynamic status of the patient with immediate intervention when signs of hemodynamic compromise are present.
- As soon as a PPH is suspected, emergent intervention with a rapid response team to ensure coordinated care and to prevent cardiovascular collapse is essential.
- Cause of hemorrhage must be identified.
- If the placenta has already been delivered, examine the placenta for missing fragments. If it has not been delivered, apply controlled cord traction. Inspect the perineum, vaginal vault, and uterine cavity.

Examination may reveal a boggy uterus, and the fundus may be palpable above the level of the umbilicus.

- Visual estimation of blood loss is associated with a significant underestimation of actual blood loss and should only be used when other objective measures are not available; use of calibrated drapes is preferred.
- Signs of a hemorrhage include heart rate >110 beats per minute, BP ≤85/45 mm Hg, oxygen saturation <95%, delayed capillary refill, decreased urine output, and pallor.
  - These changes may not be apparent until the patient develops shock.
- Signs and symptoms associated with hypovolemia include lightheadedness, palpitations, confusion, syncope, fatigue, air hunger, and diaphoresis.
- A shock index (the ratio of heart rate to systolic blood pressure) >1 indicates a significant bleeding event and requires immediate management of the patient.

▶ DIAGNOSIS

- The diagnosis of PPH is based on the physical assessment of the patient and clinical suspicion.
- Ultrasonography can be utilized to assess the pelvis for retained placenta, hematomas, or peritoneal blood.

▶ TREATMENT

- Early diagnosis and intervention are essential in reducing mortality from PPH, and a coordinated team effort must be utilized.
- Management of hypovolemia and shock and identification and treatment of the underlying cause must be undertaken simultaneously.

- Oxytocin and uterine massage are the most important initial interventions for PPH.
- Bimanual compression of the uterus can also be performed if uterine massage is ineffective.
- Foley catheter can be used to monitor urinary output and can improve uterine atony. Resuscitation measures must be implemented and include elevating the legs of the patient, administering oxygen, and infusing normal saline or Ringer's lactate.
- Early administration of tranexamic acid has been shown to reduce maternal mortality from PPH and is recommended. It should be given within 3 hours of delivery.
- Rapid transfusion of 2-4 units of packed red blood cells is recommended. Type specific is preferred, but type O Rh-negative blood may be used.
- Ergonovine, carboprost, and misoprostol may be used for PPH caused by uterine atony.
- Other interventions for uterine atony include intrauterine tamponade with a uterine balloon or gauze, B-Lynch suturing of the uterus, arterial ligation, and uterine artery embolization.
- Definitive surgical management with hysterectomy may be necessary for severe, intractable hemorrhage.

Case Conclusion

The patient is showing signs of PPH and should be treated immediately by a rapid response team. The cause of PPH should be identified. Assess the uterus for atony, begin uterine massage, and initiate resuscitative measures. Uterotonics such as oxytocin are the recommended first-line pharmacologic intervention when uterine atony is present. Careful physical examination will often reveal the source of the bleeding.

CHAPTER 367

Trauma in Pregnancy

Katherine Thompson, MCHS

A 31-year-old female patient presents to the emergency department complaining of abdominal pain after being assaulted by her spouse. She states that she is 16 weeks' pregnant. She is gravida 3, para 0, miscarriages 2, abortions 0. Before this, the pregnancy has been uncomplicated. Her previous two miscarriages, one was spontaneous and the other was initiated by prior abuse from her spouse. She endorses nausea, vomiting, vaginal spotting, and intense pelvic pain. What test will be important to perform to help determine the degree of fetomaternal hemorrhage?

▶ GENERAL FEATURES

- Trauma in pregnancy complicates 1 in every 12 pregnancies and is the primary cause of nonobstetric death in pregnant women.
- The most common causes are motor vehicle crashes, intimate partner violence, assault, and falls.
- 9 of every 10 traumas in pregnancy are classified as minor, but 60% to 70% of fetal loss result from minor trauma.

- 4-24 hours of fetal monitoring is recommended even in minor trauma.
- There are unique considerations for advanced cardiac resuscitation in pregnant patients, including positioning for CPR and considerations for the preservation of fetal life, even in the event that the mother's injuries are fatal.
- Most trauma in pregnancy is minor blunt abdominal trauma or injuries resulting from motor vehicle collisions. However, because of the likelihood of fetal demise even from cases of minor trauma, the clinical judgment should err on the side of conservative monitoring and inpatient treatment.
- Complications of trauma in pregnancy include maternal death, fetal demise, delivery complications, and, in the case of domestic violence, increase in violence following hospitalization with or without delivery.

▸ CLINICAL ASSESSMENT

- Consider transfer to a qualified trauma center for pregnant patients, following minor to major trauma.
- Notify NICU and OB/GYN team support for potential response.
- Primary assessment should examine the airway, breathing, and circulation of the mother and should follow the basic trauma assessment of nonpregnant patients. If life threats are present (cardiac arrest, unresponsive patient, hypertension or hypotension, fetal tachycardia or bradycardia), the assessment and treatment should move to advanced cardiac life support measures (see "Treatment" section).
- In the case of intimate partner violence, assessment of the patient must include safety planning for home, depression screening, and suicidality risk. Pregnant and immediately postpartum patients are at the highest risk for increased violence.
- Placental abruption is best detected via monitoring and assessment of contractions. Ultrasound has a poor sensitivity (24%) but high specificity (96%) for detecting placental abruption.
- The Kleihauer-Betke test allows identification of fetal blood cells in maternal circulation and should be performed in all women who sustain major trauma, regardless of Rh status, to determine the degree of fetomaternal hemorrhage.

▸ DIAGNOSIS

- Criteria for diagnosis of all trauma in pregnancy are based on a consideration of the mechanism of injury, presenting examination, results of monitoring, ultrasound, and Kleihauer-Betke results.

▸ TREATMENT

- If signs of major trauma are present:
  - Airway/cervical spine immobilization
  - Breathing
  - Circulation
  - Deformity/disability
  - Exposure (preserve body heat)
  - Displace uterus to left (if >20 weeks)
  - IV access (at least two large-bore access points)
  - Laboratory tests: CBC, type and screen, Kleihauer-Betke
  - Viable fetus (>23-24 weeks): continuous FHR monitoring
  - Previable fetus (<23-24 weeks): FHR via Doppler auscultation or electronic fetal monitoring
- Further assessment and treatment will depend on the mechanism of injury:
  - Falls: assess for abdominal trauma, extremity injuries.
  - Burns: aggressive fluid resuscitation, consider delivery for body surface area exceeding 50%.
  - Motor vehicle accidents (MVAs): determine seat belt utilization.
  - Intimate partner violence: assess for suicidality and depression.
  - Penetrating trauma: assess location of point of entry and base recommendations on this.
- In the case of cardiac arrest, if there is no return of spontaneous circulation within 4-5 minutes of high-quality CPR, the American Heart Association recommends considering perimortem C-section.
- Perimortem cesarean section may save the life of a viable fetus (>23-24 weeks) and has been shown to increase venous return and cardiac output in the mother by 25% to 30%. It has not been shown to be harmful.

Case Conclusion

The Kleihauer-Betke test is sensitive and specific because it can detect fetal cells in maternal circulation.

References

PART I

American College of Cardiology/American Heart Association Task Force. 2017 guideline for the prevention, detection, evaluation, and management of high blood pressure in adults. American College of Cardiology; 2017. https://www.acc.org/~/media/Non-Clinical/Files-PDFs-Excel-MS-Word-etc/Guidelines/2017/Guidelines_Made_Simple_2017_HBP.pdf

Antman EM, Loscalzo J. Ischemic heart disease. In: Kasper D, Fauci A, Hauser S, Longo D, Jameson J, Loscalzo J, eds. *Harrison's Principles of Internal Medicine*. 19th ed. McGraw-Hill; 2014. Accessed May 13, 2020. http://accesspharmacy.mhmedical.com.libproxy.lib.unc.edu/content.aspx?bookid=1130&sectionid=79743463

Bashore TM, Granger CB, Jackson KP, Patel MR. Ventricular septal defect. In: Papadakis MA, McPhee SJ, Rabow MW, eds. *Current Medical Diagnosis and Treatment 2020*. McGraw-Hill; 2019. Accessed June 4, 2020. http://accessmedicine.mhmedical.com.lmunet.idm.oclc.org/content.aspx?bookid=2683&sectionid=225039183

Bradfield JS, Boyle NG, Shivkumar K. Ventricular arrhythmias. In: Fuster V, Harrington RA, Narula J, Eapen ZJ, eds. *Hurst's The Heart*. 14th ed. McGraw-Hill. Accessed June 18, 2020. https://accessmedicine-mhmedical-com.ezpoxy.elon.edu/content.apsx?bookid=2046&sectionid=176563954

Chung MK. Vitamins, supplements, herbal medicines, and arrhythmias. *Cardiol Rev*. 2004;12(2):73-84.

Clair DG, Beach JM. Mesenteric ischemia. *N Engl J Med*. 2016;374(10):959-968. doi:10.1056/NEJMra1503884

Cutlip D, Nicolau J. Long-term antiplatelet therapy after coronary artery stenting in stable patients. In: Post TW, ed. *UpToDate*. UpToDate. Accessed May 13, 2020. https://www.uptodate.com/contents/long-term-antiplatelet-therapy-after-coronary-artery-stenting-in-stable-patients

Farber M, Parodi F. Abdominal Aortic Aneurysms (AAA). *Merck Manual Professional Version*. Updated November 2020. Accessed April 11, 2021. https://www.merckmanuals.com/professional/cardiovascular-disorders/diseases-of-the-aorta-and-its-branches/abdominal-aortic-aneurysms-aaa

Farber M, Parodi F. Aortic dissection. *Merck Manual Professional Version*. Updated November 2020. Accessed April 11, 2021. https://www.merckmanuals.com/professional/cardiovascular-disorders/diseases-of-the-aorta-and-its-branches/aortic-dissection#v940343

Farber M, Parodi F. Thoracic aortic aneurysms. *Merck Manual Professional Version*. Updated November 2020. Accessed April 11, 2021. https://www.merckmanuals.com/professional/cardiovascular-disorders/diseases-of-the-aorta-and-its-branches/thoracic-aortic-aneurysms

Freeman R, Wieling W, Axelrod FB, et al. Consensus statement on the definition of orthostatic hypotension, neurally mediated syncope and the postural tachycardia syndrome. *Clin Auton Res*. 2011;21:69.

Gale CP, Camm AJ. Assessment of palpitations. *BMJ*. 2016;352:h5649.

Gloviczki P, Comerota AJ, Dalsing MC, et al. The care of patients with varicose veins and associated chronic venous diseases: clinical practice guidelines of the Society for Vascular Surgery and the American Venous Forum. *J Vasc Surg*. 2011;53(suppl 5):2S-48S. doi:10.1016/j.jvs.2011.01.079

Gloviczki P. *Handbook of Venous and Lymphatic Disorders*. 4th ed. Guidelines of the American Venous Forum. CRC Press; 2017.

Goldman L, Schafer A. *Goldman-Cecil Medicine*. Elsevier Saunders; 2020.

Harikrishnan KN, Vettukattil JJ. Congenital heart diseases. In: Elmoselhi A, ed. *Cardiology: An Integrated Approach*. McGraw-Hill. Accessed June 9, 2020. http://accessmedicine.mhmedical.com/content.aspx?bookid=2224&sectionid=171661563

Hoit B. Cardiac tamponade. In: Gersh JB, Hoekstra J, eds. *UpToDate*. Wolters Kluwer; 2020.

January CT, Wann LS, Alpert JS, et al. 2014 AHA/ACC/HRS Guideline for the management of patients with atrial fibrillation. *J Am Coll Cardiol*. 2014;64 (21):e1-e76.

January CT, Wann LS, Calkins H, et al. 2019 AHA/ACC/HRS focused update of the 2014 AHA/ACC/HRS Guideline for the management of patients with atrial fibrillation. *J Am Coll Cardiol*. 2019;74(1):105-132.

Januzzi JL, van Kimmenade R, Lainchbury J, et al. NT-proBNP testing for diagnosis and short-term prognosis in acute destabilized heart failure: an international pooled analysis of 1256 patients: The International Collaborative of NT-proBNP Study. *Eur Heart J*. 2006;27(3):330.

John RM, Stevenson WG. Approach to ventricular arrhythmias. In: Jameson J, Fauci AS, Kasper DL, Hauser SL, Longo DL, Loscalzo J, eds. *Harrison's Principles of Internal Medicine*. 20th ed. McGraw-Hill. Accessed June 18, 2020. https://accessmedicine-mhmedical-com.ezproxy.elon.edu/content.aspx?bookid=2129&sectionid=19202879

Jone P, Kim JS, Alvensleben J, Burkett D. Cardiovascular diseases. In: Hay WW Jr, Levin MJ, Abzug MJ, Bunik M, eds. *Current Diagnosis & Treatment: Pediatrics*. 25th ed. McGraw-Hill. Accessed June 13, 2020. https://accessmedicine.mhmedical.com/content.aspx?bookid=2815&sectionid=244261246

Kusumoto FM, Schoenfeld MH, Barrett C, et al. 2018 ACC/AHA/HRS Guideline on the evaluation and management of patients with bradycardia and cardiac conduction delay. *J Am Coll Cardiol*. 2019;74(7):e51-e156.

Lin JP, Aboulhosn JA, Child JS. Congenital heart disease in adolescents and adults. In: Fuster V, Harrington RA, Narula J, Eapen ZJ, eds. *Hurst's The Heart*. 14th ed. McGraw-Hill. Accessed June 9, 2020. http://accessmedicine.mhmedical.com/content.aspx?bookid=2046&sectionid=176559711

Massera D, McClelland RL, Ambale-Venkatesh B, et al. Prevalence of unexplained left ventricular hypertrophy by cardiac magnetic resonance imaging in MESA. *J Am Heart Assoc*. 2019;8:e012250.

McNally MM, Univers J. Acute limb ischemia. *Surg Clin North Am*. 2018;98(5):1081-1096. doi:10.1016/j.suc.2018.05.002

Merkel P. Clinical manifestations and diagnosis of polyarteritis nodosa in adults. *UpToDate* Updated January 21, 2019. Accessed June 6, 2020. https://www.uptodate.com/contents/cllinical-manifestations-and-diagnosis-of-polyarteritis-nodosa-in-adults

Nakamura K, Schmidt AS. Treatment of hypertension in coarctation of the aorta. *Curr Treat Options Cardiovasc Med*. 2016;18(6):40. doi:10.1007/s11936-016-0462-x

Nishimura RA, Otto CM, Bonow RO, et al. 2017 AHA/ACC focused update of the 2014 AHA/ACC Guideline for the management of patients with valvular heart disease: a report of the American College of Cardiology/American Heart Association Task Force on Clinical Practice Guidelines. *Circulation*. 2017;135(25):e1159-e1195. doi:10.1161/CIR.0000000000000503

Page RL, Joglar JA, Caldwell MA, et al. 2015 ACC/AHA/HRS Guideline for the management of adult patients with supraventricular tachycardia. *J Am Coll Cardiol*. 2016;67(13):1-89.

Rajagopalan S, Dean SM, Mohler ER, Mukherjee D. *Manual of Vascular Disease*. 2nd ed. Lippincott Williams & Wilkins; 2012.

Sabanayagam A, Harris IS. Congenital heart disease in adults. In: Crawford MH, ed. *CURRENT Diagnosis & Treatment: Cardiology*. 5th ed. McGraw-Hill. Accessed June 13, 2020. https://accessmedicine .mhmedical.com/content.aspx?bookid=2040&sectionid=152996920

Shen WK, Sheldon RS, Benditt DG, et al. 2017 ACC/AHA/HRS Guideline for the evaluation and management of patients with syncope: a report of the American College of Cardiology/American Heart Association Task Force on Clinical Practice Guidelines, and the Heart Rhythm Society. *J Am Coll Cardiol*. 2017;136(5):e25-e59.

Stout KK, Daniels CJ, Aboulhosn JA, et al. 2018 AHA/ACC Guidelines for the management of adults with congenital heart disease. *Circulation*. 2019;139:e698-e800. doi:10.1161/CIR.0000000000000603

Sutters M. Hypertensive urgencies & emergencies. In: Papadakis MA, Mcphee SJ, Rabow MW, eds. *Current Medical Diagnosis & Treatment*. McGraw-Hill; 2021.

Torok RD, Campbell MJ, Fleming GA, Hill KD. Coarctation of the aorta: management from infancy to adulthood. *World J Cardiol*. 2015;7(11):765-775. doi:10.4330/wjc.v7.i11.76

Vahanian A. Expert review: mitral valve disease. *E-J Cardiol Pract*. 2019;16(36). Accessed June 5, 2020. https://www.escardio .org/Journals/E-Journal-of-Cardiology-Practice/Volume-16/ Expert-review-mitral-valve-disease

Varounis C, Vasiliki K, Nihoyannopoulos P, et al. Cardiovascular hypertensive crisis: recent evidence and review of the literature. *Front Cardiovasc Med*. 2016;3:51. doi:10.3389/fcvm.2016.0051

Walvick MD, Walvick MP. Giant cell arteritis: laboratory predictors of a positive temporal artery biopsy. *Ophthalmology*. 2011;118(6):1201-1204.

Wexler RK, Pleister A, Raman SV. Palpitations: evaluation in the primary care setting. *Am Fam Physician*. 2017;96(12):784-789.

Whelton PK, Carey RM, Aronow WS, et al. 2017 ACC/AHA/AAPA/ ABC/ACPM/AGS/APhA/ASH/ASPC/NMA/PCNA guideline for the prevention, detection, evaluation, and management of high blood pressure in adults. *J Am Coll Cardiol*. 2018;71(19):e1-e248.

Zipes DP, Libby P, Bonow RO, et al., eds. *Braunwald's Heart Disease: A Textbook of Cardiovascular Medicine*. 11th ed. Elsevier; 2018.

PART II

Alikhan A, Lynch PJ, Eisen DB. Hidradenitis suppurativa: a comprehensive review. *J Am Acad Dermatol*. 2009;60(4):539-561.

Bates-Jensen BM, Patlan A. Pressure ulcers. In: Halter JB, Ouslander JG, Studenski S, et al., eds. *Hazzard's Geriatric Medicine and Gerontology*. 7th ed. McGraw-Hill; 2020. Accessed May 5, 2020. http://accessmedicine.mhmedical.com/content .aspx?bookid=1923&sectionid=144522255

Centers for Disease Control and Prevention. Parasites—scabies. Accessed June 18, 2020. www.cdc.gov/parasites/scabies/health_ professionals/meds.html

Chern A, Chern CM, Lushniak BD. Occupational skin diseases. In: Kang S, Amagai M, Bruckner AL, et al., eds. *Fitzpatrick's Dermatology*. 9th ed. McGraw-Hill Education; 2019.

Clark M, Gudjonsson JE, Pityriasis R. In: Kang S, Amagai M, Bruckner AL, et al., eds. *Fitzpatrick's Dermatology*. 9th ed. McGraw-Hill Education; 2019.

Devore C, Schutze G; The Council on School Health and Committee on Infectious Diseases. Head lice. *Pediatrics*. 2015;135:e1355. Accessed June 18, 2020. https://pediatrics.aappublications.org/content/ pediatrics/135/5/e1355.full.pdf

Duran C, Baumeister A. Recognition, diagnosis, and treatment of hidradenitis suppurativa. *J Am Acad Phys Assist*. 2019;32(10):36-42. doi:10.1097/01.JAA.0000578768.62051.13

Gilbert DN, Chambers HF. Eliopoulos. In: Gilbert DN, Chambers HF, Eliopoulos GM, Saag MS, Pavia AT, eds. *The Sanford Guide to Antimicrobial Therapy 2019*. 50th ed. Antimicrobial Therapy, Inc.; 2019.

Grimes P. Vitiligo: pathogenesis, clinical features, and diagnosis. *UpToDate*. Accessed June 15, 2020. https://www.uptodate.com/contents/ vitiligo-pathogenesis-clinical-features-and-diagnosis

Grimes P, Callender V. Melasma: management. *UpToDate*. Accessed May 7, 2020. https://www.uptodate.com/contents/melasma-management

Gudjonsson JE, Elder JT. Psoriasis. In: Kang S, Amagai M, Bruckner AL, et al., eds. *Fitzpatrick's Dermatology*. 9th ed. McGraw-Hill. Accessed July 31, 2020. https://accessmedicine.mhmedical.com/content .aspx?bookid=2570&sectionid=210417798

Gunning K, Kiraly B, Pippitt K. Lice and scabies: treatment update. *Am Fam Physician*. 2019;99(10):635-642.

Handel AC, Miot LD, Miot HA. Melasma: a clinical and epidemiological review. *An Bras Dermatol*. 2014;89(5):771-782. doi:10.1590/ abd1806-4841.20143063

Hessam S, Scholl L, Sand M, Schmitz L, Reitenbach S, Bechara FG. A novel severity assessment scoring system for hidradenitis suppurativa. *JAMA Dermatol*. 2018;154(3):330-335. doi:10.1001/ jamadermatol.2017.5890

Ingram JR. Hidradenitis suppurativa: treatment. In: Dellavalle RP, Dahl MV, eds. *UpToDate*. UpToDate; 2020.

Jameson L. *Harrison's Principles of Internal Medicine*. 20th ed. McGraw-Hill; 2018:353.

Kroshinsky D, Strazzula L. Pressure ulcers. September 2019. Accessed May 5, 2020. http://www.merckmanuals.com/professional/ dermatologic-disorders/pressure-ulcers/pressure-ulcers

Kucik CJ, Martin GL, Sortor BV. Common intestinal parasites. *Am Fam Physician*. 2004;69(5):1161-1168.

Lee EY, Alhusayen R, Lansing P, Shear N, Yeung J. What is hidradenitis suppurativa. *Can Fam Physician*. 2017;63(2):114-120.

Lyford W, James W. Which physical findings are characteristic of melasma. Medscape.com. Updated April 27, 2020. Accessed June 1, 2020. https://www.medscape.com/answers/1068640-159335/which -physical-findings-are-characteristic-of-melasma

Mangold AR, Pittelkow MR. Lichen planus. In: Kang S, Amagai M, Bruckner AL, et al., eds. *Fitzpatrick's Dermatology*. 9th ed. McGraw-Hill Education; 2019.

Mimouni D, Ankol OE, Davidovitch N, et al. Seasonality trends of scabies in a young adult population: a 20-year follow-up. *Br J Dermatol*. 2003;149(1):157-159.

Patterson JW. Vascular tumors. In: *Weedon's Skin Pathology*. 4th ed. Elsevier; 2016.

Popa ML, Popa AC, Tanase C, Gheorghisan-Galateanu AA. Acanthosis nigricans: to be or not to be afraid. *Oncol Lett*. 2019;17(5):4133-4138. doi:10.3892/ol.2018.9736

Rancone K. Vitiligo: practice essentials, background, pathophysiology. Emedicine.medscape.com. Accessed April 16, 2020. https://emedicine .medscape.com/article/1068962-overview

Scleroderma Foundation. Accessed July 2, 2020. scleroderma.org

Shinkai K, Fox LP. Psoriasis. In: Papadakis MA, McPhee SJ, Rabow MW, eds. *Current Medical Diagnosis and Treatment*. McGraw-Hill; 2020. Accessed July 31, 2020. https://accessmedicine.mhmedical .com/content.aspx?bookid=2683&sectionid=225034446

Sundaresan S, Migden MR, Silapunt S. Stasis dermatitis: pathophysiology, evaluation, and management. *Am J Clin Dermatol*. 2017;18(3):383-390. doi:10.1007/s40257-016-0250-0

Thomas DR. Pressure ulcers. In: Williams BA, Chang A, Ahalt C, et al., eds. *Current Diagnosis & Treatment: Geriatrics*. 2nd ed. McGraw-Hill; 2014. Accessed May 5, 2020. http://accessmedicine .mhmedical.com/content.aspx?bookid=953&sectionid=53375672

Turrentine JE, Sheehan MP, Cruz JPD. Allergic contact dermatitis. In: Kang S, Amagai M, Bruckner AL, et al., eds. *Fitzpatrick's Dermatology*. 9th ed. McGraw-Hill Education; 2019.

U.S. Department of Health and Human Services, National Institutes of Health, U.S. National Library of Medicine. Scleroderma. Accessed July 2, 2020 https://medlineplus.gov/scleroderma.html

PART III

Alter H. Approach to the adult with epistaxis. Accessed June 12, 2020. https://www.uptodate.com/contents/approach-to-the-adult-with-epistaxis

American Academy of Ophthalmology. Blepharitis: preferred practice pattern. Accessed May 27, 2020. https://www.aao.org/preferred-practice-pattern/blepharitis-ppp-2018

American Academy of Ophthalmology. Conjunctivitis: preferred practice pattern. Accessed May 28, 2020. https://www.aao.org/preferred-practice-pattern/conjunctivitis-ppp-2018

American Academy of Otolaryngology/Head and Neck Surgery. Clinical Practice Guidelines: adult sinusitis. Accessed June 17, 2020. https://www.entnet.org/content/clinical-practice-guideline-adult-sinusitis

Bagheri N, Wajda B, Calvo C, Durrani A. *The Wills Eye Manual: Office and Emergency Room Diagnosis and Treatment of Eye Disease.* Lippincott Williams & Wilkins; 2016.

Beck RW, Cleary PA, Anderson MM Jr, et al. A randomized, controlled trial of corticosteroids in the treatment of acute optic neuritis. The Optic Neuritis Study Group. *N Engl J Med.* 1992;326(9):581-588. doi:10.1056/NEJM199202273260901

Cao Z, Zhao F, Mulugeta H. Noise exposure as a risk factor for acoustic neuroma: a systematic review and meta-analysis. *Int J Audiol.* 2019;58(9):525-532. doi:10.1080/14992027.2019.1602289

Castle JT. Cholesteatoma pearls: practical points and update. *Head Neck Pathol.* 2018;12(3):419-429. doi:10.1007/s12105-018-0915-5

Earwood J, Rogers T, Rathjen N. Ear pain: diagnosing common and uncommon causes. *Am Fam Physician.* 2018;97(1):20-27.

Guideline Central. IDSA guide to infectious disease. Accessed June 17, 2020. http://eguideline.guidelinecentral.com/idsa-guidelines-bundle/rhinosinusitis-idsa-bundle-2

Haynes JH, Zeringue M. Removal of foreign bodies from the ear and nose. In: Pfenninger JL, Fowler GC, eds. *Procedures for Primary Care.* Elsevier; 2020:1359-1364.

Kennedy KL, Singh AK. Middle ear cholesteatoma. In: *StatPearls [Internet].* StatPearls Publishing; 2019.

Koh E, Frazzini VI, Kagetsu NJ. Epistaxis: vascular anatomy, origins, and endovascular treatment. *AJR Am J Roentgenol.* 2000; 174(3):845-851.

Kucik CJ, Clenney T. Management of epistaxis. *Am Fam Physician.* 2005;71(2):305-311.

Kumar B, Pant B, Jeppu S. Infarcted angiectatic nasal polyp with bone erosion and pterygopalatine fossa involvement-simulating malignancy. Case report and review of literatures. *Internet J Pathol.* 2012;13(2). Accessed September 16, 2020. https://ispub.com/IJPA/13/2/13997

Lindsley K, Nichols JJ, Dickersin K. Non-surgical interventions for acute internal hordeolum. *Cochrane Database Syst Rev.* 2017, Issue 1. Art. No.: CD007742. doi:10.1002/14651858.CD007742.pub4

Maxson S, Yamauchi T. Acute otitis media. *Pediatr Rev.* 1996;17:191-195.

McHenry M. Cerumen impaction removal. In: Pfenninger JL, Fowler GC, eds. *Procedures for Primary Care.* Elsevier; 2020:388-392.

Morgan DJ, Kellerman R. Epistaxis: evaluation and treatment. *Prim Care.* 2014;41:63-73.

Muncie H, Sirmans S, James E. Dizziness: approach to evaluation and management. *Am Fam Physician.* 2017;95(3):154-162.

Nash SD, Cruickshanks KJ, Klein R, et al. The prevalence of hearing impairment and associated risk factors: the Beaver Dam Offspring Study. *Arch Otolaryngol Head Neck Surg.* 2011;137:432.

Papadakis MA, McPhee SJ, Rabow MW, eds. *Current Medical Diagnosis and Treatment 2020.* McGraw-Hill. Accessed June 17, 2020. https://accessmedicine-mhmedical-com.ezproxy.elon.edu/content.aspx?bookid=2683&sectionid=222924373

Park JK, Vernick DM, Ramakrishna N. Vestibular schwannoma: acoustic neuroma. *UpToDate.* Accessed June 17, 2020. https://www.uptodate.com/contents/vestibular-schwannoma-acoustic-neuroma?search=acoustic%20neuroma&source=search_result&selectedTitle=1~40&usage_type=default&display_rank=1

Riordan-Eva P, Augsburger JJ. eds. *Vaughan & Asbury's General Ophthalmology.* 19th ed. McGraw-Hill. Accessed June 19, 2020. https://accessmedicine.mhmedical.com/content.aspx?bookid=2186&sectionid=165515600

Rosenfeld R, Shin JJ, Schwartz SR, et al. Clinical practice guideline: otitis media with effusion. *Otolaryngol Head Neck Surg.* 2016;154 (suppl 1):S1-S41.

Schilder A, Bhutta MF, Butler CC, et al. Eustachian tube dysfunction: consensus statement on definition, types, clinical presentation and diagnosis. *Clin Otolaryngol.* 2015;30(5):407-411.

Sedaghat A. Chronic sinusitis. *Am Fam Physician.* 2017;96(8):500-506.

Siegel R, Bien J. Acute otitis media in children: a continuing story. *Pediatr Rev.* 2004;25:187-193.

Usatine RP, Smith MA, Mayeaux EJ, Jr, Chumley HS. eds. *The Color Atlas and Synopsis of Family Medicine.* 3rd ed. McGraw-Hill. Accessed June 19, 2020. https://accessmedicine.mhmedical.com/content.aspx?bookid=2547&sectionid=206775136

Vrablik ME, Snead GR, Minnigan HJ, Kirschner JM, Emmett TW, Seupaul RA. The diagnostic accuracy of bedside ocular ultrasonography for the diagnosis of retinal detachment: a systematic review and meta-analysis. *Ann Emerg Med.* 2015;65(2):199-203.e191.

Wajda BN, Bagheri N. *The Wills Eye Manual: Office and Emergency Room Diagnosis and Treatment of Eye Disease.* 7th ed. Lippincott Williams & Wilkins; 2017.

Walsh FB, Miller NR, Hoyt WF. *Walsh and Hoyts Clinical Neuro-Ophthalmology: The Essentials.* Lippincott Williams & Wilkins; 2016.

Wilson KF, Meier JD, Ward PD. Salivary gland disorders. *Am Fam Physician.* 2014;89(11):882-888.

PART IV

Alguire P, Dupras D; American College of Physicians. *Medical Knowledge Self-Assessment Program.* American College of Physicians; 2018.

American Diabetes Association. Standards of medical care in diabetes—2020 abridged for primary care providers. *Clin Diabetes.* 2020;38(1):10-38. doi:10.2337/cd20-as01

American Society of Clinical Oncology. Thyroid cancer statistics. Accessed June 4, 2020. https://www.cancer.net/cancer-types/thyroid-cancer/statistics

Beckers A, Petrossians P, Hansen J, Daly AF. The causes and consequences of pituitary gigantism. *Nat Rev Endocrinol.* 2018;14(12):705-720.

Center for Disease Control and Prevention. National Diabetes Statistics Report, 2020. Accessed June 12, 2020. https://www.cdc.gov/diabetes/pdfs/data/statistics/national-diabetes-statistics-report.pdf

Garber AJ, Handelsman Y, Grunberger G, et al. Consensus Statement by the American Association of Clinical Endocrinologists and American College of Endocrinology on the comprehensive type 2 diabetes management algorithm—2020 executive summary. *Endocr Pract.* 2020;26(1):107-139.

Gharib H, Papini E, Garber JR, et al. American Association of Clinical Endocrinologists, American College of Endocrinology, and Associazione Medici Endocrinologi Medical Guidelines for clinical practice for the diagnosis and management of thyroid nodules—2016 update. *Endocr Pract.* 2016;22(5):622-639.

Haugen BR, Alexander EK, Bible KC, et al. 2015 American Thyroid Association Management Guidelines for adult patients with thyroid nodules and differentiated thyroid cancer. *Thyroid.* 2016;26(1):1-133.

Kasper DL, Fauci AS, Hauser SL, Longo DL, Jameson JL, Loscalzo J, eds. *Harrison's Principles of Internal Medicine.* 19th ed. McGraw-Hill Education; 2015.

Lerma EV, Berns JS, Nissenson AR. *Current Diagnosis & Treatment*. McGraw-Hill Professional; 2009.

Smallridge RC, Ain KB, Asa SL, et al. American Thyroid Association Guidelines for management of patients with anaplastic thyroid cancer. *Thyroid*. 2012;22(11):1104-1139.

PART V

Amer T, Wilson R, Chlosta P, et al. Penile fracture: a meta-analysis. *Urol Int*. 2016;96(3):315-329.

American Urological Association. Erectile dysfunction: AUA guidelines. Published 2018. Accessed June 1, 2020. https://www.auanet.org/guidelines/erectile-dysfunction-(ed)-guideline

American Urological Association. Peyronie's disease: AUA guidelines. Published 2015. Accessed June 1, 2020. https://www.auanet.org/guidelines/peyronies-disease-guideline

Broghammer JA, Santucci RA. Urethral Strictures in Males Workup: Approach Considerations, Imaging Studies, Diagnostic Procedures. Medscape; 2020. Retrieved August 15, 2020. https://emedicine.medscape.com/article/450903-workup#c7

Burr NE, Everett SM. Management of benign oesophageal strictures. *Frontline Gastroenterology*. 2019;10:177-181.

Centers for Disease Control and Prevention. Epididymitis. http://www.cdc.gov/std/tg2015/epididymitis.htm

Dajusta DG, Granberg CF, Villanueva C, Baker LA. Contemporary review of testicular torsion: new concepts, emerging technologies and potential therapeutics. *J Pediatr Urol*. 2013;9(6):723-730. doi:10.1016/j.jpurol.2012.08.012

Domino FJ, Baldor RA, Golding J, Grimes JA, Taylor JS, eds. Bladder cancer. In: *The 5-Minute Clinical Consult 2010*. 18th ed. Lippincott Williams & Wilkins; 2009:1004-1005.

Ellsworth P, Caldamone A. Bladder cancer. In: Onion DK, ed. *The Little Black Book of Urology*. 2nd ed. Jones and Bartlett; 2007:237-239, 243-244.

Foster HE, Dahm P, Kohler TS, et al. Surgical management of lower urinary tract symptoms attributed to benign prostatic hyperplasia: AUA guideline amendment 2019. *J Urol*. 2019;202(3):592-598. doi:10.1097/JU.0000000000000319

Gill BC, Vasavada SP, Firoozi F, Rackley RR. Urethral prolapse: practice essentials, history of the procedure, problem. Medscape; 2020. Retrieved August 17, 2020. https://emedicine.medscape.com/article/443165-overview#a8

Grigorian A, Livingston J, Schubl SD, et al. National analysis of testicular and scrotal trauma in the USA. *Res Rep Urol*. 2018;10:51-56.

Koifman L, Barros R, Júnior RA, Cavalcanti AG, Favorito LA. Penile fracture: diagnosis, treatment and outcomes of 150 patients. *Urology*. 2010;76:1488-1492.

Macfarlane MT. Urothelial cancers. In: *House Officer Series: Urology*. 4th ed. Lippincott Williams & Wilkins; 2006:41-42, 251-252.

Mansbach JM, Forbes P, Peters C. Testicular torsion and risk factors for orchiectomy. *Arch Pediatr Adolesc Med*. 2005;159(12):1167-1171. doi:10.1001/archpedi.159.12.1167

National Cancer Institute, Surveillance, Epidemiology, and End Results Program. Cancer stat facts: prostate cancer. Accessed April 27, 2020. https://seer.cancer.gov/statfacts/html/prost.html

Rodriguez KM, Dao Z, Pastuszak AW, Khera M. Genitourinary disorders in primary care. In: Bhasin S, O'Leary MP, Basaria SS, eds. *Essentials of Men's Health*. McGraw-Hill; 2021. Accessed August 24, 2020.

Schade G. Testicular Cancers (germ cell tumors). In: Papadakis MA, McPhee SJ, Rabow MW. eds. *Current Medical Diagnosis and Treatment 2020*. McGraw-Hill; Accessed August 2, 2021. https://accessmedicine-mhmedical-com.proxygw.wrlc.org/content.aspx?bookid=2683&sectionid=225060139

Steinberg GD. Bladder cancer. *Medscape*. Published May 6, 2020. Accessed June 10, 2020. https://emedicine.medscape.com/article/438262-overview

Turek PJ. Prostatitis. *Medscape*. Published November 1, 2019. Accessed June 2, 2020. https://emedicine.medscape.com/article/785418-overview

Williams DA. *PANCE Prep Pearls: A Medical Study and Review Guide for the PANCE, PANRE & Medical Examinations*. 2nd ed. Create Space Independent Publishing; 2017.

PART VI

American Association for the Study of Liver Diseases—Infectious Diseases Society of America. Recommendations for testing, managing, and treating hepatitis C. Accessed May 24, 2020. http://www.hcvguidelines.org

Beck DE, Wexner SD, Rafferty JF. *Gordon and Nivatvongs' Principles and Practice of Surgery for the Colon, Rectum, and Anus*. Thieme Medical Publishers; 2018.

Blau N, van Spronsen FJ, Levy HL. Phenylketonuria. *Lancet*. 2010; 376:1417.

Castell D. Major disorders of esophageal hyperperistalsis: clinical features, diagnosis and management. In: Post T, ed. *UpToDate*. UpToDate; 2020. Accessed April 25, 2020. www.uptodate.com

Chey W, Leontiadis G, Grigorios I, et al. ACG clinical guideline: treatment of *Helicobacter pylori* infection. *Am J Gastroenterol*. 2017;112(2):212-239. doi:10.1038/ajg.2016.563

Grossi L, Ciccaglione AF, Marzio L. Esophagitis and its causes: Who is "guilty" when acid is found "not guilty"? *World J Gastroenterol*. 2017;23(17):3011-3016. doi:10.3748/wjg.v23.i17.3011

Ferri FF. *Ferri's Clinical Advisor 2020: Instant Diagnosis and Treatment*. Elsevier Mosby; 2020.

Friedman S. Irritable bowel syndrome. In: Greenberger NJ, Blumberg RS, Burakoff R, eds. *CURRENT Diagnosis & Treatment: Gastroenterology, Hepatology, & Endoscopy*. 3rd ed. McGraw-Hill Education; 2016. Accessed August 18, 2020.

Gasper WJ, Rapp JH, Johnson MD. Visceral artery insufficiency (Intestinal angina). In: Papadakis MA, McPhee SJ, Rabow MW, eds. *Current Medical Diagnosis and Treatment 2020*. McGraw-Hill Education; 2020. Accessed August 17, 2020.

Hirano I, Chan ES, Rank MA, et al. AGA institute and the joint task force on allergy-immunology practice parameters clinical guidelines for the management of eosinophilic esophagitis. *Gastroenterology*. 2020;158(6):1776-1786. doi:10.1053/j.gastro.2020.02.038

Hoversten P, Kamboj AK, Katzka DA. Infections of the esophagus: an update on risk factors, diagnosis, and management. *Dis Esophagus*. 2018;31(12). doi:10.1093/dote/doy1094

Kahrilas P. Clinical manifestations and diagnosis of gastroesophageal reflux in adults. In: Post T, ed. *UpToDate*. UpToDate; 2020. Accessed April 30, 2020. www.uptodate.com

Katz P, Gerson L, Vela M. Guidelines for the diagnosis and management of gastroesophageal reflux disease. *Am J Gastroenterol*. 2013;108(3): 308-328. doi:10.1038/ajg.2012.444

Kemp WL, Burns DK, Brown TG. Pathology of the liver, gallbladder, and pancreas. In: Kemp WL, Burns DK, Brown TG, eds. *Pathology: The Big Picture*. McGraw-Hill. Accessed October 09, 2020. https://accessmedicine-mhmedical-com.ezproxy2.library.drexel.edu/content.aspx?bookid=499&sectionid=41568298

Klarenbeek BR, de Korte N, van der Peet DL, Cuesta MA. Review of current classifications for diverticular disease and a translation into clinical practice. *Int J Colorectal Dis*. 2012;27:207-214.

Kruger D. Assessing esophageal dysphagia. *JAAPA*. 2014;27(5):23-30.

Management of benign esophageal strictures. *UpToDate*. Accessed July 20, 2020. http://www.uptodate.com/contents/management-of-benign-esophageal-strictures?source=see_link&sectionName Complex+strictures&anchor=H12

Kumbum K. Esophageal stricture. Accessed July 20, 2020. https://emedicine.medscape.com/article/175098-overview

Kwo PY, Cohen SM, Lim JK. ACG clinical guideline: evaluation of abnormal liver chemistries. *Am J Gastroenterol*. 2017;112:18-35; doi:10.1038/ajg.2016.517. Accessed May 25, 2020.

Leifeld L, Kruis W. Management des toxischen Megakolons [Current management of toxic megacolon]. *Z Gastroenterol*. 2012;50(3):316-322. doi:10.1055/s-0031-1299079

McQuaid KR. Irritable bowel syndrome. In: Papadakis MA, McPhee SJ, Rabow MW, eds. *Current Medical Diagnosis and Treatment 2020*. McGraw-Hill Education; 2020. Accessed August 18, 2020.

Poison Control: National Capital Poison Centre. Poison statistics. Accessed August 19, 2020. https://www.poison.org/poison-statistics-national

Quinlan JD. Acute pancreatitis. *Am Fam Physician*. 2014;90(9):632-639.

Schillie S, Wester C, Osborne M, Wesolowski L, Ryerson AB. CDC recommendations for hepatitis c screening among adults—United States, 2020. *MMWR Recomp Rep*. 2020;69(2):1-17.

See LS. Acute lower gastrointestinal bleeding. In: McKean SC, Ross JJ, Dressler DD, Brotman DJ, Ginsberg JS, eds. *Principles and Practice of Hospital Medicine*. McGraw-Hill; 2012: 1315-1316.

Spechler SJ. Achalasia: pathogenesis, clinical manifestations, and diagnosis. In: Post T, ed. *UptoDate*. UpToDate; 2020. Accessed April 23, 2020. www.uptodate.com

Stoffel EM, Jajoo K, Greenberger NJ. Mesenteric vascular disease. In: Greenberger NJ, Blumberg RS, Burakoff R, eds. *CURRENT Diagnosis & Treatment: Gastroenterology, Hepatology, & Endoscopy*. 3rd ed. McGraw-Hill Education; 2016. Accessed August 17, 2020.

Templeton AW, Strate LL. Updates in diverticular disease. *Curr Gastroenterol Rep*. 2013;15(8):339.

Tintinalli JE, Ma OJ, Yealy DM, et al., eds. *Tintinalli's Emergency Medicine: A Comprehensive Study Guide*. 9th ed. McGraw-Hill Education; 2020.

Tyagi S, Cappell MS. Large bowel disorders. In: McKean SC, Ross JJ, Dressler DD, Brotman DJ, Ginsberg JS, eds. *Principles and Practice of Hospital Medicine*. McGraw-Hill; 2012:1341-1343.

Vege SS. Clinical manifestations and diagnosis of acute pancreatitis. In: Whitcomb DC, Grover S, eds. *UpToDate*. Accessed October 23, 2019. www.uptodate.com/contents/clinical-manifestations-and-diagnosis-of-acute-pancreatitis?search=acute+pancreatitis

United States Preventive Services Taskforce. Recommendation: colorectal cancer: screening. Published June 15, 2016. Accessed July 24, 2020. https://uspreventiveservicestaskforce.org/uspstf/recommendation/colorectal-cancer-screening

Hande KR, Garrow GC. Acute tumor lysis syndrome in patients with high-grade non-Hodgkin's lymphoma. *Am J Med*. 1993;94:133-139.

Ishii H, Rai B, Traxer O, Kata S, Somani BK. Outcome of ureteroscopy for stone disease in patients with horseshoe kidney: review of world literature. *Urol Ann*. 2015;7(4):470-474.

Kidney Disease: Improving Global Outcomes (KDIGO) Acute Kidney Injury Work Group. KDIGO clinical practice guideline for acute kidney injury. *Kidney Int Suppl*. 2012;2: 1-150.

Kirkpatrick JJ, Leslie SW. Horseshoes kidney. *StatPearls [Internet]*. Updated May 29, 2020. Accessed 15 June 2020. https://www.ncbi.nlm.nih.gov/books/NBK431105/

Kraft MD, Btaiche IF, Sacks GS, Kudsk KA. Treatment of electrolyte disorders in adult patients in the intensive care unit. *Am J Health Syst Pharm*. 2005;62:1663-1682.

Lederer E. Regulation of serum phosphate. *J Physiol*. 2014;592:3985-3995.

Liu KD, Goldstein SL, Vijayan A, et al. AKI!Now initiative: recommendations for awareness, recognition, and management of AKI. *Clin J Am Soc Nephrol*. 2020;15(12):1838-1847. doi:10.2215/CJN.15611219

Nishikawa M, Shimada N, Kanzaki M, et al. The characteristics of patients with hypermagnesemia who underwent emergency hemodialysis. *Acute Med Surg*. 2018;5(3):222-229.

Pawar AS, Thongprayoon C, Cheungpasitporn W, et al. Incidence and characteristics of kidney stones in patients with horseshoe kidney: a systematic review and meta-analysis. *Urol Ann*. 2018;10(1):87-93.

Shah SS, Ronan JC, Alverson B. *Step-up to Pediatrics*. Lippincott Williams & Wilkins; 2014.

Talmage RV, Mobley HT. Calcium homeostasis: reassessment of the actions of parathyroid hormone. *Gen Comp Endocrinol*. 2008;156:1-8.

Turakhia MP, Blakestijin PJ, Carrero JJ, et al. Chronic kidney disease and arrhythmias: conclusions from a Kidney Disease: Improving Global Outcomes (KDIGO) Controversies Conference. *Eur Heart J*. 2018;39(24):2314-2325.

United States Renal Data System. 2019 USRDS Annual Data Report: epidemiology of kidney disease in the United States. National Institutes of Health, National Institute of Diabetes and Digestive and Kidney Diseases; 2019. Accessed August, 2, 2021. https://www.usrds.org/annual-data-report/

PART VII

Blaine J, Chonchol M, Levi M. Renal control of calcium, phosphate, and magnesium homeostasis. *Clin J Am Soc Nephrol*. 2015;10:1257.

Center for Disease Control and Prevention. Chronic kidney disease in the United States 2019. Accessed March 1, 2020. https://www.cdc.gov/kidneydisease/pdf/2019_National-Chronic-Kidney-Disease-Fact-Sheet.pdf

Chintagumpala M, Muscal JA. Presentation, diagnosis, and staging of Wilms tumor. In: Pappo AS, ed. *UpToDate*. UpToDate Inc. Updated June 17, 2019. Accessed June 6, 2020.https://www-uptodate-com

Cho JY, Lee Y H, Toi A, Macdonald B. Prenatal diagnosis of horseshoe kidney by measurement of the renal pelvic angle. *Ultrasound Obstet Gynecol*. 2005;25:554-558. doi:10.1002/uog.1904

Cohen DL, Ghosn M, Suarez J, Townsend RR. Secondary hypertension. In: Lerma EV, Rosner MH, Perazella MA, eds. *CURRENT Diagnosis & Treatment: Nephrology & Hypertension*. 2nd ed. McGraw-Hill. Accessed June 16, 2020. https://accessmedicine.mhmedical.com/content.aspx?bookid=2287&sectionid=177430098

CureSearch for Children's Cancer. About Wilms Tumor. Accessed June 4, 2020. https://curesearch.org/Wilms-Tumor-in-Children

Dirkx TC, Woodell T. Renal artery stenosis. In: Papadakis MA, McPhee SJ, Rabow MW, eds. *Current Medical Diagnosis and Treatment 2020*. McGraw-Hill. Accessed June 16, 2020. https://accessmedicine.mhmedical.com/content.aspx?bookid=2683&sectionid=225130840

Felsenfeld AJ, Levine BS, Rodriguez M. Pathophysiology of calcium, phosphorus, and magnesium dysregulation in chronic kidney disease. *Semin Dial*. 2015;28:564-577.

PART VIII

Abboud MR. Standard management of sickle cell disease complications. *Hematol Oncol Stem Ther*. 2020;13(2):85-90. doi:10.1016/j.hemonc.2019.12.007

American Psychiatric Association. *Diagnostic and Statistical Manual of Mental Disorders: Dsm-5*. American Psychiatric Association, 2013.

Beer PA, Green AR. Essential thrombocythemia. In: Kaushansky K, Lichtman MA, Prchal JT, et al., eds. *Williams Hematology*. 9th ed. McGraw-Hill; 2016:1307-1318.

Berlin NI. Polycythemia vera: diagnosis and treatment 2002. *Expert Rev Anticancer Ther*. 2002;2:330-336.

Brodskey RA. Diagnosis of hemolytic anemia in the adult. *UpToDate*. Published 2020. Updated December 13, 2019. Accessed May 4, 2020. https://www.uptodate.com/contents/diagnosis-of-hemolytic-anemia-in-the-adult?search=hemolytic%20anemia&source=search_result&selectedTitle=1~150&usage_type=default&display_rank=1

Cataland SR, Wu HF. Diagnosis and management of complement mediated thrombotic microangiopathies. *Blood Rev*. 2014;28:67-74.

DeLoughery TG. Hemolytic anemia. In: Rakel D, Kellerman RD, eds. *Conn's Current Therapy*. Elsevier; 2020:411-416.

Dhakal B, Szabo A, Chhabra S, et al. Autologous transplantation for newly diagnosed multiple myeloma in the era of novel agent induction: a systematic review and meta-analysis. *JAMA Oncol*. 2018;4(3):343-350.

Diz-Küçükkaya R, López JA. Thrombocytopenia. In: Kaushansky K, Lichtman MA, Prchal JT, Levi MM, Press OW, Burns LJ, Caligiuri

M, eds. *Williams Hematology.* 9th ed. McGraw-Hill. Accessed July 6, 2020. https://accessmedicine.mhmedical.com/content.aspx?bookid=1581&sectionid=108081041

Ebert MH, Loosen PT, Nurcombe B, Leckman JF, eds. *Current Diagnosis & Treatment: Psychiatry.* 2nd ed. McGraw-Hill Companies; 2008.

Eichenauer DA, Aleman BMP, Andre M, et al. Hodgkin lymphoma: ESMO clinical practice guidelines for diagnosis, treatment and follow-up. *Ann Oncol.* 2018;29(suppl 4):iv19-iv29.

Fenaux P, Haase D, Sanz GF, et al. Myelodysplastic syndromes: ESMO clinical practice guidelines for diagnosis, treatment and follow-up. *Ann Oncol.* 2014;25(suppl 3):57-69.

Fonseca R. Trends in overall survival and costs of multiple myeloma, 2000-2014, *Leukemia.* 2017;31(9):1915-1921.

Harrison CN, Bareford D, Butt N, et al. Guideline for investigation and management of adults and children presenting with a thrombocytosis. *Br J Haematol.* 2010;149, 352-375.

Keohane EM, Ntto CN, Walenga JM. Hemolytic uremic syndrome. *Rodak's Hematology: Clinical Principles and Applications.* 6th ed. Elsevier; 2020.

Killick SB, Bown N, Cavenagh J, et al. Guidelines for the diagnosis and management of adult aplastic anaemia. *Br J Haematol* 2016;172:187-207.

Killick SB, Carter C, Culligan D, et al. Guidelines for the diagnosis and management of adult myelodysplastic syndromes. *Br J Haematol.* 2013;164, 503-525.

Konkle BA. Disorders of platelets and vessel wall. In: Jameson J, Fauci AS, Kasper DL, Hauser SL, Longo DL, Loscalzo J, eds. *Harrison's Principles of Internal Medicine.* 20th ed. McGraw-Hill. Accessed July 16, 2020. https://accessmedicine.mhmedical.com/content.aspx?bookid=2129&sectionid=192018598

Kumar SK, Callander NS, Hillengass J, et al. NCCN guidelines insights: multiple myeloma, version 1.2020. *J Natl Compr Canc Netw.* 2019;17(10):1154-1165.

Kumar SK, Rajkumar V, Kyle RA, et al. Multiple myeloma. *Nat Rev Dis Primers.* 2017;3:17046.

Leavitt AD, Minichiello T. Increased platelet destruction. In: Papadakis MA, McPhee SJ, Rabow MW, eds. *Current Medical Diagnosis and Treatment 2020.* McGraw-Hill. Accessed July 02, 2020. https://accessmedicine.mhmedical.com/content.aspx?bookid=2683&sectionid=225044878

Moake J. Thrombotic microangiopathies: multimers, metalloprotease, and beyond. *Clin Transl Sci.* 2009;2:366-373.

Moll S. New insights into treatment of venous thromboembolism. *Hematology Am Soc Hematol Educ Program.* 2014;2014(1):297-305. doi:10.1182/asheducation-2014.1.297

Moll S. Thrombophilia: clinical-practical aspects. *J Thromb Thrombolysis.* 2015;39(3):367-378. doi:10.1007/s11239-015-1197-3

Pearson TC. Evaluation of diagnostic criteria in polycythemia vera. *Semin Hematol.* 2001;38(1 suppl 2):21-24.

Petruzziello TN, Mawji IA, Khan M, et al. Verotoxin biology: molecular events in vascular endothelial injury. *Kidney Int.* 2009;75:S17-S19.

Piel FB, Steinberg MH, Rees DC. Sickle cell disease. *N Engl J Med.* 2017;376(16):1561-1570.

Rajkumar SV. Multiple myeloma: Every year a new standard? *Hematol Oncol.* 2019;37(suppl 1):62-65.

Rajkumar SV, Dimopoulos MA, Palumbo A, et al. International Myeloma Working Group updated criteria for the diagnosis of multiple myeloma. *Lancet Oncol.* 2014;15:e538-e548.

Rose MG, Berliner N. Disorders of red blood cells. In: Benjamin IJ, ed. *Andreoli and Carpenter's Cecil Essentials of Medicine.* 9th ed. Saunders; 2016:502-514.

Sato T, Nakamura H, Fujieda Y, et al. Factor Xa inhibitors for preventing recurrent thrombosis in patients with antiphospholipid syndrome: a longitudinal cohort study. *Lupus.* 2019;28(13):1577-1582. doi:10.1177/0961203319881200

Schneidewend R, Epperla N, Friedman KD. Thrombotic thrombocytopenic purpura and hemolytic uremic syndrome. In: Hoffman R, Benz EJ Jr, Silberstein LE, et al., eds. *Hematology: Basic Principles and Practice.* 7th ed. Elsevier; 2018:1984-2000.

Sugiura T, Yamamoto K, Murakami K, et al. Immune thrombocytopenic purpura detected with oral hemorrhage: a case report. *J Dent (Shiraz).* 2018;19(2):159-163. https://www.ncbi.nlm.nih.gov/pmc/articles/PMC5960737/

Tilly H, da Silva MG, Vitolo U, et al. Diffuse large B-cell lymphoma (DLBCL): ESMO Clinical Practice Guidelines for diagnosis, treatment and follow-up. *Ann Oncol.* 2015;26(suppl 5):116-125.

Vainchenker W, Delhommeau F, Constantinescu SN, et al. New mutations and pathogenesis of myeloproliferative neoplasm. *Blood.* 2011:118(7):1723-1735.

Verhovsek M, McFarlane A. Abnormalities in red blood cells. In: McKean SC, Ross JJ, Dressler DD, Brotman DJ, Ginsberg JS, eds. *Principles and Practice of Hospital Medicine.* McGraw-Hill; 2012:1423-1442.

U.S. Department of Health and Human Services National Institutes of Health; National Heart, Lung, and Blood Institute. *The Management of Sickle Cell Disease.* 4th ed. The Institute; 2004. NIH Publication No. 04-2117.

PART IX

Adhikari EH. Syphilis in pregnancy. *Obstet Gynecol.* 2020;135(5):1121-1135. doi:10.1097/AOG.0000000000003788

American College of Obstetricians and Gynecologists. Management of genital herpes in pregnancy: ACOG Practice Bulletin No 220. *Obstet Gynecol.* 2020;135(5):1236-1238.

American College of Obstetricians and Gynecologists. ACOG Committee Opinion No. 752: prenatal and perinatal human immunodeficiency virus testing. *Obstet Gynecol.* 2018;132(3):e138-e142.

Bate SL, Dollard SC, Cannon MJ. Cytomegalovirus seroprevalence in the United States: the national health and nutrition examination surveys, 1988-2004. *Clin Infect Dis.* 2010;50(11):1439-1447.

Centers for Disease Control and Prevention. About parasites. Accessed June 19, 2020. www.cdc.gov/parasites/about.html

Centers for Disease Control and Prevention. Malaria facts. Updated April 15, 2016. Accessed January 7, 2017. https://www.cdc.gov/malaria/about/facts.html

Centers for Disease Control and Prevention. Manual for the surveillance of vaccine-preventable diseases. Accessed October 20, 2016. http://www.cdc.gov/vaccines/pubs/surv-manual/chpt16-tetanus.html

Centers for Disease Control and Prevention. Parasites—enterobiasis (also known as pinworm infection). Accessed June 19, 2020. www.cdc.gov/parasites/pinworm/index.html

Centers for Disease Control and Prevention. Tetanus Surveillance—United States, 2001-2008. Accessed October 20, 2016. https://www.cdc.gov/mmwr/preview/mmwrhtml/mm6012a1.htm

Centers for Disease Control and Prevention. Chickenpox (Varicella). Published December 31, 2018. Accessed June 1, 2020. https://www.cdc.gov/chickenpox/index.html

DHHS Panel on Antiretroviral Guidelines for Adults and Adolescents. Guidelines for the use of antiretroviral agents in HIV-1-infected adults and adolescents. Accessed June 6, 2020. https://clinicalinfo.hiv.gov/sites/default/files/inline-files/AdultandAdolescentGL.pdf

Erasmus J, McAdams HP, Farrell MA, Patz EF Jr. Pulmonary nontuberculous mycobacterial infection: radiologic manifestations. *Radio-Graphics.* 1999;19(6):1487-1505.

Gershon AA. Varicella-Zoster virus infections. American Academy of Pediatrics. Published January 1, 2008. Accessed June 1, 2020. https://pedsinreview.aappublications.org/content/29/1/5

Good RC, Snider DE Jr. Isolation of nontuberculous mycobacteria in the United States, 1980. *J Infect Dis.* 1982;146:829-833.

Hampson K, Coudeville L, Lembo T, et al. Estimating the global burden of endemic canine rabies. *PLoS Negl Trop Dis.* 2015;9(4):e0003709. doi:10.1371/journal.pntd.0003709

Center for Disease Control and Prevention. Hand, Foot, and Mouth Disease (HFMD). Updated February 2, 2021. https://www.cdc.gov/hand-foot-mouth/index.html

Hinfey PB. Tetanus. *Medscape.* Accessed October 20, 2016. http://emedicine.medscape.com/article/229594-overview#a5

Health and Human Services. National Institutes of Health. Recommendations for the use of antiretroviral drugs in pregnant women with HIV infection and interventions to reduce perinatal HIV transmission in the United States. Published December 2019. Accessed 10/8/2020. https://clinicalinfo.hiv.gov/en/guidelines/perinatal/prenatal-care-antiretroviral-therapy-and-hiv-management-women-perinatal-hiv

Honda JR, Knight V, Chan ED. Pathogenesis and risk factors for nontuberculous mycobacterial lung disease. *Clin Chest Med.* 2015;36:1-11.

Kotton C, Kumar D, Caliendo A, et al. Updated international consensus guidelines on the management of cytomegalovirus in solid organ transplantation. *Transplantation.* 2013;96:333-360.

Kucik CJ, Martin GL, Sortor BV. Common intestinal parasites. *Am Fam Physician.* 2004;69(5):1161-1168.

Montoya JG, Liesenfeld O. Toxoplasmosis. *Lancet.* 2004;363:1965-1976.

Mullins TB, Krishnamurthy K. Roseola Infantum (Exanthema Subitum, Sixth Disease) *StatPearls [Internet].* StatPearls Publishing; 2020. Updated May 4, 2020. Accessed June 16, 2020. https://www.ncbi.nlm.nih.gov/books/NBK448190/#_NBK448190_pubdet_

Nair PA. Herpes Zoster (Shingles). *StatPearls [Internet].* Published April 27, 2020. Accessed June 1, 2020. https://www.ncbi.nlm.nih.gov/books/NBK441824/

Pinninti SG, Kimberlin DW. Preventing herpes simplex virus in the newborn. *Clin Perinatol.* 2014;41(4):945-955. doi:10.1016/j.clp.2014.08.012

Philip SS. Lyme disease (Lyme Borreliosis). In: Papadakis MA, McPhee SJ, Rabow MW, eds. *Current Medical Diagnosis and Treatment 2020.* McGraw-Hill Education; 2020. Accessed August 17, 2020.

Rawlinson W, Boppana S, Fowler K, et al. Congenital cytomegalovirus infection in pregnancy and the neonate: consensus recommendations for prevention, diagnosis, and therapy. *Lancet Infect Dis* 2017;17(6):e177-e188.

Rhodes A, Evans L, Alhazzani W, et al. Surviving sepsis campaign: international guidelines for management of sepsis and septic shock: 2016. *Crit Care Med.* 2017;45(3):486-552.

Center for Disease Control and Prevention. Rocky Mountain Spotted Fever (RMSF). Accessed May 7, 2017. https://www.cdc.gov/rmsf/index.html

Saadatnia G, Golkar M. A review on human toxoplasmosis. *Scand J Infect Dis.* 2012;44(11):805-814.

Centers for Disease Control and Prevention. Shingles (Herpes Zoster). Published June 26, 2019. Accessed June 1, 2020. https://www.cdc.gov/shingles/index.html

Singer M, Deutschman C, Seymour C, et al. The Third International Consensus definitions for sepsis and septic shock (Sepsis-3). *J Am Med Assoc.* 2016;315(8):801-810.

Stamm WE. Chlamydia trachomatis infections of the adult. In: Holmes KK, Sparling PF, Mardh PA, et al., eds. *Sexually Transmitted Diseases.* 4th ed, McGraw-Hill; 2008:575.

Torriani FJ, Behling CA, McCutchan JA, et al. Disseminated Mycobacterium avium complex: correlation between blood and tissue burden. *J Infect Dis.* 1996;173:942-949.

Tremblay C, Brady MT. Roseola infantum (exanthema subitum). In: Edwards MS, Levy ML, eds. *UpToDate.* UpToDate Inc. Updated July 22, 2019. Accessed June 16, 2020. https://www-uptodate-com

Centers for Disease Control and Prevention. Trichomoniasis. Accessed April 21, 2020. https://www.cdc.gov/std/trichomonas/

Tsai S, Sun MY, Kuller JA, Rheed EHJ, Dotters-Katz S. Syphilis in pregnancy. *Obstet Gynecol Survey.* September 2019;74 (9):557-564.

United States Preventive Services Task Force. Screening for Hepatitis B virus infection in pregnant women: US Preventive Services Task Force Reaffirmation Recommendation Statement. *JAMA.* 2019;322(4):349-354. doi:10.1001/jama.2019.9365.

Curry SJ, Krist AH, Owens DK, et al. Screening for syphilis infection in pregnant women: US Preventive Services Task Force Reaffirmation Recommendation Statement. *JAMA.* 2018;320(9):911-917.

Wilkins T, Sams R, Carpenter M. Hepatitis B: screening, prevention, diagnosis, and treatment. *Am Fam Physician.* 2019;99(5):314-323.

Workowski KA, Bolan GA, Centers for Disease Control and Prevention. Sexually transmitted diseases treatment guidelines, 2015. *MMWR Recomm Rep.* 2015;64:1-137.

World Health Organization. Rabies. Accessed August 30, 2017. https://www.who.int/health-topics/rabies#tab=tab_1

PART X

Amin N, Kumar N, Schickendantz M. Medial epicondylitis: evaluation and management. *J Am Acad Orthopaedic Surgeons.* 2015;23(6):348-355.

Appelman-Dijkstra NM, Papapoulos SE. Paget's disease of bone. *Best Pract Res Clin Endocrinol Metab.* 2018;32(5):657-668.

Bouillon R. Comparative analysis of nutritional guidelines for vitamin D. *Nat Rev Endocrinol.* 2017;13(8):466-479. doi:10.1038/nrendo.2017.31

Cantini F, Salvarani C, Olivieri I, et al. Erythrocyte sedimentation rate and C-reactive protein in the evaluation of disease activity and severity in polymyalgia rheumatica: a prospective follow-up study. *Semin Arthritis Rheum.* 2000;30(1):17-24. doi:10.1053/sarh.2000.8366

Centers for Disease Control and Prevention. Human Papillomavirus. Accessed June 2020. https://www.cdc.gov/hpv/hcp/

Dejaco C, Singh YP, Perel P, et al. Arthritis & rheumatology. *Am Coll Rheumatol.* 2015;67(10)2569-2580. doi:10.1002/art.39333. VC 2015

Figueroa D, Figueroa F, Calvo R. Patellar tendinopathy: diagnosis and treatment. *J Am Acad Orthop Surg.* 2016;24(12):e184-e192. doi:10.5435/JAAOS-D-15-00703

Goldenberg DL, Schur PH, Romain PL. Clinical manifestation and diagnosis of fibromyalgia in adults. *Up-to-Date;* Accessed June 17, 2020. https://www.uptodate.com/contents/clinical-manifestations-and-diagnosis-of-fibromyalgia-in-adults?search=fibromyalgia&source=search_result&selectedTitle=1~150&usage_type=default&display_rank=1

Goldenberg DL, Schur PH, Romain PL. Treatment of fibromyalgia in adults not responsive to initial treatment. *Up-to-Date;* Accessed June 17, 2020. https://www.uptodate.com/contents/treatment-of-fibromyalgia-in-adults-not-responsive-to-initial-therapies?search=fibromyalgia&source=search_result&selectedTitle=2~150&usage_type=default&display_rank=2

Green DP. *Greens Operative Hand Surgery.* Vol. 2. 7th ed. Elsevier; 2016.

Hellmann DB, Imboden JB Jr. Fibromyalgia. In: Papadakis MA, McPhee SJ, Rabow MW. eds. *Current Medical Diagnosis and Treatment 2020.* McGraw-Hill. Accessed June 17, 2020. https://accessmedicine-mhmedical-com.ezproxy.elon.edu/content.aspx?bookid=2683&sectionid=225053184

Jo M, Gardner M. Proximal humerus fractures. *Curr Rev Musculoskeletal Med.* 2012;5(3):192-198.

Kravets I. Paget's disease of bone: diagnosis and treatment. *Am J Med.* 2018;131(11):1298-1303.

Lambert AS, Linglart A. Hypocalcaemic and hypophosphatemic rickets. *Best Pract Res Clin Endocrinol Metab.* 2018;32(4):455-476. doi:10.1016/j.beem.2018.05.009

Lineage Medical Inc. Ankle sprain. Accessed May 20, 2020. https://www.orthobullets.com/foot-and-ankle/7028/ankle-sprain

Lineage Medical Inc. Leg compartment syndrome. Accessed May 29, 2020. https://www.orthobullets.com/trauma/1001/leg-compartment-syndrome

Lineage Medical Inc. Osteomyelitis—Adult. Accessed May 23, 2020. https://www.orthobullets.com/trauma/1057/osteomyelitis--adult

Lohmander LS, Englund PM, Dahl LL, Roos EM. The long-term consequence of anterior cruciate ligament and meniscus injuries: osteoarthritis. *Am J Sports Med.* 2007;35(10):1756-1769. doi:10.1177/0363546507307396

Lundberg IE, Tjärnlund A, Bottai M, et al. 2017 European League Against Rheumatism/American College of Rheumatology classification criteria for adult and juvenile idiopathic inflammatory myopathies and their major subgroups. *Arthritis Rheumatol.* 2017;69(12):2271-2282.

Magnussen RA, Meschbach NT, Kaeding CC. ACL graft and contralateral ACL tear risk within ten years following reconstruction: a systematic review. *JBJS Rev.* 2015;3(1): 01874474-201501000-00002

Malliaras P, Cook J, Purdam C, Rio E. Patellar tendinopathy: clinical diagnosis, load management, and advice for challenging case presentations. *J Orthop Sports Phys Ther.* 2015;45(11):887-898. doi:10.2519/jospt.2015.5987

Matthews A, Smith K, Read L, Nicholas J, Schmidt E. Trigger finger: an overview of the treatment options. *JAAPA.* 2019;32(1):17-21.

MayoClinic.org. Ankylosing spondylitis. Published Mayo Foundation for Medical Education and Research 2008-2020. Accessed May 11, 2020. https://askmayoexpert.mayoclinic.org/topic/clinical-answers/cnt-20119639/sec-20312075

Munns CF, Shaw N, Kiely M, et al. Global consensus recommendations on prevention and management of nutritional rickets. *J Clin Endocrinol Metab.* 2016;101:394-415.

Myklebust G, Gran JT. A prospective study of 287 patients with polymyalgia rheumatica and temporal arteritis: clinical and laboratory manifestations at onset of disease and at the time of diagnosis. *Br J Rheumatol.* 1996;35(11):1161-1168. doi:10.1093/rheumatology/35.11.1161

O'Hanlon TP, Carrick DM, Targoff IN, et al. Immunogenetic risk and protective factors for the idiopathic inflammatory myopathies. *Medicine (Baltimore).* 2006;85(2):111-127.

Owens B, Wolf J. Lateral epicondylitis (Tennis Elbow) surgery treatment & management: approach considerations, medical therapy, surgical therapy. *Medscape.* 2017. Accessed September 17, 2017. http://emedicine.medscape.com/article/1231903-treatment#d10

Podd D. PA-C Hypovitaminosis D. *JAAPA.* 2015;28(2):20-26. doi:10.1097/01.JAA.0000459810.95512.14

Rosen HN, Drezner MK. Clinical manifestations, diagnosis, and evaluation of osteoporosis in postmenopausal women. In: Rosen CJ, Schmader KE, Mulder JE, eds. *UpToDate.* UpToDate Inc. Updated April 13, 2020. Accessed April 30, 2020. https://www.uptodate.com

Rosen HN, Drezner MK. Overview of the management of osteoporosis in postmenopausal women. In: Rosen CJ, Schmader KE, Mulder JE, eds. *UpToDate.* UpToDate Inc. Updated April 13, 2020. Accessed April 30, 2020. https://www.uptodate.com

Sankar V, Noll JL, Brennan MT. Diagnosis of Sjögren's syndrome: American-European and the American College of Rheumatology classification criteria. *Oral Maxillofac Surg Clin North Am.* 2014;26(1):13-22.

Selby PL, Davie MWJ, Ralston SH, Stone MD: Guidelines on the management of Paget's disease of bone. *Bone.* 2002;31:366-373.

Shiboski SC, Shiboski CH, Criswell L, et al. American College of Rheumatology classification criteria for Sjögren's syndrome: a data-driven, expert consensus approach in the Sjögren's International Collaborative Clinical Alliance cohort. *Arthritis Care Res (Hoboken).* 2012;64(4):475-487.

Shoback D, Rosen CJ, Black DM, Cheung AM, Murad MH, Eastell R. Pharmacological management of osteoporosis in postmenopausal women: an endocrine society guideline update. *J Clin Endocrinol Metab.* 2020;105(3):587-594. doi:10.1210/clinem/dgaa048

Stone KB, Oddis CV, Fertig N, et al. Anti-Jo-1 antibody levels correlate with disease activity in idiopathic inflammatory myopathy. *Arthritis Rheum.* 2007;56(9):3125-3131.

Vaquero-Picado A, Barco R, Antuna S. Lateral epicondylitis of the elbow. *EFORT Open Rev.* 2016;1(11):391-397. doi:10.1302/2058-5241.1.000049

Vitali C, Bombardieri S, Jonsson R, et al. Classification criteria for Sjogren's syndrome: a revised version of the European criteria proposed by the American-European Consensus Group. *Ann Rheum Dis.* 2002;61:554-558.

Wright RW, Magnussen RA, Dunn WR. Ipsilateral graft and contralateral ACL rupture at five years or more following ACL reconstruction: a systematic review. *J Bone Joint Surg Am.* 2011;93(12):1159-1165.

Yu DT, van Tubergen A. Clinical manifestations of axial spondyloarthritis (ankylosing spondylitis and nonradiographic axial spondyloarthritis) in adults. *UpToDate.* Updated January 9, 2020. Accessed May 11, 2020. https://www.uptodate.com/contents/clinical-manifestations-of-axial-spondyloarthritis-ankylosing-spondylitis-and-nonradiographic-axial-spondyloarthritis-in-adults?search=ankylosin%20spondylitis&source=search_result&selectedTitle=1~150&usage_type=default&display_rank=1#H11443893

Yu DT, van Tubergen A. Treatment of axial spondyloarthritis (ankylosing spondylitis and nonradiographic axial spondyloarthritis) in adults. *UpToDate.* Updated January 2, 2020. Accessed May 11, 2020. https://www.uptodate.com/contents/treatment-of-axial-spondyloarthritis-ankylosing-spondylitis-and-nonradiographic-axial-spondyloarthritis-in-adults?search=ankylosin%20spondylitis&source=search_result&selectedTitle=2~150&usage_type=default&display_rank=2#H44

PART XI

Abbassi N, Rossor T, Ambegaonkar G. Guillian-Barre syndrome: a review. *Paediatr Child Health.* 2019;29(11):459-462.

Attia J, Hatala R, Cook DJ, Wong JG. Does this patient have acute meningitis? *JAMA.* 1999;282(2):175-181.

Beck RW, Cleary PA, Anderson MM Jr, et al. A randomized, controlled trial of corticosteroids in the treatment of acute optic neuritis. The Optic Neuritis Study Group. *N Engl J Med.* 1992;326(9):581-588. doi:10.1056/NEJM199202273260901

Brownlee WJ, Hardy TA, Fazekas F, Miller DH, Diagnosis of multiple sclerosis: progress and challenges. *Lancet.* 2017;389(10076):1336-1346.

Doughty CT, Seyedsadjadi R. Approach to peripheral neuropathy for the primary care clinician. *Am J Med.* 2018;131:1010-1016.

Douglas VC, Aminoff MJ. Movement disorders. In: Papadakis MA, McPhee SJ, Rabow MW, eds. *Current Medical Diagnosis and Treatment 2020.* McGraw-Hill; 2020:1030-1038.

Dubosh NM, Bellolio MF, Rabinstein AA, Edlow JA. Sensitivity of early brain computed tomography to exclude aneurysmal subarachnoid hemorrhage: a systematic review and meta-analysis. *Stroke.* 2016;47(3):750-755.

Ellul M, Solomon T. Acute encephalitis—diagnosis and management. *Clin Med (Lond).* 2018;18(2):155-159.

England JD, Gronseth GS, Franklin G, et al. Practice parameter: evaluation of distal symmetric polyneuropathy: role of laboratory and genetic testing (an evidence-based review). *Neurology.* 2009;72(2):185-192.

Ettekoven CN, van de Beek D, Brouwer MC. Update on community-acquired bacterial meningitis: guidance and challenges. *Clin Microbiol Infect.* 2017;23(9):601-606.

Fusilli C, Migliore S, Mazza T, et al. Biological and clinical manifestations of juvenile Huntington's disease: a retrospective analysis. *Lancet Neurol.* 2018;17:986-993.

Goadsby PJ. Migraine and other primary headache disorders. In: Jameson JL, Fauci AS, Kasper DL, Hauser SL, Longo DL, Loscalzo J, eds. *Harrison's Principles of Internal Medicine.* 20th ed. McGraw-Hill Education; 2018.

Gregg EW, Sorlie P, Paulose-Ram R, et al. Prevalence of lower- extremity disease in the US adult population ≥40 years of age with and without diabetes: 1999–2000 national health and nutrition examination survey. *Diabetes Care.* 2004;27(7):1591-1597.

Hoffmann J, May A. Diagnosis, pathophysiology, and management of cluster headache. *Lancet Neurol.* 2018;17(1):75-83.

Jameson JL, Fauci AS, Kasper DL, Hauser SL, Longo DL, Loscalzo J. Tremor and movement disorders. In: *Harrison's Manual of Medicine.* 20th ed. McGraw-Hill Education; 2020.

Lau C, Teo WY. Overview of the management of central nervous system tumors in children. *UpToDate*. Updated November 21, 2019. Accessed July 24, 2020. https://www.uptodate.com/contents/overview-of-the- management-of-central-nervous-system-tumors-in-children

Leddy JJ, Haider MN, Ellis M, Willer BS. Exercise is medicine for concussion. *Curr Sports Med Rep*. 2018;17(8):262-270.

Logan SA, MacMahon E. Viral meningitis. *BMJ*. 2008;336(7634):36-40.

Lowenstein DH. Seizures and epilepsy. In: Jameson J, Fauci AS, Kasper DL, Hauser SL, Longo DL, Loscalzo J, eds. *Harrison's Principles of Internal Medicine*. 20th ed. McGraw-Hill. Accessed April 07, 2020. http://accessmedicine.mhmedical.com.ccmain.ohionet.org/content.aspx?bookid=2129&sectionid=192531797

Martyn CN, Hughes RA. Epidemiology of peripheral neuropathy. *J Neurol Neurosurg Psychiatry*. 1997;62(4):310-318.

McCrory P, Meeuwisse W, Dvorak J, et al. Consensus statement on concussion in sport—the 5th international conference on concussion in sport held in Berlin, October 2016. *Br J Sports Med*. 2017;51:838-847.

Meehan WP 3rd. Medical therapies for concussion. *Clin Sports Med*. 2011;30(1):115-124, ix.

Mount HR, Boyle SD. Aseptic and bacterial meningitis: evaluation, treatment, and prevention. *Am Fam Physician*. 2017;96(5):314-322.

Nold CS, Nozaki K. Peripheral neuropathy: clinical pearls for making the diagnosis. *JAAPA*. 2020;33(1):9-15.

Olanow C, Klein C, Obeso JA. Tremor, chorea, and other movement disorders. In: Jameson J, Fauci AS, Kasper DL, Hauser SL, Longo DL, Loscalzo J. eds. *Harrison's Principles of Internal Medicine*. 20th ed. McGraw-Hill; 2018:3132-3141.

Philadelphia PWEH, Wajda BN, Bagheri N. *The Wills Eye Manual: Office and Emergency Room Diagnosis and Treatment of Eye Disease*. 7th ed. Lippincott Williams & Wilkins; 2017.

Pringsheim T, Wiltshire K, Day L, et al. The incidence and prevalence of Huntington's disease: a systematic review and meta-analysis. *Mov Disord*. 2012;27:1083-1091.

Robinson J, Kothari MJ. Clinical features and diagnosis of cervical radiculopathy. In: *UpToDate*. Accessed June 14, 2020. https://www.uptodate.com/contents/clinical-features-and-diagnosis-of-cervical-radiculopathy/print#!

Rua R, McGavern DB. Advances in meningeal immunity. *Trends Mol Med*. 2018; 24(6):542-559.

Shah S, Rincon F. CNS infection. In: Lee K, ed. *The Neuro-ICU Book*. 2nd ed. McGraw-Hill. Accessed April 07, 2020. http://neurology.mhmedical.com.ccmain.ohionet.org/content.aspx?bookid=2155&sectionid=163964001

Thompson AJ, Banwell BL, Barkhof F, et al. Diagnosis of multiple sclerosis: 2017 revisions of the McDonald criteria. *Lancet Neurol*. 2018;17(2):162-173.

Walsh FB, Miller NR, Hoyt WF. *Walsh and Hoyts Clinical Neuro-Ophthalmology: The Essentials*. Lippincott Williams & Wilkins; 2016.

Ward MA, Greenwood TM, Kumar DR, Mazza JJ, Yale SH. Josef Brudzinski and Vladimir Mikhailovich Kernig: signs for diagnosing meningitis. *Clin Med Res*. 2010;8(1):13-17.

Wong ET, Wu JK. Overview of the clinical features and diagnosis of brain tumors in adults. *UpToDate*. Updated October 22, 2019. Accessed July 24, 2020. https://www.uptodate.com/contents/overview-of-the clinical-features-and-diagnosis-of-brain-tumors-in-adults

PART XII

American Psychiatric Association. *Diagnostic and Statistical Manual of Mental Disorders*. 5th ed. American Psychiatric Association; 2013.

Brown TA, Haedt-Matt AA, Keel PK. Personality pathology in purging disorder and bulimia nervosa. *Int J Eat Disord*. 2011;44:735-740.

Button EJ, Chadalavada B, Palmer RL. Mortality and predictors of death in a cohort of patients presenting to an eating disorders service. *Int J Eat Disord*. 2010;43:387-392.

Council on Children With Disabilities, Section on Developmental Behavioral Pediatrics, Bright Futures Steering Committee and Medical Home Initiatives for Children With Special Needs Project Advisory Committee. Identifying infants and young children with developmental disorders in the medical home: an algorithm for developmental surveillance and screening. *Pediatrics*. 2006;118(1):405-420. doi:10.1542/peds.2006-1231

Ebert MH, Leckman JF, Petrakis IL. *Current Diagnosis and Treatment: Psychiatry*. 3rd ed. McGraw Hill; 2019.

Fischer BA, Buchanan RW. Schizophrenia in adults: Clinical manifestations, course, assessment, and diagnosis. *UpToDate*. Accessed August 20, 2020. https://www.uptodate.com/contents/schizophrenia-in-adults-clinical-manifestations-course-assessment-and-diagnosis?search=schizophrenia%20diagnosis&source=search_result&selectedTitle=1~150&usage_type=default&display_rank=1

Hagan K, Walsh BT. State of the art: The therapeutic approaches to bulimia nervosa. *Clin Ther* 2021;43(1):40-49.

Harrington BC, Jimerson M, Haxton C, Jimerson DC. Initial evaluation, diagnosis, and treatment of anorexia nervosa and bulimia nervosa. *Am Fam Physician*. 2015;91(1):46-52.

Hyman SL, Levy SE, Myers SM, et al. Identification, evaluation, and management of children with autism spectrum disorder. *Pediatrics*. 2020;145(1):e20193447.

Maenner MJ, Shaw KA, Baio J, et al. Prevalence of autism spectrum disorder among children aged 8 years—autism and developmental disabilities monitoring network, 11 sites, United States, 2016. *MMWR Surveill Summ*. 2020;69(No. SS-4):1-12.

Magnus W, Nazir S, Anilkumar AC, Shaban K. Attention deficient disorder (ADHD). *StatPearls [Internet]*. 2020. https://www.ncbi.nlm.nih.gov/books/NBK430685/?term=adhd

Miller TR, Swedler DI, Lawrence BA, et al. Incidence and lethality of suicidal overdoses by drug class. *JAMA Netw Open*. 2020;3(3):e200607.

Mojtabai R. Brief psychotic disorder. *UpToDate*. Accessed August 20, 2020. https://www.uptodate.com/contents/brief-psychotic-disorder?search=brief%20psychotic%20disorder&source=search_result&selectedTitle=1~150&usage_type=default&display_rank=1

National Institute of Neurological Disorders and Stroke. Pervasive developmental disorders information page. Accessed August 21, 2020. https://www.ninds.nih.gov/disorders/all-disorders/pervasive-developmental-disorders-information-page

O'Carroll P, Berman A, Maris R, Moscicki E, Tanney B, Silverman M. Beyond the tower of babel: a nomenclature for suicidology. *Suicide Life Threat Behav*. 1996;26:237-252.

Posner K, Brown GK, Stanley B, et al. The Columbia Suicide Severity Rating Scale: initial validity and internal consistency findings from three multisite studies with adolescents and adults. *Am J Psychiatry*. 2011;168(12):1266-1277.

Sadock BJ, Sadock VA, Ruiz P. *Kaplan and Sadock Synopsis of Psychiatry*. 11th ed. Wolters Kluwer; 2015.

Sharma A, Couture J. A review of the pathophysiology, etiology, and treatment of attention deficit hyperactivity disorder (ADHD). *Ann Pharmacol*. 2014;48(2):209-225. doi:10.1177/1060028013510699

Tupa E, Hendrickson A, Cole K, Koch H. Suicide prevention toolkit for primary care practices. *Suicide Prevention Resource Center*. Accessed September 12, 2020. https://www.sprc.org/sites/default/files/Final%20National%20Suicide%20Prevention%20Toolkit%202.15.18%20FINAL.pdf

Westmoreland P, Krantz MJ, Mehler PS. Medical complications of anorexia nervosa and bulimia. *Am J Med*. 2016;129(1):30-37.

Wolraich ML, Hagan JF, Allan C, et al. Clinical practice guideline for the diagnosis, evaluation, and treatment of attention-deficit/hyperactivity disorder in children and adolescents. *Pediatrics*. 2019;144(4):e20192528. doi:10.1542/peds.2019-2528

PART XIII

Aggarwal V, Nicolais CD, Lee A, Bashir R. Acute management of pulmonary embolism. *J Am Coll Cardiol*. Accessed August 19, 2019. https://www.acc.org/latest-in-cardiology/articles/2017/10/23/12/12/acute-management-of-pulmonary-embolism

Chesnutt AN, Chesnutt MS, Prendergast NT, Prendergast TJ. Occupational pulmonary diseases. In: Papadakis MA, McPhee SJ, Rabow MW, eds. *Current Medical Diagnosis and Treatment 2020*. McGraw-Hill Education; 2020. Accessed August 14, 2020. accessmedicine.mhmedical.com/content.aspx?aid=1166165182

Crouser ED, Maier LA, Wilson KC, et al. Diagnosis and Detection of Sarcoidosis. An Official American Thoracic Society Clinical Practice Guideline. *Am J Respir Crit Care Med*. 2020;201(8):e26-e51. doi:10.1164/rccm.202002-0251ST

DiNisio M, van Es N, Buller HR. Deep vein thrombosis and pulmonary embolism. *Lancet*. 2016;388:3060-3073. doi:10.1016/S0140-6736(16)30514-1

Driver BE, Klein LR, Schick AL, et al. The occurrence of aspiration pneumonia after emergency endotracheal intubation. *Am J Emerg Med*. 2018;36:193-196.

Elyas A. The use of echocardiography in diagnosis of pulmonary embolism. Accessed September 8, 2020. https://www.escardio.org/static-file/Escardio/Subspecialty/EACVI/Education/Teaching%20courses/2019/Use%20of%20echocardiography%20in%20diagnosis%20of%20pulmonary%20embolism.pdf

Erasmus JJ, Connolly JE, McAdams HP, Roggli VL. Solitary pulmonary nodules: part 1. Morphologic evaluation for differentiation of benign and malignant lesions. *Radiographics*. 2000;20(1):43-58.

Europe PMC. Federal clinical practice guidelines for the diagnosis, prevention and treatment of pneumoconiosis. Accessed August 14, 2020. https://europepmc.org/article/med/27048142

Funkhouser WK. Pulmonary pathology. In: Reisner HM, ed. *Pathology: A Modern Case Study*. 2nd ed. McGraw-Hill Education; 2020. Accessed August 14, 2020. https://accessmedicine.mhmedical.com/content.aspx?aid=1173768963

Global Strategy for the Diagnosis, Management and Prevention of COPD, Global Initiative for Chronic Obstructive Lung Disease (GOLD). 2020. http://goldcopd.org

Gould M, Donington J, Lynch WR, et al. Evaluation of individuals with pulmonary nodules: with is it lung cancer? Diagnosis and management of lung cancer, 3rd ed: American College of Chest Physicians evidence-based clinical practice guidelines. *Chest*, 2013;243(5):e93-e120.

Kearon C, Akl EA, Ornelas J, et al. Antithrombotic therapy for VTE disease: CHEST guideline and expert panel report. *Chest*. 2016;149(2):315-352. doi:10.1016/j.chest.2015.11.026

Madu A, Sharman T. Bagassosis. *StatPearls [Internet]*. Accessed August 20, 2020. https://www.ncbi.nlm.nih.gov/books/NBK554444/

Martin R. Pathophysiology, clinical manifestations, and diagnosis of respiratory distress syndrome in the newborn. *UpToDate*. Accessed June 13, 2020. https://www.uptodate.com/contents/pathophysiology-clinical-manifestations-and-diagnosis-of-respiratory-distress-syndrome-in-the-newborn?search=hyaline%20membrane%20disease&topicRef=4964&source=see_link

Martin R. Prevention and treatment of respiratory distress syndrome in preterm infants. UpToDate. Accessed June 15, 2020. https://www.uptodate.com/contents/prevention-and-treatment-of-respiratory-distress-syndrome-in-preterm-infants?sectionName=Surfactant%20therapy&search=hyaline%20membrane%20disease&topicRef=5055&anchor=H23056094&source=see_link#H23056080.

Mayo Clinic Proceedings. Silo-filler's disease: a new perspective. Accessed August 20, 2020. https://www.mayoclinicproceedings.org/article/S0025-6196(12)65260-4/fulltext

McMahon H, Naidich DP, Goo JM, et al. 2017. Guidelines for management of Incidental Pulmonary Nodules Detected on CT Images: From Fleischner Society 2017. *Radiology*, 284(1): 228-243.

Metlay JP, Waterer GW, Long AC, et al. Diagnosis and treatment of adults with community-acquired pneumonia: an official clinical practice guideline of the American Thoracic Society and Infectious Diseases Society of America. *Am J Respir Crit Care Med*. 2019;200(7):e45-e67. doi:10.1164/rccm.201908-1581ST

Piazza G, Goldhaber SZ. Management of submassive pulmonary embolism. *Circulation*. 2010;122(11):1124-1129. doi:10.1161/CIRCULATIONAHA.110.961136

Rose C. Silicosis. *UpToDate*. Accessed August 20, 2020. https://www.uptodate.com/contents/silicosis?search=pneumoconiosis%20treatment&source=search_result&selectedTitle=1~125&usage_type=default&display_rank=1#H363393466

Siegel MD. Acute respiratory distress syndrome: clinical features, diagnosis and complications in adults. In: Post TW, ed. *UpToDate*. Accessed May 11, 2020. https://www.uptodate.com/contents/acute-respiratory-distress-syndrome-clinical-features-diagnosis-and-complications-in-adults

Siegel MD, Siemieniuk R. Acute respiratory distress syndrome: supportive care and oxygenation in adults. In: Post TW, ed. *UpToDate*. Accessed May 11, 2020. https://www.uptodate.com/contents/acute-respiratory-distress-syndrome-supportive-care-and-oxygenation-in-adults

Smith D. The newborn infant. In: Hay WW Jr, Levin MJ, Abzug MJ, Bunik M, eds. *Current Diagnosis & Treatment: Pediatrics*. 25th ed. McGraw-Hill. Accessed June 13, 2020. https://accessmedicine.mhmedical.com/content.aspx?bookid=2815&sectionid=244254981

Stark P. Imaging of occupational lung diseases. *UpToDate*. Accessed August 14, 2020. https://www.uptodate.com/contents/imaging-of-occupational-lung-diseases?search=pneumoconioses&-sourcesearch_resultselectedTitle=1~15&usagetype=default&display_rank=1

Tanner NT, Porter A, Gould MK, et al. 2017. Physician assessment of pretest probability of malignancy and adherence with guidelines for pulmonary nodule evaluation. *Chest*. 152(2):263-270.

PART XIV

American Cancer Society. Cancer statistics 2018. Accessed May 4, 2020. https://cancerstatisticscenter.org

American College of Obstetrics & Gynecology. ACOG Practice Bulletin No. 190: Gestational Diabetes Mellitus. 2018;131(2): e49-e64.

American College of Obstetrics & Gynecology. Practice Bulletin No. 142: cerclage for the management of cervical insufficiency. *Obstet Gynecol*. 2014:123(2 Pt 1):372-379.

American College of Obstetricians and Gynecologists. ACOG Practice Bulletin No. 193: Tubal ectopic pregnancy. *Obstet Gynecol*. 2018;131:e91-e103.

American Diabetes Association. Management of diabetes in pregnancy: standards of care in diabetes. 2021;44(suppl 1):S200-S210.

Auth PC, Kerstein MD. *Physician Assistant Review*. 4th ed. Wolters Kluwer Health/Lippincott Williams & Wilkins; 2013.

Ben-Meir A, Sarajari S. Endometriosis. In: DeCherney AH, Nathan L, Laufer N, Roman AS, eds. *CURRENT Diagnosis & Treatment: Obstetrics & Gynecology*. 12th ed. McGraw-Hill. Accessed June 01, 2020. http://accessmedicine.mhmedical.com.ezproxy2.library.drexel.edu/content.aspx?bookid=2559&sectionid=206967961

Braunstein GD, Anawalt BD. Epidemiology, pathophysiology, and causes of gynecomastia. In: Matsumoto AM, ed. *UpToDate*. UpToDate Inc. Updated February 19, 2019. Accessed June 17, 2020. https://www-uptodate-com

Braunstein GD, Anawalt BD. Management of gynecomastia. In: Matsumoto AM, ed. *UpToDate*. UpToDate Inc. Updated January 21, 2019. Accessed June 17, 2020. https://www-uptodate-com

Casper RF. Clinical manifestations and diagnosis of menopause. In: Barbieri RL, Crowley WF, Martin KA, eds. *UpToDate*. UpToDate Inc. Updated March 20, 2020. Accessed May 7, 2020. https://www.uptodate.com

Centers for Disease Control and Prevention. United States Cancer Statistics: Highlights from 2015 Incidence. USCS data brief, no 3. Atlanta, GA: Centers for Disease Control and Prevention. 2018. Accessed August 2, 2021. https://www.cdc.gov/cancer/uscs/pdf/USCS-DataBrief-No3-June2018-508.pdf

Crum C, Nucci M, Howitt B, Granter S, Parast M, Boyd T. *Diagnostic Gynecologic and Obstetric Pathology*. Elsevier; 2018. ISBN: 978-0-323-44732-4

Curtis KM, Jatlaoui TC, Tepper NK, et al. U.S. selected practice recommendations for contraceptive use, 2016. *MMWR Recomm Rep*. 2016;65(No. RR-4):1-66. doi:10.15585/mmwr.rr6504a1external icon

Cooper SM, Arnold SJ. Vulvar lichen sclerosus. *UpToDate*. 2019. https://www.uptodate.com/contents/vulvar-lichen-sclerosus?search=lichen%20sclerosus&source=search_result&selectedTitle=1~59&usage_type=default&display_rank=1#H604770996

Davis DD, Roshan A, Canela CD, et al. Shoulder dystocia. In: *StatPearls [Internet]*. StatPearls Publishing; 2020. Updated March 25, 2020. https://www.ncbi.nlm.nih.gov/books/NBK470427/

Dietz JR. Nipple discharge. In: Jatoi I, Kaufmann M, eds. *Management of Breast Diseases*. Springer: 2010:52-68.

Dixon MD. Lactational mastitis. *UpToDate*. Accessed April 30, 2020. https://www.uptodate.com

Dixon MD. Primary breast abscess. *UpToDate*. Accessed April 30, 2020. https://www.uptodate.com

Elsevier Point of Care. Clinical overview dysmenorrhea. 2020. Accessed May 6, 2020. https://www.clinicalkey.com/#!/content/clinical_overview/67-s2.0-69ca7d5c-0bd5-4318-95cb-12b42ef45eda

Goodnight W, Newman R. Optimal nutrition for improved twin pregnancy outcome. *Obstet Gynecol*. 2009;114(5):1121-1134. doi:10.1097/AOG.0b013e3181bb14c8

Hamid CA, Hoffman BL. Benign adnexal mass. In: Hoffman BL, Schorge JO, Halvorson LM, Hamid CA, Corton MM, Schaffer JI, eds. *Williams Gynecology*, 4th ed. McGraw-Hill; 2020. Accessed June 16, 2020. https://accessmedicine-mhmedical-com.proxygw.wrlc.org/content.aspx?bookid=2658&sectionid=241008530

Harris JR. *Diseases of the Breast*. Wolters Kluwer; 2010.

Hoffman BL, Schorge JO, Bradshaw KD, Halvorson LM, Schaffer JI, Corton MM, eds. *Williams Gynecology*. 3rd ed. McGraw-Hill. Accessed June 01, 2020. http://accessmedicine.mhmedical.com.ezproxy2.library.drexel.edu/content.aspx?bookid=1758&sectionid=118165490

Hoffman MS, Hochberg L. Differential Diagnosis of the adnexal mass. In: Levine D, Goff B, Chakrabarti A, eds. *UpToDate*. UpToDate, Inc; 2020. Accessed June 16, 2020. https://www.uptodate.com/contents/differential-diagnosis-of-the-adnexal-mass?search=ovarian%20cysts&topicRef=3207&source=see_link

Hofmeyr GJ. Breech presentation and shoulder dystocia in childbirth. *Curr Opin Obstet Gynecol*. 1992;4(6):807-812. https://pubmed.ncbi.nlm.nih.gov/1450343/

Kellermann R, Rakel D. *Conn's Current Therapy 2020*. Elsevier; 2020. ISBN: 978-0-323-71184-5

Legro RS, Arslanian SA, Ehrmann DA, et al. Diagnosis and treatment of polycystic ovary syndrome: an endocrine society clinical practice guideline. *J Clin Endocrinol Metab*. 2013;98(12):4565-4592. doi.org/10.1210/jc.2013-2350

Lobo R, Gershenson D, Lentz G, Valea F. *Comprehensive Gynecology*. Elsevier; 2017. ISBN: 978-0-323-32287-4

Moise KJ. Prevention of RhD alloimmunization in pregnancy. In: Lockwood CJ, Silvergleid AJ, Barss VA, eds. *UpToDate*. UpToDate Inc. Accessed September 2, 2020. https://www.uptodate.com

Moy L, Heller SL, Trikha S, et al. ACR Appropriateness Criteria® palpable breast masses. *J Am Coll Radiol*. 2017;14(5):S203-S224.

Muto MG. Management of an adnexal mass. In: Sharp HT, Goff B, Chakrabarti A, eds. *UpToDate*. UpToDate, Inc; 2020. Accessed June 16, 2020. https://www.uptodate.com/contents/management-of-an-adnexal-mass?search=management%20of%20adnexal%20mass&source=search_result&selectedTitle=1~150&usage_type=default&display_rank=1

National Cancer Institute. Cancer stat facts: ovarian cancer. Accessed May 4, 2020. https://seer.cancer.gov/statfacts/html/ovary.html

Rerucha CM, Caro RJ, Wheeler VL. Cervical cancer screening. *Am Fam Physician*. 2018;97(7):441-448.

Rogers RG, Fashokun TB. Pelvic organ prolapse in women: epidemiology, risk factors, clinical manifestations, and management. *UpToDate*. https://www.uptodate.com/contents/pelvic-organ-prolapse-in-women-epidemiology-risk-factors-clinical-manifestations-and-management?search=enterocele§ionRank=1&usage_type=default&anchor=H7156639&source=machineLearning&selectedTitle=1~16&display_rank=1#H7156639

Russo A, Calò V, Bruno L, Rizzo S, Bazan V, Di Fede G. Hereditary ovarian cancer. *Crit Rev Oncology/Hematol*. 2009;69:28-44.

Sabel MS. Overview of benign breast disease. In: Chagpar AB, ed. *UpToDate*. UpToDate Inc. Updated October 16, 2018. Accessed June 16, 2020. https://www-uptodate-com

Sabel MS. Clinical manifestations, differential diagnosis, and clinical evaluation of a palpable breast mass. In: Chagpar AB, ed. *UpToDate*. UpToDate Inc. Updated September 30, 2019. Accessed June 16, 2020. https://www-uptodate-com

Sobel J. Candida vulvovaginitis: clinical manifestations and diagnosis. *UpToDate*. 2019. https://www.uptodate.com/contents/candida-vulvovaginitis-clinical-manifestations-and-diagnosis?-search=Candidiasis%20vaginitis&source=search_result&selected-Title=2~150&usage_type=default&display_rank=2

Symonds I, Arulkumaran S. *Essential Obstetrics and Gynaecology*. 6th ed. Elsevier; 2019.

Tulandi T. Ectopic pregnancy: methotrexate therapy. In: Schreiber CA, Chakrabarti A, eds. *UpToDate*. UpToDate Inc. Accessed September 2, 2020. https://www.uptodate.com

Twin T, Higher-Order multifetal pregnancies. Multifetal gestations: twin, triplet, and higher-order multifetal pregnancies. Accessed June 25, 2020. https://www.acog.org/en/Clinical/Clinical Guidance/Practice Bulletin/Articles/2016/10/Twin Triplet and Higher-Order Multifetal Pregnancies

U.S. Preventive Services Task Force. Cervical cancer: screening. Updated August 2018. Accessed May 5, 2020. https://uspreventiveservicestaskforce.org

Welt CK Barbieri RL. Evaluation and management of primary amenorrhea. *UpToDate*. Accessed June 12, 2020. https://www.uptodate.com/contents/evaluation-and-management-of-primary-amenorrhea

Welt CK, Barbieri RL. Evaluation and management of secondary amenorrhea. *UpToDate*. Accessed June 12, 2020. https://www.uptodate.com/contents/evaluation-and-management-of-secondary-amenorrhea

Wipperman J, Neil T, Williams T. Cervical cancer: evaluation and management. *Am Fam Physician*. 2018;97(7):449-454.

Witchel SF, Oberfield SE, Pena AS. Polycystic ovary syndrome: pathophysiology, presentation, and treatment with emphasis on adolescent girls. *J Endocr Soc*. 2019;3(8):1545-1573. doi:10.1210/js/2019-00078

Comprehensive Exam

1. Which of the following is the recommended treatment for premature atrial or ventricular contractions in an asymptomatic patient without structural heart disease?
   A. β-Blocker
   B. Catheter ablation
   C. Blood thinners
   D. Reassurance and patient education

2. Which of the following is true of tetralogy of Fallot?
   A. It is the least common form of congenital heart anomalies.
   B. Because of right-to-left shunting, it is considered a cyanotic heart defect.
   C. It rarely requires surgical intervention.
   D. ECG is the diagnostic test of choice.

3. Which of the following is an ototoxic medication?
   A. Amoxicillin
   B. Ibuprofen
   C. Prednisone
   D. Propranolol

4. Your patient is 40-year-old female with no past medical history, except for near-sightedness requiring glasses. She had a minor blunt force trauma to the head yesterday. She noticed an increase in visual floaters last night and now presents with painless loss of vision in the right eye after seeing a "curtain" drop over her vision. What diagnosis is most likely?
   A. Central retinal arterial occlusion (CRAO)
   B. Central retinal venous occlusion (CRVO)
   C. Posterior vitreous detachment
   D. Retinal detachment

5. Which of the following labs should be ordered postoperatively due to potential complications of thyroidectomy?
   A. Potassium
   B. Sodium
   C. Chloride
   D. Calcium

6. Rapid correction of serum sodium can cause which of the following complications?
   A. Pulmonary embolism
   B. Myocardial infarction
   C. Pulmonary and cerebral edema
   D. Kidney stones

7. What is the mechanism of botulinum toxin?
   A. Blocks calcium channels of smooth muscle
   B. Prolongs chloride channel opening of skeletal muscle

C. Blocks cholinergic presynaptic receptors
D. Inhibits myocyte replication

8. Which ligament tear may give a false-positive Lachman examination?
   A. Medial collateral ligament
   B. Lateral collateral ligament
   C. Posterior cruciate ligament
   D. Medial patellofemoral ligament

9. A patient presents with an indeterminant sweat chloride test and symptoms concerning for cystic fibrosis (CF). What is the next step?
   A. Monitor for worsening of symptoms
   B. Genetic testing
   C. Repeat sweat chloride test
   D. CT imaging of the chest

10. A 55-year-old postmenopausal woman presents with dyspareunia and vaginal dryness for the past few months. She denies other symptoms. Her past medical history (PMH) is unremarkable, with no known medical conditions, no allergies, no medications, and no prior surgeries. On pelvic examination, her vaginal wall appears dry, pale, and lacks rugae. Which of the following is the most appropriate next step in management?
    A. Hydrocortisone cream
    B. Oral progestin
    C. Oral estrogen
    D. Vaginal estrogen
    E. Observation

11. Which of the following is the preferred therapy for patients with symptomatic sick sinus syndrome (SSS)?
    A. Atropine for the bradycardia
    B. Adenosine for the tachycardia
    C. Immediate electrical cardioversion
    D. Dual-chamber pacemaker insertion

12. Which of the following is the most appropriate recommendation for a 3-year-old female with a 4-mm diameter secundum atrial septal defect and no cardiopulmonary symptoms?
    A. Follow-up in outpatient clinic
    B. Infective endocarditis (IE) prophylaxis
    C. Limitation of physical activity
    D. Referral for surgical closure

13. Which of the following activities is associated with the development of auricular hematoma?
    A. Golf
    B. Martial arts
    C. Baseball
    D. Horseback riding

14. Which of the following is NOT a sign/symptom of optic neuritis?
    A. Pain with eye movement
    B. Dyschromatopsia
    C. Headache
    D. Relative afferent pupillary defect in the affected eye

15. What is the most common cause of primary hyperparathyroidism?
    A. Adenoma
    B. Glandular hyperplasia
    C. Familial hypocalciuric hypercalcemia
    D. Chronic renal disease

16. What is the role of exogenous calcium administration in a patient with hyperkalemia?
    A. Stimulates removal of potassium from the body
    B. Stabilizes the cardiac membrane and prevents arrhythmia development
    C. Redistributes potassium into the cells
    D. Stops RBC hemolysis and prevents potassium release

17. An 8-year-old boy presents to a clinic with a 3-day history of diarrhea and vomiting. Mom stated that he visited a petting zoo 5 days ago and played with multiple turtles in the exhibit. On examination, he is afebrile with normal vital signs. Which of the following is the best treatment for this infection?
    A. Oral rehydration solution
    B. Ciprofloxacin
    C. Dexamethasone
    D. Azithromycin

18. What imaging modality is commonly used to diagnose patellar tendonitis?
    A. CT
    B. MRI
    C. No imaging is needed
    D. Plain film radiograph

19. Which of the following is a common risk factor for foreign-body aspiration in children?
    A. Decreased cough reflex
    B. Poor hand-eye coordination
    C. Reactive airway disease
    D. Underdeveloped or immature dentition

20. A 39-year-old presents with 2 years of amenorrhea. Upon review of systems, she experiences hot flashes and night sweats. A workup reveals a negative pregnancy test, normal thyroid-stimulating hormone, normal prolactin, and an elevated follicle-stimulating hormone. Which of the following is the most likely diagnosis?
    A. Perimenopause
    B. Menopause
    C. Postmenopause
    D. Primary ovarian insufficiency

21. A 78-year-old female is found to have an asymptomatic right bundle branch block. In which leads do you expect to see prolonged, aberrant QRS complexes on an ECG?
    A. II, III, and aVF
    B. I, aVL, V_5, and V_6
    C. V_1 and V_2
    D. V_5 and V_6

22. Which of the following is true regarding diagnostic studies used to evaluate a patient in whom tetralogy of Fallot is suspected?
    A. Doppler echocardiogram is not helpful and often misses the diagnosis.
    B. ECG will show evidence of LV hypertrophy and bradycardia.
    C. Cardiac MRI is always required to establish the diagnosis.
    D. Chest x-ray (CXR) can reveal a boot-shaped heart due to prominence of the RV.

23. Which of the following physical examination findings is associated with TM barotrauma?
    A. Erythema and edema of the external auditory canal
    B. TM hypermobility
    C. Pearly TM with light reflex present
    D. Dark blue appearance of the TM

24. What would you expect to see on fundoscopic examination in a patient with retinal detachment?
    A. Retinal flap in the vitreous humor
    B. AV nicking
    C. Diffuse retinal hemorrhages with "blood-and-thunder" appearance
    D. Ischemic retinal whitening with a cherry red spot

25. What is the most common cause of hypoparathyroidism?
    A. Iatrogenic
    B. Autoimmune polyglandular syndrome
    C. Genetic mutations in calcium-sensing receptors
    D. Congenital agenesis

26. Which of the following is likely to result in a falsely elevated blood potassium level?
    A. Patient with heart failure who takes spironolactone daily
    B. Patient with acute leukemia and a WBC count of 110 000
    C. Patient with primary adrenal insufficiency
    D. Patient with diabetic ketoacidosis

27. A patient experiences pericarditis as a result of rheumatic fever. How long should prophylactic antibiotic therapy be administered?
    A. 5 years, or until age 21
    B. 10 years, or until age 21
    C. 15 years, or until age 40
    D. 20 years, or until age 60

28. A 24-year-old male presents to your office with the complaint of acute onset of left knee pain after a softball tournament. He reports he was turning third base when he stopped short and turned back. He felt a pop and immediate pain. He states over the course of the next few hours, he noted increasing swelling and decreased range of motion. On physical examination, he is only able to flex his knee to 90°. There is about 6 mm of anterior translation without a firm end point, demonstrating joint laxity. Which of the following ligaments is most likely injured?
    A. Medial collateral ligament (MCL)
    B. Lateral collateral ligament
    C. Posterior cruciate ligament
    D. Anterior cruciate ligament (ACL)

29. On ultrasound evaluation of your patient's chest, you find absent pleural sliding. What is the most likely diagnosis?
    A. Hemothorax
    B. Pneumonia
    C. Pneumothorax
    D. Pleural effusion

30. Which common cause of vaginitis shows the presence of hyphae and spores on diagnostic wet mount examination?
    A. Candidiasis
    B. Trichomoniasis
    C. Bacterial vaginosis
    D. Genitourinary syndrome of menopause

31. An 88-year-old female has paroxysmal atrial fibrillation. She also has a history of coronary artery bypass surgery, heart failure with reduced ejection fraction (EF) of 35%, hypertension, dyslipidemia, and diabetes mellitus. She has no history of peripheral arterial disease or stroke. What is her CHA_2DS_2-VASc score?
    A. 5
    B. 6
    C. 7
    D. 8

32. What is the most likely cause of myocarditis in the United States?
    A. Viral infection
    B. Bacterial infection
    C. Autoimmune disease
    D. Radiation

33. Optic neuritis is most commonly associated with which of the following?
    A. Multiple sclerosis (MS)
    B. Syphilis
    C. Lyme disease
    D. Systemic lupus erythematosus

34. Which of the following conditions would be most consistent with secondary hyperparathyroidism?
    A. Decreased PTH, decreased serum calcium, decreased urinary calcium
    B. Increased PTH, increased serum calcium, increased urinary calcium
    C. Increased PTH, normal serum calcium, decreased urine calcium
    D. Normal PTH, increased serum calcium, decreased urinary calcium

35. A 56-year-old with a past medical history (PMH) of congestive heart failure (CHF) is admitted for a CHF exacerbation. The patient undergoes several days of high-dose diuretic therapy and is feeling much better. The patient has persistent hypokalemia despite several days of potassium supplementation. What should you consider in your differential diagnosis?
    A. Hypomagnesemia
    B. Hypermagnesemia
    C. Pseudohyperkalemia
    D. Hypocalcemia
    E. Hyponatremia

36. What is the most appropriate treatment of a patient with rheumatic fever to ensure eradication of bacterial infection?
    A. Cefdinir
    B. Levofloxacin
    C. Penicillin
    D. Trimethoprim/Sulfamethoxazole (TMP/SMX)

37. Which of the following is considered a first-line treatment for patellar tendonitis?
    A. Anti-inflammatory medications
    B. Corticosteroid injection
    C. Immediate orthopedic referral
    D. Platelet-rich plasma therapy

38. A 46-year-old female undergoes core-needle biopsy for a suspicious breast mass found on screening mammography. The mass measures 1.3 cm, and there is no evidence of lymphadenopathy on imaging. The pathology report indicates the tumor is estrogen receptor positive, progesterone receptor positive, and HER-2 negative. Which of the following is the best choice for adjuvant chemotherapy after the patient undergoes lumpectomy and radiation therapy?
    A. Aromatase inhibitor
    B. Selective estrogen receptor modulator
    C. Taxane-based regimen
    D. HER-2–targeted therapy

39. A 55-year-old woman is experiencing night sweats, leading to sleep disturbances and depression. Her past medical history (PMH) is significant for a deep vein thrombosis (DVT) at age 45. She has no surgical history. Which of the following is the initial therapy of choice for her menopausal symptoms?
    A. SERM
    B. Estrogen plus progestin
    C. Venlafaxine
    D. Bioidentical hormone therapy

40. An 88-year-old female with end-stage chronic pulmonary disease and mitral stenosis is in the ED with respiratory distress. Her heart rate (HR) is rapid, and an ECG demonstrates P waves of several distinct morphologies, variable R-R intervals, and a ventricular HR of 108 beats per minute. What is the most likely diagnosis for this patient?
    A. Atrial fibrillation
    B. Atrial flutter
    C. Multifocal atrial tachycardia
    D. Transient idiopathic arrhythmia

41. A 26-year-old man presented to the ED after having survived a cardiac arrest. He had been resuscitated promptly using an automated external defibrillator. The initial rhythm was VT. He is an athlete with no significant past medical, social, or family history. The physical examination is pertinent for a forceful left apical impulse. The echocardiogram demonstrated a septal wall thickness of 32 mm. What therapeutic intervention would improve his survival?
    A. Septal myectomy
    B. β-Blocker therapy
    C. Placement of an ICD
    D. Coronary artery catheterization

42. Which of the following is NOT a symptom a patient might present to the office with for a diagnosis of a cerumen impaction?
    A. Tinnitus
    B. Ear fullness
    C. Purulent ear drainage
    D. Hearing loss

43. Which of the following would NOT be seen with sudden painless loss of vision?
    A. Angle-closure glaucoma
    B. Central retinal arterial occlusion (CRAO)
    C. Central retinal venous occlusion (CRVO)
    D. Retinal detachment

44. Which of the following is NOT a side effect of medications used to treat incontinence?
    A. Dry mouth
    B. Cognitive changes
    C. Insomnia
    D. Tachycardia

45. Which of the following ECG changes is likely to be seen with hypokalemia?
    A. Sine wave rhythm
    B. Peaked T waves
    C. Development of U waves
    D. QT segment shortening

46. A 20-year-old woman presents to the ED with complaints of a 1 week history of a high fever, constipation, abdominal pain, and rose spots. She returned from eastern Africa 2 weeks ago where she stayed in a village with poor sanitation. Which of the following is the best diagnostic test for this infection?
    A. Stool for ova and parasites
    B. Blood culture
    C. Gram stain of stool
    D. Rotavirus antigen test

47. A 45-year-old male comes into the outpatient clinic with complaints of acute-on-chronic, intermittent knee pain. He reports in high school, he was diagnosed with an anterior cruciate ligament (ACL) tear, which was surgically reconstructed. He denies mechanical symptoms, such as locking, however, does note stiffness in the morning and after prolonged sitting. X-rays were obtained and demonstrate medial compartmental joint space narrowing, but otherwise no osseous abnormalities, such as tunnel osteolysis or loose bodies. Which of the following is most likely the underlying cause of his pain?
    A. Medial meniscus tear
    B. Lateral meniscal tear
    C. Post-traumatic osteoarthritis (OA)
    D. Pigmented villonodular synovitis

48. What is the most common bacterial cause of breast abscess?
    A. *Candida*
    B. *Pasturella multocida*
    C. *Staphylococcus aureus*
    D. *Streptococcus*

49. With which of the following recurrent conditions is sick sinus syndrome (SSS) commonly associated?
    A. Atrial fibrillation or atrial flutter
    B. Asystole
    C. Ventricular tachycardia
    D. Ventricular fibrillation

50. A 68-year-old patient with a history of chronic alcohol consumption and hepatic steatosis presents with dyspnea when climbing one flight of stairs that has come on gradually over the last "several months." Labs demonstrate normal cardiac enzymes, an elevated NT-proBNP but no other abnormalities. ECG shows sinus rhythm with no ST- or T-wave abnormalities. Echo shows cardiomegaly with thin ventricular walls, an EF of 35% to 40% but adequate valve morphology and function and no wall motion abnormalities. Which treatment option is most appropriate for this patient?
    A. Alcohol cessation, loop diuretics, ACE inhibitor, and a β-blocker
    B. Biventricular pacer implantation
    C. Digoxin and loop diuretics
    D. Referral for cardiac transplantation

51. Which of the following is the best tool to use for ear foreign-body removal?
    A. Ring forceps
    B. Alligator forceps
    C. Hemostat
    D. Curved iris scissors

52. A 19-year-old female with a history of asthma presents to the ED with complaints of decreased vision and pain with eye movement in her left eye that started earlier that morning. You obtain an MRI of the brain and orbits that shows diffuse enhancement of the left optic nerve. Based on the most likely diagnosis, what treatment would you recommend?
    A. 14-day course of oral prednisone
    B. Acyclovir, azithromycin, and prednisone
    C. Supportive care, as medical management does not change the overall visual outcome
    D. 3 days of IV methylprednisone followed by an oral prednisone taper

53. Which of the following diagnostic studies is the gold standard for the diagnosis of bladder cancer?
    A. Cystoscopy with biopsy
    B. CT of the abdomen and pelvis with and without contrast
    C. Urine cytology
    D. Urinalysis

54. A patient with untreated multiple myeloma presents to the ED after routine laboratory studies demonstrated hyperphosphatemia. The patient was instructed to come into the hospital by their primary care provider. The patient is asymptomatic with a normal physical examination and no other significant laboratory abnormalities. What is the most likely cause of this patient's hyperphosphatemia?
    A. Increased phosphate excretion
    B. Pseudohyperphosphatemia
    C. Nausea, vomiting, and diarrhea
    D. Occult liver tumor
    E. Underlying type 2 diabetes

55. Which of the following organisms causes infection with fever, malaise sore throat, and formation of an adherent pseudomembrane in the posterior pharynx?
    A. *Bordetella pertussis*
    B. *Clostridium tetani*
    C. *Corynebacterium diphtheriae*
    D. *Mycobacterium leprae*

56. Which ligament in the ankle is most commonly sprained?
    A. Anterior talofibular ligament
    B. Calcaneofibular ligament
    C. Deltoid ligament
    D. Posterior talofibular ligament

57. Which of the following best describes the pathophysiology of gynecomastia?
    A. Increased androgen effects
    B. Increased estrogen effects
    C. Decreased aromatase levels
    D. Decreased estrogen-to-testosterone conversion

58. A 60-year-old woman is experiencing severe and debilitating hot flashes. She has tried lifestyle modifications. Her past medical history (PMH) is significant for depression for which she takes venlafaxine. Her surgical history is significant for a cesarean section. She wants to know if she can start hormonal therapy (HT). Which of the following is appropriate?
    A. Wait on prescribing HT, continue to observe for worsening of symptoms
    B. Discuss oral estrogen-only therapy
    C. Discuss oral estrogen plus progestin therapy
    D. Discuss vaginal estrogen cream
    E. Start a SERM alone

59. Which of the following mechanisms results in premature atrial contractions?
    A. Early depolarization of atrial tissue
    B. Late repolarization of ventricular tissue
    C. Disturbance of the Purkinje fibers
    D. Early depolarization of the ventricles

60. Which of the following interventions should be avoided in patients with cardiac tamponade?
    A. Pericardiocentesis
    B. NSAIDs
    C. Pericardiectomy
    D. Positive pressure ventilation

61. If cerumen impaction is not able to be completed during office visit, the patient may use which of the following treatments and return in 3–5 days to repeat the procedure?
    A. Saline spray
    B. Rubbing alcohol
    C. Ear wax softener drops
    D. Ear wax candling

62. Which of the following does NOT increase a patient's risk for primary open-angle glaucoma?
    A. Family history
    B. Caucasian race
    C. Elevated intraocular pressure (>21 mm Hg)
    D. Age >40

63. Which of the following is the treatment of choice for chronic mesenteric ischemia?
    A. Bowel rest
    B. Surgical revascularization
    C. Anticoagulation
    D. Symptomatic support only

64. What is the definition of hypernatremia?
    A. Potassium level >5.5 mEq/L
    B. Sodium level <145 mEq/L
    C. Sodium level >145 mEq/L
    D. Calcium level >10 mEq/L

65. An 11-year-old boy with sickle cell anemia presents with a 2-day history of worsening fever, diarrhea, and vomiting after eating raw vegetables and chicken from a local street fair. Today, he developed pain and swelling in his right femur and is walking with a limp. Which of the following is the most likely diagnosis?
    A. Hepatitis A
    B. Norovirus
    C. *Campylobacter*
    D. *Salmonella*

66. A 50-year-old female presents to the outpatient clinic with complaints of acute-on-chronic knee pain. She reports a prior history of an anterior cruciate ligament (ACL) tear 20 years ago, which was treated conservatively. She states she has been able to remain active, by avoiding high-impact activities, weight management, and leg strengthening. She states that the pain is focal along the medial joint line, and recently, she has felt some catching while flexing her knee. She denies

reoccurring instability. X-rays were obtained, which demonstrate well-perservered joint spaces without acute osseous abnormality. Which of the following is most likely the underlying cause of her pain?
    A. Medial meniscus tear
    B. MCL tear
    C. Pes anserine bursitis
    D. Patellar tendinitis

67. A 34-year-old female presents with diffuse bilateral breast pain in the upper outer breast quadrants with radiation to the axilla that increases before menses. Which of the following is the first-line diagnostic measure for this condition?
    A. Core-needle biopsy
    B. Diagnostic mammogram
    C. Targeted breast U/S
    D. U/S-guided fine-needle aspiration (FNA)

68. Polycystic ovarian syndrome (PCOS) is associated with increased risk for which of the following?
    A. Ovarian cancer (OC)
    B. Diabetes
    C. Cervical cancer
    D. Formation of ovarian cystic neoplasms

69. Which of the following is a polymorphic VT that occurs in the setting of QT prolongation, resulting in a "twisting of points" appearance of the QRS complexes?
    A. Torsades de pointes
    B. Monomorphic VT
    C. Ventricular fibrillation
    D. Nonsustained VT

70. A 42-year-old Black man presents to his primary care provider with progressive fatigue and dyspnea on exertion for 3 months. Cardiac examination is notable for a grade III/VI harsh crescendo-decrescendo murmur best heard over the left sternal border and apex. The murmur is accentuated when the patient performs a Valsalva maneuver. What findings are expected on this patient's ECG?
    A. Normal ECG
    B. Diffusely low QRS voltage
    C. Sinus tachycardia
    D. Evidence of LV hypertrophy

71. An acoustic neuroma in an elderly patient who already wears a hearing device should be treated with which of the following modalities?
    A. Watchful observation
    B. Surgical excision
    C. Stereotactic radiosurgery
    D. Chemotherapy

72. A 48-year-old patient is diagnosed with an active tuberculosis infection and was started on appropriate medical therapy, which included ethambutol. What is a potential side effect of this medication you should counsel your patient on?
    A. Aplastic anemia
    B. Optic neuritis
    C. Hepatitis
    D. Orange secretions

73. Which of the following is the safest and most timely imaging technique used in making a diagnosis of toxic megacolon?
    A. Abdominal CT scan
    B. Colonoscopy
    C. Plain radiography of the abdomen
    D. Sigmoidoscopy

74. A 65-year-old patient with a past medical history (PMH) of active tobacco abuse (2 packs per day for 40 years) presents with recurrent ventricular tachycardia. Laboratory workup is significant for hypercalcemia and an elevated parathyroid hormone–related peptide. What condition should this patient be evaluated for?
    A. Hodgkin lymphoma
    B. Hypocalcemia
    C. Pseudohypoparathyroidism
    D. Small cell lung cancer
    E. Community-acquired pneumonia

75. The description that a patient in the early localized stage of Lyme disease would give of their illness would be BEST described by which of the following statements?
    A. Vesiculopapular rash with facial weakness and fever
    B. Large swollen left knee joint with bluish red discoloration and swelling of the distal extremities
    C. "Bull's-eye" lesion progressively enlarging with arthralgias, myalgias, and fatigue
    D. Chest pain, dyspnea, and evidence of second-degree heart block on electrocardiography

76. Which of the following is true regarding the management of hip fractures?
    A. A patient who is nonambulatory does not require surgical intervention.
    B. DVT prophylaxis should be started preoperatively and continued postoperatively.
    C. Prompt surgical intervention does not improve postoperative outcomes.
    D. Total hip arthroplasty is the recommended treatment for a femoral neck fracture.

77. Which of the following is the first-line treatment for galactorrhea not associated with hormonal changes or medications?
    A. Eliminate nipple stimulation
    B. Excise the causative ducts
    C. Increase support for Cooper's ligament
    D. Use nursing pad in the breast area

78. You are seeing a sexually active 22-year-old female with reports of increased yellow to green frothy discharge and dysuria. On examination, you note cervicovaginitis (strawberry cervix). What do you suspect the diagnosis is?
    A. Candidiasis
    B. Trichomoniasis
    C. Bacterial vaginosis
    D. Genitourinary syndrome of menopause

79. You are reviewing an ECG that shows regular and rapid atrial depolarizations with "sawtooth" P waves. What is the most likely diagnosis for this patient?
    A. Atrial fibrillation
    B. Atrial flutter
    C. Multifocal atrial tachycardia
    D. Transient idiopathic arrhythmia

80. Which of the following is NOT a hallmark of cardiac tamponade?
    A. Jugular vein distention (JVD)
    B. Pulsus alternans
    C. Hypotension
    D. Pulsus paradoxus

81. A 25-year-old woman comes to the clinic with complaints of episodes of "spinning dizziness" and a sense of imbalance whenever she looks upward while changing a light bulb or painting a ceiling for the past week. It is not brought on by sound on pressure. She has no other neurologic complaints. She denies aural fullness, hearing loss, or tinnitus. Her past medical history includes well-controlled hypertension, with complaint use of hydrochlorothiazide 25 mg daily for 3 years. Which of the following physical examination components will most likely reproduce her symptoms?
    A. Dix-Hallpike maneuver
    B. HINTS examination
    C. Valsalva maneuver
    D. Weber and Rinne testing

82. An 18-year-old male comes in for evaluation of the left eye after he was skateboarding and fell. You suspect that the patient has a globe rupture of his left eye. What does the patient likely present with?
    A. Teardrop pupil
    B. Oval pupil
    C. Constricted pupil
    D. Dilated pupil

83. Which of the following endoscopic finding is associated with ulcerative colitis?
    A. Skip lesions
    B. Loss of vascularity
    C. Cobblestone appearance
    D. Esophageal ulcerations

84. A 40-year-old female presents with fever, headache, and nausea. Temperature is 100 °F. She is disoriented to place and time. Cranial nerves are intact. Neck is supple without meningismus. Petechiae and purpura are noted on the bilateral lower extremities. Laboratory studies reveal low Hb, low platelet count, high reticulocyte count, schistocytes on peripheral blood smear, and high creatinine. Which of the following is the most appropriate initial treatment?
    A. Cyclophosphamide
    B. Methylprednisolone
    C. RBC transfusion
    D. Therapeutic plasma exchange

85. What is the common incubation period of syphilis after exposure?
    A. 3 weeks
    B. 3 hours
    C. 4 months
    D. 6 months

86. Which of the following physical examination findings is most consistent with patellar tendonitis?
    A. Anterior knee laxity
    B. Large suprapatellar effusion
    C. Pain with resisted knee extension
    D. Pain with rotary stress of the knee

87. Which of the following is the most common physical examination finding for gynecomastia?
    A. Painful mound of adipose tissue located eccentric to the areola
    B. Painless concentric ring of glandular tissue extending under the areola
    C. Painless well-defined, mobile mass noted lateral to the areola
    D. Painful discoid-shaped mass located deep to the areola

88. Which of the following is TRUE regarding the diagnosis of polycystic ovarian disease (PCOS) in adults using the Rotterdam Diagnostic Criteria?
    A. Diagnosis requires sonographic evidence of PCOS.
    B. Menstrual irregularities alone, after exclusion of other causes, is sufficient for a diagnosis of PCOS.
    C. Hirsutism is considered evidence of clinical hyperandrogenism.
    D. Documentation of overweight or obesity is required for diagnosis of PCOS.

89. A 65-year-old male with a history of coronary artery disease (CAD) and heart failure with reduced ejection fraction (EF) has a left bundle branch block (LBBB). In which leads do you expect to see prolonged, aberrant QRS complexes on an ECG?
    A. II, III, and aVF
    B. I, aVL, V_5, and V_6
    C. V_1 and V_2
    D. V_5 and V_6

90. The presence of which of the following cardiac conditions would warrant a patient receiving antibiotic prophylaxis before dental procedures?
    A. Bicuspid aortic valve
    B. Hypertrophic cardiomyopathy (HCM)
    C. Bioprosthetic mitral valve
    D. Mitral valve prolapse

91. A 25-year-old pregnant woman complains of spontaneous episodes of severe vertigo and emesis for 2 days. These episodes have increased in frequency and intensity. She thinks she may have some hearing loss in her left ear but is unsure because "it sounds like the ocean" in that ear. She is asymptomatic at present. Physical examination of ENT, neurologic, and heart and lung components reveals no abnormal findings. What is the most appropriate way to treat the patient's underlying pathology?
    A. Crystal repositioning exercises
    B. Hydrochlorothiazide/triamterene
    C. Promethazine
    D. Surgery

92. What diagnostic procedure is contraindicated if you suspect a globe rupture?
    A. Slit-lamp examination
    B. CT scan
    C. Tonometry
    D. Fluorescein testing

93. Which of the following is the gold standard for the diagnosis of acute mesenteric ischemia due to an arterial thrombosis?
    A. Mesenteric angiography
    B. CT scan with contrast
    C. Barium enema
    D. Plain film of the abdomen

94. Which of the following medications is thought to precipitate the microangiopathic hemolytic anemia associated with thrombotic thrombocytopenic purpura (TTP)?
    A. Clopidogrel
    B. Prednisone
    C. Rituximab
    D. Vincristine

95. The most common peripheral nerve involvement with Lyme disease affects which of the following nerves?
    A. Facial nerve
    B. Femoral nerve
    C. Optic nerve
    D. Oculomotor nerve

96. Which is the most sensitive physical examination to diagnose an acute anterior cruciate ligament (ACL) injury?
    A. Anterior drawer
    B. Pivot shift
    C. Valgus/varus stress
    D. Lachman examination

97. A 56-year-old female is diagnosed with HER-2–negative, estrogen and progesterone receptor–positive breast cancer. Her last normal menstrual period was 3 years ago. Which of the following adjuvant oral medications should be prescribed to reduce the risk of recurrence?
    A. Selective estrogen receptor modulator
    B. Aromatase inhibitor
    C. HER-2–targeted therapy
    D. Platinum-based therapy

98. Your 38-year-old G3P2 patient, with no significant medical history, presents to your office for her routine visit but reports that she has been experiencing heavier-than-usual menstrual bleeding and cycles of longer duration over the past year. On examination, you find her uterus to be enlarged, leading you to suspect uterine fibroids, which is confirmed by TVUS. A CBC is consistent with anemia. Of the following, which treatment modality is most appropriate at this time?
    A. Gonadotropin-releasing hormone (GnRH) agonist
    B. Contraceptives containing progestin
    C. Endometrial ablation
    D. Lifestyle changes (ie, diet and exercise)

99. A 72-year-old male presents to the clinic with a complaint of palpitations and shortness of breath when ascending a flight of stairs. He has a history of hypertension, CAD, and diabetes mellitus. An ECG reveals an irregular rhythm with an atrial rate of more than 300 beats per minute and a ventricular rate of 98 beats per minute. What is the most likely diagnosis for this patient?
    A. Atrial fibrillation
    B. Atrial flutter
    C. Multifocal atrial tachycardia
    D. Transient idiopathic arrhythmia

100. A 38-year-old woman is diagnosed with hypertrophic cardiomyopathy (HCM) after initially presenting to the ED with atypical chest pain. What should subsequent management for this patient include?
    A. Treatment with a negative inotropic agent, such as a β-blocker
    B. Genetic testing for each of the patient's first-degree relatives
    C. Implementation of an intense exercise regimen to improve conditioning
    D. Emergent surgical myectomy

101. Which of the following patient symptoms would lead you to put acute otitis media (AOM) on the top of your differential diagnosis?
    A. Serous drainage from the affected ear
    B. Constant ringing in the affected ear
    C. Pressure or pain in the affected ear
    D. Sudden hearing loss in the affected ear

102. What eye muscle is more likely affected by trauma to the orbit causing a limited upward gaze on examination?
    A. Inferior rectus muscle
    B. Superior rectus muscle
    C. Lateral rectus muscle
    D. Medial rectus muscle

103. Which of the following is the gold standard for the diagnosis of Crohn disease?
    A. Colonoscopy
    B. CT scan
    C. MRI enterography
    D. Pill endoscopy

104. When investigating a new asymptomatic thrombocytosis, which of the following is NOT a useful first-line investigation?
    A. Iron studies and ferritin
    B. *JAK2 V617F*
    C. C-reactive protein
    D. Full blood count

105. The mother of one of your toddler-age patients contacts your office and notes that several children in her son's daycare have pinworms. What is your recommendation to her at this point?
    A. Wake the child nightly to look for pinworms around the anus.
    B. Watch the child for perianal itching.
    C. Wash the child's sheets and pajamas daily to prevent infection.
    D. Apply petrolatum jelly to the anus to suffocate the pinworms.
    E. Administer a one-time dose of mebendazole for prophylaxis.

106. Because her child has been scratching around his perianal area at night, a concerned parent brings in a stool sample for testing. What is your recommendation at this point?
    A. The stool sample will be helpful in determining the most likely diagnosis.
    B. A urine sample would more accurately aid in diagnosis.
    C. She should help the child perform better hygiene after bowel movements.
    D. Analysis of tape adhered and then removed from this area would be more helpful.
    E. Remove the child from his daycare because he may have gotten something there.

107. Inflammation of the patellar ligament specifically at the tibial tuberosity where the growth plate has not completely closed is best known as what condition?
    A. Jumpers knee
    B. Osgood-Schlatter disease
    C. Runners knee
    D. Salter Harris type II fracture

108. A 44-year-old male with a past medical history (PMH) of well-controlled major depressive disorder presents with bilateral breast enlargement and a thin milky breast discharge. Which of the following is the most likely cause of his current symptoms?
    A. Endocrine disorder
    B. Nipple stimulation
    C. Medications
    D. Prolactinoma

109. The diagnosis of ovarian torsion is best confirmed by which of the following?
    A. MRI with contrast
    B. CT with contrast
    C. CBC with differential
    D. U/S

110. In ventricular arrythmias, which of the following symptoms is often linked with an increased risk of sudden cardiac death?
    A. Palpitations
    B. Exercise intolerance
    C. Syncope
    D. Dizziness

111. A 38-year-old woman with a new diagnosis of hypertension was placed on hydrochlorothiazide. The following day, she presented to the ED with an episode of presyncope and hypotension. Her resting ECG is normal. After her hypotension is treated, workup for which of the following cardiomyopathies is indicated?
    A. Dilated
    B. Hypertrophic
    C. Restrictive
    D. Alcoholic

112. Which of the following is an ideal patient to perform a HINTS examination on?
    A. One who has continuous vertigo that is triggered
    B. One who has continuous vertigo that spontaneously occurs
    C. One who has episodes of vertigo that are triggered
    D. One who has episodes of vertigo that spontaneously occur

113. Which of the following treatments is the least appropriate treatment for a foreign body/corneal abrasion?
    A. Observation
    B. Topical antibiotics
    C. Topical steroids
    D. Eye protection (eg, patch)

114. Which of the following over-the-counter medications should immediately be discontinued in patients with toxic megacolon?
    A. Acetaminophen
    B. Docusate sodium
    C. Ibuprofen
    D. Loperamide

115. Which of the following is a radiographic view of the ankle?
    A. Dorsoplantar (DP)
    B. Mortise
    C. Posteroanterior (PA)
    D. Skyline

116. Which of the following is the most appropriate next step in evaluating a patient with galactorrhea and an elevated prolactin level?
    A. Clinical breast examination
    B. Diagnostic mammogram
    C. Ductography
    D. MRI

117. A 57-year-old postmenopausal woman is referred for evaluation of a 5-cm simple appearing ovarian cysts on her left ovary, found incidental during evaluation for diverticulitis. Last menstrual period (LMP) was at 50 years of age. She denies postmenopausal bleeding, bloating, or early satiety. What is the next best step in this patient's management?
    A. Immediate surgical evaluation
    B. Refer to gynecology oncologist
    C. Reassurance, no further evaluation is necessary
    D. Check CA125, if normal, repeat TVUS in 6-12 weeks

118. Which of the following is the most common cause of sick sinus syndrome (SSS)?
    A. Amyloidosis
    B. Cardiomyopathy
    C. Fibrosis of sinus node
    D. Hypothyroidism

119. Which of the following risk factors is associated with infective endocarditis (IE)?
    A. Female sex
    B. Diabetes mellitus
    C. Congenital heart disease
    D. Tobacco use

120. A 2-year-old baby is brought to the urgent care center for inconsolable crying and fever over the past 24 hours. Physical examination of the left ear reveals copious otorrhea in the left ear canal and a swollen erythematous mastoid region with a forward placed pinna on the same side. Upon culture, which of the following organisms are you the most likely to find in this patient?
    A. *Haemophilus influenzae*
    B. *Moraxella catarrhalis*
    C. *Pseudomonas aeruginosa*
    D. *Streptococcus pneumoniae*
    E. *Staphylococcus aureus*

121. A 16-year-old female presents to the ER after playing softball where she was hit in her right eye. On examination, she had a limited upward gaze. You order a CT scan because you suspect she has an orbital blowout fracture. What sign would indicate she has an orbital blowout fracture?
    A. Teardrop sign indicating a bulging optic nerve
    B. Teardrop sign indicating herniated tissue and muscle
    C. Teardrop sign indicating blockage of the ciliary body
    D. Teardrop sign indicating increased intraocular pressure

122. Definitive diagnosis of colonic ischemia is made using which of the following?
    A. Colonoscopy with biopsy
    B. CT scan with contrast
    C. Barium enema
    D. Mesenteric angiography

123. A 45-year-old female presents to the ED with a 4-hour history of sudden-onset severe RUQ pain. Physical examination reveals hepatomegaly, tenderness to the RUQ, and ascites. Bloods showed an Hb 125 g/L, platelets 650×10^9/L, WBC 14.5×10^9/L. She has a previous medical history of essential thrombocytosis. Medications include aspirin 75 mg once daily. Ultrasound shows a smooth, regular liver that is mildly enlarged and reversed flow in hepatic veins. What is the most likely diagnosis?
    A. Cholelithiasis
    B. Portal vein thrombosis
    C. Upper GI bleed
    D. Right lower lobe pneumonia

124. What is a complication of Rocky Mountain spotted fever?
    A. Third-degree heart block
    B. Encephalitis
    C. Thrombocytosis
    D. Ruptured spleen

125. What is the insertion point of the patella tendon?
    A. Inferior pole of the patella
    B. Superior pole of the patella
    C. Tibial plateau
    D. Tibial tuberosity

126. Which of the following is necessary to diagnose an adolescent with polycystic ovarian syndrome (PCOS) according to the 2015 Pediatric Endocrine Society Clinical Practice Guidelines?
    A. U/S evidence of polycystic ovaries
    B. Decreased levels of total serum testosterone
    C. Obesity
    D. Menstrual irregularities persistent 2 years after menarche

127. You diagnose a 50-year-old patient in your practice with a third-degree atrioventricular block. You recommend that he see a cardiologist immediately for a permanent pacemaker implantation. He does not want to have the procedure and asks you what the risks are if he does not get the pacemaker. Which of the following answers can be left out of this conversation with the patient?
    A. Fall due to syncope
    B. Peripheral vascular disease
    C. Sudden cardiac death
    D. Symptomatic bradycardia

128. Which of the following populations is pilonidal disease more likely to affect?
    A. Female sex
    B. Male sex
    C. Age over 30 years
    D. Physically fit

129. Which of the following statements is false concerning antibiotic treatment in otitis externa?
    A. Topical antibiotics, with or without corticosteroids, is the mainstay of treatment.
    B. Fluoroquinolone antibiotics are a superior class of antibiotics.
    C. Aminoglycoside antibiotics are known to carry the risk of ototoxicity.
    D. Treatment duration is, at a minimum, 7 days.

130. You call your local ophthalmologist or optometrist to see a patient with suspected acute angle glaucoma. Which of the following drugs is NOT appropriate to use as a temporizing measure?
    A. Topical carbonic anhydrase inhibitors
    B. Topical β-blockers
    C. Topical atropine drops
    D. Topical prostaglandin analog drops

131. What is considered first-line therapy for the management of mild inflammation in Crohn disease?
    A. Steroids
    B. Biologics
    C. Immune modulators
    D. Aminosalicylates

132. Which of the following best describes the role of plasma metalloprotease ADAMTS-13?
    A. Adheres platelets to the vessel wall
    B. Cleaves von Willebrand factor multimers
    C. Inhibits glycoprotein IIb/IIIa activity
    D. Prevents the conversion of fibrinogen into fibrin

133. A 19-year-old female presents to the office stating she has noticed a white discharge in her underwear recently, which has an odor to it. She also states that the last time she had sex 3 days ago, it was painful. On examination, there is a white, foul-smelling discharge seen on speculum examination, and a sample is taken for a wet mount. Which of the following is expected on a wet mount prep?
    A. Hyphae and spores
    B. Clue cells
    C. Protozoans
    D. Polymorphonuclear leukocytes

134. Which of the following statements is true?
    A. Coexisting traumatic brain injury (TBI) and intracranial hemorrhage is associated with poor patient outcomes.
    B. Coexisting TBI and intracranial hemorrhage is associated with better patient outcomes.
    C. TBI and intracranial hemorrhage do not overlap.
    D. TBI is unrelated to intracranial hemorrhage.

135. You are returning a phone call from a 75-year-old woman who has had a vaginal bulge for the past 72 hours. It is not painful, and she can push it back into the vagina with minimal effort. What do you recommend?
    A. Proceed immediately to the roomed.
    B. Refer her to the general surgery clinic.
    C. Tell her it is probably cancerous.
    D. Ask her to schedule an appointment for a vaginal examination.

136. Which of the following is the most appropriate management of dermoid cysts (teratoma) in a premenopausal woman?
    A. Refer for surgical evaluation, regardless of size
    B. Check CA125
    C. Expectant management unless size >5 cm
    D. Refer for MRI to confirm U/S findings

137. In a symptomatic patient with a normal ECG, which of the following initial diagnostic tests would be indicated for further evaluation of premature beats?
    A. Cardiac catheterization
    B. Cardiac MRI
    C. Holter monitor
    D. Dobutamine stress test

138. How might acanthosis nigricans be treated?
    A. Cryosurgery
    B. Curettage
    C. Weight loss
    D. Corticosteroid taper

139. Which of the following patients should be referred for mastoidectomy?
    A. Patient whose CT of the mastoid region shows coalescence of mastoid air cells
    B. Patient whose middle ear culture reveals *aspergillosis*
    C. Patient who has both mastoiditis and a positive Kernig sign
    D. Patient with mastoiditis who has a fever of 102 °F despite adequate IV antibiotic treatment after 48 hours
    E. Patient who has had multiple cases of otitis media leading up to the diagnosis of mastoiditis

140. What is the most common cause of monocular transient vision loss?
    A. Cardioembolic stroke
    B. Giant cell arteritis
    C. Papilledema
    D. Angle-closure glaucoma

141. Which of the following is the most significant risk factor for toxic megacolon?
    A. Colon polyps
    B. Diverticulitis
    C. Irritable bowel syndrome (IBS)
    D. Recent antibiotic use

142. A 50-year-old male presents to his primary care provider and is found to have a platelet count of 755×10^9/L. He has no other previous medical history. He is found to have a CALR variant mutation on peripheral blood, and a diagnosis of essential thrombocythemia is confirmed on bone marrow examination. What is the next best step?
    A. Active monitoring
    B. Cytoreductive therapy with hydroxycarbamide 500 mg once daily
    C. Low-dose aspirin 75 mg once daily
    D. Anticoagulation with rivaroxaban 20 mg once daily

143. A 23-year-old patient comes in stating he was told to come to the clinic for evaluation after a sexual contact tested positive for trichomoniasis. Which of the following would be the best treatment for him?
    A. Azithromycin 1 g PO
    B. Ceftriaxone 250 mg IM
    C. Metronidazole 2 g PO
    D. Penicillin 2.4 million units IM

144. Which of the following may help reduce the number of symptomatic days after a concussion?
    A. Light, subsymptomatic exercise
    B. Full 7 days of brain and physical rest
    C. High-dose NSAIDs early after diagnosis
    D. Head CT and brain MRI

145. Which of the following preoperative findings is most suggestive for ovarian malignancy?
    A. A unilateral ovarian mass
    B. A simple 8-cm cystic ovarian mass
    C. A complex 5-cm cystic ovarian mass that increases in size within 2 months
    D. An elevated serum CA125 in a 28-year-old woman with a stable 5-cm ovarian mass and a history of endometriosis

146. Suprapubic pressure helps to facilitate delivery in cases of shoulder dystocia by which of the following?
    A. Rotating the pubis symphysis
    B. Adducting and rotating the fetal shoulders
    C. Flattening the maternal sacrum
    D. Rotating the fetal torso extravaginally
    E. Delivering the posterior arm or shoulder first

147. Which of the following physical examination findings is expected in a small ventricular septal defect with a high gradient?
    A. Loud, harsh holosystolic murmur
    B. Palpable S2 in the pulmonic area
    C. Right ventricular heave
    D. Unequal peripheral pulses

148. Which of the following organs is most commonly involved in DRESS (drug rash with eosinophilia and systemic symptoms)?
    A. Lung
    B. Kidney
    C. Liver
    D. Heart

149. Which of the following is NOT a risk factor for otitis externa?
    A. Recent swimming
    B. Wearing hearing aids
    C. Excessive cerumen
    D. Previous radiation therapy

150. A 25-year-old female with a history of obesity and polycystic ovarian syndrome presents to her local urgent care complaining of a headache, intermittent binocular vision loss lasting a few minutes, and diplopia. An MRI of the brain is obtained and shows signs of increased intracranial pressure. Lumbar puncture reveals an opening pressure of 42 cm H_2O with normal cerebrospinal fluid studies. She is diagnosed with idiopathic intracranial hypertension. What is the most likely finding on her fundus examination?
    A. Dot blot hemorrhages
    B. Macular edema
    C. Diffuse and numerous hemorrhages with dilated and tortuous veins that resemble a "blood-and-thunder fundus"
    D. Papilledema

151. Which of the following is a risk associated with ulcerative colitis?
    A. Enteroenteric fistula
    B. Small bowel obstruction
    C. Perirectal abscess
    D. Adenocarcinoma

152. Which of the following findings suggests life-threatening bleeding in immune thrombocytopenic purpura (ITP)?
    A. Ecchymosis
    B. Hemoptysis
    C. Menorrhagia
    D. Petechiae

153. How long after ingestion of a pinworm egg might you expect a patient to exhibit symptoms?
    A. By 3 weeks after ingestion
    B. In 14 days on average
    C. Within the next couple of evenings
    D. At least 6 months after
    E. Within 2 months of ingestion

154. You are interviewing an 81-year-old patient about his psychosocial needs as part of a thorough office visit for this patient. He has a history of mild Alzheimer disease and has several family members who stay with him. He discloses that he has one family member who helps him pay some of his bills. He hesitates at this point and appears to be lost in thought. When you prompt him to continue, he says that he seems to notice that sometimes this family member makes unauthorized withdrawals from his bank account. He has questioned the family member several times, and each time, they have an excuse. This last time, though, the family member became irate and slapped your patient once. What should you do next?
    A. Because this is an adult, there is really nothing that you can do besides encouraging him to manage his own money.

B. This patient counts as a dependent adult, since he is elderly and has a disease (Alzheimer) that would prevent him from living individually. Because of this, you are a mandated reporter to your local elder abuse agency (such as the Ombudsman or others).

C. Continue with your assessment of his psychosocial needs without acknowledging the abuse. It is usually best not to engage, and he could be confabulating.

D. Insist upon confronting and speaking to the family member—there is probably been a misunderstanding.

155. A 19-year-old G0P0 female presents to her gynecology provider complaining of lower left quadrant pain with intercourse. Pelvic U/S shows an 8.5-cm complex cystic mass on the left ovary. Which of the following labs would be most helpful for diagnosing a germ cell tumor?
A. CA125
B. α-Fetoprotein (AFP)
C. Testosterone
D. Inhibin

156. A 21-year-old female, G1P1A0, is in active labor. The fetal head has been delivered but retracted back into the perineum. What is the most appropriate next step?
A. McRoberts maneuver
B. Woods corkscrew maneuver
C. Rubin's maneuver
D. Posterior axillary traction
E. Cesarean section

157. What is the association between prostaglandins and patient ductus arteriosus (PDA)?
A. Relatively high levels of prostaglandins in the preterm newborn allow for persistence of the ductus arteriosus (DA) after birth.
B. Increasing prostaglandin levels in the newborn stimulate normal closure of the DA.
C. A genetic defect in the newborn's ability to synthesize prostaglandins results in a chronically PDA.
D. Declining prostaglandin levels in the developing fetus trigger closure of the DA in the first trimester.

158. Patients with acanthosis nigricans are at increased risk for what medical condition?
A. Type 2 diabetes mellitus
B. Varicella zoster
C. Coronary atherosclerosis
D. Allergic rhinitis

159. A 7-year-old boy was diagnosed with mastoiditis 3 days ago. The diagnosis was confirmed by CT and empiric IV antibiotic treatment was initiated with a third-generation cephalosporin. Culture and sensitivity confirmed the correct antibiotic choice. The patient has maintained a temperature of 98.6 °F for the past 48 hours and reports decreased pain. Physical examination reveals a marked reduction in mastoid swelling. Which of the following represents the best next step in managing this patient?
A. Discharge the patient with a 2-week course of oral antibiotics.
B. Continue current IV treatment for an additional 48 hours and re-evaluate.
C. Confirm clearance of infection with a second CT of the mastoid region.
D. Consider repeat culture of middle ear aspirate to confirm improvement.
E. Discharge the patient with prescriptions for analgesics and oral steroids.

160. Which of the following is NOT a typical presentation of acute angle-closure glaucoma?
A. Headache
B. Vomiting
C. Halos around light
D. Purulent discharge

161. Which of the following is one of the diagnostic criteria for toxic megacolon?
A. Colonic dilation >6 cm
B. Elevated CRP
C. Intestinal pseudopolyps
D. Intraperitoneal free air

162. A 75-year-old male presents to the outpatient hematology clinic, referred for anemia and persistent thrombocytosis. Investigations reveal Hb 107 g/L, platelets 785×10^9/L, WBCs 5.5×10^9/L. Peripheral blood smear confirms thrombocytosis and dacrocytes, with no immature cells seen. He tests positive for the *JAK2 V617F* mutation. He reports 5 kg weight loss over the past 2 months and night sweats 4–5 times per week. What is the most likely diagnosis?
A. CML
B. Myelofibrosis
C. Essential thrombocythemia
D. PV

163. A 24-year-old female presents stating she has some pain with urination and itchiness "down there." She is sexually active but did not use protection during her last sexual encounter 10 days ago. On speculum examination, there is inflammation and erythema of the vaginal walls, macular lesions on the cervix, and a thick white discharge is visible. Which of the following is the most likely diagnosis?
A. Herpes simplex
B. Human papillomavirus (HPV)
C. Bacterial vaginosis
D. Trichomoniasis

164. Symptoms of generalized anxiety disorder (GAD) include all the following, except which of the following?
    A. Restlessness or feeling keyed up or on edge
    B. Intense focus
    C. Irritability
    D. Muscle tension
    E. Sleep disturbance

165. What is the most common cause of secondary dysmenorrhea?
    A. Endometriosis
    B. Polycystic ovarian syndrome (PCOS)
    C. IUD system
    D. Inflammatory bowel disease
    E. Pelvic inflammatory disease (PID)

166. Which of the following best describes moderate variability on external fetal HR monitoring?
    A. It requires maternal change of position.
    B. It is a harbinger of poor fetal outcomes.
    C. It is a reassuring finding, and no intervention is necessary.
    D. It is worrisome and plans for delivery should be undertaken.

167. When should treatment with a cyclooxygenase inhibitor be considered for a patient with a patient ductus arteriosus (PDA)?
    A. All patients with a PDA should undergo medical treatment with a cyclooxygenase inhibitor at the time of diagnosis or as soon thereafter as possible.
    B. Only preterm newborns who are experiencing functional effects of the PDA should receive cyclooxygenase inhibitor therapy.
    C. Infants and children age 3 months or older should receive a cyclooxygenase inhibitor after persistence of the PDA has been observed in multiple echocardiograms.
    D. Cyclooxygenase therapy is reserved as a preventative measure and only given to pregnant women when the fetus has confirmed presence of PDA in the third trimester.

168. A 5-year-old male presents with urticaria limited to his arms following several mosquito bites. He has intense pruritus, but no features concerning for angioedema or anaphylaxis. What is the most appropriate treatment?
    A. Oral corticosteroids
    B. Oral antihistamines
    C. Topical corticosteroid cream
    D. Intramuscular epinephrine

169. Your patient presents with right eye redness, pain, decreased vision, photophobia, and a severe headache. What is your diagnosis?
    A. Allergic conjunctivitis
    B. Bacterial conjunctivitis
    C. Consider other causes of a red eye
    D. Viral conjunctivitis

170. Benign nodules should be followed with ultrasound at which of the following periods?
    A. After 3 months
    B. After 6 months
    C. After 9 months
    D. After 12 months

171. A diagnosis of direct inguinal hernia is most often made with which of the following modalities?
    A. Clinical assessment
    B. Ultrasonography
    C. CT of the abdomen/pelvis
    D. MRI

172. Which medication is the recommended first-line treatment in Rocky Mountain spotted fever (RMSF)?
    A. Amoxicillin
    B. Ceftriaxone
    C. Doxycycline
    D. TMP/SMX

173. FDA-approved medications for autism spectrum disorder (ASD) are indicated for children with which of the following symptoms?
    A. Irritability
    B. Depression
    C. Rigid behaviors
    D. Disordered eating

174. A 40-year-old female with a FH of colon cancer has recently been diagnosed with ovarian cancer (OC). Genetic studies reveal mutations in DNA *MMR* genes. This patient is diagnosed with which of the following?
    A. Hereditary breast and ovarian cancer (HBOC) syndrome
    B. Cowden syndrome
    C. Li-Fraumeni syndrome
    D. Lynch syndrome

175. Which of the following is a common cause of secondary postpartum hemorrhage (PPH)?
    A. Placental abruption
    B. Placenta previa
    C. Uterine subinvolution
    D. Amniotic fluid embolism

176. A 10-year-old boy presents to your pediatric clinic for a well-child visit. Neither he nor his mother reports any problems with his health over the past year. On physical examination, a BP of 150/95 mm Hg

is found. Because of this finding, BP is also taken in the child's lower extremities and is found to be 100/65 mm Hg. Which of the following conditions is the most likely cause of this patient's hypertension?
A. Coarctation of the aorta (CoA)
B. Essential hypertension
C. Obstructive sleep apnea
D. Renal artery stenosis

177. A 30-year-old female present with a rash ~8 days after starting amoxicillin for streptococcal pharyngitis. She is asymptomatic aside from mild pruritis. Vital signs are within normal limits, and you note a diffuse, erythematous maculopapular rash. What is the next best step in management?
A. Discontinue amoxicillin
B. Prescribe corticosteroids
C. Prescribe topical diphenhydramine
D. No intervention necessary

178. Which of the following is NOT a risk factor for the development of cataracts?
A. Diabetes
B. Tobacco use
C. History of extensive sun exposure
D. Hypertension

179. Which of the following imaging modalities is most appropriate for evaluation of a thyroid nodule?
A. CT with contrast
B. CT without contrast
C. MRI
D. Ultrasound

180. Which of the following specialists is most critical for immediately consultation in diagnosed cases of toxic megacolon?
A. Critical care
B. Gastroenterology
C. General surgery
D. Infectious disease

181. Which of the following is the most common clinical presentation in men with gonococcal urethritis?
A. Testicular pain
B. Mucopurulent penile discharge
C. Without symptoms
D. Suprapubic pain

182. Which of the following statements is NOT true about trichomoniasis?
A. Do not take alcohol with the treatment of choice
B. Can cause cataracts and blindness in newborns
C. Can be prevented with condoms
D. May be asymptomatic is men and women

183. An adult patient with rapid-cycling bipolar disorder is treated with but has not responded to divalproex therapy. Which of the following options is the best treatment option to add at this time?
A. Clozapine
B. Escitalopram
C. Lithium
D. Lorazepam

184. Which is NOT consistent with a history of prolapse?
A. History of a reducible mass from the vaginal opening
B. Acute, severe pelvic pain
C. Difficulty emptying the bladder
D. Worsening urinary incontinence

185. Cardiotocography while a patient is laboring reveals absent variability and recurrent late decelerations. Into which category does this finding fall?
A. Category I
B. Category II
C. Category III
D. Category IV

186. In patients who have undergone total surgical repair of tetralogy of Fallot, which of the following is true regarding their ongoing care?
A. Sequelae are rare and ongoing monitoring is unnecessary.
B. Pulmonic regurgitation is common and right ventricular failure is possible.
C. Endocarditis prophylaxis is unnecessary.
D. Ventricular septal defect closure is not part of the surgical repair.

187. A 25-year-old otherwise healthy woman is diagnosed with acute pilonidal abscess without associated cellulitis. Which of the following is the most appropriate initial intervention?
A. Incision and drainage
B. IV antibiotics
C. Oral antibiotics
D. Referral for surgical excision

188. To differentiate preseptal cellulitis from orbital cellulitis, what is the imaging modality of choice?
A. Ocular ultrasound
B. CT of the orbits
C. CT angiogram of the head
D. Skull x-ray

189. Which of the following is a clinical finding in hyperparathyroidism?
A. Perioral numbness
B. Dysrhythmias
C. Muscle tetany
D. Nephrolithiasis

190. In a patient presenting with acute abdominal distention and vomiting, who is found to have an incarcerated inguinal hernia, which of the following is the most appropriate definitive treatment?
    A. Urgent surgical hernia repair
    B. IV fluids and watchful waiting
    C. Elective surgical hernia repair
    D. Manual decompression of hernia sac

191. What is the most common manifestation of rheumatic fever?
    A. Chorea
    B. Erythema marginatum
    C. Polyarthritis
    D. Prolonged QT

192. Rocky Mountain spotted fever (RMSF) is caused by which pathogen?
    A. *Borrelia burgdorferi*
    B. Parvovirus B19
    C. *Rickettsia rickettsii*
    D. *Treponema pallidum*

193. Pharmacologic treatment of conduct disorder focuses on which of the following?
    A. Decreasing depression
    B. Decreasing sleep
    C. Increasing aggressiveness
    D. Increasing anxiety
    E. Increasing energy

194. You have a 33-year-old female patient diagnosed with premenstrual dysphoric disorder (PMDD) and menorrhagia who is not interested in conceiving in the next year. She has tried exercise, a healthy diet, adequate sleep, and stress reduction, but her symptoms persist. What would you try next for her treatment?
    A. Antidepressant
    B. Oral contraception
    C. Diet change
    D. Mineral supplementation

195. A patient delivers a 9 lb 5 oz baby after a prolonged third stage of labor. Which of the following findings, if present, would lead to a diagnosis of postpartum hemorrhage (PPH)?
    A. If estimated visual blood loss is 250 mL.
    B. If the patient continues to bleed, a diagnosis of PPH can be made.
    C. If the hematocrit is <32%, the patient is considered to have a PPH.
    D. If the patient exhibits pallor, confusion, is tachycardic or hypotensive, the patient is considered to have a hemorrhage.

196. Which of the following best describes the pathophysiologic effects of coarctation of the aorta (CoA) on the heart?

    A. Backward flow of blood leads to ventricular dilation and fluid overload.
    B. Coronary ischemia caused by stenosis leads to myocardial infarction.
    C. Associated genetic defects cause hypertrophy of the septum.
    D. Stenosis of the aorta leads to ventricular hypertrophy and heart failure.

197. You have diagnosed a 40-year-old male with DRESS several weeks after he began allopurinol for recurrent gout. He has a nonproductive cough, slight hypoxia, and a modest increase in liver function tests without signs of liver failure. In addition to discontinuing the allopurinol and counseling the patient to avoid the drug for life, what treatment is indicated?
    A. Topical and systemic corticosteroids
    B. IVIG
    C. Vancomycin
    D. No treatment necessary

198. A 30-year-old female presents to the clinic complaining of right eye redness, tearing, and photosensitivity since this morning. She normally wears her contacts to sleep and changes them monthly. Corneal examination does not show corneal abrasion or ulcer, but the eye is injected, the pupil is constricted, and ciliary flush is present. You should treat her with which of the following?
    A. Lubricating eye drops
    B. Antibiotic eye drops
    C. Patching of the affected eye
    D. Anti-inflammatory eye drops

199. Fine-needle aspiration is recommended for thyroid nodules with which of the following characteristics?
    A. Microcalcifications
    B. Fully cystic
    C. <1 cm in size
    D. Regular margins

200. What would you expect to find when performing a digital rectal examination of a patient with a suspected large bowel obstruction?
    A. Empty rectal vault
    B. Rectal vault full with bloody stool
    C. Large, fungating mass
    D. Decreased sphincter tone
    E. Rectal vault with soft brown stool and normal tone

201. Following drug treatment for genital infection with chlamydia or gonorrhea, how long should patients minimally abstain from sexual intercourse after the last treatment dose?
    A. 1 day
    B. 10 days
    C. 2 weeks
    D. 1 week

202. Which of the following statements is TRUE regarding the prevention of Rocky Mountain spotted fever (RMSF)?
    A. Early detection and removal of the tick is recommended to prevent disease transmission.
    B. Vaccination is beneficial to preventing the onset of RMSF.
    C. Prophylactic therapy with doxycycline is recommended following a tick exposure.
    D. Close contacts in a patient with RMSF should be treated with doxycycline.

203. Which of the following medications should be used cautiously in a patient with a previous suicide attempt?
    A. Sertraline
    B. Venlafaxine
    C. Amitriptyline
    D. Aripiprazole

204. Histologic examination of a resected ovarian tumor suggests metastatic adenocarcinoma of the ovary. This ovarian cancer (OC) is most likely the result of metastasis from which of the following sites?
    A. Stomach
    B. Liver
    C. Lung
    D. Brain

205. A 37-year-old G1P0 is diagnosed with GDM. At what gestational age should intermittent external fetal monitoring begin?
    A. 28 weeks
    B. 30 weeks
    C. 32 weeks
    D. 36 weeks

206. A 50-year-old man presents to your clinic with complaints of generalized headache and bilateral leg pain. He denies any past medical history and does not take any medications. The patient is not in acute distress, and all vitals are within normal limits except for a BP of 180/110 mm Hg. Physical examination reveals a murmur that has not been previously documented, 2+ brachial pulses, and 1+ femoral pulses. Which of the following tests would confirm the most likely diagnosis?
    A. Chest x-ray (CXR)
    B. CT of the chest
    C. Electrocardiogram
    D. Transthoracic echocardiogram

207. Which of the following is an appropriate diagnostic test for hearing impairment in an infant?
    A. Audiometry
    B. Weber and Rinne
    C. Otoacoustic emissions
    D. Whisper test

208. Which of the following is NOT a risk factor for orbital cellulitis?
    A. Optic neuritis
    B. Bacterial sinus infection
    C. Recent history of upper respiratory infection (URI)
    D. Ocular trauma

209. Which of the following is a risk factor for thyroid cancer?
    A. Male sex
    B. History of head/neck irradiation
    C. Age <16 years
    D. History of thyroid dysfunction

210. A 48-year-old male presents to his primary care provider with complaints of right groin pain after moving his mother into assisted living last weekend. On examination, the provider notes a reducible hernia just inferior to the inguinal canal. What is the correct diagnosis?
    A. Direct inguinal hernia
    B. Indirect inguinal hernia
    C. Abdominal wall hernia
    D. Femoral hernia

211. Which of the following is the first-line antimicrobial treatment for tetanus?
    A. Azithromycin
    B. Metronidazole
    C. Penicillin
    D. Vancomycin

212. In which of the following groups should mebendazole therapy be avoided?
    A. Elderly patients
    B. Immunocompromised patients
    C. Pregnant patients
    D. Patients who are breastfeeding
    E. Pediatric patients

213. High rates of comorbidity exist between anorexia nervosa (AN) and other psychiatric disorders. What percentage of AN sufferers also have a lifelong diagnosis of major depression?
    A. 20%–30%
    B. 30%–40%
    C. 50%–60%
    D. 70%–80%

214. You have a 28-year-old female patient who complains of mood changes, such as sadness, hopelessness, irritability, anger, and anxiousness before the onset of her menses. To be considered premenstrual dysphoric disorder (PMDD), her symptoms must begin when?
    A. At the onset of menses
    B. During the follicular phase
    C. During the luteal phase
    D. At ovulation

215. You are a trauma surgery PA. Your next patient was in a motor vehicle accident. She was struck from the driver's side by a car who ran a stop sign, going ~20 MPH. She was wearing a seatbelt, and her airbags did deploy. She was able to extricate herself from the vehicle on scene, and she is not complaining of any head or neck pain. She is currently 24 weeks' pregnant, gravida 3, para 2. This has been an uncomplicated pregnancy so far. She is not complaining of any abdominal pain, cramping, vaginal discharge, or bleeding. Fetal heart tones are monitored in the ED and found to be present, and there is no sign of fetal distress. What is recommended next for this patient?
    A. Head, neck, chest, abdomen/pelvis CT scan; it is worth the risk of radiation to the fetus in order to fully examine the patient.
    B. This patient can be discharged; she is stable, and the fetus appears stable right now.
    C. It is recommended that this patient either be transferred to a hospital with maternal/fetal medicine or remain overnight for observation and fetal monitoring.
    D. Keep the patient in C-spine precautions and on a long spine board for several hours since you are not doing imaging; this way, you can determine whether there is any neck or back injury.

216. A pediatric PA is seeing a 3-year-old boy for a well-child visit. The child has coarctation of the aorta (CoA), which was fixed by open repair when he was 1 month old. The mother reports that the boy was seen about 12 months ago, and "everything was fine." She has the results of the cardiac MRI with her, and the radiologist reported that everything was normal. Does this patient need to schedule another follow-up appointment with his pediatric cardiologist?
    A. No, the patient is asymptomatic and only needs to follow up if he is having symptoms.
    B. No, the patient only needs to see the cardiologist every 2 years if he is doing well.
    C. Yes, the patient should get a cardiac MRI every year after surgical repair.
    D. Yes, the patient should get an ECG and stress test every year after surgical repair.

217. Which of the following is an activity associated with the development of TM barotrauma?
    A. Jogging
    B. Scuba diving
    C. Bicycle riding
    D. Tennis

218. Which of the following would NOT be included on the workup for an underlying etiology for central retinal arterial occlusion?
    A. ECG
    B. Echocardiography
    C. Doppler ultrasound of the legs
    D. Carotid artery imaging

219. Which of the following thyroid nodule characteristics is considered highly suspicious for thyroid cancer?
    A. Cystic texture
    B. Wider than tall shape
    C. Presence of microcalcifications
    D. Hyperechoic to surrounding thyroid tissue

220. Which of the following is the most common form of mesenteric ischemia?
    A. Chronic mesenteric ischemia
    B. Mesenteric venous thrombosis
    C. Colonic ischemia
    D. Nonocclusive mesenteric ischemia

221. Which of the following diphtheria vaccines is started at the 2-month-old well-child visit and is part of the five-dose series?
    A. Tdap
    B. DTaP
    C. DT
    D. DTP

222. What is the most common type of patellar dislocation?
    A. Superior
    B. Inferior
    C. Medial
    D. Lateral

223. Which of the following statements regarding childhood attention deficit hyperactivity disorder (ADHD) is most accurate?
    A. Symptoms of ADHD are easily understood by many and carry no negative stigma.
    B. Symptoms often progress into adulthood and lead to financial, legal, and social problems.
    C. Symptoms often regress by adulthood and cause no additional problems.
    D. ADHD is associated with good school performance and is not linked to any comorbid.

224. Which of the following initial interventions are recommended when fetal distress is evidenced on external fetal HR monitoring?
    A. Increase the rate of uterine stimulants being used.
    B. Assess for any possible disruptions in the oxygenation pathway.
    C. Plan for immediate cesarean delivery.
    D. Perform amniotomy to check for presence of meconium.

225. Increased flow across which of the following structures leads to the mid-systolic ejection murmur found in atrial septal defect?
    A. Atrial septum
    B. Pulmonic valve
    C. Tricuspid valve
    D. Ventricular septum

226. Which of the following is a common cause of hearing impairment in infants?
    A. Acoustic neuroma
    B. Presbycusis
    C. Hereditary syndrome
    D. Cholesteatoma

227. Which of the following is most likely to precipitate a case of orbital cellulitis?
    A. Bacteremia
    B. Trauma
    C. Intraorbital infection
    D. Sinus infection

228. What TSH level is appropriate for a thyroid cancer patient initially after thyroidectomy?
    A. 0.1–0.5 mU/L
    B. 0.5–1 mU/L
    C. 1–2 mU/L
    D. 0.5–2 mU/L

229. A 22-year-old male is found to have an asymptomatic indirect inguinal hernia. Which of the following is most appropriate for the provider to tell the patient about this condition?
    A. It is most likely due to excessive lifting.
    B. It has likely been there since birth.
    C. Surgical intervention is recommended at this time.
    D. It is likely related to his cigarette smoking.

230. Besides arthrocentesis, a septic joint suspicious for being gonococcal arthritis requires which of the following?
    A. A prolonged course of antibiotics
    B. Warm compresses
    C. Consultation with an infectious disease specialist
    D. Immobilization

231. A noncontrast MRI of a patient's knee reveals microtears and edema in the left medial collateral ligament (MCL). Which is NOT a reasonable treatment plan for this patient?
    A. Cryotherapy and strengthening
    B. Use of crutches and a stabilizing brace
    C. Arthroscopic allograft repair
    D. Rest with return to play as tolerated

232. A 24-year-old presents for a new patient examination. During the examination, she is visibly upset, complaining that everyone around her is incompetent, but she is grateful for you, since you are the only person who understands her. During the physical examination, you notice many fine scars on her forearms; she admits that cutting herself helps her manage anxiety. When you explain why you cannot prescribe the alprazolam she requests for anxiety, she angrily leaves the office. What personality disorder is most likely?
    A. Antisocial
    B. Borderline
    C. Histrionics
    D. Narcissistic
    E. Paranoid

233. A 50-year-old woman presents to the clinic with concerns about unpredictable menstrual cycles and night sweats. In addition to the night sweats, for ~2 minutes, multiple times per day, she becomes hot, flushed, and diaphoretic. Her past medical history (PMH) is unremarkable, and she takes no medications or supplements. Which of the following is the most likely diagnosis?
    A. Perimenopause
    B. Menopause
    C. Postmenopause
    D. Primary ovarian insufficiency

234. Your next patient in the clinic is a 15-week pregnant patient who is coming in for nonspecific pelvic pain. During the course of your interview, she discloses that the reason that she has pelvic pain this time is because her boyfriend punched her in the stomach last week. She denies any abdominal cramping or vaginal bleeding. Along with assessing her home safety, what other questions are important to ask her?
    A. Always assess patients in domestic violence situations for suicidality and depression.
    B. You do not need to ask her any questions, because you do not need to pry into people's private relationships.
    C. Ask her why she is staying in a violent relationship.
    D. Avoid questions that might trigger her or make the appointment too long, like asking about suicidal thoughts or how she is feeling about her relationship.

235. A 10-year-old girl was diagnosed with coarctation of the aorta (CoA) 1 year ago and had balloon angioplasty. Since then, she has had no problems. Upper and lower BPs are equal in the clinic today at 120/80 mm Hg. No murmur can be heard on examination, and ECG shows no LV hypertrophy. Which

of the following conditions is this patient most at risk of developing?

A. Asthma
B. Diabetes mellitus
C. Hyperlipidemia
D. Hypertension

236. What is the most appropriate management plan for a small, uncomplicated tympanic perforation that occurred 3 days ago following an episode of acute otitis media (AOM)?

A. Referral to otology for tympanoplasty
B. 14-Day course of cefdinir
C. Dry ear precautions and periodic follow-up until resolution
D. Observation, no follow-up indicated

237. A 50-year-old diabetic patient complains to his primary care provider of ocular pain and edema. Examination showed unilateral lid edema, intact extraocular muscle movements, and mild proptosis, and oral examination was notable for black discoloration, resembling eschar on the right upper hard palate. You make the clinical diagnosis of orbital cellulitis. What is the most likely pathogen?

A. *Staphylococcus aureus*
B. Group B *Streptococcus*
C. Fungi
D. *Pseudomonas aeruginosa*

238. Which of the following is a function of parathyroid hormone?

A. Increases osteoblastic activity
B. Decreases calcitriol secretion
C. Increases calcium secretion in the kidney
D. Decreases phosphate reabsorption in the kidney

239. A 47-year-old patient with ESRD on outpatient dialysis presents to the ED with shortness of breath after missing his most recent dialysis session. He is tachypneic and hypertensive, and his physical examination is consistent with volume overload. A screening ECG shows sinus tachycardia with peaked T waves. Blood sampling shows a nonhemolyzed K+ of 6.1 mEq/L. What is the most appropriate management strategy?

A. Diuretic challenge
B. 50% dextrose infusion
C. Polystyrene sulfonate administration
D. Immediate initiation of dialysis

240. What cardiac valve is most often affected by rheumatic fever?

A. Aortic valve
B. Mitral valve
C. Pulmonic valve
D. Tricuspid valve

241. Which of the following is the most common injury associated with acute compartment syndrome of the lower extremity?

A. Patellar fracture
B. Distal femur fracture
C. Tibial fracture
D. Patellar dislocation

242. A 35-year-old patient is diagnosed with group 4 PH. Which of the following is the most appropriate definitive therapy for his condition?

A. Symptomatic relief with oxygen and diuretics
B. Systemic anticoagulation and referral for surgical thrombectomy
C. Inhaled pulmonary vasodilator therapy
D. Outpatient monitoring and serial screening CT

243. Which of the following is a contraindication for combined hormonal contraception (CHC)?

A. Anemia
B. Migraine with aura
C. Thyroid disorders
D. Uterine fibroids

244. Which of the following should be initiated in all patients who present with prelabor rupture of membranes after 24 weeks' gestation?

A. Screening for Group B Streptococcus (GBS) and prophylactic treatment when appropriate
B. Prophylactic treatment of herpes simplex virus (HSV) with acyclovir
C. Magnesium sulfate for fetal neuroprotection
D. A single course of corticosteroids for fetal lung maturity

▶ ANSWERS AND EXPLANATIONS TO COMPREHENSIVE EXAM

1. **D.** Reassurance and patient education is the recommended treatment for premature atrial or ventricular contractions in an asymptomatic patient without structural heart disease.

2. **B.** Secondary to the pulmonic outflow obstruction (often in the form of pulmonic stenosis or infundibular stenosis), the hypertrophied RV shunts deoxygenated blood through the ventricular septal defect and into the left ventricle, resulting in cyanosis.

3. **B.** Many common medications are ototoxic, including aminoglycoside antibiotics, antimalarials, loop diuretics, NSAIDs, and some chemotherapy agents.

4. **D.** A retinal detachment is more likely in patients with myopia and can be caused by minor trauma. Patients will classically complain of flashes of lights and/or floaters with a "curtain" dropping across their eye. CRAO and CRVO are usually associated with cardiovascular risk factors.

5. **D.** A calcium level should be ordered postoperatively owing to potential complications of thyroidectomy.

6. **C.** Rapid correction of serum sodium can cause pulmonary and cerebral edema.

7. **C.** Botulinum toxin blocks cholinergic presynaptic receptors.

8. **C.** Posterior cruciate ligament insufficiency can result in posterior subluxation of the tibia, resulting in a perceived positive Lachman examination and exaggerated translation.

9. **B.** Genetic testing is the next step.

10. **D.** This patient has atrophic vaginitis caused by estrogen deficiency. Thus, an estrogen will be effective. Since her symptoms are localized to the vagina and she has no contraindications to HT, local application of vaginal estrogen cream is appropriate. Observation does not address the patients concern, and hydrocortisone cream is not appropriate for atrophic changes.

11. **D.** Dual-chamber pacemaker insertion is the preferred therapy for patients with symptomatic SSS.

12. **A.** Follow-up in outpatient clinic is the most appropriate recommendation for a 3-year-old female with a 4-mm diameter secundum atrial septal defect and no cardiopulmonary symptoms.

13. **B.** External ear trauma is a common sports injury. Auricular hematoma is especially common in wrestling, boxing, and martial arts.

14. **C.** Pain with eye movements, dyschromatopsia, and relative afferent pupillary defect in the affected eye are all signs and symptoms of optic neuritis. Headache is not associated with optic neuritis.

15. **A.** The most common cause of primary hyperparathyroidism is adenoma.

16. **B.** Exogenous calcium administration in a patient with hyperkalemia can stabilize the cardiac membrane and prevent arrhythmia development.

17. **A.** Salmonella (nontyphoidal type) can be transmitted after exposure to birds and reptiles. Salmonella is typically a foodborne illness and is usually caused by eating raw or undercooked meat, raw product, poultry, eggs, or egg products. Treatment is supportive for immunocompetent individuals aged >12 months and <50 years.

18. **C.** No imaging is needed to diagnose patellar tendonitis.

19. **D.** Underdeveloped or immature dentition is a common risk factor for foreign-body aspiration in children.

20. **D.** This patient is experiencing amenorrhea and vasomotor symptoms (hot flashes). An elevated FSH confirms the diagnosis of primary ovarian insufficiency since she is younger than 40 years.

21. **C.** You would expect to see prolonged, aberrant QRS complexes on ECG leads V_1 and V_2 with an asymptomatic right bundle branch block.

22. **D.** Because the RV becomes hypertrophied secondary to the pulmonic outflow obstruction and pressure from the left ventricle through the ventricular septal defect, it can result in a boot-shaped deformity of the heart that can be seen on CXR.

23. **D.** With barotrauma, otoscopy reveals a dull TM with decreased light reflex, and anatomic landmarks may be distorted. Bloody middle ear effusion gives the TM a dark blue-purple appearance.

24. **A.** The retinal tear may be visualized on fundoscopic examination as a flap in the vitreous humor.

25. **A** The most common cause of hypoparathyroidism is iatrogenic.

26. **B.** A patient with acute leukemia and a WBC count of 110 000 is likely to result in a falsely elevated blood potassium level.

27. **B.** Patients who experience rheumatic fever with carditis should continue secondary prevention with prophylactic benzathine penicillin G 1.2 million units IM monthly for 10 years, or until age 21.

28. **D.** ACL injuries occur with sudden deceleration and torsional injuries. Patients will frequently report hearing a pop and noting pain. Joint laxity will be elicited on examination by the Lachman, anterior drawer, or pivot shift test.

29. **C.** Lack of pleural sliding is often referred to as the "starry-night" sign when viewed on M-mode. Pleural effusion and hemothorax are visualized as hypoechoic fluid in the pleural space. Pneumonia is often seen with fluid accumulation within the lung parenchyma.

30. **A.** Candidiasis is diagnosed by the confirmation of spores and hyphae on wet mount. The vaginal pH is typically <4.5.

31. **C.** This patient's CHA_2DS_2-VASc score is 7.

32. **A.** In most cases, it is presumed that a viral infection is the cause of myocarditis. Bacterial causes exist, but they are far less common than viral causes in

the United States; in developing nations, bacterial causes are more common. Autoimmune disease can result in myocarditis, so that should be on the differential diagnosis in patients with a history of such a disease. In patients with a history of radiation exposure (therapeutic or otherwise), myocarditis could occur, but this is a rare complication.

33. **A.** MS is most commonly associated with optic neuritis.

34. **C.** Increased PTH, normal serum calcium, and decreased urine calcium would be most consistent with secondary hyperparathyroidism.

35. **A.** It can be difficult to fully correct a patient's hypokalemia if there is concomitant hypomagnesemia. The patient's magnesium should be normalized in conjunction with potassium supplementation.

36. **C.** Penicillin is the most appropriate antibiotic to ensure the eradication of group A *Streptococcus*.

37. **A.** Anti-inflammatory medication is considered a first-line treatment for patellar tendonitis.

38. **B.** The most commonly used selective estrogen receptor modulator in the United States is tamoxifen. Tamoxifen is an antagonist on breast tissue, and because this patient has estrogen receptor–positive breast cancer, she should respond to this therapy. An aromatase inhibitor is more appropriate for patients who are postmenopausal. A taxane-based chemotherapy regimen can be used in patients who are hormone receptor negative and HER-2 negative (called triple negative). Patients who are HER-2 positive will receive HER-2–targeted therapies.

39. **C.** Menopausal symptoms of depression and sleep disturbances can often be managed with an SSNI, such as venlafaxine. Hormone therapy (estrogen, combination estrogen/progestin, or an SERM) is contraindicated because of her history of DVT. Bioidentical hormone therapy is not recommended.

40. **C.** Multifocal atrial tachycardia is the most likely diagnosis for this patient.

41. **C.** ICD placement is warranted for secondary prevention of sudden cardiac death in patients with major risk factors, including a previous aborted cardiac arrest.

42. **C.** Purulent ear drainage is not a typical symptom associated with cerumen impaction. Tinnitus, ear fullness, and hearing loss are all symptoms associated with cerumen impactions.

43. **A.** The hallmark of CRVO, CRAO, and retinal detachment is painless vision loss. Acute angle-closure glaucoma nearly always presents with a painful red eye.

44. **C.** Drowsiness is a common side effect of antimuscarinic medications, not insomnia.

45. **C.** On ECG, development of U waves is likely to be seen with hypokalemia.

46. **B.** *Salmonella typhi* (typhoid or enteric fever) is a vaccine preventable illness that is endemic in parts of Africa. Typhoid fever is a systemic infection that is best diagnosed by blood culture, although it can be detected by stool culture if diarrhea is present after 2 weeks of infection. Humans are the only reservoir for the typhoidal types, and it is transmitted by ingestion of food and water contaminated with human feces.

47. **C.** Chronic ACL insufficiency can result in the early development of chondral damage or post-traumatic OA. The patient's symptoms are consistent with arthritis, such as stiffness after prolonged joint immobilization. Meniscal injuries would cause mechanical symptoms more so than stiffness.

48. **C.** *S. aureus* is a common cause of skin and soft-tissue infection as it resides on the skin and can enter the breast through trauma associated with breastfeeding.

49. **A.** SSS is commonly associated with recurrent atrial fibrillation or atrial flutter.

50. **A.** This patient has dilated cardiomyopathy, most likely the result from chronic alcohol consumption. Alcohol cessation should be the first recommendation as, in some cases, symptoms can be lessened or totally reversed with abstinence. Because total abstinence is difficult to achieve, treatment for heart failure is warranted. Hence, starting the patient on an ACEI, a β-blocker, and occasional diuresis with a loop diuretic would be appropriate. Digoxin is sometimes still appropriate for heart failure treatment but rarely as a first-line agent. Biventricular pacing and transplant are reserved for patients that have failed optimal medical therapy.

51. **B.** An alligator forceps is the best tool to use for this in-office procedure.

52. **D.** Treatment for optic neuritis includes IV methylprednisolone followed by an oral steroid taper.

53. **A.** Cystoscopy with biopsy is the gold standard for the diagnosis of bladder cancer.

54. **B.** Patients with hyperglobulinemia often present with hyperphosphatemia that is not real. The elevated concentration of globulin proteins interferes with the laboratory assay for phosphate. These patients need an alternative laboratory assay to measure the true serum phosphate level.

55. **C.** The upper respiratory tract is the most common site of diphtheria infection, caused by *C. diphtheriae*, in children. Nasal infection presents with serosanguinous or seropurulent nasal discharge and is often associated with whitish patches on the mucosal membrane of the septum. The posterior structures of the mouth and proximal pharynx are most characteristic for clinical diphtheria. A membrane typically develops on one or both tonsils, with extension to the pillars, uvula, soft palate, oropharynx, or nasopharynx. *C. diphtheria* multiplies on the mucous membrane surface and forms a characteristic pseudomembrane, which is initially white,

becomes gray over time, and may develop green or black necrotic patches.

56. **A.** The anterior talofibular ligament is the ligament in the ankle most commonly sprained.

57. **B.** Gynecomastia can occur for several different reasons. The first is an increase in aromatase activity (ie, such as with medications, chronic liver disease, hyperthyroidism, adrenal tumors, etc). Aromatase converts testosterone to estrogen, so any sort of a testosterone-secreting tumor (ie, testicular tumor) will increase the amount of substrate that aromatase has to convert, thus increasing the relative quantity of estrogen. Finally, any overproduction of hCG (ie, carcinoma of the lung, kidney, GI tract, or extragonadal germ cell tumors) stimulates Leydig cells to produce more testosterone, which feeds into the increased substrate pathway. Ultimately, however, an increased estrogen effect causes the breast tissue hyperplasia of gynecomastia.

58. **C.** This patient has hot flashes affecting her quality of life. Venlafaxine may be effective for hot flashes; however, she is already on this SNRI, and her hot flashes continue to be debilitating. Watching and waiting is not improving her quality of life. Systemic HT is indicated as she has no contraindications based on the information provided in the question. However, she needs both estrogen and progestin therapy since she has an intact uterus. Only patients without a uterus can be prescribed estrogen-only therapy. Vaginal estrogen cream is not indicated for hot flashes, and an SERM would need to be prescribed along with an estrogen to be effective.

59. **A.** Early depolarization of atrial tissue results in premature atrial contractions.

60. **D.** Positive pressure ventilation should be avoided in patients with cardiac tamponade.

61. **C.** Ear wax softener drops is a safe option to use to aid with repeated cerumen impaction procedure.

62. **C.** Caucasian race is not a risk factor for open-angle glaucoma. African descent is a risk factor for open-angle glaucoma.

63. **B.** Surgical revascularization is the treatment of choice for CMI.

64. **C.** Hypernatremia is a sodium level >145 mEq/L.

65. **D.** Children with sickle cell disease who are infected with salmonella are prone to developing multisystem infection such as osteomyelitis, liver and splenic abscesses, and overwhelming sepsis sometimes with fatal consequences. Sluggish blood flow through the bone and bone marrow promotes bone ischemia, necrosis, and increased susceptibility to salmonella osteomyelitis. Treatment with a third-generation cephalosporin is indicated.

66. **A.** Chronic ACL insufficiency is associated with medial meniscus tearing, whereas lateral meniscus tears are associated with acute ACL injuries. Mechanical symptoms such as catching are consistent with meniscal pathology.

67. **C.** This patient presents with classic symptoms of fibrocystic breast changes. As this presentation is commonly associated with cyst formation, this can usually be diagnosed using U/S alone. If the U/S demonstrates features of a more complicated cyst, U/S-guided FNA that demonstrates a collapse of the cyst is confirmatory of a benign lesion. If the initial U/S is noted to have a complex cyst, U/S-guided core-needle biopsy is needed to differentiate between a benign and malignant lesion.

68. **B.** Patients with PCOS should be screened regularly for diabetes as PCOS increases the woman's risk of developing diabetes.

69. **A.** Torsades de pointes is a polymorphic VT that occurs in the setting of QT prolongation, resulting in a "twisting of points" or "streamer-like" appearance of the QRS complexes.

70. **D.** ECGs in most patients with HCM are abnormal, typically showing evidence of LV hypertrophy, such as left axis deviation and diffusely prominent QRS voltage.

71. **A.** Most acoustic neuromas are very slow growing and can be observed over time with serial radiographs. The main concern is the preservation of a patient's hearing. Someone who is likely to have comorbidities and is already using hearing aids is not likely to benefit significantly from a more invasive treatment.

72. **B.** Ethambutol is known to precipitate optic neuritis.

73. **C.** Plain radiography of the abdomen is the safest and most timely imaging technique used in making a diagnosis of toxic megacolon.

74. **D.** This patient has multiple risk factors for a primary pulmonary malignancy and is presenting with ventricular tachycardia that is like due to a prolonged QT interval secondary to hypercalcemia. The elevated PTHrP, in combination with the active tobacco abuse and age, should raise suspicion for a small cell lung cancer.

75. **C.** A patient in the early localized stage of Lyme disease would describe their illness as a "bull's-eye" lesion progressively enlarging with arthralgias, myalgias, and fatigue.

76. **B.** DVT is a common potential complication of hip fractures and surgery. DVT prophylaxis is required and can be initiated preoperatively with low-molecular-weight heparin and is continued postoperatively. Surgery for hip fractures is recommended for all patients, regardless of ambulatory status. Prompt surgical intervention (within 24 hours) is recommended and will improve postoperative outcomes. A femoral neck fracture requires either hemiarthroplasty or cannulated screws depending on displacement. Total hip arthroplasty is not indicated for a femoral neck fracture unless a patient has significant OA.

77. **A.** The most common cause of galactorrhea without elevated prolactin levels is usually repeated nipple stimulation secondary to sexual intimacy, friction from clothing, or repeated expression of the discharge. Eliminating the stimulation will shut down the feedback loop to the pituitary gland and eventually stop milk production in the milk ducts.

78. **B.** Trichomoniasis presents with increased white-gray-yellow-or-green discharge, often described as frothy and odorous. It can be associated with dysuria and pruritus. A strawberry cervix (erythema of the cervix and vagina) is a classic finding with trichomoniasis.

79. **B.** Atrial flutter is the most likely diagnosis for this patient.

80. **B.** Pulsus alternans is not a hallmark of cardiac tamponade.

81. **A.** The patient's symptoms are most likely the result of BPPV as evidenced by her episodes of vertigo triggered by head movement. Dix-Hallpike testing is indicated and will reproduce the vertigo and nystagmus.

82. **A.** Patients with globe rupture typically present with teardrop pupil, which indicates an open globe injury.

83. **B.** Loss of vascularity is an endoscopic finding associated with ulcerative colitis.

84. **D.** Therapeutic plasma exchange is the most appropriate initial treatment in this patient.

85. **A.** The incubation period for syphilis is about 3 weeks but can range from 3 days to 3 months.

86. **C.** Pain with resisted knee extension is most consistent with patellar tendonitis.

87. **B.** Although gynecomastia can be painful for some adolescent males early in the breast tissue proliferation, it is does not have the consistency of adipose tissue (ie, when moving thumb and forefinger together across the tissue they touch without feeling a ridge of glandular tissue). The glandular tissue associated with gynecomastia is concentric and is found extending under the areola, not lateral to it (more descriptive of a fibroadenoma) and not deep to the areola (more likely a subareolar abscess).

88. **C.** According to the Rotterdam Diagnostic Criteria, hirsutism or moderate-severe acne is evidence of hyperandrogenism.

89. **B.** You would expect to see prolonged, aberrant QRS complexes on ECG leads I, aVL, V_5, and V_6 with an LBBB.

90. **C.** Clinical guidelines describe antibiotic prophylaxis prior to dental procedures for people with heart disease who are at increased risk for adverse outcomes of IE. Five categories of conditions are described including prosthetic cardiac valves.

91. **B.** The patient's symptoms are most likely the result of Ménière disease. The most appropriate treatment involves reducing the production of endolymph with hydrochlorothiazide/triamterene. Crystal repositioning exercises such as Epley maneuver are indicated for BPPV to fatigue the central response to moving otoliths. Promethazine will help reduce nausea and emesis, but will not ultimately treat the underlying pathology.

92. **C.** Tonometry is contraindicated in evaluation of suspected globe rupture to avoid applying pressure to an already injured globe.

93. **A.** Mesenteric angiography is the gold standard for the diagnosis of acute mesenteric ischemia due to an arterial thrombosis.

94. **A.** Clopidogrel is thought to precipitate the microangiopathic hemolytic anemia associated with TTP.

95. **A.** The facial nerve is the most common peripheral nerve involvement with Lyme disease.

96. **D.** The Lachman examination is the most sensitive physical examination finding for acute ACL injuries.

97. **B.** Women with estrogen receptor–positive breast cancer who are postmenopausal should receive an aromatase inhibitor to help reduce the risk of recurrence. Selective estrogen receptor modulators are used in premenopausal patients.

98. **B.** Oral contraceptives and IUDs containing progestin are useful as first-line treatment in the management of uterine fibroids by reducing uterine bleeding and cramps. Iron supplementation may be used to treat anemia. GnRH agonists, although helpful to shrink uterine fibroids by decreasing estrogen levels, must not be administered for >6 months because it has been shown to cause osteoporosis and other postmenopausal complications. GnRH agonists may be used short term preoperatively to decrease uterine bleeding in women choosing to undergo a hysterectomy for treatment of fibroids. Endometrial ablation is another procedure in the management of uterine fibroids, but pregnancy is impossible afterward. In this case, there is no indication the patient does not desire more children. Lifestyle changes are effective as preventative treatment for uterine fibroids but are not effective treatment for existing fibroids.

99. **A.** Atrial fibrillation is the most likely diagnosis for this patient.

100. **A.** The recommended treatment for patients with symptomatic HCM is medical therapy aimed at managing LV outflow tract obstruction and systolic anterior motion. Negative inotropic agents, such as β-blockers, non-dihydropyridine calcium channel blockers, or disopyramide typically represent the mainstay of this treatment.

101. **C.** The most common clinical presentation of AOM is ear pain or pulling on the affected ear.

102. **B.** The superior rectus muscle allows upward gaze.

103. **A.** Colonoscopy is the gold standard for the diagnosis of Crohn disease.

104. **B.** Most causes of thrombocytosis are reactive in nature from infection/inflammation or from iron deficiency. One must confirm persistent thrombocytosis first, exclude inflammatory causes with CRP, and assess iron status before sending for molecular testing (*JAK2 V617F*).

105. **E.** In situations of outbreaks, mass treatment recommended.

106. **D.** Stool samples are not helpful in diagnosis; the tape test would likely yield eggs if infected.

107. **B.** Osgood-Schlatter disease is inflammation of the patellar ligament, specifically at the tibial tuberosity where the growth plate has not completely closed.

108. **C.** The case describes both galactorrhea and gynecomastia. The patient has a history of major depressive disorder that is well controlled (presumably with medications). Antidepressants, particularly tricyclic antidepressants and SSRIs, have been associated with hyperprolactinemia and increase aromatase activity, so medications would be the first area to evaluate.

109. **D.** TVUS and transabdominal U/S is recommended for confirmation of ovarian torsion. MRI and CT can aid in detection, but MRI is time-consuming when sift intervention is needed to preserve ovarian function. CT can detect enlargement but is not specific for torsion and exposes the patient to unnecessary radiation.

110. **C.** Syncope is often linked with an increased risk of sudden cardiac death in ventricular arrythmias.

111. **B.** Diuretics are relatively contraindicated in patients with HCM because they may reduce preload, which in turn may exacerbate LV outflow tract obstruction and worsen symptoms and hypotension.

112. **B.** A HINTS examination is used to differentiate continuous, spontaneous sources of peripheral vertigo from central ones.

113. **C.** Topical steroids can cause corneal ulcer in patients with a corneal abrasion and, therefore, should be avoided.

114. **D.** Loperamide (Imodium) should immediately be discontinued in patients with toxic megacolon.

115. **B.** Mortise is a radiographic view of the ankle.

116. **D.** In a patient with galactorrhea and an elevated prolactin level, the clinician is obligated to rule out a prolactinoma or a pituitary stalk tumor with brain imaging.

117. **D.** In postmenopausal women, appropriate management for benign-appearing cysts includes evaluation of CA125 and, if normal, serial U/S.

118. **C.** Fibrosis of the sinus node is the most common cause of SSS.

119. **C.** The highest incidence of IE is reported in individuals with prosthetic valves, cardiac valves, unrepaired cyanotic heart disease, and a history of endocarditis. Additional risk factors include IV drug use, congenital or acquired structural heart diseases, and prolonged bacteremia.

120. **D.** *S. pneumoniae* is the most common cause of mastoiditis in children.

121. **B.** Teardrop sign on CT of the orbit indicates herniated tissue and muscle.

122. **A.** Definitive diagnosis of colonic ischemia is made with colonoscopy with biopsy.

123. **B.** Clinical history of a patient with known ET-MPN presenting with clinical signs and symptoms of hepatic pathology (RUQ tenderness, hepatomegaly). Ultrasound shows a smooth regular liver, and reversed flow in hepatic veins confirms most likely occlusion of portal vein. Upper GI bleed typically presents with a degree of anemia, patient has no cough or respiratory symptoms for pneumonia.

124. **B.** Rocky Mountain spotted fever can cause neurologic complications such as encephalitis. Lyme disease can cause Lyme carditis and atrioventricular conduction blocks. RMSF typically causes a lower platelet count and not thrombocytosis. A ruptured spleen is a complication found in patients with infectious mononucleosis.

125. **D.** The tibial tuberosity is the insertion point of the patella tendon.

126. **D.** In order to diagnose an adolescent with PCOS, she must have menstrual irregularities that persist 2 years after menarche.

127. **B.** Peripheral vascular disease is not a risk for this patient if he refuses to get a pacemaker.

128. **B.** Pilonidal disease is more common in sedentary, young men.

129. **B.** There is minimal clinical difference between various topical antibiotics when treating otitis externa.

130. **C.** Topical atropine drops are used to treat amblyopia, not acute angle-closure glaucoma.

131. **D.** Aminosalicylates are considered first-line therapy for the management of mild inflammation in Crohn disease.

132. **B.** The role of plasma metalloprotease ADAMTS-13 is to cleave von Willebrand factor multimers.

133. **C.** Protozoans (aka trichomonads) are diagnostic on a wet mount for trichomoniasis.

134. **A.** TBI and intracranial hemorrhage often overlap and found in conjunction in patients suffering traumatic injuries. Morbidity and mortality are both increased when TBI and intracranial hemorrhage are present.

135. **D.** Patients with a nonpainful, easily reducible prolapse should be scheduled for a vaginal examination for diagnosis and treatment.

136. **A.** All patients with teratomas should be referred for surgical evaluation.

137. **C.** In a symptomatic patient with a normal ECG, Holter monitor would be indicated for further evaluation of premature beats.

138. **C.** Skin changes related to acanthosis nigricans will improve with weight loss.

139. **D.** A patient with mastoiditis who continues to be febrile despite IV antibiotic treatment is not responding to treatment and should be referred for definitive treatment with mastoidectomy.

140. **A.** Cardioembolic stroke is the most common cause of monocular transient vision loss.

141. **D.** Recent antibiotic use is the most significant risk factor for toxic megacolon.

142. **C.** The patient has low-risk MPN-ET based on age, platelet count, and no previous thrombotic events and should be started on low-dose aspirin, then actively monitored. No indication for cytoreductive therapy at this time.

143. **C.** Metronidazole 2 g PO is the recommended treatment of choice for someone diagnosed or have sexual contact with someone diagnosed with trichomoniasis.

144. **A.** Data show that light exercise that does make any symptoms worse may be therapeutic with concussion, shortening the total days of symptom burden. Answer B is incorrect because although 7 days of rest may be needed, data show that this may actually make symptoms last longer. Answer C is incorrect because high-dose NSAIDs have not been shown to shorten the course of symptoms and, in fact, should be avoided in the first 48 hours of injury. Answer D is incorrect because neither CT nor MRI has been shown to shorten symptoms and, without neurologic symptoms, may not be needed in the evaluation of concussion.

145. **C.** A complex cystic mass that increases in size within 2 months of initial imaging is most concerning for ovarian malignancy. Bilateral ovarian masses and complex cystic masses >8-10 cm in diameter are also concerning for malignancy. Elevated CA125 in a young woman with a history endometriosis is not necessarily indicative of ovarian malignancy as CA125 can be elevated for noncancerous conditions, such as endometriosis, especially if the ovarian mass is stable (ie, not increasing in size or complexity).

146. **B.** When suprapubic pressure is applied, it works to disimpact the anterior shoulder by adducting and rotating it. This movement serves to decrease the fetal bisacromial diameter.

147. **A.** Loud, harsh holosystolic murmur is expected in a small ventricular septal defect with a high gradient.

148. **C.** The most common organ affected in DRESS is the liver. The most common form of liver involvement is an asymptomatic rise in LFTs.

149. **C.** Absence of cerumen, not excessive cerumen, is a risk factor for otitis externa.

150. **D.** Idiopathic intracranial hypertension can result in papilledema, which is swelling of the optic disc caused by increased intracranial pressure.

151. **D.** Adenocarcinoma is a risk associated with ulcerative colitis.

152. **B.** Hemoptysis suggests life-threatening bleeding in ITP.

153. **E.** It takes up to 2 months to lay eggs.

154. **B.** Elder abuse is highly underreported, likely through a combination of elders refusing or hesitating to report, being unable to report due to dementia or other conditions that affect memory and cognition and having nobody to report to. Elderly individuals often fear a loss of independence that may come from reporting elder abuse, such as losing their independent home and being forced to live in assisted living or with family. There is little utility in confronting the family members, and although there may be an element of cognitive loss in this case, that is the just of the Ombudsman and case workers to elucidate, not that of the clinician. Financial abuse can be particularly subtle, but very damaging, considering that many elderly people are on fixed incomes with narrow margins.

155. **B.** Some germ cell tumors secrete AFP, and measurement of serum levels is useful for diagnosis and surveillance. CA125 is a tumor marker for OC but is nonspecific. Testosterone and inhibins are useful markers for sex cord-stromal cell tumors.

156. **A.** McRoberts maneuver is considered a first-line maneuver in cases of traditional shoulder dystocia and involves hyperflexion of the maternal thighs toward the abdomen. All other listed maneuvers fall into the category of second-line or heroic maneuvers that should be attempted after first-line maneuvers.

157. **A.** Prostaglandins help keep the DA patent during fetal development. There are multiple sources of prostaglandins in the fetus, but the placenta is the major source. After birth and after the placenta is separated from the newborn, prostaglandin levels begin to decline. This change, in combination with increasing arterial oxygen tension levels after the newborn begins breathing, stimulates a closure response in the DA. This is accomplished within hours to days after birth. In preterm infants, particularly those under 26 weeks' gestation, prostaglandin levels are higher than they would be for the term infant, thereby keeping the DA open after birth and even after separation from the placenta. For this reason, cyclooxygenase inhibitors may be tried in preterm infants with PDA to try to artificially lower the prostaglandin levels and induce closure of the DA.

158. **A.** Patients with acanthosis nigricans are at risk for type 2 diabetes.

159. **A.** The patient is responding to treatment with culturally confirmed antibiotics and can be discharged with a 2-week course of oral antibiotics.

160. **D.** Acute angle-closure glaucoma presents with headache, vomiting, and halos around light but does not present with purulent eye discharge.

161. **A.** Colonic dilation >6 cm is one of the diagnostic criteria for toxic megacolon.

162. **B.** An elderly gentleman presenting with anemia and raised platelet count whose blood smear shows dacrocytes, in combination with *JA2 V617F* mutation and constitutional symptoms, is indicative of myelofibrosis. CML would present with raised WBC count, ET does not usually have constitutional symptoms, and PV presents with raised Hb.

163. **D.** Trichomoniasis can cause inflammation and erythema in the vagina along with a strawberry cervix. It may or may not have a clear, white, or yellow-green colored discharge.

164. **B.** GAD patients will report difficulty concentrating rather than an intense ability to focus on tasks.

165. **A.** Endometriosis is the most common cause of secondary dysmenorrhea.

166. **C.** Moderate variability is a reassuring finding and requires no further intervention.

167. **B.** Cyclooxygenase inhibitors (indomethacin and ibuprofen) prevent the production of prostaglandins in the body. This treatment is reserved for preterm newborns with a PDA that is believed to be causing respiratory compromise and/or other systemic effects. Treatment can only be given in the first few days of life when prostaglandin levels would be at their highest; treatment beyond this time would be ineffective and potentially cause harm. Surgical management (ligation) is reserved for patients that fail medical therapy or are past that window of time to use medial therapy. Percutaneous approaches are possible but limited to larger sized patients such as children and adults. Cyclooxygenase inhibitor therapy has been used as a preventative measure in utero but is not standard of care and not without risk.

168. **B.** The patient has acute urticaria, which is best managed with antihistamines to treat pruritus. Second-generation H1 antihistamines are preferred, as they cause less drowsiness and anticholinergic symptoms than first-generation H1 antihistamines.

169. **C.** This patient is presenting with many "red-flag" symptoms, and other causes of a red eye should be considered. Conjunctivitis should not present with significant pain, changes in vision, photophobia, or a severe headache.

170. **D.** Benign nodules should be followed with ultrasound after 12 months.

171. **A.** A diagnosis of direct inguinal hernia is most often made with clinical assessment.

172. **C.** Doxycycline is first-line treatment for RMSF. TMP/SMX, amoxicillin, and ceftriaxone are antibiotics not indicated in the first-line treatment of RMSF.

173. **A.** FDA-approved medications for ASD are indicated for children with irritability.

174. **D.** Lynch syndrome is characterized by an increased risk of colon cancer and OC and is associated with mutations in DNA mismatch repair (*MMR*) genes. HBOC syndrome and Lynch syndrome are the two most common syndromes with hereditary risk for OC. An association between HBOC syndrome and an increased risk for colon cancer has not been clearly defined. Cowden syndrome and Li-Fraumeni syndrome are rare hereditary syndromes associated with increased risk of colon and other cancers in women but involve different gene mutations.

175. **C.** Uterine subinvolution is a common cause of secondary hemorrhage. The other choices are the causes of primary PPH.

176. **A.** CoA is the most likely cause of this patient's hypertension.

177. **A.** The patient is showing signs of a simple drug eruption, likely because of amoxicillin use. The mainstay of treatment of a drug eruption is discontinuation of the drug. The eruption resolves spontaneously once the causative agent is removed. Oral antihistamines may be used for pruritus as needed.

178. **D.** Diabetes, tobacco use, and sun exposure are all risk factors for the development of cataracts.

179. **D.** Ultrasound is the most appropriate imaging modality for evaluation of a thyroid nodule.

180. **C.** General surgery is most critical for immediate consultation in diagnosed cases of toxic megacolon.

181. **B.** Mucopurulent penile discharge is the most common clinical presentation in men with gonococcal urethritis.

182. **B.** Trichomoniasis cannot cause cataracts and blindness in newborns, which are more typical of congenital rubella. It can cause premature labor and/or low birth weight.

183. **C.** The initial intervention in patients who experience rapid cycling is to identify and treat any underlying medical condition (eg, hypothyroidism, drug or alcohol use) that may be contributing to rapid cycling. Certain medications, such as antidepressants, may also contribute to rapid cycling and should be tapered or discontinued, if possible. Initial pharmacologic recommendations in rapid cycling generally include valproate or lithium; however, many patients require combination therapy. Another alternative therapy is lamotrigine.

184. **B.** History of prolapse is consistent with reducible mass from the vaginal opening, difficulty emptying the bladder, and worsening urinary incontinence. Acute, severe pelvic pain is not associated with a history of prolapse.

185. **C.** Category III, which is abnormal and requires prompt assessment. Category I is normal, category II does not meet criteria for category I or III but still requires further monitoring, and there is no category IV.

186. **B.** Insertion of a transannular patch to alleviate pulmonic outflow obstruction decreases the overall workload of the RV but often results in pulmonic

regurgitation that can cause the RV to fail over time. Serial echocardiograms monitoring for RV function are advised.

187. **A.** Incision and drainage is an appropriate initial intervention in otherwise healthy individuals with a first occurrence of pilonidal abscess.

188. **B.** CT of the orbits is the imaging modality of choice in suspected orbital cellulitis.

189. **D.** Nephrolithiasis is a clinical finding in hyperparathyroidism.

190. **A.** Urgent surgical hernia repair is the most appropriate definitive treatment in a patient presenting with acute abdominal distention and vomiting who is found to have an incarcerated inguinal hernia.

191. **C.** Polyarthritis is the most common manifestation, occurring in ~60% of individuals.

192. **C.** RMSF is caused by *R. rickettsii*. *B. burgdorferi* is the pathogen found in Lyme disease. Parvovirus B19 is the etiology of erythema infectiosum (fifth disease). *T. pallidum* is the bacterium causing syphilis.

193. **A.** Treatment consists of treating the comorbidities such as depression or ADHD.

194. **B.** Oral contraception is best for those patients not desiring conception and having physical symptoms, such as menorrhagia, acne, and irregular cycles. Continuous or extended regimens decrease hormonal fluctuations by suppressing ovulation.

195. **D.** This patient has two known risk factors for developing a PPH—a prolonged third stage of labor and a macrosomic infant. Visual estimation of blood loss consistently underestimates the amount of bleeding that has occurred, but PPH is present when the patient has signs and symptoms of hypovolemia, independent of visual estimations of blood loss.

196. **D.** Stenosis of the aorta leads to ventricular hypertrophy, and heart failure best describes the pathophysiologic effects of CoA on the heart.

197. **A.** First-line treatment for DRESS, once the causative medication is removed, is corticosteroids. The rash should be treated with high-potency topical steroids for 1 week. Systemic corticosteroids are used to manage visceral involvement and should be tapered gradually over 3–6 months.

198. **A.** The patient presents with symptoms of noninfectious keratitis. Lubricating eye drops are the first-line treatment along with refraining from using contact lenses until the symptoms resolve. The patient should be instructed on proper use of contact lenses.

199. **A.** Fine-needle aspiration is recommended for thyroid nodules with microcalcifications.

200. **A.** When performing a digital rectal examination of a patient with a suspected large bowel obstruction, you would expect to find an empty rectal vault.

201. **D.** Following drug treatment for genital infection with chlamydia or gonorrhea, patient should abstain from sexual intercourse after the last treatment dose for at least 1 week.

202. **A.** Early detection and removal of attached ticks are the best way to prevent RMSF. There is currently no vaccine available for RMSF. Prophylactic therapy with doxycycline is not recommened following a tick exposure in an asymptomatic patient. There are no indications that close contacts in a patient diagnosed with RMSF need antibiotic treatment for prevention.

203. **C.** Amitriptyline should be used cautiously in a patient with a previous suicide attempt.

204. **A.** Metastatic OC is most frequently from the female genital tract, breast, or GI tract.

205. **C.** It is recommended that intermittent nonstress testing should begin at 32 weeks in a patient with underlying maternal or fetal issues.

206. **D.** Transthoracic echocardiogram would confirm the most likely diagnosis.

207. **C.** Infants, toddlers, and patients unable to provide necessary feedback during audiometry may be tested by otoacoustic emissions or auditory brainstem response.

208. **A.** Bacterial sinus infection, history of URI, and ocular trauma are all risk factors for orbital cellulitis. Optic neuritis is a demyelinating process that affects the optic nerve and does not cause orbital cellulitis.

209. **B.** A history of head/neck irradiation is a risk factor for thyroid cancer.

210. **D.** This patient has a femoral hernia.

211. **B.** Metronidazole is the first-line antimicrobial treatment for tetanus.

212. **C.** Mebendazole and other pinworm meds are category C drugs.

213. **C.** 50%–60% of AN sufferers also have a lifelong diagnosis of major depression.

214. **C.** Symptoms for PMDD typically begin 5 days before the onset of menses (late luteal phase) and resolve within 4 days of onset of menses. There is a symptom-free interval during the follicular phase.

215. **C.** For both minor and major trauma, 4-24 hours of observation is recommended for fetal monitoring. CT scans are used judiciously in pregnant patients when the benefit far outweighs the risk, and there are clearly published guidelines by the American Academy of Obstetrics on this subject. No patient should be kept in C-spine precautions or on a long spine board for an extended period of time, as this increases the risk of pressure ulcers, skin breakdown, and neuropathies. In addition, pregnant patients should not be kept on their back because of the increased pressure on the vena cava by the fetus (left lateral is preferred, or a spine board that is tilted to the left).

216. **B.** No, the patient only needs to see the cardiologist every 2 years if he is doing well.

217. **B.** Activities that often result in barotrauma include diving, flying, blast injuries, and waterskiing. Hyperbaric wound care is a common iatrogenic cause of TM barotrauma.

218. **C.** A workup for central retinal artery occlusion (CRAO) seeks to determine the underlying cause. Atherosclerotic disease and cardiogenic embolism are the most common causes of a CRAO. A Doppler ultrasound of the legs would assess for a deep venous thrombosis, which will not cause retinal artery emboli.

219. **C.** The presence of microcalcifications is considered highly suspicious for thyroid cancer.

220. **C.** Colonic ischemia is the most common form of mesenteric ischemia.

221. **B.** Babies require three doses of DTaP to build up high levels of protection against diphtheria, tetanus, and whooping cough. The CDC recommends this be done at 2, 4, and 6 months. Then, young children need two booster shots to maintain that protection through early childhood, which the CDC recommends at 15–18 months and 4–6 years.

222. **D.** Lateral. This injury usually occurs when the foot is planted, and an internal twisting force is applied to a flexed knee in valgus. It can also be secondary to direct trauma.

223. **B.** Symptoms often progress into adulthood and can lead to a number of problems, including academic, financial, legal, and social.

224. **B.** The initial intervention in a patient with non-reassuring findings is to assess for disruptions in the oxygenation pathway, including checking vital signs, repositioning the laboring patient, ensuring there is no cord prolapse, and checking for signs and symptoms of placental abruption.

225. **B.** Pulmonic valve leads to the mid-systolic ejection murmur found in atrial septal defect.

226. **C.** Hearing loss in children may be hereditary or nonhereditary. Hereditary hearing loss that is syndromic occurs along with anomalies in other organ systems. Common causes of hearing impairment in adults include cholesteatoma, otosclerosis, trauma, noise exposure, and presbycusis.

227. **D.** Sinus infections are the most common cause of orbital cellulitis.

228. **A.** A TSH level 0.1–0.5 mU/L is appropriate for a thyroid cancer patient initially after thyroidectomy.

229. **B.** This patient's hernia has likely been there since birth.

230. **C.** Besides arthrocentesis, a septic joint suspicious for being gonococcal arthritis requires consultation with an infectious disease specialist.

231. **C.** This is not a reasonable plan for this patient as the majority of MCL sprains heal with conservative treatment.

232. **B.** This patient demonstrates some key features of borderline personality disorder including unstable relationships often with the perception that others are all good or all bad, lack of impulse control, sudden mood fluctuations. Patients with borderline personality often engage in self-mutilation.

233. **A.** The patient is experiencing estrogen deficiency vasomotor symptoms. She is still having menstrual cycles, although they are unpredictable. These are manifestations of perimenopause. Since she is still having cycles, she is not yet experienced menopause or postmenopause. Primary ovarian insufficiency would only apply if she was younger than 40 years.

234. **A.** Domestic violence patients commonly feel depressed, isolated, and suicidal, especially when they are pregnant. In addition, the risk of homicide for domestic violence victims who are pregnant is increased exponentially, so identifying safety risks and other homicide risk factors is crucially important for these patients. As a skilled clinician, it is important to feel comfortable asking patients uncomfortable questions, like about their relationships and their safety concerns; therefore, choice D is incorrect. Choice C is blaming and accusatory and will damage your ongoing relationship with the patient; the psychology of domestic violence relationships is complex and nuanced, and it is important to establish a supportive foundation with the patient so that she feels comfortable returning to your care even if she chooses to stay in the relationship or leave and return.

235. **D.** This patient is most at risk of developing hypertension.

236. **C.** Most tympanic perforations heal spontaneously within 3 months. Dry ear precautions and periodic follow-up until resolution are recommended.

237. **C.** The patient has symptoms of mucormycosis, which is a rare, fungal infection that commonly affects the sinuses.

238. **D.** One function of parathyroid hormone is to decrease phosphate reabsorption in the kidney.

239. **D.** Immediate initiation of dialysis is the most appropriate management strategy for this patient.

240. **B.** The mitral valve is the most affected cardiac valve, often leading to mitral regurgitation.

241. **C.** Tibial fracture is the most common injury associated with acute compartment syndrome of the lower extremity.

242. **B.** Systemic anticoagulation and referral for surgical thrombectomy is the most appropriate definitive therapy for his condition.

243. **B.** Due to stroke risk, CHC should not be prescribed to patients with migraine with aura.

244. **A.** GBS screening and prophylactic treatment is always recommended. The only exception would be if a patient had delivered a prior GBS-positive infant; in that circumstance, the patient is considered to be GBS positive and will be given antibiotics. Prophylactic treatment of HSV is recommended if the Patient has a history of genital HSV. Magnesium sulfate is indicated if the gestation is <33 weeks and delivery is imminent. Corticosteroids are recommended when the gestation is <37 weeks.

Index

A

AA. *See* Aplastic anemia (AA)
AAA. *See* Abdominal aortic aneurysm (AAA)
Abacterial prostatitis, chronic, 214
Abdominal aortic aneurysm (AAA), 11, 15, 58
    location of, 10, 14
Abdominal groans, 197
Abdominal mass in toddler, 286, 289
Abdominal obesity, 182
Abdominal pain, potential organic cause for, 233
Abdominal rescue, 648
Abdominal x-ray, 262
Abducens nerve (CN VI), 487, 490, 515
ABG (arterial blood gases), 299
ABI (ankle-brachial index), 57
Abnormal uterine bleeding (AUB)
    clinical assessment of, 613
    diagnosis of, 613
    general features of, 613
    treatment for, 613–614
ABRS. *See* Acute bacterial rhinosinusitis (ABRS)
Abscess. *See also* Breast abscess
    clinical assessment of, 89
    diagnosis of, 89
    general features of, 89
    treatment for, 89
Abuse, 519, 527–528. *See also* Child abuse;
    Domestic violence; Elder abuse; Sexual
    assault
ABVD chemotherapy, for Hodgkin lymphoma, 334
Acanthosis nigricans (AN)
    clinical assessment of, 110
    diagnosis of, 110
    general features of, 110
    treatment for, 110
ACC (adrenocortical carcinoma), 187–188
Accessory pathway disorders, 23–24
ACE inhibitors. *See* Angiotensin-converting enzyme
    (ACE) inhibitors
Acephalic migraine, 508
Acetaminophen, 151, 219, 329, 350, 357, 387, 398,
    454, 460, 462, 466, 479, 487, 492, 509,
    560, 564
    overdose, 230
Acetylcholine, 500
Acetylcholine receptor antibody (AChR-Ab), 500
Achalasia, 227, 244–245
AChR-Ab (acetylcholine receptor antibody), 500
Acid-base disorders, 283, 288
    clinical assessment of, 299–300
    general features of, 299
Acitretin, 102
ACL injury. *See* Anterior cruciate ligament (ACL)
    injury
ACLS (advanced cardiac life support), 26
Acne inverse. *See* Hidradenitis suppurativa
Acne vulgaris
    clinical assessment of, 77
    diagnosis of, 77
    general features of, 77
    treatment for, 77
Acneiform disorders, 63, 73
    acne vulgaris, 77
    rosacea, 78
Acoustic neuroma, 129
    clinical assessment of, 130
    diagnosis of, 130
    general features of, 130
    treatment for, 130
Acquired or secondary lactase deficiency, 248
Acquired thrombophilia, 325–326
Acquired thrombotic thrombocytopenic
    purpura, 340

Acromegaly
    clinical assessment of, 186
    diagnosis of, 186–187
    general features of, 186
    symptom of, 172, 176
    treatment for, 187
ACS. *See* Acute coronary syndrome (ACS)
ACTH (adrenocorticotropic hormone), 172,
    176, 184
Actinic keratosis (AK)
    clinical assessment of, 95
    diagnosis of, 96
    general features of, 95
    treatment for, 96
Active Zollinger-Ellison syndrome, 188
Acute bacterial rhinosinusitis (ABRS)
    clinical assessment of, 157
    diagnosis of, 157
    general features of, 157
    treatment for, 157–158
Acute chest syndrome, 329
Acute closed-angle glaucoma, 153
Acute coronary syndrome (ACS)
    clinical assessment of, 32–33
    diagnosis of, 33
    general features of, 32
    treatment for, 33
Acute hemolytic reactions, 342
Acute hepatitis
    clinical assessment of, 259
    diagnosis of, 259
    general features of, 259
    treatment for, 259
Acute inflammatory demyelinating polyneuropathy
    (AIDP), 493
Acute kidney injury (AKI), 281, 287–288, 335
    cause of, 281, 287
    clinical assessment of, 290
    diagnosis of, 290
    general features of, 290
    treatment for, 290
Acute lymphoblastic leukemia (ALL)
    clinical assessment of, 331–332
    diagnosis of, 332
    general features of, 331
    risk factor for, 314, 319
    treatment for, 332
Acute mastoiditis
    clinical assessment of, 139
    diagnosis of, 139
    general features of, 139
    treatment for, 139
Acute mesenteric ischemia (AMI), 273
Acute motor axonal neuropathy (AMAN), 493
Acute motor-sensory axonal neuropathy
    (AMSAN), 493
Acute myeloid leukemia (AML)
    clinical assessment of, 331–332
    diagnosis of, 332
    general features of, 331
    myelodysplastic syndrome and, 315, 320
    pathognomonic in, 314, 319
    prognostic factor in, 314, 319
    risk factor for, 314, 319
    treatment for, 332
Acute myocardial infarction (AMI), 4, 12, 45
Acute-onset unilateral testicular pain and swelling,
    202, 206
Acute open-angle glaucoma, 153
Acute otitis media (AOM)
    clinical assessment of, 128
    diagnosis of, 128
    general features of, 127–128
    treatment for, 128

Acute pharyngitis
    clinical assessment of, 164–165
    diagnosis of, 165
    general features of, 164
    treatment for, 165
Acute renal failure (ARF). *See* Acute kidney injury
    (AKI)
Acute respiratory distress syndrome (ARDS), 557,
    562
    clinical assessment of, 572
    diagnosis of, 572
    fibroproliferative stage, 558, 562–563
    general features of, 572
    severity of, 557, 562
    treatment for, 572–573
Acute stress disorder, 526, 530
Acute urticarial eruptions
    clinical assessment of, 111
    diagnosis of, 111–112
    general features of, 114
    treatment for, 112
Acyclovir, 242, 349, 356, 382, 393, 398, 496,
    621, 646
AD. *See* Alzheimer disease (AD)
Adalimumab, 102
Addictive disorders, 525, 529, 549–550
Adenocarcinoma, 611
Adenosarcoma, 614
Adenosine, 24
ADH (antidiuretic hormone), 173, 176, 184, 185,
    189
ADHD. *See* Attention deficit hyperactivity disorder
    (ADHD)
Adjuvant therapy
    for cervical cancer, 612
    for ovarian cancer, 624
Adnexal torsion, 615
Adolescent idiopathic scoliosis, 457
ADPKD (autosomal-dominant polycystic kidney
    disease), 282, 288, 293
Adrenal insufficiency, 190. *See also* Primary adrenal
    insufficiency
Adrenocortical adenomas, 187
Adrenocortical carcinoma (ACC), 187–188
Adrenocorticotropic hormone (ACTH), 172,
    176, 184
Adson maneuver, 477
Adult Treatment Panel III (ATP III) criteria, 182
Advanced cardiac life support (ACLS), 26
Aerophobia, 351, 357
AF. *See* Atrial fibrillation (AF)
Afamelanotide, 103
Age-related macular degeneration (AMD)
    clinical assessment of, 140–141
    diagnosis of, 141
    general features of, 140
    treatment for, 141
Ages and Stages Questionnaires (ASQ), 534
Agitation, acute, 536
Agoraphobia, 533
AIDP (acute inflammatory demyelinating
    polyneuropathy), 493
AIHA (autoimmune hemolytic anemia), 323–324
Airflow limitation tests, 569
Airflow obstruction, 569
Airway clearance, in cystic fibrosis, 568
AK. *See* Actinic keratosis (AK)
AKI. *See* Acute kidney injury (AKI)
Albendazole, 378
Albuminocytologic dissociation, 480, 488
Albuminuria, 40
Albuterol, 570
Alcohol abuse, 236, 240
    chronic, 311, 317